Medical-Surgical Nursing and Related Physiology

JEANNETTE E. WATSON, R.N., M.Sc.N.

PROFESSOR, SCHOOL OF NURSING, UNIVERSITY OF TORONTO,
TORONTO, CANADA

W. B. SAUNDERS COMPANY

Philadelphia, London, Toronto

W. B. Saunders Company: West Washington Square
Philadelphia, PA 19105

12 Dyott Street
London, WC1A 1DB

833 Oxford Street
Toronto 18, Ontario

Medical-Surgical Nursing and Related Physiology   ISBN   0-7216-9135-8

Print No: 9   8   7   6   5   4   3   2

Preface

Nurses are the only members of the health team who are with patients around the clock, and who are responsible for the care and health supervision of patients and families in their homes. In order to assume their responsibilities safely and effectively, nurses require an understanding of normal body functioning, the patient's disease and its impact on the individual and family. Such knowledge is basic to the identification of significant physiological, psychological and socioeconomic needs and the making of discriminative judgments as to the appropriate care. In many instances, the physician, whose time at the bedside is limited, is dependent upon the nurse to recognize and notify him of significant changes in the patient's condition that demand his attention. Nurses also require an understanding of the rationale of the therapeutic measures being used in order to understand and assess the patient's responses to his treatment. It has been with these facts in mind that the content of this book has been prepared.

The first ten chapters are not specifically related to medical-surgical nursing but are applicable to most clinical areas. Part Two relates directly to the broad area of medical-surgical nursing. The system approach has been used in these chapters, presenting first a review of the relevant physiology followed by a discussion of nursing in the more common disorders. The frequent discussions in the text of the nurse's responsibility for what happens to the patient when he leaves the hospital or clinic are intended to prompt more concern for the continuity of patient care and rehabilitation.

The book is written primarily for students and nurses giving direct patient care. The reader is reminded that the suggested care is presented as a framework or guide; it is always necessary to modify or adapt nursing to the individual patient's situation and his responses to disease and treatment.

The author gratefully acknowledges the expert contribution made to the manuscript by Miss Donna Shields, C.N.M., M.S.N., who wrote Chapter 19, Nursing in Disorders of the Reproductive System. Miss Shields is a member of the teaching staff of the University of Toronto School of Nursing.

The suggestions and comments made by those doctors and nurses who reviewed various chapters were very helpful and appreciated. The continuing encouragement and enthusiasm of the author's colleagues throughout the writing of the book were inspiring and a tremendous support and are greatly appreciated. Special thanks are due Mrs. Joan Phillips and Mrs. Elaine Broderick for the typing and editing of the manuscript.

The author is grateful to those of the staff of the New Mount Sinai Hospital who so willingly cooperated by providing photographs.

Grateful acknowledgement is given to the publisher, W. B. Saunders Company, for the splendid cooperation received in bringing this effort to completion. Special thanks go to Mr. Robert Wright, Nursing Editor, for his guidance and patience throughout the preparation of the manuscript, to Mrs. M. Lee Walters for her work as copy editor and to Mr. George Laurie for the detailed organization of activities necessary in the production of the book.

Jeannette E. Watson

Contents

9

10

11

PART II

12

13

14

Nursing in Respiratory Disorders 257

15

Nursing in Disorders of the Alimentary Canal 315

16

Nursing in Disorders of the Liver and Biliary Tract 393

17

Nursing in Disorders of the Pancreas 409

18

Nursing in Disorders of the Urinary System 416

19

Nursing in Disorders of the Reproductive System 466

by Donna Shields, B.Sc.N., C.N.M., M.S.N.

20

Nursing in Disorders of the Breast 523

21

Nursing in Disorders of the Endocrine System 532

22

Nursing in Disorders of the Nervous System............................ 581

23

Nursing in Bone Disorders 673

24

Nursing in Joint and Collagen Disease 700

25

Nursing in Skin Disorders and Burns....................................... 711

Part I

Part 1

1
Patient-Centered Care

Nursing has endeavored in recent years to broaden its goals and provide comprehensive care that encompasses consideration of the emotional, preventive and rehabilitative factors of illness as well as the curative. Much has been said and written about the need for patient-centered and family-centered nursing care and about the nurse's responsibility to teach principles of health to individuals and families. Progress in these areas has been limited, probably because of the rapid medical and technological advances, the increasing demands on nurses, and a reluctance to depart from traditional practice. If nursing is to give more than lip service to meeting patients' total needs, changes in philosophy and attitudes, accompanied by greater efforts to plan and implement care on an individual basis, are necessary.

Patients are human individuals, not just bodies with interesting disease processes. Each one has his own distinctive background, set of values, capabilities, interests and experiences. He has identity as an individual as well as a role in a family and community, all of which he maintains when he also assumes the role of a patient. All of these factors influence the meaning illness has for the patient, his responses and his needs. Because he is a human being in a social setting, the patient has psychological

and social as well as physical needs. Those of one category do not operate independently of the others; the interaction of psychological and physiological factors and their effect on health are well recognized. For example, a patient's rapid pulse, diarrhea or urinary frequency may be the effect of his fear and anxiety on his autonomic nervous system and its control of body activities.

Patients' concerns, responses and needs are more readily recognized and interpreted if the nurse appreciates the possible implications illness may have for the individual. Illness is a threat; it interferes with the patient's accustomed pattern of life and is likely to cause frustration, fear and anxiety. The type and intensity of behavioral responses vary with each individual and are influenced by such factors as the patient's total past experiences and the patterns of behavior laid down in those experiences, the nature and severity of his illness, the interference of his illness with his future plans, and by socioeconomic problems imposed by the illness. His health problem may be viewed by the patient as a threat to his life or independence. He may fear the experience of pain, or if hospitalized, he may be insecure in the strange environment which lacks familiar objects, persons and his accustomed way of life.

The patient's emotions may be expressed

verbally or they may be communicated by such manifestations as a distraught appearance, facial expressions, inability to express himself, inattention, withdrawal, depression, hostility, lack of cooperation, or overdependency. Anxiety and fear may also account for physiological changes due to increased sympathetic innervation; there may be a reduction in salivary secretion, loss of appetite, a decrease in gastrointestinal secretions, an increase in intestinal activity, urinary frequency, skin pallor and cold, moist hands and feet.

The practice of nursing requires much more than technical competence and more than the manual skills and techniques entailed in the provision of physical comfort and the giving of prescribed treatments. These latter skills, although not less important, are only a part of total nursing care and may not be as effective if his psychological and social needs are ignored. The service expected of the nurse is patient-centered, comprehensive nursing — a process that attempts to recognize and meet the physical, psychological and social needs of the patient on an individual basis. Immediate and long-term goals are directed toward having the patient achieve and maintain optimum physical and mental well-being. The setting of long-term goals implies that the nurse assumes some responsibility for the continuity of care when the patient is discharged from her service.

Many of the patient's needs may be recognized by the nurse but must be referred to and met by members of other disciplines (physician, physiotherapist, dietitian, social service worker, religious adviser, vocational adviser, and community health and welfare personnel). It is important for the nurse to have a knowledge and appreciation of the personnel and agencies who may contribute to the care of the patient, and she should be able to work cooperatively with these workers. Comprehensive nursing care may include several or all of the following activities: providing supportive, protective and comfort measures; giving psychological support and therapy; assisting with diagnostic investigations and medical treatments; working cooperatively with other health personnel who are involved with the patient's treatment; coordinating the multidisciplinary contributions; interpreting the

illness and care to the patient and his family within the limits determined by the physician; counseling and teaching the patient and his family about how their health and welfare needs may be met; and arranging for appropriate referrals.

Nurse-Patient Relationship

The nurse-patient relationship is of great importance in all phases of nursing. The relationship that is established conditions all that the nurse does with or for the patient and can profoundly affect the quality and effectiveness of his care.

Mutual acceptance is basic to the achievement of a satisfactory relationship. The nurse must accept the patient without bias or prejudice. If the patient's behavior manifests stress, emotional disturbance or unacceptance, his set of circumstances and the situation should be carefully examined to determine why he reacts as he does and if his behavior is actually an expression of some need. It is also important that the nurse be aware of behavior responses characteristically associated with persons of different cultural backgrounds and of different age groups. As the nurse conveys an appreciation of the patient's concerns and what he is experiencing, he accepts the nurse and develops trust and confidence. A sincere interest and willingness in helping the patient may be demonstrated by such things as thoughtfulness; anticipation of his needs; a patient, kindly, non-judgmental manner; and a readiness to listen to the patient and answer his questions. Frequently, the light touch of the nurse's hand conveys understanding, interest and caring. His impressions and reactions may be influenced by the way the nurse speaks, listens and acts. Recognition of his identity by addressing him by name, respect for his personal preferences, and being flexible insofar as is possible also show acceptance and contribute to a satisfactory relationship. Orienting the patient to his environment, indicating how his accustomed needs will be met, and explaining what is to take place and what is expected of him help to relieve some of his concern and tension.

Appreciation of the family's concerns and their need for an interpretation of what is happening to the patient conveys an understanding and warmth that instills confidence. The patient and family who develop confidence in the persons responsible for patient care will talk more freely about their feelings and problems. The expression and sharing of such information may prove therapeutic as well as reveal the need for appropriate nursing action. If the patient is tense, uncommunicative, complaining or uncooperative, the nurse should analyze her own reactions and feelings about the patient. She may find that she is not really accepting him but is being judgmental; she may be insecure in the situation because of lack of sufficient knowledge and skills, or she may be irritated and distracted by a personal experience and is reacting to this in the patient situation.

Basic Human Needs

A large part of nursing care consists of meeting essential basic needs which are common to all persons, sick and well.

Basic biological needs include oxygen, fluids, food, elimination of body wastes, rest and sleep, some activity and change of position, and maintenance of body temperature within a definite range. Significant psychosocial needs of each person include a sense of security, or the need to feel safe and unthreatened; the maintenance of identity as an individual; acceptance and a sense of being wanted and belonging; the opportunity for socialization; independence and, at times, dependence and interdependence; the freedom to make decisions; the opportunity to develop and use his own potentialities; interests and goals; self-respect and usefulness; and a sense of achievement. For elaboration of these points, the reader is referred to the bibliography at the end of this chapter.

The patient may or may not need assistance in meeting his requirements. When assistance is necessary, the method used must be adapted to the individual. For example, the selection of foods in meeting the fundamental need for nourishment differs in the case of an infant or young child from that of an adult. Modifications and special assistance may be necessary because of the patient's pathological problem. The patient with a respiratory condition may require special care in order to maintain an adequate supply of oxygen; such things as special positioning, suctioning to clear the airway, steam inhalations and mechanical ventilatory assistance may be necessary.

THE NURSING PROCESS

Patient-centered comprehensive nursing entails five logical steps: assessment of the patient's and his family's needs; establishing priorities and planning the most effective way of meeting those needs; implementation; recording; and evaluation. Each step is part of an ongoing process; needs change, necessitating frequent reassessments. Revisions, deletions, additions and new approaches are necessary because of changes in the patient's condition, in his responses and in prescribed treatments from day to day. New information and more understanding of the patient and his family may bring to light factors that require attention. In many instances, new needs develop when initial ones are met; for example, a patient in the acute stage of illness has different needs when he enters the convalescent stage.

Significant factors in the recognition of a patient's needs and in planning and carrying out individualized total care include:

1. Knowing who the patient is and something about his background.

2. A sincere interest in the patient, a sense of responsibility for his welfare and a sensitivity to others' needs.

3. A good nurse-patient relationship.

4. Understanding the normal needs and the potentialities of the patient. (For example, a child of 5 years has different physiological and psychosocial needs and potentialities as compared to those of an adult, aged person, or a physically or mentally handicapped person.)

5. Understanding the implications illness may have for the patient and his family and their possible reactions to these implications.

6. Knowledge of the patient's health problem for which he is seeking assistance; this includes the pathological process, effects, manifestations and severity of his disease and its possible outcome.

7. An understanding of the diagnostic and therapeutic measures used–their purpose, effect on the patient and the nurse's role.

8. Knowledge of the basic common needs of all humans, sick or well.

9. Knowledge of the available resources and facilities for providing care and assistance for the patient and his family.

Assessment of Needs

Individual patient needs are recognized by alertness and conscious effort on the part of the nurse and through obtaining information on the patient's background. What the nurse learns about the patient not only guides her activities in providing care but may be very helpful to the physician and other members of the health team in making their contribution more effective. Osler's advice to medical students was to "care more particularly for the individual patient than for the special features of the disease."[1]

The sources of pertinent information are the patient's admission record and medical history, the patient, his family and friends, other personnel caring for or who have cared for the patient, and appropriate literature.

Much information is obtained through accurate objective observation of the patient and family. The nurse tactfully, and without appearing to probe, encourages the patient to talk about himself, his family, his interests and activities, and to express his feelings and concerns about his illness. She listens attentively, and periodically comments to assure the patient of her attention and interest, or she may say something that will channel his conversation to reveal the type of information she is seeking.

Facial expressions may provide clues to the individual's feelings and emotions. Similarly, gestures and posture may indicate anxiety, tension, pain, interest or disinterest, or other reactions.

Discussions with the family, friends or other workers will frequently provide insight into some problems of the patient and his family. Also, noting attitudes and reactions when family members are with the patient may reveal something of existing relationships and may point to the source of the patient's worry.

A review of available literature relating to the individual's condition and situation will contribute to the recognition and meeting of the patient's needs.

A number of hospitals have recently introduced nursing history forms, which are used in obtaining and recording information that may be significant in the recognition of the patient's needs and in planning care. They vary markedly from one agency to another as to the amount and detail of information required. In preparing and using the nursing history form, the information asked for should be selective on the basis of its pertinence to planning and implementing care, and secondly, it should not be a repetition of that which is provided and recorded in the admission form and medical history. Examples of nursing history forms are available in a number of the references cited in the bibliography.

Planning and Implementation

When a patient's needs are expressed or recognized, consideration is then given to the course of action. Planning is more effective when it can be done cooperatively by all those participating in the patient's nursing care. When his condition and situation permit, the patient should be included in this planning. Obviously, certain problems will require immediate action; priorities and immediate and long-term goals should be established.

How the patient's needs are to be met is influenced by such factors as his condition, the seriousness of his illness, the acuteness of the need, whether he is ambulatory or not, the amount of assistance he requires, and the available facilities, resources, time and staff. In relation to time and staff, a decision should be made regarding the best use of time in the interest of the patient. The possible contribution of auxiliary workers and members of the family should be kept in mind. There is a tendency in hospitals to follow established routines rather than to make adjustments to meet the individual patient's needs. For example, if a patient is resting after having had a bad night with pain, is it not more important to let him rest than to disturb him for a bath which could just as well be given later in the day? When it is desirable for the patient to participate in self-care, the benefit of such activity is explained to him, since many patients expect to have everything done for them.

[1]Sir William Osler: Aphorisms From His Bedside Teachings and Writings. Collected by Robert B. Bean. Edited by B. Bean, New York, H. Schuman Inc., 1950, p. 93, quote No. 181.

There are several advantages to the use of a deliberate systematic approach to the planning of nursing care for each patient. Planning leads to decisions and to doing things in an orderly fashion and on time. It necessitates a more thoughtful analysis of the information pertaining to the patient and is likely to result in a better interpretation of his needs. Modifications are then more likely to be made in line with the individual's preferences, accustomed ways and particular situation.

The plan in written form is made available to all who are nursing the patient. In many instances, this may prevent frustration and annoyance for the patient since the plan would indicate his preferences, limitations and other details, making it unnecessary for him to inform each person in turn. Systematic planning also allows for more satisfactory use of personnel; activities may be delegated to appropriate members of the nursing team.

In carrying out direct nursing activities, the patient is advised about what is to be done, the purpose, what he may expect and what is expected of him. The nurse avoids rigidity and should be prepared to make adaptations to accommodate the patient as long as the principles of the treatment are observed and the maximum benefits may be derived for the patient. Awareness of factors that contribute to his comfort and safety and observation of his reactions are necessary in all that is done with or for the patient.

Recording and Evaluation

The nurse's notes are an account of significant patient reactions, behavior and verbal expressions as well as treatments and care given. Statements should be current, accurate, objective, clearly legible and concise. They keep the physician and others participating in the care of the patient informed about the patient's condition and may contribute to the diagnosis and decisions regarding the necessary treatment. The notes may also be used to assess the effectiveness of care and the patient's progress, and they may provide data for research.

A continuous evaluation is made of the patient's care. A conference of the nursing personnel involved may be used to assess the situation and consider whether the patient's needs are being recognized, whether the goals are realistic and are being met, whether the best methods are being used, what new goals should be set and what new approaches should be used. The individual nurse reflects on her role and performance; she considers her relationship with the patient and the completeness and effectiveness of her nursing; she also considers any necessary revisions.

The practice of evaluation is not only useful in improving patient care, but it can also be an educational process for the nurse. She learns that there are several approaches and methods that may be used with a single problem.

Continuity of Care

In comprehensive nursing, concern for the patient goes beyond the nurse's direct care and contact with him. Consideration of what happens to this person when he is discharged from the hospital or nursing agency is necessary. He may require continued care, adjustments in his future way of life in order to live within his functional capacity, and instruction as to specific treatments and health measures. Advice and suggestions may be indicated for the patient and family in the interest of promoting their health and preventing illness.

This part of the patient's care should not be left to the last day or two before his discharge but should receive attention throughout his illness, and early plans should be made for the necessary discussions, instruction and referrals so they may be complete and effective. Some knowledge of the situation to which the patient will return is important. This may be obtained from the family and patient, or the home situation may be assessed by a district health nurse or social service worker who may indicate the necessary adjustments.

Some teaching of the patient and his family may be incidental, but much of it involves planning and organization. Motivation and readiness for learning as well as the setting of objectives are important factors. The content of the teaching required to meet the needs may be related to the patient's present illness, the general health habits of the patient and his family or to some specific health problem of a family member. What is taught should be authentic, expressed in terms understandable to the patient, and adapted to his age, education, socioeconomic status and culture. Content related to therapeutic measures should be approved by the physician.

Teaching may be shared by the physician, dietitian or physiotherapist; it is helpful if the nurse is familiar with their instructions so she may reinforce them and be able to answer the patient's related questions.

Incidental teaching can frequently be done while giving treatments and care and may relate to what is actually being done. For some instruction, definite uninterrupted periods are arranged at a time when the patient is comfortable and rested. The periods should be relatively short; offering too much at one time may defeat the purpose and only leave the patient confused and discouraged. When the family is to be included, times are determined by when they can be present. Demonstrations of procedures such as colostomy care or the giving of insulin may be broken down into several steps and followed by opportunities for the patient or family member to carry them out under the supervision of the nurse. In some instances, group teaching may be possible if there are several patients requiring similar instruction. This is of value, as it may be followed by discussions among patients. Revelation that there are others with similar problems does much to reduce the patient's anxiety.

Time and opportunities are made available for the patient and family to ask questions and for repetition and reinforcement of the instructions. Appropriate literature, illustrations, clear simple outlines of directions and examples of improvised equipment may serve as valuable teaching aids to clarify and reinforce the content presented to the patient and family. When teaching needs are recognized they are recorded on the nursing care plan and checked off when satisfactorily accomplished.

Planning for the patient's future care or for the solution of a socioeconomic or home problem may entail referral to the social service worker or to an appropriate health or welfare agency. Any suggestions for assistance should be discussed and approved by the patient and his family before a referral is made. The patient and his family are also advised in regard to where they may get assistance or whom they should contact in certain events.

The guidance and course of action taken to ensure continuity of care should be evaluated, if possible, through some follow-up or by contacting the assisting agency personnel.

References

BOOKS

Beland, I. L.: Clinical Nursing. New York, The MacMillan Co., 1965. Chapter 1, pp. 1–32.

Bird, B.: Talking with Patients. Philadelphia, J. B. Lippincott Co., 1955.

Brown, E. L.: Newer Dimensions of Patient Care. Part 3. Patients as People. New York, Russell Sage, 1964.

Burton, G.: Personal, Impersonal and Interpersonal Relations—A Guide for Nurses. New York, Springer Publishing Co., 1958.

Kron, T.: Communication in Nursing, 2nd ed. Philadelphia, W. B. Saunders Co., 1971.

Lewis, G. K.: Nurse-Patient Communication. Dubuque, W. C. Brown Co., 1969.

Little, D. E., and Carnevali, D. L.: Nursing Care Planning. Philadelphia, J. B. Lippincott Co., 1969.

Orlando, I. J.: The Dynamic Nurse-Patient Relationship. New York, G. P. Putnam's Sons, 1961.

Peplau, H. E.: Interpersonal Relations in Nursing. New York, G. P. Putnam's Sons, 1952.

Ruesch, J., and Kees, W.: Nonverbal Communication. Los Angeles, University of California Press, 1964.

Rinehart, E. L.: Management of Nursing Care. New York, The MacMillan Co., 1969.

Skipper, J. K., and Leonard, R. C. (Ed.): Social Interaction and Patient Care. Philadelphia, J. B. Lippincott Co., 1965.

Straub, K. M., and Parker, K. S. (Ed.): Continuity of Patient Care—The Role of Nursing. Washington, D.C., The Catholic University Press, 1965.

Towle, C.: Common Human Needs. New York, National Association of Social Workers, 1952.

Wright, B. A.: Physical Disability—A Psychological Approach. New York, Harper and Brothers, 1960.

Yura, H., and Walsh, M. B. (Eds.): The Nursing Process—Assessing, Planning, Implementing, Evaluating. Washington, D.C., The Catholic University Press, 1967.

PERIODICALS

Ashton, L.: "Tortoise and Hare." Canad. Nurs., Vol. 62, No. 11 (Nov. 1966), pp. 44–45.

Cherescavich, G.: "The Expanding Role of the Professional Nurse in a Hospital." Nurs. Forum, Vol. III, No. 4, 1964, pp. 9–20.

DuMouchel, N.: "Are We Really Meeting Our Patients' Needs?" Canad. Nurs., Vol. 66, No. 11 (Nov. 1970), pp. 39–43.

Falardeau, J. C.: "The Role of the Nurse in a Changing Society." Canad. Nurs., Vol. 58, No. 3 (Mar. 1962), pp. 244–247

Hall, L.: "Nursing, What Is It?" Canad. Nurs., Vol. 60, No. 2 (Feb. 1964), pp. 150–154.

Hays, J. S.: "Analysis of Nurse-Patient Communications." Nurs. Outlook, Vol. 14, No. 9 (Sept. 1966), pp. 32–35

Henderson, V.: "The Nature of Nursing." Amer. J. Nurs., Vol. 64, No. 8 (Aug. 1964), pp. 62–68.

Ingles, T.: "Understanding the Nurse-Patient Relationship." Nurs. Outlook, Vol. 9, No. 11 (Nov. 1961), pp. 698–700.

Johnson, D. E.: "The Significance of Nursing Care." Amer. J. Nurs., Vol. 61, No. 11 (Nov. 1961), pp. 63–66.

Knowles, L. N.: "How Our Behavior Affects Patient Care." Canad. Nurs., Vol. 58, No. 1 (Jan. 1962), pp. 30–33.

Little, D., and Carnevale, D.: "Nursing Care Plans—Let's Be Practical About Them." Nurs. Forum, Vol. VI, No. 1, 1967, pp. 61–76.

McCain, R. F.: "Nursing By Assessment—Not Intuition." Amer. J. Nurs., Vol. 65, No. 4 (Apr. 1965), pp. 82–84.

Monteiro, L. A.: "Patient Teaching—A Neglected Area." Nurs. Forum, Vol. III, No. 1, 1964, pp. 26–33.

Nahm, H.: "Nursing Dimensions and Realities." Amer. J. Nurs., Vol. 65, No. 6 (June 1965), pp. 96–99.

Paulsen, F. R.: "Nursing Goals Beyond Commitment." Nurs. Outlook, Vol. 14, No. 12 (Dec. 1966), pp. 51–58.

Prince, R.: "Creating a Therapeutic Environment." Canad. Nurs., Vol. 61, No. 11 (Nov. 1965), pp. 889–894.

Schamhl, J.: "Ritualism in Nursing Practice." Nurs. Forum, Vol. III, No. 4 (1964), pp. 74–84.

Skipper, J. K., and Leonard, R. C.: "Communication and Patient Care." Canad. Nurs., Vol. 61, No. 7 (July 1965), pp. 561F–562H.

Sweet, P. R., and Stark, I.: "The Circle Care Nursing Plan." Amer. J. Nurs., Vol. 70, No. 6 (June 1970), pp. 1300–1303.

Thiessen, H.: "A Nursing Service Audit." Canad. Nurs., Vol. 62, No. 2 (Feb. 1966), pp. 57–59.

Wood, M.: Nursing Care Plan: "Guide to Better Care." Amer. J. Nurs., Vol. 61, No. 12 (Dec. 1961), pp. 61–62.

2
Rehabilitation of the Disabled

INTRODUCTION

Rehabilitation is the process by which a disabled person is assisted in developing a pattern of life that provides a sense of worth and satisfaction for him. The individual is helped to attain optimal physical, mental, social and economic independence and usefulness compatible with his abilities. There has been increasing recognition in recent years of the potentialities of disabled persons; given assistance, many can become self-reliant and be gainfully employed, taking their rightful place in society. Rehabilitation takes time, effort, money, personnel and facilities, but such expenditures can scarcely be questioned when one considers what rehabilitation means to the individual who is faced with remaining useless and dependent.

The rehabilitation process may be brief and simple for some patients, involving only a few instructions and minor adjustments. For others it may require a long period and the special techniques of a multidisciplinary team to help them develop an entirely new pattern of life. Various combinations of personnel may be necessary, depending on the type of disability and the type of person. The rehabilitation program must be individualized; two patients with a similar disability do not necessarily have the same degree of handicap, and certainly they do not have the same remaining capabilities. The team concerned with a single patient may include the physician, nurse, physiotherapist, speech therapist, psychologist, social worker, vocational counselor, educator, employment officer and recreational director. In other instances the team may be made up of the physician, nurse and physiotherapist. Each team member has a contribution to make, but these efforts have to be coordinated. Cooperative planning and an exchange of information between the workers are necessary for maximal effectiveness. Frequently, one team member has the opportunity to reinforce another's work, but this can be done only if each is familiar with the total rehabilitation plan.

Disabilities

All illness causes disability to some extent, but when the term is used in the context of rehabilitation it implies a prolonged or permanent impairment or the loss of some bodily function. The disability may be congenital or may be acquired as a result of injury or disease of any system of the body. According to Hirschberg et al., the commonest prolonged and permanent disabilities that necessitate special rehabilitative consideration are "caused by involvement of the nervous system, the musculoskeletal system and the cardiopulmonary system."[1] Handicapped persons are frequently classified according to the nature of their disability. They may be referred to as physically handicapped because their mobility is restricted or as mentally handicapped because of mental illness or a subnormal level of intelligence, which results in difficulty in the management of personal affairs or adjustment in society. The visually handicapped are those with partial or total loss of vision and those with auditory handicaps have a partial or total loss of hearing.

Unless preventive measures are instituted at the onset of a physical disability, complications and secondary disabilities may develop rapidly as the result of inactivity, pressure, injury or misuse. Immobilization and inactivity lead to muscle wasting and contracture and to stiffening of joints which limits the range of joint movement. Prolonged bed rest or confinement to a wheelchair prevents normal weight-bearing and muscle pull on the bones; this may cause a loss of calcium from the bones (osteoporosis), resulting in increased urinary excretion of calcium that predisposes to the formation of renal or bladder calculi.

Inactivity, particularly in the recumbent position, may cause a circulatory stasis. Venous drainage, especially in the lower limbs, is retarded, predisposing to clot formation (phlebothrombosis). Circulation through the lungs is slowed because of shallow respirations and reduced lung expansion; fluid may escape from the pulmonary capillaries into the alveoli and may cause hypostatic pneumonia. Respiratory function may be less efficient because of limited chest expansion, loss of respiratory muscle strength, or sedatives and narcotics which the patient may be receiving. Secretions tend to collect in the alveoli and bronchioles if the patient's position is stationary and if drugs are being used that depress the cough reflex.

Prolonged pressure on an area of the body

compresses the blood vessels in the tissues and inhibits a normal blood flow through the area. The tissue becomes necrotic and sloughs away, leaving a pressure sore. The most vulnerable areas are those over bony prominences, such as the sacral region. lateral area of the hip over the femoral trochanter, ischial region, heels, back of the head, and shoulder and scapular regions.

Constipation and fecal impaction occur frequently as a result of inactivity and the change in the patient's diet.

Occasionally, the handicapped individual may attempt to do something beyond the limitations imposed by his initial disability; as a result, he may sustain an injury that adds to his problems. For example, the patient may try to walk without the necessary assistance and fall; or a joint may be overextended, injuring ligaments or the joint capsule and causing pain, weakness and instability of the joint. Similarly, use or overexercise of a limb when a joint is acutely inflamed or when insufficient healing has taken place may cause joint damage or instability that may increase his disability and prove a hindrance to satisfactory rehabilitation.

The implications of a disability vary with each individual according to the nature and severity of the handicap and according to his personality, values, goals and responsibilities. The loss of the capacity to function as a normal, independent, productive being strikes a severe blow. It may mean dependence on others for ordinary, personal day-to-day care. A career in which a great deal of time, effort and money have been invested may be interrupted. The individual's self-image is changed, and he sees himself as different, abnormal, worthless and a burden to his family and to society.

The patient experiences bewilderment, fear, and feelings of insecurity and loneliness. The dominant emotional responses and behavior which each individual manifests are determined by his previous experiences and conditioning. The process of acceptance and adjustment will be a greater struggle for some than for others. Persons who previously possessed the capacity to meet the stresses of life successfully are usually more able to cope with this new problem; others may develop emotional and personality problems. In the initial state of conflict and turmoil, acute depression ac-

[1]Gerald G. Hirschberg, Leon Lewis and Dorothy Thomas: Rehabilitation. Philadelphia, J. B. Lippincott Co., 1964, p. 12.

companied by a lack of desire to live, denial of the existence of disability, anger, hostility and a lack of cooperation are frequent reactions met with in disabled persons. The period in which the patient overcomes the initial impact of disability, faces reality and accepts the situation may be much longer for some than for others. A change in personality may become apparent; the patient may lose interest in everything beyond himself and may tend to withdraw from the world around him, or he may become resentful and hostile.

When a member of the family becomes disabled, a change in the way of life for the whole family may be necessary. Responsibilities are shifted, financial hardships may be experienced, and plans and goals may be shattered. Their responses to the situation are also conditioned by their life circumstances, personalities and previous experiences.

The Rehabilitative Process

The rehabilitative part of the disabled person's care should start when he first comes under treatment in the hospital, clinic or home and should be continued until he has learned to live and work with his remaining abilities.

During the acute phase, treatment and care are directed toward having the patient recover from the disabling disease or injury with a minimum of dysfunction. The prevention of complications and secondary disabilities and the provision of psychological support are equally important. The acute illness is followed by the restorative and retraining phase of rehabilitation. This phase includes evaluation of the patient's functional status, potentials and persisting deficits; the setting of realistic goals; and the planning and implementing of a program of activities for realizing the goals. Who will be involved and what activities will be necessary will depend on the nature of the handicap, the extent to which the patient is damaged, his previous pattern of life, his remaining abilities and his interests. The rehabilitation program may include: measures to improve and maintain the individual's general physical condition; correction of deformities that restrict rehabilitation; passive movements and active exercises;

helping the patient to resume self-care; psychological support and therapy; special techniques for specific disabilities (e.g., speech therapy or new methods of mobility through the use of mechanical devices, such as braces, crutches or prostheses); education or vocational training; placement in employment; arranging for participation in safe, appropriate social and recreational activities; assisting the family to accept the patient and to adjust to the enforced changes in their life; teaching the family how they may best help the patient and at the same time conserve their own energy; and, if necessary, helping the family to procure welfare assistance.

In evaluation of the individual's rehabilitation potential, a history of his background is important. His education, previous interests, occupations and achievements, and role in the family and community are ascertained. His physical and mental capacity, personality and aptitudes are then assessed. An appraisal is made which should include assessment of the patient's strength; capacity for self-care; motor functions, including the ability to move from one place to another; and his communication skills. Psychological and aptitude tests may be necessary to determine his intellectual capacity and the type of vocation for which he might be prepared. Knowledge of his home, family, and the social and physical environments in which he will live is also necessary.

An interpretation of what the patient may and may not do should be made to him and his family. Then, insofar as is possible, plans for his future should respect his interests; he should be encouraged to express what he would like most to achieve within his limitations and capacity and to participate in the decisions. He is more likely to mobilize personal resources and make progress in retraining if he is working toward a goal of personal interest. If the initial rehabilitative plans and techniques are not successful, this does not preclude attempting other methods which may yield more success. Optimism, patience and persistence are necessary in those working with the patient.

There are few disabled persons who cannot be helped to some extent by rehabilitative measures. If the patient is seriously damaged and rehabilitation is not possible, care is designed to prevent further disability and regression, to reduce suffering to a minimum and to make life as tolerable as possible for the individual and his family.

Rehabilitation Nursing

Although the general medical use of the term rehabilitation is directed toward individuals with residual limitations, rehabilitation is really a part of the nursing care of all patients, for the primary objective in any patient is to restore him to optimal health and to have him return to his home and community as an independent and productive person. In this context, rehabilitation nursing is simply a part of the comprehensive care required by a patient whose illness or injury imposes some residual disability or limitations upon him.

Through her early and continuing contact with the patient, the nurse has the opportunity to contribute greatly to the patient's rehabilitation. Her attitude may have a significant influence on the patient's progress. It is important that she appreciate the impact of disability on the patient and also that she develop a positive, motivating approach which reflects an underlying belief that the situation is not hopeless and that the patient can and will be restored to a worthwhile life. Tradition and the teaching of nursing have generally emphasized doing to and for the patient, rather than encouraging, teaching and permitting self-care. As the disabled patient's condition warrants it, he is encouraged to assume more responsibility for his own care. Overprotection and doing things for him which he can do for himself only increase his dependence, passivity and feelings of inadequacy.

Nursing the disabled person should be structured from the outset to meet rehabilitative goals. Such goals include: the strengthening and maintenance of the patient's functional capacities; the prevention of further impairment and secondary disabilities; assisting the patient and his family in dealing with the psychological impact of disability; the motivation of the patient to realize his potentials; encouraging and teaching self-care; knowing and using available resources that can be of assistance in rehabilitating the patient; and helping the family to adjust to the situation and to obtain necessary assistance.

Rehabilitation measures related to disabilities associated with specific conditions are presented with the nursing care in the respective ensuing chapters. The following paragraphs include a discussion of nursing factors that are common to the care of many disabled persons, particularly in cases involving prolonged inactivity.

Positioning. The patient's position is changed every 1 to 2 hours to prevent circulatory stasis and prolonged pressure on any one part of the body, to promote expansion of the lungs and drainage of pulmonary secretions, and to contribute to his comfort. The general principles of good body alignment should be observed; overextension or strain of any joint should be avoided, and a minimum of flexion used. A firm mattress is used to prevent sagging under the patient's weight and if necessary, a bed board may be added.

In the dorsal position, the body should be in a straight line. A foot board is necessary to support the feet at right angles to the legs with the heels resting in the space between the foot board and the mattress or on some resilient material, such as sponge rubber, to avoid pressure. The space under the popliteal region is filled in to prevent strain on the knee joint, and a firm roll or sandbag is placed against the lateral surface of the thigh, extending from above the hip joint to below the knee to prevent outward rotation of the lower limb. If there is paralysis of an arm, it is abducted and a pillow is placed between the trunk and the arm to prevent adduction contracture. The forearm is slightly flexed and the wrist is supported with the fingers and thumb in extension. The thickness of the pillow under the head should be sufficient to maintain the head in line with the spine so that flexion and extension are avoided.

In the lateral position, the lower limbs are slightly flexed; the one that is uppermost is flexed to a greater degree than the other, and it is supported on a pillow to prevent strain on the hip joint. The uppermost arm is flexed and supported on a pillow in front of the patient.

When the prone position is used, the head pillow is removed, and the head is turned to one side. A flat pillow or support is placed under the patient's abdomen well below the lower border of the rib cage to prevent strain on the back. The arms are abducted and flexed at the elbows. The feet may be supported by a pillow under the ankles to keep the toes free of the bed, or the forepart of the foot may be suspended over the end of the mattress.

Skin Care. A decubitus ulcer or pressure sore will develop with startling rapidity in an area subjected to continuous pressure, but it may take weeks or months to heal. Preventive measures should be instituted promptly with all patients whose movement is restricted, who cannot shift their body weight from one area to another, and who have impaired sensory function that inhibits their awareness of the discomfort of prolonged pressure on a part. The patient's position is changed hourly, and gentle massage is used to stimulate circulation in the parts subjected to pressure. Vulnerable areas may also be protected by the use of resilient surfaces, such as foam rubber, an alternating air pressure mattress or pieces of sheep skin. The patient's skin should be kept clean and dry to prevent irritation and maceration. The undersheets should be kept dry, soft, and free of wrinkles and any irritating particles. Areas subjected to pressure are inspected with each change of position for early signs of ischemia and tissue damage. If damaged, the area may appear blanched and cool at first; then it becomes red or bluish-red, followed by darkening and then breakdown of the skin. Underlying layers of tissue may also be destroyed, and as the dead tissue is sloughed off a deep, open lesion remains and is referred to as an ulcer.

If an ulcer develops, the area is kept clean to prevent infection and is protected from pressure. Special treatment will be prescribed by the physician; any number of preparations are used in the forms of moist compresses, powders and ointments. Some of these may be for removal of the necrotic tissue (débridement); others may be to stimulate healing or to control infection. As the necrotic tissue is sloughed off, hopefully, the area fills in with granulation tissue and eventually heals over. The area around the ulcer is gently massaged to encourage an adequate blood supply to the area. A diet high in protein and vitamins B and C contributes to healing.

If the ulcer is large and the subcutaneous tissue is destroyed, the physician may consider skin grafting advisable.

As the disabled patient learns and assumes self-care, the importance of frequent change of position is explained, and he is taught to change his position at regular and frequent intervals. If he progresses to a wheelchair, a foam rubber cushion is provided, and the patient is advised to shift his weight and raise himself at frequent intervals as prolonged sitting predisposes to a pressure sore in the ischial region. When there is loss of sensation, as with the paraplegic, the individual is taught to inspect the vulnerable areas by means of a mirror at least once daily.

Psychological Reactions and Support. The disabled patient's reactions of disbelief, followed by depression and probable resentment that this has happened to him, are understandable. The nurse, knowing why he is behaving as he is, accepts his reactions; her behavior helps to convey a sense of understanding and caring. The patient is insecure, lonely and afraid; he should not be left alone for long periods. Close observation of his reactions and comments will indicate to the nurse when to encourage conversation or when it is her presence alone that is preferable to the patient. At the appropriate time, the nurse may acknowledge verbally that she knows the situation looks hopeless to him and may assure him that everything possible will be done to help him regain his strength and ability to do things for himself. Offering false hope and being over-cheerful are to be avoided. Gradually, as the patient recognizes the nurse's understanding, he may talk about his situation and, through this, begin to see things more realistically and explore possibilities for his future. His thinking is directed to the positive, to things he can do and would like to do. He is helped to become aware of his capabilities by being allowed to do things for himself as soon as possible. Early interpretation and initiation of rehabilitation measures offer hope and motivate the patient.

Periods of depression and withdrawal are to be expected from time to time, particularly when achievement of some aspect of his rehabilitation seems slow and frustrating. Such reactions are accepted, but with an attitude of expectation that he will persevere and ultimately succeed.

Frequent visits from family members may provide support and reinforce the impression that they are not rejecting him as a cripple. A bright, cheerful room is desirable, and being with others with similar disabilities may help.

Nutrition. Nutrition plays an important role in the patient's rehabilitation; a well-balanced diet is necessary for increasing the patient's strength. Anorexia may be a problem, due to the patient's emotional responses to his disability. An inadequate diet and nutritional deficiencies may predispose to complications that delay his restoration. Factors that encourage the patient to take adequate food include an environment that is physically, socially and psychologically acceptable, having the patient clean and comfortable, serving small amounts of high-calorie foods frequently, respect for his food preferences insofar as is possible, and provision of the necessary assistance. Most patients dislike having to be fed and frequently take less because of this. It improves morale and possibly increases the amount of food taken when the patient can manage self-feeding. Ingenuity on the part of the nurse is important in making minor adjustments so the food can be easily reached by the patient whose range of arm motion may be limited.

The total caloric intake is adjusted to maintain the individual's normal weight and to meet his energy expenditure. Increasing physical exercises and activity in his retraining program requires a corresponding increase in calories. Obesity should be avoided, since excess weight increases the patient's handicap and impedes rehabilitation.

A high-protein and high-vitamin diet is encouraged; the increased protein intake is necessary to maintain muscle mass and tissue resistance. The vitamins improve the patient's appetite and increase his resistance.

Calcium-containing foods may be restricted because of the predisposition to the formation of kidney and bladder calculi (see p. 647). Precipitation of the calcium occurs more readily in an alkaline urine; a diet high in foods that leave an acid metabolic waste and drugs that acidify the urine may be ordered.

Elimination. Constipation and bowel and urinary incontinence are frequently associated with disabilities. Constipation is usually the result of inactivity and changes in diet and routine. For treatment and nursing care of the patient with this problem see page 365.

Incontinence can be a serious source of emotional disturbance and discouragement for the patient. Unexpected involuntary urination or defecation when the patient has just been bathed, during meals or exercise routines, or while friends and family are visiting can be very embarrassing to him. The problem is discussed realistically with the patient; he is advised that a routine and control can be established, but it will require time and patience. The proposed plan to establish control is outlined, and the patient's role described. Mentally responsible patients are usually very anxious to cooperate.

Bowel incontinence in the disabled may be due to some damage or degenerative change of the central nervous system that causes loss of sensation of the defecation stimulus and voluntary control of the external anal sphincter.

A regular time for daily evacuation of the bowel should be decided upon, taking into consideration its convenience in relation to the day's activities and the patient's schedule when he returns home. Foods and fluids which stimulate peristalsis are included in the diet while training the bowel to empty at a specified time. One or two glycerin suppositories may be inserted into the rectum 1/2 hour to 2 hours before placing the patient on the commode or toilet, or digital stimulation may be used. It is necessary to experiment with each patient as to the type and amount of bulky foods and fluids that are most effective in bowel training. Similarly, the number of suppositories necessary and the length of time it takes for the bowel response following insertion are determined on an individual basis. Movements are likely to occur occasionally at times other than those scheduled, particularly at first. Adjustments in diet and in the use of suppositories will probably be necessary from time to time as the patient's general condition improves and his activity increases.

Bladder control is more difficult to develop than bowel control and generally requires a longer period. Incontinence due to spinal cord injury is discussed on page 648 with the care of the paraplegic patient. When it is due to degenerative disease, loss of consciousness or other illnesses an indwelling catheter may be used. The physician's instructions may be to have the catheter drain continuously at first, then to clamp it, allowing it to drain only at stated intervals of 1 to 2 hours. The interval is gradually increased to 3 to 4 hours; allowing the bladder to collect urine for longer periods encourages a more normal capacity. The catheter is removed as soon as possible, since it predisposes to bladder infection. A schedule is established for voiding; at first the patient is placed on a bedpan or commode hourly. The intervals between voidings are gradually lengthened when there is no incontinency in the shorter periods. When the intervals are short, it may be necessary to place a pad under the patient or to provide some form of drainage receptacle at night to avoid too frequent interruption of his rest. As the voidings become less frequent, the schedule becomes the same throughout the 24 hours.

A fluid intake of 2500 to 3000 ml. daily facilitates training and assists in preventing infection and calculus formation. If most of this is taken before 8 P.M., the problem of incontinency during the night is reduced. The amount voided each time is recorded, and the 24-hour volume is totaled and compared with the intake volume. This provides information as to whether the bladder is emptying completely or urine is being retained. Catheterization following a voiding may be ordered to determine if there is residual urine.

If an indwelling catheter is necessary for a relatively long period, the physician may require the bladder to be irrigated 2 or 3 times daily with an antiseptic solution to prevent infection. Disposable plastic bags may be used to receive the urine drainage; when a nondisposable drainage bottle is used it should be sterilized daily along with the drainage tubing that is connected to the catheter. The catheter is usually changed every 7 to 10 days. A urine specimen is collected every 2 to 3 days and is cultured for evidence of possible bacterial invasion. Chills, elevation in temperature and decreased urinary output may indicate urinary tract infection.

Exercises. Immobility for even a brief period causes musculoskeletal deterioration and predisposes the individual to complications that interfere with rehabilitation (see p. 618). An exercise program, approved by the physician, should be started early to maintain and increase the strength of functional muscles; to maintain the normal range of joint movement; to stimulate circulation and respirations and thus prevent complications, cramping and fatigue; and to encourage the return of function in affected muscles.

Passive exercises consist of movements of parts of the body by someone other than the patient; active exercises are carried out by the patient himself. General principles to be observed in all exercise programs are as follows: the purpose and importance of the exercises should be understood by both the patient and the person responsible for the program; the patient should be rested and in as comfortable a position as possible; in passive movements, the parts of the body are handled gently, the portion above the part being moved is stabilized, joints are supported and pressure on the body of muscles is avoided; movements should be made slowly and smoothly and kept within a pain-free range; short periods of exercise repeated at intervals are preferable to fewer long periods, which cause fatigue of the patient; and the number of times for each exercise is gradually increased.

Passive exercises are applied to the limbs to prevent muscle contracture and decreased joint movement, to stimulate normal muscle reflexes and to keep the muscle in readiness for active functioning. Each part is moved in each direction of normal movement as far as possible without causing pain.

With the pillow removed, the head may be alternately flexed forward and to each side and then, in turn, rotated left and right.

To maintain shoulder joint and arm movement, the arm is successively raised over the head as far as it will go, abducted, adducted across the chest, externally and internally rotated, and then circumducted. Flexion and extension with the upper arm stabilized are used to preserve elbow function and are followed by pronation (turning the palm downward) and supination (turning the palm upward). Similarly, the hand, fingers and thumb are moved through their normal range of movements.

With the lower limb, the hip joint and involved muscles are exercised by movement of the thigh with the knee flexed through flexion, extension, abduction, adduction, and internal and external rotation; the knee and ankle are supported in each movement. Flexion and extension of the knee may be combined with similar movements of the hip. The foot is alternately dorsiflexed and plantar-flexed, then everted and inverted with the leg stabilized. Gentle raising of the toes followed by flexion will help to maintain the phalangeal joints.

If the patient is placed in the prone position, backward movement (hyperextension) of the head, arms and lower limbs may be carried out slowly and gently.

Active exercise promotes muscle strength, maintains range of joint movement and stimulates circulation. The same series of movements cited earlier as passive exercises are performed by the patient. When he is ready for it, activities such as raising himself to the sitting position, first in bed, then to the side of the bed with legs suspended over the edge, are included.

When a set of muscles is weak, the patient may require assistance to achieve the full range of motion of the part involved. The exercise is then referred to as active assistive. Only sufficient help to complete the movement is used, and this is gradually withdrawn as the muscles strengthen.

If it is not possible to move a part through its range of motion because of an affected or immobilized joint, muscle tone may be preserved by having the patient contract his muscles in the stationary position. This "setting" of muscles is frequently used with the thigh muscles (quadriceps femoris) when a lower limb is immobilized.

In rehabilitation, the retraining of muscles may require a program of physical therapy, such as hydrotherapy or thermal treatments, and exercises involving special equipment, such as weights. These are directed by a physiotherapist and are usually done in a physical therapy department. The nurse should be acquainted with the program, since frequently some activities may be reinforced in nursing care.

A number of excellent references are available with detailed instructions and illustrations of active and passive exercises that the nurse may be expected to initiate and carry out. Examples of these are listed at the bottom of this page;[2, 3, 4] others may be found in the bibliography at the end of this chapter. It is helpful if at least one or two such references are available on the hospital ward or in the visiting nurse's office. A family member or the patient himself may be instructed to carry out an exercise program at home, and he may find a booklet with illustrations of value.

Activities of Daily Living (A.D.L.). These are the activities that are normally carried out by the individual in his daily life. Such activities include feeding oneself, personal hygiene, dressing and undressing, changing position, locomotion and basic essential hand activities. The patient's ability to carry out self-care and to move from one place to another greatly determines his degree of independence. The evaluation process will determine what he can and cannot do. Resumption of self-care may simply require being given the opportunity, motivation and encouragement, or learning new ways to accomplish it.

The nurse has the first opportunity to initiate the patient's self-help measures since the starting point is with simple activities, such as eating, washing the hands and face, combing the hair, cleaning the teeth, and cleansing oneself after going to the toilet. With the achievement of these simple initial activities the program is gradually and steadily expanded. The patient may have to learn and then practice turning in bed, rising to the sitting position, sitting on the side of the bed and transferring to a chair. Once the latter is conquered, the next goal is locomotion; he learns to pull himself up to the standing position, establish his balance and then to walk. If the patient requires a walker, cane or crutches, adjustment to the height of the patient and instruction in its use will be necessary. Each activity is made up of several motions, some of which may be difficult for the patient. Practice in the form of exercises may be used to strengthen the

---

[2]Mildred J. Allgire and Ruth R. Denney: Nurses Can Give and Teach Rehabilitation. New York, Springer Publishing Co., Inc., 1960.

[3]B. H. Fowles: Syllabus of Rehabilitation Methods and Techniques. Cleveland, The Stratford Press Co., 1963.

[4]American Heart Association: Strike Back at Stroke. New York, American Heart Association.

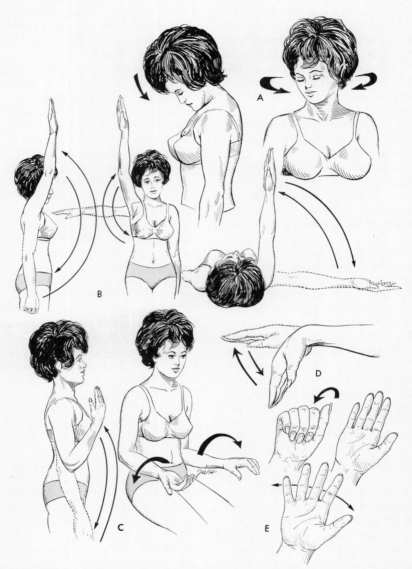

Figure 2–1 Series of line drawings illustrating some bed exercises. *A*, Flexion and rotation of head. *B*, Extension, abduction, adduction and rotation of arm. *C*, Flexion, extension, pronation and supination of forearm. *D*, Flexion and extension of wrist. *E*, Flexion, extension and spreading of fingers.

Illustration continued on opposite page.

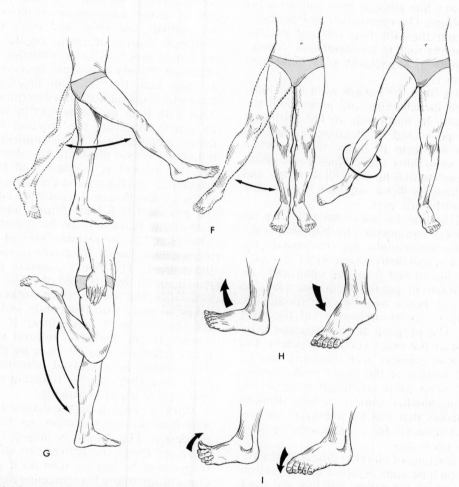

Figure 2–1 (*Continued*)   *F*, Flexion, extension, abduction, adduction and internal rotation of lower limbs. *G*, Flexion and extension of leg. *H*, Dorsiflexion and plantar flexion of foot. *I*, Flexion and extension of toes.

muscles involved in the movement that is giving trouble.

In learning to care for himself, the patient should not be rushed. Patience and restraint are required by the nurse. If the patient becomes frustrated and emotional, the nurse must guard against the sympathetic desire to take over for the patient rather than stand by and have him struggle with and solve his own problem. Overprotection and performing his activities for him will not put the patient on the road to independence. A positive attitude of expectancy of achievement is necessary.

Eliciting from the patient what he is most interested in achieving and giving him the opportunity to participate in the setting of realistic goals and in planning his activity program will help to motivate him. When he does something successfully for himself, he will realize that he can still do things and that, although difficult, self-care is a possible and a worthwhile goal.

Rehabilitation for some patients may require special equipment. Disability or paralysis of the lower limbs may necessitate the use of a wheelchair. The patient is taught transferring to and from the chair and safe management in getting from one place to another. A brace may be used to stabilize the limb or assist in support of the body weight. The purpose, application and management of the brace should be taught. For self-care in patients with disability and restricted motion of the upper limbs, special devices such as a combination knife and fork, long-handled cutlery, a long drinking tube, dishes that can be stabilized and mechanical supports for a weak wrist or grasp may be necessary.

The teaching of all rehabilitation activities should include consideration of the environment in which the patient will live and work. For example, if the person dependent on a wheelchair is to be transported to his place of work by car, he is taught not only how to accomplish the transfer from chair to car but also the management of the collapsible type of chair and the method of getting it in and out of the car.

An interest in personal grooming and appearance is encouraged; some adaptations in clothing may be necessary to facilitate normal dressing, such as front openings, zippers rather than buttons or small fasteners and shoes without laces. A few illustrated texts with many suggestions and detailed instructions for improvisations and adaptations for A.D.L. are included in the bibliography at the end of the chapter.

The Family. When a member of the family becomes disabled, it may mean a change in the way of life for the whole family. It may create financial hardships, particularly if the patient is the wage-earner; responsibilities are shifted; and plans and goals may be shattered. Varied reactions on the part of the family members to the situation may be expected. Family bonds may become greater as they face the situation together; new strengths, capabilities and a determination to cope with their problems may be revealed. In other instances, the reaction of some family members may be resentment for the individual whose disability has altered their life; the patient is rejected, and his loneliness, fear and depression are increased.

An explanation of the patient's condition, the possibilities for his future, and the rehabilitative plans is made by the physician. The nurse has the responsibility of discussing with the family their role in supporting the patient. The home situation is determined, and if there is need of socioeconomic assistance, the social service worker may be asked to meet with the family and arrange for the necessary assistance. If a social worker is not available, referral to appropriate resources may be made by the nurse. This should be discussed with the family first, since they may be reluctant to accept any type of social assistance.

Marked concern for the disabled member may lead to overprotection that fosters dependence. The family is helped to realize there are things the patient can still do and others that he can learn to do if given the opportunity to use his remaining capabilities. Members of the family are encouraged to talk to the nurse about their situation, express their concerns and fears, and to ask about the patient's condition and care. They are advised how they may best help him and themselves. In the initial, acute stage, having someone of his own with him who displays a realistic optimistic attitude will provide support for the patient. This person may be taught how to assist the nurse in some aspects of the patient's care. As the patient's condition improves, it may be helpful if the family discusses their plans for their adjustments with him so he is made to feel he is still an integral part of the family.

The rehabilitative plans will include informing the family what the patient can and cannot do and what care and adaptations are necessary in his future. An assessment of the home in preparation for the patient's return is necessary. Some changes may be necessary in the environment to accommodate the patient and allow him to be as independent as possible. Appropriate reading material may be given them so they will have a better understanding of the disabled person's condition and necessary care. For example, an illustrated outline of the exercise routine that is to be continued or illustrations of a wall-bar or raised toilet seat may prove very helpful. A referral may be made to the district visiting nurse who will give them more direct assistance in the home with the planning for the necessary adjustments and care.

When the family is being taught how to care for the patient at home, consideration should also be given to how they may conserve their energy, protect their health and live a normal life. They can be guided in the sharing of various aspects of the patient's care and can be shown that each has a part to play.

The family is advised that former associates and friends of the patient should be encouraged to visit and maintain a contact with him. They may be surprised to learn that he still has an interest in many things and may still participate in some. All too often, frequent visits are made at first and then, as weeks and months go by, tend to diminish, and the individual's life becomes needlessly narrowed to the institution or home with limited outside contacts.

References

BOOKS AND MONOGRAPHS

Allgire, M. J., and Denney, R. R.: Nurses Can Give and Teach Rehabilitation. New York, Springer Publishing Co., Inc., 1960.
*American Heart Association: Strike Back at Stroke. New York, American Heart Association.
*_____: Up and Around. New York, American Heart Association.
*_____: Do It Yourself Again. New York, American Heart Association.
Fowles, B. H.: Syllabus of Rehabilitation Methods and Techniques. Cleveland, The Stratford Press Co., 1963.
Gordon, E. E.: A Home Program for the Care of Bed Patients. New York, National Multiple Sclerosis Society, 1952.
_____: A Home Program for Patients Ambulatory With Aids. New York, National Multiple Sclerosis Society, 1952.
_____: A Home Program for Independent Ambulatory Patients. New York, National Multiple Sclerosis Society, 1952.
Heather, A. J.: Manual of Care for the Disabled Patient. New York, The MacMillan Co., 1960.
Hirschberg, G. G., Lewis, L., and Thomas, D.: Rehabilitation. Philadelphia, J. B. Lippincott Co., 1964.
Institute of Physical Medicine and Rehabilitation: A Bladder and Bowel Training Program for Patients with Spinal Cord Disease. June 1952.
Lawton, E. Buchwald: Activities of Daily Living. New York, The Institute of Physical Medicine and Rehabilitation, Bellevue Medical Center, 1956.
_____: Activities of Daily Living for Physical Rehabilitation. New York, The Blakiston Division, McGraw-Hill Book Co., Inc., 1963.
Morrissey, A. B.: Rehabilitation in Nursing. New York, G. P. Putnam's Sons, 1951.
Public Health Nursing Section, Colorado State Department of Public Health; Elementary Rehabilitation Nursing Care. Washington, United States Department of Health, Education and Welfare, Public Health Service, Division of Nursing, 1966.
Rusk, H. A.: Rehabilitation Medicine. St. Louis, C. V. Mosby Co., 1958.
Rusk, H. A., and Taylor, E. J.: Living With a Disability. New York, The Blakiston Division, McGraw-Hill Book Co., Inc., 1953.
Sorenson, L., and Ulrich, P. G.: Ambulation, A Manual for Nurses. Minnesota, American Rehabilitation Foundation.
Travis, G.: Chronic Disease and Disability. Berkeley, University of California Press, 1961.

*Distributed in Canada by the Canadian Heart Foundation, Toronto.

PERIODICALS

Canadian Nurse: "Series on Rehabilitation." Canad. Nurse, Vol. 59, No. 3 (Mar. 1963), pp. 225–262.

Deaver, G.: "Rehabilitation." Amer. J. Nurs., Vol. 59, No. 9 (Sept. 1959), pp. 1278–1281.

Drake, M. F.: "Rehabilitation, an Added Dimension in Nursing Care." Amer. J. Nurs., Vol. 60, No. 8 (Aug. 1960), pp. 1105–1106.

Hastings J. E. F.: "Rehabilitation and Public Health." Canad. J. Publ. Health, Vol. 53 (July 1962), pp. 279–283.

Henderson, I., and Henderson, J. E.: "Psychological Care of Patients with Catastrophic Illness." Canad. Nurse, Vol. 61, No. 11 (Nov. 1965), pp. 899–902.

Hunt, T. E.: "Care and Rehabilitation of Patients in Their Homes." Canad. J. Publ. Health, Vol. 53 (Jan. 1962), pp. 22–27.

Kottke, F. J., and Blanchard, R. S.: "Bedrest Begets Bedrest." Nurs. Forum, Vol. 3, No. 3, 1964, pp. 57–72.

Larkin, J. M.: "Assessment of the Disabled; Rehabilitation in Canada." Queen's Printer, Ottawa, Issue No. 14, Summer 1966, pp. 18–25.

Madden, B. W., and Affeldt, J. E.: "To Prevent Helplessness and Deformities." Amer. J. Nurs., Vol. 62, No. 12 (Dec. 1962), pp. 59–61.

Olsen, E. V., et al.: "The Hazards of Immobility." Amer J. Nurs., Vol. 67, No. 4 (Apr. 1967), pp. 779–794.

3
Causes and Effects of Disease

THE NORMAL CELL

The material of which all living matter is composed is referred to as protoplasm. It is organized in discrete microscopic units called cells. There are many different types of cells in the human body; they vary in size, shape, composition and function, but they all have certain common characteristics in structure and activity.

A knowledge of the organization of the basic structural and functional unit contributes to an understanding of the structure and functions of the body and its component parts. An appreciation of the normal is necessary for recognition of the abnormal as well as for an awareness of the effects of disease and the necessary supportive measures.

Structural Features of a Cell

All cells have three main structural parts at some time in their life cycle: a surface membrane, cytoplasm and a nucleus.

Cell Membrane. The cell is enveloped by a very thin membrane which gives delineation, support and protection to the cell substance. Its semipermeability, because of minute pores, allows the passage of water and small molecular solutes in and out of the cell, but it also displays an active, discrim-inative role in relation to what passes in and out.

Cytoplasm. Cytoplasm forms the bulk of the cell. Its composition varies according to the specialized function of the cell. For example, the cytoplasm of mature red blood cells features the hematin-protein compound hemoglobin for the purpose of transporting oxygen; muscle cell cytoplasm consists of compounds responsible for chemical reactions that bring about a thickening and shortening of the cell (contraction).

Cytoplasm is in a fluid state and contains several functional structures or organelles: the endoplasmic reticulum, Golgi apparatus, mitochondria, lysosomes and the centrosome.

The endoplasmic reticulum is a network of tubules that is connected with the nuclear and cell membranes. On the outer surfaces of the tubules are small granular particles called ribosomes which consist of ribonucleic acid (RNA) and protein. The ribosomes are considered to be responsible for the synthesis of protein substances characteristic of the particular type of cell. The products may be for cell use (e.g., enzymes, structural components) or for secretion.

The Golgi apparatus is a series of small vesicles associated with the endoplasmic reticulum. It is prominent in cells which are involved with secretion, and it is suggested that secretions formed by the ribosomes are collected in these vesicles.

The mitochondria are small, flexible bodies which vary in number in different cell types. They contain oxidative enzymes to catalyze reactions that liberate energy which is needed for cellular functions.

Lysosomes contain hydrolytic enzymes that break down particles that are useless or harmful to the cell. Leukocytes contain an unusual number of these minute bodies in order to destroy organisms and other foreign substances taken into the cells by phagocytosis.

The centrosome consists of a pair of cylindrical bodies called centrioles and is situated close to the nucleus. This body is concerned with cell division.

Nucleus. The nucleus is a spherical or ovoid body enclosed in a membrane and, in most cells, lies centrally within the cytoplasm. This structure is the vital control center of the cell; without it the cell cannot reproduce, and its activities cease. An exception to the latter point is the erythrocyte produced by the red bone marrow cells; as the cell matures, its nucleus is extruded, hemoglobin is formed, and the cell is released into the circulation where it functions as a transport for oxygen for approximately 120 days.

The nucleus contains the chromosomes, which determine cell characteristics and transmit the heredity of the cell and the organism from one generation to the next. All human somatic cells contain 23 pairs of chromosomes. When the cell is not in the reproductive phase the chromosomes are scattered throughout the nucleus as long, drawn-out threads. They are readily stainable and may be referred to as chromatin material. Each chromosome consists of a chain of units called genes. The gene is a large, complex molecule of a protein compound known as deoxyribonucleic acid (DNA), and each gene has a specific location on a particular chromosome. The DNA of each gene has similar constituent elements, but the structural arrangement of these may vary from one gene to another; this arrangement determines the specific genetic information. The gene exerts its control on the cell through directing specific protein synthesis (including enzymes) by the cytoplasm. In other words, the DNA determines the

cell properties by directing the essential cytoplasmic composition associated with the particularities of the cell's function. It is suggested that each gene is responsible for the formation and nature of one enzyme which acts as a catalyst.

A second protein found in the nucleus is ribonucleic acid (RNA). It is produced by the DNA and transmits the encoded information of the genes to the ribosomes of the cytoplasm. Within the nuclear material, minute spherical bodies called nucleoli appear. They contain RNA and other proteins, and it is thought they may be concerned with the synthesis of RNA molecules which correspond in molecular structure to the RNA derived from the chromosomes.

Physiological Activities of the Cell

Metabolism. Intracellular activities are chemical reactions which are referred to collectively as metabolism. The metabolic processes are of two types: catabolism refers to reactions in which there is a chemical breakdown of compounds into simpler compounds or atoms; this breakdown is accompanied by a release of energy. New compounds are synthesized from simpler substances during the anabolic process, or anabolism. Both types of processes go on to some extent at all times to maintain the cells and perform the functions that contribute to the overall activities and maintenance of the body as a whole. At times the rate of anabolism may exceed that of catabolism and cell substances accumulate; at times of increased body activity, catabolism proceeds more rapidly and cell substances may be markedly reduced.

A requisite to cellular health and normal functioning is the provision of adequate amounts of essential nutrients such as proteins, carbohydrates, minerals and vitamins. The substances used in metabolism are taken into the cell from the immediate extracellular fluid environment. A constant supply of oxygen is necessary for metabolism. Cellular activities cannot be sustained without the products of oxidative processes. The catabolism of many compounds to release energy results in the production of carbon dioxide, which is eliminated from the cell; this elimination of carbon dioxide and the absorption of oxygen comprise cellular respiration. In addition to carbon dioxide, various substances may be formed during metabolism which are of no use to the cell and, if retained, inhibit cellular functions. These waste products are passed out of the cell and eliminated from the body through an excretory channel. Substances called secretions are formed by some cells to serve a specific useful purpose when discharged. For example, some cells secrete mucus to protect cells from irritating materials; cells of the thyroid secrete thyroxin, which influences the rate of metabolism, particularly the oxidative process, of practically all cells in the body.

The cellular chemical reactions are catalyzed by enzymes which are produced by the ribosomes under the direction of the genes via RNA. These catalytic protein compounds are specific; that is, there is a particular enzyme for each type of chemical reaction. The reaction may be to break down a compound, transfer an atom or molecule from one compound to another or to rearrange component atoms within a molecule. The breakdown of a complex compound involves a series of reactions and a specific

enzyme for each reaction. If one enzyme is lacking, the normal metabolism of the substance is arrested at that level. For example, a specific enzyme is necessary to convert galactose to glucose so it can be catabolized to carbon dioxide and water and release required energy. If the gene that directs the production of the necessary enzyme is abnormal or absent, the galactose accumulates, resulting in an abnormally low blood sugar level, weakness due to the lack of energy production and mental deficiency as a result of an inadequate supply of glucose to the brain cells. The condition is known as galactosemia and is classified as an inborn error of metabolism; this implies an inherited enzyme abnormality or deficiency. Similarly, the condition known as phenylketonuria is due to a congenital deficiency of the enzyme that promotes a reaction to convert the amino acid phenylalanine (a component of many proteins) to tyrosine. Phenylalanine accumulates in the blood and spinal fluid and is damaging to the brain, resulting in mental retardation. The absence of the enzyme is detected through its excretion in the urine as phenylpyruvic

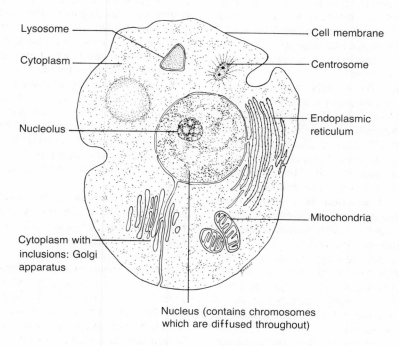

Lysosome

Cytoplasm

Nucleolus

Cytoplasm with inclusions: Golgi apparatus

Cell membrane

Centrosome

Endoplasmic reticulum

Mitochondria

Nucleus (contains chromosomes which are diffused throughout)

Figure 3-1 Diagram of a typical cell.

acid—hence, the name phenylketonuria. If detected soon after birth, a diet low in proteins containing phenylalanine may prevent mental deficiency.

Cellular Movement. Cellular content is in fluid form. Movement of the whole or a part of a cell may occur by the flow of cytoplasm from one part to another in a manner similar to that observed in the amoeba. Leukocytes move in this way in their migration out of the blood stream into extracellular spaces and when they surround and engulf an organism or particle. The movement of a muscle cell (contraction) is achieved by a shortening of the cell with a corresponding increase in the thickness; this action is the result of a series of chemical reactions within the cytoplasm. Some cells have cilia, which are fine, hair-like processes of the cytoplasm which quickly swing in one direction and then slowly resume their former position. They move particles along a surface in the direction of their initial lashing motion. Organized movement of definite parts of the cell occurs as the cell proceeds through the reproductive process.

Irritability. Cells are sensitive and will react to changes in their immediate environment. A change which will initiate a cellular response is referred to as a stimulus. The type of reaction or response of the cell will vary with the type of stimulus and the characteristic of the particular type of cell. Cells may be more irritable to a specific type of stimulus than to others.

Reproduction. New cells are necessary for growth of the organism and for replacement of worn-out cells. They are produced by a cell dividing into two cells, each having a nucleus with 23 pairs of chromosomes as well as cytoplasm with the same properties as those of the parent cell. This process of cell division is referred to as mitosis, and it involves a series of changes in which there is a rearrangement of the centrioles and chromosomes and a subsequent division of the nucleus and the whole cell.

The interval between the end of one mitosis and the beginning of the next is referred to as the interphase, or the amitotic or intermitotic phase. The changes characteristic of reproduction are described as they occur in the following 4 phases:

1. *Prophase.* Preceding this initial phase, cell substance is increased, and the DNA duplicates itself. Each chromosome divides longitudinally into two chromatids which remain attached by a centromere. The chromosomes coil spirally, becoming shorter and thicker, and appear as distinct entities. The two centrioles move away from each other to opposite poles of the cell and develop fibrils stretching out between them. The nucleoli and nuclear membrane disappear.

2. *Metaphase.* The fibrils of the centrioles grow into the nuclear region to become attached to the centromeres of the chromosomes, which arrange themselves in a line between the two centrioles.

3. *Anaphase.* The two chromatids of each chromosome separate at their centromere; one is attracted by a fibril toward one centriole. This results in an equal number of chromatids—corresponding to the original number of chromosomes (46)—being located in either half of the cell.

4. *Telophase.* The final phase involves nuclear re-formation in order to enclose each group of chromatids and constriction of the cytoplasm by indentation of the cell membrane through the center. The spindle formed by the fibrils disappears, a typical nucleus forms in each half of the cell, and the chromatids lengthen (uncoil) and diffuse irregularly throughout the nucleus. Each centriole divides to form a centrosome, and final division of the cytoplasm produces two separate cells which are identical in structure to the original parent cell.

Meiosis (Reduction Division). A new organism is conceived by the union of a female gamete (ovum) and a male gamete (sperm). The union forms a single cell from which all the cells of the body are derived. Obviously, the characteristic number of chromosomes (46) must be established in the initial single cell.

Initially, when both the female and male germ cells are produced by the sex glands they contain 23 pairs of chromosomes. During a maturation process, a special type of cell division takes place in which the number of chromosomes is reduced to half. This cell division process is referred to as meiosis, or reduction division. In meiotic cell division, one of each pair of chromosomes passes to an opposite end of the cell. When the two halves of the cell separate, each daughter cell contains only 23 single

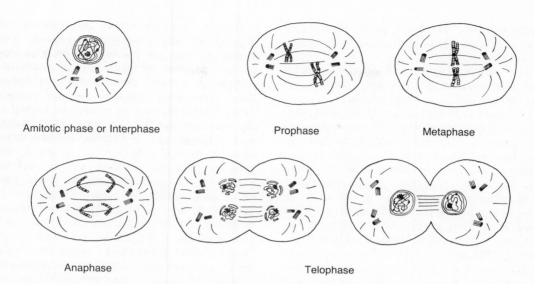

Amitotic phase or Interphase   Prophase   Metaphase

Anaphase   Telophase

Figure 3–2 Phases of mitosis.

chromosomes (haploid chromosomes). At conception, the union of the sperm with haploid chromosomes and an ovum with a corresponding number establishes the distinctive 23 pairs of chromosomes. The resulting cell rapidly reproduces by mitosis, which continues in order to form the new organism.

Homeostasis

For normal functioning, cells require the maintenance of a relatively constant internal environment, which is referred to as homeostasis. This means that each cell, in order to preserve its normalcy, must be surrounded constantly by a fluid with certain definite physical and chemical properties.

Homeostasis is not an absolute constancy but is rather a dynamic balance that varies within narrow limits. Derangements beyond these limits are not compatible with normal cell functioning. The extracellular environment must be within a definite temperature range; it must be capable of supplying the cells with oxygen and essential materials, as well as removing their secretions and waste products. Cellular activities tend to produce changes, but under normal conditions body mechanisms operate continuously to restore and maintain a suitable environment. To quote Guyton: "The functions of all the organs in the body are directed toward a single goal, to maintain constant conditions in the fluids that surround the cells, thereby allowing the cells to continue living, growing and reproducing."[1]

Movement of Substances Across the Cell Membrane. There is a continuous passing of substances in and out of the cells by physical passive processes and by cellular action. The membrane, being semipermeable, permits water and small molecular substances, such as potassium and sodium, to pass through by physical processes. Active transportation by the cell moves large molecular particles, such as protein and fat, across the membrane and may move various substances against a pressure gradient. The latter is an important mechanism in maintaining normal cell composition. For example, a much higher concentration of potassium is required within the cells than in the extracellular fluid; however, the reverse is true of sodium. In order to maintain these conditions, the cells actively transport potassium in and sodium out. One method of active transportation used with large molecular substances is pinocytosis. This process involves invagination of the cell membrane at the site of contact with the particle. The molecule sinks into the invaginated area and is surrounded by the membrane. A vesicle is formed which sep-

---

[1]Arthur C. Guyton: Function of the Human Body, 2nd ed. Philadelphia, W. B. Saunders Co., 1964, p. 4.

arates from the membrane and is moved into the cytoplasm where it disappears, releasing its contents.

The physical processes concerned with the movement of substances in and out of the cell are diffusion and osmosis.

Diffusion is the tendency of the molecules of a substance to disperse equally throughout a space. It is the result of the natural, spontaneous movement of particles from a higher to a lower concentration. Water, gases and some solutes diffuse readily through a semipermeable membrane; if the distribution is equal on both sides, the constant random motion of particles results in the movement of as many particles in one direction as the other. The diffusion of more molecules of a substance in one direction than in the opposite is dependent upon a concentration gradient.

Diffusion is responsible for the movement of gases between the alveolar air of the lungs and the blood and between the blood and the cells. Similarly, many substances absorbed from the intestine create a pressure gradient between the blood and the interstitial fluid and between the interstitial fluid and the intracellular content; this results in the diffusion of these substances from the blood to the interstitial fluid and on into the cells. In the opposite direction, products of metabolism diffuse from the cells into the interstitial fluid and then into the blood.

Osmosis is the movement of water through a semipermeable membrane from an area of lesser concentration of solutes to that of a greater concentration. It occurs only when there is a difference between the concentration of solutes on one side of the membrane and that on the other.

Osmotic pressure is the attraction or pull exerted by the particles of solutes. The degree of osmotic pressure is proportional to the number of particles of contained solutes. A greater concentration of potassium, phosphate, magnesium and protein exists within the cell as compared to that of the extracellular fluid. Sodium, bicarbonate and chloride are in higher concentration outside the cell than within. Normally the osmotic pressure created by the solutes remains relatively constant on both sides of the cell membrane, and water diffuses in and out of the cell without a net loss or gain on either side of the membrane. Under such circumstances, the fluids are said to be isotonic; that is, the fluid on each side of the membrane has the same osmotic pressure.

When the osmotic pressure within the cell becomes greater than that of the interstitial fluid, osmotic equilibrium is quickly restored by the movement of water into the cell. Conversely, when the solutes of the extracellular fluid become concentrated, water passes out of the cell. This latter situation may occur in dehydration, which may be due to an excessive loss of extracellular fluid from the body or to an inadequate fluid intake. Unless the extracellular fluid volume is restored, the loss of water from the cells may interfere with normal cell functioning.

Solutions administered intravenously may be classified as isotonic, hypertonic or hypotonic. An isotonic solution has the same osmotic pressure as the plasma.

A hypertonic solution has a greater concentration of solutes than the plasma. When such a solution is given intravenously, the increased osmotic pressure of the plasma

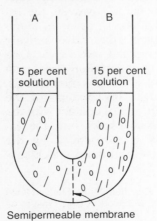
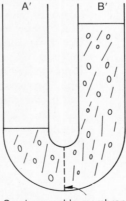

A   B   A'   B'

5 per cent solution | 15 per cent solution

Semipermeable membrane

O = Solute particle

Figure 3–3 Osmosis. *A,* Solution has fewer solute particles (lower osmotic pressure). *B,* Solution has three times as many solute particles as *A* (higher osmotic pressure). *A'* and *B',* Water moves from *A* to *B* until the osmotic pressure is equal on both sides of the semipermeable membrane.

Figure 3–4 Isotonic, hypertonic and hypotonic solutions. *A,* Isotonic solution. Osmotic pressure of fluid introduced is same as that of the plasma and intracellular fluid. No net gain or loss to the cell. *B,* Hypertonic solution. Osmotic pressure of fluid introduced is greater than that of the plasma and intracellular fluid. Water moves out of the cell. *C,* Hypotonic solution. Osmotic pressure of fluid introduced is less than that of the plasma and intracellular fluid. Water moves into the cell, causing it to swell.

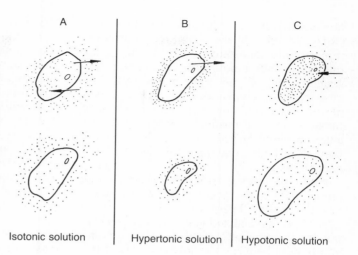

causes water to pass out of the blood cells and from the interstitial spaces across the capillary membranes. A hypertonic solution of glucose or a preparation of urea may be given to a patient with cerebral edema. The increased osmotic pressure of the blood draws fluid into the capillaries in the brain, thus reducing the edema.

A hypotonic solution has a lower osmotic pressure than the plasma. When given intravenously it reduces the plasma osmotic pressure, and water passes into the blood cells, causing them to swell and burst (see Fig. 3–4).

GENERAL ORGANIZATION OF THE BODY

Going from the simplest to the more complex, the structural units of the body are the cells, tissues, organs and systems.

Tissues. As cited previously, the cell is the basic structural and functional unit of the body. Those similar in structure and function are held together by an intercellular substance to form a tissue. The distinctive features of a tissue are determined by the special characteristics of the constituent cells and intercellular substance. Just as the cells of one type of tissue vary in composition, size, shape and arrangement from those of another, the intercellular substance varies in nature and amount. It may be dense and hard, fluid or gel, or may occur in the form of fibers. It may be rigid or pliable, elastic or nonextensible, and tough or fragile. In certain tissues, the intercellular substance

is minimal; in these cases the cells provide the bulk and the particular function of the tissue. In other tissues there is more intercellular substance which plays a major role.

There are four major types of tissues: epithelial, connective, muscular and nervous. Variations occur in the tissues of these major categories as the cells and intercellular substance are adapted to meet the various needs of the body.

Epithelial tissues function in protection, secretion, absorption and filtration. They are found covering all external and internal surfaces as well as in secreting structures and consist mainly of cells with a minimal amount of intercellular substance. The cells reproduce readily, which is essential to the maintenance of surface and lining tissues. Examples of epithelial tissues are the skin, mucous and serous membranes, and the endothelial lining of the blood and lymph vessels and heart chambers.

Connective tissues are concerned mainly with the physical form and mechanical activities of the body rather than with its physiological activities. They provide an internal supporting framework, protection for other structures and connections between parts of the body so they become a functional unit. The intercellular substance predominates in connective tissues and gives them their special characteristics. Examples are bones, tendons, ligaments, cartilage, fascia and adipose tissue. Blood is classified as a connective tissue; in this instance the cells have an equally significant role as that of the intercellular substance, plasma.

Muscular tissue is responsible for all

movements of the body and its organs. The elongated cells (fibers) with their contractile property are important functional units; the relatively small amount of intercellular substance serves only as retaining material. The cytoplasm of muscle cells is called sarcoplasm. Muscle fibers, with the exception of those of visceral muscle, are not capable of cell reproduction; when severely damaged they degenerate and are replaced by connective tissue.

Nervous tissues form the brain, spinal cord and the network of nerve fibers throughout the body. There are two types: one consists of specialized cells (neurons) which initiate and transmit impulses to control and coordinate the physical and mental activities by which the body adapts itself to changes in its external environment. The neurons are incapable of cell division; if a cell process (nerve fiber) outside the brain or cord is injured, it may regenerate only if the cell body is uninjured (see p. 590). The other type of nervous tissue is made up of neuroglial cells and is found in the brain and spinal cord. It serves to support and protect the nervous tissue proper.

Organs. A combination of different types of tissues which are arranged to work in conjunction with one another forms an organ, such as the heart, liver, or stomach. Each organ has a definite form and location in the body and performs specialized activities which are dependent upon the functional contribution of each constituent tissue.

Systems. Several organs are arranged and correlated to form a system, which performs an overall major body function. For example, the digestion of food is dependent upon the coordinated activity of the alimentary tract and accessory organs of the digestive system. The skeletal, muscular, circulatory, respiratory, digestive, excretory, nervous, endocrine and reproductive systems comprise the major complex structural units. Total body functioning is dependent upon the coordinated activities of its various systems. No system functions independently of the others.

DISEASE

Health and disease are relative terms which are difficult to define precisely. The condition of the organism is the result of interaction between the cells within the body and between the body and its environment. As long as the interaction and adaptive mechanisms can maintain normal structure and optimal functional efficiency accompanied by a sense of well-being, the individual is said to be healthy. Disease is a departure from health due to an interruption or disorder of function. There are varying degrees of departure from normal; it may be severe enough to cause incapacity of the individual, or it may be less serious, allowing the individual to remain active but without a sense of well-being.

In some instances, a disturbance in function may develop without becoming apparent to the patient or to others; examples of this may be seen in the early stages of some heart diseases, cancer, tuberculosis and cirrhosis of the liver. This may be due to a sufficient number of normal cells which maintain an adequate degree of functioning, or it may be due to compensatory mechanisms, such as hypertrophy. The effects of a disturbance in function of one part of the body is likely to be reflected in the functioning of other or all parts because of the dependence of each system on the others for its oxygen, nutrients, elimination of wastes and other essentials.

Abnormal cellular structure causes abnormal function, but functional disturbances may occur without any observable change in structure. In other instances, a disturbance in cellular activity may lead to changes in tissue structure. Structural changes resulting from disease in tissues are called lesions. The presence of lesions classifies a disease as being organic rather than functional; functional disease is characterized by a disturbance in function without demonstrable lesions. The manifestations of changes in function and structure are referred to as signs and symptoms.

Pathology is the study of the cause (etiology), developmental process, and the effects of disease. Knowledge of these factors is useful in all aspects of nursing. An appreciation of the cause and factors that favor the development and progress of disease may be applied in preventive nursing. Some understanding of the disease process and its effects on structure and function provides the basis for supportive and therapeutic measures and may alert the nurse to possible complications.

CAUSES OF DISEASE

The cause of some diseases is unknown, and a continuous study goes on searching for the etiologic factor in such conditions as cancer, multiple sclerosis, rheumatoid arthritis, leukemia and psychosis. Recognized causes of disease include the following:

Heredity

An abnormal cellular structure or function may be the result of an abnormal gene in the sex cell of one or both parents. A gene for each trait is received from each parent; in some instances, the new organism may receive only one defective gene, and the manifestation of disturbance will depend on whether the gene is dominant or recessive. If it is dominant, the abnormality will be expressed, but if it is recessive the normal gene will dominate, resulting in normal structure and functioning. If each parent contributes a defective recessive gene for a particular trait, the abnormality is expressed as an hereditary disease.

Developmental Defects

Some abnormal structural and functional defects that are present at birth are due to a failure or an abnormality in the developmental process during the embryonic or fetal stage. The cause in most cases is unknown; in a few instances, the abnormality is associated with an abnormal chromosome pattern in the cells; this is attributed to a faulty reduction-division of the chromosomes in one of the germ cells. For example, an extra chromosome is present in the cells in mongolism. Developmental defects are seen in some infants born to mothers who have had German measles during the first trimester of pregnancy. It is suggested that the rubella virus may pass through the placenta and into the developing tissues of the embryo, thus interfering with normal tissue development. Similarly, toxic chemicals, such as the drug thalidomide, taken during pregnancy may disturb normal fetal development.

Biological Agents

One of the commonest causes of disease is the invasion of the body by bacteria, viruses, fungi or parasites. They harm or destroy the tissues by their direct action on the cells or by the toxins they produce.

Physical Agents

Mechanical injury may damage tissues to the extent of impairing or completely interrupting their function. Cells may be destroyed when subjected to extreme heat or cold. Exposure to excessive sun rays and to radiation from x-rays or radioactive material may alter cell structure and activity or may actually cause destruction of the cells.

Chemicals

When some chemicals are introduced into the body they have an injurious effect on tissue cells. The chemical may disrupt normal cellular chemical reactions either by forming incompatible compounds or by interfering with normal enzymatic action within the cells.

Deficiencies and Excesses

An inadequate supply of materials essential to normal tissue structure and activity may cause a variety of diseases. The deficiency may be due to an insufficient intake of nutritional substances or a specific element, lack of absorption from the intestine, or an interference in the delivery of the essential substances to the cells by the circulatory system.

The lack of a normal oxygen supply to any tissue seriously impairs its function. If the supply is completely cut off, the cells quickly die. The deficiency may be local or general; local hypoxia may be due to a blockage of the vessels supplying the area. General oxygen deprivation may be due to respiratory insufficiency or a disturbance in the oxygen carrying or delivery mechanisms.

An excess of nutrients may also create problems such as increased demands on body function and the storage of excess fat. Morbidity statistics indicate a higher incidence of hypertension, cardiovascular diseases and diabetes in obese persons.

Emotions

Psychological reactions to stressful situations may influence a person's autonomic nervous system and alter its control of the viscera. Changes in autonomic innervation may increase or decrease the function of certain structures; this may have marked effects on total body functioning.

Tissue Responses

Illness may be caused by the responses or reaction of tissues to an injury or irritation. Examples of this are inflammation and allergic reaction, both of which are discussed in ensuing sections of this chapter.

EFFECTS OF DISEASE AGENTS UPON CELLS

When tissue cells are subjected to adverse conditions they may exhibit one or more of the following responses: inflammation, regeneration and repair, degeneration, necrosis, atrophy, hypertrophy, hyperplasia, metaplasia, neoplasia or allergy.

Inflammation

The process of inflammation is a local defensive tissue reaction to injury or irritation. It is designed to remove or destroy the injurious agent (inflammant), keep the injury localized and repair the damage.

The causes of inflammation are many, but they may be broadly classified as: physical (e.g., mechanical agents, extreme heat and cold, radiant energy), chemical (e.g., strong acids and alkalies, irritating gases, poisons, products of necrotic tissue, products of altered metabolism), biological (e.g., microorganisms) and immunological (e.g., antigen-antibody and autoimmune reactions).

The process of inflammation consists of three phases: (1) the cellular and vascular responses, (2) the formation of the inflammatory exudate and (3) the repair of the tissues. In the initial phase, there is a momentary constriction of the blood vessels at the site of injury; this is followed by their dilation in response mainly to the chemical histamine that is released by the injured cells. A marked increase in the blood supply to the area occurs (hyperemia) and causes the characteristic redness and heat at the site.

The rate of blood flow decreases in the dilated vessels, and the blood cells, particularly the leukocytes, move out of the central portion of the stream and collect along the vessel walls. The relaxed capillary walls become more permeable and leukocytes, plasma, erythrocytes and blood platelets escape into the interstitial spaces.

The leukocytes attack the inflammant and assist in disposing of the cellular debris by phagocytosis. The plasma brings antibodies to the site. This action may make the offending agent more susceptible to phagocytosis; it may also neutralize toxins. It dilutes and carries away toxins and debris, brings macrophages (reticuloendothelial cells) to the site which aid the leukocytes in phagocytosis, and transports fibrinogen (a blood protein) into the area to form an interlacing network of fine fibers (fibrin) that walls off the area and forms a framework for reparative tissue.

In the exudative phase, the fluid and blood elements that escape from the vessels, the dead tissue cells, products released by the dead and injured cells, and the inflammant comprise the inflammatory exudate. The nature and amount of exudate depend upon the intensity and duration of the inflammant and the tissue involved.

A serous exudate consists chiefly of fluid with few cells and little or no fibrin. It is seen in the early stages of inflammation or when the injury is mild. An example is the fluid in a blister or that which accumulates when a serous membrane, such as the pleura or the peritoneum, is irritated. Much of the fluid is an increased secretion of serum by the affected membrane.

Purulent exudate, or pus, is a thick fluid made up of leukocytes, dead and living microorganisms which caused the injury, liquefied dead tissue cells, and the fluid and blood elements that escaped from the vessels. The formation of pus may be referred to as suppuration, and organisms that cause it are classified as pyogenic. A localized collection of purulent exudate is called an abscess. The localization is maintained by surrounding the area with leukocytes and fibrin. If the organisms emigrate into the surrounding tissues, the infection spreads and is called cellulitis.

Fibrinous exudate indicates a vascular permeability that allows a greater amount of fibrinogen to leak into the interstitial area. The protein is precipitated by tissue extract (thromboplastin), which is released by injured cells and blood platelets and forms fibrin. An excessive amount of fibrin may form a membranous coating over a tissue surface, and its stickiness may cause the surfaces to adhere. The fibrin may be replaced by fibrous tissue, and bands of fibrous adhesions may form between two surfaces. Adhesions develop most frequently on serous surfaces such as the pleura, pericardium and the intestines.

A hemorrhagic exudate contains a large number of erythrocytes and may be described as sanguinous.

The collection of inflammatory exudate distends the interstitial spaces, producing swelling and pressure on nerve endings and thereby causing pain. Some of the pain may also be due to irritation of the nerves by chemicals released by the injured cells or the inflammatory agent.

In the reparative phase, once the inflammant has been overcome and the debris cleared away by leukocytes, macrophages and lymphatic drainage, the space is returned to normal or is filled in by the regeneration of tissue cells or fibrous scar tissue or by a combination of the two. A description of this phase of the inflammatory process follows on page 34.

Systemic Reactions Associated with Inflammation. Toxic products of the inflammatory process may be absorbed into the blood stream at the site of injury or may be carried away in the lymph. Solid particles in the lymph may be arrested in lymph nodes where they may be destroyed by phagocytic cells. Soluble products of the reaction may pass through the lymph nodes and be delivered into the blood stream to be circulated throughout the body, causing general body irritation and responses. These give rise to the systemic or general body manifestations of inflammatory disease, which are headache, fever, increased respiratory and pulse rates, general malaise, loss of appetite, lethargy and weakness. An examination of the blood may reveal an increase above the normal in the number of leukocytes and an increase in the blood sedimentation rate. If the inflammant is a microorganism, a serum titer may demonstrate a significant increase in the number of antibodies.

The severity of general body symptoms depends upon the amount and toxicity of the absorbed inflammatory products, which in turn are determined by the nature and intensity of the inflammant.

Classification of Inflammation. Inflammation may be classified in a variety of ways:

ACCORDING TO THE DURATION OF THE REACTION. It may be termed acute if it has a sudden onset and progresses quickly to recovery, permanent injury or death. Chronic inflammation usually has an insidious onset and persists over a period of months to years. A subacute inflammatory process is usually considered intermediary to the foregoing types in both severity and duration.

ACCORDING TO THE STRUCTURE AFFECTED. The suffix -*itis* is used to denote inflammation of the particular tissue or structure indicated by the preceding part of the word. For example: myocarditis implies inflammation of the muscle fibers of the heart; pneumonitis, inflammation of the lung tissue; laryngitis, inflammation of the larynx; peritonitis, inflammation of the peritoneum, and so on.

ACCORDING TO THE NATURE OF THE EXUDATE. Fibrinous inflammation indicates that a relatively large amount of fibrin is formed. Purulent inflammation implies suppuration.

ACCORDING TO THE ETIOLOGIC AGENT. Another basis of classification that may be used occasionally relates to the nature of the inflammant. The terms traumatic, chemical, bacterial or allergic may be used as descriptive terms.

Nursing in Inflammation. Much of the care of the patient with an area of inflammation is determined by the site of the process, the function which is disturbed and the nature of the inflammant. The following general principles apply:

The affected part is placed at rest, and when this is not possible, demands upon it should be reduced to a minimum.

If a limb is involved, the patient may receive some relief from pain by elevation of the part. This encourages venous and lymphatic drainage which may reduce the swelling, and it also increases the flow of a fresh supply of blood into the area with more elements to combat the offending agent and restore the tissue to normal.

Hot or cold applications may be ordered. Heat favors an increased blood supply to the part and relaxation of muscle tissue, which may be in spasm because of the injured cells. Cold applications cause constriction of the vessels and thus reduce the volume of exudate and diminish the swelling which is responsible for the pain. Cold also reduces the sensitivity of the pain nerve endings, and when bacteria are the causative agent their activity and multiplication may be delayed.

If the inflammant is known to be microorganisms, antimicrobial drugs such as antibiotics, sulfonamide, antitoxin or specific preparations are prescribed.

General rest is beneficial in increasing the patient's ability to combat the disease, particularly if constitutional symptoms are manifested. The patient is encouraged to take plenty of fluids to promote dilution and elimination of absorbed toxic products.

Repair of a Lesion

When tissue is damaged several processes may occur to repair the area. The processes are recovery, regeneration and replacement with fibrous tissue.

When the injury is slight, cell changes may be reversible, and a complete recovery occurs. If the irritant caused the inflammatory response without cellular necrosis, the exudate is removed and the area returns to normal; this result is called resolution.

In the case of a more severe injury, the damage to some cells may be irreversible and they die. The area is healed by replacement of the destroyed tissue by living cells. The healing is by regeneration if the new cells produced by the surrounding cells are similar in structure and function to the cells being replaced. The ability to reproduce cells varies greatly from one type of tissue to another. Nervous, muscular and elastic tissues have very little or no regenerative capacity after structural growth is completed. Epithelial, fibrous, osseous, lymphoid and bone marrow tissues exhibit a much greater ability to reproduce like cells.

When regeneration is not possible, repair occurs by replacing the lost tissue with fibrous tissue. The fibrin of the inflammatory exudate, which was formed in response to the injury, provides a framework in which granulation tissue develops. The latter is formed by the ingrowth of capillaries from surrounding vessels and by fibroblasts from marginal connective tissue. The formation of granulation tissue in an injured area is sometimes referred to as "organization." At this stage, the tissue appears as a very soft, gelatinous-like red mass because of its many newly formed capillaries and large immature fibroblasts around which collagen fibers develop. As the fibroblasts and collagen fibers mature, the tissue shrinks, many capillaries are constricted and obliterated, and an area of firm fibrous tissue remains which is known as a cicatrix or scar. Marginal surface epithelium (e.g., skin) proliferates to form a surface covering.

The fibrous tissue substitution for the original specialized cells may reduce the functional capacity of the affected structure or may cause mechanical interference because of its firm, constricting nature, such as is seen in pyloric obstruction when a peptic ulcer heals. Factors which delay healing include:

1. *Tissue trauma and a reduced blood supply.* The more serious the tissue injury and interference with the blood supply to the affected area, the longer will be the period required to replace the destroyed tissue.

2. *Infection.* Invasion of the wound by microorganisms may increase tissue destruction and impede the formation of granulation tissue.

3. *Nutritional deficiencies.* A deficient intake of protein results in a lack of the essential amino acids from which new tissue is constructed. An insufficient supply of vitamin C prevents the formation of collagen fibers that support the developing fibrous tissue.

4. *Mechanical factors.* Friction on a wound destroys the soft granulation tissue. The presence of a foreign body that prevents the apposition of wound edges retards healing.

5. *Adrenocortical hormones.* An excess of these hormones inhibits inflammation and, as a result, the formation of granulation tissue.

Degenerative Changes

Degeneration of cells is characterized by changes in the chemical reactions and composition of the cytoplasm as well as a corresponding decrease in cell function. It may be due to a diminished blood supply, inadequate oxygen or nutrients, trauma, infection, toxic substances, or an alteration in the enzyme systems within the cells. The cells may contain an accumulation of an abnormal substance or an excess of normal materials which they cannot metabolize or extrude.

Descriptive terms such as fatty, cloudy swelling, hyaline (translucent), amyloid (waxy, starch-like) and mucoid may be applied to degeneration according to the changes observed in the composition and the appearance of the cells.

Necrosis

Necrosis is the death of cells or tissue within a living organism. It may be caused by a lack of essential materials for cell activity, mechanical injury, extreme heat or cold, chemical or bacterial poisons or radiation. The dead cells may be liquefied by their contained enzymes. They may disintegrate and coagulate to form a relatively firm dry mass or may disintegrate to form a mass of caseous material which is grayish white and soft and cheesy in consistency. The latter is characteristic of cells destroyed by tuberculous infection.

Gangrene is the death of a relatively large area of tissue; it may involve a part or the whole of an organ or limb. Infarction is a term used to denote necrosis of an area of tissue caused by ischemia (inadequate blood supply to the part).

Atrophy

A decrease in the size of a structure may be due to a reduction in the size of the individual tissue cells or a decrease in the number of constituent cells. The latter is due to a failure of the replacement of cells to keep pace with cells destroyed or worn out; this is commonly seen in the later years of life. The cause of atrophy may be nutritional deficiency, a reduced blood supply, excessive functional demands on the tissue, disuse, interruption of the nerve supply to the part, toxic substances or physiologic aging mechanisms (e.g., atrophy of the uterus and breasts after menopause due to a change in the concentration of sex hormones).

Hypertrophy and Hyperplasia

A frequent response of a tissue to increased demands placed upon it is hypertrophy, which is achieved by an increase in the size of the individual cells. It may be observed in the enlargement of skeletal muscles with increased work and exercise.

An increase in the volume of tissue due to an increased number of cells is called hyperplasia.

Hypertrophy and hyperplasia are beneficial in cases in which an increase in function is necessary. The heart, for example, may compensate for increased resistance to the flow of blood from a chamber by the hypertrophy of the myocardial fibers of the walls of that chamber. Hyperplasia of the bone marrow and lymphoid tissues increases the number of leukocytes and is helpful in severe infection. In other instances, an increase in the size of a structure may be harmful. Hypertrophy of the heart muscle may require a greater blood supply than the coronary arteries can supply. An enlarged organ may cause pressure or obstruction in some situations. A frequent example of this is hyperplasia of the prostate gland; the enlarged gland imposes upon the urethra, causing retention of urine.

Metaplasia

This tissue response to adverse conditions is the replacement of tissue by cells that are different from their predecessors. For example, following repeated injury and irritation, the normal, ciliated, mucus-secreting epithelial lining of the respiratory tract may be replaced by a thicker, nonsecreting squamous epithelium. This substitution reduces the normal, protective cleansing mechanisms and predisposes to infection.

Neoplasia

This term means new formation or growth. Normally, the production of cells is a regulated process allowing for growth of the organism in early life and for replacement of worn-out or damaged cells throughout the total life span. Occasionally the control of cell reproduction is lost in some tissue and an excessive production occurs. The cells are usually atypical, serve no useful purpose, develop at the expense of surrounding tissues and continue their characteristics through successive generations of cells. The resulting mass is referred to as a new-growth or neoplasm.

When the neoplasm produces an evident swelling, it may be called a tumor. If it is confined by a capsule, remains localized and the rate of growth of the cells is relatively slow, the new growth is said to be benign. Malignant neoplasms (cancers) grow more rapidly, are not encapsulated and spread into surrounding tissues. Some of their cells may be carried from the site of their origin and may set up colonies of the malignant cells (metastases) in other areas of the body. The proliferative growth of malignant cells with their invasion and destruction of normal tissue eventually ends in death of the patient. Cancer is discussed more fully in Chapter 8.

Allergy (Hypersensitivity)

The term allergy implies an altered state of tissue reactivity. Some persons have an unusual sensitivity to certain substances and, upon contact with them, manifest an adverse reaction not seen in most people. The substance that causes the abnormal reaction is called an allergen or may be referred to as an antigen, since it causes the body to produce antibodies.

The allergen is usually a protein; in the few exceptions in which it is nonprotein, it becomes linked to a protein in the body and forms a compound to which the tissues are sensitive. The reaction-producing substance is specific to the individual and may be a food, an animal or plant emanation (e.g., horse dander, pollen), a chemical (e.g., dye) or a drug. It may reach the tissues by inhalation, ingestion, parenteral injection, or by direct contact with the skin. In the case of ingestion, the allergen may have a local effect on the gastrointestinal tissues or may be absorbed unchanged and carried by the blood to sensitive tissues.

Antibodies are usually considered an asset, but in allergic persons the body develops antibodies that cause adverse reactions and a disease state in defense against the substance to which its tissues are sensitive. The first contact with the allergen may not produce manifestations of an allergic reaction, but antibodies are formed that attach or remain close to the sensitive cells. Subsequent contacts produce an interaction between the allergen and antibody (antigen-antibody reaction). The tissue cells are injured and release harmful substances such as histamine, acetylcholine and serotonin which may be circulated through the body, producing adverse effects on other tissues. The inflammatory process may also develop at the site of the injured cells.

Allergic disorders include hay fever, asthma, eczema, urticaria, dermatitis, specific drug sensitivity (e.g., penicillin, sulfonamide, aspirin), specific food sensitivity (e.g., shellfish, milk, wheat, eggs, mushrooms), serum sickness and anaphylaxis. An antigen-antibody reaction is also considered to be the causative factor in rheumatic fever and nephritis. Currently one finds an increasing number of references that suggest a similar etiologic basis for rheumatoid arthritis and collagen diseases such as disseminated lupus erythematosus, polyarteritis and scleroderma.

The cells in which a sensitivity is most frequently manifested appear to be those of epithelial, connective and smooth muscle tissues. The areas of the body most frequently involved are the respiratory tract, skin and gastrointestinal tract. The reactions may take the form of itching, excessive secretion and edema of the nasal pharyngeal mucous membrane (hay fever); spasmodic constriction of the muscle tissue of the bronchial tubes and swelling and edema of their mucosa (asthma); erythematous, vesicular and inflammatory eruptions of the skin (urticaria, eczema, dermatitis); vomiting and diarrhea (food sensitivity); increased permeability of blood vessels and generalized edema; or vasodilation leading to circulatory failure manifested by a weak pulse, sharp fall in blood pressure and collapse (anaphylaxis). Combinations of these may occur in the same patient. One allergen may cause a reaction in more than one area of the body; for example, a person with a hypersensitivity to a particular food may develop both gastrointestinal and skin reactions, or he may develop asthma and a gastrointestinal reaction. The reaction varies in different persons, depending on their tissue sensitivity.

Reactions may occur immediately or may

be delayed. In the immediate type, manifestations appear within minutes to a few hours of receiving the allergen. When the reactions are delayed, a period of several days or weeks may elapse between the contact and the onset.

Changes in the blood may occur; an increase in the eosinophil leukocytes is frequently seen. In immediate reactions, an increase in polymorphonuclear leukocytes (neutrophils) may be evident; however, it may be the monocytes that are increased in a delayed reaction.

Genetics are considered to play a role in allergic reactions; it is thought that the capacity to develop a hypersensitivity can be inherited. Antigen-antibody reactions have a tendency to occur in families. The disorder may differ from one family member to another. One may exhibit a skin reaction; another may suffer from asthma. At the same time, siblings or offsprings of the affected person may not manifest any hypersensitivity. When there is a history of an allergy on both the maternal and paternal sides, a greater number of the offspring become affected, and reactions appear at an earlier age.

Identification of the Allergen. An effort is made to learn of any allergic disorders in the family, and a detailed history is taken of the patient's personal, occupational, and recreational activities and environment.

The allergen may be readily identified by the patient, family or nurse when repeated reactions are associated with the inhalation, ingestion or injection of a certain substance. For example, the patient may become ill each time he eats a particular food, or the nurse may note that certain signs and symptoms are manifested whenever he receives a certain drug.

Sensitivity to a substance may be detected by an intradermal or scratch skin test in which extracts of common allergens (dust, molds, feathers, animal danders, pollens, cosmetics, dyes, wool, synthetic clothing material and various foods) are used. The intradermal method involves the injection of a minute dose of each extract into the superficial layers of the skin. A small amount of normal saline is injected and used as a control or comparison. In the scratch test, a drop of each allergen is applied at areas along a superficial scratch.

The arm or the upper back may be the site used for the test; the former is preferable so that at early signs of a reaction a tourniquet can be applied to slow absorption and prevent anaphylaxis. Emergency equipment and drugs that are used in the treatment of anaphylactic shock (see p. 38) should be readily available for immediate use.

The sites are observed 15 to 30 minutes after the administration of the allergens. A positive reaction is indicated by itching and the appearance of erythema and a wheal (a blanched elevation surrounded by redness).

When food is suspected of being the excitant, an elimination diet may be used to identify the specific food. Common or suspected food allergens (e.g., wheat, milk, eggs) are omitted from the diet until the reaction subsides, and then they are added one at a time and the patient's tolerance is noted.

Treatment and Nursing in Allergy. Treatment includes avoidance of the allergen, drug therapy and hyposensitization.

Avoidance of the allergen may involve such things as moving to another geographical area, a change of occupation, air conditioning to reduce pollen and dust inhalation, the elimination of a particular food from the diet, the use of foam rubber pillows instead of those filled with feathers, the use of non-allergenic cosmetics, avoiding clothing of certain synthetic material, or the removal of certain pets from the environment.

Drugs used to relieve allergic reactions include the following: antihistamines (e.g., Chlor-Trimeton, Pyribenzamine, Benadryl); aminophylline, which is especially valuable in relaxing bronchospasm; adrenal corticoids (e.g., Hydrocortisone, Prednisone); ephedrine preparations (e.g., Neo-Synephrine, Privine), which may be used locally to shrink the nasal mucous membrane; isoproterenol (e.g., Isuprel), which may be nebulized and inhaled or may be given orally; and epinephrine hydrochloride (Adrenalin), which is used in severe reactions and allergic emergencies where quick action is necessary.

Hyposensitization, or desensitization, consists of a series of subcutaneous injections of the specific allergen(s). The doses are very small but are progressively increased over an extended period of time. The exact mechanism by which this procedure reduces the patient's hypersensitivity is not understood. One author suggests that with the resulting increase in antibodies, a larger dose of the allergen is required to elicit a reaction, or antibodies may be formed that block the antigen-antibody reaction.[2] Another reference states that the free serum antibodies are so increased that they block the access of the allergen to the sensitive cells.[3]

The nurse may play an important role in helping the patient to accept and make the adjustments that will help to prevent reactions. If the allergen is a food, the patient is advised as to what should be eliminated from his diet and what substitutions may be made in order to meet his nutritional requirements. When the exciting substance is an inhalant, methods to reduce dust and pollens in the air are suggested. These may include such things as damp dusting; vacuum cleaning rather than sweeping; the removal of flowers, drugs, drapes and dust catchers from the environment; and the use of a mask in certain situations. The importance of avoiding physical and mental exhaustion, emotional upsets, infections and malnutrition is discussed with the patient since these influence his hypersensitivity and predispose to a reaction.

The allergic person is advised to carry a card in his wallet that indicates his allergy and to register with Medic Alert. This organization provides the person with an identification pendant or bracelet that immediately alerts contacts to the fact that he has an allergy.

Anaphylaxis. This is an immediate and serious allergic reaction manifested by acute respiratory distress and circulatory collapse. The patient's breathing becomes difficult because of severe bronchial constriction and probably laryngeal edema; there is a sharp fall in the blood pressure, and the pulse is rapid and weak and may quickly become imperceptible. Urticaria may also become evident. The picture is one of shock; this accounts for the term anaphylactic shock, which is synonymous with anaphylaxis.

The exact mechanism is not understood but present knowledge attributes this severe reaction to the release of large amounts of histamine, acetylcholine and other toxic substances by tissue cells injured by the antigen-antibody reaction. These substances are known to cause the contraction of bronchial muscle, vasodilation, and increased permeability of the capillaries.

Urgent treatment is necessary to prevent the reaction from proving fatal. Whenever a substance that is a possible antigen is given, the injection should be administered in a limb so that a tourniquet may be applied to reduce absorption if early signs of anaphylaxis appear. Epinephrine hydrochloride (Adrenalin) 1:1000 is given intramuscularly or intravenously to relax bronchial contracture and to constrict the blood vessels. If given intramuscularly, the epinephrine should be administered as close to the site of injection of the exciting substance as possible. The patient is placed in the shock position, which is dorsal recumbent with the lower limbs elevated. Clothing at the neck should be loosened. An oropharyngeal or an endotracheal tube may be introduced to establish an airway. If the larynx is edematous, a tracheotomy may be necessary. If cardiac arrest occurs, external cardiac massage is instituted (see p. 229).

Aminophylline is administered intravenously to promote bronchial dilation. An intravenous infusion of plasma or some other solution may be started to increase the intravascular volume. A vasopressor such as levarterenol (Levophed) may be added to the intravenous solution to raise the blood pressure.

The blood pressure, pulse and respirations are checked and recorded at frequent intervals, which are lengthened as the patient improves. The patient is kept under close observation for several days for possible recurrence of reactions and for irreversible damage from the anaphylactic shock.

Slower acting drugs to counteract further antigen-antibody reaction are prescribed for several days. These may be corticoid preparations (e.g., prednisone) or antihistamines (e.g., Chlor-Trimeton). A corticoid preparation may be given intravenously at first, then orally when the patient's condition has improved.

[2]T. R. Harrison et al., (Eds.): Principles of Internal Medicine, 4th ed. New York, The Blakiston Division, McGraw-Hill Book Co., Inc., 1962, pp. 1258–59.

[3]Sir Stanley Davidson: The Principles and Practice of Medicine, 7th ed. London, E. & S. Livingstone Ltd., 1965, p. 26.

Prevention of Serious Allergic Reactions.
Observation of the following precautions may avert a serious reaction in some instances. Patients should be questioned as to allergy and drug and food sensitivity on admission to the hospital and clinic and also when an initial home visit is made. If such is indicated, it should be reported to the doctor and clearly and conspicuously marked on the front of the patient's chart and nursing care plan.

Before administering the first dose of a drug that is known to be a common allergen, it is advisable to ask the person if he has ever taken it before; this may elicit a history of a previous reaction. The patient is observed closely after the first two or three doses of any of these drugs for signs of an untoward reaction. The common offenders include penicillin, streptomycin, animal serum (e.g., antitoxin), acetylsalicylic acid and iodide preparations used as contrast media in x-rays. Penicillin and serums are responsible for the greatest incidence of anaphylaxis. Before giving the initial dose of either of these, a small test dose should be given intradermally. A sensitivity is manifested by the appearance of itching, erythema and a wheal at the site within 15 to 20 minutes. When the initial dose of a drug known to cause adverse reactions is given in a clinic or doctor's office, the patient is asked to remain for 20 to 30 minutes.

An emergency tray or cart should be kept fully equipped and quickly available, and it should be familiar to all staff in the event of a serious reaction. Minimal equipment on such a tray would be tourniquets, nasopharyngeal airway, endotracheal tube, sterile syringes and needles, alcohol sponges, and a drug box containing ampules of epinephrine and aminophylline.

Early signs of anaphylaxis are redness and itching at the site of injection, repeated sneezing, pallor, and complaints of a peculiar sensation in the throat, a tightness of the chest or faintness. Reactions may be prevented if the patient carries a notice of his allergic problem in his wallet or pocket, or if he is wearing a Medic Alert tag.

Serum Sickness. This is an antigen-antibody reaction that occurs one to two weeks after the injection of a foreign serum such as tetanus or diphtheria antitoxin. The signs and symptoms are urticaria (hives), fever, headache, joint swelling, pain and the enlargement of lymph nodes. The condition is treated by the administration of an antihistamine or corticoid preparation.

Autoimmune Disease

The body differentiates between its own protein and exogenous or foreign protein. Generally, antibodies are formed only in response to an exogenous antigen. Occasionally, an antigen may be developed within a person (autoantigen) which stimulates the formation of antibodies (autoantibodies). The antigen may be produced by the entrance of a foreign nonantigenic substance which combines with an endogenous protein, altering it and making it antigenic. The formation of antibodies by the body against its own protein is known as autoimmunization. The antigen-antibody combination may cause a reaction, and the resulting disease is classified as autoimmune.

Tissue Transplantation

The transplantation of tissue or an organ from one person to the body of another has received a great deal of attention. As cited previously, the body distinguishes between its own protein and foreign protein. Foreign tissue is treated as an antigen, and the body rejects it by producing antibodies which attack it. An exception to this is the case in which the transplant is from one identical twin to the other.

Some degree of success has been achieved in the transplantation of a kidney from one person to another. Tolerance for the transplant is developed by total body irradiation or the administration of cortisone, which suppress the formation of antibodies. The latter, however, increases the risk of infection; the patient is unable to produce antibodies which would normally overcome invading organisms which are prevalent in his environment.

Laboratory research and experimentation continue to search for a means by which the antigen-antibody mechanism can be controlled so that a healthy organ of one person may be transplanted to another person and be accepted.

References

BOOKS

Anthony, C. P.: Anatomy and Physiology, 7th ed. Saint Louis, C. V. Mosby Co., 1967. Chapter 2.

Beeson, P. B., and McDermott, W. (Eds.): Textbook of Medicine, 13th ed. Philadelphia, W. B. Saunders Co., 1971, pp. 786–806.

Boyd, Wm.: An Introduction to the Study of Disease, 5th ed. Philadelphia, Lea and Febiger, 1962, Part 1.

Davidson, S.: The Principles and Practice of Medicine, 7th ed. Edinburgh, E. & S. Livingstone Ltd., 1965, pp. 20–26.

Guyton, A. C.: Function of the Human Body, 3rd ed. Philadelphia, W. B. Saunders Co., 1969. Chapters 2, 3 and 4.

Harrison, T. R., et al. (Eds.): Principles of Internal Medicine, 4th ed. New York, The Blakiston Division, McGraw-Hill Book Co., Inc., 1962, pp. 1257–1274.

Hopps, H. C.: Principles of Pathology, 2nd ed. New York, Appleton-Century-Crofts, 1964. Chapters 1, 3, 5, 6 and 11.

Jacob, S. W., and Francone, C. A.: Structure and Function in Man, 2nd ed. Philadelphia, W. B. Saunders Co., 1970. Chapters 2 and 3.

Smith, A. L.: Microbiology and Pathology, 8th ed. Saint Louis, C. V. Mosby Co., 1964. Chapters 39, 42 and 44.

Walter, J. B., and Israel, M. S.: General Pathology, 2nd ed. Boston, Little, Brown & Co., 1965. Chapters 3 to 15.

PERIODICALS

Brachet, J.: "The Living Cell." Sci. Amer., Vol. 205, No. 3 (Sept. 1961), pp. 51–61.

Hildreth, E. A.: "Some Common Allergic Emergencies." Med. Clin. North Amer., Vol. 50, No. 3 (Sept. 1966), pp. 1313–1323.

Miller, M. W.: "The Comprehensive Approach to the Allergic Patient." Med. Clin. North Amer., Vol. 49, No. 5 (Sept. 1965), pp. 1415–1424.

4
Infection

The term infection implies entrance into the body of pathogenic (disease-producing) organisms which may or may not produce a disease state. The latter depends on the particular organism, its virulence and the host's resistance.

Pathogens

The organisms capable of producing disease are called pathogens and include bacteria, viruses, fungi, protozoa and parasitic worms.

Bacteria are forms of plant life which are microscopically visible and are broadly classified according to their shape as cocci (spherical), bacilli (rod-shaped) or spirochetes (spiral). They may be found almost anywhere. They are present in the soil, air, water, food and refuse and are also found in the body cavities and on the body surface.

Bacteria are a major cause of disease, although many types are nonpathogenic. Some species normally inhabit a particular area of the body without causing disease and are referred to as the normal bacterial flora of that area or commensals. For example, the skin is a normal habitat of staphylococci; colon bacilli are always present in the intestine; and lactobacilli inhabit the vagina. Commensals may play an essential role in the body; for instance, the main source of

vitamin K, which is necessary for blood-clotting, is the bacterial action in the intestine. The bacterial flora may be potential pathogens if they gain access to other areas of the body.

Viruses are the smallest pathogenic organisms and may only be seen under electron-microscopic magnification. They produce disease by entering the host's cells and may cause proliferation, degeneration or destruction.

Fungi are multicellular, mold-like organisms which produce interlacing filaments or chains. A disease caused by a fungus is called a mycosis, or it may be indicated by the suffix -osis preceded by the name of the causative fungus. Thrush, ringworm and histoplasmosis are examples of mycotic disease.

Protozoa are single-celled organisms that belong to the animal kingdom and are more complex in structure and activity than bacteria. Diseases that are caused by protozoa include malaria, sleeping sickness, amoebic dysentery and trichomoniasis.

Infection may be caused by parasitic worms, which may be referred to as helminths. The helminthic infections most commonly seen are those caused by the roundworm, pinworm, tapeworm and trichinella spiralis. The latter causes trichinosis.

The filarial worm (fluke) that causes filariasis or elephantiasis and the hookworm are more prevalent in tropical areas.

Invasion by Pathogenic Organisms. Sources of pathogens are infected human beings, infected animals, water, soil, and decaying animal and vegetable matter. The infecting agents may enter the host through the respiratory tract, the alimentary tract, a break in the skin or the genitourinary tract. A fetus may become infected by transplacental transmission. Normally the placenta is an effective barrier, but certain organisms (the spirochete that causes syphilis; viruses which are present in the mother) are likely to cross into the fetus.

Many microorganisms have an affinity for certain tissues and organs. For example, the virus that causes mumps has a predilection for the parotid glands. Similarly, the pneumococcus readily affects the lungs, and the meningococcus prefers the meninges.

Disease may or may not develop when pathogenic organisms invade body tissues. This depends on the virulence of the organisms and the host's resistance. Virulence refers to the capacity of the organisms to survive, multiply and injure the host's tissues. It is greater in some types and in certain strains of the same type. A serious influenza epidemic occurs because the prevalent organism is so virulent that practically everyone whom it invades becomes ill. An organism of weaker virulence may be quickly destroyed by the host's defense mechanisms; or in some instances the organism may remain alive within the host but is unable to multiply to the number necessary to overcome the defenses and injure tissues sufficiently to produce disease. In the latter situation, the host may become a carrier who is capable of transmitting the organism to others whose defenses may be weaker.

The major way in which infecting agents cause disease is by their production of harmful chemical substances called toxins. The toxin may be liberated by the organism while it is alive (exotoxin), or it may be released with its disintegration (endotoxin). Toxins may injure the cells at the site of their release and may also be absorbed into the blood and affect other structures throughout the body. In most instances, a toxin is specific as to the tissues it affects; for example, the exotoxin produced by diphtheria

bacilli injures cardiac muscle cells and may cause myocarditis.

Host Defenses

Defenses against pathogens are natural (innate) or acquired.

Innate Defenses. Normal body structure and activities provide the individual with considerable protection against infection. Externally, the skin is an effective barrier against the entry of organisms as long as it remains intact. The acidity and fatty acid content of its glandular secretions tend to destroy or inhibit the growth of many pathogens. Microorganisms are ever present on the skin; they penetrate the hair follicles and the ducts of the sweat and sebaceous glands. Thorough washing and scrubbing under running water reduce their number but do not produce a sterile surface. This makes the use of sterile gloves necessary when handling sterile equipment if asepsis is to be maintained.

The mucous membrane of the respiratory tract plays an important protective role. Its secretion traps and carries away organisms; the cilia filter the air and sweep out offenders. The mucus may also induce coughing, which forcefully expels material bearing organisms from the tract. Drying of the membrane, destruction of the cilia and loss of the cough reflex reduce the protective mechanism.

The mucus secreted in the gastrointestinal tract protects the mucous membrane lining from the hydrochloric acid and digestive enzymes. Absence of the mucus could result in ulceration that would permit the entrance of pathogens. The acidity of the gastric secretion destroys many organisms that are ingested.

The microorganisms that are normal inhabitants of some areas of the body may play a defensive role. For example, the reaction of the natural flora of the secretions of the vaginal mucosa produces an acidity that creates a resistance to infective agents.

Another important natural defense mechanism is phagocytosis; pathogens that invade the body may be engulfed and destroyed by leukocytes and macrophages. In many infections the number of leukocytes in circulation is rapidly increased, and they migrate to the site of invasion. Changes in the proportion of different types of leukocytes are characteristic of infection by certain types of organisms. Lymph nodes are strategically situated along the course of the lymphatics and filter out bacteria to be destroyed by phagocytosis.

The inflammatory process is a protective mechanism and is described on page 32.

Body fluid contain some substances that are antibacterial. One of these is an enzyme (lysozyme) that destroys bacteria by breaking down their cell walls. Plasma contains gamma globulin which forms antibodies in response to infective agents or their toxins.

Good health habits such as optimal nutrition and hydration, adequate rest and exercise, and the avoidance of fatigue and stress promote the body's natural resistance to infection.

Some persons have what is referred to as a natural immunity to certain diseases. Immunity may be defined as the resistance of the body to pathogenic organisms. Natural immunity to certain pathogens varies with species, races and individuals. A species of animal may be very susceptible to infection by a certain type of organism which is incapable of producing disease in humans. Persons of the Negroid race exhibit a poor resistance to tuberculosis as compared with Caucasians, but the exact reverse is apparent in relation to malaria. A natural resistance to certain infections may be present in some individuals; this is evident when a family or group is equally exposed to an infectious disease and all but one become ill. Age is considered to be a factor in natural immunity; certain infections have a higher incidence in children and rarely occur in the elderly, and infections characteristic of the later years of life have a lesser incidence in younger persons.

Acquired Defenses. Immunity to an infection may be acquired by an individual as a result of contact with the infecting agent or its products. The host develops an immunity by forming substances that are capable of destroying the invading organisms or neutralizing their toxins. The organism or toxin that stimulates the formation of the defensive substances is known as an antigen; the substances formed in response to the antigen are called antibodies or immune bodies.

Antibodies are molecules of gamma globulin that "have been modified by the presence of an antigen so that they are highly specific for that particular antigen."[1] Gamma globulin is a fraction of the blood protein globulin; a person deficient in gamma globulin is very susceptible to infections and is said to have agammaglobulinemia. Gamma globulin and antibodies are formed by cells of the reticuloendothelial tissues (e.g., lymph nodes and spleen).

Antibodies combine with or attach to the antigens and are classified according to their effect on them. Bacteriolysins bring about dissolution of the infecting agents; opsonins make the organisms more vulnerable to phagocytosis; antitoxins neutralize toxins; agglutinins cause the organisms to aggregate, or clump; and precipitins cause precipitation of antigens that are in solution. Antibodies are specific to the antigen; for example, antitoxins formed in response to tetanus toxin are incapable of neutralizing the toxin liberated by diphtheria bacilli.

Acquired immunity may be active or passive. Active immunity develops when the host forms his own antibodies in response to an antigen. He may develop this immunity naturally from having had the disease, or it may be produced artificially by injections of the antigen. The antigen used in artificially acquired immunity may be a solution of dead or attenuated organisms (e.g., smallpox vaccine) or a solution of weakened toxin (e.g., diphtheria toxoid). The length of time active immunity lasts varies; it may be very brief, or it may remain with the person throughout life. Many of the communicable diseases, such as measles, chickenpox, smallpox, diphtheria, poliomyelitis and scarlet fever, usually confer a lifelong immunity. Artificially induced active immunization may require booster doses of specific antigens at intervals of a few years.

Passive acquired immunity may also be natural or artificial. Natural passive immunity occurs in the newborn infant. Antibodies developed by the mother pass through the placenta to the fetus. These maternal antibodies only protect the infant through the first few months of life. Artificial passive immunity is developed by the injection of serum taken from an animal

[1]H. C. Hopps: Principles of Pathology, 2nd ed. New York, Appleton-Century-Crofts, 1964, p. 210.

which has actively produced the antibodies. This type of immunity is rapidly established but is of short duration. The foreign antibodies are destroyed by the recipient in a relatively short period. It takes time to produce antibodies; serum that contains specific antibodies formed by an animal is given to those who already have the infection, or who have been exposed. The foreign antibodies provide an immediate defense during the period the recipient is forming his own antibodies. Diphtheria antitoxin and tetanus antitoxin are the most commonly used immune serums.

A preparation of human gamma globulin may be used to protect susceptible contacts of certain viral diseases, such as measles.

Immunization Program. Artificially induced active immunity for certain diseases is recommended for every child. A discussion with the mother of a newborn infant concerning her discharge from the hospital and any follow-up home visits should include an explanation of immunization procedures for the prevention of diphtheria, tetanus, whooping cough, poliomyelitis, measles, and smallpox. The infant should be taken to the doctor or a clinic in the third month for the initial injection.

The vaccine used is a combination of diphtheria toxoid, tetanus toxoid, measles vaccine, pertussis vaccine, and poliomyelitis vaccine. Three doses, each of 1.0 ml., of the combined vaccine are administered subcutaneously at monthly intervals. The child should also receive vaccination for smallpox during the first year. This involves the introduction of smallpox vaccine into a superficial scratch or several minute punctures. The area is left exposed; later, if a vesicle forms and breaks, it is covered with a sterile dressing. The reaction is checked in 6 to 7 days.

Artificially induced immunity becomes weaker over a period of months to years; it varies in relation to the different diseases. As a result, reinforcing doses are necessary. The physician may recommend a booster dose of measles vaccine 6 to 12 months after the initial series is completed. This may be followed by a reinforcing dose of a combined vaccine for diphtheria, whooping cough, tetanus and poliomyelitis 6 to 12 months following the first series. The latter is usually repeated before the child starts school.

The combined vaccine is not used for older children or adults since there is a greater possibility of a sensitivity reaction. Immunization for each disease is done separately. A record of the immunization received and the date is issued for each individual and should be kept safe for future reference. A pamphlet with information about the vaccine and directions for administration and storage accompanies each vial and should be carefully read by the nurse. See Table 4–1 for a sample immunization program.

There is always the possibility that the person may be hypersensitive to a vaccine and will develop a serious reaction. For this reason, he may be asked to remain for 20 to 30 minutes for observation. Epinephrine hydrochloride (1:1000) and sterile equipment for administration should always be readily available in the event of an undesirable reaction.

Factors Predisposing to Infection

Factors that influence the host's resistance and susceptibility to infection include the following:

Nutrition. Poorly nourished persons have an increased susceptibility to infection, particularly if their diet has been deficient in protein and vitamins. Their natural tissue resistance and ability to form antibodies are reduced.

Age. Infants, children and elderly persons are less able to resist infection.

Occupation. Certain occupations provide increased exposure to infecting agents or may reduce the efficiency of one's protective mechanisms. For example, persons working with cattle may be exposed to undulant fever; those working in mines are more susceptible to tuberculosis.

Exposure to Cold. A lowering of the body temperature below normal is thought to decrease the ciliary movement in the respiratory tract, reduce the blood supply to superficial tissues and suppress antibody formation.

Metabolic Disturbances and Other Diseases. The person who already has some abnormality in function within the body is less able to resist or cope with an infection. For instance, the diabetic is prone to infection.

Corticoid Medication. The patient re-

TABLE 4–1 SAMPLE IMMUNIZATION PROGRAM FOR INFANTS AND PRESCHOOLERS*

AGE	IMMUNIZING AGENT	DOSES
Beginning at 3 months	Quint vaccine (diphtheria toxoid, tetanus toxoid, pertussis vaccine, measles vaccine, poliomyelitis vaccine) or Quad vaccine (diphtheria toxoid, tetanus toxoid, pertussis vaccine, poliomyelitis vaccine)	Three doses at monthly intervals (initial series)
Six months or over	Smallpox vaccine	One dose initially; then repeat every 4 to 5 years
Twelve to 18 months	Quad vaccine (as above)	One booster dose following initial series of Quint vaccine or Quad vaccine; repeated once just before child starts school
Twelve months or as soon after as possible	Measles vaccine Type A (Rubeovax) live attenuated measles virus vaccine Type B (Lirugen) live attenuated measles virus vaccine	One dose given only to children who have had initial series of Quint vaccine One dose given only to children who have had Quad vaccine and not had measles or any other measles vaccine

*For older children and adults, immunization for each disease is done separately.

ceiving corticoid therapy exhibits a marked susceptibility to infection. The steroids suppress the protective inflammatory response and the production of antibodies.

Radiation. Exposure to large doses of radiation, particularly total body irradiation, reduces the patient's defense mechanisms. Leukocyte and antibody production are suppressed.

Types of Infections

Certain terms may be used to describe infection. Local or focal means the infection remains confined to one area. A generalized or systemic infection is one in which the organisms are disseminated throughout the body. A mixed infection is due to more than one type of pathogen. If a person becomes infected by another type of organisms during the course of an infection, it is termed a secondary infection, and the initial one is referred to as primary. An infection may be acute or chronic.

The presence of bacteria in the blood produces bacteremia. Septicemia means organisms have entered the blood stream and are actively multiplying and producing toxins. Toxemia implies a concentration of bacterial toxins in the blood. Pyemia is a type of septicemia in which the organisms are clumped together or incorporated into small thrombi (bloot clots). The clumps, or thrombi, may become deposited at various sites throughout the body and may cause small, scattered abscesses.

Manifestations of Infection

Manifestations common to many infections include the following: fever, which may be preceded by chills; an increase in the pulse and respiratory rates; anorexia; nausea and vomiting; headache; apathy and fatigue; joint and muscle pain; and general malaise. The patient may appear hot and flushed, and the tongue is frequently furred and dry. There may be enlargement and tenderness of the lymph nodes. If the infection is local, the area becomes red, swollen, hot and painful. In addition to these common signs and symptoms, specific features characteristic of a specific infection may be present and may play an important role in the diagnosis.

Diagnostic Procedures Used in Infections

Leukocyte Count and Differential. Some infections cause an increase in the white blood cells well above the normal, while in others there may be a decrease below the normal.

Normal:

7000 to 9000 per cu. ml.

Normal differential:

neutrophils — 60 per cent of all leukocytes

eosinophils — 1 to 3 per cent of all leukocytes

basophils — 0.5 per cent of all leukocytes

monocytes — 3 to 7 per cent of all leukocytes

lymphocytes — 25 to 35 per cent of all leukocytes

Erythrocyte Sedimentation Rate. The rate at which the red blood cells settle in a specimen of blood is increased in infection.

Normal:

Westergren — male, 0 to 15 mm. in 1 hour; female, 0 to 20 mm. in 1 hour

Wintrobe — male, 0 to 9 mm. in 1 hour; female, 0 to 15 mm. in 1 hour

Antibody Tests. A specimen of blood may be examined to determine the concentration of antibodies present; this is referred to as an antibody titer. Tests may also be done to detect the presence of certain antigens or antibodies; a known antibody may be used to determine the presence of an antigen, or a known antigen may be used to detect antibodies.

Identification of the Causative Organism. The infective agent may be identified by direct microscopic examination, culture or animal inoculation.

In direct examination a specimen of sputum, blood, spinal fluid, urine, feces, or the discharge or scrapings from a lesion may be stained and examined under the microscope for organisms. Appearance, shape, and certain staining characteristics assist in identifying different organisms.

A culture involves the sterile collection of suspect material from the patient and the introduction of the material to cultural media (food materials). The media are observed for a period of time for the growth of organisms. The material to be cultured may be sputum, nasal or throat secretions, blood, urine, feces, wound discharge or spinal fluid.

Animal inoculation may be used for the identification of the organism of a few diseases such as tuberculosis and mycotic infections. Appropriate material from the patient is injected into a laboratory animal. The animal is killed after a certain period and examined for evidence of the suspected disease.

All specimens collected to determine the presence and type of pathogenic organism must be collected with sterile equipment and placed in a sterile container. Special sterile containers are usually provided by the laboratory for particular specimen materials along with directions as to the necessary precautions to be observed in collection. The specimen should be delivered promptly to the laboratory to avoid drying; if this is not possible, it is recommended that it be stored in the refrigerator until it can be cultured or examined.

Skin Tests. Two commonly used skin tests are the tuberculin (Mantoux) and Schick tests. In the tuberculin test, a small dose of old tuberculin or purified protein derivative tuberculin is injected intradermally on the flexor surface of the forearm. A positive reaction is indicated by swelling and edema at the site of injection and a surrounding redness in 2 to 3 days; this result means the individual has or has had an infection by tubercle bacilli. The test is considered negative if there is no reaction. If the first test is negative, the test may be repeated with a larger dose of tuberculin.

The Schick test is used to determine susceptibility to diphtheria. A small dose of diphtheria toxin is administered intradermally into a forearm, and a dose of inactivated toxin is given intradermally in the opposite arm. The latter is used as the comparative control. In a positive reaction, the site of the active toxin injection manifests redness in 48 hours which persists for 1 to 2 weeks. The control shows no reaction. A positive reaction indicates that the recipient of the toxin does not have antibodies to neutralize the toxin and is considered susceptible. A negative Schick test shows no reaction on either arm and indicates the person has sufficient antitoxin antibodies to protect him.

Skin tests to identify specific allergens are discussed on page 37.

Nursing in Infection

Nursing measures in infection are directed toward increasing the patient's resistance and toward the prevention of the transmission of the infecting agent to others.

Increased rest is planned for the patient in order to minimize the demand on body structures. A diet high in protein and vitamins plays an important role in the production of antibodies and support of natural tissue resistance. Anorexia may be a problem; frequent small amounts of concentrated foods may be necessary if tolerated. The fluid intake is increased to a minimum of 2500 to 3000 ml. unless contraindicated; fluids promote the dilution and excretion of toxins and are also necessary because of the fever.

Antimicrobial drugs (antibiotics and sulfonamide) are prescribed; it is important that these drugs be given promptly at the times specified by the physician in order to maintain an effective blood concentration.

In the case of a localized infection, warm, moist applications (compresses or soaks) may be ordered. The area may have to be opened to provide drainage if suppuration develops. The wound receives aseptic care to prevent a secondary infection. A local application of an antimicrobial preparation may be prescribed; the wound should be cleansed of pus and tissue debris before the application to ensure contact of the preparation with the living infective agents.

The nurse caring for a patient with an infection should have a knowledge of the means by which his infective agents may leave his body and be transmitted. With this understanding, appropriate precautionary measures are used to prevent transmission of the organisms to other persons and to guard against reinfection of the patient.

Pathogenic organisms leave the body of an infected person via respiratory tract exhalations and secretions, bladder and bowel excreta, and wound discharge. Transmission may be direct (from one person to another) or indirect (via contaminated persons and articles). For example, the infected patient may cough out organisms, which become airborne and are inhaled by others. Obviously, a precautionary measure that one would institute here would be to teach the patient that, when coughing, he should cover his nose and mouth with a tissue, which is then disposed of in a paper bag.

Infective excreta or wound discharge may be deposited on the patient's clothing and bedding or may be transferred from his hands to articles handled by him. Organisms may be picked up from these possible sources by a nurse, family member or other personnel, who may become infected or may transfer the pathogens to another person. A constant awareness of the source of infection and of what is likely to be contaminated as well as the observance of precautionary measures to avoid the spread of infection are necessary.

Since medical asepsis, surgical asepsis and isolation techniques are topics introduced early in the nursing student's preparation, details are not presented here. If a review is necessary, the reader is referred to texts that present the introduction to basic principles and practice of nursing.

References

BOOKS

Hopps, H. C.: Principles of Pathology, 2nd ed. New York, Appleton-Century-Crofts, 1964. Chapter 7.
Perez-Tamayo, R.: Mechanisms of Disease. Philadelphia, W. B. Saunders Co., 1961. Chapter 7.
Smith, A. L.: Microbiology and Pathology, 8th ed. Saint Louis, C. V. Mosby Co., 1964. Chapters 12, 13–17, 34.
Thomas, C. G.: Bacteriology. London, Bailliere, Tindall and Cox, 1964.
Young, G. G.: Witton's Microbiology, 3rd ed. New York, Blakiston Division, McGraw-Hill Book Co., Inc., 1961.

5

Fluid and Electrolyte Balance;
Acid-Base Balance

FLUID AND ELECTROLYTE BALANCE

Normal body functioning demands a relatively constant volume of water and a definite concentration of certain chemical compounds known as electrolytes. An electrolyte is a compound that dissociates in solution; it breaks up into separate electrically charged atoms or radicals called ions. For example, sodium chloride (NaCl) in solution forms sodium ions (Na^+) and chloride ions (Cl^-); sodium bicarbonate ($NaHCO_3$) breaks up into sodium ions (Na^+) and bicarbonate radicals (HCO_3^-); and calcium chloride ($CaCl_2$) yields calcium ions (Ca^{++}) and two chloride ions (Cl^-) for each calcium ion because calcium is bivalent. The ions that carry a positive charge are called cations, and those that are negatively charged are anions. The number of cations in a solution equals the number of anions so that the electrical chemical balance is maintained.

BODY WATER

Water is essential for all body processes; it transports substances to and from the cells, promotes necessary chemical activities, and maintains a physicochemical constancy that is important in normal cellular functions.

Approximately 60 to 65 per cent of the total body weight of an average adult is water. In the newborn infant, water comprises about 77 per cent of the body weight but progressively decreases with age to adult levels. Since fatty tissue is practically free of water, the proportion of water to body weight is less in an obese individual.

Distribution of Body Water

Body water is contained within two major physiological reservoirs—the intracellular and extracellular compartments. The extracellular fluid, which is about 20 per cent of the total body weight, is subdivided into the intravascular and interstitial fluids. The intravascular fluid is that contained within the blood vessels; the interstitial fluid is that contained in the tissue spaces between the blood vessels and the cells. The latter provides an internal environment for all cells as well as an exchange medium between the blood and the cells. The three fluid compartments are separated by semipermeable membranes.

TABLE 5–1 DISTRIBUTION OF BODY WATER

TOTAL BODY WATER (60 TO 65 PER CENT OF ADULT BODY WEIGHT)

Extracellular water (approximately 20 per cent of body weight)	Intracellular water (approximately 40 per cent of body weight)
1. Intravascular fluid (approximately 5 per cent of body weight) 2. Interstitial fluid (approximately 15 per cent of body weight)	

Electrolyte Composition of the Fluids

Although the extracellular and intracellular fluids are separated by the cellular semipermeable membrane, marked differences exist between the electrolyte concentrations in the two compartments. The difference is maintained by the cells, which actively reject certain electrolytes and retain others. For example, sodium is in much higher concentration in the extracellular fluid; the difference is maintained by cellular action referred to as the "sodium pump."

The major ions of cellular fluid in order of their quantity are potassium (K^+), phosphate (PO_4^{--}), magnesium (Mg^{++}) and protein (Pr^-). Much lesser amounts of sodium (Na^+), sulfate (SO_4^{--}), bicarbonate (HCO_3^-) and chloride (Cl^-) are also present.

In the extracellular compartments, sodium (Na^+), chloride (Cl^-) and bicarbonate (HCO_3^-) are of greatest abundance; calcium (Ca^{++}), potassium (K^+), magnesium (Mg^{++}), phosphate (PO_4^{--}) and sulfate (SO_4^{--}) occur in much lesser amounts. A significant difference between the intravascular and interstitial fluids is the greater quantity of protein in the former. The other electrolytes diffuse readily between the two compartments, but the large particles of protein are unable to pass through the capillary membrane.

Movement of Water Between Fluid Compartments

A continuous exchange of fluid takes place between the intravascular and interstitial fluids and between the cellular and interstitial fluids. The net exchange is dependent on two principal forces: the osmotic pressure created by the electrolytes and the blood proteins; and the hydrostatic pressure of the blood. When the osmotic pressure changes in one compartment, water moves across the semipermeable membrane from the lesser osmotic pressure to the greater until an equilibrium is established (see p. 28). Hydrostatic pressure is the driving force that causes filtration of fluid through a semipermeable membrane.

Exchange Between Intravascular and Interstitial Compartments

The total volume of fluid that moves across the capillary membranes is enormous because of the vast number of capillaries, but the net exchange between the intravascular and interstitial compartments is very small. Fluid moves out at the arterial end of the capillary and is drawn back in at the venous end.

Two opposing forces exist within the vascular compartment: the hydrostatic pressure of the blood, which forces fluid out through the semipermeable membrane, and the osmotic pressure of the blood proteins which is a holding or pulling force. The volume and direction of movement of fluid depends on the difference between these two opposing forces. When the blood enters the arterial end of the capillaries the hydrostatic pressure is greater than the protein osmotic pressure, and fluid filters out of the vessels. The movement of fluid out is also opposed by the hydrostatic pressure exerted by the volume of interstitial fluid, which is negligible if lymphatic drainage is normal. The effective filtrative force which moves fluid from the vascular compartment to the interstitial spaces may be expressed as the following equation:

Blood hydrostatic pressure (B.H.P.) − protein osmotic pressure (Pr. O.P.) − interstitial hydrostatic pressure (Int. H.P.) = effective filtrative pressure.

These pressures are approximately:

B.H.P. 34 mm. Hg − Pr. O.P. 24 mm. Hg − Int. H.P. 2 mm. Hg = filtrative pressure 8 mm. Hg.

The blood hydrostatic pressure is reduced as the blood flows through the capillaries and becomes less than the protein osmotic pres-

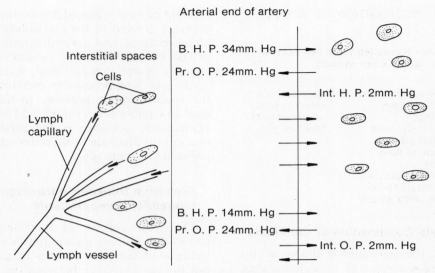

Figure 5–1 Exchange of water between intravascular and interstitial compartments. B.H.P. = Blood hydrostatic pressure; Pr.O.P. = protein osmotic pressure; Int.H.P. = interstitial hydrostatic pressure; Int.O.P. = interstitial osmotic pressure.

sure. As a result, fluid is drawn into the vascular compartment from the interstitial spaces at the venous end of the capillaries. The effective osmotic pressure may be expressed as follows:

Pr. O.P. 24 mm. Hg – B.H.P. 14 mm. Hg – Int. O.P.* 2 mm. Hg = vascular osmotic pressure 8 mm. Hg.

Exchange Between Extracellular and Intracellular Compartments

The net exchange of water between the cellular and interstitial fluids is governed by differences in the osmotic pressure in the two compartments. In the extracellular fluid, the principal osmotic forces are exerted by the sodium and chloride ions. Potassium,

---

*A small amount of blood protein may escape in the filtrate into the interstitial spaces.

magnesium and phosphate are mainly responsible for the osmotic pressure within the cells. Normal electrolyte concentrations maintain equal osmotic pressures in both compartments, and water diffuses freely between the compartments without net gain or loss in either. A decrease in the volume of extracellular water causes an increase in the concentration of ions and a corresponding increase in the osmotic pressure. This results in the movement of water from the cellular compartment into the interstitial space to establish an equilibrium. Conversely, if the osmotic pressure within the cells exceeds that of the interstitial fluid, water moves into the cells.

Fluid Balance

A minimum daily intake equal to certain obligatory fluid losses is necessary to maintain the optimal volume and distribution of

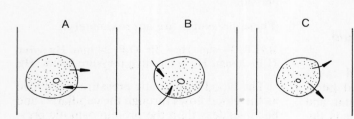

Figure 5–2 Exchange of water between cellular and interstitial compartments. *A,* Osmotic pressure of interstitial fluid is equal to that within the cell. Water passes freely between the compartments without net gain or loss. *B,* Osmotic pressure of interstitial fluid is less than that within the cell. Water passes into the cell. *C,* Osmotic pressure of interstitial fluid is greater than that within the cell. Water passes out of the cell.

TABLE 5–2   AN AVERAGE DAILY WATER INTAKE AND OUTPUT

INTAKE		OUTPUT	
Fluid ingested	1300 ml.	Urine	1500 ml.
Water content of ingested food	1000 ml.	Feces	150 ml.
Water of oxidation	250 ml.	Via lungs and skin	900 ml.
Total intake	2550 ml.	Total output	2550 ml.

body fluid. The daily obligatory losses total approximately 1300 ml., which include the water evaporated from the skin and lungs and the volume required by the kidneys to excrete the solid metabolic wastes. Approximately 900 ml. are lost in perspiration and respiration, and 400 ml. is considered the minimum quantity required by normal kidneys to eliminate the metabolic wastes.

Sources of body fluid are the ingested fluid and foods and the cellular oxidation processes. The average fluid and food intake by healthy persons usually provides a volume well in excess of the obligatory losses.

A balance is maintained between the intake and output by certain mechanisms in order to preserve a constancy in fluid volume. When the intake is reduced or if there is an excessive loss as in vomiting or diarrhea, the urinary output is decreased and one is prompted to increase the intake by the sensation of thirst. Conversely, if there is an increase in the intake, a corresponding increase in the urinary output occurs.

When the intake volume does not equal that of the obligatory loss, body fluid is drawn upon, and the normal volume is reduced. One then develops a negative fluid balance (dehydration) which may seriously affect body functioning if not corrected promptly. Electrolyte concentrations and osmotic pressures are altered, resulting in abnormal fluid shifts between compartments. Faulty excretion with a continued intake may result in an excessive volume in the fluid compartments, producing a positive fluid balance. Electrolyte concentrations are changed, and harmful wastes are retained.

Mechanisms that adjust intake and output to preserve fluid balance include the following:

Thirst.   This is a sensation which one interprets as a need for fluid. The fluid may be needed to cover a loss or to reduce an elevated osmotic pressure of the extracellular fluid which may be due to a salt excess. A group of cells in the hypothalamus is sensitive to variations in the osmotic pressure of the extracellular fluids. An increase results in impulses that evoke the sensation of thirst. Dryness of the oral and pharyngeal mucous membrane and a decrease in the intravascular volume, as in hemorrhage, also initiate the thirst sensation.

Adjustment of Kidney Output.   The kidneys perform the most important role in regulating the volume and chemical composition of body fluids. Certain factors from outside the kidneys influence them in the amount of fluid and electrolytes they should reabsorb or eliminate in the urine to preserve homeostasis.

A large amount of water and solutes are filtered out of the blood into the renal tubules. The production of the filtrate depends upon the hydrostatic pressure of the blood; if there is a fall in blood pressure, there is a corresponding decrease in the volume of filtrate. About 80 per cent of the filtrate is quickly reabsorbed in the proximal portion of the renal tubules. Absorption of water and salts in the distal portion is adjusted to the amount necessary to maintain normal volume and osmotic pressure of the body fluids.

The tubules are governed as to how much water to reabsorb by the antidiuretic hormone (ADH). This hormone is secreted by the hypothalamus and is delivered to the posterior lobe of the pituitary gland (neurohypophysis) where it is stored and released as required. Within the hypothalamus are cells (osmoreceptors) that are sensitive to variations in the osmotic pressure of the extracellular fluid. An increase in the osmotic pressure above the normal results in impulses being delivered to the posterior pituitary lobe, which bring about the release of ADH. The increased osmotic pressure may be due to a water deficit or to an increased intake of sodium chloride. The hormone stimulates the tubules to reabsorb water from the filtrate. This increases the extracellular water and reduces the osmotic pressure. Conversely, a fluid intake that lowers the osmotic pressure results in ADH being withheld, and the kidneys then allow a greater loss of water.

A second hormone that indirectly influences water balance is aldosterone, which is secreted by the adrenal cortex. It stimulates the renal tubules to reabsorb sodium and excrete potassium. Sodium is chiefly responsible for the osmotic pressure of the extracellular fluid; an increased absorption brings about the release of ADH and a resulting decrease in the water loss. The control of the amount of aldosterone secreted is not understood.

Water loss via the kidneys is also affected by the load of solid wastes they are required to eliminate. There is always a certain amount of solid metabolic wastes to be excreted, but it may vary with diet and cellular activities. If there is an increased amount, the kidneys may require more water to eliminate them. An example of this is seen when the blood sugar exceeds the normal; the person excretes a greater volume of water in order to eliminate the excess sugar. This accounts for the increased urinary output and excessive thirst which are characteristic of diabetes mellitus.

DISTURBANCES IN FLUID BALANCE

Dehydration

Dehydration is a negative fluid balance; the fluid loss exceeds the intake and there is a reduction in the normal volume of body fluid. A negative water balance does not only imply changes in the water volume; it involves changes in electrolyte concentrations. The latter may exceed the normal if the fluid intake is reduced or if the water loss exceeds the rate of electrolyte loss. The osmotic pressure of the extracellular fluid

is increased, water shifts from the cells and intracellular dehydration develops. In other instances, the electrolytes may be depleted by excessive losses with the fluids; for example, a loss of gastrointestinal secretions involves losses of certain electrolytes as well as water.

Causes of Dehydration. A negative fluid balance may be caused by an excessive loss of fluid from the body, an insufficient fluid intake or a deficiency of electrolytes.

EXCESSIVE LOSS. Abnormal losses of body fluid may be from: (a) the gastrointestinal tract by vomiting, diarrhea, aspiration, or fistula or ileostomy drainage; (b) the skin by excessive perspiration in fever or exposure to a high environmental temperature; (c) the lungs when there is an increased respiratory rate; (d) the vascular compartment by hemorrhage or by loss of plasma in severe burns; (e) the kidneys because of a deficiency of the antidiuretic hormone (diabetes insipidus) or adrenal cortical secretion (Addison's disease), chronic renal disease in which the kidneys cannot concentrate the wastes, or an increased load of solid wastes which demands more water for elimination (e.g., excess blood sugar in diabetes mellitus); and (f) wounds which are draining.

INSUFFICIENT FLUID INTAKE. An inadequate intake of fluid may be due to the inability to swallow, a lack of available fluid or negligence in taking fluid.

DEFICIENCY OF ELECTROLYTES. A reduction in body fluid may occur with a lowered electrolyte concentration because body mechanisms operate to restore a normal concentration and osmotic pressure by eliminating water. This is seen in Addison's disease in which a deficiency of aldosterone results in an inadequate reabsorption of sodium by the renal tubules. The osmotic pressure of the extracellular fluid is reduced; this in turn results in ADH being withheld, and less water being reabsorbed in the kidneys.

A relative deficit of electrolytes may develop when an excessive amount of water is ingested or a nonelectrolyte solution is administered intravenously. The concentration of the body electrolytes is lowered; also, as the excessive water is eliminated, electrolytes may be washed out with it.

Effects of Dehydration. The effects of dehydration depend on the volume of the fluid deficit and the rate at which it develops. Effects are more acute when it develops rapidly, when the patient is an infant, a young child or an elderly person, and if the patient's general condition is poor.

Interstitial fluid is depleted first; it becomes hypertonic and causes water to move out of the cells. Cellular dehydration alters cellular concentrations and eventually disrupts normal cellular metabolism.

If the fluid deficit is not corrected, the intravascular volume is eventually depleted; the blood pressure falls, the pulse becomes progressively weaker and the patient presents a picture of shock. Anuria (absence of urine formation) develops and leads to the retention of metabolic wastes. The patient is disoriented, eventually lapses into coma and death may ensue.

Implications for Nursing. It is important that the nurse realize the significance of normal amounts of water and electrolytes in body functioning and the need for recognition of early deficits.

OBSERVATIONS. The patient's daily fluid intake and output volumes should be known to the nurse. If the output exceeds the intake, there is an immediate need for an increased fluid intake unless the patient previously has had a positive fluid balance and edema. A urinary specific gravity in excess of 1.030 should be noted also as a need for an increased fluid intake unless contraindicated.

The condition of the patient's mouth and skin is also a good source of information as to the patient's hydrational status.

When a fluid deficit is known to exist a frequent check should be made of the patient's vital signs (temperature, pulse and blood pressure), general appearance and responses.

FLUID REPLACEMENT. The necessity to restore normal hydration is urgent in order to restore normal metabolism, circulation and renal function. The method used for the administration of replacement fluids will depend on the patient's condition. Intravenous infusion is used to re-establish a satisfactory balance quickly. When ordering the quantity and type of solution to be given the physician considers the cause, source and volume of the losses as well as the general condition of the patient. Blood chemistry studies are done to determine possible electrolyte imbalances.

Once the intravenous infusion is started, the nurse is responsible for maintaining the desired rate of flow, detecting any difficulties and noting the patient's reactions. If the patient is an infant, young child, an elderly person or a patient with a cardiac or pulmonary condition, the rate of flow must be carefully controlled. Too rapid infusion may overload the circulatory system and lead to pulmonary edema and cardiac dilatation.

If the patient is permitted oral fluids, some persuasion and resourcefulness may be necessary on the part of the nurse. Small amounts are given at frequent intervals, preferences for certain fluids should be ascertained and respected if possible, and the necessary assistance in taking a drink should be provided. The patient may be too sick or too weak to reach out and take the fluid himself; holding the glass and elevating his head will prove more effective than simply placing the fluid at the bedside with instructions to the patient to take it.

MOUTH CARE. The mouth requires frequent cleansing and rinsing. Oil, vaseline or cold cream may be applied to the lips to relieve the dryness and prevent cracking.

SKIN CARE. Frequent bathing or temperature sponges may help to reduce the fever as well as provide comfort for the patient. The amount of bedding and the room temperature should be adjusted to the patient's temperature.

HEADACHE. Cold compresses to the forehead and a quiet environment with subdued lighting may relieve the patient's headache to some extent.

REST. The patient is encouraged to rest as much as possible in order to lessen the demand on cellular activities. Nursing care is planned so that there will be a minimum of disturbance for the patient.

SAFETY PRECAUTIONS. Crib sides and close observation are necessary to protect the patient if there are indications of confusion and disorientation.

Edema

Edema is the accumulation of an excessive amount of fluid in the interstitial spaces locally or generally. If it occurs generally, it implies a positive fluid balance in which the fluid intake has exceeded the output.

Causes. The mechanisms of formation of edema include the following:

INCREASED VENOUS PRESSURE. If for any reason there is an increase in the hydrostatic pressure of the blood in the venous end of the capillaries in excess of the blood protein osmotic pressure, the return of interstitial fluid into the capillaries is inhibited. This mechanism contributes to the formation of edema in cardiac failure and in cases in which there is obstruction to venous flow.

OBSTRUCTION TO LYMPHATIC DRAINAGE. Interference with the drainage of interstitial fluid that is normally carried away in the lymphatic vessels results in edema. This produces a localized edema and may be seen in the arm of a patient who has had a radical mastectomy which involves resection of the axillary lymphatics and lymph nodes that drain the arm. This type of edema is also seen in elephantiasis, in which the filarial worms cause an obstruction in the lymphatics.

DEFICIENCY OF BLOOD PROTEINS. A decrease in the amount of blood proteins (albumin, globulin and fibrinogen) reduces the osmotic pressure of the intravascular fluid. Much of the fluid that is filtered out of the arterial end of the capillaries remains in the interstitial spaces because the protein osmotic pressure is not sufficient to return it at the venous end. This may be seen in nephrosis, a kidney disease in which albumin escapes from the glomeruli into the renal tubules and is lost to the body in urine. It may also occur in malnutrition, in which a lack of protein results in decreased formation of blood proteins.

INCREASED CAPILLARY PERMEABILITY. An excessive amount of fluid in the interstitial spaces may be due to permeable capillaries. An example of this type of edema is that which is seen in inflammation and hypersensitivity reactions.

RENAL INSUFFICIENCY. Diminished kidney filtration may cause an insufficient output of water, resulting in an accumulation in the interstitial compartment. This may be due to disease in the kidneys (e.g., acute nephritis) or to a decreased blood flow through the kidneys (e.g., heart failure, shock).

EXCESSIVE HORMONES. An excessive concentration of adrenal cortical secretions, particularly aldosterone, increases the reabsorption of sodium by the renal tubules. In turn, the excess of sodium and the corresponding increase in extracellular osmotic pressure causes an increased release of ADH. More water is reclaimed in the kidney tubules and eventually accumulates in the interstitial spaces.

If for any reason there is an abnormal release of ADH, an excess of water is conserved and forms edema.

Manifestations of Edema. Indications of the presence of edema include weight gain, swollen tissues which pit on finger pressure, weakness, apathy, slowness or absence of responses, anorexia and a decreased urinary output. There may be moist gurgling sounds with respirations, indicating fluid accumulation in the alveoli (pulmonary edema).

A gain in weight is one of the earliest symptoms of water retention. A person may accumulate approximately 10 pounds of water before it becomes apparent on the surface. If the person is ambulatory, edema may be observed first in swelling of the feet and ankles. The bed patient usually exhibits signs of fluid accumulation in the sacral region. Localized edema according to the patient's position is referred to as dependent edema. Later, as the total interstitial compartment becomes overloaded, a generalized edema is evident.

Implications for Nursing. The treatment and nursing care of the patient depends on the cause of edema. Only a few general principles are cited here.

An accurate record is made of the fluid intake and loss. The patient is weighed daily or every other day if possible. This should be done at the same time each day, with the patient wearing the same amount of clothing, and on the same scale each time.

Specific orders should be received from the physician as to the patient's fluid and salt intake. With the exception of localized edema, salt is usually restricted. Fluid restrictions are governed by the patient's circulatory status and urinary output.

The skin requires special attention since edematous tissue is poorly nourished and breaks down readily. The patient's position is changed frequently. Vulnerable pressure areas are examined, bathed and gently massaged every two to three hours. The skin may also be protected by placing the patient on a resilient surface; an alternating pressure air mattress, foam rubber or a sheepskin may be used. Gentle handling is also very important.

The excess of fluid in generalized edema may cause mental confusion and disorientation. Safety precautions such as crib sides and a closer attendance to the patient may be necessary.

If a diuretic is ordered, an accurate record is made of the volume of urine excreted. If the patient is ambulatory, he should be close to a bathroom. Frequent use of a urinal or commode will be necessary for the bed patient. He should not be kept waiting or receive an impression that his demands are excessive. The frequent voiding can be quite exhausting for the patient; the necessary assistance in getting on and off the pan and allowing the patient to rest undisturbed between voidings help to conserve his energy.

In the case of pulmonary edema, the patient is usually placed in the semirecumbent position. This helps to decrease the venous return to the heart and lungs and may reduce the pulmonary edema.

Water Intoxication

This is a fluid imbalance in which there is an increase in the body water without a comparable increase in the body sodium. The osmotic pressure of the extracellular fluid is less than that of the intracellular fluid. As a result, water leaves the interstitial spaces and enters the cells, disturbing their normal concentrations and activities. The amount the cells will hold is limited, so an excess may also remain in the interstitial spaces.

The cause of water intoxication is a decreased urinary output with a continuing intake of water or an excessive intake of water without salt.

The signs and symptoms are similar to those seen in the person with a sodium deficiency. The patient experiences headache, muscle cramps, nausea and vomiting, and excessive perspiration. Cerebral disturbances are manifested in drowsiness, confusion and loss of coordination. Convulsions and coma may develop if the condition is not corrected in the early stages.

Water intoxication is treated by stopping the fluid intake and the administration of a diuretic.

ELECTROLYTES

As cited previously, normal body functioning requires the presence of certain electrolytes in definite concentrations. The electrolytes are responsible for creating the osmotic forces that control the volume and location of fluid in the body. Certain ones have a specific role in the maintenance of an optimal alkaline reaction (acid-base balance) and in vital cellular activities.

Fluid balance and electrolyte balance are interdependent; a disturbance in one is immediately reflected in the other. A loss or gain in any one of the major compartmental ions alters the osmotic pressure, and a subsequent water shift occurs; changes in their concentration also alter cellular activities.

A deficit in an electrolyte concentration may result from a decreased intake, an excessive loss or dilution by an excessive water retention. An excessive concentration may be due to an excessive intake, reduced excretion or a water deficiency.

Measurement of Electrolyte Concentration

In clinical investigation of the electrolyte composition of body fluids, the physician is interested in the effective chemical activity of the electrolyte concentration. For this reason, the concentration is expressed in the number of milliequivalents per liter of body fluid. A *milliequivalent* (mEq.) represents a unit of chemical activity or combining power of a substance. Information as to the number of units available for physiological chemical activity is more meaningful than a statement of the weight of the substance in mg. or Gm. per cent. A small amount of one substance may react or combine with a much larger amount of another. For instance, 1 mg. of hydrogen may replace 23 mg. of sodium or may combine with 35 mg. of chloride. When chemicals react or combine each does so in a certain, definite unvarying proportion. The proportion is related to the atomic weight of the substance and, in the case of electrolytes, to the number of electrical charges each ion carries. The latter is known as the valence of a substance. Ions which carry one charge are termed monovalent, and those with two charges are divalent. An ion with one positive charge will combine with an ion with one negative charge (e.g., $Na^+ + HCO_3^- \rightarrow NaHCO_3$; $H^+ + Cl^- \rightarrow HCl$). An ion with two positive charges will react with two ions, each having a negative charge, or with one ion that carries two negative charges (e.g., $Ca^{++} + Cl^- \; Cl^- \rightarrow CaCl_2$; $Ca^{++} + SO_4^{--} \rightarrow CaSO_4$). From this it may be seen that the chemical activity of an electrolyte is proportional to the total number of electrical charges carried by the ions in a given volume of fluid.

To determine the number of milliequivalents (chemical combining units) of an electrolyte, the weight in mg. in 100 ml. of blood serum is established. This figure is then divided by the atomic weight of the particular electrolyte which yields the number of ions in 100 ml. of serum. Since the chemical activity depends on the valence, the above figure is then multiplied by the valence of the electrolyte to obtain the number of milliequivalents in 100 ml. In clinical practice it is customary to express the number of milliequivalents present in a liter (1000 ml.) of body fluid, so the number in 100 ml. must be multiplied by 10. The formula may be written as follows:

Milliequivalents per liter (mEq./L.) =
$$\frac{\text{mg. per cent}}{\text{atomic weight}} \times \text{valence} \times 10$$

To illustrate:

1. A solution contains calcium 20 mg. per cent (20 mg. per 100 ml.). Calcium is divalent and has an atomic weight of 40. Using the formula:

$$\text{mEq./L.} = \frac{20}{40} \times 2 \times 10 = \frac{400}{40} = 10$$

TABLE 5–3. MILLIEQUIVALENTS PER LITER OF ELECTROLYTES IN BLOOD SERUM

ELECTROLYTE	MEQ./L.
Sodium	142
Chloride	103
Potassium	5
Calcium	5
Magnesium	2
Bicarbonate	27

2. A solution contains sodium 207 mg. per cent (207 mg. per 100 ml.). Sodium is monovalent and has an atomic weight of 23. Using the formula:

$$\text{mEq./L.} = \frac{207}{23} \times 1 \times 10 = \frac{2070}{23} = 90$$

Sodium

The greatest proportion of sodium is contained within the extracellular fluids, and its concentration is maintained relatively constant within a narrow range. It plays an important role in maintaining the osmotic pressure of the extracellular fluids, which in turn influences the volume and movement of body water. It is necessary for normal nervous and muscular tissue functioning, and for the regulation of the acid-base balance.

The average diet contains sodium well in excess of the body's requirement. It occurs in natural foods, and much is added in the form of sodium chloride in the preparation and preservation of foods. The excess is eliminated mainly in the urine, but some is also lost in the feces and sweat.

A sodium deficiency (hyponatremia) is usually the result of an excessive loss, but may also occur because of a decreased intake. Body sodium may be depleted by: excessive sweating in fever or a high external temperature; loss of gastrointestinal secretions as in vomiting, diarrhea, and gastrointestinal suctioning; a deficiency of adrenal cortical secretion which results in too little sodium being reabsorbed by the kidney tubules (Addison's disease); impaired kidney tubule function due to renal disease; or loss of intravascular fluid as in hemorrhage and burns. The concentration may also be reduced to below the normal by intravenous infusion of a nonelectrolyte solution.

A decreased intake may be due to a prolonged therapeutic low sodium diet or to insufficient food intake.

Manifestations of a sodium deficiency may include: dehydration because the kidneys attempt to maintain a normal osmotic pressure in the extracellular fluids by excreting more water; apathy; headache; weakness; muscular cramps which may progress to twitching and convulsions; abdominal cramps; diarrhea; and nausea and vomiting. If the deficiency persists, the symptoms become progressively more severe, the patient lapses into unconsciousness and manifests circulatory failure.

A sodium deficit is not uncommon among persons working in a high environmental temperature. The increased sweating causes an excessive loss of water and sodium; the person experiences thirst and usually drinks large amounts of water without replacing the salt. The extracellular sodium becomes diluted. In such situations, sodium chloride tablets are provided which the workers are advised to take to prevent sodium deficiency.

An excess of sodium in body fluids (hypernatremia) may develop as a result of an excessive intake or a decreased excretion. The excessive intake may be by intravenous infusion or by ingestion. Decreased excretion may be caused by an excessive secretion of aldosterone by the adrenal cortex or by the administration of corticoid preparations; reabsorption of sodium ions by the kidney tubules is increased. Retention may also occur in renal disease, particularly if the intake is not reduced.

The signs and symptoms of an excess of sodium are edema (accumulation of fluids in the tissue spaces), mental confusion and decreased urinary output (oliguria). The oral mucous membrane becomes dry and sticky, and the tongue is rough and dry. If the condition remains uncorrected, the patient is likely to become comatose.

Potassium

As with other electrolytes, the amount of potassium in the body is kept relatively constant; deviations in concentration in either fluid compartment have serious physiologic effects. It is present in the extracellular fluids in small amounts, but it is especially abundant and active within the cells. Potassium is particularly important for the normal functioning of all muscle tissue. The kidneys provide the chief regulation of concentration, particularly if an excess occurs in the extracellular fluid, but they are less efficient in conserving this ion when a deficiency occurs. Considerable potassium is excreted in the feces since there is a high content in gastrointestinal fluids.

A potassium deficiency (hypokalemia) may be caused by: a decreased intake, decreased intestinal absorption or an increased loss.

Potassium is widely distributed in foods; a deficiency is unlikely if there is an adequate intake of food unless there is reduced absorption in the intestine. The latter may occur in disease of the intestine, such as regional ileitis and steatorrhea, and in cases in which a portion of the intestine has been removed.

An increased loss may be via the kidneys, stomach or intestine. Aldosterone promotes reabsorption of the sodium ions and excretion of potassium by the kidneys. Obviously, an excessive secretion of this hormone may account for a potassium deficit. Chronic renal disease in which there is impaired tubular reabsorption may also result in an increased loss in urine. Loss of gastrointestinal secretions incurred by vomiting, aspiration, fistula or ileostomy drainage, or diarrhea may cause an extensive loss of potassium.

Muscle tissues are very sensitive to a reduced potassium concentration, and the predominant symptoms of a deficit are the result of altered skeletal, smooth and cardiac muscle activity. The effect on the heart produces a rapid weak pulse, and as the deficiency becomes more severe, cardiac dilatation and failure develop. Skeletal muscles become weak and flabby (loss of tone), and the patient experiences generalized weakness. If the potassium deficiency becomes progressively greater, paralysis of the arms, legs and respiratory muscles may occur. Smooth muscle disturbance is manifested by diminished peristalsis in the gastrointestinal tract, leading to abdominal distention, nausea and vomiting, and an absence of bowel elimination.

When the potassium concentration of the extracellular fluid is depleted, potassium tends to move out of the cells, creating an intracellular deficit. The cells retain sodium and hydrogen ions in an effort to establish an ionic balance. These ionic shifts seriously affect normal cell functioning, and the normal alkalinity of the extracellular fluid is altered because of its loss of sodium and hydrogen ions.

An excessive concentration of potassium (hyperkalemia) may be the result of decreased renal excretion, increased catabolism or the administration of excessive amounts.

A decreased output of urine from any cause (e.g., renal diseases, dehydration, shock) reduces the normal excretion of potassium. Decreased renal excretion of potassium in a normal volume of urine may be caused by an insufficient adrenal cortical secretion. Reabsorption of an excessive amount of potassium by the kidney tubules is promoted in the absence of the corticoids.

The rapid breakdown of tissue cells in trauma or disease releases a large amount of intracellular potassium, raising the extracellular levels to above normal. This may occur with severe burns and crushing injuries, and is particularly serious if at the same time there is a diminished urinary output.

The administration of excessive amounts of potassium either by oral medication or intravenous solution could result in hyperkalemia.

The manifestations of a potassium excess include apathy, mental confusion, numbness and tingling of the extremities, abdominal cramps, diarrhea, a progressively decreasing pulse rate and eventual cardiac arrest.

Calcium

Most of the calcium in the body is in the bones and teeth (approximately 99 per cent); a relatively small amount is present and essential in the body fluids. The latter plays an important role in neuromuscular irritability and blood coagulation. It also influences membrane permeability. The principal regulation of calcium concentration in the body fluids is the hormone parathyrin, which is secreted by the parathyroid glands. A fall in the extracellular calcium stimulates the secretion of parathyrin, which causes a withdrawal of calcium from bone tissue, an increased reabsorption of calcium ions by the kidneys, and probably an increased absorption of the mineral from the intestine. When the concentration is increased above the normal, parathyrin is not released, less calcium is added to the body fluids and more calcium is excreted by the kidneys.

A constant intake of calcium is necessary to maintain normal concentrations within the bone tissue and body fluids. The food sources are limited mainly to milk and milk products; vegetables and fruits are the second best sources, but in the average diet they provide only about one-quarter of the calcium requirement. The minimum daily requirement is estimated to be about 850 mg., which is the equivalent of about three 8-ounce glasses of milk. Demands are greater during the growth period and during pregnancy and lactation.

Absorption of calcium from the intestine is largely dependent upon the presence of vitamin D. It is also influenced by other contents of the diet; a high phosphate concentration tends to reduce absorption and fatty acids may cause the formation of insoluble, nonabsorbable calcium salts. Also, an increased pH of intestinal fluid slows calcium absorption.

A reciprocal relationship exists between the levels of calcium and phosphorus in the extracellular fluids. An elevation of one accompanies a decrease in the other, but their functions are not comparable. Phosphate is the principal anion in the intracellular fluid; it is essential to the energy-producing activities of the cell, and in the extracellular fluid it is necessary for the maintenance of a normal acid-base balance.

A deficiency of calcium in the extracellular fluid (hypocalcemia) may be due to a dietary deficiency, decreased intestinal absorption, hypoparathyroidism or impaired kidney function.

Calcium is the mineral most likely to be deficient in the human diet because of its limited sources. Decreased intestinal absorption may result from a deficiency of vitamin D, increased alkaline or fatty acid intestinal content or disease of the intestine. Absorption may also be reduced if the content is hurried through the small intestine and eliminated, as in diarrhea, or if it is lost via a fistula.

A decrease in the secretion of parathyrin produces an abnormally low concentration. This may occur as a result of a new growth in the parathyroid glands or because of trauma during a surgical procedure such as thyroidectomy.

A calcium deficit may also develop in chronic renal disease because of impaired reabsorption of the ions from the filtrate or because abnormal amounts of phosphate are being retained, resulting in a compensatory decrease in calcium.

A lowered calcium concentration in body fluids produces symptoms that are known as tetany in which there is a nervous and muscular hyperirritability. The patient may experience "pins and needles," numbness in the extremities and twitching of the facial muscles. In more severe deficits, painful tonic spasms of skeletal muscles occur and may be followed by convulsions. Spasm of the larynx and respiratory muscles may interfere with breathing.

Hypocalcemia may also inhibit normal blood coagulation. Bleeding of the mucous membranes or into the tissues or excessive bleeding of a wound may result. Calcium ions are necessary in the conversion of prothrombin to thrombin in the clotting process.

A deficiency may be quickly corrected by intravenous administration of calcium chloride 5 per cent or calcium gluconate 10 per cent in 5- to 20 ml. doses. Calcium gluconate or calcium chloride and vitamin D may be prescribed for oral administration. These should be given one-half to three-quarters of an hour before meals to insure maximum absorption.

An excess of calcium in the extracellular fluid (hypercalcemia) occurs with an excessive administration of vitamin D, hyperparathyroidism, thyrotoxicosis, the breakdown of bone tissue by malignant metastases (secondary cancer), prolonged immobilization, multiple myeloma (tumors in bones), the ingestion of large amounts of milk accompanied by alkaline medication, and impaired renal function.

Manifestations of hypercalcemia include loss of muscle tone, weakness, anorexia, nausea and vomiting, and increased urinary output with resulting thirst. The high urinary content of calcium may lead to the formation of kidney or bladder stones. The patient may also experience pain in bones as their structure is weakened by the withdrawal of calcium.

ACID-BASE BALANCE

Cellular chemical processes produce relatively large amounts of acids, but body fluids are normally kept slightly alkaline.

The acidity or alkalinity of a solution depends upon the concentration of hydrogen (H^+) and hydroxyl (OH^-) ions. Hydrogen ions in excess of hydroxyl ions make a solution acid; hydroxyl ions in excess of hydrogen ions produce an alkaline solution. When they are equal the solution is neutral. A compound that completely dissociates its hydrogen ions is referred to as a strong acid; for example, hydrochloric acid which completely dissociates when placed in water is a strong acid ($HCl \rightarrow H^+ \ Cl^-$). One that only partially frees its hydrogen ions is referred to as a weak acid; for example, a molecule of carbonic acid dissociates into one hydrogen ion and a bicarbonate ion ($H_2CO_3 \rightarrow H^+ \ HCO_3^-$) and therefore is termed a weak acid.

The symbol pH is used to express the hydrogen ion concentration, or the degree to which a solution is acidic or alkaline. It represents the negative logarithm of the hydrogen ion concentration. For example, a neutral solution, such as water, with a pH of 7 contains 10^{-7} or $\dfrac{1}{10,000,000}$ or 0.0000001 gram of hydrogen ions per liter. A solution with a pH of 6 contains 10^{-6} or $\dfrac{1}{1,000,000}$ or 0.000001 gram of hydrogen ions per liter; it contains 10 times as many hydrogen ions as a solution with a pH of 7. A pH of 8 indicates a hydrogen ion concentration per liter of 10^{-8} or $\dfrac{1}{100,000,000}$ or 0.00000001 gram. Since a solution of pH_7 is neutral, as the pH decreases below 7, the hydrogen ion concentration increases, and the solution becomes acidic. Conversely, as the pH increases above 7 and hydrogen ion concentration decreases, the solution becomes alkaline. In other words, a pH of 7 denotes neutrality. Less than 7 indicates acidity, and the smaller the figure, the greater the degree of acidity; a pH greater than 7 denotes alkalinity, and the greater the figure, the greater the degree of alkalinity.

Obviously the use of the symbol pH is less cumbersome than the expression of the hydrogen ion concentration by fraction or decimal.

Acid-Base Regulation

Body fluids normally have a pH of approximately 7.4. Certain mechanisms operate to maintain the normal pH within a very narrow range; a variation of a few tenths in either direction is incompatible with normal cellular activity.

The chief acid resulting from metabolism is carbonic acid, which is formed by the chemical combination of water and carbon dioxide ($H_2O + CO_2 \rightarrow H_2CO_3$). The combination is promoted by the enzyme carbonic anhydrase within the cells. In addition to carbonic acid, cellular activity produces a substantial quantity of stronger acids such as sulfuric, phosphoric, lactic, uric, aceto-acetic, β-hydroxybutyric and hydrochloric acid. The acids must be rapidly neutralized or weakened by chemical reactions, and since their production is continuous, there must be a constant elimination of them from the body. The volatile carbonic acid is removed by the lungs by eliminating carbon dioxide; the nonvolatile acids are excreted by the kidneys.

Control Mechanisms. The optimum pH of body fluids is maintained by acid-base buffer systems in the body fluids, respiratory excretion of carbon dioxide, and selective excretion of hydrogen ions or bases by the kidneys.

BUFFER SYSTEMS. Buffers are substances which tend to stabilize or maintain the constancy of the pH of a solution when an acid or a base is added to it. They do this by rapidly converting a strong acid or base to a weaker one which does not dissociate as rapidly to yield free hydrogen or hydroxyl ions.

A buffer system consists of two substances—a weak acid and a salt of that acid. The buffer systems of body fluids include the following pairs:

carbonic acid / bicarbonate	$\dfrac{H_2CO_3}{NaHCO_3 \text{ or } KHCO_3}$
acid phosphate / alkaline phosphate	$\dfrac{NaH_2PO_4}{Na_2HPO_4}$
acid plasma protein / proteinate	$\dfrac{HPr}{Na \text{ proteinate}}$
hemoglobin / potassium hemoglobinate	$\dfrac{Hb}{KHb}$
oxyhemoglobin / potassium oxyhemoglobinate	$\dfrac{H \cdot HbO_2}{KHbO_2}$

The principal buffer pair of the plasma is the carbonic acid–sodium bicarbonate system. Maintenance of a normal pH is greatly dependent upon the ratio of carbonic acid concentration to that of bicarbonate, which normally occurs as 1:20. As long as there are 20 bicarbonate ions to one carbonic acid molecule, the pH will remain within normal range regardless of the actual amounts of the two substances.

When a strong acid is added to a fluid that contains the carbonic acid–bicarbonate system, it combines with the bicarbonate ion to form carbonic acid. Thus, the strong acid which dissociates readily to yield many hydrogen ions is replaced by a weaker acid which frees fewer hydrogen ions. This reaction may be illustrated by the following equations: hydrochloric acid + sodium bicarbonate yields carbonic acid + sodium chloride ($HCL + NaHCO_3 \rightarrow H_2CO_3 + NaCl$); lactic acid + sodium bicarbonate yields carbonic acid + sodium lactate ($HLa + NaHCO_3 \rightarrow H_2CO_3 + NaLa$). If a strong base is added to a fluid containing this buffer system, the base combines with the carbonic acid to form bicarbonate (weaker base) and water as shown in the following: sodium hydroxide + carbonic acid yields sodium bicarbonate + water ($NaOH + H_2CO_3 \rightarrow NaHCO_3 + HOH$).

When an acid is added to a solution with the acid phosphate–alkaline phosphate system, it combines with the alkaline phosphate to form acid phosphate. To illustrate, hydrochloric acid + sodium alkaline phosphate yields sodium acid phosphate and sodium chloride ($HCl + Na_2HPO_4 \rightarrow NaH_2PO_4 + NaCl$); and carbonic acid + sodium alkaline phosphate yields sodium acid phosphate and sodium bicarbonate ($H_2CO_3 + Na_2HPO_4 \rightarrow NaH_2PO_4 + NaHCO_3$). The phosphate system is especially active in the kidneys where the acid phosphate that has been formed is eliminated.

Oxyhemoglobin and reduced hemoglobin act as the acids of buffer pairs in the erythrocytes, and the potassium salt of the hemoglobin forms the other part of the systems. Oxyhemoglobin is a stronger acid (i.e., it dissociates its hydrogen ions more freely) than reduced hemoglobin and carbonic acid, and the latter is a stronger acid than reduced hemoglobin. When carbon dioxide diffuses into the red blood cells carbonic acid is formed ($CO_2 + H_2O \xrightarrow{\text{carbonic anhydrase}} H_2CO_3$); this is also a reversible reaction. The carbonic acid is buffered by potassium

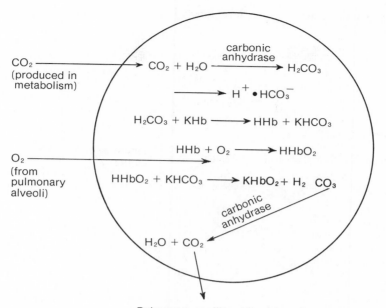

Figure 5–3   Role of the red blood cell in pH regulation.

hemoglobinate to form the weak acid hemoglobin and potassium bicarbonate (H_2CO_3 + KHb $\rightarrow$ HHb + $KHCO_3$). When the acid hemoglobin is oxygenated to oxyhemoglobin in the lungs it becomes a stronger acid and is rapidly buffered by potassium bicarbonate to form potassium oxyhemoglobinate and carbonic acid ($HHbO_2$ + $KHCO_3$ $\rightarrow$ $KHbO_2$ + H_2CO_3). Carbonic anhydrase reverses its action and the carbonic acid is broken down into carbon dioxide and water; the carbon dioxide diffuses out of the cells into the blood and into the alveoli of the lungs (see Fig. 5–3).

RESPIRATORY REGULATION. A second important factor in the maintenance of the normal pH of body fluids is the elimination of carbon dioxide in respiration. Carbon dioxide is constantly produced in cellular metabolism and diffuses from the cells into the blood and erythrocytes. As a result, carbon dioxide is in greater concentration in the blood when it enters the pulmonary capillaries than in the air in the alveoli of the lungs. The pressure gradient results in some carbon dioxide diffusing from the blood into the alveoli from which it is exhaled. This reduces the amount available to form carbonic acid in the body fluids.

The neurons of the respiratory control center in the medulla are extremely sensitive to the concentration of carbon dioxide and hydrogen ions in body fluids. An increase in either stimulates the center to increase the rate and volume of respirations so more carbon dioxide may be eliminated. Conversely, a decrease in the concentration of carbon dioxide or hydrogen ions below the normal results in slower shallow respirations so that carbon dioxide is retained to form carbonic acid.

Obviously any condition that impairs the capacity of the lungs to eliminate carbon dioxide from the body predisposes to an increase in the carbonic acid level and a decrease in the pH of body fluids; on the other hand, increased pulmonary ventilation may increase the pH of the body fluids by the excessive loss of carbon dioxide.

KIDNEY REGULATION. The kidneys play an important role in maintaining the acid-base balance by excreting hydrogen ions and forming bicarbonate in amounts as indicated by the pH of the blood. The cells of the distal portion of the renal tubules are sensitive to changes in the pH; when there is a decrease below the normal, hydrogen ions are excreted and bicarbonate is formed and retained. Conversely, when there is an increased alkalinity above the normal, hydro-

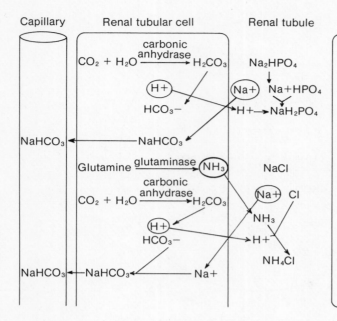

Figure 5–4 The role of the kidneys in pH control.

gen ions are conserved and base-forming ions are excreted. In other words, the kidneys may excrete many or few hydrogen ions and form more or less bicarbonate according to the need.

The elimination of acid ions and the formation of bicarbonate involve the following processes:

1. Within the renal tubular cells, carbon dioxide and water form carbonic acid $(CO_2 + H_2O \xrightarrow{\text{carbonic anhydrase}} H_2CO_3)$ which ionizes to release hydrogen and bicarbonate ions (H^+ HCO_3^-). The hydrogen ion moves out into the renal tubule.

2. Alkaline sodium phosphate (Na_2HPO_4) in the tubular fluid is converted to acid sodium phosphate (NaH_2PO_4) by accepting a hydrogen ion and releasing a sodium ion (Na^+). The acid sodium phosphate is excreted in the urine.

3. The sodium ion passes into the tubular cell in exchange for the hydrogen ion that moved out. There it combines with the bicarbonate ion to form sodium bicarbonate ($NaHCO_3$), which diffuses into the blood.

4. Additional hydrogen ions may be eliminated by the kidneys forming ammonia and eliminating it as an acid salt. Within the tubular cells, the amino acid glutamine is broken down and ammonia (NH_3) is re-

leased into the tubule. Sodium chloride in the tubular fluid ionizes ($NaCl \rightarrow Na^+$ Cl^-); the ammonia combines with a hydrogen ion and a chlorine ion to form ammonium chloride ($NH_3 + H^+ + Cl^- \rightarrow NH_4Cl$), which is eliminated in the urine. The sodium ion passes into the tubular cell to form sodium bicarbonate, which passes into the blood.

In summary, to preserve the normal pH the kidneys secrete hydrogen ions into the renal tubules in exchange for sodium ions, acidify alkaline phosphate, form and retain sodium bicarbonate and form an ammonium acid salt (see Fig. 5–4).

Acid-Base Imbalance

Normally the pH of body fluids is maintained within the narrow range of 7.35 to 7.45. When the alkalinity falls below 7.35 the condition is known as acidosis or acidemia; when it is above 7.45 the condition is referred to as alkalosis or alkalemia.

Significant blood tests used in determining the acid-base imbalance include the following:

1. Carbon dioxide content. The carbon dioxide represented in this test includes that in the blood in solution, carbonic acid and bicarbonate. The normal is expressed at

50 to 70 volumes per cent, or 21 to 30 mEq./L.

2. Carbon dioxide-combining power. This provides information as to the amount of carbon dioxide carried in the blood as bicarbonate. The normal is expressed as 50 to 65 volumes per cent, or 21 to 28 mEq./L.

3. Carbon dioxide pressure (pCO_2). This test indicates the partial pressure of carbon dioxide dissolved in the blood and is of value in detecting acid-base imbalance associated with disturbances of respiration. The normal pCO_2 is 35 to 45 mm. Hg. An increase indicates a greater concentration of carbonic acid.

4. Serum concentration of various electrolytes. See page 56 for normal levels.

Urinalysis may also provide useful information. Significant factors are:

a. The pH of the urine. The normal range is 5 to 8, depending on the diet and drug therapy.

b. Total volume. Normally a minimum of 1000 to 1500 ml. are excreted in 24 hours.

c. Amounts of various solids; ammonia, bicarbonate, calcium, chloride, ketones and potassium.

Acidosis

When the hydrogen ion concentration is increased in body fluids, the three control mechanisms (buffer systems, respiration, and kidney activity) endeavor to re-establish a normal pH. If the carbonic acid–bicarbonate ratio can be kept normal by increased respiratory elimination of carbon dioxide and by increased kidney elimination of hydrogen ions and formation of sodium bicarbonate, the pH is kept within normal range. The condition is then said to be compensated acidosis. If the mechanisms cannot compensate adequately, a decrease in the carbonic acid–bicarbonate ratio develops, the pH falls below normal, and a state of uncompensated acidosis exists.

Acidosis may be classified according to the cause as respiratory or metabolic.

Respiratory acidosis develops as a result of hypoventilation; the elimination of carbon dioxide does not keep pace with the production and the carbonic acid concentration of the blood increases. Inadequate elimination of carbon dioxide by the lungs may be caused by acute or chronic respiratory disease (e.g., pneumonia, emphysema, fibrosis of the lungs) or depression of the respiratory center by drugs or disease.

Metabolic acidosis may develop as a result of the production or ingestion of an excessive amount of acid, the retention of nonvolatile acids or an excessive loss of base from the body.

An excessive production may be seen in uncontrolled diabetes mellitus and starvation in which there is an excessive catabolism of fat by the cells as a source of energy. Ketone bodies, viz., aceto-acetic acid, β-hydroxybutyric acid, and acetone, are produced in abnormally large amounts and at a greater rate than that at which the cells can complete their oxidation to energy, carbon dioxide and water. The acids deplete the bicarbonate buffer, and the pH of the body fluid falls.

Overdosage or prolonged administration of ammonium chloride, acetylsalicylic acid or acetazolamide (Diamox) may give rise to acidosis. With ammonium chloride, the ammonium radical is converted to urea, leaving hydrochloric acid, which uses up bicarbonate in buffering. Acetazolamide may depress the ability of the renal tubular cells to form sodium bicarbonate and secrete hydrogen ions to acidify urine.

A decreased urinary output, whether due to renal disease or a condition such as severe dehydration or shock, will obviously result in the retention of nonvolatile acids which are constantly produced in metabolism. Respirations and the buffers can compensate for a period of time, but eventually the bicarbonate is depleted as the acids accumulate and no bicarbonate is being formed by the renal tubular cells. In chronic kidney disease, the tubular cells may be damaged and their ability to secrete hydrogen ions and form sodium bicarbonate and ammonia is impaired. As a result, acidification of the urine is diminished and excessive amounts of hydrogen ions are retained.

A frequent cause of metabolic acidosis is an abnormal loss of alkaline secretions that are normally reabsorbed. The secretions that comprise the intestinal juice have a high sodium and potassium bicarbonate concentration; diarrhea, an intestinal fistula, or the vomiting or suction of fluids from the intestine may deplete the body's bicarbonate.

Effects and Manifestations of Acidosis. A decrease in the pH causes a depression of the central nervous system; mental responses are slow and dulled. The patient may complain of headache, become drowsy and disoriented, and lapse into coma. Anorexia, nausea and vomiting are common. In metabolic acidosis, respirations increase in rate and depth (hyperpnea). The urinary output may be increased in an effort to excrete excess acids; dehydration develops rapidly because of the associated vomiting, diuresis and decreased intake.

The plasma bicarbonate is reduced in metabolic acidosis but remains normal or may be elevated in respiratory acidosis. The pCO_2 is increased in respiratory acidosis. The urinary pH is decreased in acidosis, and disturbances in electrolyte concentrations develop.

Implications for Nursing. The patient with acidosis is critically ill and requires close observation of vital signs, fluid balance, orientation and level of consciousness. Frequent collection of urine specimens may be required and may necessitate the use of a retention catheter. Blood specimens are taken at frequent intervals; the required equipment is kept readily available and the necessary assistance is provided in the collection of the blood.

If the patient is conscious, oral fluids are encouraged. The fluids permitted may vary with the cause of the acidosis. For example, salted broth, orange juice and milk may be given in diabetic acidosis, but in the case of acidosis associated with renal failure these may be contraindicated because of the potassium content. Parenteral fluids are administered; the solutions given are based on the blood chemistry reports and kidney function. The rate of flow should be defined by the physician; frequently a limited amount is given fairly rapidly if the patient is dehydrated; then the rate is slowed.

Frequent mouth care is especially important because of the hyperpnea, mouth-breathing, vomiting and dehydration that commonly accompany acidosis.

Safety precautions are necessary if the patient manifests disorientation. If comatose, all the points applicable to the care of an unconscious patient will require consideration (see p. 103).

Alkalosis

This is an acid-base imbalance in which there is an increase in the pH in excess of 7.45 due to a carbonic acid deficit or an excessive amount of bicarbonate. It may be classified as respiratory or metabolic.

Respiratory alkalosis is due to an excessive loss of carbonic acid by hyperventilation. Carbon dioxide is being excreted by the lungs in excess of its production. The rapid deep breathing may be caused by an anxiety state, hysteria or central nervous system disease that is producing overstimulation of the respiratory center, high fever or hypoxia.

The pH of the blood and the ratio of carbonic acid to bicarbonate are increased. If the condition is prolonged, large amounts of base are excreted by the kidneys, resulting in increased losses of sodium and potassium. There is a corresponding decrease in the excretion of chloride and hydrogen ions.

The patient frequently complains of dizziness. Tetany may develop as a result of increased neuromuscular irritability; signs and symptoms of this are tingling in the distal portions of the extremities, cramps, and tonic spasms of muscles which may progress to convulsions.

If the condition is of psychological origin, an explanation of the overbreathing and its effects may lead to voluntary correction. An effort is also made to help the patient resolve his concerns. Having the patient rebreathe his own carbon dioxide by breathing into a paper bag is helpful. Inhalation of 5 per cent carbon dioxide in oxygen may be ordered.

Oxygen inhalation may be ordered if the respiratory alkalosis is caused by hypoxia, and if the latter is due to anemia, a transfusion of whole blood or packed cells may be administered.

Metabolic alkalosis may develop as the result of an abnormal loss of hydrochloric acid from the stomach in vomiting or gastric suction, excessive ingestion of alkaline substances (e.g., sodium bicarbonate) or a potassium deficit. The plasma concentration of bicarbonate is elevated with a corresponding increase in the pH and carbonic acid–bicarbonate ratio.

Respirations become slow and shallow

in an effort to increase the carbonic acid content of the blood. If the hypopnea is prolonged, it may produce an oxygen deficiency, and the patient becomes cyanotic.

Kidney compensation is by conservation of hydrogen and chloride ions and by increased excretion of bicarbonate. If the alkalosis is caused by vomiting, there is likely to be an associated dehydration which leads to decreased urinary output and reduced renal compensation.

Tetany may ensue with the patient exhibiting the signs and symptoms cited in respiratory alkalosis.

An intravenous infusion of normal saline is usually ordered immediately in the treatment of metabolic alkalosis. The plasma concentration of potassium is determined, and if there is a deficit, potassium in some form is prescribed. It may be administered orally or intravenously; if the latter method is used, the rate of flow is specified by the physician. It is usually given very slowly and limited to a definite amount in a certain number of hours. The patient receiving a potassium solution intravenously is observed closely for signs of hyperkalemia, which include a slow, weak pulse, restlessness and muscular weakness. Ammonium chloride may be prescribed intravenously or by mouth, especially if the alkalosis is due to vomiting, which depletes the chloride ions. Precautions similar to those mentioned above in relation to parenteral potassium administration are necessary if ammonium chloride is given intravenously.

References

BOOKS

Anthony, C. P.: Anatomy and Physiology, 7th ed. St. Louis, C. V. Mosby Co., 1967. Chapters 15 and 16.
Beeson, P. B., and McDermott, W. (Eds.): Cecil-Loeb Textbook of Medicine, 13th ed. Philadelphia, W. B. Saunders Co., 1971, pp. 1618–1639.
Brooks, S. M.: Basic Facts of Body Water and Ions. New York, Springer Publishing Co., 1960.
Dutcher, I. E., and Fielo, S. B.: Water and Electrolytes, Implications for Nursing Practice. New York, The MacMillan Co., 1967.
Guyton, A. C.: Function of the Human Body, 3rd ed. Philadelphia, W. B. Saunders Co., 1969. Chapter 18.
Harper, H. A.: Review of Physiological Chemistry, 6th ed. California Lange Medical Publications, 1957. Chapters 18 (pp. 273–277) and 10 (pp. 145–151).
Harrison, T. R. et al. (Eds.): Principles of Internal Medicine. New York, The Blakiston Division, McGraw-Hill Book Co., 1962. Chapter 51.
Langley, L. L.: Outline of Physiology, 2nd ed. New York, The Blakiston Division, McGraw-Hill Book Co., 1965. Chapter 26.
Metheny, N. M., and Snively, W. D., Jr.: Nurses' Handbook of Fluid Balance. Philadelphia, J. B. Lippincott Co., 1967.
Sodeman, W. A., and Sodeman, W. A., Jr.: Pathologic Physiology, 4th ed. Philadelphia, W. B. Saunders Co., 1967, Chapter 7.
Statland, H.: Fluid and Electrolytes in Practice, 3rd. ed. Philadelphia, J. B. Lippincott Co., 1963.

PERIODICALS

Burgess, R. E.: "Fluids and Electrolytes." Amer. J. Nurs., Vol. 65, No. 10 (Oct. 1965), pp. 90–95.

6
Body Temperature

Body temperature depends on the difference between the amount of heat produced and the amount lost. Normally, the body maintains a relatively constant temperature within the range of 36° to 37° C. (97° to 98.6° F.) regardless of the environmental temperature. For this reason, man is classified as homoiothermic, or warm-blooded, as opposed to the poikilothermic, or cold-blooded, species whose body temperature fluctuates with variations in the environmental temperature.

Heat Production and Dissipation

Constancy of a temperature of 36° to 37° C., which favors normal cellular activity, is maintained by physiological processes that preserve a balance between heat production and heat dissipation. An increased production of heat is compensated by increasing the loss; conversely, a decrease below normal body temperature initiates a decrease in the heat loss as well as an increase in the production of heat.

Heat is generated in the body by the catabolic chemical reactions within the cells. The more active the tissue, the greater is its production of heat; as a result, especially large amounts are produced by the muscles and liver. A small amount may be acquired

from external sources by radiation and conduction.

Normally, an excess of heat is produced within the body and must be eliminated to maintain a normal temperature. The excess is dissipated by the physical processes of radiation, conduction, convection and vaporization. Most of it is lost through the skin, and the remainder is eliminated in respirations and excreta.

Radiation is the process by which radiant energy is transmitted from one object to another without direct contact. Conduction is the transfer of heat between two objects that are in contact. Convection is the process by which heat is carried away from a surface by air currents passing over it. Evaporation of one gram of water from the surface of the skin and respiratory tract utilizes about 0.58 calorie. Some vaporization takes place constantly, but the amount taking place on the skin varies. If there is a need to increase the heat loss, the sweat glands increase their secretion and more heat is used in evaporation. If there is a need to conserve body heat, less moisture is released on to the skin surface to prevent the use of heat in vaporization.

Heat loss by radiation, conduction and convection depends on a temperature gradient. If the environmental temperature is equal to or greater than that of the body, these processes are ineffective and heat dissipation becomes dependent on the evaporation process.

Temperature Regulation

Responses to changes in body temperature are evoked by sensory nerve impulses that originate in the skin and by the direct effect of the blood temperature on the hypothalamus.

Receptor cells that are sensitive to heat and cold are located in the skin. When changes in the cutaneous temperature occur, the receptors give rise to nerve impulses that are delivered to the cerebral cortex and hypothalamus of the brain. Those that reach the cerebral cortex make the individual conscious of the temperature change. He may then produce voluntary responses to aid in correcting the change. For example, if he experiences the sensation of cold, he may voluntarily increase muscle activity to generate more heat, seek a warmer environment and add clothing to reduce the heat loss. In a hot environment, the voluntary responses might be to decrease activity in order to lower the heat production and to change to lighter clothing to permit more radiation.

In the anterior portion of the hypothalamus is a group of neurons that is referred to as the thermostatic or heat-regulating center. This center responds to cutaneous temperature impulses and to changes in the temperature of the blood. When the body temperature rises above normal, impulses are discharged that cause dilation of the cutaneous blood vessels and stimulation of the sweat glands. Heat loss is increased by evaporation of the additional sweat as well as by radiation from the larger volume of blood brought to the surface.

If the normal body temperature is threatened by a reduction in body heat, the center initiates impulses which reduce heat loss and increase the production of heat. Superficial blood vessels constrict, secretion by the sweat glands is inhibited, and shivering occurs.

Variables Within the Normal

The body temperature shows slight variations within the normal range from one individual to another and under certain circumstances. Variables within the normal include:

Time of Day. The temperature is higher in the late afternoon and evening following the activities of the individual's day. It falls during the night with decreased activity, being lowest about 4 to 6 A.M. If the individual is active during the night and sleeps during the day, the times of higher and lower temperatures are usually inverted.

Age. Infants and young children have a higher normal temperature. Their heat production is greater owing to their growth and activity. Also, the ability to regulate heat loss and production is not sufficiently developed in the early years to efficiently regulate a constancy of temperature.

Older people have a somewhat lower normal temperature because of their slower metabolic rate and reduced muscular activity.

Exercise. Strenuous exercise may cause an elevation of $0.5°$ to $1°$ C. in temperature, but it quickly returns to normal when the activity ceases. Women in labor frequently show an increase in temperature which is attributed to the increased muscular activity.

Menstrual Cycle. A variation in temperature is characteristic of certain phases of the menstrual cycle. There is an increase of $0.3°$ to $0.5°$ C. when ovulation occurs, which is usually about the middle of the cycle. The slight increase is maintained until a day or two before the onset of menstruation when it falls to the previous level.

Pregnancy. A slight increase in temperature occurs in the first 3 to 4 months of pregnancy and is followed by a gradual fall of $0.5°$ to $1°$ C. The lower temperature continues to full term and returns to the individual's normal level after parturition.

Thermometer Scales

The thermometers for measuring body temperature may be scaled in Fahrenheit (F.) or Centigrade (C.), and it may be necessary at times to know the equivalent of one in the other system.

The difference between the freezing point ($0°$ C.) and the boiling point ($100°$ C.) on the Centigrade scale is 100 degrees; on the Fahrenheit scale the difference is 180 degrees ($32°$ F. = freezing point; $212°$ F. = boiling point). This indicates that 100 Centigrade degrees equal 180 Fahrenheit degrees, or one Fahrenheit degree equals 5/9 of a Centigrade degree. The freezing point on the Fahrenheit scale is 32 degrees, but on the Centigrade scale it is 0 degrees; therefore, when converting to Centigrade the 32 must first be subtracted in order to find the number of degrees to be converted. When converting to Fahrenheit the 32 must be added to the product so that the result will be adjusted for the Fahrenheit scale. The following formulas may be used when conversion from one system to the other is necessary.

The formula to convert Fahrenheit degrees to Centigrade is:

$$(\text{F. degrees} - 32) \times \frac{5}{9} = \text{C. degrees}$$

Example: The conversion of 100° F. to C. degrees.

$$(100° \text{ F.} - 32) \times \frac{5}{9} = 37.7° \text{ C.}$$

The formula to convert Centigrade degrees to Fahrenheit is:

$$\left(\text{C. degrees} \times \frac{9}{5}\right) + 32 = \text{F. degrees}$$

Example: The conversion of 39° C. to F. degrees.

$$\left(39° \text{ C.} \times \frac{9}{5}\right) + 32 = 102.2° \text{ F.}$$

ABNORMAL BODY TEMPERATURE

FEVER

Fever, or pyrexia, is an elevation of the body temperature above normal due to a disturbance of the heat-regulating center. There is an increase in heat production that exceeds the rate of dissipation. Fever is considered a reliable indication of a pathological process within the body.

The disturbance in the heat-regulating center may be caused by the direct action of brain disease or increased intracranial pressure or by the action of some substance that is released into the blood at the site of tissue injury or disintegration anywhere in the body. The substance, which may be referred to as a pyrogen, is thought to be the product of the injured or disintegrating cells or of leukocytes which invade the area. In recent years, on the basis of experimental work, there is increasing support for the theory that the pyrogen is released by the leukocytes.[1, 2, 3]

Stimulation of the hypothalamic heat center by the pyrogen is analogous to the setting of the thermostat of an automatic heating system to a higher level; heat is produced until the set level of temperature is achieved. The higher temperature is maintained as long as the pyrogen is present. As the concentration of the pyrogen is reduced, the level of the thermostat is lowered, and there is a corresponding decrease in the fever by activation of the heat-dissipating responses—peripheral vasodilation and sweating.

Manifestations and Effects of Fever

The initial manifestations of fever vary with the degree of disturbance in the thermostatic center. If the elevation is moderate and gradual, the patient may experience slight chilliness for a brief period, general malaise, headache and anorexia. With a sudden and greater degree of stimulation of the center, the patient has a chill in which he shivers and feels very cold, even though his temperature may already be above normal. His skin becomes pale and is cold to the touch because of the peripheral vasoconstriction. The shivering is increased muscular activity for the purpose of producing heat; it may be severe enough to cause chattering of the teeth and shaking of the whole body. The chill lasts until the temperature reaches the level set by the stimulated thermostatic center in the hypothalamus. Then, as long as the pyrogen is effective, a balance between the heat production and dissipation maintains the temperature at approximately this higher level.

[1]C. M. MacBryde (Ed.): Signs and Symptoms, 4th ed. Philadelphia, J. B. Lippincott Co., 1964, p. 451.

[2]W. A. Sodeman and W. A. Sodeman, Jr.: Pathologic Physiology, 4th ed. Philadelphia, W. B. Saunders Co., 1967, pp. 203–204.

[3]A. C. Guyton: Medical Physiology, 4th ed. Philadelphia, W. B. Saunders Co., 1971, p. 841.

Frequently, the onset of fever in infants and young children is accompanied by a convulsion which is due to the immaturity and instability of their nervous systems.

With subsidence of the chill, the patient's skin becomes hot and flushed, and he complains of being hot. Disorientation and delirium are not uncommon when the fever is high, especially in older persons.

The basal metabolic rate is increased in proportion to the elevation of temperature. With a fever of 40.5° C. (105° F.) there is an increase in metabolism of approximately 50 per cent. A negative nitrogen balance develops with the increased destruction of body protein in metabolism, and there is a loss of weight. Respirations and the heart rate are accelerated. There is a greater loss of fluid by evaporation from the hot skin and in the increased respirations.

If the temperature rises above approximately 40.5° C. (105° F.), there is danger of cellular damage. The hypothalamus may lose its capacity for temperature regulation, resulting in a progressive increase in fever until death occurs. The limit to which the temperature may rise before causing death is about 43.3° to 44.4° C. (110° to 112° F.).

When the pyrogenic factor is suddenly removed, the mechanisms that contribute to heat loss are set in operation. There is marked peripheral vasodilation and profuse sweating (diaphoresis); heat is lost rapidly by radiation and vaporization. This sudden lowering of the temperature is referred to as the crisis of fever. If the temperature returns to normal gradually over a period of several days, the process is known as lysis.

Fever is thought to serve a useful purpose in some infections. A high temperature will destroy a large number of the causative organisms in gonorrhea and neurosyphilis. Other pathogenic organisms may be made less virulent by a high fever. It is also suggested that the increased metabolism supports an increased production of antibodies since patients who fail to develop a marked febrile response in a severe infection usually do less well.

Types of Fever. Fever may be classified according to its variation within 24 hours or 2 or 3 days. An intermittent fever is one in which the temperature falls to normal and rises again within the 24-hour period; a remittent fever manifests a variation of one or two degrees, but does not reach normal within the 24 hours. A relapsing fever occurs when there are alternating periods of one or several days of normal and elevated temperature.

Heat Stroke

A heat stroke occurs with relatively long exposure to extreme heat. At first the individual may experience headache, visual disturbances, nausea and vomiting. Weakness, flaccidity of the muscles, a rapid bounding pulse and rapid respirations are manifested. The individual becomes delirious, collapses, and lapses into coma. The skin is hot and dry, and there is an absence of sweating due to central nervous system damage. The temperature progressively rises to 40.6° to 43.3° C. (105° to 110° F.).

Unless the condition is discovered in the early stages and the body is rapidly cooled, circulatory failure develops and the patient dies. The patient may be immersed in a cold bath, given a cold sponge followed by the application of ice bags, or a cooling blanket that is used to induce hypothermia may be applied.

Nursing in Fever

The care of the fever patient depends largely on the causative condition, but the following points require consideration.

Rest. Fever produces an increased metabolic rate, so the patient is advised to decrease his activity. With an elevation of 37.7° C. (100° F.) or higher, bed rest is usually recommended.

Observations. The temperature, pulse and respirations are usually noted every 4 hours; they may be checked oftener in high fever and when these vital signs may indicate complications. For example, when caring for a patient with brain disease or trauma, it may be necessary to record the temperature, pulse and respirations hourly. An increase in temperature and a decrease in pulse and respirations may indicate increasing intracranial pressure.

If the fever is of unknown origin, the nurse observes the patient closely for the development of signs and symptoms which may be helpful to the physician in making a diagnosis.

Care During a Chill. If the patient experiences a chill at the onset of the fever, several light covers are used and tucked in closely to the body to prevent heat loss. If heat applications in the form of hot water bottles or an electric heating pad are employed, extreme precautions are necessary to avoid burning the patient. As soon as the chill is over, heat applications and the extra covers are removed to prevent loss of body fluid and sodium by excessive sweating.

Fluids and Food. Unless contraindicated by the patient's disease, the fluid intake in fever is increased to a minimum of 2500 to 3000 ml. for an adult because more fluid is lost by evaporation from the skin and in the increased respirations. The inclusion of broths and soups is recommended for their salt content. A record is made of the fluid intake and output.

Since fever is accompanied by an increase in metabolism and in destruction of body protein, an increase in the caloric and protein intake is necessary. This may be difficult during the acute stage owing to the anorexia and the patient's condition, but it should be effected as soon as possible. When the patient's intake consists mainly of fluids, calories and protein may be increased by giving milk drinks, eggnogs, and gruel, and by adding cream, glucose, or lactose to a commercial preparation such as Sustagen or Protinol.

Cooling Procedures. To prevent the temperature from reaching the level at which tissue damage may occur, a cooling procedure may be employed in the form of sponging the surface of the body with a cool solution of approximately 35 per cent alcohol in water, or one may apply ice bags to the head, axillae, along the sides of the trunk and to the groins. Covers should be kept to a minimum, and the room kept cool and well ventilated.

Medications. If the temperature approaches the dangerous levels, a drug that lowers the sensitivity of the heat-regulating center and produces diaphoresis may be ordered. The antipyretic drug most commonly used is acetylsalicylic acid (Aspirin) in doses of 0.3 to 0.6 Gm. for an adult every 3 or 4 hours.

Comfort Measures. The mouth becomes very dry and a source of discomfort to the fever patient. It should be cleansed and rinsed with a mild antiseptic solution every 2 hours. Vaseline, oil or cold cream may be applied to the lips to prevent cracking.

Herpes simplex (fever blister, cold sore) may develop about the mouth. The lesion appears first as a sore, burning papule; then a vesicle forms, followed by encrustation and scab formation. It is due to a virus which has probably been latent in the cells and becomes activated by the higher body temperature. An ointment may be prescribed to inhibit the spread and soften the encrustation. If the lesions occur within the mouth, they may discourage the taking of fluids and nourishment; a mouthwash containing a topical anesthetic may be ordered.

Frequent back rubs, changes of position and changes of linen may help to reduce the patient's discomfort. Frequent bathing is necessary because of the increased perspiration.

An enema may be necessary to relieve constipation, which is frequently associated with fever.

HYPOTHERMIA

Hypothermia means a subnormal body temperature and is encountered much less frequently than fever. The cause may be prolonged exposure to cold, reduced metabolism as occurs in hypothyroidism (myxedema) or depression of body activities by alcohol intoxication, heavy sedation or circulatory failure. Clinically, the term hypothermia is used most often to indicate deliberate cooling of a patient for therapeutic purposes.

Prolonged Exposure to Cold

When an individual is accidentally exposed to extreme climatic cold, the first physiological responses are peripheral vasoconstriction, increased heat production by shivering and accelerated metabolism, and an increase in the pulse and respiratory rates. With continued exposure, the internal body temperature is gradually lowered. The cooling of the brain results in a depression of the heat-regulating center in the hypothalamus, and the ability to protect the body temperature is lost. There is a progressive depression of metabolism and a slowing of mental and muscular responses. The individual becomes drowsy, eventually lapses into coma, and may develop respiratory and circulatory failure.

The patient suffering cold exposure is treated by immersion in a warm bath of 42° to 43° C. (107° to 110° F.) for 10 to 20 minutes; this warms the peripheral blood and tissues. It is not prolonged since superficial vasodilation would reduce the blood supply to the vital centers. Rewarming is then continued at normal room temperature. Some instability in body temperature control is likely for 7 to 10 days, so the patient is usually kept at rest and under observation during that period.

Induced Hypothermia

Purpose and Effects. Hypothermia may be intentionally produced to decrease the rate of metabolism and oxygen utilization. The low temperature may be maintained for an hour to several days, depending on the purpose and the patient's condition. It may be employed during surgery on the heart, large blood vessels or brain which necessitates a temporary interruption of the blood flow in the area. It may also be used following cerebral surgery or severe head injuries in order to prevent or reduce severe cerebral edema or hyperthermia. Cooling of the cells reduces their activity and prevents the damage that would normally ensue with a decreased oxygen supply.

The temperature most frequently used in induced hypothermia is within the range of 32° to 26° C. (89.6° to 78.8° F.). The decrease in cellular activity and oxygen requirement is proportional to the decrease in temperature. A decline to 30° to 28° C. reduces metabolism by approximately 50 per cent. The pulse and respiratory rates are slowed and are accompanied by a fall in blood pressure. The patient becomes stuporous and may lose consciousness with lower hypothermic levels. There is a loss of the gag reflex and corneal and pupillary reactions, and there is a diminished response to pain. The viscosity of the blood increases. The urinary output may not be markedly reduced at first, but it progressively decreases and has a low specific gravity.

Methods of Induction. Hypothermia may be produced by the application of cold to the surface of the body or by extracorporeal cooling of the blood.

Surface cooling methods include immersion in an iced-water bath, enclosure of the patient in large plastic sheets filled with crushed ice, placing the patient between electrically controlled blankets with coils through which a cold fluid is circulated, and the application of ice bags over the body surface. The latter may be combined with the circulation of cool air over the body by fans.

The blanket method is the most satisfactory; it is simpler and provides better control. The temperature of the fluid flowing through the coils is maintained at the level at which the gauge on the accompanying refrigerating unit is set. The blankets may also be used to rewarm the patient following hypothermia.

The extracorporeal method of cooling is used during surgery. The blood is diverted from a large vessel, circulated through a cooling coil outside the body, and returned to another blood vessel. The heart-lung machine (pump-oxygenator), which is used in cardiac and vascular surgery as a mechanical pump to maintain circulation and to add oxygen to the blood, is also equipped with a heat-exchanger that may be used to either cool or warm the blood. The extracorporeal circulation of the blood through a heat exchanger has certain advantages; the patient may be cooled more quickly, better control of the body temperature is provided, and the patient may be quickly rewarmed on completion of the surgical procedure.

Reduction of the body temperature can only take place when heat production does not compensate for heat loss. Before hypothermia induction is commenced, the patient receives a drug that depresses the heat-regulating center and prevents the shivering response. Shivering must be avoided because of the associated heat production and the marked increase in the utilization of oxygen. The sedative effect of the drug also reduces the unpleasantness of the cooling for the conscious patient. Examples of the drugs used are chlorpromazine (Thorazine), promethazine hydrochloride (Phenergan), and meperidine hydrochloride (Demerol), all of which may be administered intramuscularly or intravenously.

The internal body temperature is monitored continuously during hypothermia by special electric thermometers. Probes which record the temperature are placed in the esophagus and rectum. These are connected to a transducer that converts the heat energy to electrical energy which is registered on a scale. When the temperature is within 1 or 2 degrees of the desired level, the cooling procedure is discontinued or reduced, and a downward drift of 1 or 2 degrees will continue. Obese persons cool more slowly and manifest a greater tendency to drift.

Rewarming. Following surgery, the patient may be rewarmed before leaving the operating room. As cited above, if extracorporeal cooling was used, the heat-exchanger of the heart-lung machine may be used to rewarm the patient. If the blanket method was used, warm water may be circulated through the coils. In many instances, the patient is simply covered with blankets and allowed to rewarm at his own rate.

Nursing Responsibilities in Hypothermia

Preparation. The conscious patient and the patient's family may have considerable apprehension when advised that hypothermia is to be used. The purpose and method to be used should be explained, and their questions answered to reduce their anxiety.

The skin should be clean and inspected for discolored areas and lesions. If the hypothermia is to be prolonged, a light protective application of oil or lanolin is usually made to the entire body surface.

Collapse of the peripheral veins occurs with the cooling; for this reason, an intravenous infusion is started prior to induction so fluid and electrolytes may be administered during the treatment. An indwelling catheter is inserted so that renal function and the fluid output may be checked.

The pre-induction medication is given as ordered, and the patient's blood pressure, pulse, respiratory rate, level of consciousness and responses are noted for a comparative baseline later.

Emergency equipment that should be assembled and readily available includes an intermittent positive pressure respirator, oxygen, tracheotomy set and an emergency drug tray with vasopressors and cardiac and respiratory stimulants.

Care During Hypothermia. A nurse remains in constant attendance. Frequent observations and recordings are made of the pulse rate and rhythm, respirations and blood pressure. Cardiac irritability may increase with cooling, and fibrillation may develop. Suctioning may be necessary to clear the airway, and respirations may have to be assisted by a respirator. A constant check of the temperature is necessary; any change in the level of temperature or indication of shivering is reported promptly to the physician. There is danger of cardiac arrest if the temperature falls too low.

The skin is inspected every 1 to 2 hours; discolored or firm, immovable areas may indicate frostbite, in which case there is a crystallization of the tissue fluid, or fat necrosis. If ice bags are being used, they are moved from one area to another frequently. When cooling blankets are used, frequent turning of the patient is necessary. The use of a ripple (alternating air pressure) mattress also helps to protect the skin. To prevent contractures and hyperextensions, good body alignment is kept in mind when positioning the patient; passive range-of-motion exercises are used to preserve normal joint movement.

The fluid intake and output are accurately recorded; the daily fluid intake is determined by the 24-hour output. Frequent urine specimens are collected for analysis.

The mouth is cleansed and moistened every 2 to 3 hours, and the nasal passages are kept clear of secretions. Since the corneal reflex may be absent and the secretions diminished, the eyes may have to be irrigated and protected with eye pads.

Rewarming. During the rewarming period, constant observation of the patient is just as important as during the hypothermic phase. As the temperature approaches normal, the extra blankets used in rewarming are gradually removed to prevent it from rising above the normal level. Frequent checking of the pulse, respirations and blood pressure is still necessary.

After the patient is rewarmed, the special

thermometer probes are removed, but recording of the temperature every 3 or 4 hours continues for 2 or 3 days as there may be some instability of the hypothalamic heat-regulating center. Frequent checking of the pulse continues for the first 24 to 48 hours since the patient may still develop cardiac irregularity or fibrillation.

The indwelling catheter is removed when a normal urinary output is established. Oral fluids are administered in small amounts and progressively increased as tolerated.

References

BOOKS

Anthony, C. P.: Textbook of Anatomy and Physiology, 7th ed. Saint Louis, C. V. Mosby Co., 1967, pp. 424–428.

Guyton, A. C.: Textbook of Medical Physiology, 4th ed. Philadelphia, W. B. Saunders Co., 1971. Chapter 71.

MacBryde, C. M. (Ed.): Signs and Symptoms, 4th ed. Philadelphia, J. B. Lippincott Co., 1964. Chapter 22.

Sodeman, W. A., and Sodeman, W. A., Jr.: Pathologic Physiology, 4th ed. Philadelphia, W. B. Saunders Co., 1967, pp. 202–205 and 228–235.

PERIODICALS

Hickey, C. H.: "Hypothermia," Amer. J. Nurs., Vol. 65, No. 1 (Jan. 1965), pp. 116–122.

Lewis, F. J.: "Hypothermia – Physiology and Clinical Application," Surg. Clin. North Amer., Vol. 42, No. 1 (Feb. 1962), pp. 69–76.

Michenfelder, J. D., et al.: "Induced Hypothermia: Physiologic Effects, Indications and Techniques." Surg. Clin. North Amer., Vol. 45, No. 4 (Aug. 1965), pp. 889–897.

Nugent, G. R.: "Prolonged Hypothermia." Amer. J. Nurs., Vol. 60, No. 7 (July 1960), pp. 967–969.

7
The Patient with Pain

PAIN

Pain is a distressing sensation which warns the sufferer of some disturbance or undesirable change in the body and reflexes that attempt to remove or produce withdrawal from the cause. It plays an important protective role; one progressively learns from early childhood to avoid and correct the situations which cause pain. When the sensation is lost in an area of the body as it is in spinal cord injury or leprosy, the lack of awareness of injury and the absence of normal protective responses may lead to extensive tissue damage. Pain is one of the most impelling symptoms that prompts a person to seek medical advice. It should be remembered, however, that there are serious diseases, such as cancer and heart disease, which may be painless at the onset; as a result, persons may delay seeing a physician until the disease is in an advanced stage.

Pain Mechanism

The structures essential for the pain sensation are receptors that are sensitive to pain stimuli, an impulse pathway to and within the central nervous system (brain and spinal cord), and areas within the brain for perception, interpretation and the initiation of responses.

Stimuli that cause pain sensation are received by freely branching bare nerve endings which form a diffuse network in the tissue. The concentration of these receptors varies throughout the body; they are abundant in the skin and on joint surfaces, but there are relatively fewer in the deeper tissues and viscera.

A wide variety of stimuli evoke pain; these stimuli include mechanical agents (e.g., cutting, blow, friction, distention), thermal agents (extremes of heat and cold), chemicals (e.g., chemicals released by injured cells or microorganisms), electric current, ischemia and sustained muscle contraction. Many are nonspecific but elicit pain through their intensity. For instance, light pressure produces an awareness of touch, but increasing the intensity of the pressure causes pain. similarly, heat and cold must reach a certain intensity to stimulate pain receptors.

The sensory, or afferent,* nerve fibers, whose bare terminal branches form the pain receptors, provide a peripheral pathway to conduct the impulses into the spinal cord or brain stem. These sensory nerve fibers

---

*Sensory, or afferent, nerve fibers carry impulses towards the central nervous system (brain and spinal cord). Motor, or efferent, nerve fibers transmit impulses away from the central nervous system to peripheral structures.

74

are of two types: some are larger and have a fatty insulating sheath (myelinated); the others are smaller and nonmyelinated. The myelinated fibers transmit the impulses very rapidly and produce the sharp pain that is felt immediately when the injury occurs. The nonmyelinated fibers conduct more slowly and are responsible for the more diffuse, throbbing pain or ache that follows the immediate sharp pain associated with the initial injury.

When pain impulses enter the spinal cord some may pass to motor neurons, which initiate impulses that are carried out of the cord along motor or efferent nerve fibers to skeletal muscles. These motor impulses produce a reflex response, such as withdrawal of the injured part from the object producing the pain stimulus (as seen in the withdrawal of the finger that receives a pin prick or touches a very hot object). The other pain impulses that enter the cord ascend the lateral spinothalamic tract to the thalamus in the brain. From here they are relayed via a thalamocortical pathway to the appropriate sensory area of the cerebral cortex, and the individual becomes aware of the pain. Interpretation also takes place as to the site of the pain, its quality and intensity. In addition to producing perception and interpretation of pain, the impulses received at the cortical level initiate impulses which activate the physical and psychological responses to pain.

Pain Perception and Reactions

The pain sensation has two components: perception and reactions.

Perception is the awareness or feeling of pain. The severity of the pain perceived depends upon the intensity and frequency of the pain impulses. Qualifying the type of pain and relating it to various stimuli are learned experiences. The child gradually learns to associate the unpleasant feeling with objects and situations that cause pain.

The point at which a stimulus first elicits the awareness of pain is referred to as the pain threshold. Some authors indicate that the threshold is fairly constant and uniform for all persons,[1, 2] and that differences occur mainly in the responses. Others claim that the pain threshold may vary from one person to another and also that it varies from one time to another and under differing conditions for a given individual.[3, 4] The threshold may be elevated by such things as distraction, strong stimuli in other parts of the body (e.g., pain in one part of the body raises the threshold in other parts) and pathological conditions which involve the pain receptors, impulse pathways or cortical sensory areas. Depressed activity of the cerebral cortex due to certain drugs, alcohol, shock or debilitation may also raise the threshold.

A lowering of the pain threshold (hyperalgesia) may occur with inflammation or injury of structures concerned with the pain sensation or of neighboring tissues to such structures. The pain threshold may also be lowered by a reduction of other stimuli. The latter accounts for a patient's increased pain during the night when ordinary stimuli are at a minimum.

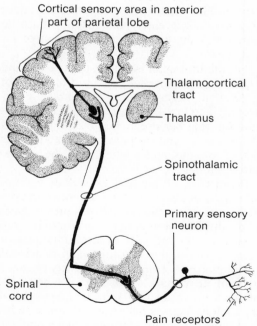

Cortical sensory area in anterior part of parietal lobe

Thalamocortical tract

Thalamus

Spinothalamic tract

Primary sensory neuron

Spinal cord

Pain receptors

Figure 7–1 Diagram illustrating pathway of pain impulses.

[1] A. C. Guyton: Textbook of Medical Physiology, 4th ed. Philadelphia, W. B. Saunders Co., 1971, p. 578.
[2] C. M. MacBryde (Ed.): Signs and Symptoms, 4th ed. Philadelphia, J. B. Lippincott Co., 1964, p. 74.
[3] Ibid., p. 75.
[4] N. B. Taylor and M. G. McPhedran: Basic Physiology and Anatomy. Toronto, The Macmillan Co. of Canada Ltd., 1965, p. 273.

The reaction component of pain is comprised of all the psychological, physical, voluntary and involuntary responses that are made when pain is perceived.

The physical reactions include those of skeletal muscles and the involuntary physiological responses implemented through the release of adrenalin and stimulation of the sympathetic nervous system. Skeletal muscle reaction may be the immediate withdrawal reflex (cited previously), involuntary contraction, or increased tone in an attempt to splint or immobilize the affected part (e.g., rigidity of the abdomen). Voluntary muscle activity may also be involved in correcting the situation when the individual removes the offending object, treats the site or seeks assistance.

The physiological responses are superficial vasoconstriction, an increased blood supply to the brain and skeletal muscles, a decrease in salivary secretion, reduced gastrointestinal action, increased secretion of perspiration and dilatation of the pupils. As a result, the patient manifests pallor and an increase in blood pressure, pulse and respirations. The skin becomes cold and clammy, and the lips and mouth are dry.

If the pain is deep, severe and prolonged, the above defense reactions may not develop and the patient may exhibit shock and extreme weakness; the blood pressure falls, the pulse weakens and nausea and vomiting may occur.

Even when the intensity and the nature of the pain stimulus are the same for several persons, the type and degree of reactions are likely to vary considerably because of individual differences in psychological make-up. The nature of a person's reactions is determined, to a large extent, by his past experiences and the degree of threat and frustration inherent in the pain for him. Some may audibly complain by moaning, crying or verbal expression of suffering and fear and may further indicate their distress by restlessness and purposeless movements. Others may be very stoical, remain still and suffer in silence.

Factors which may influence patients' responses include the following:

Sociocultural Background. An individual's responses become conditioned by social and cultural attitudes to pain. Some learn from those around them that pain is to be endured without obvious emotional reactions. If others have been accustomed to persons in pain exhibiting outward responses which are accepted and which receive attention, they consciously or unconsciously develop a similar pattern of response.

Emotional State. If the patient is in an emotional state to begin with, his evaluation of pain is likely to be exaggerated. If the illness has disrupted plans, created financial or home problems or the origin of the pain is the heart or a common site of cancer, the patient is threatened to a greater degree and is more fearful.

Physical Condition. Psychological reactions are usually greater in weak and fatigued persons. For instance, the obstetrical patient whose labor is prolonged may be quite calm and uncomplaining at first, but as she becomes fatigued and fearful that something is wrong, her pain becomes less tolerable.

Previous Pain Experience. Responses may be either increased or decreased by the memory of previous pain. Fear of a repetition of former severe suffering may produce marked outward reactions. With some a greater tolerance and resignation may develop.

Significance of the Pain. Apprehension is always greater when a situation is not understood or when one does not know what to expect. The patient who fears he has cancer may manifest greater pain reaction until he learns that the biopsy report is negative for malignancy.

To children, pain is a new, unpleasant and frightening experience which they cannot understand; overt expressions may be expected. The labor patient who has been prepared during her pregnancy by explanations of the source and purpose of the labor pains is less anxious and calmer than the unprepared patient.

Distraction. Reactions as well as perception are influenced by the amount of the patient's attention that is focused on the pain. If a situation commands considerable concentration on the part of the individual or creates pleasurable emotion, pain responses are minimized. The person actively engaged in competitive sports may not even be aware of the pain of an injury he receives. But if the patient focuses his whole attention on his discomfort, reactions are more pronounced.

Intensity and Duration of Pain. If the pain

stimulus is very intense, the individual feels more threatened. He may find it difficult to control his emotional responses and may even become quite disorganized. Similarly, pain of long duration is wearing and may initiate more overt reactions; on the other hand, the patient may become more resigned to the pain and take the attitude that he has to live with it.

Types of Pain

Some of the more common terms used to classify pain are as follows:

Superficial pain occurs when the receptors in surface structures are stimulated. Conversely, deep pain arises from deeper tissues, such as muscle, periosteum and viscera.

Localized pain arises directly from the site of the disturbance. Referred pain is that which is felt in a part of the body which is remote from the actual point of stimulation. The impulses usually arise in an organ, but the pain is projected to a surface area of the body. A classic example of referred pain is that associated with angina pectoris; the pain originates in the heart muscle as a result of ischemia, but it may be experienced in the midsternal region, the base of the neck and down the left arm. Pain arising in the gallbladder or bile ducts may be referred to the epigastrium and the right scapular region.

The mechanism of referred pain is not clearly understood. Several explanations are offered;[5, 6, 7] the one most commonly accepted appears to be one which states that the area of stimulation and that in which the pain is felt are both innervated by nerve fibers that arise from the same segment of the spinal cord. Each spinal nerve contains sensory fibers that are distributed to certain viscera, skeletal muscles and an area of superficial tissues. The pain impulses from all of these areas are delivered to the same segment of the spinal cord from which they ascend via a common spinothalamic tract to

the thalamus and are relayed to the cerebral cortex. It is suggested the faulty localization in the brain may be attributed to the infrequency of visceral pain impulses as compared with the frequency of impulses arising in cutaneous areas.

Another theory suggests that the fibers carrying the pain impulses from the viscera and those from peripheral tissues converge upon the same neuron at some point in the pain pathway within the central nervous system. The impulses are then interpreted as coming from the superficial area because of previous experience.

Projected pain occurs when impulses are set up at some point along the pain pathway beyond the peripheral pain receptors. The pain is perceived as arising at the site of the pain receptors served by the pathway in which the pain originated. A person who has had an amputation may experience what is referred to as phantom limb pain. Stimuli arising from the stump may be localized on the basis of the previously established body image, and as a result the pain is projected to the portion of the limb that was removed.

Persistent, severe pain that cannot be effectively controlled by the usual medications is referred to as intractable pain.

Nursing the Patient with Pain

The nurse plays an important role in the relief and support of a patient who is experiencing pain and may also make a significant contribution to the diagnosis and treatment through accurate observations.

A person may mention to a nurse that he has a pain but doesn't consider it severe enough to consult a doctor. The nurse, without alarming the patient, should urge him to see his physician, since pain is an indication of some disturbance, which, if recognized early, may be corrected before causing more severe suffering and inconvenience.

Important considerations in the care of a patient with pain are:

Attitude of the Nurse. When acceptance, gentleness and a desire to provide relief are evident in the nurse's response to his suffering, the patient senses an emotional warmth and understanding that allay much of his fear and make the pain more tolerable.

The nurse guards against forming personal

[5]N. B. Taylor and M. G. McPhedran: Basic Physiology and Anatomy. Toronto, The Macmillan Co. of Canada Ltd., 1965, p. 274.

[6]C. M. MacBryde (Ed.): Signs and Symptoms, 4th ed. Philadelphia, J. B. Lippincott Co., 1964, pp. 77–78.

[7]T. C. Ruch and H. D. Patton (Eds.): Physiology and Biophysics. 19th ed. Philadelphia: W. B. Saunders Co., 1965, pp. 356–358.

opinions as to whether the patient really has pain of the intensity expressed. Criticism of the patient's behavior is avoided; past experience and circumstances condition each person's emotional responses. Whether or not the intensity of the pain is due entirely to the physical disturbance or is aggravated because of anxiety or sociocultural factors, it is real to the patient and requires attention.

Observation. Certain information about the pain is obtained from the patient and his family and is objectively recorded. Alert observations are made of the patient for associated symptoms and the effect of the pain. Failure to recognize a patient's pain and its characteristics could lead to a delay in diagnosis and necessary treatment.

Pain is wholly subjective; only the person experiencing the pain knows the nature, intensity and location of it. Information that should be elicited from the patient includes:

Location. This should be as specific as possible. For example, abdominal pain may be localized to the lower or upper right or left quandrant, epigastrium or mid-abdomen.

Type. Crampy; stabbing; sharp; dull; throbbing; burning; aching; boring.

Intensity. Mild; severe; excruciating.

Onset. Sudden or gradual. Note the time it began.

Duration. Persistent; intermittent.

The nurse also takes note of:

Changes in the Site. Tenderness; swelling; discoloration; firmness; rigidity.

Position assumed. Knees drawn up; resting on his knees; sitting up; refuses to change position; clasping or holding a part.

Emotional responses. Crying; screaming; restless; thrashing about; anxious.

General appearance. Color (flushed, pale, gray, cyanosed); distressed; pinched facies; weak; prostrated.

Vital signs. Pulse, respirations, blood pressure and temperature.

Any provoking or relieving factors. Is its occurrence or relief related to meals, medication, activity, a certain position, treatment, or coughing? Does it occur or become worse at any particular time of the day?

Associated symptoms. Nausea and vomiting; profuse perspiration; fainting; inability to perform usual functions; disorientation; inability to rest and sleep.

Patient's history and circumstances. Is the patient worried about the diagnosis and outcome of his illness or about a family or financial problem? Is he lonely and fearful in the strange new environment?

Positioning. A change of position may provide some relief for the patient by reducing the pressure and tension on the affected area. Venous and lymphatic drainage are promoted in order to decrease the accumulation of fluid in the tissue and thereby relieve pain. Adequate assistance and extreme gentleness are necessary when turning or moving the patient. It is done slowly, and support is provided for the painful area. It is often helpful to ask the patient how the movement can be made least distressing for him. Good body alignment contributes to comfort by eliminating tension and hyperextension. Support and elevation of a painful limb on a pillow may be helpful. Immobilization and support by mechanical devices may ease the patient's pain and lessen the discomfort associated with moving. Examples of such devices are a fracture board and firm mattress, a splint applied to a limb, an abdominal or chest binder, and a Stryker or Foster bed.

Rest. Care is planned so that the patient is disturbed as little as possible. Consideration should be given to his location in the ward. Noise in the environment should be kept to a minimum; the more the patient is alerted, the more acutely he is aware of his pain.

Reducing Anxiety. Relief of worry may substantially contribute to the relief of pain. If the patient is overly anxious about his illness and its outcome, it may be helpful to encourage him to talk about it. His concern could be brought to the attention of the doctor, who will then talk with the patient about his condition. An understanding of the cause of the pain and its probable duration may reduce the patient's anxiety. Pain may become less severe if the patient knows that the nurse has taken care of a worrisome home problem by arranging for assistance from a social worker or visiting nurse.

The patient who is advised ahead of time that he is likely to experience some pain (e.g., the surgical patient) may suffer less if he knows it is expected and is not an indication that he is not progressing favorably. When explaining the pain, the doctor assures the patient that everything possible will be done to provide relief and minimize his discomfort.

Diversion. In some instances, depending on the nature of the illness and on the particular individual, some diversion which is acceptable to the patient may reduce his concentration on the pain. A brief visit and chat with someone, a few moments with his religious adviser, reading or listening to a radio may prove beneficial.

Local Applications. The application of moist or dry heat or cold (subject to the approval of the physician) may produce relief of pain. The effects of heat are the relaxation of muscle tension or spasm and the increased rate of blood flow through the area. Precautions against burning are necessary, since the patient in pain may be less sensitive to excessive heat.

Cold applications stimulate constriction of the local blood vessels and reduce the amount of blood in the area and the accumulation of tissue fluid (lymph). This diminishes the painful swelling and congestion in the affected area. Cold also reduces the sensitivity of the pain receptors.

Supportive Care. Remaining with the patient, holding his hand or placing a hand on his arm or shoulder, and making an occasional comment that acknowledges his suffering or offers encouragement all convey to the patient that someone understands and cares. Such support may make the pain more tolerable. Simple nursing measures such as bathing the face and hands with cool water, rinsing of the mouth or offering sips of fluid, gentle massage of the back or tense muscles and change of position may contribute to relaxation and may lessen the discomfort.

Analgesics. The drugs used to relieve pain include those that depress pain perception, reduce the patient's response to pain or relax muscle spasm.

It is important that the nurse be familiar with the action of the prescribed drug, the usual dosage, factors that influence the dosage and effectiveness, the frequency with which it may be given and the possible side effects. A knowledge of the condition of the patient who is to receive the analgesic is also necessary. Frequently the administration is left to the discretion of the nurse

since the order may be "give when required" (P.R.N.). The prescribed analgesic should be used judiciously and under conditions that will contribute to maximum benefit for the patient. Treatments and nursing measures are done before or immediately following the administration of the drug so the patient may remain undisturbed as much as possible. The administration of the drug should not be withheld unnecessarily since pain may initiate harmful physiological responses and may contribute to shock. Also, the longer the patient suffers, the more fearful and apprehensive he becomes, making it more difficult to achieve relief. In other words, pain is easier to control if it can be relieved soon after the onset. When persistent, severe pain, such as that often associated with terminal malignancy, is being experienced, the patient is observed closely to determine the duration of the effect of an analgesic; the nurse's observations are then discussed with the doctor. Administration at more frequent and regular intervals may be ordered to prevent the pain from reaching severe intensity.

At no time should an analgesic replace nursing measures that, in many instances of less severe pain, may provide relief.

The drugs commonly used to reduce pain perception include the opiate preparations of morphine, codeine, Pantopon and papaverine; meperidine hydrochloride (Demerol): and, for mild aching pain, acetylsalicylic acid (Aspirin).

If the patient is apprehensive, regular doses of a sedative, such as sodium amytal or phenobarbital, or a tranquilizer, such as prochlorperazine (Compazine) or methaminodiazepoxide hydrochloride (Librium), may be ordered as an adjunct to an analgesic in order to decrease the patient's fear and tension and reduce his pain responses. A sedative may enhance the effectiveness of a smaller dose of an analgesic.

When the cause of pain is known to be muscle spasm, a preparation that produces relaxation of the muscle tissue may be prescribed. For example, spasm of the smooth muscle tissue of the gastrointestinal tract, the urinary tract and biliary tract may be relieved by antispasmodic preparations, such as tincture of belladonna, atropine sulfate, methantheline bromide (Banthine) and propantheline bromide (Pro-Banthine). These drugs are effective by reducing the para-sympathetic impulses to the visceral muscle. Pain due to spasm of the blood vessels may be relieved by vasodilators, such as nitro-glycerin, papaverine and tolazoline hydro-chloride (Priscoline).

The analgesic drugs may produce side effects, the incidence and nature of which vary from one patient to another. Nausea and vomiting are two of the most common reactions. The time relationship between the administration of the drug and the onset of the nausea or vomiting should be noted and brought to the physician's attention. Fre-quently, patients who are upset by morphine and codeine may tolerate Pantopon or me-peridine.

The more potent analgesics, such as opiates and meperidine, cause some de-pression of the respiratory center. The rate and volume of respirations should be noted following the administration of these drugs, particularly in the cases of older patients and those known to have respiratory dys-function.

One must be always alert to the possi-bility of addiction when a patient is receiving repeated doses of analgesics or sedatives. It is not likely to become a problem if given over a period of a few days when the pa-tient's condition is such that pain may be expected. If the patient requests the drug for relief beyond this period, it is brought to the physician's attention. If a patient is experiencing intractable pain, he may de-velop a decreasing response to the pre-scribed dose. The rate at which the patient increases his tolerance for an analgesic may be slowed by giving him a tranquilizer or sedative as well as regular doses of an anal-gesic.

Constipation, a dry mouth, impaired ability to make decisions and occasionally disorientation are also side effects of anal-gesics that may occur and for which the nurse must be alert.

Neurosurgery to Relieve Pain

In some instances, intractable pain which cannot be effectively controlled by anal-gesics is relieved by surgical interruption of the pain pathway either outside or within the central nervous system. The procedure is usually reserved for patients with an in-curable disease such as cancer and those who suffer the excruciating pain of tic douloureux (trigeminal neuralgia).

When the source of the pain is localized to a relatively small area of the body a neurectomy may be done. This involves severing or crushing the peripheral sensory nerve fibers to the affected area.

A second neurosurgical procedure used is a rhizotomy, in which the sensory path-way which carries impulses from the affected area is interrupted just before it enters the spinal cord. (The area of fibers that is severed or crushed lies between the asso-ciated dorsal ganglion and the cord.) The disadvantage of a rhizotomy is that it causes the loss of the sense of touch and position in the area, so it is used principally to relieve pain in the upper part of the trunk.

When intractable pain is in the lower part of the trunk and in the lower limbs or if it involves a large part of the body which is supplied by several spinal nerves, a chor-dotomy may be done. This entails division of the bilateral spinothalamic tracts in the spinal cord. The temperature sense is also lost in the affected area since the impulses responsible for the sensations of heat and cold take the same pathway as those for pain.

References

BOOKS

Guyton, A. C.: Textbook of Medical Physiology, 4th ed. Philadelphia, W. B. Saunders Co., 1971, pp. 577–591.
MacBryde, C. M. (Ed.): Signs and Symptoms, 4th ed. Philadelphia, J. B. Lippincott Co., 1964. Chapter 3.
Ruch, T. C., and Patton, H. D. (Eds.): Physiology and Biophysics, 19th ed. Philadelphia, W. B. Saunders Co., 1965. Chapter 16.

Taylor, N. B., and McPhedran, M. G.: Basic Physiology and Anatomy. Toronto, The MacMillan Co. of Canada, 1965, pp. 272–275.
Way, E. L. (Ed.): New Concepts in Pain and Its Clinical Management. Philadelphia, F. A. Davis Co., 1967.

PERIODICALS

Livingstone, W. K.: "What is Pain?" Sci. Amer., March, 1953.
Programmed Instruction: Pain
    Part 1. "Basic Concepts and Assessment." Amer. J. Nurs., Vol. 66, No. 5 (May 1966), pp. 1085–1108.
    Part 2. "Rationale for Intervention." Amer. J. Nurs., Vol. 66, No. 6 (June 1966), pp. 1345–1368.

8
The Patient with Cancer

NEOPLASMS

Normally, the production of cells is a regulated process which allows for growth in early life and for the replacement of worn-out or damaged cells throughout life. Occasionally the control of cell reproduction is lost in some cells in a particular area of the body and an excessive production occurs, forming an abnormal mass that is referred to as a newgrowth or neoplasm. It may be benign or malignant (Table 8–1).

Growth of a benign neoplasm is slow and tends to be expansive rather than invasive; the mass remains localized, frequently is encapsulated, and the cells may show little abnormality from those of the normal tissue from which they originated. When excised, it rarely recurs. Since a benign newgrowth is a space-occupying lesion, it may cause serious effects on neighboring structures, depending on its size and location. In some instances it may obstruct blood vessels or a passageway or may cause pressure on vital

TABLE 8–1 DIFFERENCES IN BENIGN AND MALIGNANT NEOPLASMS

	BENIGN	MALIGNANT
Cells	Relatively normal and mature.	Little resemblance to normal; poorly differentiated, atypical in size and shape, and immature.
Growth	Slow and restricted. Expansive, pushing aside normal tissue.	Usually rapid and unrestricted. Invasive of surrounding tissue.
Spread	Remains localized. Usually encapsulated.	Metastasizes via blood and lymph streams.
Recurrence	Rarely recurs.	Frequently recurs.
Threat to host	Depends on size and location. May cause pressure on vital organs or obstruct a passageway.	Threatens life by reason of its local destructive proliferation and formation of secondary neoplasms in other structures.

TABLE 8–2 CLASSIFICATION OF MALIGNANT AND BENIGN NEOPLASMS

TISSUE OF ORIGIN	BENIGN NEOPLASMS	MALIGNANT NEOPLASMS
Epithelium		Carcinoma
Surface epithelium	Papilloma	Epithelioma (squamous or basal cell carcinoma)
Glandular epithelium	Adenoma Polyp	Adenocarcinoma
Connective Tissue		Sarcoma
Fibrous tissue	Fibroma	Fibrosarcoma
Embryonic fibrous tissue	Myxoma	Myxosarcoma
Bone	Osteoma	Osteosarcoma
Cartilage	Chondroma	Chondrosarcoma
Fat	Lipoma	Liposarcoma
Muscle Tissue		
Smooth muscle	Leiomyoma	Leiomyosarcoma
Skeletal muscle	Rhabdomyoma	Rhabdomyosarcoma
Endothelial Tissue		
Blood vessels	Hemangioma	Hemangioendothelioma Hemangiosarcoma
Lymph vessels	Lymphangioma	Lymphangio-endothelioma
Hematopoietic (bone marrow), Lymphoid and Reticulo-Endothelial Tissues		Leukemia Hodgkin's disease Multiple myeloma Lymphosarcoma
Nerve Tissue		
Nerve	Neuroma Neurofibroma	Neurogenic sarcoma
Ganglion	Ganglioneuroma	Neuroblastoma
Brain	Glioma	Glioblastoma Astrocytoma Medulloblastoma
Melanoblasts (pigmented cells)	Nevus	Melanoma
Placental Tissue	Hydatid mole	Choriocarcinoma (Chorionepithelioma)
Gonads	Teratoma (e.g. dermoid cyst of ovary)	Malignant teratoma
Adrenal Medulla	Pheochromocytoma	Malignant pheochromocytoma

tissues leading to serious malfunction. Some benign lesions tend to become malignant if left untreated; examples are polyps in the stomach and intestine, papilloma of the bladder and larynx, and pigmented moles.

A malignant growth destructively proliferates into surrounding tissue and may spread to other parts of the body. Some of the cells become detached from the primary mass and are carried via the blood or lymph to a distant area of the body where they set up colonies of the malignant cells (metastases). The cells tend to grow and reproduce rapidly; they lack normal cellular differentiation and are atypical in size, shape and staining properties.

As well as being classified as malignant or benign, a neoplasm is also named according to the type of tissue involved. A classification of the more common neoplasms is found in Table 8–2.

CANCER

Cancer is a term commonly used to designate any disease that is a malignant neoplasm. As cited previously, malignant neoplasms have certain common characteristics, but there are also marked differences from one type to another because of the type of tissue involved, the location, and the degree of departure from normal of the cells of the newgrowth. They differ as to signs and symptoms, effects on the host, rate of growth, metastases, form of treatment used and their response to treatment.

Incidence and Trends

Cancer accounts for a large number of deaths each year. In Canada in 1966 cancer claimed 134.1 lives per 100,000 of the population.[1] In the United States 303,000 died of cancer in 1966, and it is estimated that 309,000 lost their lives as a result of the disease in 1967.[2] Statistics indicate that in recent years cancer has accounted for an increasing number of deaths. Factors which have probably influenced the increase include a decrease in deaths from other diseases such as pneumonia, diphtheria and scarlet fever; a greater number of persons living to an older age, which increases cancer susceptibility; and the increased risk of developing certain cancers because of greater exposure to specific carcinogens (e.g., cigarette smoking).

Statistics also show significant changes in the incidence of the disease in the two sexes. The death rate was about equal for males and females in 1945, but since then there has been a notable difference; the rate for females has shown a decrease which is mainly due to a lesser incidence of uterine and gastric cancer. The rate for males has increased and is attributed mainly to the rise in cancer of the lung and prostate.[3]

Other important trends reported are the changes in the occurrence of certain types of cancer. Gastric and uterine cancer have both shown a decrease, but the mortality rates for leukemia and cancer of the respiratory system, urinary system and breast have increased.[4] Such changes in incidence may provide clues to predisposing factors and causes in relation to environment, occupations, health habits and customs and may also indicate the value of preventive and early detection programs. For instance, the decrease in uterine cancer may be correlated to the increasing practice of an annual Papanicolaou vaginal smear. The increase in cancer of the respiratory tract, particularly the lungs, in attributed to increased cigarette smoking.

The incidence of cancer varies with age. It occurs in infants and children as well as adults but increases with advancing age. Leukemia and neoplasms of the central nervous system account for many of the malignancies occurring in children up to five years of age. Between the ages of five and fifteen years there is a lesser incidence, but from fifteen on there is a steady increase.[5]

Etiology

The intensive study of cancer cells has led to the belief that the uncontrolled multiplication of atypical cells which is characteristic of cancer is due to a change in the structure of the deoxyribonucleic acid (DNA) in the nucleus of a cell. Certain chemical and physical agents are recognized as having a role in the cause of some cancers, but with many cancers the etiological factor in the transformation of a normal cell into malignant cells is not known. Once the atypical cells develop, the abnormal characteristics are continued in the cells that result from their mitosis. A large number of chemical carcinogens (factors which incite cancer) have been identified and include coal tar and its derivatives, soot, arsenic, chromates, asbestos, nickel, and aniline dyes. Many of these have been recognized through the high incidence of cancer associated with prolonged occupational exposure to a specific chemical. For example, persons working with an aniline dye, which may be absorbed through the skin and excreted in the urine, show a high incidence of urinary bladder cancer.

[1]The National Cancer Institute of Canada, Toronto.

[2]American Cancer Society: 1968 Cancer Facts and Figures. New York, American Cancer Society Inc., 1967, p. 3.

[3]Ibid., pp. 4 and 13.

The National Institute of Canada: Cancer Mortality Trends in Canada and the Provinces 1944–1963. Toronto, National Cancer Institute of Canada, 1965, pp. 5–7.

D. Schottenfeld and R. W. Houde: The Changing Pattern of Cancer Morbidity and Mortality and Its Implications. Med. Clin. North Amer., Vol. 50, No. 3 (May 1966), pp. 627–628.

[4]The National Cancer Institute of Canada, op. cit., pp. 6–7.

[5]Ibid., p. 13.

A significant relationship between cigarette smoking and the sharp rise in lung cancer has been shown in several studies. There is also considerable concern about the increasing amount of industrial air pollution from the combustion of coal and petroleum; this may also prove to be a source of a chemical that causes lung cancer.

Excessive exposure to sun rays may lead to skin cancer. X-rays and radioactive substances have proven beneficial to the diagnosis and treatment of disease, but repeated and heavy radiation may lead to cancer. The adverse effects may not be evident for quite a long period following the irradiation, since the effects are cumulative. Repeated exposures to an amount that is considered harmless may eventually be pathologically significant. This was evident in personnel working with x-ray equipment before the need for more adequate protection was recognized; many of them developed leukemia or cancer of the skin.

Viruses are currently receiving considerable attention. It is known that a number of viruses are capable of inducing cancer in a variety of animals. As yet, no causal association between them and cancer in humans has been definitely established.

Chronic irritation of an area and repeated tissue destruction and repair are thought to be contributing factors in the development of malignant neoplasia. For example, the incidence of cancer of the lip is greater in pipe smokers; similarly, cancer of the cervix is more prevalent in women with unrepaired cervical lacerations.

Other contributory or predisposing factors are considered to be individual intrinsic characteristics such as heredity, host resistance or susceptibility, sex, and hormonal balance. Genetic factors are thought to be responsible for a predisposition to develop cancer. Hopps states that "the incidence of cancer in siblings born of parents both of whom have (or get) cancer is approximately four times greater than that of siblings neither of whose parents have (or get) cancer."[6] Familial occurrence of some neoplasms such as retinoblastoma, premalignant polyps in the colon, and neurofibromatosis has been recognized, but an hereditary relationship has not been established for all neoplastic disease. Some persons may have an actual susceptibility to cancer because of their genetic or general constitution; others may have adequate resistance or defense mechanisms which prevent or terminate the characteristic lawless growth of cells or which wall them off to keep them localized. The concentration of certain hormones appears to influence the change of some normal cells to malignant ones and their subsequent growth. Such cancers are said to be hormone dependent and manifest changes in growth activity when the concentration of certain hormones is altered. For instance, estrogen favors the growth of some breast cancers while androgens tend to suppress their progress. On the other hand, androgens are associated with the growth of prostatic cancer, and by reducing their secretion by castration or by counteracting them with the administration of female hormones, growth may be suppressed. Whether the hormone is the primary incitant in hormone-supported cancers or it simply produces a tissue susceptibility to a primary factor is not known. Cancer has been produced experimentally in mice by the injection of estrogen.

There are striking differences in the incidence of some cancers related to sex. The fact that breast cancer is frequent in females and rare in males may be explained on the basis of hormonal differences. But why there is a much higher incidence of cancer of the stomach and urinary system in males than in females is not understood. Hopps cites the unusual difference in the sexes in relation to cancer of the ear; the middle ear is more commonly the site in females, but in males the inner ear is more frequently the part involved.[7]

Prevention and Early Detection

The public requires a better understanding of the cancer problem, and every nurse has an obligation to participate in disseminating the necessary knowledge. Every opportunity should be taken to advise uninformed persons of the importance of

[6]H. C. Hopps: Principles of Pathology, 2nd ed. New York, Appleton-Century-Crofts, 1964, p. 341.

[7]Ibid., p. 338.

avoiding exposure to carcinogenic agents and of the role of early detection and treatment. A more hopeful and constructive attitude is needed; many persons have an abnormal fear and a fatalistic point of view of cancer. Many do not realize that some cancers can be cured in the early stage and that some may be recognized in an asymptomatic phase by certain examinations (e.g., vaginal or cervical smear).

The National Cancer Society has instituted intensive campaigns to alert the public to the "seven danger signals" and to urge prompt investigation of any one of them. The early signs stressed are unusual bleeding or discharge; a lump or thickening in the breast or elsewhere; a sore that does not heal; a persistent change in bowel or bladder habits; a persistent hoarseness or cough; persistent indigestion or difficulty in swallowing; and a change in a wart or mole. The presence of any one does not necessarily mean that a person has cancer, but early recognition increases the possibility of successful treatment. It should be known that frequently at the onset, cancer does not cause pain. Emphasis is placed on the role of regular periodic examinations. The nurse has many opportunities to discuss with her patients and friends the importance of regular self-examination of the breasts and the annual Pap smear (see section in this chapter on Exfoliative Cytologic Tests). The breast self-examination procedure should be explained, and the excellent pamphlet, published by the National Cancer Society, which clearly outlines and illustrates the examination steps should be made available. The nurse also has a responsibility to inform people that cigarette smoking causes lung cancer and to help them break the habit.

In some instances, a person delays seeking medical consultation because he does not have a private physician or because he cannot afford it. The nurse can be of help in advising him of a clinic or out-patient department to which he may go. If these are not available, a referral may be made to the local health department or local branch of the National Cancer Society where arrangements will be made for him to see a physician.

In order to assume her role in the cancer prevention and early detection program, the nurse must keep informed as to the trends in the incidence of cancer and the current advances made. She should be familiar with the work and the publications of the National Cancer Society. An important contribution can be made by advising the public of the organization and work of the National Cancer Society and its local branches. Support of these organizations makes possible continuous cancer research, education and treatment as well as a variety of services to cancer patients and their families. The nurse should know that films, pamphlets and speakers are available for cancer education for both professional and lay groups.

Effects of Cancer

The manifestations and effects of cancer depend on the location of the neoplasm, its stage, and whether there are secondary conditions such as ulceration, hemorrhage, infection and metastases. Cancer is a space-occupying lesion. It may obstruct a passageway; compress blood vessels; exert pressure on regional nerves, causing pain or even paralysis; or it may produce malfunctioning by its invasion and replacement of normal tissue.

As the lesion grows, there is an insufficient blood supply and inadequate nutrition to maintain it and the normal tissue. Necrosis of a portion of the normal tissue results with subsequent ulceration. Vessels may be eroded, leading to chronic hemorrhage and anemia. Frequently there is a marked loss of weight and strength as the rapidly growing cells compete with normal cells for nutrients, and disturbances develop in the normal metabolic and physiological processes throughout the body. Disfigurement and infection may be serious problems if superficial tissues are involved.

An important effect of malignant disease is the emotional disturbance it creates. All ill persons usually experience some psychological stress as well as physical, but it is especially true of those who are advised or even suspect they have cancer. The person's anxiety may be concerned with a belief that all cancer is incurable, fear of a prolonged painful illness, unfulfilled goals, or with the distress that his illness or death will create for the family. The behavioral response will vary from one person to another, depending on each one's circumstances and his previous attitude and pattern of responses to stressful situations. Some patients become very depressed and give up; others may withdraw and avoid any discussion or mention of the problem but may manifest their anxiety in other ways, such as restlessness, inability to sleep and loss of interest in everything and everyone. Certain patients may be resentful that this should happen to them, and a few become completely disorganized.

Diagnostic Procedures

The diagnostic procedures used vary according to the site of the lesion being investigated.

Biopsy. This is the removal of a small section of suspect tissue for laboratory staining and microscopic examination to determine if there are cells with malignant characteristics. Depending on the site, the tissue specimen may be obtained by excision, a special hollow punch or biting forceps, aspiration, or by scraping a surface (curettement). Before examination, the specimen is made firm usually by immersion in a chemical substance such as formalin. Sometimes a tissue specimen is frozen just as soon as it is obtained for a quick examination. This "frozen section" method is used during an operation when an immediate report is necessary in order to determine the extent of the surgery. If the specimen indicates a malignant neoplasm, more radical surgery is done.

Pathologists frequently grade malignant neoplasms according to the degree of differentiation and abnormal appearance of the cells and whether the malignant cells have invaded lymph or blood vessels in the tissue specimen. Usually the more primitive the cells (anaplasia), the more rapid are the growth and spread of the neoplasm. Grade I indicates that the neoplastic cells have a higher degree of differentiation and a closer resemblance to normal cells. In grade IV the cells show little differentiation and are markedly atypical. Grades II and III are intermediate to I and IV. One must guard against making any definite decision as to the prognosis because of the grade given to a cancer. The important factor is whether the cancer is still localized; a cancer classified as grade IV may be cured if

treated early; on the other hand, a grade I may prove fatal if treatment has been delayed, because metastases will most likely have developed.

Radiologic Examination. Internal parts of the body may be examined for form and density by x-ray. A radiopaque substance may have to be administered before the examination to provide a contrast medium. For instance, the patient may receive barium by mouth if the esophagus, stomach or intestine is to be viewed (see p. 333); for kidney and ureter x-ray a radiopaque dye (an iodide preparation) is given intravenously (see p. 425).

Radioactive Isotopes. Radioactive isotopes and compounds are also used in diagnosing some cancers. A specific isotope or radioactive tagged compound is given according to the tissue being investigated; some tissues are known to absorb and concentrate a certain chemical. If a radioactive substance is administered, special instruments may then be used to detect and record the localization, distribution and concentration of the substance in the body. This process of detecting radiation within the body is known as scanning. The first radioactive isotope used for this purpose was iodine[131] to detect disease of the thyroid. Since then a number of radioactive isotopes have been introduced for both diagnostic and therapeutic purposes. Scanning may be used to detect both primary and secondary cancerous lesions.

Examples of some radioactive chemicals used in diagnosis are: iodine[131] (I^{131}) in thyroid disease; iodine[131] rose bengal in liver disease; gold[198] (Au^{198}) in liver disease; radioiodinated serum albumin (RISA) in brain disease and for tracing circulation in the lung; chromium[51] (Cr^{51}) in red blood cell studies; iron[59] (Fe^{59}) in iron absorption and hemoglobin studies; calcium[47] (Ca^{47}) in bone disease; and strontium[85] (Sr^{85}) in bone disease. For a discussion of the nature of radioisotopes and the nursing care of patients who receive a radioactive isotope, please see the section on Internal Radiotherapy in this chapter (p. 91).

Exfoliative Cytologic Tests. These tests involve the microscopic examination of smears of secretion or fluid taken from a body cavity. Cells are continuously shed from the epithelial surface tissue of the body cavities; this process is referred to as exfoliation or desquamation. Normally, cell replacement by the basal layer of epithelium parallels the exfoliation. Cancer may attack the epithelial lining of organs or body cavities, and some of the neoplastic cells become separated from the tissue and appear in the secretions found on the internal surface of the cavity. Cancer may be detected through recognition of these malignant cells before there are any other recognizable signs or symptoms, resulting in early successful treatment. Specimens may be taken from the cervix, vagina, respiratory tract, mouth, esophagus, stomach, urinary tract, prostate and the pleural and peritoneal cavities. The examination may be referred to as a Pap smear; "Pap" is derived from Papanicolaou, the name of the physician who introduced the use of smears for cytological examination. An annual vaginal or cervical Pap smear on all women over 30 years of age is recommended by the National Cancer Society. The increase in this practice has led to early recognition and treatment of cancer of the uterus in many women and may be correlated to the recent decline of deaths due to uterine cancer.

Endoscopy. This is the introduction of a lighted tube (endoscope) into a body passage or organ for direct inspection of the area. At the same time a biopsy may be obtained by means of a biting forceps passed through the endoscope. This method of examination may be used in the larynx (laryngoscopy), bronchi (bronchoscopy), esophagus (esophagoscopy), stomach (gastroscopy), sigmoid (sigmoidoscopy) and rectum (proctoscopy). These are discussed in Part II of this book in connection with the specific sites.

Treatment

Cancer may be treated by surgery, ionizing radiation, drugs or a combination of these.

Surgery. Surgical excision is considered the most effective therapy provided the disease has not already metastasized. The operation may be simple, as in the case of a basal cell cancer of the skin, or it may be quite radical and probably disfiguring. The lymphatics and lymph nodes which drain the area are also removed in the hope of preventing metastases.

In some instances, surgery may involve the removal of unaffected glands which secrete hormones that are supportive of the so-called hormone-dependent neoplasms (breast and prostatic cancer). For instance, the ovaries and adrenal glands may be removed in some breast cancers.

Radiotherapy. X-rays, or rays and particles which emanate from radioactive materials may be used alone or in conjunction with surgery or chemotherapy to treat cancer. Radiation has become increasingly useful in the diagnosis and treatment of disease, but it is also potentially harmful unless it is carefully controlled and certain precautions are observed. Just as with most drugs, an excessive amount can be very damaging and may prove fatal. Even an x-ray for diagnostic purposes involves the absorption of a small amount of x-radiation by the patient. Most of the cells exposed recover, but there is a small residual injury which is irreversible—so small that it is insignificant. With many such exposures though, the irreversible damage adds up, or is cumulative. For this reason, x-rays are used discriminately and with precautions.

In radiation, the x-rays, gamma rays or alpha and beta particles which are emitted have an ionizing effect on the cells of the tissues through which they pass. The structure of the atoms of the chemicals which compose the cells is altered. If the amount of radiation is high, the resulting chemical changes lead to destruction of the cells. Some types of tissue cells are more susceptible to ionizing radiation than others; hematopoietic cells of the bone marrow, lymphocytes, gonadal cells (ovaries and testes) and the cells of the mucous membrane of the mouth and gastrointestinal tract are the most sensitive. These are cells which divide and reproduce rapidly. Malignant neoplastic cells, which also reproduce rapidly and are poorly differentiated, are more susceptible than normal cells.

No one would dispute the value of radiation, but, as cited previously, it can be biologically harmful. Like many other things in our environment, it has both positive and negative potentials. The latter depend mainly on whether certain precautions are observed. When involved with either external or internal diagnostic or therapeutic radiation, three basic facts in relation to protection should be kept in mind. One is that the shorter the period of time one spends in an area where x- or gamma rays are being emitted, the less hazardous is the exposure. When caring for a patient who contains a radioactive substance, necessary treatments and care should be well planned and expedited to minimize the time spent at the bedside. A monitoring badge is worn so that the amount of exposure can be estimated. If it should approach what is considered the maximum level for safety, the personnel caring for the patient are changed.

The second basic fact that is important in radiation protection is that the greater the distance from the source, the less radiation will be received. When the distance is doubled, the intensity decreases by a factor of four. For instance, at four feet from the source there is only one-sixteenth of the exposure that there would be at one foot.

Thirdly, effective shielding materials are available for protection. Ionizing rays lose energy when coming in contact with matter. The denser and thicker the matter, the fewer are the rays that will pass through it. Because of its density, lead is used extensively in providing shielding. One-eighth of an inch of lead will provide as much protection as several feet of concrete.

Therapeutic radiation may be derived from an external source, or from a radioactive substance placed within the body.

EXTERNAL RADIOTHERAPY. This may be provided by an x-ray machine or by a radioactive substance such as cobalt[60] or cesium[137] which emits gamma rays. X-rays are electromagnetic waves produced in a special vacuum tube (x-ray tube); an electric current is passed into a wire filament at one end, freeing electrons which rapidly travel through the tube. At the opposite end, they are absorbed by a metal plate of tungsten or molybdenum; this results in the emission of x-rays. The higher the voltage of the electrical current applied to the tube, the more penetrating are the x-rays produced. As a result, high- or super-voltage machines are used in the treatment of cancer in deep-lying structures. Lower-voltage machines which produce low-energy rays are used in diagnostic procedures and in the treatment of superficial neoplasms. Patients undergoing external radiation treatment receive a series of exposures (fractionated doses) rather than one massive dose, which would produce excessive damage that might cause death. The number and spacing of the treatments are determined according to each individual by the radiologist.

The use of gamma rays emitted by a radioactive substance in external irradiation is referred to as teletherapy. Radioactive cobalt[60] (or cesium[137]) is encased in a large lead container which only allows the escape of gamma rays through a controlled aperture. The patient is placed at a considerable distance from the source in order to reduce the skin damage. Mechanical devices permit rotation of the radiation beam or of the table on which the patient is placed. The beam is directed at an angle that results in its continuous penetration of the affected area but which reduces the amount of exposure of any one area of the skin.

The teletherapy unit differs from the x-ray machine in that the latter does not give off rays once the electricity is turned off. The radioactive cobalt[60] continuously emits rays, and the opening through which the rays exit must be closed by heavy shielding shutters when it is not being used for treatment. Both the x-ray machine and the teletherapy unit are housed in rooms with specially constructed walls through which x-rays and gamma rays cannot pass. While treatment by either is in progress no one but the patient remains in the room. A means of communication between the patient and the radiologist or technician is provided, and a window is available through which the patient may be observed.

The objective is to deliver sufficient radiation to destroy the malignant tissue with a minimum of damage to normal tissue. The x- or gamma rays are directed to a circumscribed area of the body. The parts of the patient's body not being treated are usually protected by lead sheets. Particular attention is given to the protection of the patient's gonads to prevent genetic mutations. The patient is positioned by the radiologist and asked to remain immobile during the treatment. Patients who cannot be relied upon to maintain the desired position may receive a sedative before going to the treatment unit, and straps or sand bags may also be necessary.

The dose of external radiation may be expressed as a number of roentgens. A roentgen (r) is a unit of gamma or x-rays emitted and indicates the amount to which the patient was exposed. If the amount of radiation absorbed is expressed, the rad is the unit of measurement used.

NURSING RESPONSIBILITIES IN EXTERNAL RADIOTHERAPY. It is important that the patient receive an explanation before the initial treatment as to what he may expect. A brief explanation of the machine, which may appear rather ominous, will help to reduce his fears. He is advised that although he will be alone in the room, he will be under constant observation by the radiologist or technician, with whom he may communicate. He is also told that the treatment period will be brief. He should know that he will not experience any pain or sensation as the rays penetrate, and that it is important that he maintain the position he is placed in by the radiologist. The patient and his family may have some erroneous ideas about radiation; time should be taken to talk with them, answer questions and reassure them that the treatments are well controlled and adequate protection is used. If the patient is allowed to go home, the importance of keeping the appointments for his treatments is stressed.

The skin of the area to be treated is thoroughly but gently cleansed and dried. The radiologist may outline the area to which the radiation beam is to be directed with a marking pencil; this must not be removed until the series of treatments is completed.

Following the treatment, the patient is observed for possible reactions which vary with each individual's ability to tolerate radiation, the dosage received, and the area of the body treated.

Some local skin reaction may be expected; it may be mild, exhibiting only a slight redness for a brief period with transitory epilation (loss of hair), or a more pronounced erythematous response with a temporary suppression of sweat gland activity in the area may develop, followed by dry desquamation. With larger doses and more sensitive skin, more severe reactions may be manifested; marked erythema may be followed by purple discoloration, blister formation and moist desquamation. Healing is slow in severe reactions and leaves the skin dark, atrophied, thin and very sensitive to heat, cold and trauma; there is also per-manent epilation and destruction of sweat glands in the area.

Instructions as to the care of the skin are given by the radiologist and usually include the following suggestions. The area is gently cleansed with tepid water and patted dry. Soap is not used and brisk rubbing is avoided. Markings circumscribing the area are to remain. Alcohol, powders, oils, lotions, creams and ointments are not used unless prescribed by the doctor. If the axillae have been irradiated, deodorants must not be applied. The site is kept dry and may be covered lightly with smooth cotton. Adhesive tape is never applied; scotch tape may be used to secure a protective covering if necessary. Pressure is prevented by avoiding any restricting clothing and prolonged periods of lying on the area. No hot or cold applications are used on the site, which must also be protected from exposure to direct sunlight. In the case of a male, if the face is involved, shaving with an electric razor may be permitted after a few days if necessary.

If itching and irritation accompany the erythema, the radiologist may suggest applications of plain calamine lotion (i.e., without phenol) if the area is dry. Cornstarch may be used in some situations. Later, lanolin or a light oil may be used when the skin is dry and desquamating.

If the mucous membrane of the mouth, pharynx or esophagus has been irradiated, dryness due to suppression of mucus secretion and ulceration may cause discomfort and dysphagia (difficulty in swallowing). Modification of the diet to bland, soft or liquid foods will be necessary. The mouth is rinsed frequently with a mild alkaline mouthwash, and to avoid injury to the mucous membrane, the teeth are gently cleansed with absorbent cotton or gauze rather than with the usual brush.

When the larynx is treated by radiation, the patient is hospitalized for three or four days following each treatment and is closely observed for any sign of difficult breathing. Edema may develop and occlude the airway, necessitating prompt intubation or a tracheostomy.

Many patients experience anorexia and a sense of fatigue following a treatment. Some are nauseated and vomit, particularly if thoracic or abdominal tissue has been exposed; an antiemetic drug such as dimenhydrinate (Dramamine) may be ordered for oral, intramuscular or rectal administration. Frequent blood cell counts are done because the hematopoietic tissue (blood cell forming tissue) is extremely sensitive to radiation. Anemia, leukopenia and thrombocytopenia may develop. Contact with persons with an infection is avoided, especially those with a respiratory infection, because of the patient's lowered resistance.

General supportive care applicable to all patients receiving radiotherapy include extra rest, an increased fluid intake and a high-calorie, high-protein, high-vitamin diet. Maintaining an adequate nutritional and fluid intake may be a problem because of anorexia and nausea. An explanation of the importance of food and fluids should be made to the patient, and small amounts of those foods preferred by him should be offered at frequent intervals throughout the day.

When reactions develop, the patient may need reassurance that they are not unexpected and are not an indication of a recurrence or worsening of his cancerous disease.

INTERNAL RADIOTHERAPY. Radioactive isotopes may be introduced into the body to deliver radiation to an affected part. A solution of the radioactive isotope may be administered orally or intravenously, or it may be injected into a body cavity. In some cases the isotope may be enclosed within a nonradioactive metal and implanted in a tissue or body cavity.

Before discussing internal radiotherapy, a brief explanation of the nature of radioactive isotopes may be necessary. Varying forms of the same element may occur as the result of differences in atomic weights and are referred to as isotopes. The isotopes of an element have identical atomic numbers and similar chemical properties, but they have a difference in the number of neutrons in the nuclei; this results in the variance in atomic weights. To illustrate, there are two isotopes of hydrogen (H) — deuterium (H^2) and tritium (H^3). They have an atomic number of 1, which is the same as hydrogen. The nucleus of the hydrogen atom contains one proton and no neutrons. The deuterium nucleus has one proton and one neutron, making the atomic weight 2, and the atomic weight of tritium is 3 because its atomic

nucleus contains one proton and two neutrons. Uranium is another example of an isotope; some of its atoms may have an atomic weight of 235 (U^{235}) and others occur with an atomic weight of 238 (U^{238}).

Those elements which have an atomic weight greater than 209[8] and in which the ratio of neutrons to protons is over 1.5[9] have a tendency to be unstable. For example, radium, an unstable element with an atomic weight of 226, has 88 protons and 138 neutrons in its atomic nucleus. The atoms of unstable elements constantly undergo some disintegration or decay until stability is established. The disintegration gives rise to the emission of particles and high-energy electromagnetic waves, and the element or isotope is said to be radioactive. The particles are of two types. The alpha particles, which are comprised of protons and neutrons, are capable of penetrating only a few centimeters of air and a fraction of a millimeter of tissue and therefore are of little value in therapy. The second type of particulate emitted is referred to as the beta particle; it is identical to an electron and is capable of penetrating surface tissue. The waves of energy released in radioactivity are known as gamma rays, which are similar to x-rays. They are highly penetrating and are capable of passing through concrete of several feet in thickness. A dense metal such as lead is required for shielding from gamma radiation.

The selection of a radioactive isotope which is to be administered orally or intravenously is based on the affinity of the affected tissue or organ for a particular ele-

---

Atomic Structure. The atom of an element consists of electrons (negatively charged particles), protons (positively charged particles) and neutrons (neutral particles). The protons and neutrons form a dense core, or nucleus, around which the electrons revolve in rings or orbits.

Example: One atom of oxygen consists of 8 electrons, 8 protons and 8 neutrons.

Atomic Number. The atomic number of an element is equal to the number of protons or the number of electrons since both are the same.

Atomic Weight or Mass. Protons and neutrons are the heavy particles of the atom. The atomic weight, or mass, of an element is equal to the sum of the protons and neutrons in an atom.

[8]Hessel H. Flitter: An Introduction to Physics in Nursing, 5th ed. Saint Louis, The C. V. Mosby Co., 1967. p. 208.

[9]Ibid., p. 205.

ment. The uptake and concentration of the radioactive isotope is comparable to that of the nonradioactive isotope of the element. For instance, radioactive phosphorus (P^{32}) which emits beta rays is administered orally or intravenously and is concentrated in bone tissue from which its radiation readily penetrates to the bone marrow. This accounts for its use in treating polycythemia vera and myelogenous leukemia. Radioactive iodine (I^{131}) is taken up by the thyroid tissue and is concentrated in the thyroid gland. It may be used in the diagnosis and treatment of thyroid disease.

Colloidal radioactive gold[198] (Au^{198}), which emits both beta and gamma radiation, is used principally in the treatment of pleural or peritoneal effusion due to cancer of the lung or cancer within the abdomen. The suspension of gold is injected into the pleural or peritoneal cavity and the patient is turned every 15 minutes (side, prone, opposite side, back, and sitting positions) for two hours, then every half hour for 2 hours and hourly for 3 hours to provide even distribution within the cavity. The gold preparation that is injected is purple; as a result, leakage at the site of injection is readily detected and special precautions are taken in the changing and disposal of the dressing and linens to protect the handler from radiation. A patient who receives radioactive gold is usually very ill; should death occur, the body is conspicuously tagged as having had the radioisotope, and the mortician is advised as to the necessary precautions.

The curie (Ci) is a unit of measurement of radioactivity, but it is too large a unit for use in medicine. The dosage of isotopes is usually expressed in millicuries (mCi) (1/1000 of a curie) or in microcuries (μCi) (1/1,000,000 of a curie).

NURSING RESPONSIBILITIES IN INTERNAL RADIOTHERAPY. Nursing responsibilities associated with the use of liquid radioisotopes will vary with the different isotopes and with the dosage used. Tracer or diagnostic dosage is smaller than that used for therapeutic effects. The nurse is concerned with the patient's reactions and with the precautions necessary to protect herself and others from radiation that may be emitted from the patient or his body discharges. There is also the danger of direct contam-

ination from the accidental spilling of the radioisotope. Some understanding of the nature of the radioisotope used is necessary. The radioisotope laboratory is consulted as to the precautions to be used with each patient who receives a radioactive isotope.

The patient is usually placed in isolation in a single room and a notice placed on the door indicates that no visitors are permitted to enter. Preferably, the room has a window through which the patient can be observed and an intercommunication system so that the time spent in the room is minimized. An explanation to the patient of the procedure and the precautions is necessary. The patient is likely to be apprehensive or resent his isolation unless he is oriented to the plan of treatment and understands it is temporary as well as necessary for the protection of others. It is helpful if he has a telephone during his isolation so he can talk with his family and friends. A radio or television and reading material may also help to relieve his boredom and anxiety.

The nurse's time in the room is restricted to a minimum, and when doing anything for the patient that brings her in close contact, she wears a gown and rubber gloves. She works quickly and remains only long enough to give the necessary care, having thoughtfully anticipated the patient's needs and planned ahead of time what observations should be made as well as the details of care to be carried out. All nurses participating in the patient's care are required to wear a monitoring badge which records the amount of radiation received. Long periods of total isolation are avoided; brief visits from the doorway will let the patient know he has not been forgotten.

The radioactive isotope is eliminated in the urine or feces, but some may also be present in vomitus or wound discharge. Specific directions are necessary as to the disposal of excreta and contaminated dressings. For instance, radioactive iodine is eliminated in the urine, so it is collected in a lead-encased container and taken to the laboratory where it is stored until the radioactivity has decayed. In addition to wearing gloves, the nurse should wash her hands very thoroughly with soap and running water after any contact with the patient or handling of bedding, bedpan, dressings, syringes, needles and other equipment. If an area of the nurse's skin becomes contaminated, it is washed with soap and water and monitored. If contamination is still indicated, the washing and monitoring are repeated. Linen is usually put in metal containers and stored until monitoring indicates it is safe. Dishes may have to be washed and kept in the room. Syringes, needles and other treatment equipment are thoroughly washed with soap and water and kept in the room until monitoring indicates their safety before being returned to general stock.

When the isolation is terminated, the room and remaining equipment are monitored, cleansed by persons who are adequately protected with gloves, gown and shoe covers, and then monitored again. The room is left to air for 24 to 48 hours.

The patient is advised as to the elimination of the isotope so he will not think he is a continuing source of danger to his family and others.

Another method of delivering radiation internally is by the implantation of radium, or radon (a gas produced by the decay of radium), which is enclosed within a metal such as gold, silver, platinum or brass. It may be used in the form of a tube, needle, plaque or wire which is placed within the tissue or cavity. Interstitial implants are used principally in the treatment of cancer of the skin (rodent ulcer), lip, tongue and mouth. Intracavitary implantation is used to treat cancer of the cervix or endometrium. The alpha and most of the beta particles are absorbed by the enclosing metal while the gamma rays pass through and penetrate surrounding tissues.

The implant procedure is carried out in the operating room or in a radiation unit. Most of the implants are sterilized by immersion in a germicide for a stated period. Following the implantation, the patient is placed in a private room; if he is placed in a ward he is put in an end bed which is six to seven feet from the adjacent bed to reduce possible radiation exposure to others. A sign is placed on the patient's bed and chart to inform the hospital personnel that the patient is receiving radiation therapy. The ambulatory patient is advised to remain within his own unit.

In the case of mouth, lip or tongue therapy, specific orders are received as to mouth care. Following a mouth wash, the emesis

basin is examined to make sure no implants have escaped. The nurse need not wear gloves since the container prevents direct contact with the radioactive substance. If an implant is displaced, it should be handled with a long forceps, placed in a designated lead container, and the radiologist is promptly notified. All dressings and bedding that are removed are examined before disposal to make sure no radiation material has been displaced. This is important because it could be a source of danger to others; also, most of these implants are very costly and are reusable.

In the case of uterine implantation, the radium tube may be held in place by an applicator and gauze packing. The patient is usually required to remain in the dorsal recumbent position. A small pillow to fill in the space in the small of the back may relieve some discomfort. A retention catheter is passed at the time the radium is inserted since the patient will not be able to use a bedpan because of the applicator which protrudes from the vagina. A low residue diet may be ordered so that the patient will be less likely to have a bowel movement. Any shifting or displacement of the applicator should be reported at once. The radium is removed at a specified time by the surgeon, cleaned in a germicide and placed in a lead container.

Occasionally, implantations of radon seeds are permanent. This is possible because radon has a short half-life (four days), but the patient must remain in the hospital until the radioactivity has decreased to a safe level. This permanent type of implantation may be used in the treatment of cancer of the urinary bladder; the seeds are placed in the cancerous tissue. All urine is collected and checked for radioactive material during the period the radon is active.

Some general basic rules to follow in caring for a patient who is being treated by radioactive implantations include the following. The patient should receive a simple explanation of the procedure and necessary precautions so he will know what to expect and what is expected of him. Time is taken to answer his questions and dispel misconceptions; understanding is a defense against fear. Following the insertion of the implant, specific orders as to the necessary precautions and care of the patient are received from the physician or radiologist. The temperature is taken every four hours; an elevation over 38° C. (100° F.) is reported. The nurse works quickly when caring for the patient, keeping the time spent at the patient's bedside to a minimum without neglecting him.

Any displacement or loss of the radioactive implant(s) is promptly reported to the physician or radioisotope laboratory. Any radioactive implant is handled with a long forceps, never with the hands. All dressings and bedding are checked before disposal in case they contain dislodged implants. The patient is usually allowed to have visitors, but they are required to maintain a distance of three feet from the patient.

The nurse should know the time at which the radioactive implant is to be removed; she should have the necessary equipment ready in advance and, if necessary, remind the person responsible for the removal.

Chemotherapy. Drug therapy has assumed increasing importance in recent years in the treatment of some cancers, particularly those which are too widespread to be treated by surgery or radiation (e.g., leukemia, metastatic cancer). It may be used alone or in conjuction with surgery or radiation. Unfortunately, the drugs used are nonspecific in action and many of them are highly toxic and damaging to normal cells as well as to neoplastic cells. As in radiation, the cells that proliferate rapidly are the most suceptible to the toxicity, and patients may experience irritation and ulceration of the mouth and gastrointestinal tract and suppression of the hematopoietic tissues. Most of the drugs used may be classified as alkylating agents, antimetabolites or hormones.

The alkylating agents also known as antimitotic drugs act within the nucleus of the cell and alter the deoxyribonucleic acid (DNA) molecules, resulting in an inhibition of cell growth and reproduction. The antimetabolites interfere with normal cellular reactions and the formation of certain chemicals essential in the structure and functioning of the cells. Hormones change the chemical environment of the cancer cells and may counteract the hormone which is favoring the growth of the neoplastic cells. A few miscellaneous drugs which do not fit into the above categories are also used.

Table 8–3 lists some of the drugs used in cancer therapy and indicates the method(s) by which they may be administered, the cancer disease in which it may be used and the possible toxic effects.[10] New drugs are introduced frequently, and the search continues for a drug that will be selective and prove toxic to malignant cells without damaging normal tissue.

The channels by which anticancer drugs are administered are intravenous, oral, intramuscular, intracavity and intra-arterial. The latter method of administration may be intra-arterial infusion or perfusion.

In intra-arterial infusion, the drug is introduced directly into the artery that supplies the malignant area. The drug circulates through the affected part in high concentration before it becomes diluted in the general circulation. For instance, in liver cancer, the organ may be infused with the drug of choice via a small catheter introduced into the hepatic artery. Since it is intra-arterial, pressure is required to overcome the arterial blood pressure. A small mechanical pump may be used which delivers a certain amount of the drug at a prescribed rate.

Intra-arterial perfusion is a more complex procedure, involving an extracorporeal circulation. It is carried out in an operating room and requires the use of a pump oxygenator (heart-lung machine). The venous blood from the affected part is diverted into the tube of the pump where the anticancer drug is added. The blood is returned to the artery that supplies the structure to be treated. The isolated circuit is maintained for one-half to one hour. This method of treatment prevents the circulation of the toxic drug through the total body and maintains a higher concentration in the malignant tissue for a longer period. In some instances, on completion of the perfusion,

[10]Compiled from the following sources:

T. F. Nealon Jr. (Ed.): Management of the Patient with Cancer. Philadelphia, W. B. Saunders Co., 1965. Chapter 10.

M. W. Falconer, M. R. Ralston and H. R. Patterson: The Drug, the Nurse, the Patient, 4th ed. Philadelphia, W. B. Saunders Co., 1970, pp. 358–367.

D. A. Karnofsky and G. O. Clifford: Selection of Anticancer Drugs for Inclusion in Memorial Hospital Formulary. Med. Clin. North Amer., Vol. 50, No. 3 (May 1966), pp. 857–868.

B. M. Livingstone: Cancer Chemotherapy Research. Amer. J. Nurs., Vol. 67, No. 12 (Dec. 1967), pp. 2549–2550.

TABLE 8-3 DRUGS USED IN CANCER CHEMOTHERAPY

Drug	Channel of Administration	Malignant Neoplastic Diseases	Toxic Effects
Alkylating Agents Mechlorethamine (nitrogen mustard, Mustargen)	Intravenous Perfusion	Leukemia Hodgkin's disease Lymphosarcoma Multiple myeloma Polycythemia vera Cancer of breast, ovary and lung	Nausea and vomiting Anorexia Depression of hematopoietic cells of the bone marrow leading to anemia, leukopenia and thrombocytopenia Amenorrhea
Triethylenethiophosphoramide (thio-TEPA)	Intravenous	Same as above, Melanoma	Same as above
Bulsulfan (Myleran)	Oral	Chronic myelogenous leukemia	Same as above (nausea and vomiting rare)
Chlorambucil (Leukeran)	Oral	Chronic lymphocytic leukemia Hodgkin's disease Lymphosarcoma	Same as above (nausea and vomiting rare)
Melphalan (Alkeran)	Oral	Multiple myeloma	Same as above (nausea and vomiting rare)
Cyclophosphamide (Cytoxan)	Oral Intravenous	Leukemia Lymphosarcoma Multiple myeloma Hodgkin's disease Wilms' tumor (malignant tumor of kidney in young children) Neuroblastoma Cancer of lung Rhabdomyosarcoma	Same as above Stomatitis Skin rash Alopecia (loss of hair) Hemorrhagic cystitis Diarrhea

Table continued on following page.

TABLE 8-3   DRUGS USED IN CANCER CHEMOTHERAPY *(Continued)*

DRUG	CHANNEL OF ADMINISTRATION	MALIGNANT NEOPLASTIC DISEASES	TOXIC EFFECTS
Antimetabolites			
Amethopterin (methotrexate)	Oral Infusion	Leukemia Choriocarcinoma Cancer of testicle	Nausea and vomiting Stomatitis Gastrointestinal ulceration Bone marrow depression—anemia, leukopenia and thrombocytopenia
6-Mercaptopurine (Purinethol)	Oral	Leukemia	Nausea and vomiting Bone marrow depression—anemia, leukopenia and thrombocytopenia
5-Fluorouracil (5-FU)	Intravenous Infusion	Cancer of colon, pancreas, ovary and breast	Nausea and vomiting Stomatitis Bone marrow depression—anemia, leukopenia and thrombocytopenia
Thioguanine	Oral	Leukemia	Bone marrow depression—anemia, leukopenia and thrombocytopenia
Hormones			
Estrogens Diethylstilbestrol, ethinyl estradiol (Estinyl)	Oral	Cancer of prostate, cancer of breast in women over 60 years	Feminization of male; fluid retention; uterine bleeding
Progestins Hydroxyprogesterone (Delalutin)	Intramuscular	Cancer of endometrium	
Androgens Testosterone proprionate, thioxymesterone, Halotestin	Intramuscular, oral	Breast carcinoma	Masculinization, fluid retention

Table continued on opposite page.

	Route	Indications	Side effects
Corticosteroids Cortisone, hydrocortisone, prednisone	Oral	Leukemia, Hodgkin's disease, lymphosarcoma, multiple myeloma	Fluid retention, susceptibility to infection, hypertension, gastric ulcer
Miscellaneous Actinomycin (an antibiotic)	Intravenous	Wilms' tumor Rhabdomyosarcoma	Nausea and vomiting Stomatitis Alopecia Bone marrow depression—anemia, leukopenia and thrombocytopenia
Vinca alkaloids Vinblastine (Velban)	Intravenous	Hodgkin's disease Choriocarcinoma Lymphosarcoma	Gastrointestinal disturbances Muscle weakness Loss of reflexes Paresthesia
Vincristine (Oncovin)	Intravenous	Leukemia Wilms' tumor	Same as above
Urethane	Oral	Multiple myeloma	Nausea and vomiting Bone marrow depression
Quinacrine (Atabrine)	Intracavity	Effusion due to malignancy (pleural, peritoneal)	Fever Pain
o,p'-DDD	Oral	Adrenal cortex carcinoma	Nausea and vomiting Anorexia Skin eruptions Diarrhea

the blood may be replaced by transfusion blood to prevent the toxic drug from entering the general circulation. Since some blood containing the drug may escape into the systemic circulation, the patient must still be observed for possible toxic reactions. For details of the intra-arterial infusion and perfusion procedures, the reader may consult the references cited below.[11]

Nursing Problems Common to Patients with Cancer

The nursing related to cancer of specific sites is considered in the appropriate sections in Part II. Only some general factors that are commonly associated with most cancers are discussed here.

Psychological Impact. Cancer has become one of the most dreaded diseases, and the majority of persons believe that once a diagnosis of the disease has been made, a death warrant has been issued. Certainly not every patient with cancer can be cured, but neither can all patients with heart conditions. Something can be done for almost every cancer patient; some can be cured, and the survival rate has shown a steady improvement (one in three[12]). Many patients whose disease is not cured live normal useful lives, symptom-free for long periods. It is necessary for the nurse to see the disease in its proper perspective and to develop a hopeful, positive attitude if she is to help the patient and his family with the emotional burden imposed by cancer.

The decision as to whether or not the patient is told he has cancer rests with the physician and the patient's family. It is influenced by the patient's circumstances, his responsibilities and obligations, the anticipated course of the disease, and by knowledge of the patient's philosophy of life and death and how he has accepted or coped with crises in the past. It may be necessary to tell the patient so he can deal with business affairs and make arrangements to pre-

vent difficulties and hardships for the family. At present, with the prevalence of cancer and the amount of publicity given to it, it is difficult for a patient not to suspect the possibility. In many instances, evasion of answers and deception on the part of those around him only reinforce the patient's suspicions. The uncertainty of not knowing may cause more continuous anxiety and agitation than actually knowing the diagnosis. On the other hand, some patients do not ask because they do not want their suspicion verified.

The nurse must know what the doctor has told the patient and the family in order to be prepared for their questions and discussions. When she knows that the patient has been told, his reactions are observed, and if he wishes to talk about the problem, the nurse should listen and not try to avoid the situation. At times, the nurse will probably need the assistance of the physician or the patient's spiritual adviser to reinforce the support she is endeavoring to give the patient and his family. His religious faith frequently proves a source of comfort and peace that helps him to accept the situation.

The nursing student or recent graduate may need assistance from the head nurse or clinical supervisor in these difficult situations. She may have had little or no experience with death and may not yet have developed a philosophy or acceptance that it must come to all at some time. It may be helpful if she is given an opportunity to talk about the situation and her feelings and explore how she can be supportive to the patient and family. A continued, sincere interest in his welfare and attention to details of his physical, mental and social needs assure the patient of support and confidence that help to reduce his despair and keep hope and faith alive.

Nutrition and Fluids. The fluid intake for cancer patients may have to be increased by 1000 to 1500 ml. above the normal, particularly if they are receiving radiotherapy. The products of the rapid cellular breakdown place additional demands on the kidneys. For example, the uric acid concentration increases, and unless it is well diluted and eliminated it may crystallize in the kidney tubules, leading to renal insufficiency or shut-down. The patient's cooperation is sought by advising him that plenty of fluids

[11] B. Clarkson and W. Lawrence: Perfusion and Infusion Techniques in Cancer Chemotherapy. Med. Clin. North Amer. Vol. 45, No. 3 (May 1961), pp. 689–708.
P. Edwards: Regional Cancer Chemotherapy. Canad. Nurse, Vol. 63, No. 4 (April 1967), pp. 41–43.
[12] American Cancer Society: 1968 Facts and Figures. New York, American Cancer Society Inc., p. 4.

are important, and a supply is kept at the bedside. For the person who is weak and finds even taking a drink an effort, the necessary assistance is provided. If sufficient fluids cannot be taken by mouth, intravenous infusions are administered.

Anorexia and severe weight loss are common problems with many cancer patients. Every effort and considerable ingenuity may be necessary on the part of the nurse to tempt the patient and to help him maintain a satisfactory nutritional intake. The form of food given will depend on the location of the neoplasm. If the patient is unable to eat, tube feeding may be necessary. For the patient who can take food in the regular form, preferences (consistent with his condition) are considered, the family is encouraged to bring in his favored dishes, protein concentrates (e.g., Sustagen) are used in drinks, and small amounts of high-calorie foods offered at frequent intervals rather than at three regular full meals. Vitamin supplements may be ordered to meet deficiencies and to improve the patient's appetite.

Pain. The patient may be free of pain in the early stages of his disease, but later as the neoplasm invades surrounding tissues and metastasizes it causes pressure and involves sensory nerves. Nursing measures such as a change of position, a back rub, the use of pillows to provide support to a part, and a little time spent at the bedside listening and talking to the patient should be used to reduce the amount of analgesic needed and to enhance the effectiveness of that given. Initially, the patient's pain may be relieved by mild analgesics such as aspirin or aspirin compound. Later a more potent drug, in progressively larger doses, may be necessary as the patient develops a tolerance for the analgesic and the pain becomes more severe. Prompt response to the complaint of pain means a great deal to the patient. Knowing that relief of pain is quickly available reduces his apprehension and may even lessen the amount of drug needed. If a patient is kept waiting while in pain, he may develop the habit of registering his complaint well before the hour he knows the drug may be repeated.

Skin Care. Frequently, the cancer patient becomes emaciated and his tissue has less vitality and resistance. Pressure sores readily develop unless preventive measures are used. Frequent turning, gentle massage, cleanliness and dryness are very necessary. An air or alternating pressure mattress or a sheepskin placed under the areas subjected to pressure is helpful. The vulnerable areas are inspected frequently; any discoloration is brought to the physician's attention, and pressure on the site is avoided as much as possible.

Odor. The sloughing of tissue in cancer and secondary infection are likely to cause an offensive odor which may produce considerable embarrassment for the patient and family. Dressings must be changed frequently, and the patient and bedding must be kept scrupulously clean. Irrigations or dressings of potassium permanganate 1:10,000 to 1:5000 may be helpful, and a number of commercial deodorants are available. The patient will be less embarrassed if he is in a private room which can be kept well ventilated.

Activity. Just as with other patients, those with cancer are encouraged to resume their normal pattern of life if they are able. Going back to work is good for the patient's and his family's morale, and being occupied prevents concentration on his disease. Independence within his physical limitations is encouraged and guidance as to the care required will be necessary. If the patient has a colostomy or tracheostomy or requires a prosthesis, the necessary instruction for care and adaptation to daily living is given. (Specific problems such as these are discussed in the related sections in Part II.)

The patient who cannot return to work may still be well enough to go home. As well as receiving instruction as to the necessary care at home, the patient and his family are advised of the available resources for assistance. A referral may be made to the visiting nurse association, welfare department or local branch of the National Cancer Society according to the need. When necessary, local branches of the National Cancer Society will provide dressings, colostomy equipment and drugs, loan certain equipment such as a wheelchair or hospital bed, and arrange for nursing and housekeeping services. The National Cancer Society may also have volunteer workers who make home visits and transport patients to the clinic or physician's office.

The patient is kept active and independent as long as possible; inactivity and prolonged bed rest only add to the problems by promoting circulatory stasis, muscular atrophy and weakness, pressure sores and elimination difficulties. Judgment is needed; activity should not be unduly urged beyond the patient's actual physical capacity. Details in good grooming, such as shaving, a shampoo, and a haircut or hair-do, are encouraged and arranged. This type of attention conveys a sense of worth and hope to the patient. Some form of diversion which may interest the patient is made available. Visitors, association with others and participation in social activities are advocated as long as the patient is well enough. Oversolicitous family members may need suggestions as to how to spare themselves and protect their own physical and mental health.

If the patient is in the advanced stage of his disease, the goal may simply be to keep the patient as comfortable as possible and to provide emotional support for the family. Thoughtful attention to small details which may appear rather insignificant to the nurse may assume great importance to the dependent patient.

The Role of the Visiting Nurse in Cancer

The visiting nurse has a responsible role to play in disseminating factual knowledge that will help the public develop a more optimistic attitude toward cancer. More people need to learn that many kinds of cancer are preventable and by what means and that many persons with cancer are cured. They should be alerted to the "seven danger signals" and the importance of diagnosis and treatment while the disease is still localized.

During her home visits and health discussions in clinics, the nurse has the opportunity to stress regular periodic examinations and monthly breast self-examination. National Cancer Society pamphlets which explain the hazards of cigarette smoking and excessive exposure to sun rays and certain chemicals may be distributed and discussed. An early sign or symptom which a person ignores or considers insignificant may be recognized and prompt investigation urged. In some instances, it may be necessary for the visiting nurse to make an appointment with the doctor or clinic for the patient. A follow-up visit is made to see if the patient kept the appointment and if further assistance is required. Should the patient be scheduled for hospital admission for further investigation or treatment, an explanation is made as to what may be expected. There may be questions to answer which could help to allay unrealistic fears on the part of the patient and his family. The home situation may be such that the patient feels that he or she cannot leave to go to the hospital. The nurse explains that any delay should be avoided, and she may be able to make suggestions or arrange for assistance that will solve the immediate home problems.

The cancer patient and his family frequently require the assistance of the visiting nurse after discharge from the hospital. Contributions which she may make include recognition of the needs of the patient and his family, the actual giving of care, instruction as to treatment and activity, provision of emotional support, and arrangements for necessary socioeconomic help.

References

BOOKS

Bouchard, R.: Nursing Care of the Cancer Patient. St. Louis, The C. V. Mosby Co., 1967.

Falconer, M. W., Norman, M. R., and Patterson, H. R.: The Drug, the Nurse, the Patient, 4th ed. Philadelphia, W. B. Saunders Co., 1970.

Flitter, H. H., and Rowe, H. R.: An Introduction to Physics in Nursing, 5th ed. Saint Louis, The C. V. Mosby Co., 1967, pp. 151–153 and 202–219.

Gius, J. A.: Fundamentals of General Surgery, 3rd ed. Chicago, Year Book Medical Publishers Inc., Chapter 9.

Hopps, H. C.: Principles of Pathology, 2nd ed. New York, Appleton-Century-Crofts, 1964. Chapter 12.
Nealon, T. F., Jr. (Ed.): Management of the Patient With Cancer. Philadelphia, W. B. Saunders Co., 1965.

PERIODICALS

American Cancer Society: "1968 Cancer Facts and Figures," New York, American Cancer Society Inc., 1969.

Boeker, E. H. (Ed.): "Symposium on Radiation Uses and Hazards." Nurs. Clin. North Amer., Vol. 2, No. 1 (March 1967), pp. 3–113.

Burt, A. L.: "The Role of the Public Health Nurse in the Care of the Cancer Patient." Nurs. Clin. North Amer., Vol. 2, No. 4 (Dec. 1967), pp. 683–689.

Clarkson, B., and Lawrence, W.: "Perfusion and Infusion Techniques in Cancer Chemotherapy." Med. Clin. North Amer., Vol. 45, No. 3 (May 1961), pp. 689–708.

Edwards, P.: "Regional Cancer Chemotherapy." Canad. Nurse, Vol. 63, No. 4 (April 1967), pp. 41–43.

Henderson, I. W. D.: "Current Status of Cancer Chemotherapy." Canad. Nurse, Vol. 63, No. 4 (April 1967), pp. 37–40.

Karnofsky, D. A., and Rawson, R. W. (Eds.): "Symposium on Medical Advances in Cancer." Med. Clin. North Amer., Vol. 50, No. 3 (May 1966).

Lewison, E. F.: "The Nurse's Role in Early Detection of Cancer of the Breast." Nurs. Forum, Vol. 4, No. 3, 1965, pp. 83–86.

Livingstone, B. M.: "Cancer Chemotherapy Research." Amer. J. Nurs., Vol. 67, No. 12 (Dec. 1967), pp. 2549–2550.

Miller, A.: "The Patient's Right to Know the Truth." Canad. Nurse, Vol. 58, No. 1 (Jan. 1962), pp. 25–29.

Moore, G. E.: Cancer—100 Different Diseases. Amer. J. Nurs., Vol. 66, No. 4 (April 1966), pp. 749–756.

Rogers, A.: "Pain and the Cancer Patient." Nurs. Clin. North Amer., Vol. 2, No. 4 (Dec. 1967), pp. 671–682.

The National Cancer Institute of Canada: Cancer Mortality Trends in Canada and the Provinces 1944–1963. Toronto, The National Cancer Institute of Canada, 1965.

9

The Unconscious Patient

CONSCIOUSNESS

Consciousness may be defined as an awareness of one's external environment. It depends upon the activation of a normal cerebral cortex by a stream of impulses from the reticular activating system. This system is a central core of neurons in the brain stem and midbrain and receives branches from all the sensory pathways that enter the brain. Tracts ascend from the reticular formation to the cerebral cortex, transmitting impulses which activate the cortical neurons and induce a state of alertness. This arousal prepares the cortex for the reception and interpretation of the ingoing sensory impulses. The excited cerebral cortex gives rise to impulses which are conducted to the reticular formation, which in turn initiates further stimuli to the cortex, thus setting up a cycle that maintains wakefulness and cerebral alertness.

Normal sleep is physical and mental inactivity from which a person can be roused to consciousness. It is thought it occurs as a result of eventual fatigue of the neurons and a decrease in the impulses arising in the reticular formation. Usually, activity may be quickly increased by the reception of sensory stimuli, such as noise or pain, resulting in cerebral arousal and wakefulness.

UNCONSCIOUSNESS

Interruption of impulses from the reticular activating system or failure of the cerebral cortical neurons to be alerted produces a loss of consciousness. Other than destruction of the cortical or cortical activating cells (reticular formation) by trauma, the basic factors contributing to unconsciousness are considered to be oxygen and glucose deprivation. Neurons require a constant supply of both these substances for cellular activity. A deficiency of oxygen for even a few seconds decreases neuronal metabolism to a point that unconsciousness ensues.

Causes

Impaired consciousness may result from a variety of intracranial or systemic conditions. These include: (1) a head injury involving concussion, depressed skull fracture, hemorrhage or a penetrating wound; (2) cerebral vascular disease such as ruptured aneurysm, thrombosis, hemorrhage and embolism; (3) compression of brain tissue by a space-occupying lesion, which may be a newgrowth, abscess or a hematoma, or by an elevated intracranial pressue due to an increased volume of cerebrospinal fluid; (4) a deficiency in the oxygen supply to the brain as occurs in respiratory failure, shock, hemorrhage and severe deficiency of red blood cells and hemoglobin; (5) a deficiency of glucose to the brain cells due to hypoglycemia (insulin shock); (6) the effects of certain drugs (e.g., anesthetic) or toxic substances (e.g., retained metabolic wastes in renal failure or toxins produced in an infection); and (7) epileptic seizures.

Levels of Unconsciousness

Unconsciousness is described in terms of depths or levels according to the type of responses that are elicited by various types of stimuli. Loss of consciousness may be preceded by a period of excited confusion or apathy. Stupor is the level in which the person can be roused and may respond to some extent. His answers to questions are likely to be incoherent. Light coma is a state of unconsciousness from which the patient cannot be roused but in which peripheral reflexes (e.g., corneal, plantar, withdrawal from painful stimuli) are present and some restlessness may be manifested. Deep or profound coma is the level at which there is no arousal and peripheral reflexes and movement are absent. Deep coma may progress to involvement of the vital centers (respiratory, cardiovascular) in the medulla with ensuing respiratory and circulatory failure.

Effects of Unconsciousness

The normal person has a variety of sensory and response mechanisms which enable him to be aware of his environment and to protect himself. Even during sleep many of these are preserved; for example, discomfort prompts one to change his position, and pain awakens him. With loss of consciousness, the awareness and responses essential to comfort, protection and self-preservation no longer operate. Protection and self-preservation become the responsibility of those caring for the patient.

Loss of skin sensation and immobility may lead to pressure sores or to burns if heat applications are used. The absence of certain reflexes poses a threat. Loss of the corneal reflex and depression of lacrimal secretion may result in prolonged exposure, drying and injury of the cornea and may lead to ulceration. Respiration is threatened by the absence of the pharyngeal and laryngeal reflexes that normally prevent the aspiration of mucus, food and vomitus. Secretions and foreign material are retained in the respiratory tract when there is depression of the cough reflex. Obstruction of the airway may occur as a result of relaxation of the lower jaw and tongue, and respirations may be infrequent and weak because of depression of the respiratory center.

Immobility and the loss of skeletal muscle tone predispose to circulatory stasis and thrombosis. Metabolic activity is usually depressed throughout the body, resulting in a reduced heat production unless there is an infection or involvement of the heat-regulating center in the hypothalamus.

Nursing Responsibilities

Establishment and Maintenance of a Patent Airway. The comatose patient is placed in a lateral or semiprone position with the neck aligned with the spine. Either position facilitates the drainage of mucus and vomitus and prevents obstruction of the airway by the relaxed tongue and jaw. If mucus is troublesome, frequent suctioning with a flexible catheter may be necessary. The catheter has several holes, is moistened before being introduced and is handled gently to avoid trauma of the mucous membrane. The doctor may suggest that the foot of the bed be elevated to further promote pulmonary drainage.

If the patient's condition restricts him to the dorsal position, an oropharyngeal airway may be necessary in order to maintain an airway, or a tracheostomy may be done to facilitate respirations and the removal of secretions. See page 281 for the care of a patient with a tracheostomy.

Positioning. When the patient is placed in the lateral or semiprone position (as cited above) attention is given to good body alignment and to the prevention of contractures, foot and wrist drop, muscle strain, joint injury, and interference with circulation and chest expansion. A small, firm pillow is placed under the head and the neck aligned with the spine. The arm that is uppermost is flexed at the elbow and rests on a pillow to prevent a drag on the shoulder and wrist drop. The arm that is down is drawn slightly forward, flexed at the elbow, and lies on the

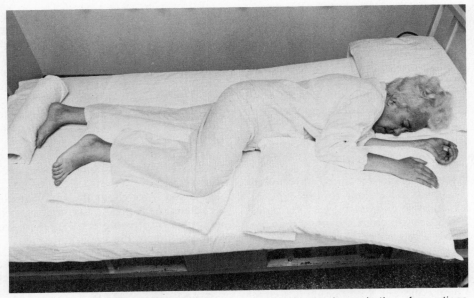

Figure 9-1 Positioning of the unconscious patient to prevent the aspiration of secretions.

bed parallel with the neck and head. The lower limb that is uppermost is flexed at the hip and knee and supported on a firm, plastic-covered pillow; the other lower limb is extended. Dorsiflexion of the feet is maintained by the use of firm pillows, sandbags or a footboard (see Fig. 9–1).

The patient is turned hourly to promote circulation and to prevent the accumulation of pulmonary secretions and the development of pressure sores. A minimum of two or three persons is necessary to turn the unconscious patient in such a manner that hyperextension and joint and muscle strain are avoided. Turning is facilitated if the patient is nursed on a Foster or Stryker frame.

The extremities are passively moved through their normal range of motion at least twice daily to preserve joint function and prevent circulatory stasis.

In some conditions (e.g., cerebral injury and following some brain operations), the patient may have to remain on his back. The arms are slightly adducted and supported on pillows. Trochanter rolls are used to prevent outward rotation of the lower extremities, and the space under the knees may be filled in by a folded towel or small pillow. The feet are supported in the dorsiflexion position.

Observations and Recording. Important observations of the unconscious patient include the following. The temperature, pulse, respirations and blood pressure are recorded frequently, the interval depending on the patient's condition and the medical order. For example, if the coma is due to a head injury or intracranial disease, the nurse may be required to record the pulse and blood pressure every 15 or 30 minutes and the temperature every 1 to 2 hours. Any change in the level of consciousness which may be manifested by a response to an external stimulus or by spontaneous behavior such as movement of the limbs is recorded. The reaction, size and equality of the pupils are noted, and the eyes are examined for retracted lids, discharge and edema. The skin is checked for discoloration and dryness or moisture. Increased spasticity or flaccidity of muscles and rigidity and hyperextension of the head are recorded. The fluid intake and output are measured and the fluid balance determined.

Protection from Injury. Crib sides are always used unless someone is in constant attendance on the patient. He could suddenly regain consciousness, be confused and fall out of bed. It may be necessary to pad the sides of the bed if the patient is restless and thrashing about.

Skin Care. The unconscious patient is predisposed to the rapid development of pressure sores. Precautions are taken to keep the skin clean and dry and the bedding free of wrinkles. Besides a complete daily bath, pressure areas are bathed and gently massaged frequently to stimulate the circulation. Alcohol and powder may be used, but if the skin is dry an oily preparation or lanolin is indicated. A resilient, soft material, such as sponge rubber or sheep-skin, is placed under the pressure areas, or an alternating air pressure (ripple) mattress may be used. If a pressure sore develops, it is treated aseptically, just as any wound, and as little pressure as possible is placed on the area.

Fluids and Nutrition.   No attempt is made to give the comatose patient food or fluid by mouth; the absence of the swallowing reflex could lead to the aspiration of either into the respiratory tract. The patient is sustained on intravenous infusion or feedings given via a nasogastric tube (see p. 339). The liquid tube feeding contains the essential food elements and may provide 1500 to 2500 calories per day. A feeding of 100 to 200 ml. may be given every 2 to 3 hours. If there is any regurgitation (fluid welling up around the tube into the mouth), the volume given at one time is decreased, and the frequency of the feedings is increased. If the patient's condition permits, it is helpful to slightly elevate the head of the bed during the feeding. The tube is rinsed with 30 to 45 ml. of water after each feeding.

The presence of the tube in a nostril tends to irritate the mucous membrane and stimulate mucus secretion. The area is cleansed twice daily with applicators which have been moistened with normal saline, and the area is also lightly lubricated. The tube is secured loosely enough so that it does not continuously press on any one area of the nostril.

Care of the Eyes.   If the corneal reflex is absent and the eyelids are retracted, eyeshields or eyepads are applied to protect the cornea from possible injury and continuous exposure. A daily irrigation with sterile normal saline and the instillation of a drop of mineral oil or ophthalmic ointment may be ordered to provide moisture and protection.

Care of the Mouth and Nose.   Dentures are removed in case they become displaced and interfere with breathing. The mouth and tongue tend to become dry and coated, necessitating cleansing every 2 hours with swabs which have been moistened in an antiseptic. An application of mineral oil to the tongue and of oil, vaseline or cold cream to the lips helps to prevent drying and encrustations.

The nostrils are examined daily for accumulated secretions, which are removed by moist applicators.

Elimination.   The comatose patient has urinary incontinence or may have retention with incontinent overflow. An indwelling catheter is usually passed to lessen the danger of skin irritation and ulceration. The catheter may be clamped for specified intervals to maintain normal bladder tone and capacity. It is taped to the thigh or secured to the bed to prevent undue traction. If a retention catheter is not used, frequent attention is necessary to protect the skin. Pads are used to absorb the urine and are changed promptly after voiding. The bed may be protected by a square of absorbent material (such as cellucotton) with an undersurface of plastic. The skin is washed after each voiding, dried thoroughly and a protective powder (e.g., zinc stearate) or ointment (e.g., zinc oxide ointment) is applied.

The patient may have involuntary stools, particularly if he is receiving tube feedings. Prompt cleansing and changing of soiled pads and bedding are necessary. If the bowels do not move, a cleansing enema may be ordered every second day.

Other Considerations.   The hair is combed and kept tidy, the nails are kept clean and short, and the male patient is shaved if possible.

It may be necessary to place mittens on the hands if the patient is restless and pulls at the nasogastric tube or catheter. These are removed twice daily; the hands are bathed, and the fingers are passively exercised and put through their normal range of motion.

At all times, the patient is protected from unnecessary exposure.

Conversation is guarded in the presence of the patient; nothing should be said that would not ordinarily be said if the patient were conscious. Occasionally things that have been said are recalled when the patient regains consciousness.

The temperature of the environment and the number of covers are controlled according to the patient's temperature.

The family and their concern for the patient requires some consideration. Time should be taken to talk with them and answer their questions. It may be helpful to them if a family member is allowed to remain at the bedside and participate in some aspects of the care. For example, the relative might assist with the turning and positioning of the patient. Family socioeconomic problems may have resulted from the illness; a referral to the social or welfare service may provide the necessary assistance.

Recovery of Consciousness. When a patient recovers consciousness, he is likely to experience a period of confusion and bewilderment. He is unable to appreciate what has happened and where he is. The presence of a familiar face and voice will mean much to the patient at this time. He is reoriented and advised as to what has taken place.

There may be some residual disability that necessitates the planning and the initiation of a rehabilitation program.

References

BOOKS

Harrison, T. R., et al. (Eds.): Principles of Internal Medicine, 4th ed. New York, The Blakiston Division, McGraw-Hill Book Co., Inc., 1962, pp. 311–321.

MacBryde, C. M. (Ed.): Signs and Symptoms, 4th ed. Philadelphia, J. B. Lippincott Co., 1964, pp. 619–632.

Nash, D. F. E.: The Principles and Practice of Surgical Nursing, 2nd ed. London, Edward Arnold Publishers Ltd., 1961. Chapter 11.

PERIODICALS

Brooks, H. L.: "The Golden Rule for the Unconscious Patient." Nurs. Forum, Vol. 4, No. 3, 1965, pp. 12–18.

Locke, S.: "The Neurological Aspects of Coma." Surg. Clin. North Amer., Vol. 48, No. 2 (April 1968), pp. 251–256.

Luessenhop, A.: "Care of the Unconscious Patient." Nurs. Forum, Vol. 4, No. 3, 1965, pp. 6–11.

Olmstead, R. W., and Murtagh, F.: "The Unconscious Patient." Pediat. Clin. North Amer., Vol. 9, No. 1 (February 1962), pp. 3–16.

10
Preoperative and Postoperative Nursing

Surgery is defined in Webster's dictionary as being "the treatment of disease, injury or deformity by manual or instrumental operations."[1] This indicates the special feature that categorizes the patient as being surgical, but the care that contributes to the restoration and maintenance of optimum physiological status before and after the operation comprises a large portion of the total surgical treatment and is extremely important in determining the patient's progress and recovery.

Surgical operations may be classified as elective, essential or emergency. An elective operation is not necessary for the patient's survival but is expected to improve the patient's comfort and health. Essential surgery is considered necessary to remove or to prevent a threat to the patient's life. An emergency operation is one which must be done with a minimum of delay in the interest of the patient's survival.

PREOPERATIVE NURSING

The preoperative period, which begins with the decision that surgery is to be performed, may extend over an hour to several

days or weeks. Whenever possible, sufficient time is taken to assess and treat the patient so that he goes to the operation in the best condition possible. Intelligent, conscientious preoperative nursing may contribute much to having the patient achieve an optimum condition that favors a satisfactory postoperative progress and minimizes the possibility of complications. During the period that the patient is at home awaiting admission to the hospital, a visiting nurse may contribute to the patient's physical and psychological preparation. She may answer some questions of the patient and his family, provide psychological support, advise the patient on such things as nutrition and rest, and assist with social and economic problems precipitated by the impending surgery.

Psychological Preparation

Few patients face surgery without some degree of anxiety. The concerns and fears vary from one person to another; some may be anxious about the pain and discomfort, possible disfigurement and incapacity, or death. Others may be worried because of the expense being incurred, absence from work, lack of support for dependents, lack of care for the family or disruption of plans. Many are disturbed because they simply don't know what to expect. The patient's emotional state and physical condition should

---

[1]Webster's New World Dictionary of the American Language (College Edition). Cleveland, The World Publishing Co., 1956, p. 1467.

receive equal consideration. Psychic stress evokes physiological responses that may impair health; the emotionally disturbed patient may experience a greater problem with vomiting, urinary retention, pain and restlessness during the postoperative period.

Through her more prolonged and intimate contact with the patient, the nurse has the opportunity to assess his perception of the situation and his attitudes. Many of his and his family's fears may be unrealistic—based on misinformation and misconceptions about the surgery. The surgeon, in a limited time, will have discussed the operation with the patient and family as to what it involves, why it is necessary and the expected results. Frequently, the patient and his family are so emotionally overcome at the time that they do not grasp all that has been said. Later, they want clarification and usually have a number of questions. The nurse should determine what information was given them by the doctor and, in simple understandable terms, answer their questions. Tact is necessary in order to avoid increasing their anxiety. The patient is encouraged to reveal his fears and concerns which are accepted by the nurse as reasonable and to be expected. The problems are explored, and, through verbalizing them and receiving some explanation or available assistance, some of the apprehension may be allayed. The fact that someone expects him to have some qualms and is sufficiently interested to listen to him is in itself a comfort to the patient. Some patients may be reluctant to express their fears because they think of them as a personal weakness in themselves, but they may be manifesting their insecurity in other ways as tenseness, restlessness or withdrawal. The nurse, recognizing the problem, may initiate a discussion by saying, "I am sure you are concerned about your operation; there may be something I could clarify for you if you would like to talk about it." There may be the occasional patient who displays a total lack of concern; this person may have considerable deep underlying concern which for some reason he is denying. His reaction is brought to the surgeon's attention.

The patient receives an explanation of why several days of hospitalization are necessary before the actual operation. He is kept informed as to the purpose and what is involved in the investigative and preparatory procedures. What he may expect on the day of operation and in the postoperative period is discussed. Ignorance of what is going to happen usually causes more fear and mental suffering than being advised of the facts. Any anticipated permanent change in body function or appearance is explored, and the patient is advised as to the available assistance and how he may manage his life; emphasis is placed on the positive aspects. For instance, a woman who is to have a mastectomy may be concerned about her appearance but is relieved when she learns that special prosthetic brassieres are available. A patient who is being prepared for a permanent colostomy may be encouraged to see and talk with a person who has had the same operation and is living a relatively normal, active life.

Consideration is given to placement on the ward by selecting a unit that is quiet and nearer to those less likely to increase anxiety in the patient. Long periods in which the patient is entirely alone should be avoided; relatives are encouraged to visit and the nurse should "drop in" at frequent intervals. Some form of diversion in which he is interested may be provided. The patient may find his religious adviser a source of strength and courage, but one must be cautious about suggesting such a visit. The patient may request it, or the nurse might tactfully suggest it to the family without increasing their anxiety. In some instances help beyond that which the nurse can provide is needed to reduce the patient's fear. It may be necessary to consult the surgeon or anesthetist and have one of them talk further with the patient.

Family members are kept informed, and time is taken to talk with them, answer their questions, and advise them as to how they can offer support to the patient.

Physical Preparation

Observations. Common concerns with all surgical patients are cardiac, pulmonary and renal function; blood volume and composition; nutritional status; and fluid and electrolyte balance. Basic laboratory tests for all preoperative patients include urinalysis, hematocrit, hemoglobin, leukocyte count, and bleeding or clotting time. Other laboratory tests, functional studies and x-rays may be done as well as specific investigative procedures relevant to the patient's particular surgical condition. These studies should be understood by the nurse so she can provide the necessary explanation and support for the patient, and make the necessary adaptations in nursing.

The patient's history and physical examination records are reviewed for significant information that may influence both preoperative and postoperative care. The nurse should be constantly alert for signs and symptoms that might indicate a condition or change in the patient which could interfere with the patient's progress and predispose to complications. Such factors as the following are promptly reported to the physician: an elevated temperature; change in pulse, respirations or blood pressure; a rash; a cough, complaint of sore throat or nasal discharge that might point to a respiratory infection; bleeding gums, which may indicate a vitamin C deficiency; onset of menstruation; diarrhea; nausea and vomiting; and a deficient food or fluid intake.

Nutrition. The patient who is malnourished tolerates surgery less well. Protein deficiency delays healing and decreases the resistance to infection by resulting in a slower response in antibody formation. Vitamin C also plays an important role in healing since it is necessary for the laying down of collagen fibers. Optimal amounts of the vitamin B complex are necessary for normal glucose metabolism and for the maintenance of cellular enzymes. A deficient intake of carbohydrate depletes the liver glycogen, leaving the body without a reserve source of glucose, which leads to catabolism of the body tissues.

If the patient can tolerate it, he is given a high-calorie (3000 to 4000 calories), high-carbohydrate diet and vitamin supplements. The patient is more likely to cooperate if he is advised of the significant role nutrition plays in his postoperative progress. Feeding the patient or providing some assistance may be necessary if he is weak or uncomfortable. Frequent small feedings may prove more successful than three large meals. When possible, the patient is consulted as to foods that he would prefer.

If the patient's condition is such that the ordinary solid food cannot be taken, fluids containing commercial protein concentrates and glucose may be tolerated. When oral intake is insufficient or not possible, intravenous solutions of glucose, protein preparations, plasma or whole blood may be administered.

There is considerable increase in the risk in surgery on obese persons. They have a greater tendency to develop cardiovascular, pulmonary and wound complications. The excessive fat tissue frequently makes the operative procedures more difficult. The patient who is overweight is advised of the need to lose weight before his operation and is placed on a diet of 500 to 1200 calories.

Fluids and Electrolytes. A normal fluid balance is extremely important in the surgical patient; dehydration predisposes to shock, a retention of metabolic wastes, and disturbances in the electrolyte concentrations. The patient who has been ill for some time, particularly if his disorder is gastrointestinal, frequently has a fluid deficit. A record of the fluid intake and output is kept, and the patient is observed for signs of dehydration (see p. 52). A minimum intake of 2500 to 3000 ml. is encouraged unless contraindicated. Blood chemistry studies are done to determine electrolyte concentrations, and deficiencies should be made up by oral or parenteral preparations.

Rest and Exercise. The patient awaiting an operation may find it difficult to rest and sleep because of decreased activity and anxiety. It is brought to the doctor's attention, and regular small doses of a mild sedative (e.g., amytal sodium, phenobarbital) may be prescribed to provide relaxation and the necessary rest.

When the patient is well enough, he is usually kept ambulatory and encouraged to get some exercise. This prevents general weakness and diminishes the probability of circulatory complications later.

Information and Instruction. Deep breathing and coughing at frequent intervals will be necessary after the operation. These are to prevent pulmonary complications by fully expanding the lungs and removing secretions. The purpose is explained to the patient, and he is taught how they are done and encouraged to practice. Assurance is given that the necessary assistance and support will be provided. Smoking is discouraged; any irritation of the respiratory tract predisposes to pulmonary complications.

Postoperative lower limb exercises to prevent circulatory stasis and thrombosis are described and demonstrated. The patient is also advised that he will be assisted in getting out of bed for brief periods in the early postoperative period as this promotes normal body processes and reduces problems such as vomiting, gas pains and difficulty with voiding. He is also told that he need not be alarmed by the nurse's frequent checking of his pulse and blood pressure; they are checked on all patients to provide information as to their condition. If the use of drainage tubes (e.g., chest or gastric) or special equipment is anticipated, these are also mentioned so that he won't think his condition is worse than had been expected.

Specific Therapy. Certain treatments to correct secondary physiological disturbances or coexistent disease may comprise a large part of the preoperative preparation. The patient who has developed anemia because of a loss of blood or nutritional deficiency may receive one or more blood transfusions (see p. 119). A course of an antimicrobial drug may be necessary to clear up some infection. A diabetic patient may require dietary and insulin therapy to bring his disease under control, lower the blood sugar, and have the urine free of sugar and ketone acids. The purpose of any such treatments and their significance to the surgery are explained to the patient and his family.

Operative Consent

Before any operation, it is necessary to obtain the patient's signature to a statement which gives consent for the anesthetic and operation.* The purpose is to protect the hospital, surgeon and anesthetist against claims of unauthorized anesthesia and surgery. The statement indicates that the nature of the anesthetic and operation have been explained and that consent is given. A clause is usually included that permits further or alternative procedures that are deemed necessary during the operation. Exceptions may be added at the patient's request. When asked to sign the consent the patient must be

rational, alert and not under the influence of any drug that might impair comprehension and judgment. Preferably, the signing is done a day or two before the day of operation, not just before bedtime the night before the operation or the morning of operation as it is likely to increase the patient's anxiety at such a time.

The signing of an operative consent must be witnessed by a person authorized to do so by the hospital; in some institutions only a doctor is permitted to act as a witness, in others it may be either a doctor or a nurse. The witness attests to the fact that in his presence the statement has been read and explained to the signatory who stated that he or she understood and then signed the consent.

If the patient is a minor, the permit must be signed by a parent or legal guardian. If he is a minor but is married or earning his own living, he may sign the consent. When a relative of a minor is not close by, consent by telephone, letter or telegram may be accepted. In the case of an emergency involving a minor or an unconscious patient, consent may have to be obtained by telephone. If a relative cannot be reached and immediate surgery is necessary in the interest of the patient's life, a brief statement explaining the circumstances may be signed by two physicians.

For operations that are likely to permanently alter the patient's functional ability or appearance, the signature of a close relative is required as well as the patient's. For instance, when a hysterectomy is to be done, the husband's consent may also be necessary. Other examples of cases in which two signatures may be required are operations on the brain and amputations. It is advisable for the nurse working in a new or unfamiliar situation to determine the policies pertaining to consents of the particular hospital and surgeons.

Immediate Preoperative Preparation

The following preparatory measures receive consideration the day before and on the day of operation.

Food and Fluids. The patient's stomach should be empty when he goes to the operating room to prevent the possibility of

---

*A consent signed by the patient is also necessary for major diagnostic procedures.

aspiration of vomitus. No solid food is given after a light evening meal on the day before operation. Clear fluids are permitted and encouraged up to six hours before the scheduled hour for the surgery. An explanation is given as to why food and fluid are withheld. If the patient's mouth becomes dry and uncomfortable, he is given a mouthwash. Parenteral fluids may be ordered the morning of operation, particularly if the surgery is scheduled for late in the day. When a patient inadvertently takes food or fluid, the surgeon or anesthetist is promptly notified. It will probably necessitate a postponement of the operation or the passing of a gastric tube to evacuate the stomach content.

When the patient is a child, the doctor may stress the giving of clear sweetened fluids for 24 hours up to four to six hours before operation. This is to promote an optimal glycogen reserve in the liver since it is normally proportionately less than in the adult and will be depleted quickly.

Elimination. The physician's orders may or may not include an enema. If the patient has had a normal bowel movement the day before operation, it may not be considered necessary. Some surgeons prefer all patients having major surgery to have a cleansing enema to prevent possible incontinency during operation that might occur with the relaxation of the sphincters. It may also avoid serious constipation following the operation when diet and activity are restricted.

The bladder should be empty when the patient goes to the operating room in order to prevent incontinence during the anesthetic induction and operation. In the case of low abdominal or pelvic surgery, a full bladder may interfere with the surgical procedure by making the site less accessible, and it may also increase the risk of accidental injury to the bladder wall. The patient is asked to void just before the preoperative sedative takes effect. If the patient is unable to void, or to be certain that the bladder is empty, catheterization may be ordered. The doctor may want an indwelling catheter passed and attached to a drainage system if the patient is receiving continuous intravenous infusion or if he wants the bladder to remain collapsed throughout the operation.

Local Preparation. Although the details of the preparation of the site of the operation

vary according to the area and the surgeon's preference, the principles are the same. The site is treated to have it as free as possible of dirt particles, hair, desquamated cells, secretions and organisms.

When the skin is to be prepared, the site of the incision and a generous surrounding area are carefully shaved and thoroughly cleansed with water and a detergent the afternoon or evening before operation (see Fig. 10–1 for areas). In some instances, the cleansing is followed by an application of a disinfectant such as benzalkonium chloride (Zephiran chloride) 1:1000. Further cleansing and the application of a disinfectant are done in the operating room.

If a patient is discovered to have acne or infected lesions, the operation may be delayed until the condition is corrected. Daily antiseptic baths or the application of an antimicrobial preparation may be prescribed.

Special preparation extending over several days may be ordered by the surgeon for some operations such as skin grafts and orthopedic procedures. Specific instructions for local preparation are received for any surgery on the head, face and eye.

When vaginal surgery is to be done, in addition to shaving and cleansing the area surrounding the vaginal orifice, a cleansing antiseptic douche may be ordered.

For rectal and lower bowel surgery, the patient may be required to have water or saline enemas until the return is clear. These are given high and slowly, and the patient is allowed to rest following each one. They should also be given early enough to make sure all fluid is expelled before the patient is taken to the operating room. The perineum and surrounding area are thoroughly cleansed with water and detergent following the final evacuation.

In the case of operations on the mouth or throat, unless specific preparatory instructions are given, the teeth are cleaned and the mouth rinsed well with an antiseptic mouthwash the night before and the morning of the day of operation.

Personal Care. Depending on the patient's condition, he has a tub bath, shower, or bed bath on the morning of operation. If the surgeon approves, the patient who is able is encouraged to do this for himself, since the ambulation and activity stimulate circulation and deeper respirations. If the operation is

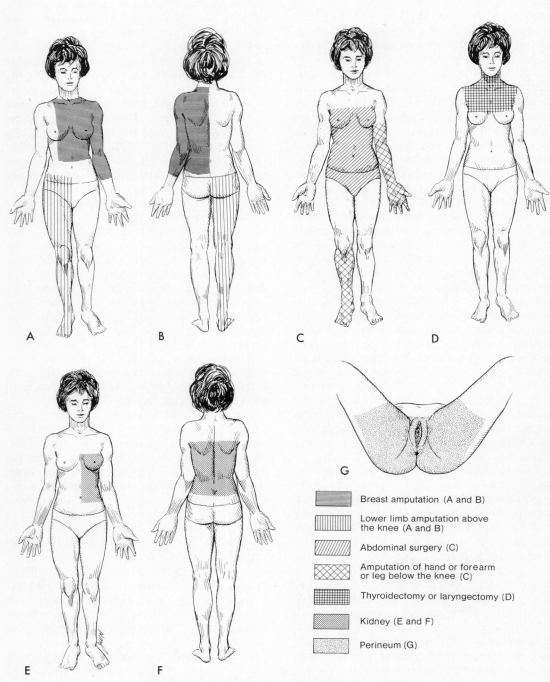

Figure 10–1 Areas of the skin prepared for surgery.

Breast amputation (A and B)

Lower limb amputation above the knee (A and B)

Abdominal surgery (C)

Amputation of hand or forearm or leg below the knee (C)

Thyroidectomy or laryngectomy (D)

Kidney (E and F)

Perineum (G)

scheduled for an early hour, the bath is taken the night before so the patient is disturbed as little as possible in the morning. A clean hospital gown is provided.

The teeth are cleansed and an antiseptic mouthwash is used the night before and the morning of the day of operation to make sure all food particles are removed. Dentures are removed because they may become displaced and interfere with respirations. They are placed in an appropriate container in the patient's locker. Occasionally, the anesthetist may ask to have the dentures left in place so the anesthetic mask will fit more closely to the face. Any prosthesis, such as an artificial eye or limb, is removed and safely stored.

The hair is combed, neatly braided if long enough, left free of hair pins, and secured under a turban so that it does not become soiled or interfere with the anesthetic. Colored nail polish and make-up are removed since checking of the patient's color and of the lips and nail beds for cyanosis is necessary. All jewelry is removed for safekeeping. If the patient does not wish to remove a wedding ring, it is securely taped or tied to the hand. The identification wristlet is checked to make sure it is clearly legible and secure.

Special Procedures. Some special procedures may be ordered preceding certain operations. A nasogastric or duodenal tube may have to be passed, an intravenous infusion started, or an intravenous cut-down done and a cannula inserted for the administration of intravenous solution or whole blood. The nurse sees that the necessary equipment is available at the bedside so that the procedure may be completed by the time the patient receives the preoperative sedation.

Medication. When the immediate preoperative orders are given, it should be clarified as to whether there are any preceding orders for medications. The patient may have been receiving digitalis, insulin or other important drugs and the omission of such could have serious effects.

A sedative is usually given the night before operation to ensure a good night's sleep for the patient. A barbiturate such as phenobarbital (Luminal), amytal sodium, pentobarbital sodium (Nembutal), or secobarbital sodium (Seconal) is commonly used.

The patient is advised not to get up after taking the drug but to signal for the nurse if he wishes something or is unable to sleep. Frequently, simple nursing measures such as a back rub, change of position, turning the pillow or staying with the patient briefly may reduce tension and apprehension and promote sleep. Since an older person sometimes becomes confused after receiving a barbiturate, crib sides are placed on his bed.

Approximately 45 to 90 minutes before operation, the patient usually receives an injection of a drug to produce relaxation and allay anxiety. The preparations commonly used include meperidine hydrochloride (Demerol), morphine sulfate, codeine and phenobarbital sodium. The physician's choice of drug is based mainly on the patient's condition and age. For example, if the patient is known to readily develop respiratory problems, morphine is not used because of its depressing effect on the respiratory center. Milder sedatives such as phenobarbital are used for children.

If a general anesthetic is to be given, the patient may also receive atropine or hyoscine hydrobromide (Scopolamine) to reduce salivary and respiratory secretions. Scopolamine tends to make the respiratory secretions less tenacious than atropine. It may be administered alone without a sedative to young children since it depresses mental activity as well as secretions.

All preparatory procedures should be completed before the preoperative sedative is given. The patient is then left undisturbed, and quietness is maintained. A relative may remain in the room to provide comfort and security for the patient.

A final check and recording are made of the pulse, respirations and blood pressure about one-half hour after the preoperative drug has been given.

Patient's Chart. Treatments and any pertinent reactions of the patient are recorded, and the complete chart including the nurses' notes, diagnostic reports, progress notes, patient's history and the operative consent are put together and taken to the operating room with the patient. A sheet on the front of the chart should list any factors that may be considered particularly important for the anesthetist, surgeon and operating room staff to note. Examples are allergies, drug sensitivity, coexistent disease and limitation of joint movement in a limb. The latter may be significant in relation to positioning the patient on the operating room table. The patient's blood type is also noted.

Patient's Family. The family is notified when the operation is to take place and usually one or two members come to the hospital before the operation. They are allowed to visit the patient briefly before the preoperative sedation is given. As cited previously, one may remain quietly in the room as long as the patient is not disturbed.

After the patient is taken to the operating room, the relatives are directed to a place where they may wait and are advised that they will be notified as soon as the patient returns. The nurse stops to speak to them occasionally and may provide a cup of coffee or suggest where they may go to get refreshments. During a long operation, the surgeon may send someone from the operating room to advise them of the progress. He usually sees them as soon as the operation is completed to inform them of the patient's condition.

Emergency Preoperative Preparation

Preoperative preparation in emergency surgery is limited to basic essentials. When the patient is in shock or is bleeding, the hemoglobin is checked and the blood typed immediately. An intravenous infusion is started using normal saline or a plasma expander (Dextran 6 per cent) until compatible whole blood is available.

If the patient is to have an inhalation anesthetic and has most likely taken food and fluid within the last six to eight hours, a gastric tube is passed to evacuate the stomach content. In the case of hemorrhage from a peptic ulcer, perforation of an ulcer or intestinal obstruction, a nasogastric or duodenal tube is passed and intermittent suction-siphonage started in order to keep the stomach or duodenum free of fluid and gas.

As soon as possible, the patient is asked to void to obtain a specimen for urinalysis and to have the bladder empty for the surgery. If the patient is unable to void, catheterization is usually ordered as it is important to know before operation whether the urine contains sugar or abnormal constituents that might indicate impaired renal function.

The skin at the site of operation is shaved and thoroughly cleansed, the permit for operation is signed, and preoperative medication is given. Any dentures or prosthesis and jewelry are removed, and the hair is covered with a turban.

If the patient has just been admitted and is not accompanied by a relative, the nurse makes sure she obtains the name and telephone number of a family member and notifies the person as soon as possible.

Transportation of the Patient to the Operating Room

At the appropriate time, the patient is taken to the operating room either in his bed or on a stretcher. If the bed is used, the woolen blanket is replaced with a flannelette sheet to prevent the possibility of creating static electricity in the operating room since many of the anesthetic drugs are explosive and inflammable. The bedding is tucked in along the sides, and a name tag is attached to the bed so the patient will be returned to his own bed postoperatively. When a stretcher is used, sufficient covers are used to protect the patient from exposure and drafts. The covers are tucked in and either crib sides or straps used to guard against the patient falling off the stretcher.

The nurses or a nurse and an orderly accompany the patient. A nurse remains with the patient until a member of the operating room staff takes over. If the patient is awake, the ward nurse leaves him with a cheerful reassuring word that indicates a genuine interest in his welfare. He should not be left alone or exposed to the commotion and conversations that are frequently common to an operating room corridor. Such experiences only arouse the patient's anxiety. If he has to wait for a period of time, it should be in a quiet room.

POSTOPERATIVE NURSING

All surgery has certain common effects that vary in extent and intensity with each particular individual and each specific operation. It produces tissue trauma, pain, psychological reactions and loss of blood. There is an increased possibility of invasion of body tissues by pathogenic organisms through a break in the continuity of the skin, or by the introduction of foreign objects into the body. In addition, there are disturbances in body functions which are due directly to the surgical procedure or indirectly to the responses of the autonomic nervous system and the adrenal glands to the associated psychic and physical stresses.

The nurse who is caring for a patient following an operation must possess knowledge and understanding of the implications of the particular surgery for the patient, its possible effects on the patient's body functions, and the care and support required to assist in his return to normalcy with a minimum of discomfort and pain. A constant watchfulness of the patient's clinical progress is necessary. Adverse changes and their possible significance must be recognized promptly and the surgeon alerted. If it is possible, the nurse who is to care for the patient in the postoperative period has had an opportunity to become acquainted with the patient and learn something of his condition before the operation. The patient may be more confident with a nurse who is not a complete stranger, and the nurse, knowing something of the patient, is better able to evaluate his reactions and condition.

Preparation to Receive the Patient

Most hospitals have a recovery room, either within the operating room department or adjacent to it, to which the patient is taken on completion of the surgery. In a few instances, the patient may be returned directly to his ward unit. The recovery room has several distinct advantages: constant surveillance is provided by a staff who are experienced in immediate postoperative care and whose attention is undivided; proximity to the operating room reduces the distance the patient is transported in this critical period; equipment necessary for emergencies is concentrated in the area and is in immediate readiness; and one nurse may care for two or three patients—a situation which would not be possible on the ward where each patient is in a different location. The patient remains in the recovery room until he fully regains consciousness and his vital signs are stabilized.

Some hospitals have intensive care units in which critically ill patients and patients with a special problem, such as respiratory insufficiency, receive care. The patient who has had major surgery or who has developed serious complications may be transferred directly from the operating room to the intensive care unit where the type of care given in the recovery room may be extended for several days or weeks. The advantages of such a unit are similar to those of the recovery room, but the latter provides a briefer period of care. In a few situations, the two units may be combined, using the same staff and equipment.

In the unit, to which the operative patient is to go, certain basic preparations are made to receive the patient. The bed is made up with two flannelette sheets to provide warmth and absorption of skin moisture. The top bedding is fan-folded to one side to facilitate the transfer of the patient. A piece of waterproof material is placed at the head of the bed over the bottom flannelette sheet and covered with a towel or draw sheet; if it becomes soiled with vomitus it can be changed with a minimum of disturbance to the patient. If drainage from any area of the body is anticipated, the same precaution is taken. Side rails are attached to the bed and are ready for use as the patient may be restless and confused during recovery from the anesthesia.

Basic equipment to be assembled at the bedside includes: a sphygmomanometer, stethoscope, oropharyngeal airway, tongue depressor, tongue forceps, two emesis basins, tissues, face towel, recording sheets and infusion pole. A suction apparatus, a portable emergency respirator (ambu bag with oxygen), and an emergency tray with cardiac and respiratory stimulants, sterile syringes and needles, tourniquet and alcohol swabs should be quickly available.

Equipment most likely to be needed because of the nature of the surgery is also assembled in readiness for prompt use. For instance, if the patient is having gastric surgery, equipment for gastric suction-siphonage drainage will be necessary; if the operation is an amputation, tourniquets must be at the bedside.

The room or unit is ventilated and tidied; unnecessary equipment and objects are removed, and the daily cleaning is done in order to prevent disturbance of the patient later. The light signal is tested to make sure it is in order should assistance be required.

Transportation of the Patient from the Operating Room

On completion of the operation, the patient is dried if the skin is moist with perspiration, and a clean gown and flannelette sheet are applied. He is then lifted gently and without unnecessary exposure by a mechanical lifting device or by a sufficient number of persons to provide adequate support and prevent strain on any part, particularly the operative area. When the bed is used the patient is placed in the lateral or semiprone position, and the side rails are raised. If the transfer is to a stretcher, the dorsal recumbent position is more likely to be used, and straps are placed over the patient (one above the elbows, the second above the knees) and secured for safety. Side rails may also be used. Sufficient covers are used to ensure warmth and protection from drafts. The head is extended and an oropharyngeal airway is probably in place to facilitate breathing. If the patient is on his back and an airway is not used, the lower jaw must be held up and forward to prevent the tongue from obstructing breathing. The anesthetist and a nurse accompany the patient to the recovery room or the ward. Along with immediate treatment orders, the nurse taking over receives a report on what was done, the patient's condition and anything special for which she should be alert.

Postoperative Care

The discussion presented here deals with general postoperative considerations applicable to most surgical patients. Modifications and additional care as related to specific surgery are included in the various sections in Part II.

A nurse remains in constant attendance until the patient fully regains consciousness, is oriented to his surroundings and his vital signs are stabilized.

Observations and Recording. When the patient is received, an immediate check is made of the respirations, pulse, blood pressure, color, condition of the skin (warm or cold, dry or moist) and the level of consciousness. The wound area is examined for bleeding and drainage. These initial observations and the patient's preoperative vital signs serve as a comparative base line which assists the nurse in recognizing favorable and unfavorable changes and in making decisions as to action.

The vital signs are recorded every 15 minutes for 2 hours; if they are satisfactory, the intervals are then progressively extended to every half hour, every hour and then every 2 hours over the next 12 to 24 hours; then they are recorded every 4 hours.

Observation of the patient's color, skin condition, and operative site for any untoward signs continues, and the patient's responses are noted. The fluid intake and output are accurately recorded until normal fluid and food intake and normal urinary elimination have been resumed.

Treatments. The physician's orders are noted immediately for specific treatments. For instance, oxygen, intravenous infusion, appropriate drainage system, special positioning and observations, and drug therapy may be indicated by the doctor's orders.

Any drainage tubes that are to be connected to appropriate bottles or a suction-siphonage system must receive prompt attention as they are usually clamped during transit from the operating room. If drainage is not quickly established, the tube may become plugged, or sufficient pressure may be built up within the body cavity to cause serious effects. For example, if a gastrointestinal tube remains clamped following gastric or duodenal surgery, distention may cause a leakage of secretions into the peritoneal cavity and may result in peritonitis.

Positioning. During unconsciousness, unless contraindicated by the nature of the surgery, the patient is placed in a lateral or semiprone position without a pillow under the head. This facilitates respirations and lessens the danger of aspiration of mucus and vomitus. A pillow may be placed at the patient's back and front if necessary to maintain the desired position. The knees are flexed to reduce strain. If it is necessary to keep the patient on his back, an oropharyngeal tube may be necessary during the unconscious period to prevent occlusion of the airway by the tongue. The head must be turned to one side when vomiting occurs, and suctioning is used to make sure the pharynx and mouth are cleared.

When the patient has had a spinal anesthetic the foot of the bed is elevated. The

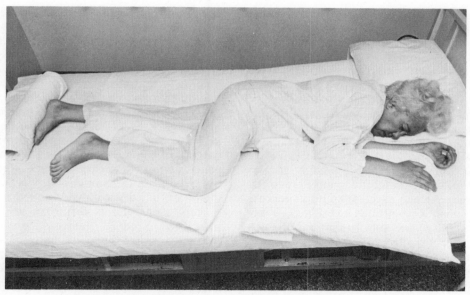

Figure 10–2 Positioning of unconscious patient after surgery.

patient will be conscious but is not permitted a pillow and is advised to keep his head down. This is necessary because there is usually an associated fall in blood pressure due to the effect of the anesthetic on the vasomotor nerves, causing vasodilatation. This position is maintained until sensation and motor ability have returned to the toes and the systolic blood pressure is over 90 mm. Hg.

Postoperatively, the patient's position is changed every 2 hours (side – side – back – side) to promote full expansion of both lungs and to prevent circulatory stasis and pressure. If any one position is restricted, it will be indicated by the surgeon. To illustrate, a patient who has had a pneumonectomy (removal of a lung) is not usually permitted to lie on the nonoperative side since it diminishes the expansion of his remaining lung. Specific orders for positioning are necessary following cerebral surgery.

Two nurses are necessary for turning the patient until he is alert and responsive. During the first 24 to 48 hours, changes of position are made slowly since the vascular reflexes which adjust the distribution of blood with postural changes may be dulled and slower.

Recovery from Anesthesia. While the patient is emerging from anesthesia, he may be restless. Other than crib sides and a splint to the arm that has a needle in a vein for intravenous infusion, restraints are not used. The nurse protects the patient from injuring himself and prevents the tubes from being dislodged. As the patient regains consciousness, he is reassured that someone is with him.

Should the patient not respond within an hour or two, the physician is notified of the delay. It may be because of slow elimination or metabolism of the drugs and anesthetic agents, or it may be due to shock or depressed brain activity due to a lack of oxygen.

When consciousness is regained, a few simple nursing measures may lessen the patient's discomfort. The flannelette sheets are removed if the body temperature is within normal range; excessive perspiration is avoided since it may deplete body fluids. The face and hands are bathed, the mouth rinsed with a cool mouthwash, the back rubbed, and the position changed. The environment should be quiet and ventilated without exposing the patient to drafts. The direct shining of light in the patient's eyes is avoided by lowering the window shade or adjusting the lamp.

Common Postoperative Discomforts. Discomforts common to many postoperative patients include pain, nausea, and vomiting, gas pains and apprehension.

Complaints of pain in the operative area are to be expected because of the unavoidable tissue trauma in surgery. Inadequate control of postoperative pain may cause restlessness and contribute to shock and injury to the operative site. The surgeon usually orders an analgesic such as meperidine hydrochloride (Demerol), morphine or codeine to be given every 4 hours if required (p. r. n.) for the first 24 or 48 hours. The patient should be kept relatively free of pain, but excessive use of the drug is to be avoided. Careful judgment is required of the nurse, since narcotics tend to depress respirations. Respirations are checked before and after the administration of each dose, especially of morphine. If the respirations are only 12 or less per minute, the narcotic is not given until the physician is consulted. The use of narcotics is more hazardous with older persons, patients with some respiratory insufficiency (example: patients with chronic bronchitis or emphysema) and with young children. The patient's position is changed, and deep breathing, coughing and necessary treatments are done just before or immediately following the drug injection so that the patient may derive maximum benefit. After the first day or two, the dose of the analgesic is usually reduced or a milder drug is substituted. When the doctor has not specified a time limit on the drug, the question is raised by the nurse after 48 hours.

Prevention of strain on the operative site by good positioning and support with a pillow or binder contribute to the prevention and relief of pain. For instance, a patient with a pendulous abdomen who has had abdominal surgery may suffer less discomfort if the strain on the wound is relieved by the use of an abdominal binder.

Occasionally, a patient may complain of a backache or pain in a shoulder which may have been caused by prolonged immobilization during surgery. Gentle massage may provide relaxation and relief. If the lower limbs are causing discomfort, massage is never used, but a change of position and support under the full length of the limbs may be helpful. Massage of the lower limbs is discouraged because of the danger of dislodging a thrombus that may have formed because of venous stasis.

The majority of surgical patients experience some nausea and vomiting immediately after the operation as a result of the toxic effects of the anesthetic and the handling of viscera in abdominal surgery. Assistance is provided by having the basin available, holding the patient's head, providing a mouthwash and wiping the patient's mouth. If the patient is still under the influence of the anesthetic or drugs, precautions are taken to prevent aspiration by turning the patient's head to the side and if necessary using suction to make sure the vomitus is removed from the mouth and pharynx. Oral fluids are usually withheld, and the patient is kept quiet and is disturbed as little as possible. Emesis basins are emptied promptly, soiled linen is changed, and the room is ventilated. Vomiting that persists beyond 24 hours after operation is reported as it may indicate a complication or intolerance to the analgesic being used. (For a fuller discussion of nausea and vomiting see p. 329.)

Patients who have had abdominal surgery may experience some pain and distention which are caused by an accumulation of gas in the gastrointestinal tract. Most of the gas is air that is swallowed during nausea or when the patient is tense and fearful. The depressing effects of anesthetics and drugs, handling of the intestine during surgery, and the lack of food intake in the tract may contribute to a reduction in peristalsis. The discomfort may be relieved by the insertion of a rectal tube for a brief period or by an enema. When the distention is high, a nasogastric tube may be passed and suction-decompression used (see p. 338). If the distention persists, it may indicate a serious complication such as a paralytic ileus, bowel obstruction or peritonitis (see p. 370). Frequent turning, early ambulation, and normal fluid and food intake are helpful in re-establishing normal peristalsis and preventing distention and gas pains.

The postoperative patient may be apprehensive and concerned about his condition; this anxiety is likely to cause restlessness and aggravate discomfort and pain. An explanation of what has taken place and what he may expect may relieve some of his concern. He is also told that the nurse is close by and will be in and out frequently to check on him. Having a family member visit or remain quietly in the room may be helpful. It may be necessary for the nurse to remain at the bedside until the patient regains sufficient confidence and control. If he is worried about the findings at operation, it may be helpful to have the surgeon advise him as to his condition and the prognosis.

Fluids and Nutrition. A blood transfusion will probably be given during a major operation or immediately after to replace the blood loss or to combat shock if the blood pressure falls below 90 mm. Hg. Before the transfusion is started, the blood is checked by two persons to be certain that the label bears the patient's name. The blood bank labels the blood with the patient's name after making sure it is the right type and is compatible. The blood should be at room temperature or cooler when given. The patient is observed for signs or symptoms of untoward reactions which may be a chill, fever, dyspnea, pain in the lumbar region or chest, or a fall in blood pressure. Later, the urine may contain hemoglobin and hematin crystals because of hemolysis of red blood cells. The rate of flow is set by the doctor; initially, it may be introduced very slowly (2 to 3 ml. per minute): symptoms of a reaction are usually manifested during the infusion of the first 50 to 100 ml. of each bottle or unit of blood. After 100 ml., the rate may be increased to 4 to 10 ml. per minute. The rate of flow will depend on the reduction in the patient's vascular volume, blood pressure and cardiac function. It is usually considerably slower in an elderly person.

If a reaction is manifested, the transfusion is stopped and the doctor is notified immediately. In some situations, the blood and equipment are then returned to the blood bank for examination to determine the cause of the reaction.

Oral fluid and food are restricted during the period of nausea and vomiting and following abdominal operations. Intravenous infusions of electrolyte and glucose solutions are given to meet the patient's daily requirements and maintain a normal balance. Frequent rinsing of the mouth and cool, moist compresses laid over the lips will help with the patient's discomfort of thirst.

As soon as fluids are permitted, sips of water are given and gradually increased in amount. The intake is then progressively increased as can be tolerated through fluids and soft, bland diet to general diet. The resumption of a normal diet as soon as possible promotes normal gastrointestinal functioning. The patient is less likely to experience abdominal distention, gas pains and constipation. Normal nutrition also favors wound healing, maintenance of strength and a sense of well-being.

In the case of a patient who has had surgery on the alimentary tract (gastric or intestinal), all oral intake is withheld until specifically ordered by the physician.

The postoperative patient may be rather indifferent to food, but he may be encouraged to take more by the offering of small amounts of those foods for which the patient has indicated a preference. Frequently food and fluids are not taken simply because the patient is weak and finds the effort expended in reaching and feeding himself too exhausting. The necessary assistance should be provided until the patient regains sufficient strength. The amounts of food and fluid taken are recorded until a normal diet is resumed.

Elimination. The postoperative patient may have a temporary inability to void because of a depression of the bladder sensitivity to distention; the impulses that produce the desire to void and the reflex emptying are not initiated. The inhibition may be due to the anesthetic, drugs or trauma in the region of the bladder. The recumbent position, nervous tension and fear of pain may also contribute to urinary retention. The patient may have the desire to void but is unable to do so because of spasm of the external sphincter. When the bladder becomes distended, a small amount may be voided frequently, but the bladder is not emptied; this is referred to as retention with overflow. Restlessness, complaints of pain or of a feeling of pressure in the pelvic area, and a palpable fullness above the symphysis pubis are associated with retention.

Distention and stagnation of urine predispose to inflammation and infection of the bladder. If the patient has not voided for 8 to 10 hours, efforts are made to induce voiding by leaving the patient alone on the bedpan or with the urinal, opening taps to produce the sound of running water, pouring warm water over the vulva of the female, and by elevating the head of the bed unless contraindicated. The unnatural position of being in bed is one of the common problems; the surgeon may allow the patient to get out of bed and use a commode or a bedpan placed on a chair. The male patient may be permitted to stand at the side of the bed to use a urinal. If the patient is permitted up, someone must remain with him in case he becomes faint.

Difficulty in voiding may have been anticipated by the physician and an order left to catheterize the patient if necessary in 10 to 12 hours. If there is no order and the patient has not passed urine for 10 hours, a report is given to the doctor. The amount of fluid the patient has had since last voiding should be noted. Strict asepsis and gentleness are necessary in the passing of a catheter to avoid trauma of the mucous membrane and the introduction of infection.

In major abdominal and pelvic surgery, an indwelling catheter may be passed and left in place for 2 or 3 days to avoid repeated catheterization as well as pressure from a full bladder on the internal operative site. An indwelling catheter may also be used to determine hourly secretion of urine if the patient is in shock or has some renal insufficiency due to disease. There is concern if the output is less than 30 ml. per hour.

Since the bowel is usually empty at the time of surgery and food intake is restricted for 2 or 3 days, bowel elimination is not an immediate postoperative concern. The patient, probably accustomed to a daily bowel movement, may be worried unless he is advised that the delay is to be expected and will not be harmful.

If a normal diet is quickly re-established, a laxative or enema may not be necessary. Some doctors order a mild laxative, glycerine suppository, or a small enema 2 days after operation. Early ambulation and being allowed to go to the toilet or use a commode help in re-establishing normal bowel elimination.

Deep Breathing, Coughing and Leg Exercises. As soon as the patient regains consciousness, he is required to do supervised deep breathing and voluntary forced coughing every 2 hours to fully expand the lungs and remove tracheobronchial secretions. Many anesthetic agents cause some irritation of the respiratory tract and increased secretions. If the latter are retained, a bronchial

tube may become plugged, resulting in the collapse of a segment of the lung (atelectasis) and reduced oxygen and carbon dioxide exchange. Bronchitis or pneumonia may develop, since retained secretions provide an excellent medium for the growth of pathogenic organisms.

Even though the patient received instruction and practiced these procedures before the operation, he may be very reluctant to carry them out because of the fear of pain. He must be assisted to the sitting position and given the necessary encouragement and support. One hand is placed at the patient's back, the other may be placed over the wound site to provide support during the coughing. The deep breathing and coughing are repeated 8 to 10 times every 2 hours. If the patient is very weak or complains of dizziness, it may be necessary to start with fewer deep breaths and progressively increase them as the patient's tolerance improves.

Bed rest and inactivity tend to produce venous stasis, particularly in the lower limbs. To minimize the stasis and the resulting danger of thrombus formation, circulation is stimulated by foot and leg exercises. These are usually commenced 8 to 10 hours after the operation and done every 2 to 3 hours until the patient is up and walking. Alternating active flexion and extension of the toes, dorsal and plantar flexion of the feet, and flexion and extension of the legs and thighs are carried out under the direction of the nurse. If early ambulation is not possible and the surgeon approves, self-care and the following exercises are included as soon as the patient's condition permits: flexion and extension of the head; flexion and extension of the fingers, hands, forearms and arms; abduction, adduction and external rotation of the arms at the shoulders; and contraction of the abdominal muscles. These activities stimulate circulation and respirations and prevent contractures and loss of strength.

Early Ambulation. Within 24 to 48 hours after surgery, if his vital signs are stable and his general condition satisfactory, the patient is assisted out of bed and encouraged to walk about. At first the patient may take only a few steps, but movement can be progressively increased as the patient feels stronger and more secure. This early ambulation promotes the return of normal physiological activities such as gastrointestinal peristalsis, reduces the incidence of respiratory and circulatory complications, prevents the loss of muscle tone, improves the patient's morale, and shortens the period of hospitalization and convalescence.

The patient is likely to be very fearful and helpless the first time he gets out of bed, and he will need assistance and support. The head of the bed is lowered, and he is turned to a lateral position near the edge of the bed with his legs and thighs flexed. The patient is then slowly assisted to the sitting position and his legs are put over the side of the bed. After a brief rest in this position while the nurse puts his slippers and dressing gown on him and notes his reactions, the erect position is assumed. Then, with help, he is encouraged to take a few steps. This is repeated 2 or 3 times each day and the walking is increased. Sitting in a chair for prolonged periods is discouraged since it favors venous stasis in the lower limbs.

The patient is encouraged to use a commode or go to the toilet while up to promote normal bladder and bowel elimination. Precautions against overactivity are necessary when the patient is up more frequently for longer periods because the reparative processes are still going on within the body.

Early ambulation is contraindicated or delayed when there is shock, hemorrhage, infection, cardiac insufficiency, and in the case of feeble, elderly persons.

Wound Care. The objectives in wound care are to have it remain uninfected and heal firmly with a minimum of scar tissue. On completion of the surgery, the incision is covered with a sterile gauze dressing and the area is inspected frequently during the immediate postoperative period for signs of drainage or bleeding. If the dressing becomes moist with serous drainage, it is reinforced by the application of sterile pads without disturbing the initial dressing. Should bright blood be evident, the doctor is notified promptly. In 2 or 3 days, the surgeon may order the dressing removed and the wound left exposed or covered with a thin layer of gauze. This is to eliminate warmth and moisture, which favor infection and maceration of the wound edges, and the use of adhesive, which can be irritating to the skin. The sutures are removed in 5 to 7 days.

A drain may have been inserted at the time of surgery to allow the escape of serum, pus or a body fluid such as bile. The tube may pass through the incision or a separate small stab wound. Specific orders are given as to the required care and when the tube is to be removed. Precautions are necessary when moving or bathing the patient in order to prevent dislodgement of the tube, particularly when it is attached to a drainage system.

Preparation for Discharge from Hospital. Surgical patients remain in the hospital for a much shorter period now than they did a few years ago. Early ambulation, self-care, and early resumption of a normal diet hasten recovery and help to maintain the patient's strength, making a shorter period of hospitalization possible. Since the reparative processes continue, the patient and his family receive instructions as to the amount of activity permitted and the necessary rest. If dressings or treatments are required, the patient and a family member are taught how these are carried out, or a referral may be made to a visiting nurse organization. The nurse discusses with the doctor when he wants to see the patient for an examination and arranges a clinic or office appointment. The doctor may give the patient some idea of when he may return to work before he leaves the hospital, or it may not be decided until he has his initial follow-up examination.

Postoperative Complications

Only the more common complications are presented here; specific complications that may be associated with particular operations are presented in the ensuing respective chapters.

Shock. This is a circulatory insufficiency due to a disproportion between the intravascular volume and the vascular capacity. It may develop during or immediately following the surgery, or it may develop more slowly and become evident several hours after operation. Early manifestations are a fall in blood pressure, rapid weak pulse, subnormal temperature, grayish pallor and cold clammy skin. The condition is serious and immediately life-threatening; prompt action is necessary to prevent irreversible shock. See the section on Shock (p. 237).

Hemorrhage. Postoperative bleeding may occur as a result of a slipped ligature or from an increase in the blood pressure, opening up previously collapsed vessels or dislodging the clot that plugged a severed vessel.

The hemorrhage may become evident externally at the site of operation, or it may be concealed internally and only manifested and recognized by changes in the vital signs, the patient's general appearance and complaint of weakness. Loss of blood causes a fall in blood pressure; a rapid, thready pulse; deep, rapid respirations, which are referred to as air hunger; pallor; apprehension; restlessness; and weakness.

Any suspicion of hemorrhage must be immediately reported. The patient is kept as quiet and undisturbed as possible; morphine or meperidine hydrochloride (Demerol) is usually ordered to allay his apprehension and reduce restlessness. The head is lowered to prevent cerebral ischemia. The dressing is reinforced as required. If the bleeding is from a limb, a tourniquet and pressure dressings are applied, and the part is elevated. An intravenous infusion of a plasma expander (e.g., Dextran 6 per cent) may be given while blood is being obtained for a transfusion. The patient may have to be returned to the operating room to have the blood vessel ligated.

Secondary hemorrhage may occur several days or weeks after the operation because of the erosion of a blood vessel by infection or malignant disease.

Respiratory Complications. Depression of the respiratory center by drugs or the anesthetic agent may occur and is manifested by slow, shallow respirations and cyanosis. An intermittent positive pressure respirator (see p. 286) may be used to overcome the insufficient ventilation and gas exchange. A respiratory stimulant such as nikethamide (Coramine) or caffeine sodium benzoate may be given. The use of narcotics (e.g., morphine or meperidine) for the relief of pain is limited in these patients because of their depressing effect on respirations.

Respiratory distress in the immediate postoperative period is often due to an obstruction of the airway by the relaxed lower jaw and tongue or to aspiration of mucus and vomitus. The latter may produce a laryngeal spasm or cause bronchitis or pneumonia.

Obstruction of a bronchial tube by aspirated material or a plug of mucus results in atelectasis, which is the collapse of the portion of the lung distal to the obstruction. If the collapsed area is large, the patient becomes dyspneic and cyanosed; his respirations are rapid and shallow, the pulse rate and temperature are elevated and chest expansion is decreased on the affected side. On examination there is percussion dullness and rales in the area. The trapped secretions tend to harbor organisms leading to infection (pneumonia) in the collapsed area.

A chest x-ray may be ordered to determine the extent of the area involved. Frequent deep breathing, coughing and turning are required. An increased fluid intake, steam inhalations and the administration of an expectorant such as potassium iodide may be ordered to liquefy the secretions, making them easier to raise. Percussion of the chest by a physiotherapist to dislodge the mucus is done several times a day. If the mucus plug cannot be dislodged, bronchoscopic aspiration may be necessary. An antibiotic is prescribed to combat the infection.

Pneumonia may develop independently of atelectasis. Any retained secretions in the alveoli and bronchial tubes readily become infected. The patient's temperature, pulse and respirations are elevated, and the sputum becomes purulent and blood streaked. See page 296 for a detailed discussion of pneumonia.

Prevention of postoperative respiratory complications begins with the preoperative preparation. Recognition of even a very mild respiratory infection is important and should be reported. Unless the surgery is an emergency, the operation is deferred until the infection is cleared up. A good nutritional status contributes to the patient's resistance, and smoking should be discouraged. It is extremely important that the patient's stomach is empty when receiving an anesthetic to decrease the danger of aspiration of vomitus.

Postoperative nursing measures that contribute to the prevention of respiratory complications include the following: lateral or semiprone positioning of the patient during recovery from anesthesia to prevent obstruction of the airway and promote drainage of secretions and vomitus to prevent aspiration; use of the suction when necessary to remove secretions from the pharynx and mouth; frequent deep breathing, coughing and change of position; protection of the patient from chilling and exposure to persons with a respiratory infection; ambulation as soon as ordered; and prompt recognition and reporting of adverse signs and symptoms.

Cardiac Arrest. Rarely, sudden heart failure occurs in the postoperative patient and demands rapid emergency treatment. External cardiac massage and artificial respirations by the mouth-to-mouth method are initiated immediately. The cardiac arrest is due to failure of the heart muscle to contract or to ventricular fibrillation. In the latter, the normal synchronized contractions of the muscle fibers of the ventricles are replaced with irregular uncoordinated contractions that result in incomplete filling and emptying of the chambers and insufficient blood being pumped into the systemic circulation. A defibrillator may be used by which one or two electric shocks are delivered to the heart.

Drug therapy may include epinephrine hydrochloride (Adrenalin) 1:1000, calcium chloride 10 per cent for direct intracardiac injection to stimulate contractions, and sodium bicarbonate (44.6 mEq. per ampule) intravenously to combat the metabolic acidosis that develops rapidly with the oxygen deficiency in the tissues. For details of cardiac massage see page 229.

Phlebothrombosis and Thrombophlebitis. Phlebothrombosis is the formation of a clot in the veins due to a stasis of the blood. It develops most often in the lower limbs. Pressure on the calves of the legs and prolonged flexion of the legs should be avoided. Although the patient may find a pillow under the knees or the elevation of the gatch frame at the knees very comfortable, these are hazardous since they promote venous stasis. Frequent foot and leg exercises play an important role in the prevention of phlebothrombosis in the bed patient.

The thrombus formation is a "silent" process; there may be some tenderness in the calf of the leg that is accidentally discovered on pressure, but generally there are no evident signs or symptoms. If phlebothrombosis is suspected or recognized, the patient is placed at rest with the foot of the bed elevated. An anticoagulant (e.g., heparin) may be prescribed to prevent enlargement of the thrombus. The condition is very dangerous because the clot may be carried along in the blood stream and eventually may block a vital blood vessel, causing what is called an embolism which may prove fatal. Since venous stasis is more likely to occur in varicosed veins, as a precautionary measure the surgeon may order the application of elastic bandages to the lower limbs from the foot to the thigh before surgery. These usually remain until just before the patient is discharged or resumes a normal amount of activity. The nurse removes and reapplies them twice daily to give the necessary skin care.

Thrombophlebitis is due to trauma, infection or chemical irritation of the wall of a vein initiating a local inflammatory reaction and clot formation. In this instance the clot is fairly firmly attached to the wall of the vein. The condition is quickly recognized because the surrounding tissue becomes edematous, reddened and painful, and there is an elevation of temperature and pulse.

The patient is kept on bed rest with the affected limb elevated. External heat may help to relieve the pain caused by vasospasm, and an anticoagulant may be ordered to prevent enlargement of the thrombus. The affected limb is handled very gently and is never massaged, in order to avoid dislodging the clot and the possibility of an embolism.

Wound Complications. Infection in the operative site is manifested by fever, increased pulse rate, general malaise and redness, swelling and tenderness of the wound area. Spontaneous purulent drainage occurs unless the infection is deep in which case the surgeon may remove a suture and probe the area to facilitate drainage. A swab of the first discharge is taken for culture to determine the causative organism. An antimicrobial drug (antibiotic or sulfonamide) is administered and frequent application of hot, moist dressings may be ordered to increase the blood supply to the area and to promote drainage of the exudate. Even though the wound is infected, strict aseptic dressing technique is used to prevent the introduction of a secondary infection. When the soiled dressings are removed, they are immediately placed in a paper bag for disposal, and precautions are taken to avoid contamination of the bedding and other objects in the environment to prevent the transmission of the infection to others.

Excessive strain on a wound as occurs in prolonged abdominal distention or severe coughing, wound infection, malnutrition, and general debilitation may cause separation of the edges of the incision; this separation is called dehiscence. Re-suturing or the application of adhesive straps may be used to pull the edges together.

If there is some separation of all the tissue layers (skin, fascia and peritoneum) in an abdominal wound, protrusion of a loop of intestine on to the surface of the abdomen may occur. This is referred to as evisceration. It is usually sudden, and the patient experiences "something giving way" and a warm sensation on the skin surface due to the escape of peritoneal fluid and the viscera. The surgeon is notified and sterile dressings moistened with sterile normal saline are applied to the exposed intestine. If a large portion of the bowel is eviscerated, a sterile towel moistened with the saline will provide better protection. A binder may be applied for support. The patient is requested to lie very still and the head and shoulders and the lower limbs are slightly elevated to reduce the strain on the abdominal wall. Someone remains with the patient to provide reassurance, and a sedative may be ordered to allay fear. Since the patient will most likely be returned to the operating room, an anesthetic and operative consent is signed after the surgeon has explained what is necessary, and the family is notified. The anesthetist or surgeon is advised as to when the patient last took food and fluid so that necessary precautions are taken to prevent aspiration. Lavage or induced vomiting are contraindicated since intra-abdominal pressure would be increased and more intestine eviscerated.

Gastrointestinal Complications. Persistent vomiting beyond 24 hours after operation causes concern. It may be due to the patient's sensitivity to the drugs which have been given, or it may be caused by acute dilatation of the stomach which can occur after almost any surgery if there is shock. Gastric dilatation is characterized by frequent vomiting of small amounts without effort, and upper abdominal distention which imposes on the diaphragm, causing dyspnea. A nasogastric tube is passed and suction-decompression established (see p. 338).

Mechanical intestinal obstruction, paralytic ileus and peritonitis are serious complications that may develop following abdominal surgery. These conditions are discussed in Chapter 15.

HICCUPS (SINGULTUS). Hiccups may occur as a troublesome, exhausting, postoperative complication, particularly after abdominal operations. They are paroxysmal, intermittent contractions of the diaphragm with the glottis closed. The cause is mechanical or chemical irritation of the phrenic nerve or its site of origin in the cervical spinal cord. They may be associated with gastric dilatation, abdominal distention, peritonitis, pleurisy, pneumonia, uremia or the ingestion of very hot or cold fluids.

The hiccups may cease spontaneously as the cause is corrected. If persistent, the inhalation of carbogen (carbon dioxide 5 per cent in oxygen) for 5 minutes at frequent intervals to stimulate deep regular respirations may provide relief. Rebreathing the air in a paper bag held closely over the mouth and nose may be used.

PAROTITIS. Dehydration, lack of oral intake and the omission of frequent hygienic mouth care predispose the patient to infection of the parotid gland. Normally, parotid salivary secretion is stimulated with fluid and food intake; this secretion washes out any organisms that may have found their way into the parotid ducts (Stensen's ducts). In the absence of secretion and adequate mouth care, organisms multiply in the mouth and have access to the glands. A painful swelling appears at the angle of the jaw on the side of the infected gland, and the patient develops a fever and systemic signs of infection. Older persons seem to have a greater predisposition to parotitis, and it may prove fatal when secondary to surgery or other illnesses.

Prevention involves keeping the mouth clean and moist and encouraging the patient to take fluids and food as soon as permitted. Chewing gum or sucking a sour fruit candy may be helpful in stimulating salivary secretion.

Treatment involves local heat applications and antimicrobial drug administration. If suppuration develops, surgical drainage may be necessary.

References

BOOKS

American College of Surgeons, Committee on Pre and Postoperative Care: Manual of Preoperative and Postoperative Care, 2nd ed. Philadelphia, W. B. Saunders Co., 1971. Part 1.

Davis, L. (Ed.): Christopher's Textbook of Surgery, 9th ed. Philadelphia, W. B. Saunders Co., 1968. Chapter 11.

Gius, J. A.: Fundamentals of General Surgery, 3rd ed. Chicago, Year Book Medical Publishers, Inc., Inc., 1966. Chapters 10 and 12.

LeMaitre, G., and Finnegan, J.: The Patient in Surgery, 2nd ed. Philadelphia, W. B. Saunders Co., 1970. Chapters 5, 6 and 8.

PERIODICALS

Carnevali, D.: "Preoperative Anxiety." Amer. J. Nurs., Vol. 66, No. 7 (July 1966), pp. 1536–1538.

Dumas, R. G.: "Psychological Preparation for Surgery." Amer. J. Nurs., Vol. 63, No. 8 (August 1963), pp. 52–55.

11
Age—Implications for Nursing

INTRODUCTION

Significant structural, physiological and psychosocial differences exist between children and adults and between these groups and senescents. The differences influence nursing needs, how they are expressed by the patient, and the ways in which they should be met. Medical-surgical nursing references usually relate to the mature patient, but many diseases and dysfunctions are common to infants, children and elderly persons. Adaptations in the care cited are necessary because of existing variants due to age.

FACTORS IN ADAPTING CARE TO CHILDREN

The following paragraphs include some important considerations in the care of the sick child. They are certainly not all-inclusive, but they may serve to indicate that differences do exist and to prompt the reader to refer to pediatric nursing texts for details. Although children may experience any of the illnesses to which adults are subject, infections, dysfunctions associated with congenital defects, nutritional problems and accidents have a much higher incidence. Neoplastic, metabolic and degenerative diseases occur much less frequently in the earlier years of life.

Illness and Hospitalization

To a young child, illness and pain are new and frightening experiences of which he has no understanding. If hospitalization is necessary, it imposes separation from the parents, strangeness and loneliness, which may have adverse effects on the child. Anything that is strange and unknown is potentially threatening; in addition to physical care he requires attention that will develop a sense of trust and security.

If the child is old enough, it is helpful if the parents prepare him for hospitalization. A simple truthful explanation is made as to what a hospital is, why boys and girls are there, and why he must go. If he is not prepared, hospitalization may be interpreted as desertion or punishment. It is helpful if the child receives a general description of his hospital bed, how he will receive his meals, what he will wear, the use of the bedpan, and the personnel who will care for him. A number of picture and story books are available that are useful in preparing the child for hospitalization.[1] A copy of one of

---

[1] Examples: Margaret and H. A. Rey: Curious George Goes to the Hospital. Boston, Houghton-Mifflin Co., 1966.

The Hospital for Sick Children, Toronto: Billy Goes to Hospital. Toronto, Women's Auxiliary of the Hospital for Sick Children.

these may usually be obtained from the local children's hospital or the library. It is comforting if one or two favorite toys are taken along so that he will have something familiar close to him. When possible, the child is placed in a room or ward with children of his own age.

Individual differences in responses to frightening situations occur and depend largely on previous experiences and training. For example, although some preparation is still necessary, hospitalization for the child of school age is less difficult. He has had the experience of separation from his mother and home for part of each day and has usually developed some degree of independence. Some children may fight and resist the nurse, while others may withdraw and become listless, probably because of feelings of being forsaken by their parents. Understanding and accepting the child's fears and insecurity, the nurse provides the attention and care that hopefully leads to his recognition of her as a source of affection and security.

The child needs the mother's support in adjusting to the strange environment and situation. She is encouraged to remain close to the child, to undress him and to participate in the admission procedure. The nurse takes over gradually, and the child, seeing the mother's approval of this, becomes more accepting of the nurse. When the child is old enough to understand, the parents should tell him that they are leaving but will return and will take him home as soon as he is better. The nurse accepts the child's concern and behavior when they leave, gives him attention and tries to introduce new interests. Although an occasional child may be inconsolable, the nurse should patiently persist in her efforts to provide comfort and emotional support. To give up and leave him alone only adds to his despair.

Parents

The young child is totally dependent on his parents, particularly his mother. His security and source of satisfaction in relation to his physical and emotional needs are vested chiefly in her or the person who mothers him. The mother as well as the child usually experiences considerable emotional disturbance on separation, and she needs the understanding support of the nurse. She may fear the outcome of the illness or be concerned about the child suffering. She may develop feelings of inadequacy and guilt and may attribute the situation to some neglect on her part. Some of the parents' anxiety may be due to the expenses being incurred by the illness; a referral to the social or welfare service may be necessary for the provision of assistance.

The nurse assesses the mother's reactions and, on recognizing anxiety, makes an effort to avoid giving the impression she is taking over the child. The mother is encouraged to talk about the child, remain with him as much as possible, especially at first, and to participate in his care. Her participation reassures the child, provides an outlet for the mother and establishes a better nurse-parent relationship in that it acknowledges the normal mother-child relationship. The nurse enquires as to whether there is anything special she should know about the child's accustomed care, such as food likes and dislikes, how he communicates his need to go to the toilet, his sleeping habits (his usual bedtime and whether he has a nap during the day), patterns of play, and what independent behavior he has developed. As well as providing information to be used in nursing, this manifests an interest in the child and respect for the care he has received from his mother.

Free visiting is permitted by many pediatric units now. The mother is usually anxious to spend a good deal of time with her sick child but may require guidance in the interest of the care of other children at home. In participating in the child's care, she should not be required to do more than she desires or she may think the nurse does not want to care for him. The nurse is still responsible for his total care and should know what takes place. Working with the mother provides an excellent opportunity for teaching and improving health practices which are favorable to the child's health and development. The mother may learn much simply by observing the care given.

Growth and Development

An important factor that influences the nursing of children is that the patients are in a period of physical growth and psychological and social development. It is necessary for the nurse to be familiar with the norms for the age of the child in her care. She has a responsibility to foster normal growth and developmental processes and recognize abnormalities and regression as well as to meet the physical needs incurred by the child's illness. The amount of attention related to this aspect of nursing will vary with the age of the child, the nature and length of his illness, and the parents' understanding of his needs.

Until one has had considerable experience with children and the application of knowledge of growth and development, it is usually necessary to refer to texts to determine the norms for the age of the child for whom care is being planned and implemented. It is not the intention to present a review of the characteristics of normal development here since there is an abundance of literature in this field. Several suitable textbooks are included in the references at the end of this chapter.

Illness frequently produces some regression in young children, particularly those in the preschool age group. Earlier patterns of behavior and greater dependency may be manifested; for example, the child may not indicate a need to go to the toilet and may revert to bed-wetting, or he may make no attempt to feed himself. Information as to the child's independent and self-care activities is obtained from the parents, and opportunities are provided for their continuance within the limits imposed by his illness. If the need to learn and "to do for himself" is ignored, overdependency develops, motor skills regress, and the child is less able to cope with the situation.

The child also requires opportunities to play, explore, learn, express himself, and achieve in association with his peers if he is to develop. This cannot be left to chance but takes planning, patience and time on the part of the nurse. A variety of toys and amusements are necessary and are selected according to the child's age, condition, interests and level of development. A play room or section of the ward is made available for ambulatory and wheelchair patients and is staffed by trained workers. For the children confined to bed, games may be organized that will involve several patients. Toys or games may be selected from carts which are taken through the wards, or as part of nursing care a story may be read to the bed patient. It should be remembered that a child has a short attention span; new interests and stimulation are needed. Most pediatric nursing texts include a chapter on play in which specific suggestions are made for play and amusement suitable for the various age groups. Play activities which promote motor coordination and dexterity, perception, and self-expression are also indicated.

A person tends to develop responses that are satisfying to him, but these may not always be acceptable to society. It is important the child develop patterns of behavior that are acceptable to those around him. Group play provides opportunities for socialization and the learning of appropriate acceptable behavior.

If the school child is in the hospital or is confined to bed at home for a prolonged period, his school work is continued by a visiting teacher provided by the local school board. His diet will probably require periodic adjustment to meet his growth requirements.

Signs, Symptoms and Observation

Signs and symptoms of illness in an infant or child differ somewhat from those in a mature patient because of the effect of the disease on immature developing tissues and organs. The onset of an illness is frequently more abrupt and acute. An evident change in behavior, fussiness, refusal of food, vomiting, diarrhea and fever are common to many conditions in children and do not point to the specific nature or site of the problem. A convulsion is common at the onset of a fever, and the temperature rises to higher levels than in an adult. Serious dehydration leading to shock may develop with startling rapidity as a result of vomiting, diarrhea, fever and reduced intake. The child loses weight and becomes debilitated quickly because of the lack of nutritional reserves. The provision of fluids and nourishment become an immediate concern with any sick child.

Observation is an important part of all nursing, but it plays an even more significant role in the care of children. The infant and the young child are unable to verbalize and describe their discomforts and needs; the physician and nurse are dependent on objective signs. Many nonverbal communications in the form of behavioral manifestations have meaning that is just as important as the vital signs. The diagnosis and treatment may be greatly influenced by the nurse's accurate, objective description of the child's physical, mental and emotional responses.

Pertinent factors that should be noted and recorded include the following: crying— whether it is the normal strong vigorous cry or is shrill and piercing, feeble, or a whimper; body movements and positions— whether restless, making purposeless movements, abnormally still and favoring one position, cries and protests when a particular part or area is moved or touched or when he is picked up; abnormal loss or increase in muscle tension (e.g., rigidity and hyperextension of the neck); frequent brushing or rubbing of a part (e.g., face or ear); apathy— passive, withdrawn, indifferent to environment; increased dependency—appears fearful and bewildered, clings to the nurse or parent; failure to eat and drink; change in the number and character of stools; change in the volume and character of urine; skin eruptions; facial expression and color— drawn, aged appearance, pallor, eyes sunken, shadows under the eyes, mottling or cyanosis; and any behavior that differs from that expected for the age and level of development or from that which was previously exhibited. Excessive sweating is not normal and is brought to the physician's attention since it may indicate some autonomic nervous system dysfunction.

Continuity of care by the same nurses is important so that physical and behavioral changes will be recognized promptly. It is also better for the child as he becomes accustomed to the same nurses to whom he can relate; lack of a continuing warm relationship causes anxiety in the child and later a cold indifference to everyone.

Physical Factors

Significant physiological and structural differences between the child and adult include the following factors.

Resistance. Children are more susceptible to infection, and the younger the child, the greater the susceptibility. As he becomes older he develops antibodies and some immunity following repeated infections. The infant is born with a natural passive immunity to some infections through having received antibodies from the mother's blood. Measles, diphtheria, poliomyelitis, smallpox, and streptococcal and pneumococcal infections are relatively rare in infants up to six months of age. The antibodies which diffused across the placenta from the mother's blood into the fetus gradually diminish over the first five to six months of life, and the child begins to manufacture his own antibodies after repeated exposures to invading pathogenic organisms (antigens). The principal defense mechanisms and the reticuloendothelial tissues concerned with antibody formation are immature and slower to respond in the child, contributing to the high incidence of childhood infections.

Parents should be urged to consult their physician as to the recommended schedule for active immunization for their infant (see p. 45).

When it is learned that a hospitalized child has had no inoculations, it should be brought to the doctor's attention.

Because of their lower resistance, children should be protected from contact with known and suspected sources of infection. The child with an infection requires prompt attention and treatment; his immaturity and lack of antibodies and reserves may lead rapidly to an overwhelming infection.

Fluids. There is a proportionately greater volume of water in the body of the child than in the adult; approximately 70 to 80 per cent of body weight is water as compared to approximately 60 per cent of the adult's weight. The water in the young is used more rapidly; the increased heat production results in a greater amount being vaporized and the urinary output is proportionately greater since the immature kidneys are less efficient in conserving water and concentrating wastes.

Serious dehydration, acid-base imbalance and shock can develop with startling rapidity when there is a reduced fluid intake or an increased loss of fluid as in vomiting, diarrhea and fever. Unfortunately all of these latter factors commonly occur together in childhood illnesses. An early assessment of the ill child's state of hydration is necessary. Vomiting, diarrhea, high fever and failure to take fluids should be reported promptly so that body fluids may be brought up to the optimal level. Signs of dehydration are dry mouth with thick stringy saliva, loss of tissue turgor, sunken eyes, depressed fontanelles in the infant, apathy and loss of weight. If it is allowed to progress to greater fluid depletion, the reduced intravascular volume causes shock, which is manifested by pallor, cold skin, rapid weak pulse and an abnormally low blood pressure.

Resourcefulness and patience are necessary on the part of the nurse in getting the child to take an adequate amount of fluid by mouth. A pleasant positive approach, assuming the child is going to take the fluid, rather than a demanding, urgent manner is helpful. Over-urging may only result in the child vomiting. Allowing the young child to choose between two or three fluids and to select a colored straw may capture the child's cooperation. An accurate record of the intake and output is necessary.

When sufficient fluid cannot be given orally, parenteral fluids are administered by intravenous or interstitial infusion (hypodermoclysis). Sites used for intravenous infusion in the young include a vein on the medial side of an ankle and a scalp vein. If the latter is used, the area is shaved in preparation. A cut-down may be necessary in which a local anesthetic is injected into the skin at the site and a small incision is made to expose the vein. A cannula or needle is then introduced into the vein and secured by suture material. The area is protected by a sterile dressing. Adequate restraint is necessary during the starting of intravenous infusion and later to prevent dislodgement of the needle or cannula. The mummy restraint which encloses the arms, trunk and lower limbs, and immobilization of the head with sand bags are used if the scalp vein is the site of the infusion. When a limb is used, clove-hitch restraints, and a splint on the particular arm or leg may be applied. The volume and rate of flow of the intravenous fluid are indicated by the physician and carefully controlled. If the fluid is given more rapidly than it can pass from the intravascular compartment into the tissues, the cardiovascular system may become overloaded, leading to serious and even fatal results.

In interstitial infusion (hypodermoclysis) a quantity of fluid is introduced slowly into the subcutaneous tissues. Sites which may be used are the anterior aspects of the thighs and the scapular and pectoral areas. The rate at which the solution is administered is regulated according to the rate of absorption. If it is allowed to run too rapidly it will cause considerable local swelling and discomfort. Hyaluronidase, an enzyme, may be added to the fluid to promote absorption.

Nutrition. Infants and children require more calories in proportion to size and weight than adults in order to support their growth process, higher metabolic rate and physical activity. The daily requirement is approximately 110 to 120 calories per kilogram of body weight during the first two years of life and gradually declines to 40 to 60 calories per kilogram at maturity. Malnutrition is manifested quickly in a child with an inadequate caloric intake as his reserves are very limited.

The sick child frequently presents nutritional problems; food may be refused because of a loss of appetite, the strange environment, despair at being separated from his parents, or because the food is not what he is accustomed to at home. The nurse needs to know the nutritional requirements of the child according to his age, the necessary restrictions because of his condition, how much he is actually taking and changes in his weight. As with the giving of fluids, resourcefulness and patience are frequently necessary to have the patient receive sufficient nourishment. The following suggestions may be helpful: a positive approach, assuming the child is going to take the food; he should not be hurried or bribed and is commended when he eats what is offered; milk may be withheld until later if he is inclined to drink it all and then refuse the solid foods; and similarly, only the more important food principles (eggs, meat, vegetables) may be offered and carbohydrates, such as bread and desserts, withheld so he doesn't satisfy his appetite on those first. Giving him a choice when possible may add some enticement. Self-feeding is permitted and encouraged unless it is contraindicated by his illness. When the condition permits, the child usually eats better when at a table with others.

In some instances, it may be beneficial to have the mother visit at mealtime, provided she does not become overanxious and aggravate the problem. Her presence may provide a situation with which the child is familiar. Normally, parents are discouraged from bringing in home-cooked food, but occasionally it may be of value to permit them to bring the child some food which he likes, is accustomed to receiving at home, and which is compatible with his condition.

If the child is obese, fats and starches are reduced. In long-term illness, it is important that adjustments be made from time to time in the number of calories and diet according to the child's age and progressive growth requirement.

Nausea and Vomiting. Vomiting frequently occurs with any illness in a child. Nausea may precede the vomiting but cannot be verbalized by the young. In some instances it may be suspected and vomiting anticipated when the child manifests pallor, increased salivation, restlessness and sweating.

Regurgitation, which is nonforceful, effortless vomiting that occurs without abdominal muscle contraction, is common in infants because of the incomplete development of the cardiac sphincter. The cause of this type of vomiting is more often the swallowing of air or gastric distention due to overfeeding.

The immaturity of the neuromuscular system, which results in less efficient reflexes, increases the possibility of aspiration of vomitus; the infant or child must be quickly turned to the prone position to promote drainage from the pharynx and mouth. The nursing observations and responsibilities cited in the care of the patient who is vomiting (p. 329) will also apply to the child. It must be remembered, though, that the child lacks the reserve which the adult is likely to have and, in vomiting, will develop serious dehydration and malnutrition more rapidly.

Elimination. The normal infant has an average of two stools per day; after one year, bowel elimination is usually decreased to one stool per day. Stools are examined for changes in volume, color, composition and consistency. The characteristics of the stool normally are determined by the food; changes from the normal may indicate a necessary dietary adjustment, particularly in infants.

Elimination which is too frequent or is absent, excessive straining at stool, and abnormality of the stool are reported and recorded. An abnormal stool is saved for the physician's inspection and for possible laboratory examination. An enema or laxative is only administered when ordered by the physician since either causes loss of fluid.

Rest and Sleep. The increased activity, higher metabolic rate and lesser reserve of the young result in their need for more rest and sleep than mature persons. Nursing includes plans for regular rest periods and naps during the day as well as a regular early bedtime hour at night. Special bedtime rituals are determined from the parents and followed as much as possible; for example, the child may be accustomed to saying his prayers to someone or to having a certain toy or blanket to cuddle.

Vital Signs. The young child's temperature-regulating mechanism is not fully developed, and as a result fever rises to higher levels than in adolescents or adults. He tolerates exposure to cold less well because his ability to conserve body heat by vascular constriction is less efficient.

The temperature is taken rectally up to the age of seven to eight years. The thermometer is held and the other hand is placed on the child during the recording to prevent sudden movement and possible breaking of the thermometer in the rectum. For a fever over 38.8° C. (102° F.), temperature-reducing measures such as a tepid sponge bath and the administration of antipyretic drugs (e.g., acetylsalicylic acid) may be ordered. The tepid sponge bath is discontinued if cyanosis, weak pulse or slow respirations are manifested.

The pulse and respirations vary with age, activity, emotions and crying. The volume and rhythm of the pulse are more significant than the rate. More accurate information may be obtained if they are checked when the child is sleeping and before the temperature is taken, since the insertion of the rectal thermometer may disturb the child and cause variation. The pulse rate gradually decreases, reaching adult levels by adolescence. The average normal range for different age groups is as follows:

Infant	140 to 120 per minute
1 to 5 years	120 to 90 per minute
5 to 10 years	90 to 80 per minute
10 to 16 years	90 to 74 per minute

The respirations are more rapid and shallow in the infant and preschooler than in the older child and adult. They vary from 30 to 50 per minute in infancy and gradually decrease to adult levels of 16 to 20 per minute by the age of ten to twelve years.

The blood pressure is considerably lower in infancy and childhood than in maturity; it gradually increases with weight. The width of the cuff used in determining the blood pressure varies with the size of the child. If the cuff is too narrow, the blood pressure recorded will be higher than it actually is; if it is too wide, a lower reading is obtained. The cuff used should be approximately two-thirds the length of the upper arm. Cuffs usually appropriate for different ages are as follows:

Infants	cuff of 1 to 1½ inches
2 to 8 years	cuff of 3 inches
8 to 12 years	cuff of 4 inches
12 to 14 years	cuff of 5 inches

The child should be at rest for an accurate recording of blood pressure; fear, restlessness and excitement are likely to produce an erroneously high systolic pressure. The average normal blood pressures according to age are found at the bottom of this page.

Urinary System. The urinary output in infants and young children is proportionately larger than in children over eight or nine years and adults. The immature kidneys have less discriminatory ability; they are unable to conserve water and regulate the output according to the intake and to concentrate wastes to the same extent.

Pyelonephritis (infection of the kidney pelvis and tissue) due to colon bacillus is relatively common in young females because of the short urethra. Prevention necessitates prompt changing of soiled diapers or underclothing and thorough cleansing following defecation. In cleansing, precautions are taken to avoid the possibility of transmitting contamination toward the urethral meatus.

Respiratory System. In early years, on inspiration the chest cavity is enlarged mainly by the contraction and lowering of the diaphragm. The infant's and young child's ribs are horizontal and the intercostal muscles have a lesser role in respiration. As a result, the rise and fall of the chest wall during respiration is less noticeable than in the older child and adult, and movement of the abdomen is more evident.

The lumen of the respiratory tract is smaller and so is more readily occluded in inflammatory conditions and aspiration. The larynx is sensitive, and irritation or inflammation may quickly cause spasmodic contraction, making breathing difficult. The nasal passages, being small, obstruct easily in respiratory infections, making sucking difficult. The cough reflex is absent in the infant and less efficient while developing in the young child; as a result, they do not get rid of secretions or a foreign body as readily as older children and adults. Because of these several differences, infants and children with respiratory infection require prompt treatment and close observation for respiratory insufficiency. Sternal and intercostal retraction and flaring of the nostrils frequently accompany severe respiratory difficulty and must be reported promptly to the physician. Prolonged rapid respirations exhaust a young child more rapidly than an older child or adult. Mucus should be wiped away quickly or removed by nasopharyngeal suctioning to prevent aspiration. The patient is kept on his side or in the semiprone position as much as possible to promote drainage of secretions. Cool moist air and increased fluid intake are provided to liquefy the mucus and facilitate its removal.

If oxygen or air is administered directly under pressure into the child's respiratory tract, the pressure must be kept lower for a child up to twelve years so that the lungs are not damaged by overdistention. Similarly, caution is also necessary if mouth-to-mouth resuscitation is used.

Middle-ear infection (otitis media) is a common complication of respiratory infec-

	Systolic pressure	*Diastolic pressure*
Infancy	85 mm. Hg	50 mm. Hg
1 to 6 years	85 to 90 mm. Hg	50 to 60 mm. Hg
6 to 10 years	90 to 100 mm. Hg	60 to 65 mm. Hg
10 to 16 years	100 to 118 mm. Hg	65 to 70 mm. Hg

tion in children. The incompletely developed eustachian tube is straighter and wider, making it a more accessible pathway to the middle ear from the pharynx.

Nervous System. The child's developing nervous system is unstable. As a result, convulsions frequently accompany illness in children up to four to five years of age, especially if there is a fever. A nurse should remain with the child during the seizure to protect him from injury. A padded tongue depressor may be placed between the teeth to prevent biting of the tongue; suction is quickly made available to remove excess oral secretions. The seizure should be reported promptly and the following observations recorded: child's condition and activity immediately preceding the seizure; the parts of the body involved; whether the movements are jerky (clonic) or whether the body or involved parts remain contracted and rigid (tonic); the patient's color, secretions, eye movements and pupillary changes; the length of the seizure and period of unconsciousness; incontinence; temperature, pulse, and respirations as well as any changes in behavior and awareness following the seizure. It must be remembered that convulsions may not always be due to the immaturity of the central nervous system; they may be associated with metabolic or central nervous system disorders.

Immature reflexes and lack of complete muscular coordination predispose the developing child to falls and accidents, necessitating greater protective measures on the part of those responsible for him. Blows to the head are more serious because of the open fontanelles and incompletely developed suture lines in the skull.

Blood Values. Normal blood values for the infant and the child up to twelve years differ from those for adults. Erythrocytes (red blood cells) are more numerous at birth and gradually decrease to a lower level over the first two or three months; adult levels are usually reached by the age of twelve years. The leukocyte count is higher in the infant and in the child up to about twelve years with a higher percentage of lymphocytes. In Table 11-1 Blake and Wright present the normal blood values for various ages.

Safety Measures

The child's normal curiosity, desire to explore, and lack of experience and understanding necessitate special precautions and constant alertness on the part of the nurse to reduce the possibility of injury from falls, the swallowing or aspiration of foreign bodies, burns, suffocation and poisoning. Essential protective measures include the following: crib sides must be kept up and securely fastened unless the nurse or a parent is right at the bedside, facing the child. If the nurse must turn from the child to get something during direct care or if the child is on a treatment table, she keeps a hand on the child. The sides should also be kept up on empty cribs to discourage ambulant children from climbing.

Young children, whether in bed or up, are not left unattended for long periods.

If a restraint is necessary, that applied to the trunk must fit closely enough to remain in position and prevent the child from wiggling out of it. When restraints are applied

TABLE 11–1 NORMAL BLOOD VALUES FOR CHILDREN[2]

	BIRTH TO 3 MONTHS	12 WEEKS	6 MONTHS	2 YEARS	12 YEARS
Erythrocytes (millions per cu. mm.)	4.5 to 5.5	3.5 to 4.5	4 to 4.5	4.3 to 4.7	4.5 to 5.0
Leukocytes (per cu. mm.)	20,000	12,000	12,000	10,000	8,000
Hemoglobin (grams per cent)	15.5 to 18.5	10 to 12	11 to 13	12 to 13.5	13.5 to 15
Thrombocytes (per cu. mm.)	350,000	300,000	300,000	300,000	300,000

[2]F. G. Blake and F. H. Wright: Essentials of Pediatric Nursing, 7th ed. Philadelphia, J. B. Lippincott Co., 1963, p. 557.

to the limbs, precautions are necessary to avoid interference with the circulation.

The use of soft pillows and plastic sheeting is avoided; if either is used, it must be secured to the bed to prevent the possibility of the child pulling it over his face and smothering. All of the windows should have screens firmly secured in position. Radiators, electrical outlets and fans are covered, and doorways and the entrances to stairways are guarded by gates if children are ambulatory. Sharp-edged toys and those with loose or detachable small parts that might be swallowed or aspirated are removed. Safety pins are kept closed and out of reach.

Medications are kept in a locked cupboard and never left at the bedside or within reach of a child. During administration, the nurse must not turn her back on a medicine tray or cart that has a medication on it. Use of the term "candy" should not be used as a means of persuasion when giving the child a pill as it may lead to his taking an overdose of available pills at a later date.

A positive identification of the child by checking the necklace or bracelet and the bassinette or crib card is necessary before administering a treatment and medication since the infant or child is not capable of questioning or advising the nurse that he is the wrong patient.

Medications, fluids and foods are not to be forced because of the possibility of causing aspiration as well as fear and resentment in the child. Infants' feeding bottles must not be propped because of the danger of aspiration.

Extreme caution is necessary with the use of steam inhalations and applications of heat. With the former, the kettle and the steam outlet are screened and kept out of reach. Hot water bottles must not be more than 44° to 46° C. (110° to 115° F.) and must be tightly stoppered and covered. Taps must be turned off tightly; bath water is tested with a thermometer before placing a child in it.

Sufficient assistance should be available during treatments to provide adequate restraint to ensure safety.

Whenever the opportunity presents, the child who is old enough to understand is taught what is safe and unsafe. The nurse also has a responsibility for educating parents and others as to their role in the prevention of accidents.

Medication

Drug dosage for children is based on their weight and age, and must be very accurate. Children and particularly infants are observed closely for the effects of drugs given since their immature enzyme systems, liver and kidneys may not completely metabolize and excrete the drugs. Although the doctor prescribes the dose of the drug to be given, the nurse should be familiar with how a dosage is determined. If she is not familiar with the drug or has reason to question the dosage she may make a quick check before administering the drug. In many instances, the label or brochure accompanying the drug will indicate the dosage or the amount to be given per kilogram of body weight. Or the dosage may be checked by using Clark's rule which is:

$$\text{Infant's or child's dose} = \frac{\text{weight of child in pounds} \times \text{adult dose}}{150 \text{ (which is the average adult weight)}}$$

Occasionally for older children, Young's rule may be used:

$$\text{Child's dose} = \frac{\text{age of child in years} \times \text{adult dose}}{\text{age of child in years} + 12}$$

When administering drugs to children, a positive, firm approach is used. The nurse's attitude and comment reflect no doubt about the child's cooperation. The child's questions are answered honestly. For infants and children up to five or six years, tablets and pills are crushed and put into solution. Medications should not be disguised in food as it may cause future refusal of that particular food. Many medications are placed in fruit flavored syrups which disguise any disagreeable taste. As cited under safety measures, special precautions are taken by the nurse to be sure she has the right child. Care is taken to avoid force in administering oral medication. The head and shoulders are elevated during the taking of oral medicine to avoid possible aspiration.

Infants and children tolerate opiates poorly, and a smaller dose than might be expected according to the previously mentioned rules is always prescribed.

When children are to receive hypodermic or intramuscular injections, if they are old enough to be frightened and resist, they should receive some preparation. Sufficient assistance should be available to hold the child securely and provide support. Needles are selected according to the child's size and should be sharp and in good condition. Afterwards, the child's crying and protestations are accepted; the nurse advises him that she knows it hurt and tries to comfort the child by picking him up or, in the case of an older child, by staying with him.

Nursing Procedures

The child's size must always be considered, since it dictates variations in certain procedures. Oversized equipment such as tubes or needles can be traumatizing to the child's tissues and interfere with effectiveness of the treatment.

Procedures are described in simple terms to the child who is old enough to understand even part of what is being said. Sometimes it is possible and helpful to let the child explore the equipment, see illustrations, or in some instances demonstrate to some extent on the child's doll or toy animal. Resourcefulness is needed to devise approaches and methods. The child should be approached with a patient, positive attitude rather than a domineering, demanding manner that threatens him. It is helpful if the child is involved and is asked to do something that contributes. Whenever possible, the same nurse gives the treatment. Sufficient assistance must be available to provide the restraint necessary to make the treatment safe. The temperature of treatment solutions must be tested by a thermometer and should not be used if over 40.5° C. (105° F.) unless specified by the physician.

When positioning an infant or young child it should be remembered that prolonged pressure from remaining in one position for a long period may alter the shape of young developing bones. It is particularly significant in relation to the skull because of the fontanelles and developing suture lines. Freedom of movement is necessary to promote muscular development and coordination.

When possible, the infant and young child should be held during feeding and some nursing care procedures; physical contact is reassuring and tends to make the situation less frightening.

THE ADOLESCENT

Adolescence is the period of transition from childhood to adulthood and extends roughly from the thirteenth to the nineteenth year. It is characterized by marked structural, physiological, emotional and social behavioral changes. There is an increased secretion of the sex and somatotropic (growth) hormones, producing structural and physiologic changes which include a spurt in physical growth (an increase in both height and weight), the appearance of secondary sex characteristics, the onset of menstruation in girls and the production of sperm in boys. The physical growth occurs more rapidly than nervous control can be established, resulting in some awkwardness or ungainliness in the young adolescent. The secondary sex characteristics evident in the female are an enlargement of the breasts and hips, a broadening of the pelvis, the growth of pubic and axillary hair, and the onset of menstruation which indicates increased concentrations of sex hormones, ovulation and the ability to reproduce. In boys, the secondary sex developments include enlargement of the genitals; a general increase in skeletal muscle mass; the growth of hair on the pubis, axillae, chest and face; and an increase in the size of the larynx which produces voice changes. The activity of the sebaceous and sweat glands is increased in both sexes, giving rise to the common adolescent problem of acne.

Adolescents are faced with the body changes, new feelings and reactions that puberty brings. They become very self-conscious and sensitive and frequently display mood shifts and emotional instability. Their responses to situations are unpredictable; interests, moods and attitudes may vacillate between extreme opposites. For example, teen-agers tend to be ambivalent, alternately displaying acceptance and resistance to authority, content and discontent, and independence and dependence. They frequently go through a phase of rebelling against adult opinions and conventional society in general; on the other hand, they place tremendous importance on identification and conformity with their peers. They want to make their own decisions but are generally not sufficiently experienced to sever dependence and parental control entirely. Adults often make the problem more difficult by telling an adolescent he is old enough to know that or do that and in the next breath tell him he is too young to know or decide what is best. In this period of life, the decision must also be made as to a vocation or career for the future. Adolescents facing the changes, problems and necessary adjustments characteristic of this period of life require understanding and unobtrusive guidance from adults.

Illness is disturbing to the adolescent for different reasons than for the child; he resents the interference with his freedom and school and social activities and feels threatened by the imposed dependence. He becomes the focus of his parents' attention at a time when he has been trying to be independent of them. If hospitalization is necessary, the adolescent is likely to be humiliated if placed in a children's ward. If no adolescent ward is available, careful consideration should be given to placement in an adult ward because the impressionable teen-ager is readily influenced by conversation and behavior of the adults.

In many instances a student nurse may be assigned to care for the patient and, being an adolescent herself, has problems similar to those of the patient. She may find the situation difficult and require the guidance and support of a mature, understanding instructor or head nurse. The patient's ever-changing moods and attitudes must be accepted, and the nurse's approach should be adapted to elicit cooperation.

The nurse should be prepared to listen to the adolescent's opinions and concerns, treat them confidentially, and give advice or explanations when the opportunity presents but should avoid an authoritarian manner. For example, the patient may need assistance in understanding the physical changes in his or her body.

Because the adolescent is very sensitive and easily humiliated, it is important that precautions be taken to avoid any unnecessary exposure, and adequate privacy should be provided. Procedures are carefully explained as he is likely to show more interest in detail than either younger or more mature patients.

The nutritional and energy requirements of the teen-ager are markedly increased; the daily intake to meet the needs may vary from 2200 to 3000 calories depending on his activities and rate of growth. Protein content should be kept high—80 to 100 grams per day. Emphasis is placed on the inclusion of meat, fish, eggs, cheese, fresh vegetables and fruits, whole grain cereal and milk. When planning the diet during illness, it is important to consider the growth needs of the adolescent as well as the cause of his illness.

SIGNIFICANT FACTORS IN NURSING THE SENESCENT

Aging and life's stresses result in structural and functional changes which appear throughout the later years of the life span. The changes are regressive and degenerative in nature, and the age at which they appear and their rate of progression are individual factors. Chronological age and the degree of change do not necessarily correspond for all persons. It is important for the nurse to know that, although there is marked individual variation, there are certain changes which may be expected in the advanced years and that elderly people are structurally and functionally different persons than they were in their youth and maturity. Their needs, the ways in which these are expressed and should be met, and their responses to illness differ.

Illness and Hospitalization

Illness is usually more threatening to the older person simply because of his age and his recognition of a difference in his body efficiency. If hospitalization is necessary, he may be very apprehensive and pessimistic in regard to the outcome of his illness. In some instances, the older person becomes resentful at being transferred to a hospital or nursing home because it is interpreted by him as an indication that the family does not want to look after him. Adjustment to the hospital is likely to be difficult; the unfamiliar environment and personnel and the change in the patient's accustomed routine and way of life produce insecurity. The stress may bring about confusion and marked behavioral changes necessitating special precautions to protect him. Frequently, the older person has experienced the loss of his spouse and a number of his contemporaries, and illness and hospitalization seem to further emphasize his aloneness. He is accustomed to having familiar personal possessions around him and to suddenly have all of these except a few toilet articles removed may be very distressing and frequently initiates protests and restlessness.

If the illness necessitates confinement to bed, the enforced activity is very hazardous and must be kept to a minimum with senescents. Circulatory stasis, hypostatic pneumonia, decubitus ulcers and loss of strength become immediate concerns. The slowing-up of the circulation to the brain predisposes to disorientation and confusion. Many of the older citizens have an income inadequate for the present cost of living. Expenses incurred by illness and dependence only add to their financial worries.

Repeated orientations to the situation are needed because the senescent forgets quickly. Explanations are necessary about such things as to why he is in bed and in the hospital, how his regular needs (e.g., meals, toilet) will be met, the whereabouts of his family members and when they will come, and the location of his personal belongings. Rigid adherence to routines may be very disturbing to the elderly. In many instances, the practice of some hospital customs could be delayed and introduced gradually.

Consideration in regard to the placement of the older person in the hospital ward is necessary; proximity to patients with infections is avoided because of his lowered resistance. If ambulatory, being near the bathroom is important. He should not be left unobserved or alone for long periods.

Structural and Functional Changes — Implications for Nursing

General Changes. Some basic cellular changes develop gradually as part of the aging process. The rate of cell division (reproduction), growth and repair becomes slower. In some areas, regeneration becomes less than the rate of cell destruction, resulting in tissue atrophy and, in the case of injury or disease, diminished recovery and healing ability. There is also less specialization in the cells being produced; in many instances, cells are replaced by those of a less specialized order, such as fibrous or fatty tissue cells. These less specialized cells require less oxygen and nutrients but are incapable of the specialized activities of the cells replaced.

There is a reduction in the fluid maintained within the cells and their environment. An inadequate fluid intake or an excessive loss of fluid may quickly lead to serious dehydration. The rate of metabolism decreases with advancing years and reduces the amount of energy and heat produced. The homeostatic mechanisms become less efficient in maintaining the normal constancy of the internal environment (e.g., chemical concentrations, fluid volume, pH, temperature). The reduced efficiency in regulation leaves a decrease in the body's reserves and a lesser margin of safety.

Such general changes obviously influence the functional ability of various organs and systems and must be kept in mind when caring for the elderly.

Cardiovascular System. The heart is one of the few organs which do not atrophy. More often, it is found to hypertrophy because of the increased demands on it created by vascular changes and hypertension. It no longer has as great a capacity for increasing the rate and strength of contractions to meet increased demands as incurred by physical exercise.

The walls of the arteries become less distensible because of a loss of elastic tissue and the development of patchy areas of fatty and calcium deposits in the walls. The intima becomes thicker, and the lumen of the vessels narrows. Resistance is offered to the flow of blood, the blood pressure is elevated and there is a diminished blood supply to organs and tissues, lowering their level of function.

The walls of veins are thinner and weaker, predisposing to the slowing of venous drainage and the pooling of blood.

The blood itself has greater constancy than most other tissues in the body. Unless an actual blood dyscrasia develops or dietary deficiencies are experienced, the plasma volume and blood composition show little change.

IMPLICATIONS FOR NURSING. Changes in the cardiovascular system necessitate a reduction in the physical demands on the patient. He is cautioned to move more slowly to avoid sudden increases in cardiac demands and output. A large part of the animal fat in the diet should be replaced by vegetable fat, which may reduce the blood cholesterol and the formation of atherosclerotic plaques in the walls of the arteries.

If an intravenous infusion is to be administered, the rate of flow is slower than that used with a younger person. The less elastic arteries and weaker heart may not be capable of accommodating a rapidly increasing intravascular volume. The rate of flow and the volume to be given in 24 hours are usually stated by the physician.

Immobility and prolonged bed rest are avoided, since they predispose to circulatory stasis and thrombosis. When bed rest is necessary, a change of position every 1 to 2 hours and passive and active exercises, particularly of the limbs, are important to promote venous drainage and circulation.

Respiratory System. In later years, the respiratory system is likely to be less efficient and less resistant to infection. The bronchial walls become thinner. The cough is weaker and less effective in clearing the tract, leaving retained secretions which favor infection. A reduction in the vital capacity and the slower circulation of the blood through the lungs result in a decreased oxygen concentration in the blood which encourages degenerative changes throughout the body. When the older patient is at rest, the shallow breathing and slower pulmonary circulation predispose to the escape of fluid into the alveoli and ensuing coughing, dyspnea and hypostatic pneumonia.

IMPLICATIONS FOR NURSING. In order to encourage better oxygenation and prevent respiratory complications, it is necessary to have the patient breathe deeply 5 to 10 times, cough and change position every 1 to 2 hours. One should be sure that the position assumed allows for free chest expansion for better ventilation. Early ambulation and activity within the limitations imposed by the illness are encouraged. Protection of the elderly patient from exposure to persons with an infection is necessary because of the lowered resistance. Respiratory infection in the older person should receive prompt attention; otherwise, it may become serious very quickly.

Digestive System and Nutrition. The stomach of the elderly person loses muscular strength and tone and takes longer to empty. There is usually some decrease in secretions and acidity; some persons may have a reduced tolerance to certain foods, such as fats. Fewer active taste buds combined with decreased activity contribute to a decrease in appetite. The loss or neglect of teeth may interfere with the taking of essential foods.

Loss of muscular tone in the intestine reduces peristalsis; the content is moved along more slowly, causing constipation.

The metabolic rate is reduced so that fewer calories are necessary than in previous years. If the person continues the same caloric intake, obesity is likely to develop; this should be avoided since it increases the demands on the cardiovascular system and on the weight-bearing joints.

IMPLICATIONS FOR NURSING. Nutritional deficiencies are frequently found in older persons and may be due to living alone or a reduced interest in and desire for food. In others, the malnutrition may be attributed to an inadequate income, limited cooking facilities and refrigeration, ill health or the lack of dentures.

In order to keep tissue destruction to a minimum, emphasis is placed on high-protein foods, fresh fruits and vegetables in the older person's diet. Vitamin supplements and a protein concentrate preparation added to liquids may be necessary for a period of time to make up deficiences and meet the daily requirements. The nurse may have to combat anorexia with frequent small servings, by determining and respecting the patient's food choices if possible, and by feeding the patient. If he is ambulatory, the meals may be more appealing and pleasant if arrangements are made to have him eat with others. If dentures are posing a problem, the dietary department is advised so that the meat is minced and other foods are appropriately prepared.

The inadequate fluid intake which is common in illness and the somewhat decreased salivary secretion in the aged readily lead to dryness of the mouth and tongue and an accumulation of tenacious offensive matter (sordes). Frequent care is necessary to keep the mouth moist and clean and to prevent parotitis. Infection and inflammation of a parotid gland is a complication that may occur, particularly in older persons, if good oral hygiene is not maintained.

If constipation is a problem, more roughage, bulky foods and fluids are gradually introduced in the diet to regulate bowel elimination. If a laxative is needed, the patient receives a bulk-forming laxative, such as a psyllium seed preparation (Metamucil), or a lubricant, such as mineral oil. The latter preparation is used for only a brief period, since it may prevent the absorption of the fat-soluble vitamins. Dependence upon the continuous use of any laxative should be discouraged.

In preparation for the patient's discharge from the hospital, he should receive counseling as to his nutritional needs and the selection, purchase and preparation of foods in accordance with his circumstances. Since it is difficult for an older person to remember, written suggestions and pamphlets on recommended dietary allowances should be provided. A referral may be made to the local welfare department or Visiting Nursing Association so that some guidance may be provided when he goes home.

As cited previously, the elderly person may develop dehydration very quickly. An explanation of the importance of fluid, the frequent offering of small amounts and giving the patient his choice may be helpful in having him take an adequate amount. The older person will often take twice as much water if it is not ice cold.

Urinary System. Sclerosed areas in the kidneys may develop as a result of a decrease in the renal blood supply. The ability of the kidneys to concentrate wastes may be reduced, and they require solids to be well diluted for elimination. The bladder loses some of its tone and may not be completely emptied during voiding. The residual urine undergoes some decomposition which predisposes to bladder inflammation and infection; the urea releases ammonia which accounts for the ammoniacal odor which is characteristic of some old persons' urine. Frequency and incontinence are common problems, particularly in illness, and can be embarrassing to the patient and may lead to social withdrawal.

IMPLICATIONS FOR NURSING. The reduced ability of the kidneys to concentrate wastes indicates the need for a minimum of 1500 to 2000 ml. of fluid per day. Because of the urgency and frequency of urination, the ambulatory patient should be placed near the bathroom. If incontinency develops, it may be necessary to introduce an indwelling catheter in order to protect the patient's skin and to keep him comfortable. Prolonged use of the retention catheter is discouraged, since it is likely to cause irritation of the urethral and bladder mucosa. While it is being used, the fluid intake is increased to 2500 to 3000 ml. daily, unless contraindicated, to reduce the predisposition to infection and the formation of urinary calculi. The catheter is usually kept clamped and opened only at stated intervals for drainage. Continuous drainage of the bladder promotes loss of muscle tone, making re-establishment of normal voluntary control more difficult. When the catheter is removed, the patient is placed on the bedpan or the toilet at regular, frequent intervals to avoid incontinence. The intervals are gradually increased, and as the patient's general condition improves and he is more secure, the normal conditioned reflex and voluntary control are likely to be resumed.

Understanding and patience are necessary on the part of the nurse with the patient who experiences frequency or incontinence. Manifestations of displeasure and impatience only create more anxiety for the patient which in turn further aggravates the problem.

When the patient is incontinent, the skin should be cleansed and the bedding changed promptly. The skin may be protected by the application of a protective cream or lotion or a moisture repellant powder following each voiding and cleansing.

Reproductive System. The earliest senescent changes in the female occur in the reproductive organs. Ovulation and menstruation cease and there are changes in the concentrations of sex hormones. The vaginal mucosa becomes thinner, dry and less resistant to infection.

Reproductive ability persists to a much later age in the male; atrophy of the testicles occurs at a later age than atrophy of the ovaries. The older male may experience hypertrophy of the prostate gland which leads to difficulty in voiding and incomplete emptying of the bladder.

IMPLICATIONS FOR NURSING. Careful cleansing and frequent bathing of the female perineal area provides protection against infection. Patients are urged to have a complete physical examination annually and given assistance in arranging for it if necessary.

Skin. The older person's skin is dry, thin and wrinkled and, as a result, is easily damaged by pressure, chemicals and trauma. Loss of elastic and subcutaneous fatty tissue causes flabbiness and wrinkles. Diminished secretions due to atrophy of the sebaceous and sweat glands contribute to the dryness. Pigmented areas frequently appear on exposed areas. The superficial blood vessels are less efficient in dilating and contracting to regulate body temperature. As a result, in hot weather heat dissipation is poor, and when exposed to cold, the body is not as capable of conserving heat. Local sensation of heat, pressure and painful stimuli may be less acute and are not as reliable in initiating protective reflexes and responses.

Fingernails and toenails tend to thicken and become brittle. The hair loses its color and tends to become dry and thin.

IMPLICATIONS FOR NURSING. The skin of the elderly patient requires special attention because of the changes associated with the aging process. Daily bathing may be inadvisable because of the dryness. A mild soap is used sparingly, and lanolin or an oil is applied after bathing. Bony prominences and pressure areas are massaged gently every 2 or 3 hours and are examined for any indication of pressure sores or trauma. Frequent changes of position, prompt changing of soiled linen and cleansing of the patient following incontinence, placement of a sheepskin pad under pressure areas, and the use of an alternating air pressure mattress (ripple mattress) contribute to keeping the skin intact and in good condition when the patient is confined to bed.

Soaking of the feet in warm water followed by an application of lanolin or oil will soften and remove much of the hard, dry scaly skin that tends to accumulate. The oil softens the nails, making it easier and safer to cut them.

If local heat applications are used, special precautions are necessary to avoid burns because of the reduced sensitivity. Exposure to extremes of temperature should be avoided. In hot weather, the patient's activity is kept to a minimum, and the room temperature is controlled as much as possible. The older person is more sensitive to cold; he produces less body heat and is less able to conserve body heat. In a room temperature which others find comfortable, he may be chilly. For this reason, the older patient usually requires warm clothing and more bed covers, which should be of light weight.

Skin wounds heal more slowly and are more easily infected in the aged because of the reduced blood supply to the area and the lower general resistance. Aseptic care of wounds and good nutrition play an important role in preventing infection and promoting healing.

Musculoskeletal System. The bones become more brittle in the later span of life. There is a reduction in the organic material and some demineralization usually takes place as a result of the changes in the concentration of some endocrine secretions. These alterations in bone structure increase the incidence of fractures in older people. Joint action may become restricted to varying degrees because of degeneration of the cartilage on the ends of weight-bearing bones, arthritis, the formation of adhesions or calcium deposits. The intervertebral discs undergo some atrophy and the vertebrae tend to flatten. As a result the older person loses height.

There is a decreased strength and some slowing of response in the muscles. If the person remains active, the muscle tissue shows some atrophy but remains relatively strong. Disuse of the muscles leads to fatty infiltration and marked weakness.

IMPLICATIONS FOR NURSING. Since the elderly tend to fall more readily and their bones fracture easily, their environment and activities are controlled as much as possible to prevent accidents. The patient should be well oriented to his surroundings, which should be well lighted. A light left burning at night so that he can readily find his way to the bathroom if ambulatory or the provision of a commode at the bedside may prevent a fall. Crib sides on the bed may be necessary to lessen the danger of the patient falling out of bed or getting up when his condition does not permit ambulation. Lowering of the bed and removal of the casters also contribute to preventing accidents. The use of scatter rugs is avoided and foot stools or other pieces of furniture over which the patient might trip or stumble are removed.

Overweight in the elderly is to be avoided, as cited previously. As well as hastening degenerative changes in the joints, it can make mobility and activity practically impossible for the patient.

The nurse has to be understanding and patient with the slower responses and movements of the older person and also help the family to accept the change.

Exercise and activity are encouraged within the limitations imposed by the older patient's physical condition. The family and friends frequently require guidance in relation to this; with the very best intentions, they may foster inactivity and its undesirable results by waiting on the older person and discouraging self-care and participation in other forms of activity. If left to simply rest in bed or a chair, the person regresses mentally and physically.

Muscle contractures, deformities and restricted joint movement will develop rapidly in the older patient unless emphasis is placed on daily exercises. Passive movement of the head and limbs through their normal range by the nurse may be necessary if the patient is too ill or weak to carry out the exercises. It must be remembered that in taking the joints through their range of motion the movement is not forced beyond the range of comfort. Many of these patients may have some permanent joint changes which restrict the range of motion.

Special Senses. The refractive ability of the eyes is reduced because of changes in the lens. The elderly person develops farsightedness and experiences narrowing of the visual field and diminished visual acuity. Adaptation in dimly lit and darkened rooms is lost and may lead to the person tripping over objects, such as stools or chairs, and injury.

Atrophy of the auditory nerve occurs in varying degrees. Acuity for higher pitched tones is lost first. As the ability to communicate is progressively impaired; the older person's interests become limited and he tends to isolate himself socially.

A dulling of temperature perception and a decrease in the speed of the withdrawl reflex may result in burns. For example, an older person may not recognize that a hot water bottle that has been applied is excessively hot. Similarly, pain perception may be decreased; for this reason, lack of the complaint of pain or the severity of pain described is not always dependable for it may not necessarily correspond to the degree of severity of the causative pathological process. For example, a myocardial infarction may occur in an aged person without any complaint of the chest pain which is considered practically a classical characteristic of such an episode in a middle-aged person.

IMPLICATIONS FOR NURSING. Impaired vision places further emphasis on the need for repeated and thorough orientation of the patient to his surroundings. Good lighting is necessary, particularly for any close work or reading. For suggestions as to how those with impaired vision or hearing may be helped, please see Chapters 26 and 27.

In relation to the possible decrease in perception of temperature and pain, greater precautions are necessary in the use of heat applications and baths, and it must be kept in mind that the patient's condition may be more serious than is indicated by his complaints.

Psychological Changes. Some degree of organic cerebral change is associated with the aging process, but any change in personality or regression in cerebral activity varies greatly from one individual to another. Most aging minds show some loss of memory for recent events, slower comprehension, and a shorter span of concentration. Learning ability may be sustained to a surprising level if the person's interest and desire to learn are high.

One sees many variants; in addition to the pleasant, alert, elderly persons who adjust readily, there are some who are unhappy, irascible, complaining and aggressive. Many of the emotional disturbances and personality differences seen are functional and are not due to organic brain changes. In many instances, they are due to the unfortunate social and economic conditions imposed on the elderly by present-day society. Forced retirement, inadequate income, the current social attitude of society which depreciates the worth of older citizens, and the loss of close family members and friends are factors that contribute to changes in the behavior of many elderly persons. They may not be consulted or allowed to make decisions in spite of the fact that many older persons have developed greater understanding, foresight and a more balanced senses of values through the experiences in years of living. Occasionally one hears an elderly person say, "No one cares what I think or how I feel. I am completely ignored and expected to passively accept others' decisions." Just as in earlier years, these persons have the need for recognition, affection, achievement and some degree of independence. Enforced dependence and loss of self-esteem often lead to introversion; the person withdraws, isolates himself and lives in the past. Most older people tend to feel secure in their established pattern of living and resist new ideas and changes.

IMPLICATIONS FOR NURSING. Physical care alone is not adequate for the elderly; they require respect, a voice in matters which concern them and meaningful activity to contribute to an incentive for living. It is important that the nurse understand that many of the emotional disturbances seen in older persons are due only in part to organic aging changes.

As with all patients, each aged person is assessed carefully by the nurse; his reactions to the circumstances, interests and mental and physical capacities are noted. The psychological status, obviously, will influence the amount of protective care required and the necessary precautions for safety. An atmosphere of acceptance and respect is reassuring to the patient. When change is necessary, it is explained, discussed, and when possible introduced gradually. The older person's wishes and pattern of living are given consideration, and unnecessary rigidity in routines should be avoided. By discussing his care with him, respect for the patient's years and individuality is manifested; by showing this respect, the nurse may avoid the reaction of resentment toward the young taking over. Enforced and abrupt change threatens and antagonizes the older patient. Use of the proper form of address and using the patient's name indicate respect for his identity.

When his physical condition permits, an effort is made to promote the patient's interests and to encourage activity and socialization with others.

Medications and the Elderly

Reduced efficiency in metabolism, renal excretion and circulation in older persons results in a decreased tolerance for many drugs, particularly when they are given in the average adult dosage. Detoxification of drugs by the liver may be incomplete and may occur at a much slower rate. The products may be retained in the blood for a longer period before being eliminated in the urine. A cumulative effect develops more often in the elderly, and they may build up a concentration that exceeds the maximum dose. In some instances, a delayed reaction occurs as the result of impaired circulation.

Drug reaction is less predictable than with younger persons. For this reason, these patients are observed closely following the administration of drugs. Sedatives, such as barbiturates, and analgesics, such as opiates, may cause excitement and confusion in some while others may experience respiratory depression and such sound sleep that the resulting immobility predisposes to circulatory stasis and pressure sores. Usually smaller doses of narcotics and sedatives are used for the aged.

Older patients are frequently required to continue drug therapy at home following discharge from the hospital. Schwartz et al. found a high incidence of errors in self-administration of drugs among elderly patients. They found an average of 1.5 errors were made by each of the 178 older persons studied.[3] The errors included omission of the drug and incorrect dosage, frequency and timing. Many of the patients lack accurate knowledge as to the purpose of the drug; others may have wrong information. Self-medication presents a problem among older patients; the dangers and ineffectiveness of patent and unprescribed medicines need greater emphasis. Their use usually results in a serious delay in getting proper attention. These factors have implications for the hospital and visiting nurses. Hospital patients who are to continue a medication after discharge should receive a clear, simple explanation of its purpose, the importance of taking it as prescribed, what may happen if it is omitted and how the supply may be renewed if it is to be continued. Labels and directions for dosage, frequency and method of taking the drug should be clearly written and reviewed with the patient. Some patients

[3]D. Schwartz, B. Henley, and L. Zeitz: The Elderly Ambulatory Patient—Nursing and Psychosocial Needs. New York, The MacMillan Co., 1964, pp. 110–113.

responsible for self-administration of drugs require a calendar and time sheet drawn up that will be helpful in reminding them to take the medication. Encouraging the patient to immediately record the taking of his drug may avoid repetition and a toxic dose. If there are family members, one of them should also receive the instructions. A referral may be made to the Visiting Nurse Association so that the patient will receive supervision.

Convalescence and Rehabilitation

The convalescent period following an illness is likely to be longer for the aged than for younger persons. The patient is likely to become discouraged because it takes him longer to regain his strength. As well as to counteract the undesirable physiological effects of bed rest, early ambulation is promoted to improve the older person's morale. Once he is allowed up he is likely to be more optimistic about his recovery.

Many of the elderly persons seen by nurses have been socially isolated and emotionally starved prior to their illness. As the patient's physical condition improves, nursing care is planned and implemented to promote activities and mental and physical independence within the limits imposed by aging and health status. Interests are determined, and mobility and socialization are encouraged. Suggestions are made to the patient and family as to the activities, interests and sources of assistance that may help to make the older person's life more useful and satisfying and to counteract the apathy, depression and complete dependence so frequently seen. A few simple adjustments such as hand rails on the wall and the side of the bathtub and a seat in the tub may permit self-care. Most communities now have organized health and social services for senior citizens, but many older persons require information about these services and assistance in making the initial contact with them.

References

NURSING CHILDREN

BOOKS

Armstrong, I. L., and Browder, J. J.: The Nursing Care of Children. Philadelphia, F. A. Davis Co., 1964. Chapters 1, 2, 3, 4 and 5.

Blake, F. G., and Wright, F. H.: Essentials of Pediatric Nursing, 7th ed. Philadelphia, J. B. Lippincott Co., 1963.

Bowley, A. H.: The Psychological Care of the Child in Hospital. London, E. & S. Livingstone Ltd., 1961.

Clements, F. W., and McCloskey, B. P.: Child Health, Its Origins and Promotion. London, Edward Arnold (Publisher) Ltd., 1964.

Dimock, H. G.: The Child in Hospital. Toronto, MacMillan Co. of Canada, 1959.

Latham, H. C., and Heckel, R. V.: Pediatric Nursing. Saint Louis, The C. V. Mosby Co., 1967. Chapter 13.

Marlow, D. R.: Pediatric Nursing, 3rd ed. Philadelphia, W. B. Saunders Co., 1969. Chapters 2, 3, 4 and 26.

Nelson, W. E. (Ed.): Textbook of Pediatrics, 9th ed. Philadelphia, W. B. Saunders Co., 1969. pp. 1–13 and 186–194.

Robertson, J.: Young Children in Hospitals. New York, Basic Books Inc., 1958.

PERIODICALS

Gallagher, J. R. (Ed.): Symposium—"The Medical Care of the Adolescent." Med. Clin. North Amer., Vol. 49, No. 2 (March 1965).

Lovelock, P. A.: "Sick Children at Home." Canad. Nurse, Vol. 61, No. 8 (August 1965), pp. 623–627.

Sparks, L.: "Humpty Dumpty Goes to Hospital." Canad. Nurse, Vol. 64, No. 3 (March 1968), pp. 34–36.

NURSING OLDER PEOPLE

BOOKS

Moss, B. B.: Caring for the Aged. New York, Doubleday & Co. Inc., 1966.

Newton, K., and Anderson, H. C.: Geriatric Nursing, 4th ed. Saint Louis, The C. V. Mosby Co., 1966.

Rudd, T. N.: The Nursing of the Elderly Sick, 5th ed. London, Faber and Faber Ltd., 1966.

Schwartz, D., Henley, B., and Leitz, L.: The Elderly Ambulatory Patient—Nursing and Psychosocial Needs. New York, The MacMillan Co., 1964.

Stieglitz, E. J.: The Second Forty Years, 3rd ed. Philadelphia, J. B. Lippincott Co., 1952.

PERIODICALS

Bier, R.: "Motivation of the Chronically Ill Aged Patient." (Clinical Session—American Nurses' Convention, 1962.) New York, American Nurses' Association.

Hulicka, I. M.: "Fostering Self-Respect in Aged Patients." Amer. J. Nurs., Vol. 64, No. 3 (March 1964), pp. 84–89.

Lane, H. C. (Ed.): "Symposium on Care of the Elderly Patient." Nurs. Clin. North Amer., Vol. 3, No. 4 (December 1968), pp. 649–748.

MacDonald, R. I.: "The Care of Older People." Med. Clin. North Amer., March 1952, pp. 569–583.

"The Aged in Our Society." (A series of articles.) Nurs. Outlook, Vol. 12, No. 11 (November 1964).

Part II

12
Nursing in Blood Dyscrasias

COMPOSITION AND PHYSIOLOGY OF BLOOD

Blood is a red fluid tissue that is pumped through the vascular system by the heart. It transports cellular requirements and products from one part of the body to another. There is a continuous exchange between the fluid surrounding the cells and the blood; this exchange serves to maintain a suitable cellular environment that varies only within narrow limits.

Blood is opaque and has a viscosity about 3 to 4 times that of water. Its color is dependent on the pigment in the hemoglobin of the red blood cells and varies with the amount of oxygen combined with the hemoglobin. A higher concentration of oxygen produces a brighter red. Blood has a slightly alkaline reaction, with a pH of 7.35 to 7.40. The average volume in the adult is 5 to 6 L. or approximately 70 to 75 ml. per kg. of body weight. The volume remains remarkably constant.

FUNCTIONS OF THE BLOOD

The blood performs several main functions:

1. Transportation of oxygen from the lungs to the cells and carbon dioxide from the tissues to the lungs for excretion.

2. Transportation of absorbed nutrients from the alimentary tract to the cells.

3. Conveyance of metabolic wastes from the cells to the organs of excretion (kidneys, lungs, liver and skin).

4. Maintenance of a normal interstitial fluid volume. The interstitial fluid is the medium of exchange between the blood and the cells. Unless its volume is kept relatively constant, the concentration of solutes may be so altered that the passage of substances in and out of the cells is affected.

5. Distribution of hormones and other endogenous chemicals that regulate many body activities.

6. Transference of heat from the site of production to the surface of the body where it can be dissipated.

7. Protection of the individual against excessive loss of blood by coagulation and against injurious agents, such as bacteria and toxins, by its leukocytes and antibodies.

BLOOD COMPONENTS

Fifty-five per cent of the blood is a straw-colored fluid called plasma in which the formed elements of the blood (blood cells and platelets) are suspended.

145

Plasma

The constituents of plasma are water (90 to 91 per cent) and a wide variety of solutes. The latter include all the substances which cells take in and use as well as many substances produced by the cells. Examples are the nutrients (amino acids, glucose and lipids); the gases (oxygen and carbon dioxide); electrolytes and salts; and cell products such as hormones, enzymes, urea, uric acid and creatinine. In addition, there are also blood proteins, anticoagulants, clotting factors and antibodies.

The concentration of the solutes remains relatively constant even though water and solutes are continually being added and removed. There are temporary variations, but under normal conditions, certain complex interactions and mechanisms function quickly to restore the plasma to normal. A good example of a quick readjustment that is made to preserve constancy is the maintenance of the plasma concentration of glucose between 80 to 120 mg. per cent. Following a meal, the blood sugar becomes elevated, but within one to two hours the level returns to normal, owing mainly to liver cells removing glucose, converting it to glycogen and storing it. Conversely, much of the plasma glucose may be removed into the cells to be oxidized to produce energy, but a normal concentration in the plasma is maintained by the conversion of glycogen to glucose in the storage depots and its release into the blood.

Four types of proteins comprise the greater part of the solutes of the plasma. These are referred to as the plasma or blood proteins and are serum albumin, serum globulin, fibrinogen, and prothrombin. The normal concentration of the plasma proteins is about 6 to 8 Gm. per cent. They are large in molecular structure and do not readily diffuse through the capillary walls. The resulting concentration of these nondiffusible substances within the capillaries is responsible for what is referred to as the colloidal osmotic pressure of the plasma. A pressure gradient results between the tissue fluid and the blood that promotes the movement of the fluid from the interstitial spaces back into the capillaries (see p. 50). An abnormal decrease in the plasma proteins, especially albumin, reduces the colloidal osmotic pressure, resulting in an accumulation of fluid in the tissues known as edema. The proteins contribute to the viscosity of the blood which influences circulation and blood pressure.

The plasma proteins are formed from the amino acids of ingested foods but in protein starvation they may be synthesized from tissue protein. Serum albumin, fibrinogen and prothrombin are formed by the liver. Albumin, because of its greater molecular weight, functions mainly in producing the colloidal osmotic pressure. Fibrinogen and prothrombin are concerned with the blood clotting process; their role in this is discussed on page 155.

Serum globulin is produced by reticuloendothelial cells (phagocytic cells of spleen, lymph nodes, liver and bone marrow) and may be separated into three fractions—the alpha, beta, and gamma globulins. The gamma globulin fraction contains antibodies. For this reason it may be administered to provide a temporary immunity against measles or other infections.

In summary, the functions of the plasma proteins are as follows:

1. They exert an intravascular osmotic pressure that influences fluid exchange between the interstitial and intravascular compartments.

2. Fibrinogen and prothrombin play a role in blood coagulation which protects the individual from an excessive loss of blood.

3. Serum globulin provides antibodies protecting the individual against microbial agents and their toxins.

4. At the site of inflammation or injury, fibrinogen forms a medium in which the various tissues can grow and repair themselves. (See Tissue Repair, p. 34).

5. Plasma proteins provide viscosity to the blood.

6. In starvation, the plasma proteins may be broken down and used as a source of amino acids for the tissues.

7. Plasma proteins will combine with both alkalis and acids and can act as buffers to maintain a normal pH of body fluids. They may accept hydrogen ions from acids or, when necessary, donate hydrogen ions to reduce excessive alkalinity.

Formed Elements of the Blood

The formed elements include the red blood cells (erythrocytes), the white blood

TABLE 12–1 COMPOSITION OF BLOOD

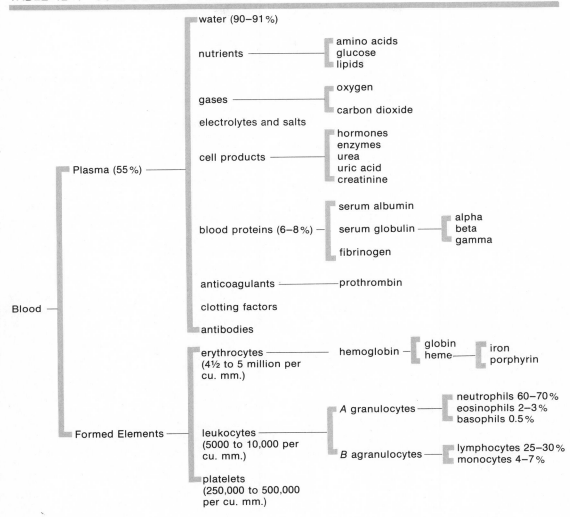

cells (leukocytes) and the blood platelets (thrombocytes).

Erythrocytes. The normal red blood cell is an elastic biconcave disk. The blood nor-

TABLE 12–2 NORMAL VALUES OF THE PLASMA PROTEINS

	GRAMS PER CENT
Total plasma proteins	6–8
Albumin	4.05
Globulins	2.5
alpha globulin	0.46
beta globulin	0.86
gamma globulin	0.75
Fibrinogen	0.3

mally contains approximately 4.5 to 5.0 million erythrocytes per cu. mm. Each cell has a nucleus when first formed, but the normal mature circulating erythrocyte is devoid of a nucleus.

The function of red blood cells, by virtue of their composition, is the transportation of oxygen and carbon dioxide between the tissues and the lungs. The major constituent of the cell is hemoglobin, which is made up of the protein globin and an iron-containing pigment called heme. Heme is formed by the union of iron and the pigment porphyrin; four molecules of heme combine with one molecule of globin to form hemoglobin. Oxygen has an affinity for this compound; four molecules of oxygen combine

TABLE 12–3 FORMATION OF RED BLOOD CELLS (ERYTHROPOIESIS)

STAGES OF DEVELOPMENT	DESCRIPTION
Stem cell ↓	
Hemocytoblast ↓	A large, undifferentiated, nucleated cell that divides by mitosis into 2 proery-throblasts.
Proerythroblast ↓	A nucleated cell with no hemoglobin that divides into 2 smaller nucleated cells.
Early normoblast ↓	A nucleated cell with no hemoglobin that divides into 2 cells. The nucleus is smaller than it was in the previous stage and the cytoplasm is more abundant.
Intermediate normoblast ↓	A nucleated cell that does not divide. The nucleus becomes smaller and more dense, and a small amount of hemoglobin appears.
Late normoblast ↓	A cell in which the nucleus becomes fragmented and disintegrates as the hemoglobin content of the cytoplasm increases.
Reticulocyte ↓	A non-nucleated cell with an increased amount of hemoglobin. The cytoplasm has a reticular (network of strands) appearance due to the products of the disintegrated nucleus.
Erythrocyte	The mature red blood cell from which the nuclear remnants have disappeared. It is almost completely filled with hemoglobin and is released into the blood stream.

with one molecule of hemoglobin to form oxyhemoglobin. Approximately one Gm. of hemoglobin combines with 1.3 ml. of oxygen. This is a loose combination, so when there is little or no free oxygen in the red cells' environment (plasma), oxygen is freed from the red blood cell and diffuses out of the cell into the plasma, leaving what is known as reduced oxyhemoglobin.

Hemoglobin is produced by the red blood cells themselves before they are released into the circulation from their source of production, the red bone marrow. Because of its pigment content, the hemoglobin gives the red color to the blood. The normal concentration of hemoglobin is 14 to 16 Gm. per 100 ml. of blood. It is slightly higher in men than in women.

PRODUCTION OF ERYTHROCYTES (ERYTHROPOIESIS*). After birth, erythrocytes are produced exclusively by the red bone marrow. Prenatally, in the developing organism, they are first produced by the yolk sac and then by the liver in the second to fifth months. During the remaining months the red bone marrow develops and gradually takes over the role. During infancy and childhood most of the bones contain red bone marrow that participates in erythropoiesis. When the growth process is completed, the red blood cells are produced by

the red bone marrow of the skull bones, vertebrae, ribs, sternum, pelvis and proximal ends of the femora and humeri.

The red blood cells, and the white blood cells produced by the marrow, develop from common primitive stem cells which differentiate to become either red or white blood cells. In erythropoiesis, the stem cell forms a hemocytoblast which goes through a series of nuclear and cytoplasmic changes, becoming progressively smaller. These changes are outlined in Table 12-3 and comprise what is referred to as the maturation process of red blood cells.

FACTORS IN ERYTHROPOIESIS. Under normal conditions the rate of production and maturation of red blood cells approximates the rate of removal of the old cells from the circulation and their destruction. The red blood cell count and the amount of hemoglobin remain relatively constant — sufficient to meet the tissues' oxygen needs but, at the same time, controlled in order to prevent a concentration of cells that would impede the blood flow.

The oxygen concentration of the blood is the essential factor regulating the production of erythrocytes. If the rate of cell destruction is increased or if there is a loss of red blood cells as in hemorrhage, there is a prompt increase in erythropoiesis if the bone marrow is normal and the essential substances are available. At high altitudes where the oxygen concentration of the air is

---

Poiesis is the Greek word meaning formation or production.

low, the body compensates by producing more red blood cells. The red bone marrow does not respond directly to the hypoxemia (lowered concentration of oxygen in the blood). The stimulation is mediated through a substance called erythropoietin, or hemopoietin, that is produced by body tissues in response to the hypoxemia. The exact source of erythropoietin is not known, but both the kidneys and the liver have been suggested.

Protein, iron, vitamin B_{12} (cyanocobalamin), folic acid (pteroylglutamic acid—a member of the vitamin B complex) and traces of copper must be available to the bone marrow to insure an adequate production of normal erythrocytes. Protein is a necessary element in the structure of the cell and its hemoglobin. Iron is essential for the formation of hemoglobin. Only a limited amount of iron is absorbed from the small intestine; it is then loosely combined with a protein (apoferritin) to form ferritin which is stored in the intestinal mucosa and liver. Ferritin is released as iron is needed by the bone marrow. Much of the iron used in the formation of hemoglobin is derived from the breakdown of worn-out erythrocytes. Only a small amount of dietary iron is necessary to maintain that required under normal circumstances. Since an excess of absorbed iron cannot be eliminated, its absorption is controlled by the small intestine; that is, the mucosa rejects or absorbs iron according to the rate of use. If erythropoiesis is increased—as it is in hemorrhage, pregnancy or other conditions causing hypoxemia—more iron is absorbed. In persons who have a normal hemoglobin concentration and a normal amount of iron in storage, extra dietary iron and medicinal iron preparations do not increase the absorption; the excess iron is simply eliminated in the feces. With increased demands on the bone marrow, the iron stored in the intestinal mucosa and liver is reduced, and absorption by the intestine is increased accordingly.

Vitamin B_{12}, which is referred to as the extrinsic factor or antianemic factor, is essential to normal erythropoiesis. It acts as a catalyst, promoting the synthesis of nucleic acids to form normal red blood cells. It is especially abundant in liver and red meats and is only absorbed in the presence of a factor or enzyme which is secreted by the gastric mucosa and is known as the intrinsic factor. The vitamin is then stored in the liver and released as it is needed. In the absence of either the extrinsic factor or the intrinsic factor, the number of erythrocytes is reduced, and many that are in circulation are abnormal. Normoblasts do not divide as many times but grow larger and may contain a greater amount of hemoglobin than normal. These large cells are called macrocytes. There may also be large, primitive, nucleated cells in circulation that are known as megaloblasts.

Folic acid (pteroylglutamic acid), acting as a catalyst, also influences the production and maturation of erythroblasts and is sometimes used in the treatment of a deficiency of red blood cells. The richest dietary sources of this vitamin are liver, kidney and fresh green vegetables.

Traces of copper are essential to serve as a catalyst for the absorption of iron and its utilization in the formation of hemoglobin.

LIFE SPAN AND NORMAL DESTRUCTION OF ERYTHROCYTES. The average length of life of the red blood cells is 120 days. As the cell ages, the continuous friction between the blood cells and against the vessel walls weakens the cell membrane, and it eventually ruptures. The cell fragments are engulfed by macrophages (large phagocytic cells of the reticuloendothelial tissues) in the liver and spleen. The hemoglobin, which comprised most of the cell substance, is broken down; the globin and iron fractions are reclaimed for use. The porphyrin molecules are converted to bilirubin and excreted in bile.

Leukocytes. The white blood cells are less numerous and larger than the erythrocytes, and they have nuclei. There are several types, which differ in structure, origin, function and staining reaction. Normally, the blood contains 5000 to 10,000 per cu. mm. The count tends to be lower after a period of rest and increases following a meal or activity. There is a rapid increase to above normal in most infections in defense of the body. The term leukocytosis is applied to an increase above the normal number of white blood cells. A decrease in the white blood cells below the normal is called leukopenia.

TYPES OF LEUKOCYTES. The leukocytes may be divided into two major groups on the basis of whether their cytoplasm is granular or nongranular.

Granulocytes. The granulocytes are formed in the red bone marrow and have lobulated nuclei. Three types are recognized by the staining quality of their cytoplasm. The neutrophils stain with a neutral dye, and their nuclei may have several lobes. The latter characteristic results in the neutrophils also being called polymorphonuclear leukocytes. They may comprise 60 to 70 per cent of the total white blood cells.

Eosinophils stain with eosin, a red acid dye, and normally constitute about 2 to 3 per cent of the white blood cells.

About 0.4 per cent of the total leukocytes stain with basic dyes and are called basophils.

Agranulocytes. The white blood cells with agranular cytoplasm are of two types — lymphocytes and monocytes. The lymphocytes are smaller than the granulocytes and have a large spherical nucleus that fills most of the cell. They are produced in the lymphoid tissue (lymph nodes, spleen, tonsils and thymus). Twenty-five to 30 per cent of the total white blood cells are lymphocytes.

The monocytes are larger than the lymphocytes and have a kidney-shaped nucleus. Differing opinions exist regarding their origin; Guyton states that they are produced by lymphoid tissue,[1] Green attributes their production to bone marrow,[2] and Chaffee and Greisheimer indicate that both marrow and lymphoid tissue (especially the spleen) are responsible for the origin of monocytes.[3] They form 4 to 7 per cent of the leukocytes.

LEUKOCYTE COUNT. When a white blood cell count is requested, an estimation is made of the total number of cells per cu. mm. (as cited previously, the normal is 5000 to 10,000 per cu. mm.). Frequently, a differential white cell count is done, since it is known that certain types of cells are increased in certain disease conditions. For example, in acute infections, the neutrophils increase rapidly; in chronic infections, the lymphocytes are increased; the number of monocytes are increased in protozoal infections such as malaria; and the eosinophil

---

[1] A. C. Guyton: Textbook of Medical Physiology, 4th ed., Philadelphia: W. B. Saunders Co., 1971, p. 110.

[2] J. H. Green: An Introduction to Human Physiology, 2nd ed. London, Oxford University Press, 1968, p. 14.

[3] E. E. Chaffee, and E. M. Greisheimer: Basic Physiology and Anatomy, 2nd ed. Philadelphia, J. B. Lippincott Co., 1969, p. 305.

TABLE 12–4 TYPES AND AVERAGE PERCENTAGES OF LEUKOCYTES[4]

	PER CENT
Granulocytes	
Neutrophils	62.0
Eosinophils	2.3
Basophils	0.4
Agranulocytes	
Lymphocytes	30.0
Monocytes	5.3

[4]Guyton, op. cit.

count is known to rise in allergic reactions and with parasitic invasion of the body. In a differential count the percentage of the various types of leukocytes is determined.

The various types of white blood cells are produced by the stem cells in the blood cell-forming organs in three primitive forms — the myeloblasts, monoblasts and lymphoblasts. The myeloblast is nongranular and the nucleus is not divided into lobules. Successive changes occur and are characterized by the appearance of granules in the cytoplasm and differentiation of the cell into a neutrophil, basophil or eosinophil. Following this, nuclear changes develop, resulting in lobulation and the release of the cell into the blood. The monoblast undergoes mitotic division to form the promonocyte. The cell remains large and nongranular, but the nucleus changes, becoming oval and then kidney-shaped.

The lymphoblast, although produced in lymphoid tissue, goes through developmental phases comparable to the other leukocytes. The lymphoblast divides by mitosis and the cells progressively become condensed to form mature, small lymphocytes.

FACTORS IN LEUKOPOIESIS. Little is known about the physiological stimulus responsible for the production and maturation of leukocytes. It has been observed that the breakdown of white blood cells is followed by the appearance of numerous young white blood cells in the blood. This suggests that a chemical which stimulates leukopoiesis may be released from the disintegrated cells.

Increased leukopoiesis occurs in infection, hemorrhage and tissue destruction. The nutrients, protein and vitamins which are essential to all cells of the body are necessary for the production of leukocytes. Some

TABLE 12–5   FORMATION OF WHITE BLOOD CELLS (LEUKOPOIESIS)

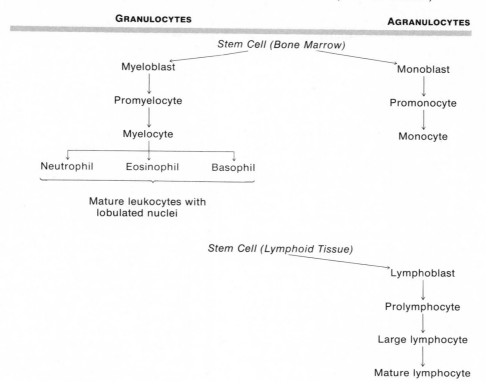

drugs may depress the production of leukocytes; for example, sulfonamides, gold, thiouracil and cortisone preparations may result in a low white blood cell count.

CHARACTERISTICS AND FUNCTIONS OF LEUKOCYTES.   The leukocytes serve as an important body defense. They destroy many injurious factors such as microorganisms and the products of degenerating tissues. This is made possible by certain special properties the cells possess—namely, diapedesis, mobility, chemotaxis and phagocytosis.

Diapedesis is the ability of the leukocytes to squeeze through the capillary walls and escape into the tissues. They are capable of ameboid movement* which takes them through the tissues to the source of irritation. The neutrophils are especially mobile; they are attracted by a chemical substance which is liberated by bacteria or by the irritated tissue cells.

Phagocytosis is the engulfing and digesting

of particles and is the most important function of the neutrophils and monocytes in protecting the body against microorganisms.

LIFE SPAN AND DESTRUCTION OF LEUKOCYTES.   The life span of the white blood cells varies greatly with the body's protective needs and with the types of white cells, ranging from a few hours to as long as 200 days. The granulocytes survive a shorter period than do the agranulocytes. Guyton suggests 14 days as the average life span for granulocytes, but this may be much shorter if there is infection to combat. Many of the lymphocytes have been found to survive 100 to 200 days.[5]

It is thought that the white blood cells that are destroyed or die are disposed of by phagocytosis by the macrophages of the reticuloendothelial tissues.

Blood Platelets (Thrombocytes).   The third and smallest of the formed elements of the blood is the platelet. They are oval, nonnucleated structures, numbering 250,000 to 500,000 per cu. mm. of blood. They are

---

*Ameboid movement is achieved by the cell protruding a protoplasmic extension into which the remaining cell substance streams.

[5]Guyton, op. cit., p. 112.

produced in the red bone marrow by giant cells (megakaryocytes). These large marrow cells extend a part of their membrane, which separates from the parent cell to form a platelet. The platelets tend to adhere readily to foreign substances. Their membrane is thin and fragile and has a negative charge on its outer surface. Normally, the intima of the vessels is also negatively charged; this repels the platelets and keeps them from adhering. When a vessel wall is injured, the endothelial lining at the point of injury loses its charge, platelets strike the area, rupture and adhere, initiating coagulation of the blood at that site.

Platelet production is increased following tissue trauma and destruction and in hypoxemia. It is suggested that, as well as a reduced oxygen concentration of the blood, chemical substances liberated by degenerating or injured tissue stimulate the bone marrow to increase platelet formation.

FUNCTIONS OF BLOOD PLATELETS. The platelets initiate the blood clotting process through their disintegration and release of thromboplastin (platelet-factor) which activates prothrombin (see Coagulation of the Blood, p. 155). On disintegration, they also liberate serotonin (5-hydroxytryptamine) which causes vasoconstriction that, in turn, contributes to reducing the loss of blood when a vessel is interrupted.

With any slight damage to the inner surface of blood vessels, the platelets clump and stick together at the site, helping to plug leaks and prevent loss of blood.

BLOOD GROUPS

Blood may differ from one individual to another according to the presence or absence of specific antigens (agglutinogens) in the red blood cells and the presence or absence of specific, naturally occurring antibodies (agglutinins) in the plasma. For this reason, the blood of a person taken at random cannot be used in transfusion, since the bloods might be of different types and could cause a serious reaction. The blood groups of greatest clinical significance are the ABO and Rh (Rhesus) types.

ABO Blood Groups

In the ABO system, an individual's blood is typed as A, B, AB, or O, depending on the presence or absence of agglutinogens termed A and B in his erythrocytes. If a person has A or B or both A and B agglutinogens, his plasma will not contain antibodies that will agglutinate his own erythrocytes.

In blood that is typed as A, the erythrocytes contain agglutinogens A. The plasma has Anti-B agglutinins which only cause clumping of erythrocytes that have agglutinogens B. Blood that is typed as B has erythrocytes containing agglutinogens B and, in the plasma, Anti-A agglutinins, which only cause clumping of red blood cells with agglutinogen A. In blood that is typed as AB, the erythrocytes bear both agglutinogens A and B. The plasma is free of Anti-A and Anti-B agglutinins; otherwise, the individual's own red cells would be attacked. In blood that is typed as O, both agglutinogens are absent, but the plasma contains both Anti-A and Anti-B agglutinins.

The type of blood is determined by adding specially prepared sera, containing either Anti-A or Anti-B antibodies. The procedure is as follows:

Anti-A serum is added to a sample of the blood to be typed, and if clumping of the red blood cells occurs, the blood is type A.

Anti-B serum is added to a sample of the blood to be typed, and if clumping occurs, the blood is type B.

If clumping of the red cells occurs with the addition of Anti-A and Anti-B sera, the presence of both A and B agglutinogens is indicated, and the blood is type AB.

When there is no agglutination with the addition of either Anti-A or Anti-B serum, it indicates the absence of both A and B agglutinogens in the erythrocytes. The blood type is O.

BLOOD TYPE	AGGLUTINOGEN IN ERYTHROCYTES	AGGLUTININS IN PLASMA	PERCENTAGE OF POPULATION
A	A	Anti-B	42
B	B	Anti-A	9
AB	A and B	—	3
O	—	Anti-A and Anti-B	46

The blood type of a person is determined genetically; a gene received from each parent influences the type of blood of the offspring. The genes for A and B agglutinogens are equally dominant. The genotype of an individual of type A may be AA or AO. With type B, it may be BB or BO. In the case of type AB, it is AB.

Blood Transfusion

When the volume of circulating blood is reduced, the clinical value of the administration of blood donated by another individual is well recognized. The blood used must be of the same type as that of the recipient. If the bloods are not of the same type, the recipient's plasma may contain agglutinins that will clump the red blood cells of the donor's blood. The agglutinated cells may block blood vessels and could prove fatal if the occluded vessels supply vital areas. In a few hours, the clumped cells are destroyed by macrophages (large phagocytic cells) of the reticuloendothelial system, releasing hemoglobin into the plasma. The disintegration of the red cells is referred to as hemolysis. The free hemoglobin in the plasma is treated as foreign protein and is excreted by the kidneys.

The important precaution to be observed in a blood transfusion is to prevent the donation of red blood cells that will be agglutinated by agglutinins in the recipient's plasma. Since type O has neither A nor B agglutinogens, this blood may be given to a recipient of any one of the four types. For this reason, the person of type O is referred to as a universal donor.

Conversely, since an AB type does not have either Anti-A or Anti-B antibodies in his plasma, the individual is considered to be a universal recipient.

The following table indicates possible donors for each blood type in the ABO system.

RECIPIENT	POSSIBLE DONOR
Type A	Types A and O
Type B	Types B and O
Type AB	Types AB, A, B, and O
Type O	Type O

Whenever possible, it is considered safer to use a donor with blood of the same type as that of the person requiring the transfusion. To ensure compatibility of the donor's and recipient's blood, cross-matching is done. A small quantity of each of the bloods is centrifuged in separate tubes. Some of the recipient's cells are added to the donor's serum and vice versa. If no agglutination occurs in 15 minutes, the bloods are considered compatible.

Rhesus (Rh) Blood Groups

This system involves six red blood cell antigens (agglutinogens) which are designated C, D, E, c, d, and e. Varying degrees of antigenicity exist in the group of factors. The D factor is the strongest antigen and is of greatest clinical significance. Approximately 85 per cent of Caucasians possess the D factor and are usually classified as Rh positive. The remaining 15 per cent are said to be Rh negative.

Plasma antibodies (agglutinins) against the D factor do not occur naturally. They only develop in the plasma of Rh(D) negative blood when the D factor is introduced. The Anti-D agglutinins will clump erythrocytes containing the D factor. The formation of Anti-D antibodies may be evoked within an Rh negative person receiving a transfusion of Rh(D) positive blood, or by the development of an Rh(D) positive fetus within an Rh(D) negative mother. In the case of the blood transfusion, usually no clumping of the Rh positive donor's cells in the Rh negative recipient's blood occurs with the first transfusion, because the Anti-D antibodies are developed slowly and may not reach sufficient concentration before the foreign positive cells are terminated. If a second transfusion of Rh(D) positive blood is given, a reaction occurs, causing agglutination of the donor's cells.

When an Rh positive fetus develops within an Rh negative mother, some of the fetal red blood cells, or D factors released by worn-out erythrocytes, pass through the placenta into the maternal circulation. The mother forms Anti-D agglutinins which diffuse into the fetal circulation and cause agglutination of the fetal erythrocytes. The clumped cells are ultimately disintegrated, and the hemoglobin is broken down and converted to bilirubin, causing jaundice (yellowness of the skin and conjunctivae). This condition is known as erythroblastosis fetalis. The destruction of red blood cells may prove fatal to the fetus, depending on the concentration of antibodies that reach

TABLE 12–6 Rh FACTOR: GENETIC POSSIBILITIES FOR AGGLUTINOGEN D

		RH NEGATIVE MOTHER		
		X	X	
RH POSITIVE FATHER (HOMOZYGOUS)	X^D	X^DX	X^DX	OFFSPRING: All heterozygous Rh positive
	Y^D	Y^DX	Y^DX	

		RH NEGATIVE MOTHER		
		X	X	
RH POSITIVE FATHER (HETEROZYGOUS)	X^D	X^DX	X^DX	OFFSPRING: 50 per cent chance of Rh positive; 50 per cent chance of Rh negative
	Y	YX	YX	

		RH NEGATIVE MOTHER		
		X	X	
RH NEGATIVE FATHER (HOMOZYGOUS)	X	XX	XX	OFFSPRING: All Rh negative (The mother will not form antibodies.)
	Y	YX	YX	

Note: The Rh factor (agglutinogen D) is dominant. If the father is Rh positive and the mother is Rh negative, the offspring will be Rh positive and the mother will form antibodies.

the fetal circulation. If the fetus goes to term, at birth the infant will exhibit jaundice, anemia, edema and enlargement of the spleen and liver. Prompt treatment by a series of exchange transfusions is necessary. Compatible Rh negative blood is given. The exchange is made by alternate withdrawal and injection of equal amounts of blood. The first baby sensitizes the Rh negative mother but usually escapes the hemolytic disease. With subsequent pregnancies, the Anti-D agglutinins progressively increase if the fetuses are Rh positive. Immunization of Rh negative persons seems to vary; some develop antibodies more readily than others.

The Rh blood group factors are inherited, and the gene for the D agglutinogen is always dominant. One who is Rh positive may be homozygous (DD), having inherited a gene for the D factor from each parent, or may be heterozygous (D–), having inherited a gene for D from one parent only. The child of an Rh positive father who is homozygous and an Rh negative mother will always be Rh positive because of the dominance of the D factor. The child of an Rh positive father who is heterozygous and an Rh negative mother has a 50 per cent chance of being Rh positive. If the developing organism in utero is Rh negative, there is no problem.

HEMOSTASIS AND BLOOD COAGULATION

Any rupture or severance of a blood vessel is normally followed by certain responses in an effort to reduce the loss of blood. These responses are local vasoconstriction and coagulation of the blood and the formation of scar tissue to close the opening in the vessel. These defense responses occur frequently in the body without the individual being aware of them. During normal day-to-day activities and in minor injuries, minute blood vessels are ruptured and the loss of blood is controlled by these mechanisms. If it is a large vessel, especially an artery, that is interrupted, coagulation and vasoconstriction may not be adequate in checking the bleeding. Ligation, pressure or cautery may have to be used.

Vasoconstriction in Hemostasis

Local vasoconstriction reduces the blood flow to the injured site and is brought about by direct vascular muscular tissue reaction to the injury and by reflex nerve impulses that occur as a result of the trauma to the vessel. In the latter, sensory impulses arising in the injured vascular wall are transmitted into the central nervous system causing impulses to be sent to the musculature of the vessel stimulating contraction. This vascular spasm is augmented by the release of serotonin (5-hydroxytryptamine) by the disintegrating platelets at the site of injury. Serotonin has a local stimulating effect on the vascular muscle.

Blood Coagulation

Coagulation of the blood is the formation of a jelly-like mass in the blood by the conversion of the soluble plasma protein fibrinogen to an insoluble mass of fine threads called fibrin. Blood cells are enmeshed in the fibrin to form the mass known as a clot. The conversion of fibrinogen to fibrin is dependent upon the enzyme thrombin. This enzyme is normally present in the circulating blood in an inactive form known as prothrombin. Vitamin K is essential for the formation of prothrombin by the liver. Its conversion to thrombin depends on the presence of calcium ions and on the enzyme thromboplastin, which is released by disintegrating platelets and damaged tissue cells.

The essential major steps in coagulation are:

1. The release and activation of thromboplastin.

2. The conversion of prothrombin to thrombin by thromboplastin (prothrombin activator) in the presence of calcium ions.

3. The conversion of fibrinogen by thrombin to fibrin.

Blood Clotting Factors. Blood coagulation is a complex process and a large number of factors have been recognized as having some role. The exact function of some factors is not clearly understood, but the absence of any one produces a bleeding tendency. The factors have been numbered to provide a common international nomenclature, but certain synonyms are also applied. The first four factors are the older, well established essentials in coagulation and are still referred to by the names of long standing.

A list of the factors and their role in the blood clotting process is found in Table 12–7.[6]

Normal Anticoagulants. A remarkable property of blood is its ability to remain fluid in the blood vessels; this is necessary

---

[6]Guyton, op. cit., p. 141.

Green, op. cit., p. 15.

E. E. Selkurt (Ed.): Physiology. Boston, Little, Brown and Co., 1963, p. 198.

TABLE 12–7 BLOOD CLOTTING FACTORS AND THEIR ROLES IN BLOOD COAGULATION

Factor	Synonym	Role in Blood Coagulation
I	Fibrinogen	Forms fibrin
II	Prothrombin	Forms thrombin which converts fibrinogen to fibrin
III	Thromboplastin	Converts prothrombin to thrombin
IV	Calcium	Serves as a catalyst in conversion of prothrombin to thrombin
V	Labile factor (accelerator globulin Ac-G, proaccelerin)	Necessary in the formation of active thromboplastin
VII	Proconvertin (stable factor, serum prothrombin conversion accelerator SPCA)	Accelerates the action of tissue thromboplastin
VIII	Antihemophilic factor AHF (antihemophilic globulin AHG)	Promotes the breakdown of thrombocytes and the formation of active platelet thromboplastin
IX	Christmas factor (plasma thromboplastin component PTC)	Similar to Factor VIII
X	Stuart factor	Promotes the action of thromboplastin
XI	Plasma thromboplastin antecedent PTA	Promotes clumping and breakdown of thrombocytes and the release of thromboplastin
XII	Hageman factor	Similar to Factor XI

TABLE 12–8 SCHEMA OF THE CLOTTING PROCESS

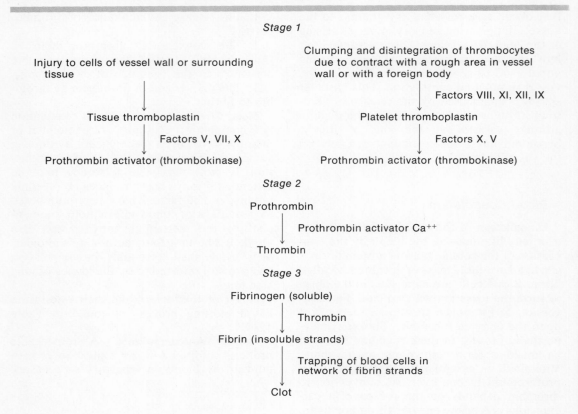

for its circulation. Under normal circumstances, small amounts of thromboplastin are released by the disintegration of some thrombocytes and tissue cells and could initiate coagulation. In order to counteract this, coagulation inhibitors—heparin and antithrombin—are normally present in the plasma.

Large granular cells in the pericapillary connective tissue that are known as mast cells are the principal source of heparin. It inhibits the formation and action of thrombin. If thrombin is produced in relatively small amounts, it is neutralized by antithrombin, an alpha globulin, and the conversion of fibrinogen to fibrin does not take place. The presence of antithrombin and heparin prevent coagulation under normal conditions, but with increased tissue and platelet destruction, the greater concentration of thromboplastin is sufficient to initiate spontaneous coagulation.

Blood that is collected from one person for administration to another is prevented from clotting by the addition of sodium citrate. The citrate combines with the calcium to form insoluble citrate of calcium. Certain blood examinations require that the blood remain fluid; an oxalate, which combines with the calcium, is usually added.

Clot Retraction and Organization. After a clot forms, the fibrin strands shrink and the plasma that was trapped along with the blood cells is extruded. This fluid differs from normal plasma because it lacks fibrinogen; it is referred to as serum. The fibrin strands of the clot attach to the edges of the injured area of the blood vessel; as they shrink, they pull the edges of the opening closer together, helping to check the loss of blood.

The opening in the vessel is repaired by a process called clot organization. Fibroblasts proliferate the clot, and as they mature, the area is filled in by fibrous tissue. Macrophages (large reticuloendothelial phagocytes) clear away the trapped blood cells. Endothelial cells of the intima proliferate to replace the vessel lining in the area.

BLOOD DYSCRASIAS AND DISEASES OF BLOOD-FORMING ORGANS

Blood disorders (dyscrasias) may affect the erythrocytes, leukocytes or the coagulation process. The problem may be due to a defect originating in the blood-forming organs, the deficiency of an essential element, or the abnormal destruction of cells. The disorders may be primary or secondary to another disease.

Blood Investigation Procedures

Common blood studies used in erythrocyte disorders include the following tests:

Red Blood Cell Count. Normal: 4½ to 5 million per cu. mm.

Hemoglobin Content of Erythrocytes. Normal: males, 13 to 15 Gm. per 100 ml.; females, 13 to 14 Gm. per 100 ml.; children (3 months to puberty), 10 to 14 Gm. per 100 ml.

Hematocrit (Packed Cell Volume). The volume of red blood cells in 100 ml. of blood. Normal: males, 45 to 50 ml. per cent; females, 40 to 45 ml. per cent.

Erythrocyte Indices. Mean corpuscular volume (MCV)—average size of individual red cell. Normal: 82 to 92 cu. microns. Mean corpuscular hemoglobin (MCH)—average amount of hemoglobin per red cell. Normal: 29 to 32 micromicrograms. Mean corpuscular hemoglobin concentration (MCHC)—average Gm. of hemoglobin in 100 ml. packed cells. Normal: 30 to 38 Gm. per 100 ml. packed red cells.

Reticulocyte Count. The percentage of circulating red blood cells that are reticulocytes. Normal: 0.5 to 1.0 per cent.

Leukocyte Count. Normal: 5000 to 10,000 per cu. mm.

Differential Leukocyte Count. An estimation of the percentage of the various types of white blood cells that constitute the leukocytes in circulation. Normal: Neutrophils (polymorphonuclear leukocytes) 60 to 70 per cent; Eosinophils 2 to 3 per cent; Basophils 0.4 to 3 per cent; Monocytes 4 to 7 per cent; Lymphocytes 25 to 30 per cent.

Thrombocyte (Blood Platelet) Count. Normal: 250,000 to 500,000 per cu mm.

Urinary Urobilinogen. An estimation of the urobilinogen that is excreted in the urine. It is increased in excessive red blood cell destruction (hemolytic anemia) and liver disease. Normal: present in very small amount (0 to 4 mg. in 24 hours).

Fecal Urobilinogen. An estimation of the amount of urobilinogen that is excreted in the feces. It is increased in excessive red blood cell destruction. Normal: 50 to 300 mg. in 24 hours.

Erythrocyte Fragility. Red blood cells are observed for their reaction and hemolysis in a series of hypotonic sodium chloride solutions of graded tonicity. Some normal cells begin to hemolyze in a solution of approximately 0.5 per cent and practically all are hemolyzed in approximately 0.3 per cent salt solution.

Cells characteristic of a certain hemolytic anemia (spherocytosis) rupture in a higher concentration than do normal cells, indicating increased osmotic fragility.

Bone Marrow Biopsy. The investigation of most blood dyscrasias includes the examination of a specimen of red bone marrow. Smears are made of the marrow specimen and the cells are examined. The number of cells in the various developmental and maturational phases and the size, shape and characteristics of cell content are noted.

The sites used most frequently for marrow biopsy are the sternum and iliac crest. Preparation of the patient involves an explanation of the procedure and its purpose and the shaving and cleansing of the skin over the site to be used.

The area receives an application of an antiseptic and is draped with sterile towels. The physician injects a local anesthetic before introducing the aspiration needle. Considerable pressure is necessary to pass the needle through the cortex of the bone into the marrow space. The stylet is then removed from the needle, and a syringe is attached for the collection of 1 to 2 ml. of marrow. On completion of the procedure, a small sterile dressing is applied to the puncture site.

Coombs' Test. The erythrocytes are examined for the presence of immune bodies (agglutinins) that adhere to the red blood cells and lead to clumping and hemolysis. This is referred to as the direct Coombs test. An indirect method is done on serum to test for the presence of the antibodies to the erythrocyte antigens.

The Coombs' test may be used in identifying a hemolytic anemia or erythroblastosis fetalis.

Lymph Node Biopsy. A tissue specimen of a lymph node that has undergone some change is obtained.

Coagulation Tests. Coagulation or clotting time is the time it takes the blood to clot. Normal: 7 to 12 minutes. Bleeding time: the time it takes bleeding to stop naturally. Normal: 2 to 5 minutes. Prothrombin time: the time it takes for coagulation following the addition of thromboplastin and calcium to the specimen. Normal: 12 to 20 seconds. Fibrinogen level: Normal: 200 mg. per 100 ml. of blood.

Descriptive Terms

Variations in the size, shape and hemoglobin content may occur in red blood cell disorders. Certain descriptive terms are used to denote some of these characteristics.

Erythrocytes that are larger than the normal are referred to as being macrocytes; if they are smaller than the normal, they are microcytes. Cells that possess a normal amount of hemoglobin are said to be normochromic, but if they are deficient, they are described as hypochromic. Those with a volume of hemoglobin greater than the normal are hyperchromic. If the cells present abnormal shapes, they are described as poikilocytic.

Anemia may sometimes be classified according to the characteristics of the erythrocytes. For example, in anemia which is due to an iron deficiency, the cells are hypochromic and microcytic; the disease may be referred to as hypochromic-microcytic anemia.

ERYTHROCYTE DISORDERS

A deficiency or an excess may occur in the number of circulating red blood cells, or the cell composition may be abnormal.

Anemia

The term anemia implies a reduction in the oxygen-carrying capacity of the blood as a result of fewer circulating erythrocytes than is normal or a decrease in the concentration of hemoglobin.

TABLE 12–9 TYPES OF ANEMIA

1. Anemia due to decreased erythropoiesis
   a. Deficiency anemia
      Iron deficiency anemia
      Vitamin B_{12} deficiency anemia (pernicious anemia)
      Folic acid deficiency anemia
   b. Aplastic anemia (anemia due to depressed bone marrow activity)

2. Anemia due to excessive rate of hemolysis
   Hemolytic anemia
   a. Due to intracorpuscular defects
      Congenital hemolytic jaundice (hereditary spherocytosis)
      Hemoglobinopathy
         Sickle cell anemia
         Thalassemia (Mediterranean anemia or Cooley's anemia)
   b. Due to extracorpuscular factors, such as
      Hemolytic streptococcus infection
      Immune bodies
      Certain drugs

3. Anemia due to blood loss

The abnormal reduction in the number of erythrocytes may be due to decreased erythropoiesis, excessive red blood cell destruction or hemolysis, or loss of blood. Anemia due to decreased erythropoiesis may be caused by a deficiency of factors essential for normal production or by depressed bone marrow activity. An abnormal rate of destruction of the red blood cells may be associated with intracorpuscular defects or extracorpuscular factors.

Table 12–9 outlines the principal types of anemia according to cause.

General Effects and Manifestations of Anemia. Although there are various causes and types of anemia, they present a common problem—that of a decreased capacity of the blood to transport oxygen. The patients, regardless of the cause or type of their anemia, manifest signs and symptoms attributable to tissue and organ hypoxia and the ensuing reduced metabolism. The occurrence and severity of these manifestations depend on the degree of anemia present.

The person experiences general fatigue, lassitude, shortness of breath on exertion, and anorexia. The mucous membranes (e.g., conjunctivae) and skin become pale. Complaints of headache, dizziness, faintness, and tingling or "pins and needles" in the extremities are common. The pulse rate is increased, and frequently palpitation is experienced. In severe anemia, the circulation or renal function may be sufficiently impaired to cause some edema and, probably, some fluid in the bases of the lungs. In the older person, angina pectoris which is due to the myocardial hypoxia may occur. There is a general reduction in efficiency throughout the body and a lowered resistance to infections.

Deficiency Anemias. An essential nutrient for erythrocyte production, such as iron, vitamin B_{12}, folic acid, ascorbic acid and protein, may be lacking in the diet, or there may be defective absorption of an essential factor. In some instances, there may be an increased demand within the person which the normal supply cannot meet.

IRON DEFICIENCY ANEMIA. Anemia due to a deficiency of iron is characterized by small red blood cells with less than the normal content of hemoglobin (microcytic-hypochromic). There is usually some slight reduction in the total number of red blood cells. The deficiency of iron may be due to an insufficient dietary intake, chronic or acute blood loss, or gastric hypochlorhydria, which diminishes the absorption of ingested iron. Iron deficiency is seen frequently in children because of their increased requirements for growth. It is not uncommon in women during their reproductive years because of the menstrual blood loss and because of the increased demands during pregnancy and lactation. Anemia due to an iron deficiency is uncommon in adult males unless there has been a loss of blood or the development of hypochlorhydria secondary to gastric disease or atrophy of the gastric mucosa.

In addition to the general symptoms of anemia (see p. 158), the patient with iron deficiency anemia may experience soreness and inflammation of the mouth and tongue. The tongue may be very red and may have a smooth, glazed appearance due to atrophy of the papillae. Rarely, the patient with a severe anemia complains of dysphagia (difficulty in swallowing). The combination of dysphagia, stomatitis (inflammation of the mouth) and atrophic glossitis (inflammation of the tongue with atrophy of papillae) in anemia may be referred to as the Plummer-Vinson syndrome. Changes in the fingernails are common in prolonged iron deficiency.

They become brittle and concave or spoon-shaped.

A well-balanced diet containing an adequate quantity of iron-rich foods is important in the prevention of this type of anemia. It may be necessary to supplement the dietary intake with medicinal iron during periods of increased demands, such as pregnancy and lactation. A supplement may also be necessary for the woman with an excessive menstrual flow.

Unless there is an obvious reason for an iron deficiency anemia, the patient is investigated to determine the primary cause. For example, malabsorption of iron may be the result of a reduced secretion of hydrochloric acid.

Medicinal iron is the principal form of treatment and is usually given orally in the form of a ferrous salt. Examples of preparations commonly used are ferrous sulfate and ferrous gluconate. Oral iron medications may cause gastrointestinal irritation and crampy pain. If the patient complains of distress, the drug is administered with the meal or with a snack. The physician may recommend that it be given with a glass of orange juice, since it is suggested that vitamin C promotes iron absorption. The patient is advised that his stools will be black and tarry. He may experience some diarrhea or, with some preparations, may develop constipation, necessitating a mild laxative. Ferrous salt in a syrup or an elixir may be used for children. Any liquid product containing iron is given well diluted through a drinking tube to prevent staining of the teeth.

For patients who cannot tolerate oral preparations or if oral administration is contraindicated because of some gastrointestinal disturbance or malabsorption, iron may be given parenterally. Injections of iron dextran (Imferon) or dextriferron may be given intramuscularly and, occasionally, intravenously. The patient is observed for toxic reactions, which are manifested by headache, dizziness, joint pains and fever. Rarely, an anaphylactic reaction may occur; the patient complains of dyspnea and chest pain, the pulse is rapid and weak and the blood pressure falls.

The patient with iron deficiency anemia is encouraged to take an adequate diet that contains iron-rich foods. These are red meats, organ meats (especially liver), eggs, fish, green leafy vegetables, enriched whole grain cereals and bread, and dried fruits.

VITAMIN B$_{12}$ DEFICIENCY ANEMIA. Vitamin B$_{12}$ (cyanocobalamin) is essential for normal maturation of the red blood cells and may be referred to as the antianemic factor. When it is not available to the red bone marrow, excessively large cells called megaloblasts are formed. The number of red blood cells produced is less than normal and they show marked variation in size and shape. The megaloblasts contain a greater than normal amount of hemoglobin, but the deficiency in the total number of erythrocytes results in an inadequate oxygen-carrying capacity of the blood. The condition may be referred to as megaloblastic anemia.

The causes of Vitamin B$_{12}$ deficiency anemia may be an inadequate dietary intake; non-absorption of the vitamin because of a deficiency of the intrinsic factor, resulting from a gastric secretory defect, gastrectomy, or intestinal disease; or disease of the liver, resulting in its inability to store sufficient vitamin B$_{12}$ to meet the normal erythropoietic needs.

The commonest vitamin B$_{12}$ deficiency anemia is that due to a failure of the gastric mucosa to secrete sufficient intrinsic factor. It is known as pernicious anemia or Addisonian pernicious anemia. The incidence is greater in persons between 35 and 65 years, and there appears to be some familial tendency.

In addition to the general symptoms of anemia, the patient may experience gastrointestinal and nervous system changes. The tongue is sore and has a smooth, raw, beefy red appearance. There is a loss of appetite and some intolerance for food, but the person does not always show a corresponding loss of weight. The lack of vitamin B$_{12}$ (antianemic factor) may cause myelin and nerve fiber degeneration in the spinal cord and peripheral nerves. As a result of this degeneration, the patient may develop tingling or "pins and needles" or coldness and numbness in the extremities. Unless the deficiency is corrected, motor disturbances may develop in the form of muscular weakness, ataxia (loss of coordination and staggering) and paralysis. In prolonged, severe deficiencies, degeneration of the optic nerves may occur, resulting in serious impairment of vision. When degenerative changes occur in the spinal cord, the condition is referred to as subacute combined degeneration of the cord.

In severe pernicious anemia, the skin may show some jaundice, a result of increased hemolysis. Laboratory examination of the blood reveals a deficiency of erythrocytes. The cells are unusually large with more than the normal amount of hemoglobin (macrocytic-hyperchromic). Gastric analysis demonstrates hypochlorhydria even after stimulation with histamine (see p. 334). Bone marrow aspirated by sternal puncture shows hyperplasia of the bone marrow and failure in normal erythropoiesis.

Pernicious anemia is treated by intramuscular injections of vitamin B$_{12}$. A daily dose may be prescribed for a period of time; then, the interval between injections is gradually increased, and the dosage is reduced to a maintenance level according to the patient's response. The patient will require regular maintenance doses of vitamin B$_{12}$ for the rest of his life. The majority of persons with pernicious anemia require 50 to 1000 micrograms monthly to maintain normal hemoglobin and erythrocyte levels. Regular red cell counts and hemoglobin estimations are necessary. Initially, the rapid regeneration of erythrocytes in response to treatment may deplete the iron stores, resulting in insufficient hemoglobin production. Ferrous sulfate may be prescribed in addition to the vitamin B$_{12}$.

If the anemia is very severe with a hemoglobin as low as 4 to 5 Gm. per cent, a blood transfusion may be considered advisable. If used, the blood is administered very slowly because a sudden increase in the blood volume might precipitate sudden heart failure. The patient is usually kept on bed rest if the hemoglobin is less than 7 Gm. per cent. The recommended diet is light, easily digested, and rich in protein, iron and vitamins. Highly seasoned and coarse foods are avoided if the mouth is sore.

Regular medical examinations are necessary so that early and insidious regressive changes may be recognized before serious degenerative changes develop.

In contrast to pernicious anemia, the anemia associated with a dietary deficiency of vitamin B$_{12}$, intestinal disease and liver disease does not manifest a hypochlorhydria or degenerative changes of the nervous system. The dietary deficiency of vitamin B_{12} (extrinsic factor) usually occurs when the diet lacks animal protein and consists mainly of carbohydrates and vegetables. Impaired absorption may occur in regional ileitis, steatorrhea and parasitic infections. Blind or stagnant loops in the small intestine may result following intestinal surgery or with multiple diverticula (sacs or out-pouchings in the walls) and may cause a proliferation of bacteria that use up the available vitamin B_{12} before it can be absorbed. The treatment of these anemias includes treatment of the initial cause and parenteral administration of vitamin B_{12}. Oral or parenteral preparations of folic acid may also be used.

ANEMIA DUE TO DEFICIENCY OF FOLIC ACID AND VITAMIN C. A lack of folic acid or ascorbic acid may interfere with the production of normal erythrocytes. Either deficiency may result from inadequate intake or a malabsorptive problem. Folic acid (Folvite) may be given orally or intramuscularly to treat anemias other than pernicious anemia. It cannot replace vitamin B_{12} in treating pernicious anemia since it does not arrest degeneration of the nervous system, despite the blood picture returning to normal.

Vitamin C enhances the catalytic action of folic acid in erythropoiesis. If the folic acid dietary intake is satisfactory, the administration of vitamin C in anemia will assist in increasing red cell production.

Aplastic Anemia. This type of anemia is the result of insufficient bone marrow activity. There may be an actual reduction in the amount of blood-forming marrow, or the marrow may have a functional defect. Aplastic anemia usually results in a deficiency of leukocytes and thrombocytes as well as insufficient red blood cells. When all three formed elements of the blood are reduced, the condition is referred to as pancytopenia.

Depression of bone marrow activity may be the result of the toxic action of certain drugs or industrial chemicals, excessive exposure to radiation, chronic infection or crowding by tumors or neoplastic tissue. Drugs capable of suppressing bone marrow function include sulfonamides, antineoplastic agents (e.g., nitrogen mustard, busulfan, cyclophosphamide, methotrexate, mercaptopurine), gold salts (e.g., Myochrysine), chloramphenicol (Chloromycetin) and phen-

ylbutazone (Butazolidin). Benzol, lead, mercury and arsenic (possible industrial chemicals) may also be offenders in bone marrow failure. In relation to radiation, drugs and chemicals, there appears to be no direct correlation between the dosage and the development of the anemia. Sensitivity of the individual seems to be a contributing factor.

The person with aplastic anemia is critically ill, and as well as suffering severe hypoxia, he is susceptible to infection because of the deficiency of leukocytes (leukopenia). Spontaneous bleeding is a problem due to the lack of thrombocytes. The onset of the anemia may be sudden and prostrating, or it may be insidious and gradual. The patient manifests the general symptoms of anemia (p. 158), oral and throat lesions, fever, infection and hemorrhagic areas.

Treatment includes removal of the cause, frequent transfusions of whole blood, antibiotic administration to control infection and a corticoid preparation such as prednisone. Supportive nursing care is very important. Close observations are made for infection, hemorrhage and increasing hypoxia. Precautions are necessary to prevent infection (reverse isolation).

Hemolytic Anemia. Excessive hemolysis (disintegration of red blood cells) causes anemia if the rate of destruction exceeds the erythropoietic ability of the red bone marrow. Premature hemolysis may result from an intracorpuscular (intrinsic) defect that reduces the ability of the cells to survive the normal life span in circulation, or it may be due to an extrinsic (outside of the erythrocytes) factor or mechanism.

The patient's symptoms depend on the rate, severity and duration of the cell destruction. As well as the symptoms produced by the anemia, there is an increased concentration of bilirubin in the blood; this may cause jaundice, which is evident first in the sclerae, an increased amount of urobilinogen in the urine and feces and, rarely, free hemoglobin in the plasma and urine. The laboratory examination of the blood reveals an increased number of reticulocytes in circulation (reticulocytosis) because of the constant demand for new cells, as well as a deficiency in the total number of red cells. Examination of a bone marrow specimen demonstrates hyperplasia and hyperactivity of the marrow. Acute hemolytic anemia may cause a chill followed by a high temperature, prostration, headache and pain in the back and legs.

The hemolytic anemias caused by a congenital corpuscular defect include hereditary spherocytosis, sickle cell anemia, and thalassemia.

HEREDITARY SPHEROCYTOSIS. This type of hemolytic anemia is also known as congenital hemolytic jaundice, familial hemolytic anemia, and acholuric jaundice. The intracellular abnormality in metabolism causes the mature cells to be spherical, predisposing them to entrapment and hemolysis in the spleen. Being spherical rather than shaped as a biconcave disc, the surface area of a cell is less than that of a normal red cell. An increase in the cell content by osmosis (which would be tolerated by the normal cell) causes the spherical cell to rupture. For this reason, the spherocytes are said to have an increased osmotic fragility. The disorder is inherited from an affected parent. The gene with the abnormal trait is dominant; that is, to have the disorder expressed, one need only receive a gene for the trait from one parent. The age at which the disease is recognized varies, depending on its severity. The patient may have little difficulty and go undiagnosed until adulthood. The enlarged spleen may be discovered during a routine examination. It is usually the jaundice or the symptoms of anemia that prompt the patient to seek medical assistance. Occasionally, the increased bilirubin leads to the development of gallstones.

Removal of the spleen reduces the excessive destruction of the abnormal red blood cells and relieves the anemia. The abnormal erythrocytes persist, but the majority survive a normal life span in the absence of the spleen.

HEMOGLOBINOPATHY. Hemoglobin occurs in several types because of slight variations in the globin fraction of the compound. The type is genetically determined. The normal hemoglobin that develops after birth is known as type A(Hb-A). The hemoglobin in the red blood cells of the fetus is type F(Hb-F) and is normally replaced by Hb-A during the first 6 months of life. Several abnormal types have been identified and are designated S, C, D, E, G, H, I, J, K, L, M, N, O, P, and Q.[7] The term hemoglobinopathy indicates the presence of red blood cells with an abnormal type of hemoglobin, which may be Hb-F. Abnormal hemoglobin may cause an excessive hemolysis. Sickle cell anemia and thalassemia are the commoner hemoglobinopathies that lead to hemolytic anemia.

Sickle Cell Anemia. This anemia is characterized by erythrocytes that contain Hb-S. This abnormal hemoglobin is less soluble, particularly when it gives up its oxygen and becomes reduced oxyhemoglobin and when the pH is below normal. It crystallizes, resulting in a cell which assumes a sickle or crescent shape. Sickling results in (1) a life span which is shorter than that of normal red cells and (2) in the cells stagnating and clumping in the smaller blood vessels. The vessels may become occluded, leading to a greater reduction of the oxyhemoglobin and local metabolic acidosis (reduced pH); these results promote more sickling and tend to set up a vicious circle.

Hemoglobin-S is an inherited trait seen chiefly in Negroes. If a person is heterozygous (i.e., he inherited a gene for sickling from only one parent), a greater number of his erythrocytes contain normal hemoglobin (Hb-A), and he remains asymptomatic unless exposed to severe hypoxia. When a person is homozygous, having received a gene for sickling from each parent, the majority of his red blood cells have Hb-S, and he manifests signs and symptoms characteristic of sickle cell anemia.

There is a continuous premature destruction of red blood cells, resulting in a hemoglobin level of approximately 7 to 8 Gm. per cent, an enlarged spleen and liver, increased bilirubin in the blood, an excessive number of reticulocytes in circulation and hyperplasia of the red bone marrow. Frequent sites of stagnation of red blood cells and vascular obstruction are the lower limbs, lungs, kidneys, joints, mesenteric arteries and the brain. The patient experiences pain and impaired function in whatever area suffers the interrupted blood supply. For example, occlusion of a kidney vessel may result in hematuria and renal insufficiency;

---

[7]R. B. Thompson: Haematology, 2nd ed. London, Pitman Medical Publishing Co. Ltd., 1965, p. 96.

obstruction of a cerebral artery may cause some paralysis.

Symptoms do not usually appear in the first six months of life. The person may have symptom-free periods alternated with exacerbations. The latter may be referred to as crises and are frequently precipitated by infections, especially those of the respiratory and gastrointestinal tracts. During quiescent periods, care is directed toward the prevention of infections. A well-balanced, nutritious diet and plenty of regular rest are important. Intramuscular injections of gamma globulin may be given to promote antibody production, and antimicrobial drugs such as a sulfonamide or antibiotic preparation may be used as a prophylactic measure. Regular visits to the clinic or the doctor are necessary for physical and blood examinations. Since the majority of these patients are children, the nature of the disease and the importance of prophylactic care during remissions must be carefully explained to the parents.

Care during a crisis includes bed rest, analgesics for the relief of pain and increased fluid intake. Clear fluids are given orally, but if they are not tolerated, intravenous infusions are used. A close check is kept on the vital signs and urinary output and for the appearance of "new" signs and symptoms. If the anemia is severe, the patient may receive blood transfusions and oxygen. The latter is only used during the acute emergency period since prolonged use and the ensuing high oxygen concentration in the blood may cause suppression of erythropoiesis.

Thalassemia. Synonyms that may be used for this type of anemia are Mediterranean anemia, Cooley's anemia and hereditary leptocytosis.

This disease occurs in two forms, major and minor, and is seen most frequently in persons of the mediterranean countries and Southeast Asia. Both forms have the common feature of a genetically determined defect in the cellular synthesis of the globin fraction of the hemoglobin. The red blood cells are thinner than normal, fragile, irregular in shape and deficient in hemoglobin. A large percentage of the hemoglobin is of the fetal type (Hb-F).

Thalassemia major, also referred to as Cooley's anemia, is homozygous and is manifested in infancy or early childhood. Fortunately, this form of the disease is of lesser incidence. It produces very severe anemia and marked hyperplasia of the red bone marrow and may cause pain in the bones. Reticulocytosis occurs and immature nucleated red blood cells may appear in the circulation. The spleen and liver are enlarged as a result of the rapid hemolysis, and jaundice may be apparent. Growth and development are retarded, and the child does not usually survive beyond early childhood. Treatment consists mainly of blood transfusions.

Thalassemia minor is heterozygous and is less severe. The red blood cells are smaller than normal but are less deficient in hemoglobin than those of the major type, and there is less hemolysis. The degree of anemia varies greatly in affected persons; some may be asymptomatic and live a normal life with their disease only being detected by a blood cell examination. Others may be handicapped to some degree by anemia.

HEMOLYTIC ANEMIA DUE TO EXTRACORPUSCULAR FACTORS. Extrinsic mechanisms that may cause hemolysis include some infections, immune bodies, and certain drugs and chemicals.

An increased rate of erythrocyte destruction may be associated with severe infections caused by the hemolytic streptococci, *Staphylococcus aureus*, pneumonoccus, *Bacillus welchii* and some viruses. Excessive hemolysis may also accompany malaria. The red blood cells may be damaged by the pathogenic organisms or their toxins.

Hemolytic anemia may be caused by antibodies which may be acquired or may be developed in response to an endogenous or exogenous antigen. Erythroblastosis fetalis is an example of hemolytic anemia occurring as a result of acquired antibodies (see p. 153).

When a person develops antibodies that result in the destruction of his own erythrocytes, the condition is referred to as auto-immune hemolytic anemia. Frequently, the cause of this condition is not known. In many instances, it is secondary to a collagen disease (e.g., lupus erythematosus) or to a disease involving lymphoid tissue (e.g., Hodgkin's disease). The agglutinins adhere to the red blood cells, predisposing them to entrapment and destruction, especially in the spleen and liver.

Hemolytic jaundice may develop in some persons receiving preparations of quinine, sulfonamide, salicylic acid and phenacetin. Incidence has also been reported in persons exposed to insecticides, arsenic, and coal tar products such as analine dyes and toluene. The mechanism by which certain drugs and chemicals produce hemolysis in some persons is not known.

Treatment of autoimmune hemolytic anemia includes blood transfusions, splenectomy to reduce the trapping and destruction of the red blood cells, and the administration of a corticoid preparation such as prednisone to decrease antibody formation.

Anemia due to Blood Loss. The loss of blood removes erythrocytes from the circulation, reducing the oxygen-carrying capacity of the blood. A blood count taken immediately after a hemorrhage does not reflect the degree of anemia since the total intravascular volume is reduced. Over a period of 24 to 48 hours, the intravascular volume is restored by the entrance of extracellular fluid into the vascular compartment and probably by intravenous infusion. The red blood cells at this time are those that were in the blood previous to the blood loss and are now dispersed in a greater volume of plasma. The count (per mm.) now gives a more accurate indication of the severity of the anemia.

Normally, the bone marrow responds quickly to the tissue hypoxia, and the erythrocyte count returns to normal over a period of 4 to 5 weeks. At first, more than the normal number of reticulocytes are in circulation and some immature nucleated normoblasts may also be released. Since considerable iron is lost from the body in hemorrhage, hemoglobin production may lag behind red blood cell production. The administration of an iron preparation may be necessary to bring the hemoglobin concentration back to normal.

If the blood loss is 20 per cent or more of the total blood volume, rapid replacement by means of a blood transfusion is necessary. This quickly increases the total circulating volume as well as the number of erythrocytes to carry oxygen.

In cases of chronic blood loss in which there is a continuous loss of a relatively small amount over a long period, the bone marrow may keep the erythrocyte count close to normal. The continuous loss of iron, however, creates a deficiency of that essential element, and the erythrocytes in circulation are small and lack a full complement of hemoglobin. The anemia may be described as microcytic-hypochromic. Treatment includes correction of the cause of the bleeding and the administration of an iron preparation such as ferrous sulfate.

Nursing in Anemia. The care required by the anemia patient varies with the severity and cause of his disease. The anemia may not be severe enough to necessitate bed rest or hospitalization. It may be chronic, as in pernicious and sickle cell anemia, resulting in the patient's need for continuous treatment and supervision and modification in his way of life. With some, their anemia may be entirely cured by correction of the cause. Depending on the etiologic factor, there may be symptoms and problems besides those attributable to anemia. For example, in hemolytic anemia there may be the problem of jaundice; in the sickle cell type there is the serious problem of vascular obstruction. Regardless of the type of anemia, the patients have one common difficulty, namely, a decreased capacity of their blood to transport to oxygen.

Care is directed toward eliminating the cause, increasing the oxygen-carrying capacity of the blood, reducing the demand for oxygen, alleviating the discomforts experienced, preventing complications and, when the disease is chronic, helping the patient to live a life that is as useful and satisfying as his condition will permit.

The following considerations are not necessarily applicable to all anemia patients nor are they all inclusive. As well as adapting the care to the individual, the severity and type of his anemia must be considered.

REST. Energy expenditure is reduced in order to decrease the demand for oxygen. The anemic patient fatigues quickly, may complain of light-headedness or may faint on exertion. The ambulatory patient is encouraged to lighten his activity load and rest at intervals throughout the day. With severe anemia bed rest is necessary until the red blood cells and hemoglobin increase and there is less evidence of hypoxia. An explanation of the basis of the fatigue and weakness and the importance of rest may help the patient through this difficult period. Nursing care is planned to conserve the patient's energy; uninterrupted periods of rest, assistance in turning, feeding, and a restricted number of visitors for brief periods only are important factors. Activity short of fatigue and breathlessness is encouraged.

OBSERVATIONS. The patient with pernicious anemia is observed for signs of degenerative changes in his nervous system. Any complaint of tingling, numbness and sensations of "pins and needles" in distal portions of the extremities, loss of finer movements, difficulty in holding small objects, weakness of limbs, ataxia and impaired vision are immediately brought to the doctor's attention. The patient's tolerance for activity is noted.

NUTRITION. Diet has an important role in erythropoiesis. It should be light, easily digestible and selected to provide the protein, iron, vitamins and other elements for the production of red blood cells and hemoglobin. Anorexia frequently poses a problem. It is helpful to discuss with the patient the importance of foods in increasing the red cells and hemoglobin and to determine his food preferences. Small portions offered 5 or 6 times a day may be more acceptable than the usual 3 meals. If the patient's mouth, tongue and esophagus are sore, roughage and hot and spiced foods are avoided. Mouth care just before the food is served, remaining with the patient, provision of the necessary assistance if weakness is a problem, and a well-ventilated, neat environment which is free of commotion and disturbing sights are conducive to having the patient take his food.

MOUTH CARE. In pernicious and iron deficiency anemias, a common problem is the sore mouth and tongue. Frequent cool, mildly alkaline mouthwashes are necessary. A soft-bristled toothbrush or an absorbent applicator is used to clean the teeth. The mouth is cleansed before and after taking nourishment.

SKIN CARE. The skin is more susceptible to pressure and breaks down readily because of the reduced oxygen supply in the tissues. If the patient is confined to bed, his position is changed every 1 to 2 hours; pressure areas receive frequent, gentle massage and are protected by the use of sponge rubber, sheepskin or an alternating air pressure mattress (ripple mattress).

If the anemia is hemolytic, there may be jaundice and pruritus (itching of the skin). Slightly warm or tepid water is used for bathing. Sodium bicarbonate is added to the bath water, or oatmeal that is tied in a gauze bag and squeezed through the water may help to relieve the irritation. The use of soap in avoided. Calamine lotion or caladryl may be applied for relief. The patient's fingernails are kept short and clean to prevent excoriation and infection of the skin should the patient scratch the irritated areas.

WARMTH. As a result of the reduced amount of oxygen available for metabolism, the anemia patient produces less body heat. He may require extra clothing and bedding and a warm, ventilated room. Local heat applications are not used, especially with the pernicious anemia patient since he may have some sensory loss.

PREVENTION OF INFECTION. The patient with severe anemia is more susceptible to infections. Consideration is given to his placement in the hospital ward to avoid contact with a patient with infection. Visitors and personnel with any infection, such as a cold or sore throat, should not be permitted contact with the patient. The person with aplastic anemia is placed in reverse isolation since he is lacking leukocytes to provide him ordinary protection.

MEDICATIONS. Various medications are used in the treatment of anemia. The drug used depends on the cause and type of the anemia. These drugs have been cited in the preceding discussion of the various types of anemia. The principal antianemic drugs are preparations of iron, vitamin B_{12} and folic acid.

BLOOD TRANSFUSION. In severe anemia the patient may require a blood transfusion. Unless the anemia is due to blood loss, there is a danger of overloading the circulation if whole blood is given. It must be given very slowly and the patient's pulse and respirations checked frequently. In most instances, unless there has been a blood loss, a small volume of concentrated (packed) cells is given.

INSTRUCTION. The patient and his family are advised of the important role of good nutrition. Meal planning and foods that should be included to promote red blood cell and hemoglobin production are discussed.

If the anemia is chronic, regular visits to the doctor or clinic are stressed. The necessity of maintenance doses of vitamin B_{12} is explained to the pernicious anemia patient; even though he feels well he must not omit the prescribed vitamin B_{12}. If the disease is severe and a weekly injection is prescribed, a referral may be made to the visiting nurse organization so the patient may receive the drug at home rather than having to go to the clinic so frequently.

In the case of sickle cell anemia, the parents receive an explanation of the disease and factors that predispose to crises, and instruction is given as to the care of the affected child (see p. 163).

SPLENECTOMY. The spleen is removed in some hemolytic anemias. Preparation of the patient for surgery is similar to that for any abdominal surgery (see p. 107). The postoperative care includes that which is necessary for any patient who undergoes intra-abdominal surgery (see p. 114). The close proximity and attachment of the spleen to the diaphragm may temporarily affect diaphragmatic function and may result in reduced expansion of the left lung. Regular deep breathing and turning are important in preventing respiratory complications. Since the spleen exerts some influence on the production and liberation of cells from the marrow, there may be a marked increase in the number of thrombocytes in circulation following splenectomy, predisposing to thrombus formation. Optimal hydration to avoid hemoconcentration, frequent change of position, bed exercises and early ambulation to prevent stasis are important considerations in the postoperative nursing.

Polycythemia (Erythrocythemia)

An excessive number of erythrocytes and a corresponding increase in the concentration of hemoglobin is referred to as polycythemia or erythrocythemia. The red blood cell count may be 8 to 12 million per cu. mm. with a hemoglobin concentration of 18 to 25 Gm. per cent. The condition may be primary or secondary.

Secondary polycythemia is a physiological compensatory increase in the number of erythrocytes by the red bone marrow in response to a low concentration of oxygen in the blood. It occurs normally at high altitudes, where the atmospheric oxygen tension is low, and in pathological conditions in which there is inadequate oxygenation of the blood. Examples of the latter are congenital malformations of the heart which lead to blood by-passing the pulmonary-circulatory system and pulmonary conditions that interfere with normal gas exchange (e.g., emphysema).

Primary polycythemia is a rare proliferative disorder of the red bone marrow in which there is an uncontrolled production of an excessive number of red blood cells and hemoglobin. It is usually accompanied by some overproduction of myelocytes (leukocytes produced by the marrow) and thrombocytes. The cause is unknown. The onset is usually in middle-aged persons, with a higher incidence in males and Jewish persons.

Polycythemia greatly increases the total volume and viscosity of the blood. The blood pressure is elevated and the work load of the heart is increased. The rate of flow through the vessels is reduced and, with the increased number of thrombocytes and blood viscosity, predisposes to the development of thrombi. Occlusion of a vessel may occur, causing a cerebral vascular accident, coronary thrombosis, pulmonary infarction or gangrene. Heart failure may develop as a result of the increased cardiac demands. The spleen enlarges because of the increased number of red blood cells to be destroyed.

Symptoms may include complaints of headache, dizziness, a full feeling in the head, pruritus, and pain in the limbs. The patient manifests ready fatigue, dyspnea, a lowered heat tolerance and a high dusky red complexion. These patients also have a tendency to develop a peptic ulcer. This is attributed to an associated increase in gastric secretions.

Treatment and care of the patient with polycythemia are aimed at decreasing the activity of the red bone marrow and at reducing the volume and viscosity of the blood. Radioactive phosphorus (P^{32}), which is taken up by the bone marrow cells, may be administered to suppress the bone marrow. Irradiation of the long bones by x-rays may be used. Drugs such as nitrogen mustard, busulfan (Myleran) and cyclophosphamide (Cytoxan) may also be given to inhibit erythropoiesis. A phlebotomy (venesection) may be done periodically to provide a temporary reduction in the blood volume. Five hundred to 1000 ml. may be withdrawn each time. The regular blood bank equipment for the collection of blood is used, and the blood is donated to the bank. Red and glandular meats and iron-containing foods are restricted in the patient's diet.

These persons are not usually hospitalized until a complication such as thrombosis, peptic ulcer or cardiac insufficiency develops. A reasonable amount of activity is encouraged to prevent circulatory stasis. They are advised of the need for regular, frequent visits to their physician or the clinic for close supervision. The family and patient are alerted to early indications of impending complications and advised of the importance of promptly getting in touch with the physician.

LEUKOCYTE DISORDERS

Alterations in the number of leukocytes may involve an increased or decreased production of the cells.

Leukocytosis

The number of leukocytes in circulation normally increases to a level in excess of the normal (7000 to 10,000 per cu. mm.) in defense of the body in most infections and in response to necrotic tissue. This increase is referred to as leukocytosis and is usually predominant in one type of white cell. Information as to which type of leukocytes are in excess of the normal provides significant information for the physician, since some leukocytoses are known to be associated with certain pathological conditions. For instance, neutrophil leukocytosis normally develops quickly in response to most infections (e.g., appendicitis, pneumonia) and tissue destruction (e.g., myocardial infarction); lymphocytosis is characteristic of certain infections such as measles, mumps, pertussis, and infectious hepatitis; and an increase in eosinophils (eosinophilia)

accompanies many allergic conditions. The white blood cell count returns to normal when the infection is checked, the necrotic tissue is disposed of, or the initiating factor, such as an allergen, is removed.

Leukemia

This is a disease of the tissue that forms the cellular elements of the blood. It causes a persisting, uncontrolled and abnormal proliferation of leukocytes comparable to the uncontrolled production of cells in malignant neoplastic disease. For this reason, leukemia is sometimes referred to as cancer of the blood. There is a marked increase in the number of leukocytes in circulation and many of these are immature and abnormal. It may be the lymphoid tissues that are affected, resulting in an excessive production of lymphocytes; or uncontrolled production may occur in the red bone marrow, causing an excessive generation of granulocytes or monocytes.

The leukemic cells invade other tissues and many organs of the body, causing dysfunction in these areas. Hyperplasia of the bone marrow and the accumulation of white blood cells hamper the production of erythrocytes and thrombocytes, leading to anemia and thrombocytopenia. Enlargement and impaired function of the lymphoid tissues and the liver occur. The enlargement may interfere with neighboring structures; for example, an increase in the size of the mediastinal nodes may cause pressure on the respiratory tract. An enlarged spleen and liver may crowd the stomach, reducing its capacity.

The marked overproduction of leukocytes and the rapid rate of their destruction result in an increase in the body's rate of metabolism. The use of substances in the proliferation of these cells deprives other cells of essential metabolic elements, and the increased amount of cell destruction increases the concentration of metabolic wastes.

Types of Leukemia. Leukemia may be classified according to the predominant type of leukocyte and whether the process is acute or chronic. The disease may be acute or chronic myelogenous or granulocytic leukemia, the excessive cells being granulocytes which are produced by the bone marrow. It may be acute or chronic lymphocytic leukemia in which there is a proliferation of lymphocytes; or it may be acute or, rarely, chronic monocytic leukemia in which there is a marked overproduction of monocytes.

The chronic form of the disease progresses more slowly and is of greater duration, the acute having the reverse characteristics. The patient with acute leukemia may survive only a few weeks or months; the person with a chronic leukemia may live several years.

Any type of leukemia may occur at any age, but there is a higher incidence of acute leukemia in children and young adults. Chronic leukemia is seen more often in persons over 40 years of age, and there is a greater frequency of the chronic form of the disease, especially lymphocytic, in males.

Etiology. Leukemia is a fatal disease of unknown etiology in most instances. There is significant evidence that overexposure to ionizing radiation is the causative factor in some cases. This is substantiated by the high incidence of leukemia in the survivors of the Hiroshima and Nagasaki atomic bombs, radiologists, and patients with ankylosing spondylitis (arthritis of the spine) who were treated by x-ray radiation. Viruses and absorption of the chemicals benzol, pyridine and aniline dyes have been strongly suspected of being leukemogenic. Regardless of the initial cause, Guyton states that the uncontrolled production of leukocytes is the result of a "cancerous mutation of a myelogenous or a lymphogenous cell."[8]

Manifestations. Acute leukemia usually has an abrupt outset that is frequently accompanied by an upper respiratory infection. The onset of a chronic form is insidious; the signs and symptoms are less intense and less incapacitating in the early stages.

Fever, excessive perspiration, lowered heat tolerance, tachycardia and weight loss are seen in the patient with an acute form of leukemia because of the increased metabolic rate. Bone marrow dysfunction and the resulting anemia are manifested by pallor, shortness of breath, extreme fatigue and weakness, and palpitation. External and internal bleeding may occur due to the reduced production of thrombocytes. Bleeding of the gums, nose and gastrointestinal tract is common. Petechiae or ecchymoses may appear as further evidence of the reduced ability of the blood to coagulate. The patient with myelogenous leukemia will most likely complain of tenderness and pain in the long bones and sternum from the hyperplasia and crowding in the bone marrow.

Although there is an excessive number of leukocytes, they are immature and do not provide the normal defense against infection; the patient may complain of a sore mouth and throat which exhibit infected necrotic ulcers. An acute infection such as pneumonia, septicemia or perirectal abscess may develop. The spleen and liver enlarge, and in the later stages, infiltration of the leukemic cells into the kidneys may cause renal insufficiency. Sensory and motor disturbances, severe headache, convulsions or disorientation may occur, indicating central nervous system involvement. In lymphatic leukemia, the lymph nodes enlarge and are tender.

The blood picture is one of an excessively high white blood cell count and a large percentage of the cells are primitive. The erythrocyte and thrombocyte counts are abnormally low. A specimen of aspirated bone marrow demonstrates the proliferation of leukemic cells.

Treatment and Nursing. The treatment and care of the patient with leukemia are directed toward suppressing the abnormal cell production and supporting the patient physiologically and psychologically.

Some of the anticancer drugs, such as methotrexate, cyclophosphamide, 6-mercaptopurine, busulfan and vincristine sulfate, have been effective with some patients in producing temporary remissions, especially in acute lymphocytic leukemia. In chronic forms of leukemia, radiation therapy (by x-ray) to long bones, spleen and areas of lymph nodes or the administration of radioactive phosphorus (P^{32}) may be employed. See Chapter 8 for reactions to anticancer drugs and radiation.

Blood transfusions are given to relieve the anemia and deficiency of thrombocytes. The patient may also receive an antimicrobial preparation to prevent or treat infection.

Nursing care of the patient who suffers from acute leukemia or who is in the late stages of the chronic form of the disease is supportive and symptomatic.

REST. Rest and the prevention of un-

---

[8]Guyton: op. cit., p. 116.

necessary expenditure of energy are important because of the increased metabolic rate and the hypoxia. The acutely ill patient requires assistance in turning and moving.

OBSERVATIONS. The patient is observed for regressive changes which are likely to progressively appear as various organs are invaded by excessive numbers of leukocytes. The fluid balance is recorded, the vital signs are checked frequently, and the patient is observed for indications of disorientation, infection and hemorrhage.

NUTRITION AND FLUIDS. A fluid intake of 2500 to 3000 ml. is encouraged because of the fever and to promote elimination of the increased uric acid by the kidneys. This waste results from the rapid cell destruction and, unless well diluted, may crystallize in the renal tubules, impairing kidney function.

Nutrition is a problem with the acute leukemic patient; he has anorexia and his mouth is likely to be sore. A high-calorie, high-vitamin diet is desirable. The patient's preferences and what can be tolerated are determined from day to day. Concentrated foods and nutritious fluids are used whenever possible. When there is stomatitis, rinsing the mouth with an anesthetic mouthwash just before each meal may reduce the discomfort associated with eating.

ORAL HYGIENE. Because of the patient's susceptibility to infection and the hemorrhagic tendency, special care of the mouth is very important. It is cleansed gently and frequently with a mildly alkaline mouthwash. A very soft-bristled toothbrush is used to gently clean the teeth. An oil or cream may be applied to the lips to prevent "cracking," and adherence.

SKIN CARE. Because of the fever, weakness, and susceptibility to infection, the patient's skin requires special attention. Frequent bathing is necessary to remove the perspiration and provide comfort.

A mild antiseptic soap may be used for its antibacterial effect. The patient's position is changed frequently to prevent pressure sores and other complications. The alternating air pressure mattress (ripple mattress) is very helpful here. Extreme gentleness is required when doing anything for the patient to avoid pressure that might precipitate bleeding into the tissues. Following an injection, pressure is applied to the site for several minutes to reduce the amount of bleeding and the formation of a hematoma.

PAIN. Local applications of ice packs may be used over the painful areas. The administration of an analgesic may be necessary to provide relief, particularly as the disease becomes progressively more severe.

ENVIRONMENT. Placement of the patient on the hospital ward requires consideration. Whether the patient should be in a single room or not depends on the particular individual and his age. Children and young adults are usually more secure and less fearful with others. Obviously, he should not be placed near a patient with an infection, and no one with an infection should be allowed to visit or care for him.

Because of the patient's lowered heat tolerance, fever and shortness of breath, a cooler well-ventilated environment is more comfortable for him.

PSYCHOLOGICAL SUPPORT. One is faced with the ever burning question as to whether the patient should be told that he has this fatal disease. The reader is referred to the former discussion relevant to this on page 98. The nurse must be familiar with what information the patient has received from his doctor.

The family will be very distressed and will require sympathetic understanding and emotional support from the nurse. Their fears and concern are acknowledged, and they are encouraged to talk about them. They are permitted to be with the patient and to participate in his care as much as possible without overtaxing themselves and neglecting other members of the family. They may find support from a visit from their religious adviser.

If the patient's condition improves and a remission of the disease occurs that permits the patient to go home, the family is given direction as to the necessary care and health supervision. This will include instruction concerning the amount of rest and activity recommended by the physician, the high-calorie, high-vitamin diet that the patient should receive, how to protect him from exposure to infection, the administration of prescribed medications and signs and symptoms that should prompt the immediate seeking of medical attention.

Leukopenia

Leukopenia may be defined as a reduction in the number of white blood cells below the normal limit of 5000 per cu. mm. It is almost always due to a decreased production or excessive destruction of neutrophils, resulting in the condition known as agranulocytosis or neutropenia. Lymphopenia (a decrease in the lymphocytes to below normal) may be seen occasionally in patients receiving ACTH or an adrenocorticoid preparation and in those with uremia.

Neutropenia

In most instances, this blood disorder is the result of the toxic effects of certain drugs in persons with a sensitivity or idiosyncrasy. The drugs found most frequently to be offenders include gold salts, sulfonamides, aminopyrine (Pyramidon), phenylbutazone (Butazoladin), chlorpromazine (Thorazine) and thiouracil preparations. The condition may also be associated with typhoid fever, malaria, miliary (widespread throughout the body) tuberculosis or any severe, overwhelming infection (e.g., septicemia).

Neutropenia may be an integral part of the aplastic anemia that may develop with radiation and anticancer drug therapy, or it may be due to an excessive destruction of the neutrophils by the spleen (hypersplenism). The disease has a higher incidence in females than in males.

Manifestations. Neutrophils play an important role in defending the body against infection because of their ability to ingest and destroy organisms. Neutropenia lowers the normal resistance to infection, resulting in prompt invasion of the mucous membranes and skin by pathogenic organisms.

The disease usually has a sudden onset and is manifested by chills, fever and prostration. Infected, ulcerated areas appear on the mucous membrane in the mouth, throat, rectum and vagina. Skin and respiratory infections may develop. Some patients complain of severe joint pain (arthralgia).

Treatment and Nursing. Treatment of neutropenia includes prompt elimination of any suspected cause. Antibiotic therapy in large doses is commenced promptly to prevent infection and check that which may be established. If the neutropenia is a part of pancytopenia, a blood transfusion may be given to relieve the anemia, but it does not alter the white blood cell count since transferred leukocytes are quickly removed from the circulation. A corticoid preparation such as prednisone may be prescribed, especially if the deficiency of neutrophils is thought to be the result of an excessive destruction of the patient's cells. If the infection can be controlled and supportive care provided, a gradual increase in the number of neutrophils and improvement in the patient's condition may be expected in 1 to 2 weeks.

The patient is protected from infection by reverse isolation. Only sterile linen and equipment are used. Personnel contacting or caring for the patient are screened for possible infection and are required to wash their hands thoroughly under running water before attending to the patient. A clean coverall type of gown and a mask are worn at the bedside. Visitors are restricted to one or two immediate family members who are free of infection. They are also required to wear a gown and mask and are requested not to go within 3 to 4 feet of the bedside. The floor is wet mopped, and the furniture is washed frequently to reduce the number of contaminated dust particles.

More effective isolation may be achieved by the use of a plastic isolator tent or "life island." This equipment completely encloses the patient and bed, creating a barrier to outside organisms. Air entering the enclosure is filtered by a mechanical ventilator. Sterile gloves are used when giving care through the sleeves or portholes in the sides of the tent.

Care of the mouth is extremely important. It is rinsed or irrigated every 1 to 2 hours with normal saline or a mild, antiseptic mouthwash. The patient should receive 2000 to 2500 ml. of fluids per day and a high-protein, high-vitamin diet. Because of the oral lesions, the patient may have difficulty taking adequate food. Nutritious fluids, soft bland foods, protein concentrates and vitamin supplements may be used.

Constipation is avoided; the hard stool may injure the intestinal mucosa, making it more vulnerable to infection.

Prevention of Neutropenia. In some instances, neutropenia might have been prevented if the affected person had understood the danger inherent in self-medication. Whenever the opportunity presents, the nurse has the responsibility to inform lay persons that drugs should only be taken under medical supervision and according to the specific directions of the physician. It is not uncommon to learn of someone who has been taking a potentially dangerous drug on his own over an abnormally long period of time. Equally dangerous is the situation in which a family member, neighbor or friend shares a drug or suggests one that has been prescribed for him and has proved helpful. They do not appreciate that a drug may affect one person quite differently from another and that it is prescribed by the doctor on an individual basis following a careful study of the patient's condition. Reactions and side effects are unpredictable; some supervision is necessary to recognize early toxic manifestations.

Multiple Myeloma

This is a rare, malignant disease in which multiple, small, solid tumors develop in the bone marrow. It is seen chiefly in persons over 50 years of age. The patient experiences severe pain in the affected bones and develops anemia. The tumors are composed of abnormal plasma cells. The function of normal plasma cells is the production of globulins; cells of the myeloma produce an abnormal globulin (Bence-Jones protein) which may be detected in the blood and urine. A marked increase in the serum globulin reverses the normal albumin-globulin ratio. A bone marrow biopsy demonstrates the presence of numerous plasma cells which normally are not found in the marrow. An x-ray may reveal areas of rarefaction (osteoporosis) in the affected bones.

The patient is treated with radiation and an anticancer drug. Blood transfusions are given because of the anemia, and analgesics are usually required to control the pain. Precautions are necessary to avoid falls and possible fracture of the affected bones.

DISORDERS AFFECTING LYMPHOID TISSUE

Infectious mononucleosis, Hodgkin's disease and lymphosarcoma are diseases affecting lymphoid tissues.

Infectious Mononucleosis

This disease is characterized by enlargement of the lymph nodes and spleen, fever, sore throat, headache and malaise. Blood tests reveal a lymphocytosis and the presence of atypical lymphocytes.

Infectious mononucleosis has a higher incidence in young adults and is thought to be due to a virus. Although infectious, direct transmission of the disease to others is rare. Diagnosis is confirmed by a positive Paul-Bunnell test (heterophile agglutination test). This examination indicates the presence of antibodies that cause the agglutination of sheep red cells and are known to develop in infectious mononucleosis.

The disease usually runs a self-limited course of 2 to 3 weeks. The treatment is symptomatic. The patient is kept in bed until the temperature is normal and a high-calorie, high-protein diet is recommended. Irrigations may be helpful if the throat is sore. Convalescence is usually prolonged. The patient is warned that fatigue and less than his accustomed strength may be expected and that his previous activities should be resumed very gradually.

Hodgkin's Disease (Lymphadenoma)

Hodgkin's disease is a fatal condition of unknown etiology. It has an insidious onset and is manifested by painless enlargement of one group of lymph nodes (usually cervical at the beginning). Progressively, the disease spreads to other lymphoid tissues throughout the body, and a variety of symptoms develop, depending upon the lymphoid tissue involved. The enlarging lymph nodes may cause pressure on nerves, resulting in pain, or may impose on neighboring organs, causing dysfunction. Axillary and inguinal nodes frequently interfere with venous and lymph drainage, leading to edema in the arms and legs. Enlarged mediastinal nodes may produce a distressing cough, dyspnea or difficulty in swallowing (dysphagia).

Constitutional symptoms are not prominent until the later stages. The patient gradually develops fatigue, weakness, fever, anorexia, loss of weight and pruritus. These are likely to be seriously aggravated by the treatments used (radiation, chemotherapy). Fluctuations in the symptoms and the size of the nodes may occur.

Hodgkin's disease has a higher incidence in males. It may develop at any age but is seen more often in those between 20 and 40 years of age. The average length of time the patient survives is 2 to 5 years, but a few live as long as 10 to 15 years. Diagnosis of the disease is established by a biopsy of an affected lymph node. Large atypical cells known as Reed-Sternberg cells are characteristic of Hodgkin's disease.

Treatment and Nursing Care. The patient is treated with radiation and an anticancer drug such as nitrogen mustard and cyclophosphamide (Cytoxan). The reader is referred to Chapter 8 for the nursing care of the patient receiving these forms of therapy.

In the early stages when the constitutional symptoms are absent or mild and the patient is free of pain, he is encouraged to remain active and to live a normal, useful life. The family, and perhaps the patient, receive an explanation of the nature and prognosis of the disease and the treatment involved. The patient's and his family's socioeconomic situations are assessed; referrals for assistance may be necessary.

Lymphosarcoma

This is a malignant tumor of lymphoid tissue characterized by a proliferation of lymphocytes. Unlike leukemia, the cells are confined within the lymphoid tissues until the later stages of the disease. It occurs more often in males and in those over 40 years of age.

The disease progresses similarly to Hodgkin's disease; usually only one area of lymphoid tissue is affected at first, but there is a gradual dissemination to other regions. The symptoms are largely dependent upon the location of the tumors. They reflect the pressure and interference imposed on neighboring structures by the enlarging lymphoid tissues. Fever and progressive debilitation accompany the extension and increasing severity of the disease. The patient may live 1 to 2 years. The treatment employed is the same as that used for Hodgkin's disease.

HEMORRHAGIC DISORDERS

An abnormal tendency to bleed may be due to a disorder of the clotting mechanism, an excess of anticoagulant or a vascular defect. A hemorrhagic disorder is characterized by prolonged bleeding following tissue damage; spontaneous bleeding into mucous membrane, skin and organs; and bleeding in more than one area of the body.

Failure of the clotting mechanism may result from a deficiency of any of the essential factors in the coagulation process (see p. 155). These disorders include hemophilia, hypoprothrombinemia and thrombocytopenia.

Hemophilia

This is a bleeding tendency that occurs in males as a result of a deficiency of Factor VIII, the antihemophilic factor. It is inherited as a sex-linked recessive trait. The defective gene is carried on an X chromosome and is transmitted from mother to son.

The female has two X sex chromosomes, and the male has one X and one Y. If a female inherits an X chromosome bearing the hemophilic gene from her father, she becomes a carrier. The disorder is not manifested in her because the X with the abnormal gene is dominated by the normal X chromosome. If the carrier marries a nonhemophiliac, there is a 50 per cent chance her daughters will be carriers. Her male progeny have a 50 per cent chance of being hemophilic (see Table 12–10). The sons of a hemophilic father only receive a Y chromosome from him so the disorder is not passed on to them or their descendants. All daughters of a hemophiliac male carry the trait since the father's genetic contribution to each is an X chromosome, which in his case bears the defective gene (see Table 12–10).

Hemophilia is usually recognized within the first year or two of life. Excessive bleeding from the umbilical cord does not occur because of the transplacental transfer of the mother's Factor VIII (AHG) to the fetus. Occasionally, persistent bleeding when the infant is circumcised leads to early diagnosis of the disorder.

The severity varies in individuals; some bleed excessively with a very slight trauma, others only with a more severe injury or during incidents such as tooth extraction or surgery. Most children experience some bleeding into joints, especially the knees, ankles and elbows. With some, this may be so severe that, as well as causing pain, it

TABLE 12–10   GENETIC POSSIBILITIES IN HEMOPHILIA

NORMAL MALE

		X	Y
FEMALE	X	XX	XY
CARRIER	X^h	X^hX	X^hY

XX Normal female
XY Normal male
X^hX Female carrier
X^hY Male with hemophilia

MALE WITH HEMOPHILIA

		X^h	Y
NORMAL	X	XX^h	XY
FEMALE	X	XX^h	XY

XX^h Female carrier
XY Normal male

produces crippling deformities. Early death may occur as a result of the pressure of a hematoma (collection of blood within tissue) on a vital structure or from the loss of blood. The latter is rarely fatal since blood and plasma have become so readily available.

Treatment and Nursing Care.   An episode of bleeding is treated by the intravenous infusion of fresh whole blood or frozen plasma to supply Factor VIII(AHG). Local measures used to control the hemorrhage include the application of gentle pressure, cold and hemostatic agents (e.g., thrombin) to the site.

The hemophiliac must be protected from trauma as much as possible. The severity of his disease determines the restrictions placed on his activities. He may be able to attend a regular school but is advised against certain forms of play. For the child whose disease is severe, arrangements may be made for him to pursue his education at home or to attend special classes. The condition must be kept in mind in the selection of toys.

Every person with hemophilia should always carry some form of identification that indicates his disorder and his blood type. His dentist is advised of the condition on the initial visit so that the necessary precautions may be taken. A very soft brush is used to clean the teeth to prevent bleeding from the gums. If a tooth extraction is necessary, the hemophiliac is hospitalized.

Hypoprothrombinemia

Hypoprothrombinemia is a deficiency of prothrombin chiefly resulting from a de-

ficient supply, impaired absorption or defective utilization of vitamin K. The vitamin is essential in the formation of prothrombin and Factor VII by the liver. If the diet does not supply an adequate amount, it is synthesized by the bacteria that normally inhabit the intestinal tract. The bleeding tendency in the newborn is attributed to the lack of bacterial synthesis of vitamin K during the first 2 to 3 days of life when the tract is free of organisms. Sterilization of the bowel by the oral administration of sulfonamides or antibiotics may also produce a vitamin K deficiency.

Bile salts are essential in the intestine for the absorption of vitamin K. A frequent cause of a deficiency of prothrombin is obstruction of the flow of bile into the small intestine. An insufficient production of prothrombin may also occur in liver disease such as chronic cirrhosis.

Hypoprothrombinemia due to impaired synthesis or absorption is treated with a synthetic preparation of vitamin K (menadione) which may be administered parenterally or orally. When the deficiency is due to liver disease, the patient may receive blood transfusions to supply prothrombin.

Thrombocytopenia (Thrombocytopenic Purpura)

Failure of the coagulation process may be due to a deficiency of circulating blood platelets. The reduced number of thrombocytes may be primary or secondary. Primary or idiopathic thrombocytopenia is of unknown etiology. An antigen-antibody reaction has been suggested in which the person develops antibodies (agglutinins) which destroy his thrombocytes. The disease is manifested by bleeding in any site. Petechiae and purpuric areas may appear in the skin or mucous membrane, and bleeding from the nose or the gastrointestinal or urinary tract may occur. Children and young adults, especially females, are more often affected. The severity of the disease varies, and alternating remissions and relapses may occur. The patient is kept at rest and is treated with a corticoid preparation (e.g., prednisone) and transfusions of fresh blood. If the patient does not respond favorably to these, splenectomy may be done.

A reduction in the blood platelets may be secondary to a number of conditions. It is frequently the result of depressed bone marrow activity which is associated with radiation exposure, anticancer drugs and drug sensitivity. Thrombocytopenia also occurs in hypersplenism, leukemia and lupus erythematosus.

Excess of Anticoagulant

Hemorrhage may be a complication of excessive anticoagulant drug therapy. The products commonly used are heparin and preparations of coumarin (e.g., Dicumarol) and phenindione, or Danilone. Heparin inhibits the conversion of prothrombin to thrombin. The other anticoagulants prevent the utilization of vitamin K to form prothrombin. If bleeding occurs, administration of the drug is stopped. Whole blood transfusions may be necessary, and in the case of heparin, protamine sulfate is used as an antidote. If the bleeding is due to the other two anticoagulants cited above, parenteral injections of vitamin K are administered as well as blood transfusions. See page 219 for nursing responsibilities during anticoagulant therapy.

Vascular Purpura

In some instances, bleeding into tissues and organs occurs because of damage to, or a defect in, the small blood vessels. The result may be increased permeability or inadequate vasoconstriction, predisposing to blood loss. This type of disorder may be associated with an allergic reaction, septicemia or a vitamin C deficiency (scurvy).

A rare hereditary bleeding disorder known as hereditary hemorrhagic telangiectasia is characterized by dilated, thin-walled vessels that lack the normal amount of muscular tissue. Angiomas (tumors composed of blood vessels) appear on the skin and mucous membrane surfaces, and normal vasoconstriction does not take place in the affected vessels.

Nursing Patients with a Tendency to Bleed

Specific nursing needs of patients with hemorrhagic disorders vary with each individual and with the cause, associated symptoms, and severity of the disease, but there are some common problems and general considerations applicable to all.

OBSERVATIONS. The skin and mouth are checked for the appearance of petechiae and purple patches. Excreta are examined for blood. A constant alert is necessary for symptoms of internal bleeding such as pallor, weakness, air hunger (rapid deep respirations), rapid weak pulse, fall in blood pressure and signs of disturbed organ function (e.g., cerebral dysfunction due to bleeding into the brain).

PROTECTION FROM TISSUE TRAUMA. The patient is handled gently and tissues are subjected to a minimum of pressure. If confined to bed, he is turned every 1 to 2 hours, and a soft resiliant material such as sponge rubber or sheepskin is placed under the patient. As well as receiving an explanation of the importance of avoiding falls, bumps, scratches, cuts and pressure, the patient and his family receive suggestions as to how tissue trauma may be prevented during the time between bleeding episodes.

MOUTH CARE. A very soft toothbrush is used for cleaning the teeth. The mouth is rinsed frequently with a mild, cool mouthwash. Very hot, rough and highly seasoned foods are avoided in order to prevent damage to the oral and gastrointestinal mucosa.

REST. The patient is kept at rest in bed during a bleeding episode. Since he may not be experiencing any particular discomfort, he may find it difficult to remain inactive. The important role that rest plays is explained, and some suitable diversion should be found for the patient.

PREVENTION OF CRIPPLING DEFORMITIES. Bleeding into joints is a common problem and causes severe pain. In many instances, bone and joint damage and contractures result. The affected joint is immobilized in optimal alignment and protected from the weight of bedding by a cradle. When the bleeding is under control, exercises and physiotherapy are prescribed to restore as full function as possible to the joint(s).

PARENTERAL INJECTIONS. If subcutaneous and intramuscular injections are necessary, a small gauge needle is used. Gentle pressure is applied to the site for several minutes following the administration.

IDENTIFICATION. Every person with an hemorrhagic disorder should at all times bear some form of identification (card or Medic Alert bracelet or pendant) that clearly indicates his bleeding problem and his blood type.

PATIENT AND FAMILY INSTRUCTION. The nature of the disease and the limitations it imposes are explained to the family and to the patient if he is old enough to understand. The restrictions and constant precautions that are necessary usually produce psychological reactions. It is very difficult for a child to refrain from participating in the activities and games of his playmates. He may become resentful and seek undesirable outlets. The nurse emphasizes positive activities and helps parents and the patient to plan for his development and education as well as for appropriate safe recreation. They are advised of the constant need to be alert to early signs of bleeding and of the necessary prompt action.

References

BOOKS

de Gruchy, G. C.: Clinical Haematology. Oxford, Blackwell Scientific Publications, 1960.
Linman, J. W.: Principles of Hematology. New York, The Macmillan Co., 1966.
Thompson, R. B.: A Short Textbook of Hematology, 2nd ed. London, Pitman Medical Publishing Co. Ltd., 1965.

PERIODICALS

Crosby, W. H. (Ed.): "Symposium on Hematologic Disorders." Med. Clin. North Amer., Vol. 50, No. 6 (Nov. 1966).
Lunceford, J. L.: "Leukemia—Disease Process, Chemotherapeutic Approach and Nursing Care." Nurs. Clin. North Amer., Vol. 2, No. 4, pp. 635–647.
McElfresh, A. E.: "Congenital Microspherocytosis." Pediat. Clin. North Amer., Vol. 9, No. 3 (Aug. 1962), pp. 665–670.
Miller, R. W.: "Etiology of Childhood Leukemia." Pediat. Clin. North Amer., Vol. 13, No. 2 (May 1966), pp. 267–275.
Scott, R. B.: "Sickle Cell Anemia." Pediat. Clin. North Amer., Vol. 9, No. 3 (Aug. 1962), pp. 649–661.
Seidler, F. M.: "Adapting Nursing Procedures for Reverse Isolation." Amer. J. Nurs., Vol. 65, No. 6 (June 1965), pp. 108–111.

13
Nursing in Cardiovascular Disease

CIRCULATION

Normal cellular activity is dependent upon a constant supply of oxygen, nutrients, and certain chemicals as well as the removal of metabolic by-products. The unicellular organism is in direct contact with the outside environmental source of its essentials, but in complex multicellular organisms, cell needs are not as simply met. Specialized organs are necessary for the processes of oxygenation, nutrition and excretion as well as a transportation system between these organs and the cells throughout the body. This transportation of materials to and from tissue cells by the propulsion of blood through a closed system of tubes is the process referred to as circulation.

CIRCULATORY STRUCTURES

The circulatory system consists of the heart and the vascular system.

Heart

The heart is a hollow, conical-shaped, muscular organ lying obliquely in the thoracic cavity. Approximately two-thirds of it is situated to the left of the midline. The upper border (or base) lies just below the second rib; the apex, which is directed downward, forward and to the left, lies on the diaphragm at the level of the fifth intercostal space in the midclavicular line. These boundary locations are significant in determining any abnormal enlargement and in counting the apical pulse. The structural organization of the heart includes the pericardium, heart walls, chambers, orifices, valves and coronary system.

Pericardium. The pericardium is a strong, nondistensible sac which loosely encloses the heart and attaches to the large blood vessels at the base of the heart and to the diaphragm at the apex. It consists of two layers. The outer one forms the fibrous pericardium, and the inner one, the serous pericardium, is divided into two layers also; one layer lines the sac, and the other is reflected over the surface of the heart as the epicardium, or visceral pericardium. The space formed between the sac and the heart is normally only a potential space. The surfaces are in close contact, and sufficient serum is secreted to keep them moist so that adhesion and friction between the heart and the sac are prevented. The fibrous pericardium, because of its inextensible nature, averts overdistension of the heart. It also supports the heart, preventing change of its position during postural changes. Although the pericardial sac is firm and considered

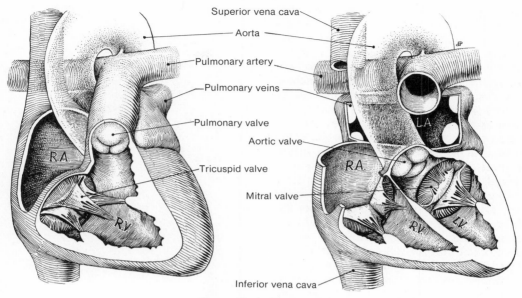

Superior vena cava

Aorta

Pulmonary artery

Pulmonary veins

Pulmonary valve

Aortic valve

Tricuspid valve

Mitral valve

Inferior vena cava

Figure 13–1 The heart.

nonextensible, it does extend in response to the gradual, sustained stretching imposed by enlargement of the heart (hypertrophy).

Heart Walls and Chambers. From shortly after birth, the human heart is divided longitudinally by a partition into two halves between which there is no direct communication. The cavity of each side is divided horizontally by an incomplete partition which results in two upper chambers, called the right and left atria, and two lower ones, which are the right and left ventricles (see Fig. 13–1).

The walls of the heart consist of three layers—the epicardium, myocardium and endocardium. The myocardium (heart muscle) comprises the main functional part of the heart wall; its rhythmic contractions provide the pumping force which maintains circulation. It is formed of involuntary striated muscle fibers which interlace, branch, anastomose and coalesce. This arrangement produces a very firm, closely related mass of tissue through which an excitatory impulse for contraction spreads very quickly. The muscle fibers of the atria are continuous and behave as a single mass. Similarly, those of the ventricles are also continuous and act as a single mass. Atrial

muscle fibers are completely separated from those of the ventricles by fibrous tissue.

The atrial myocardium is much thinner than that of the ventricles, and the left ventricular wall is thicker than that of the right. This difference can be correlated with the force that must be given to the contained blood. The atria are receiving chambers and are only required to deliver the blood to the ventricles, which discharge blood from the heart. The right ventricle pumps blood through the lungs to the left atrium, forming the circuit referred to as the pulmonary circulatory system. The left ventricle must provide sufficient pressure to carry blood through all parts of the body and return it to the right atrium. This latter circuit is referred to as the systemic circulatory system.

Special Structures. Two small masses of specialized tissue lie within the atrial myocardium—the sino-atrial (S-A) node and the atrioventricular (A-V) node. The S-A node is located in the upper part of the right atrium near the superior vena cava and is responsible for initiating the impulses for the rhythmic heart beats.

The A-V node lies in the lower part of the interatrial septum and is a part of the system that conducts impulses from the atria to the ventricles. A bundle of fibers called the bundle of His proceeds from junctional tissue at the A-V node into the ventricular septum where it divides into two, forming the left and right bundle branches. As it descends, each bundle branch gives rise to a network of fine fibers which are known as the Purkinje fibers. They are distributed to the ventricular myocardial cells.

Orifices in the Chambers. The right atrium has three inlets and one outlet. Blood is received from two large veins, the superior and inferior venae cavae, and the coronary sinus. The outlet channels the blood into the right ventricle. The right ventricle has two openings—the inlet from the right atrium and an outlet into the pulmonary artery.

The left atrium has four inlets, which are the terminations of the four pulmonary veins, and one outlet into the left ventricle. The blood received from the left atrium is discharged by the left ventricle into the aorta.

Endocardium. The endocardium is the smooth endothelial lining of the heart chambers. It covers the valves and is continuous with the lining of the blood vessels entering and leaving the heart. Its smooth surface reduces friction between the blood and the vessel.

Cardiac Valves. Normal circulation requires the flow of the blood in one direction only. This is maintained in the heart by a set of four valves—two atrioventricular and two semilunar.

The atrioventricular valves are formed of fibrous cusps, or leaflets, which derive from the fibrous ring that encircles each atrioventricular opening. They are covered with endothelial tissue which is continuous with the endocardium. The right atrioventricular valve has three cusps and is referred to as the tricuspid valve; the left one has two cusps and is called the mitral valve. These valves open into the ventricles but are prevented from opening into the atria by fine tendinous cords (chordae tendineae) which insert on the free border of the leaflets and originate in small pillars of muscle projecting from the ventricular walls (papillary muscles). When the ventricles fill, the valve flaps are forced up in the direction of the atrioventricular opening. They meet, closing off the opening, and with the contraction of the papillary muscles sufficient tension is

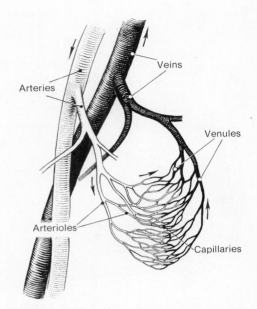

Figure 13–2 Artery—arteriole—capillary—vein sequence in circulation.

exerted by the chordae tendineae to prevent the valves from opening into the atria (see Fig. 13–1).

The semilunar valves guard the openings from the ventricles into the pulmonary artery and aorta. These consist of three pocket-like pouches arranged around the origin of the artery, with the free borders being distal to the ventricle (see Fig. 13–1). During the contraction of the ventricles and ejection of blood under considerable pressure into the aorta and pulmonary artery, the valve flaps lie free in the stream, offering no resistance to the flow of the blood. When the ventricles relax and there is a reversal in the direction of pressure, blood fills out the semilunar pouches, bringing their surfaces together. This closes off the aperture into each ventricle, preventing a backflow.

Cardiac Blood Supply (Coronary System). The myocardium receives its blood supply from the right and left coronary arteries, which arise from the aorta just beyond the aortic semilunar valve. The left coronary artery divides into the anterior descending artery and the circumflex artery. The anterior descending branch is distributed to the anterior part of the left ventricle and portions of the right ventricle. The circumflex artery carries blood to the lateral and lower posterior, left ventricular walls and to the left atrium. Branches of the right coronary artery supply the remaining portions of the myocardium. The large arteries divide and subdivide to form a network of smaller arteries and capillaries throughout the heart muscle. The blood is returned to the right atrium through a system of progressively enlarging veins which terminate in the coronary sinus.

The myocardium requires a large blood supply since it must work continuously and adapt its activity to the varying needs of tissues throughout the body. The coronary vessels dilate to increase the supply when demands are increased. They also dilate when there is an increase in the carbon dioxide concentration of the blood and a decrease in the pH.

The flow of blood through the coronary system is dependent upon the pressure of the blood in the aorta; a reduction in blood pressure will result in a lesser volume entering the coronary arteries. The coronary volume is greater during myocardial relaxation. In systole, with the myocardium contracted, the vessels are compressed and their volume is reduced. When a person is at rest, the blood entering the coronary system is approximately 4 per cent of the total cardiac output. The coronary blood supply can be increased, but to a lesser degree than the cardiac output. That is, the work of the myocardium can be increased to a greater extent than its blood supply can be.

Vascular System

The blood travels from the heart successively through arteries, arterioles, capillaries and veins back to the heart. The structure of each type of vessel is modified according to its function and location. One common structural characteristic of all the vessels is the smooth, endothelial lining known as the intima. The arteries and arterioles form a high-pressure distributing system; the capillaries are structured and organized for exchanging substances between the blood and interstitial fluid; the venules and veins serve as a low-pressure collecting system which returns the blood to the heart.

Arteries. The large arteries carry blood away from the heart and branch and subdivide many times. Their structure varies with their size, the larger ones being more elastic and less muscular. Elasticity is an important property of these vessels; with the ejection of blood from the heart, the vessel distends and on recoil exerts a slight pressure on the contained fluid, helping to force it forward. If resistance is offered to the flow of the blood, normally the arteries can stretch to accommodate the increased volume of blood, and the pressure of the blood remains within the normal range. Reduced elasticity and a thickening of the arterial walls with a narrowing of the lumen, as seen in arteriosclerosis and atherosclerosis, result in a rise in the arterial blood pressure.

Arterioles. The smallest arteries emerge as arterioles which have walls composed mainly of a well-developed muscular coat over the endothelium. The muscle tissue may contract or relax to decrease or increase the amount of blood through the arterioles. This feature of the arterioles gives them an important role in determining arterial blood pressure and in controlling the blood supply to tissues.

Capillaries. Each arteriole channels its content into microscopic endothelial tubes, the capillaries, which anastomose with each other to form a capillary bed. These vessels are the principal functional unit of the cardiovascular system. The functions of the other structures (heart, arteries and veins) are contributory to that of the capillaries. The exchange of substances to maintain and regulate cell activity takes place as the blood passes through these minute, semipermeable vessels.

Not all the capillaries are open at all times. There are wide variations in the amount of activity in some tissues (e.g., skeletal muscle), while in others a more constant blood supply is necessary, as in brain tissue. Similarly, when an area is irritated, more blood is brought to that part in its defense (e.g., inflammation). The number of capillaries through which blood is passing at any given time is adjusted locally to meet the needs of the tissues in the area. Blood volume in the capillaries increases as tissue activity increases. Ruch and Patton state that in some resting structures only $1/20$ to $1/50$ of the capillary bed may be open to circulation.[1] This adjustment is made possible by the fact that some capillaries have at their origin a ring of plain muscular tissue which forms a precapillary sphincter.

Venules and Veins. The collecting part of the vascular system originates in venules which drain the capillaries and progressively unite and enlarge to form the veins. They differ from arteries in several ways: they carry blood toward the heart; their walls are much thinner and less elastic with the result that they collapse when empty; the contained blood is under a much lower pressure; and many of the veins have valves.

The structure of veins changes as they increase in size; more muscle and fibrous tissue appear in the walls, but in comparison with arteries, the muscle fibers are sparse. Most of the pressure of the blood created by the heart is dissipated in the arterioles and capillaries, and in order to maintain the flow in one direction, valves similar in structure to the semilunar valves of the heart occur at intervals in many of the veins. They are particularly numerous in the lower extremities where the blood is flowing against gravity. The thinner walls of the veins are readily compressed by skeletal muscle contraction; this assists the blood along its course toward the heart, since backflow toward the capillaries is prevented by the valves.

PHYSIOLOGY OF CIRCULATION

Normal circulation through the cardiovascular system is dependent upon an appropriate pressure gradient throughout the system, an adequate volume of blood, a closed system of unobstructed tubes and a set of valves to ensure flow in one direction only.

Principles Applicable to the Flow of Fluids through Tubes

Since circulation is the continuous flow of blood in a pressure system comprised of a pump and a series of tubes filled with the blood, it might be well at this point to consider some physical factors which govern the flow of any liquid through tubes. The

[1]Theodore C. Ruch and Harry D. Patton: Physiology and Biophysics, 19th ed. Philadelphia, W. B. Saunders Co., 1965, p. 619.

rate at which a fluid moves through a tube depends upon the pressure gradient and the resistance to flow.

Pressure Gradient. Fluids flow from an area of high pressure to one of lower pressure. The pressure of the fluid at any given point in the system must be greater than that in the succeeding area into which it is to flow. This difference is referred to as the pressure gradient, or driving force. If the pressure should become the same throughout the system, no movement of the fluid takes place.

The pressure gradient which maintains the normal flow of blood through the vessels is the difference between the pressure of the blood in the arterial system and that of the venous system. The main source of the driving force is the pumping action of the heart which produces a relatively high pressure in the arteries.

Resistance to Flow. The amount of resistance offered to the flow of fluid is determined by the dimensions of the tube and the viscosity of the fluid.

The pressure of a fluid progressively decreases as it flows through a tube because of the friction between the fluid and the walls of the tube. This friction, which is referred to as peripheral resistance, causes a loss of energy. Fluid flows more slowly through a tube of smaller diameter since more friction is created between the walls and the fluid, resulting in an increase in resistance. As the blood flows through the blood vessels having a lesser radius (arterioles and capillaries), resistance is increased, causing a decrease in the rate of flow and blood pressure.

Similarly, resistance is increased as the length of the tube increases, since the greater amount of surface provides more friction.

If the volume of fluid remains the same in a system of tubes, the rate of flow decreases as the tubular space (capacity) increases. This factor contributes to the marked decrease in the velocity of the blood in the capillaries. Although the radius of the capillaries is extremely small, the total cross-sectional area of the vast number of these minute tubes exceeds the total area of all the other vessels combined.

The viscosity of a fluid is an internal resistance to flow created by the friction between the molecules of the fluid and their tendency to cohere. Obviously, a greater concentration of particles in a fluid produces an increased internal resistance. For example, an excessive number of blood cells, particularly erythrocytes, increases the viscosity of the blood and retards its rate of flow.

In summary, resistance to flow is inversely proportional to the diameter of the tube, directly proportional to the length of the tube, and directly proportional to the viscosity of the fluid. If the volume of fluid remains the same, the rate of flow decreases as the diameter of the tube increases.

The preceding principles are based on the flow of fluids through rigid tubes. Some modification is necessary in applying them to circulation. The blood vessels are not rigid tubes and their diameters are variable. Branches, divisions and curves occur at frequent intervals in the blood vessels. Blood is viscous, and its flow is pulsatile rather than steady in a large part of the circulatory system.

THE ROLE OF THE HEART IN CIRCULATION

The pressure that keeps the blood in continuous movement through the circulatory system originates in the heart and is augmented slightly by the elastic recoil of the large arteries. A continuous succession of alternate myocardial contractions and relaxations, occurring rhythmically on an average of 60 to 70 times per minute, pumps the blood through the body.

Impulse Origin and Conduction in Heart Contraction

The cells of the myocardium are of two types—those which contract when stimulated and those which originate and conduct impulses. The contractile muscle fibers have an absolute and a relative refractory period. The fibers are unresponsive to any stimulus during the absolute refractory period which immediately follows a contraction. The relative refractory period is the interval in which the muscle fibers gradually recover their excitability (ability to respond to a stimulus) but will respond to a stimulus if it is stronger

than the usual. The refractory period in cardiac muscle is longer than in other muscle tissue. Excitability is more slowly regained, giving the heart chambers time to fill effectively.

Contraction of the myocardium is dependent upon impulses which arise within the myocardium itself. The structures capable of generating and conducting impulses within the myocardium form the conduction system. They are the sino-atrial (S-A) node, tracts of conducting fibers originating with the S-A node, the atrioventricular (A-V) node, the bundle of His, bundle branches and the Purkinje fibers. Several areas of the conduction system are capable of the spontaneous generation of impulses—namely, the S-A node, the junctional tissue where the conducting fibers join the A-V node, the bundle of His and the Purkinje fibers. The rates at which impulses are normally fired vary in the different areas: the S-A node originates approximately 60 to 80 impulses per minute; the junctional tissue, 50 to 60 impulses per minute; the bundle of His, 40 to 50 impulses per minute; and the Purkinje fibers, 30 to 40 per minute. If the S-A node is discharging at a normal rate, the impulses which are fixed at a slower rate

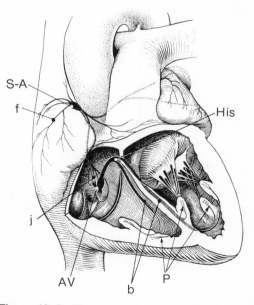

Figure 13–3 The conduction system of the heart.

by the other areas arrive at the contractile fibers following their contraction when they are refractory. Since the region which is producing the highest rate of impulses sets the heart rhythm (number of contractions per minute), the S-A node is referred to as the normal pacemaker.

Impulses arising in the S-A node are quickly conducted through the atria, initiating their contraction. At the same time, they are transmitted to the A-V node where they are delayed; this delay allows for completion of atrial emptying and ventricular filling. From the A-V node and junctional tissue they travel through the bundle of His and along the right and left bundle branches and the widely distributed Purkinje fibers to the ventricular contractile fibers.

The Cardiac Cycle

The succession of events which occurs with each heartbeat is called the cardiac cycle. It consists of the relaxation and contraction of the atria and ventricles and the opening and closing of the cardiac valves in a sequence that permits the filling and emptying of the heart chambers. Contraction of the atria or ventricles is called systole; their relaxation is known as diastole. In referring to contraction or relaxation of the atria or ventricles, the terms used are atrial or ventricular systole or atrial or ventricular diastole respectively. If systole or diastole is used alone, it refers to ventricular performance only.

The sequence of events of the cardiac cycle is as follows: The atria in diastole fill with blood received from their inlet vessels. In the early part of the relaxation period, the atrioventricular (A-V) valves are closed; but as pressure builds up in the atria, it becomes greater than that in the ventricles, forcing the A-V valves open, and the blood starts to flow through into the ventricles. Atrial diastole is followed in a fraction of a second by contraction to complete the emptying of the two upper chambers, and the atria again enter their diastole.

During the filling and contraction of the ventricles, the blood floats the A-V valvular flaps up, closing off the A-V openings and preventing a regurgitation of blood into the atria. In order to receive the blood from the atria, the ventricles must be in diastole and

at this time, the semilunar valves are closed. With ventricular filling, the intraventricular pressure builds up until it exceeds that in the aorta and pulmonary artery with the result that the semilunar valves open, allowing blood to flow into the arteries. The ventricular muscle contracts, and the ventricles are emptied.

During ventricular systole, the papillary muscles also contract, exerting tension on the fine tendons (chordae tendineae) inserted on the A-V valvular flaps. This prevents the flaps from opening into the atria. If this control was not placed on the A-V valves, there would be a backflow into the atria, especially with the ventricular contraction. The ventricles relax following their systole and emptying. This results in the pressure being greater in the arteries than in the ventricles, thus favoring the backflow of blood into the ventricles. But flow in the direction of the heart brings about the closure of the semilunar valves by the filling of the semilunar pouches; their free borders are brought together, preventing the blood from re-entering the ventricles from the arteries. The cardiac cycle is now completed.

The cycle in a heart beating approximately 70 times per minute is completed in 0.7 to 0.8 of a second. The length of each phase of the cycle varies; atrial diastole lasts approximately 0.7 second, while its systole is approximately 0.1 second. Ventricular diastole is about 0.4 to 0.5 second, and its systole takes about 0.3 second. Following the ventricular contraction there is a brief period, approximately 0.4 second, in which the entire myocardium is relaxed. The ventricular diastole overlaps the atrial diastole.[2]

Heart Sounds

Two sounds are produced in quick succession in each cardiac cycle. These are followed by a brief pause before being repeated in the next cycle. The first is a prolonged, low-pitched sound ("lubb"), heard best over the apex. It is produced mainly by the closure of the A-V valves and may be referred to as the systolic sound.

---

[2] N. T. Taylor, and M. G. McPhedran: Basic Physiology and Anatomy. Toronto, The MacMillan Co. of Canada Ltd., 1965, p. 361

The second, or diastolic, sound is briefer and higher pitched ("dup"). It follows ventricular systole and is produced by the closure of the semilunar valves.

Cardiac Output

The volume of blood ejected from each ventricle in a minute is known as the cardiac output. The output of each ventricle with each contraction is called the stroke volume. In an adult, the cardiac output varies from 3000 to 5000 ml. per minute, and the stroke volume is about 60 to 70 ml. If it were 60 ml. in a person with a heart rate of 60, the cardiac output would be 3600 ml. (Stroke volume × heart rate = cardiac output per minute.)

The volume of blood that the normal heart pumps out each minute is increased in any situation that increases the body demands and activity. This is readily seen in physical exercise. In strenuous exertion the cardiac output may increase to a volume 13 times the output during rest. This is achieved by an increase in the heart rate and the stroke volume. An increase in the cardiac output also occurs in high environmental temperature, emotional responses such as fear, anger or other excitement, after a heavy meal and in the later months of pregnancy.

Physiologically, the cardiac output is contingent upon the efficiency of the heart as a pump and upon the venous return. Obviously, normal heart structures, absence of disease, and an adequate supply of nutrients and oxygen are important factors in the heart's ability to produce the necessary force to eject the contained blood. If the heart is undamaged and is in a condition to respond, the strength of the heartbeat is determined mainly by the length of the muscle fibers when contraction begins. Stretching of muscle fibers, within limits, increases the strength of their contraction. The length or stretching of the myocardial fibers is dependent upon the volume of blood entering the heart. This principle is known as Starling's law of the heart and may be expressed in this manner: "the energy of contraction is proportional to the initial length of the cardiac muscle fiber."[3]

---

[3]Stanley W. Jacob and Clarice A. Francone: Structure and Function in Man, 2nd ed. Philadelphia, W. B. Saunders Co., 1970, p. 320

The volume of the venous return to the heart is influenced by several factors: the volume and pressure of the blood, resistance to the blood flow, physical exercise and respirations. A decrease in the volume or pressure of the blood in the systemic circulation causes a decrease in the venous return. This is seen in hemorrhage, in which the volume is reduced, and in shock, which is characterized by a fall in blood pressure. Certain areas of the body normally contain a relatively large volume of blood which may be moved out when the normal circulating volume is threatened. These areas are referred to as blood reservoirs and are the liver, spleen, large abdominal veins and venous plexuses of the skin. When necessary, the liver will increase its output into the hepatic vein, and the spleen will contract to empty as much as three-quarters of its contained blood into the circulation. Similarly, when the total circulating volume is reduced, the large abdominal veins constrict to increase their outflow. The venous plexuses of the skin which normally contain a considerable volume of blood will also constrict when necessary to provide a greater flow to the heart.

Increased resistance to the blood flow anywhere in the circulatory system may reduce venous return to the heart and cause a corresponding decrease in cardiac output.

Muscular exercise is one of the most significant factors in promoting venous return. When skeletal muscles contract, veins are compressed, and more blood is forced out of them. It must move toward the heart since the valves prevent a backward flow. Also, the increased metabolism in the muscles during exercise increases their need for oxygen and nutrients, resulting in local vasodilation of the arterioles and capillaries which reduces resistance to the flow of blood in the muscles. Since exercise usually involves a large number of muscles, this causes an appreciable decrease in the total resistance in the systemic circulation, favoring an increased venous return and cardiac output.

The rate and depth of respirations also have a marked effect on venous return; increased respirations increase the volume of blood entering the right atrium. On inspiration, the diaphragm descends, compressing the abdominal cavity and increasing the pressure on the veins in that area. At the same time, the thoracic cavity enlarges and the pressure on regional veins is reduced. This increases the pressure gradient between the blood in the abdominal veins and that in the thoracic veins so that a greater volume flows from the abdominal veins into the thoracic vena cava and on into the heart.

The foregoing explanation of the effects of exercise and respirations on the venous return and cardiac output explains the importance of having inactive and bed patients breathe deeply at frequent intervals and do some physical exercises. These activities promote circulation and help to prevent complications that may occur with circulatory stasis.

Sympathetic nervous innervation may augment the volume of blood in circulation, and thus the venous return, by causing organs such as the liver and spleen to reduce their intrinsic volume.

The ability of the heart to increase its output commensurate with increased tissue activity and needs is referred to as cardiac reserve. The normal heart is capable of forwarding the volume of blood delivered to it and of responding to an increased demand without difficulty. It does this without causing breathlessness, tachycardia or palpitation beyond 5 to 10 minutes. It can do approximately 13 times what it does at rest if its reserve is normal.

Heart Rate

The number of heartbeats per minute varies in different persons and under different conditions. The average normal rate for an adult is 70, but it may range from 60 to 90 beats per minute. Several factors influence the heart rate. In the infant a rate of 110 to 130 is normal. It becomes progressively slower as the child grows older; by the early teens it is usually about 80. Muscular exertion will produce a marked increase, especially if one is unaccustomed to physical exercise. The rate usually increases during emotional reactions, fever, and in the lower atmospheric pressures found at high altitudes.

Regulation of Cardiac Activity

Certain nervous, chemical and mechanical factors play an important role in the action of the heart.

Nervous Influence. The heart muscle is capable of generating its own impulses for contraction, but nerve impulses from the parasympathetic and sympathetic divisions of the autonomic nervous system may modify the rate and strength of the contractions. Nervous regulation is mediated by impulses with arise in the medulla oblongata in a group of neurons known as the cardiac center. Parasympathetic impulses reach the heart by way of branches of the vagus nerve (10th cranial nerve) and are delivered to the S-A and A-V nodes and to the atrial muscle. Vagal or parasympathetic innervation has an inhibitory effect on cardiac activity; it slows the heart rate and decreases the force of the atrial contraction by reducing the excitability of the pacemaker (S-A node) and the conductivity of the A-V node and conducting system.

Sympathetic impulses enter the heart by the cardiac accelerator nerves, originating in a cervical ganglion. These impulses are transmitted to the S-A node, the conducting system, and the atrial and ventricular muscle. Sympathetic stimulation increases the heart rate and the strength of the heart contractions.

Parasympathetic innervation predominates in heart action. Normally, it exerts a fairly constant check on the heart rate, thus conserving the heart's strength.

The cardiac center may be stimulated by impulses originating in higher levels of the brain or in some part of the body which is outside the central nervous system (brain and spinal cord). One need only recall the change experienced in one's own heart action during fear, anger or other excitement. The response of increased or decreased heart activity is due to impulses being discharged by the cerebral cortical level to the cardiac center.

Sensory impulses from outside the central nervous system enter the cord or brain and may be relayed to the cardiac center, resulting in innervation of the heart. The response of the heart to peripheral sensory impulses may be referred to as a cardiac reflex. The most significant of these are the vasosensory impulses originating in the pressoreceptors and chemoreceptors. A group of sensory nerve endings in the aortic arch and in the carotid artery at its bifurcation are sensitive to changes in the blood pressure and are called pressoreceptors. In the same areas are nerve endings that are sensitive to changes in the carbon dioxide and oxygen concentration and the pH (hydrogen ion concentration) of the blood. These are known as the chemoreceptors. Impulses initiated in these receptors enter the brain or cord and are relayed to the cardiac center.

An increase in blood pressure produces a response in the cardio-inhibitory center. Vagal stimulation of the heart is increased and the heart rate decreases.* A decrease in the oxygen concentration, an increase in carbon dioxide concentration and a decrease of the pH of the blood result in stimulation of the cardio-accelerator center and in elevation of the heart rate.

Chemical Influence. Normal, rhythmic heart contractions are greatly dependent upon an optimal concentration of potassium, sodium and calcium in the extracellular fluid.** These minerals play an important role in the excitability of the cardiac muscle cells and their contraction.

If potassium is increased above the normal concentration in the extracellular fluid, an impairment in conduction and contraction occur. It causes a prolonged relaxation of the heart with abnormal dilation of the chambers. The pulse becomes slow. A decrease below the normal concentration of sodium results in weaker contractions. The pulse is rapid and weak, and there is a fall in blood pressure. An excess sodium concentration does not directly affect cardiac action. An excess of calcium produces a stronger and prolonged systole. Conversely, a lack of calcium prolongs the diastole.

Other chemicals of significance in heart action are oxygen and carbon dioxide. Any deficiency of oxygen is quickly reflected in a weakening of heart action. The myocardium is much more sensitive to oxygen lack than skeletal muscle; it will stand only one-fifth as much oxygen deficiency as skeletal muscle. The pulse becomes rapid, weak and irregular. With an excess of carbon dioxide in the blood, as may occur in respiratory insufficiency, heart action is impaired. Conduction is slowed, the relaxation period is prolonged and the contraction is briefer than normal.

Mechanical Influence. The principal mechanical influence on cardiac activity is the stretching of the myocardial fibers by the volume of blood entering the chambers. As previously stated, stretching of muscle fibers increases the strength of their contraction (Starling's law of the heart, p. 183). An increase in arterial blood pressure also demands a greater force of contraction; the heart muscle must release a greater amount of energy to perform its function because of meeting greater resistance.

BLOOD PRESSURE AND PULSE

Blood Pressure

Blood pressure may be defined as the pressure exerted laterally on the walls of the blood vessels. It varies in different parts of the circulatory system, being greatest in the large arteries, with a progressive decrease as the blood continues on through the smaller arteries, arterioles, capillaries and veins. The pressure is highest in the aorta and lowest in the large caval veins which enter the heart. Blood pressure at any point in the vascular system is dependent upon the force with which the heart pumps the blood out of the ventricles, the volume of blood in the system, the elasticity of the arteries and the amount of resistance to the flow of the blood from one portion of the circulatory system to the next.

Arterial Blood Pressure. The blood pressure of greatest clinical interest is that in the arteries. The pulsatile nature of heart activity causes fluctuations in the pressure. With each contraction of the left ventricle, a volume of blood is pumped into the aorta, which is already filled with blood. This causes an appreciable increase in the pressure of the blood and stretches the aortic walls. If the aorta were not elastic, the rise in pressure would be much higher and sharper. During the ventricular diastole, the elastic walls of the aorta recoil, exerting a pressure on the contained blood. If the aorta were a rigid tube which did not recoil, the pressure of the blood would fall more rapidly and to a much lower level than it does normally. The higher pressure produced by the ventricular systole is referred to as the

---

*Marey's law. The pulse rate is inversely related to the arterial blood pressure.

**Optimal serum concentrations:

K+	3.5 –	5.0 mEq./L.
Na+	135.0 – 145.0 mEq./L.	
Ca++	4.5 –	5.5 mEq./L.

systolic blood pressure. The lower pressure that occurs during the ventricular diastole is dependent upon the recoil of the large arteries and is known as the diastolic blood pressure. The difference between the systolic pressures is called the pulse pressure. Pulse pressure varies inversely with the elasticity of the arteries. Rigid vessels with a loss of ability to distend and recoil produce a higher systolic pressure and a lower diastolic pressure, resulting in a higher pulse pressure.

MEASUREMENT. Arterial blood pressure is most frequently measured in millimeters of mercury (mm. Hg) by means of a sphygmomanometer and a stethoscope using the brachial artery. The rubber cuff of the blood pressure apparatus is applied to the upper arm just above the elbow and is inflated with air which compresses the brachial artery. The pressure in the cuff is transmitted to the column of mercury of the manometer. The stethoscope is applied over the brachial artery just below the cuff.

When the cuff pressure becomes greater than the blood pressure, no pulse is heard. The air in the cuff is slowly released and the height of the mercury on the manometer noted when the pulse is first heard. This corresponds to the systolic blood pressure.

With further slow deflation of the cuff, the pulse gradually becomes softer and fades. The level of the mercury is again noted just before the pulse becomes inaudible; this represents the diastolic blood pressure. If the blood pressure is recorded as 100 mm. Hg, it simply means that the pressure of the blood on the walls of the vessel is sufficient to raise a column of mercury to a height of 100 mm. The normal systolic pressure in a healthy young adult in a sitting position is 100 to 135 mm. Hg; the normal diastolic pressure is 60 to 80 mm. Hg. Blood pressure may also be determined by a more direct method. A needle or a cannula is placed in an artery and connected to a mercury manometer on which the blood pressure is indicated. For continuous monitoring of blood pressure, the needle may be connected to a transducer for electronic recording.

FACTORS WHICH DETERMINE ARTERIAL BLOOD PRESSURE. Arterial blood pressure is influenced by the strength of the heartbeat, volume of blood, elasticity of the vessels and the resistance offered to the flow of blood.

If the myocardial strength is weakened by disease, lack of essential materials or a deficiency in stimulation, it follows that the pressure under which the blood is ejected into the arteries would be reduced as well as the volume of blood emitted. The arterial pressure is directly proportional to the cardiac output.

Any reduction in the intravascular volume will reduce the head of pressure and the stretch and recoil of the arteries, resulting in an appreciable decrease in the pressure of the blood. Small decreases in the volume are compensated for by the contraction of vessels, but in some conditions (e.g., hemorrhage, severe dehydration, burns) the loss may be beyond compensation. In some instances, vasodilation may occur (e.g., shock, anaphylaxis), increasing the capacity of the system beyond that of the contained volume, and the blood pressure falls. A disproportion between the volume of blood and the capacity of the vascular system due to widespread vasodilatation or a diminished blood volume, as in hemorrhage, reduces the venous return to the heart. This is an important factor in determining the cardiac output, the strength of the heartbeat and the blood pressure.

Aldosterone, a hormone secreted by the adrenal cortex, produces an increase in the intravascular volume and a corresponding increase in blood pressure by its effect on kidney activity. It promotes absorption of sodium by the kidney tubules. The increased sodium concentration of the blood in turn causes more water to be absorbed by the renal tubules, increasing the total vascular volume and, as a result, the blood pressure. Conversely, a reduction in aldosterone secretion will reduce the intravascular volume, and the blood pressure falls. The mechanism that regulates the amount of aldosterone secreted by the adrenal cortices is not yet established.

The elastic quality of the large arteries has an important role in determining blood pressure. It allows for an increase in the capacity of the arteries when the blood is ejected by each heartbeat. The stretch factor reduces the resistance offered to the flow of blood from the heart, thus reducing somewhat the demand on that organ. With ventricular diastole and the run-off of blood into succeeding vessels, the elastic arterial wall recoils. This provides some pressure on the contained blood to augment its forward movement and helps to maintain a continuous flow of blood between ventricular contractions. The pressure of the blood at this time (i.e., during arterial recoil and between ventricular contractions) represents the diastolic blood pressure. If the elasticity of the arteries is reduced, as in arteriosclerosis, the blood is pumped into rigid, nondistensible tubes; the systolic pressure is increased because of the lack of vascular stretching and the diastolic pressure is reduced because of the reduced recoil force.

The amount of resistance with which the blood is met as it flows through the vascular system depends mainly on the caliber of the arterioles and the viscosity of the blood.

The relatively large lumen of the arteries offers little peripheral resistance to the flow of blood, but their subsequent branching into numerous arterioles introduces more surface contact for the blood which increases friction and resistance to the flow. This resistance determines the rate at which blood can flow from the arteries into the arterioles, which in turn influences the volume of blood confined in the arteries and, hence, the arterial blood pressure.

Normally, the arterioles are in a constant state of partial contraction referred to as the basic level of tone, but the caliber of the vessels may be modified by contraction or relaxation of the well-developed, circular, smooth muscle in the walls in response to various factors. Obviously, with relaxation, the increased diameter of the arterioles will offer less resistance, more blood will pass from the arteries through the arterioles to the capillaries and the arterial blood pressure will tend to be normal or below normal. Conversely, with contraction of the arterioles, the decreased diameter increases the resistance to the blood flow, less blood escapes from the arteries and arterial blood pressure is maintained at a normal or above normal level. The caliber of the arterioles is controlled by nerve impulses delivered to the musculature of the arterioles and by certain chemical changes in the extracellular fluids. The latter may exercise their influence directly on the vessels or indirectly through the autonomic nervous system.

Neural control of vasotone is exerted by the autonomic nervous system. The vessels are supplied by two types of nerve fibers: those whose impulses cause contraction of the muscle tissue of the vessel are the excitatory or vasoconstrictor nerves, and those which cause relaxation are the inhibitory or vasodilator nerves. All vasoconstrictor nerves derive from the sympathetic division of the autonomic nervous system. Vasodilation may be initiated by a decrease in sympathetic innervation which allows a relaxation of the smooth muscle of the vessel or, in some instances, dilation results from impulses delivered by nerves to the vessel walls. The vasodilator, or inhibitory, nerves in some areas of the body belong to the parasympathetic division; in others the vasodilator as well as the vasoconstrictor nerves originate in the sympathetic nervous system. Sympathetic vasodilators are distributed to the vessels of skeletal muscles, the intestines, the genitalia, the coronary system and some areas of the skin. Parasympathetic vasodilators supply the vessels in the pharynx, tongue, sweat and salivary glands and brain.[4]

The principal source of the impulses that regulate the caliber of the blood vessels is the vasomotor center in the medulla. Some may arise from spinal cord neurons in the thoracolumbar areas. These areas may be influenced by impulses received from the blood vessels themselves, the pressoreceptors and chemoreceptors of the carotid sinus and aortic arch, the cerebral cortex, the hypothalamus and various other regions of the body such as the skin, muscles and viscera.

Chemical influence of the smooth muscle in the vessels may be direct or may be indirect through the nervous system. Certain chemical changes in the composition of the extracellular fluid may result in the initiation

---

[4]Facts relating to the innervation of the blood vessels are not well established. Some controversy appears between several authoritative references (listed).

Arthur C. Guyton: Textbook of Medical Physiology, 4th ed. Philadelphia, W. B. Saunders Co., 1971, p. 272.

Ewald E. Selkurt (Ed.): Physiology. Boston, Little, Brown and Co., 1963, p. 331.

Charles H. Best and Norman B. Taylor: The Physiological Basis of Medical Practice, 7th ed. Baltimore, The Williams and Wilkins Co., 1961, p. 256.

L. L. Langley: Outline of Physiology, 2nd ed. New York, The Blakiston Division, McGraw-Hill Book Co., 1965, pp. 225–26.

of nerve impulses which influence the blood vessels. Increased carbon dioxide or decreased oxygen tension results in vasoconstriction and a corresponding increase in resistance. Similarly, an increase in the hydrogen ion concentration (decreased pH) causes vasoconstriction.

A direct effect on the arterioles may be produced by metabolites and hormones. Metabolites produce the opposite effect locally to that caused indirectly through the nervous system. An increase in the concentration of hydrogen ions and carbon dioxide and a diminished oxygen tension in an area cause dilatation of the arterioles in that area. The indirect action of the nervous system produces a more general vasoconstriction and a rise in blood pressure, increasing the rate of flow through the locally dilated arterioles where there is an increased need for more oxygen, nutrients and for more metabolites to be removed.

When tissue cells are irritated or injured, chemical substances are released which produce relaxation in the local arterioles and capillaries, resulting in more blood in the area. One of these substances is identified as histamine, a strong vasodilator.

Still another chemical substance, renin, stimulates vasocontriction and increases arterial blood pressure. It is produced by kidney tissue in response to a diminished blood supply (renal ischemia). Renin is a proteolytic enzyme which, when released into the blood stream, acts upon a globulin fraction, producing the vasoconstrictor angiotonin (hypertensin) that acts directly on the arterioles. It would appear that angiotonin has no significant role in the maintenance of normal blood pressure as it is quickly destroyed in the healthy person. It remains active for a longer period in persons with a blood pressure higher than normal and is receiving some attention in relation to the disease hypertension.

The hormones associated with vasomotor activity are epinephrine and pituitrin. Epinephrine, secreted by the adrenal medulla or administered parenterally, has a direct vasoconstricting effect on the arterioles in the skin, mucous membranes and the splanchnic area. At the same time, it inhibits the tone in the arterioles of the skeletal muscles and the coronary system. Ruch and Patton suggest that the effect of epinephrine on the coronaries may be indirect, since the hormone stimulates metabolism which results in oxygen need and an accumulation of metabolites.[5]

Pituitrin, which is secreted by the neurohypophysis or posterior lobe of the pituitary gland, contains a principle, vasopressin. It excites the smooth muscle of most blood vessels, but its effect is slower than that of epinephrine.

It may be seen from the foregoing discussion of vasomotor regulation that peripheral resistance is a complex affair. Resistance is directly proportional to the length of vessels and inversely proportional to the diameter, and many factors may influence the diameter. A moderate degree of vasoconstriction is essential; most of the arterioles must be in a partial state of constriction at all times. If too many vessels relax at one time, blood pressure falls to dangerously low levels, and circulation becomes seriously impaired.

Frequent and quick readjustments in the caliber of the arterioles are necessary to maintain a relatively constant level of blood pressure and to meet the changing needs of tissue cells. Increased activity of structures or areas demands more blood in those parts and vasodilation occurs. To compensate for the increased volume in one area, vasoconstriction must occur in other parts of the body to maintain a forward movement of the blood and a normal cardiac output and blood pressure. For example, when a person moves from the recumbent to the upright position, because of gravity the blood tends to collect in the lower part of the body. This causes a decrease in the blood pressure in the aorta and carotid arteries, and the pressoreceptors then initiate the reflex response of vasoconstriction in the arterioles. This response maintains an adequate circulation throughout the upper parts of the body.

The second factor on which the resistance to the flow of blood depends is the viscosity of the blood. It is a much less significant factor than the caliber of the arterioles. Viscosity is the resistance to flow created within the fluid itself by the friction and cohesiveness between its molecules. Re-

[5]Theodore C. Ruch and Harry D. Patton: Physiology and Biophysics, 19th ed., Philadelphia, W. B. Saunders Co., 1965, p. 610.

sistance of a fluid is directly proportional to its viscosity.

Blood viscosity is mainly dependent on the concentration of the red blood cells and blood proteins. It is approximately 2.5 to 5 times the viscosity of water. An increase above the normal number of red blood cells (polycythemia) impedes the flow of blood and may cause an appreciable increase above normal in the arterial blood pressure. The caliber of the arterioles is subject to frequent fluctuations, but usually viscosity only changes when blood is diluted or when there is an increase or decrease in the number of red blood cells.

NORMAL VARIATIONS IN ARTERIAL BLOOD PRESSURE. Age, exercise, emotions and weight influence blood pressure.

Blood pressure changes with age. During infancy and childhood, blood pressure is lower than later in life. In the newborn infant systolic pressure is approximately 55 to 90 mm. Hg; the diastolic is approximately 40 to 55 mm. Hg. This gradually increases throughout childhood, reaching adult level about puberty. Usually in the fifties, the systolic pressure begins to show a slight increase which progresses with age, corresponding to the loss of elasticity and to the thickening of the walls of the arteries characteristic of the aging process.

Physical exertion is accompanied by a rise in the arterial blood pressure due to the increased venous return and the increased production of metabolites such as carbon dioxide and lactic acid. The systolic pressure may increase as much as 60 to 70 mm. Hg in strenuous exercise.

Emotions may also cause an elevation in blood pressure; the more excited, anxious, angry or fearful a person becomes, the higher the blood pressure goes. Vasoconstriction is increased due to sympathetic innervation and the release of epinephrine into the blood stream.

Blood pressure increases with increased body weight, especially after middle age. This is of significance in our present-day society in which overweight and hypertension have a high incidence.

Capillary Blood Pressure. The pressure of the blood on entry to the capillaries is approximately 20 to 35 mm. Hg. This varies with the constriction and dilation of the arterioles. It is this pressure that is responsi-ble for the movement of fluid and dissolved particles through the semipermeable capillary walls into the interstitial spaces, making them available to cells. The volume of fluid that moves out into the interstitial spaces is dependent upon the capillary blood pressure and the opposing pressure exerted by the interstitial fluid. The capillary blood pressure is quickly reduced by this loss of fluid and to some extent by the resistance of the minute vessels. As a result, by the time the blood leaves the capillaries, the pressure is reduced to approximately 10 to 20 mm. Hg. The movement of fluid across the capillary walls is more fully discussed under Fluids and Electrolytes, p. 49.

Venous Blood Pressure. The pressure of the blood is reduced slowly but progressively from the time it leaves the capillaries and reaches the right atrium.

Venous blood pressure is influenced by cardiac strength, blood volume, respirations and posture. Venous pressure is actually the force that remains of that created by the left ventricular contraction. The blood enters the venous system under a pressure of approximately 10 mm. Hg. The walls of the veins continue to offer some resistance and the blood, particularly in the lower parts of the body, must travel a considerable distance before reaching the heart.* As a result, the pressure is dissipated progressively, and by the time it reaches the right atrium is very low—0 to 1 mm. Hg. Obviously, if the left ventricular systole is weak and the blood starts out at a lower than normal arterial pressure, it will tend to move more slowly in the veins toward the heart.

Maintenance of normal pressure and flow of the venous blood are influenced by the ability of the right heart chambers to empty sufficiently to receive the volume of blood being forwarded by the large veins. If the heart cannot pass on the blood it receives, the normal volume cannot enter and there is a damming back in the veins. The resulting increased volume causes an increase in the blood pressure. Normal emptying of the right atrium actually promotes venous flow; in diastole, the empty right atrium tends to produce an aspirating effect on the large veins.

---

*Pressure is inversely proportional to frictional resistance and the length of the tube.

The greater the volume of blood flowing into the veins from the arterioles and capillaries, the greater will be the venous pressure. If the arterioles are constricted, the pressure in the veins will be lower. If the arterioles are dilated, as in muscular exercise, the greater volume escaping into the veins will increase the venous pressure. Normally, marked changes do not occur since the veins have the ability to adjust by either venoconstriction or dilation to the volume of blood being received. This is accomplished mainly in the smaller veins.

On inspiration there is a decreased intrathoracic pressure and an increased intra-abdominal pressure. Abdominal venous pressure increases while that in the thoracic veins is lowered, causing a larger volume of blood to move into the thoracic veins. On expiration, intrathoracic pressure increases, compressing the veins and raising the pressure within them, thus helping to move the blood into the atria.

Due to gravity, the upright position favors an increase in venous pressure in the lower parts of the body, but continuous venous return is preserved by compensatory mechanisms. The pressoreceptors initiate reflex vascular constriction which usually preserves an adequate blood pressure. In spite of the compensatory vasoconstriction, a greater volume of blood is likely to accumulate in the lower veins during long periods of standing. This may be seen in persons who faint when required to stand for a relatively long period.

MEASUREMENT OF VENOUS BLOOD PRESSURE. Venous blood pressure is an important parameter in the care of seriously ill patients. It reflects the intravascular volume and the ability of the heart to forward the blood it receives. Measurement of the venous pressure may be made in a peripheral vein, such as the medial basilic, or in a large central vein, such as the superior vena cava. To record peripheral venous pressure a needle is inserted into a superficial vein (usually the medial basilic in the antecubital region) and is attached to a water manometer. The patient is placed in the supine position if possible with the arm level with the right atrium. The level to which the water rises in the manometer is noted. The pressure may be recorded in millimeters of Hg but is so small that it is usually expressed in millimeters of centimeters of water.*

The normal venous pressure in an arm or leg vein in an adult who is supine is approximately 8 to 10 cm. of water. It is slightly lower in females and in children.

Central venous pressure is more reliable than the peripheral and is being used clinically more and more in assessing the patient's condition. An intravenous catheter is passed into the superior vena cava via a basilic or jugular vein or into the inferior vena cava via a femoral vein. The catheter is attached to a three-way stopcock which is also connected to a water manometer and intravenous flask and tubing. In setting up the CVP line, the physician positions the zero level of the manometer at the level of the right atrium which is approximately in line with the midaxillary and suprasternal notch. What is most important is that the equipment be at the same level for each determination so the initial level is usually marked on the patient's skin. In most instances, the changes in the venous pressure are more significant than the actual level. The patient should be flat, if possible, and in the same position for each reading. The pressure is generally recorded hourly. When the catheter is introduced, the stopcock is adjusted to allow fluid to flow to the patient. Then, to determine the venous pressure, the stopcock is turned to direct the fluid up into the manometer to a level of 30 to 35 cm. The valve is then adjusted to close off the flow from the intravenous bottle and establish a flow line between the manometer and the catheter. When the fluid reaches the level of the venous pressure, it remains at a relatively stationary level, rhythmically rising and falling 1 to 2 cm. with respirations. Following the recording, the stopcock is readjusted to allow the intravenous solution to flow to the patient.

The normal central venous pressure is approximately 5 to 10 cm. of water. This varies with the patient's size, position and state of hydration. The significance of the pressure is determined in conjunction with the arterial blood pressure, the hourly output of urine, pulse rate and volume and electrocardiograph. The nurse requires a directive as to the levels at which the physician should be notified and the rate and volume of intravenous infusion adjusted.

---

*Mercury is approximately 13 times as heavy as water.

Pulse

Each ventricular contraction ejects a volume of blood into the aorta, producing an increase in the blood pressure which causes an expansion of the artery. During ventricular diastole, the elastic recoil of the aorta moves the blood into the next portion of the artery, which stretches and then recoils. This alternating expansion and recoil spreads along the whole arterial system, producing a pulse wave. Each pulsation corresponds to a heartbeat and is the result of the impact of the ejected volume of blood on the arterial wall. The pulsations occur in the arteries of the pulmonary circulatory system as well as in the systemic circulation.

A pulse may be felt in arteries near the surface of the body and is a valuable source of information about the heart and vessels. The radial artery at the wrist is the most convenient site for feeling the pulse, but it may also be felt in the temporal, carotid, brachial, external submaxillary, abdominal aorta, femoral, popliteal and dorsalis pedis arteries. When palpating a pulse, the observer notes the following: the frequency per minute, which represents the number of left ventricular contractions that are strong enough to produce pulse waves that will reach the peripheral artery being used; the volume, which indicates the strength of the heart contraction; the rhythm, or regularity, of the intervals between pulsations; and the tension and thickness of the arterial wall, which give some indication of the resistance.

The loss of pressure of the blood in arterioles and capillaries effaces pulse in the veins. There is one exception; a feeble venous pulse may be palpated in the internal jugular veins while the subject is in a recumbent position. It is caused by the atrial systole. Since no valves guard the openings of the vena caval veins into the right atrium, a small amount of blood is regurgitated into the large veins with atrial contraction, producing a weak pulse.

FETAL CIRCULATION

The circulatory pathway in the fetus differs from that established at birth. This is a necessity, since the developing organism is dependent upon the maternal blood for its oxygen and nutrients as well as for the elimination of its metabolic wastes.

Special Circulatory Structures

Several special structures are developed in the fetal circulatory system, and they function to support the developing organism during intrauterine life. Two umbilical arteries arise from the fetal hypogastric or internal iliac arteries and deliver fetal blood from the aorta to the placenta. One umbilical vein originates in the placenta. The blood which is transported has taken on oxygen and nutrients in the placenta in exchange for carbon dioxide and other metabolic wastes. The placenta is a mass of finger-like projections (chorionic villi) which penetrate deeply into the thick endometrium early in pregnancy. The villi become highly vascularized and lie in close contact with the maternal blood in the wall of the uterus to allow for an exchange of substances. The ductus venosus is a vein formed by a continuation of the umbilical vein along the undersurface of the liver. It receives blood from the portal vein and gives rise to a few small vessels which enter the liver. The ductus venosus terminates in the inferior vena cava. The ductus arteriosus is a short vessel between the pulmonary artery and the descending thoracic aorta. Blood flowing through this vessel bypasses the pulmonary system. The foramen ovale is an opening between the right and left atria. A valve permits blood to flow from the right atrium into the left atrium, thus bypassing the pulmonary system.

The Circulatory Pathway in the Fetus

With these special structures in mind, the course which fetal blood takes may be outlined.

Starting with the left ventricle of the fetal heart, the blood is received into the aorta and continues on the usual route. A supply is distributed through aortic branches to structures in the thoracic and abdominal regions. Some of the blood continues on to the lower limbs via the external iliac arteries, but the greater volume of it is delivered to the placenta by the two umbilical

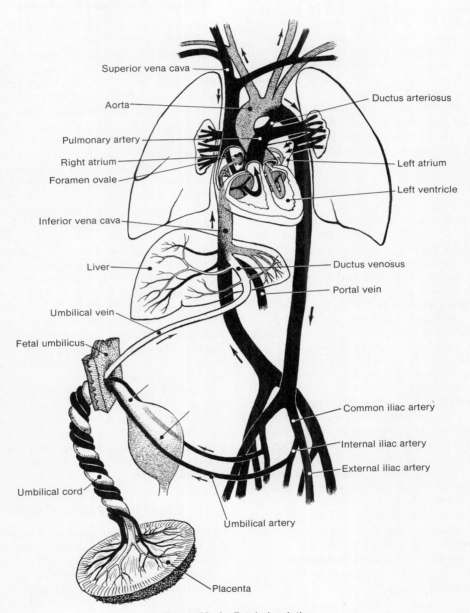

Figure 13–4 Fetal circulation.

arteries which derive from the hypogastric arteries (internal iliac arteries). The umbilical arteries leave the fetus in the umbilical cord and pass to the placenta where they divide and subdivide into thin-walled capillaries contained in the villi of the placenta. The semipermeable walls of the capillaries permit the movement of oxygen and nutrients into fetal blood from maternal blood and movement of wastes from fetal blood to maternal blood. Since this exchange is through capillary walls, there is no direct mixing of the fetal and maternal bloods.

The fetal blood is collected in the placenta into the umbilical vein and passes via the umbilical cord to the fetus. Within the fetal body, the umbilical vein proceeds to the liver where it becomes the ductus venosus. Most of the blood bypasses the liver, continuing on into the inferior vena cava by which it enters the right atrium.

A volume of the blood in the right atrium passes through the foramen ovale into the left atrium because the pressure of the blood in the right atrium is greater than that in the left atrium. The remainder of the blood flows into the right ventricle and out into the pulmonary artery. Only a small portion of this blood continues on through the lungs and is eventually delivered to the left atrium by the four pulmonary veins. The larger portion is shunted through the ductus arteriosus into the aorta, thus bypassing the lungs.

The shunting of the blood through the foramen ovale and the ductus arteriosus into the aorta greatly reduces the volume of blood in the pulmonary circulation. This particular pathway would seem to be so designed because the lungs of the fetus are not functioning, and no purpose would be served by having all the blood pass through the pulmonary system.

The blood in the left atrium passes into the left ventricle and out into the aorta to join that received from the ductus arteriosus. The circuit is now completed.

Changes in Fetal Circulation at Birth

After birth, the new organism must function independently, so the special structures are no longer useful. With the cutting of the umbilical cord, no blood enters either the umbilical vein or arteries. The portion of these vessels within the body contract, thrombose and eventually become fibrous cords. The ductus venosus, now nonfunctional, also becomes fibrous. All the blood in the portal vein is now directed into the liver.

When the lungs expand and become functional, a greater volume of blood enters the pulmonary circulation and flows into the left atrium. The pressure of the blood in the left atrium is now higher than that in the right atrium and the foramen ovale in the atrial septum is closed. A gradual constriction and atrophy of the ductus arteriosus take place, and its closure is usually complete within a few weeks of birth.

TABLE 13–1   SCHEMATIC OUTLINE OF FETAL CIRCULATION

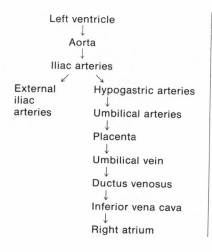

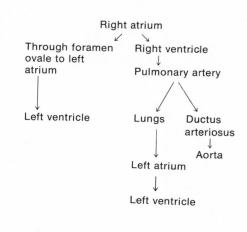

NURSING IN IMPAIRED CARDIAC FUNCTION

Heart disease is a national health problem of considerable proportions. It is the leading cause of death in Canada and in the United States, and despite medical advances, the figures continue to climb. In Canada 52,576 persons died of heart disease in 1964; in 1967 75,000 deaths were attributed to this cause.[6] In the United States 711,604 deaths were due to heart disease in 1965.[7]

Many nursing hours in hospitals, homes and clinics are devoted to patients with heart disease. Cardiac patients comprise almost 4 per cent of the caseload of hospitals in Ontario.[8]

Nurse's Role in Prevention of Heart Disease

The nurse has many opportunities to contribute to the prevention of cardiac insufficiency. Whether her work is in the hospital, clinic, home, industry or school, she may participate in case-finding, education and provision of care. In order to recognize and fulfill her responsibilities in the preventive program, the nurse must be informed and must make a personal effort to keep abreast of new knowledge. As well as an understanding of the role of the heart in supplying all the cells throughout the body with materials essential to their survival and activities, a knowledge of how this function may be impaired by various pathological processes is necessary. This information serves as the basis for the recognition of excessive demands on the heart, significant signs and symptoms and the need for medical attention. It also provides the basis for explanations and appropriate health education as well as for the planning and giving of safe and effective care.

People are urged to secure an early diagnosis and treatment of illnesses which may damage the heart. Examples of such conditions are rheumatic fever, hypertension, syphilis and hyperthryoidism. The promo-

tion of immunization for diphtheria contributes to the prevention of heart disease because the toxin produced by the causative organisms may have a serious effect on the heart muscle.

Opportunities arise many times for the nurse to discuss the hazards of obesity and its possible effects on the heart. Similarly, the advantages of such things as moderate exercise, annual physical examinations and the reduction of animal fat in the diet are stressed. Avoidance of unaccustomed strenuous physical activities and overexcitement, particularly by persons past middle age, are stressed in health education in relation to the prevention of heart disease. All too often one reads of sudden deaths due to a heart attack suffered while shovelling snow or while participating in competitive sports. The nurse has an important role in helping both adults and children to develop good health habits and to live a balanced life of physical activity, rest, work and recreation.

Recent studies have indicated a higher incidence of coronary heart disease among cigarette smokers. Established smokers are encouraged to stop or at least reduce the number of cigarettes smoked per day. Every effort should be made to discourage young persons from starting the smoking habit.

The nurse is ever alert to the possible significance of shortness of breath, cyanosis, edema and chest pain on exertion. Recognition leading to an early diagnosis and treatment may prevent irreparable damage and eventual incapacitation of the person.

It must be understood that much heart disease can be and is cured. Many persons with a heart condition or reduced cardiac efficiency live useful, satisfactory lives by readjusting their activities. The nurse must appreciate these facts to develop an optimistic, encouraging attitude with cardiac patients. Any pessimism on her part may readily be conveyed to a patient or family who, generally, tend to be overpessimistic about heart disease. Motivation, instruction and planning to have the heart patient live within the functional ability of his heart may prevent progression of his heart disease and possible heart failure. Follow-up of patients to provide guidance in following the doctor's suggestions may prevent problems and relapses. For example, visits to the child who has had rheumatic fever may ensure

---

[6]Canadian Heart Foundation.

[7]Demographic Year Book, 1966, United Nations, p. 510.

[8]A. H. Sellers: "The Problem of Cardiovascular Disease in Ontario." Canad. J. Publ. Health, Vol. 52, No. 5 (May 1961), p. 200.

the continuation of prescribed prophylactic doses of penicillin or sulfonamide.

Manifestations of Impaired Heart Function

Any impairment in circulation due to an abnormal heart condition is reflected in signs and symptoms which are produced by two main factors: a reduced blood supply to tissues throughout the body, causing a reduced nutrient and oxygen supply and an accumulation of metabolic wastes; and the inability of the heart to forward the blood it receives. The latter results in an excessive volume in the venous system, creating congestion and increased pressure that interfere with the function of tissues and organs.

The signs and symptoms of cardiac conditions vary with the degree to which circulation is impaired and with the form and location of the heart condition. Those which are discussed here do not necessarily all occur in every patient, nor are they all inclusive but are the more common problems presented by cardiac patients.

Abnormal Pulse. The pulse rate may be abnormally fast or slow and the intervals between the heartbeats may be unequal. The volume may vary.

Blood Pressure. Arterial blood pressure is an important indicator of the patient's circulatory status. The systolic pressure depends on the cardiac output and, obviously, will fall with a reduced output by the left side of the heart. Venous pressure is frequently used to assess the ability of the heart to accept the inflow into the right side of the heart. A venous pressure in excess of the normal may indicate cardiac insufficiency or failure or an excessive intravascular volume.

Dyspnea. The patient may experience shortness of breath or labored breathing only on exertion, or it may be present even at rest. This is due to pulmonary congestion. The left side of the heart may not be forwarding all the blood it receives, and the blood is dammed back in the pulmonary veins. The pulmonary congestion and hypertension resist alveolar expansion, increasing the work of breathing and decreasing the vital capacity. If the congestion is of long-standing, alveolar tissue changes occur; the elastic tissue is replaced with fibrous tissue, and normal gas exchange is disturbed.

Cough. Fluid escapes into the alveoli from the capillaries in the congested pulmonary system and acts as a cough stimulus. This collection of transudate in the alveoli may be referred to as pulmonary edema. The fluid may be raised as a frothy sputum and in severe heart failure may contain blood.

Hypoxia. Any impairment in circulation will create an oxygen deficiency in tissues. The cardiac output may be reduced, or a disturbance in pulmonary circulation may reduce the exchange of gases in the lung. Symptoms of an oxygen deficiency are many and varied since the function of all structures is affected. The brain quickly reflects oxygen deprivation and reduced mental efficiency, apathy and disorientation are manifested. If the deficiency is severe, consciousness is lost and, unless the supply to the brain is promptly re-established, there is likely to be permanent tissue damage.

Severe pain occurs when muscle tissue, such as the myocardium, is deprived of adequate oxygen. Hypoxia may also cause cyanosis, a bluish color, which is usually seen first in the lips and nail beds.

Edema (see p. 53). Excess fluid accumulates in the interstitial spaces of the tissues in cardiac disease when the heart cannot forward the blood it receives. The blood backs up in the veins and venules, raising the venous blood pressure. Normally, at the venous end of the capillaries the colloidal osmotic pressure exceeds the hydrostatic pressure of the blood, and interstitital fluid moves into the capillary. But if the hydrostatic pressure of the blood in the distal portion of the capillaries exceeds the blood protein osmotic pressure, interstitial fluid will not be moved into the capillaries.

The retention of sodium ions also contributes to the formation of edema in the cardiac patient. The decreased sodium excretion is favored by the reduced blood flow through the kidneys which results from the impaired circulation. It is also suggested that some mechanism may exist which causes an increased secretion of aldosterone by the adrenal cortices. This hormone promotes reabsorption of sodium in the kidney tubules.

Edema is a very characteristic sign of some weakening in heart function. Considerable fluid accumulates before the edema becomes apparent; a person may retain 10 to 15 pounds of excess fluid before the edema becomes evident. It appears first in the dependent parts of the body where the venous and capillary blood pressures always tend to be greater. If the patient is ambulant, it becomes evident first in the ankles and feet; but if he is in bed, it appears initially in the sacral region.

Pain. The chest pain which cardiac patients experience is usually due to the deficiency of oxygen in the myocardium. Pain in the abdomen may be due to venous congestion in the viscera.

Palpitation. Change in heart function may cause the person to be conscious of his heartbeats. Palpitation may be due to the apex of the enlarged heart striking the chest wall with each contraction, or it may occur with an increased stroke volume in extrasystole, or ectopic beat (see Arrhythmias, p. 200).

General Debilitation, Loss of Strength and Decreased Mental and Physical Efficiency. Weakness, loss of appetite and weight, general apathy and reduced efficiency occur as the results of the reduced nutrient and oxygen supply, venous congestion and the accumulation of metabolic wastes. In a child, growth and development may be retarded.

Abnormal Heart Sounds. Cardiac murmurs are abnormal sounds caused by small jets of blood which create eddies in the blood stream. Movements of these currents produce audible vibrations which are referred to as murmurs. The most frequent causes of heart murmurs are stenosed and insufficient valves and openings between the right and left sides of the heart. Murmurs may also occur in an aneurysm, a localized saccular dilation of an artery.

The physician, in determining the significance of a murmur, considers when it occurs in the cardiac cycle, its intensity, quality of sound, duration, factors (such as respiration and change of position) which alter the sound and the patient's history. Murmurs in some persons may have no great significance.

Occasionally in tachycardia, a third heart sound becomes audible, producing then a quick sequence of three sounds during each cardiac cycle. This phenomenon is referred to as gallop rhythm and is an unfavorable sign since it indicates a weakening and dilatation of the heart and often precedes heart failure.

Friction rub is a sound produced by the contact between the two pericardial surfaces with each heartbeat. Because of disease, the surfaces are rough, causing audible vibrations.

Diagnostic Procedures

In determining the cause of a circulatory disturbance, the physician considers the patient's history, makes a detailed examination and may require special studies of heart function and structure. Although the diagnostic procedures are mainly the concern of the attending physician, the nurse requires some understanding of them in order to meet the associated nursing needs.

Blood Tests. Various blood tests are used in investigating heart disease. Those used will depend on the presenting signs and symptoms.

LEUKOCYTE COUNT. The number of white blood cells may be of significance since these will be increased if there is an inflammatory process as occurs in bacterial endocarditis and rheumatic fever. Leukocytosis also occurs following a myocardial infarction as a result of the necrotic tissue.

Normal: 5000 to 10,000 per cu. mm.

ERYTHROCYTE COUNT AND HEMOGLOBIN CONCENTRATION. These are observed to determine the oxygen-carrying capacity of the patient's blood. In congenital cardiac defects which establish an abnormal blood pathway, the red blood cells and hemoglobin may be increased as a compensatory mechanism, since areas of the body are deficient in oxygen.

An increase in the erythrocytes increases the viscosity of the blood, adding to the work of the heart and predisposing to thrombus formation.

In those with rheumatic fever or bacterial endocarditis, there may be fewer erythrocytes and less hemoglobin than normal.

Normal:

Erythrocytes, $1\frac{1}{2}$ to 5 million per cu. mm.

Hemoglobin, 12 to 16 Gm. per 100 ml. (varies with age and sex).

Hematocrit, males 45 to 50 volumes per cent; females 40 to 45 volumes per cent.

ERYTHROCYTE SEDIMENTATION RATE. The rate at which erythrocytes settle in a blood sample is increased in inflammatory conditions and in myocardial infarction. Periodic checking of the sedimentation rate gives information as to the progress of the disease; as the inflammatory process subsides or as the infarcted area heals, the rate decreases.

Normal:
> Westergren, male, 0 to 15 mm. in 1 hour; female, 0 to 20 mm. in 1 hour.
> Wintrobe, male, 0 to 9 mm. in 1 hour; female, 0 to 15 mm. in 1 hour.

BLOOD CULTURE. Studies may be made to determine the causative organism in bacterial endocarditis.

PROTHROMBIN TIME. This test reflects the amount of prothrombin in the blood. Some heart patients receive anticoagulant therapy and a frequent check must be made of the concentration of prothrombin which serves as a guide to the dosage of the drugs.

Normal: 11 to 12 seconds.

SERUM ENZYMES. Certain intracellular enzymes known to be present in myocardial cells are released into the blood when the cells are damaged or destroyed. Determination of the serum concentration of these various enzymes provides information that assists in confirming myocardial infarction (coronary occlusion) and the extent of the damage.

The enzymes tests include: serum glutamic oxaloacetic acid (SGOT), serum lactic dehydrogenase (SLDH), serum creatine phosphokinase (SCPK) and serum alpha-hydroxybutyrate dehydrogenase (SHBD).

The concentration of SGOT rises quickly after a myocardial infarction, reaching a peak in 24 to 48 hours and usually returning to normal within 4 to 7 days.

Normal range: 10 to 40 units.

Following an infarction the SLDH level begins to rise after 6 hours, reaching a peak in 48 to 72 hours. The increase persists for 5 to 10 days and then gradually returns to normal.

Normal range: 100 to 300 units.

SCPK begins to show a postinfarction increase in approximately 2 to 5 hours, reaching its peak within 24 hours of the infarction. It usually returns to normal within 2 to 3 days.

Normal range: 0 to 20 units.

An increase in SHBD occurs within 12 hours of an acute myocardial infarction. The elevation persists for 1 to 3 weeks.

Normal range: 50 to 200 units.

BLOOD GASES. The circulatory status of a patient is reflected in the blood concentrations of oxygen and carbon dioxide. The volumes differ in arterial and venous blood for obvious reasons. The amount is usually expressed as the oxygen tension (pO_2) in mm. Hg. Rarely, the volumes per cent are recorded.

Normal:
> pO_2, arterial, 95 to 100 mm. Hg.
> O_2, arterial, 15 to 23 vol. per cent.
> pO_2, venous, 35 to 40 mm. Hg.
> O_2, venous, 10 to 16 vol. per cent.

The partial pressure of carbon dioxide in the blood provides information about the pH of the body fluids and is usually reported in mm. Hg. The carbon dioxide combining power indicates the available alkali and reflects the amount of carbon dioxide in the blood available to form carbonic acid.

Normal:
> pCO_2, arterial, 35 to 40 mm. Hg.
> pCO_2, venous, 40 to 45 mm. Hg.
> carbon dioxide combining power, 50 to 58 vol. per cent.
> bicarbonate (alkali), 22 to 28 mEq. per L.

Electrocardiography. Electrocardiography is the study of the electrical activity associated with heart contractions. The electrocardiogram, which produces a visible record of heart activity, provides one of the most dependable aids to physicians in assessing heart function and in diagnosing heart disease.

Each heart contraction generates electrical currents which spread from the heart through the body to its surface. These currents, which reflect the activity of the heart, are picked up from the body surface. An electrocardiograph makes a photographic tracing of the variations in intensity of the electrical currents.

The electrocardiogram is obtained by placing electrodes on the extremities and chest, which lead the currents to the electrocardiograph. An application of contact jelly is made to the skin beneath the electrodes in order to facilitate conduction. A characteristic series of waves occurs on the graph during each cardiac cycle. The waves for each cycle are divided into five segments, and each segment, which represents a particular phase in the heart cycle, is given an identifying letter—namely, P, Q, R, S and T. The base line of the graph represents zero electrical potential. Three of the waves

(P, R and T) appear above the base line, and two (Q and S) appear below.

The P wave represents the activity of the atria. The Q R S complex is a tracing of the impulse transmission from the atria to the ventricles and the ventricular contraction. The time between P wave and R represents the time of conduction from the atria to the ventricles (P=R interval). The S T segment is an interval of zero potential when activity of the ventricles is completed. The T wave is correlated with the recovery of the ventricular muscle.

The tracing is studied for deviations by comparing it to a tracing that would be made by a normal heart; the direction, contour and timing of the waves and segments are noted. Information is obtained that is related to impulse formation and conduction and to the condition and response of the myocardium.

A nursing responsibility associated with this diagnostic procedure is to give the patient a brief explanation of the test. Some patients are fearful that they will receive a shock from the electrodes. The patient is advised that he should simply relax and that he will not feel anything as the instrument records his heart's action. If digitalis or quinidine has been prescribed for the patient, it must be noted on the requisition as well as on a conspicuous place on the patient's chart, as either drug may influence the interpretation of the tracing.

If the patient is very ill, the nurse remains with him during the test. Should he be receiving oxygen, this will have to be discontinued because of the danger of using electrical instruments in the presence of oxygen. The oxygen flow may be discontinued when the technician is ready to start the recording. The patient's reaction to this withdrawal must be observed closely.

Roentgenograms. An x-ray of the chest may be made to note the size and shape of the heart. Visualization of the lungs may show a density that may indicate an increased volume of blood in the pulmonary circulation and fluid in the alveoli. The size and shape of the pulmonary artery and aorta may also be noted.

Fluoroscopic examination allows the physician to observe the heart in action. The functioning of different chambers and large vessels may be noted.

A brief explanation of the patient's role may be necessary if he is apprehensive and completely unfamiliar with x-ray procedure.

Angiocardiogram. In this test, also known as a cardiopulmonary angiogram, visualization of the heart and vessels is made possible by the injection of a radiopaque dye into a vein or artery or directly into a heart chamber. The site depends on the type of abnormality suspected. A series of x-ray pictures is taken, or a fluoroscopic study is made, as the blood flows through the heart and pulmonary system. The pathway of the blood is followed, and the size, shape, and the filling and emptying of the various structures are noted. This examination is of particular importance in identifying congenital defects of the heart and large vessels.

Preparation of the patient includes an explanation of the test so that he will have some idea of what to expect. This may be given by the doctor, but if it is not, the nurse must have sufficient understanding of the procedure to be able to prepare the patient and reduce his fear.

In may be necessary to obtain a written consent for an angiocardiogram, depending on the policy of the particular hospital. Food and fluids are withheld for 6 to 8 hours previous to the hour of the test, and a sedative may be ordered thirty minutes to an hour before the patient is taken to the x-ray or cardiology department.

The physician usually administers a test dose of the radiopaque dye before proceeding with the angiocardiogram in case of a hypersensitivity to such substances. This examination is not done on a person with a history of asthma or allergic reaction. A reaction to the dye might be manifested

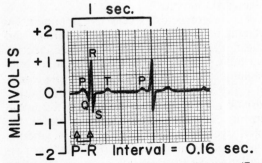

Figure 13–5 A normal electrocardiogram. (From Guyton, A. C.: Textbook of Medical Physiology, 4th ed. Philadelphia, W. B. Saunders Co., 1971, p. 173.)

by respiratory distress, fall in blood pressure, shock, urticaria, and nausea and vomiting. Antihistamines, adrenalin and oxygen should be quickly available in the event of a reaction. Post-examination care involves close observation for signs of delayed reaction. The site of injection should be examined for a few days for signs of irritation or thrombosis.

Circulation Time. This test measures the time it takes the blood to flow from one part of the body to another. A substance with a characteristic taste may be injected into the antecubital vein, and the time interval between the injection and when the patient first tastes the substance is noted. This interval represents the time the blood took to pass from the arm through the right side of the heart, pulmonary system and left side of the heart, into the aorta and out to the taste buds via the lingual artery. There are several different substances which may be used. A saccharin preparation may be injected to produce a sweet taste, or a bitter-tasting preparation of bile salts (Decholin) may be used. Accuracy of the test depends largely on the patient's alertness and senses.

Another method of determining circulation time is by the injection of a radioactive material into the vein of one arm. A Geiger counter is placed over the other arm and the time noted when the radioactive material is registered.

The normal time for these circuits varies from 10 to 20 seconds.

Nursing responsibilities involve an explanation of the test and what will be expected of the patient, preparing for and assisting with the injection of the test substance, and establishing the circulation time.

Vital Capacity. Vital capacity represents the maximum volume of air that a person can exhale after inhaling to the maximum. The normal is approximately 2500 to 5000 ml. It is normally higher in males than females and will be greater in those accustomed to regular and fairly strenuous activity.

In the procedure, the patient is required to take a maximum breath and then exhale into the mouthpiece of a spirometer which makes a graphic record of the volume of air exhaled.

Lung capacity may be reduced in heart conditions by an excessive volume and pressure of blood in the pulmonary circulatory system. Expansion of the lungs meets with resistance, and fluid escapes into the alveoli and reduces respiratory efficiency.

The nurse advises the patient as to the value of the test and what will be required of him.

Phonocardiography. Heart sounds may be picked up, amplified and recorded by a microphone placed on the chest. A study of the phonocardiogram is helpful in cases in which the physician has difficulty in distinguishing the heart sounds and murmurs by the usual auscultation.

Cardiac Catheterization. In this procedure, a long radiopaque catheter is passed into either the right or left side of the heart under a fluoroscope to detect congenital defects, determine the pressure in the different heart chambers and obtain blood specimens for estimation of oxygen concentration in certain chambers. For example, an atrial septal defect results in an oxygen tension higher than normal in the right side. A contrast material or radiopaque dye may also be introduced into the heart through the catheter.

Right heart catheterization provides information about the right side of the heart and the pulmonary circulation. The catheter is introduced through a cutdown in the basilic vein of the right arm and, under a fluoroscope, is passed through the right subclavian vein and superior vena cava into the right atrium. It may then be guided through the tricuspid valve into the right ventricle and on into the pulmonary artery. An x-ray may be taken with the catheter in various positions for future studies.

In left heart catheterization, one of two approaches may be used. One method is the retrograde passage of the catheter into a femoral artery through the aorta and aortic valve to the left ventricle. It may then be advanced through the mitral valve into the left atrium. The other approach is transeptal. The catheter is passed through a peripheral vein into the right atrium and from there through the interatrial septum into the left atrium. In some instances, the catheter may then be guided under the fluoroscope into the left ventricle.

Preparation of the patient for a cardiac catheterization includes some explanation of the procedure and obtaining a written consent. Although the doctor usually talks with the patient and family, the nurse should be conversant with the procedure. It is understandable that the patient and relatives are generally apprehensive. The nurse encourages them to verbalize their fears and is prepared to answer questions about the procedure.

Food and fluid are withheld for a stated number of hours preceding the catheterization. Some patients, especially young children, may have to receive a general anesthetic. A sedative may be ordered.

The patient's reaction must be observed closely during the procedure. Heart action is constantly observed on the oscilloscope of an instrument which visibly registers and traces the electrical activity of the heart. Irritation of the myocardium by the catheter may precipitate fibrillation, so a defibrillator is close at hand. The patient experiences little discomfort, but may complain of a fluttering or irritation in the chest, especially during movement of the catheter. He is advised that this is a temporary sensation.

Following the catheterization, which may have taken two or three hours, the patient is given fluids and nourishment and is allowed to rest. The pulse is checked at frequent intervals—every 15 minutes for the first hour and then at gradually increased intervals if it remains normal. An irregular, rapid or weak pulse is promptly reported to the physician. If the catheter was passed through a femoral artery, the patient remains flat for 24 hours, and the site where the catheter was inserted is examined frequently for possible bleeding.

The site at which the catheter was introduced is observed for several days for possible irritation or phlebitis, evidenced by redness and tenderness.

Cardiac Arrhythmias

Normally, the rate and rhythm of the heart contractions are established by impulses generated in the S-A node. A disorder in the rate or rhythm is referred to as a cardiac arrhythmia and is due to some disturbance in the formation or conduction of impulses. The arrhythmia may be of short duration or persistent and may be functional in origin, result from organic heart disease or be associated with an electrolyte imbalance (e.g., potassium).

Common irregularities include paroxysmal tachycardia, bradycardia, ectopic beats (extrasystoles), fibrillation and heart block. The initial site of the disorder may be in the S-A node or may be elsewhere in the conduction system.

Paroxysmal Tachycardia. This is an abrupt onset of a very rapid heart rate, usually 150 to 250 beats per minute. It may last a few seconds or days. Such attacks cannot be explained in some; in others, they may be related to organic disease of the heart. Such a rapid heart rate is serious if imposed upon a diseased heart.

The patient is advised to rest, and the physician is notified. If the patient is subject to recurring attacks, he is encouraged to recognize and avoid possible precipitating factors, which might be fatigue, emotional stress, reaching, or excessive smoking or coffee drinking. In some instances, an attack may be relieved by measures that increase parasympathetic (vagal) innervation to the heart. Among those suggested is pressure on the carotid sinus or eyeballs. Caution must be used in relation to the latter as too frequent and too heavy pressure may predispose to retinal detachment in the eye. Some subjects of paroxysmal tachycardia find that it may be checked by assuming a certain position, such as flexion of the trunk or holding the arms over the head.

The Valsalva maneuver, which involves an inspiration followed by voluntary closure of the glottis and an effort to exhale, may prove helpful. Intra-abdominal and intrathoracic pressures are increased; this reduces the venous return from the extremities and head, thus reducing the volume of blood entering the heart. This in turn decreases the cardiac output and the arterial blood pressure. On expiration, an increased volume of blood enters the heart and the output is increased with a corresponding rise in the blood pressure. The latter causes the pressoreceptors to elicit vagal impulses which slow the heart.

An antiarrhythmic drug such as procainamide hydrochloride (Pronestyl) or quinidine may be prescribed. These drugs reduce the myocardial excitability and slow the rate.

Bradycardia. This is the term used for an abnormally slow pulse rate. It is applied when the pulse rate is below approximately 54 per minute in the adult, less than 80 in the child and less than 100 in the infant.

Circulation may be adequately maintained by an increased stroke volume in a person with bradycardia. With fewer contractions more blood collects in the heart chambers, producing greater stretching of the myocardial fibers and resulting in a stronger contraction and an increased output. Obviously, this can only occur if the myocardium is in good condition. If the heart rate is less than 30 to 40 minute, circulatory insufficiency is likely to occur, especially with physical activity.

Bradycardia may be caused by a weakness of the myocardium due to coronary insufficiency, toxic conditions or tissue damage in the heart. Circulatory reflexes may initiate a compensatory increase in the heart rate, but if the cause persists and becomes progressively severe, the heart muscle may gradually become depressed and less responsive, producing fewer contractions. Any disturbance which initiates an increase in vagal nerve impulses to the heart will produce a decrease in the heart rate; an example of this may be seen in older persons who frequently develop arteriosclerotic changes in the carotid sinus region. Their pressoreceptors become hypersensitive, and with even slight pressure on the neck, the circulatory reflex may be initiated, resulting in increased vagal innervation to the heart. Other examples of conditions in which slowing of the heart rate may be secondary are increased intracranial pressure and myxedema (a deficiency of thyroid secretion).

The pulse rate may be normally slower in those with a well-developed cardiac reserve. In such persons, the venous return is of greater volume and the myocardium develops a greater strength, producing an increased stroke volume with each contraction. The resulting increased blood pressure initiates the pressoreceptor reflex which reduces the heart rate.

Ectopic Beats. When impulses which influence the heart rate and rhythm are generated elsewhere than in the S-A node, the contractions are called ectopic or premature beats, or extrasystoles.

The ectopic or premature beat occurs when the myocardial fibers are in the relative refractory period* following a normal

contraction. The impulses from the S-A node for the succeeding normal contractions are ineffective since they arrive when the muscle fibers are in the absolute refractory period* following the premature beat, and no contraction takes place. This causes a longer than normal pause before the next normal contraction and the heart "misses" a beat. The next normal contraction may be stronger because of the prolonged filling period. The time between the normal heart contraction which preceded the extrasystole and the one that follows, is equal to two normal cardiac cycles. The subject usually describes the experience as his heart "missing a beat," followed by a thud.

Extrasystoles, or premature beats, may be due to ischemic areas in the heart muscle, a small scarred or calcified area pressing on neighboring fibers or to inflammation. The fibers may also become irritated and hypersensitive as a result of some toxic condition, such as can occur with the excessive use of tobacco, coffee, tea or alcohol. The extrasystoles may occur irregularly with varying lengths of time between them. The incidents may be so rare as to have no clinical significance, but they should be investigated if persistent even though they occur irregularly and at relatively long intervals. Premature beats may arise regularly and at a rate in excess of that of the normal S-A pace, resulting in paroxysmal tachycardia.

Fibrillation. This is an arrhythmia in which the normal rhythmic contractions of the myocardium of either the atria or ventricles are replaced by extremely rapid (250 to 500 per minute), ineffective contractions, irregular in force and rhythm. Some area of the heart gives rise to very rapid and irregular impulses, and the myocardial contractile fibers do not achieve contraction and relaxation that permit normal emptying and filling of the chambers.

Atrial fibrillation is a fairly common and serious arrhythmia. It is due to some myocardial weakness or disease which may be the result of coronary insufficiency, rheumatic heart disease, thyrotoxicosis or acute infection. The atria are never completely empty, and normal filling cannot take place.

---

*See page 181 for information concerning refractory periods.

*See page 181 for information concerning refractory periods.

Since little pressure is created by the atrial contractions, the flow of blood into the ventricles is mainly due to the pressure created by the volume of blood. Circulation may become seriously impaired. Only a proportion of the impulses arising in the atria are conducted through the A-V node to the ventricles, but those that do pass through far exceed the normal in frequency and are irregular. Normal filling and emptying of the ventricles do not take place, cardiac output is reduced, arterial blood pressure falls and the blood is backed up in the large veins. The pulse is very rapid, weak and irregular. With some ventricular contractions, the stroke volume may be so reduced that radial pulsation does not occur. This sets up a pulse deficit which is defined as the difference between the apical and radial pulses. To determine a pulse deficit accurately, the ventricular rate is counted for a full minute, using a stethoscope placed over the apical region. At the same time, a second person counts the radial pulse for a full minute. If two people are not available, one may count one pulse and then the other, each for a full minute.

Atrial fibrillation may be treated with a digitalis preparation or quinidine sulphate. Digitalis slows the heart rate by depressing the impulse conduction through the myocardium and by increasing vagal nerve stimulation. The myocardial contractions are strengthened which brings about more efficient emptying of the heart chambers. Quinidine prolongs the refractory period of the myocardial fibers and is used to restore normal sinus rhythm. The latter drug is less predictable as to the patient's reaction; close observation of the patient and frequent checking of the heart action are necessary. Procainamide hydrochloride (Pronestyl) may be ordered instead of quinidine as an anti-fibrillatory drug. It has the same effect as quinidine on the myocardium.

A complication that may follow atrial fibrillation is embolism. The blood that was not forwarded during fibrillation may have formed a thrombus in an atrial chamber and then, when normal heart action is re-established, the thrombus may be moved out into the circulation.

In ventricular fibrillation, very rapid asynchronous contractions arise in the ventricular myocardium. The fibrillating contractions are so ineffective in pumping that the condition may prove fatal very quickly. The pulse and blood pressure become unobtainable in a few seconds, the patient quickly loses consciousness, his pupils dilate and his reflexes are lost. Prompt emergency treatment may re-establish circulation. Cardiac massage accompanied by artificial respirations may sustain life and restore circulation (see Cardiac Arrest, p. 229). Ventricular fibrillation may occur in mechanical injury or irritation of the heart, coronary occlusion, hypothermia and electrical shock.

A defibrillator may be used to treat ventricular fibrillation. Although an electrical shock may cause fibrillation, it can also be used to stop fibrillation. Two electrodes ("paddles") are placed on the chest wall, one on each side of the heart or one on the ventral wall with the second on the dorsal wall. A strong current (approximately 400 volts) is passed through the electrodes for a brief period. All the muscle fibers of the myocardium are thrown into contraction together and then enter a refractory period simultaneously. This quiescent period may give the normal pacemaker, the S-A node, an opportunity to take over. It is important to make sure that no one is touching the bed or the patient during the electrical discharge.

Frequently, ventricular fibrillation is preceded by premature ventricular contractions (PVC) which may be recognized on an oscilloscope tracing when a patient's heart action is being continuously monitored. Prompt administration of an antiarrhythmic drug such as lidocaine (Xylocaine) or procainamide (Pronestyl) may prevent serious ventricular tachycardia or fibrillation.

Heart Block. This is a condition in which impulse formation is depressed or impulse conduction is blocked.

Conduction may be interrupted between the S-A node and the atria, but interruption occurs more often as a result of failure of the A-V node or a portion of the atrioventricular conducting system. If sino-atrial impulses are not received by the atria, the latter will respond to those arising from the A-V junctional tissue. If impulses do not pass along the pathway from the atria to the ventricles, impulses in the lower part of the conduction system will be responsible for the contractions of the ventricles. The atria will continue at the rhythm set by the S-A node (approximately 70 per minute) while the ventricles will contract approximately 30 to 40 times per minute.

Heart block occurs in varying degrees of severity. Conduction may simply be delayed through the A-V node and the intervals between the atria and ventricular contractions are lengthened. In a second degree or partial heart block, the ratio of atrial to ventricular contractions may be 2:1 or 3:1. A complete block in the A-V node or the A-V junctional tissues results in the ventricles contracting 30 to 40 times per minute, while the atria continue to contract at the pace set by the S-A node.

The S-A node, or the conduction pathways, may be damaged by inflammatory disease such as rheumatic fever, coronary insufficiency, pressure from scarred or calcified tissue, or surgical trauma.

Heart block may be a temporary or permanent condition. If it is permanent, the independent ventricular rhythm may become firmly established and with some restriction of activities, the patient may live a fairly normal life. In some instances, the ventricular rhythm may be irregular and episodes of cardiac arrest may threaten the patient. Cardiac asystole lasting 10 seconds or longer may occur, reducing the cardiac output to a level that causes cerebral ischemia. The patient becomes dizzy and may faint or convulse, or sudden death may occur. This type of episode is referred to as a Stokes-Adams attack or syndrome.

Heart block may be treated by the administration of isoproterenol (Isuprel) and an electrical pacemaker. During a Stokes-Adams episode, isoproterenol may be administered intravenously, intramuscularly or directly into the heart muscle. Regular doses sublingually or subcutaneously may be prescribed to increase cardiac contractions and prevent a Stokes-Adams seizure.

In serious conduction defects and cardiac arrest, an electrical pacemaker may be employed to stimulate ventricular contractions. It is a device which delivers a prescribed number of electrical charges per minute into the heart to stimulate it to contract. The electrodes may be applied externally to the chest wall over the heart or internally, directly to the heart.

External pacemaking is used for quick emergency stimulation of the ventricles. The electrodes are placed on the chest wall over the heart and held in position by a rubber band which is applied around the chest. To promote conduction an application of contact paste is made to the skin beneath the electrodes. The physican adjusts the machine to deliver an effective voltage and sets the rate or "pace" of the electrical discharges into the heart. Effectiveness is determined by checking a peripheral pulse.

The length of time an external pacemaker may be used is limited because of the discomfort to the patient. The relatively high voltage of electricity necessary to stimulate the heart through the chest wall causes pain in skeletal muscle and may burn the skin. The patient must be kept immobile and precautions used to avoid dislodging the electrodes. If the stimulation is prolonged, it is necessary to cleanse and dry the skin area under the electrodes and apply fresh contact paste every three hours to lessen the danger of burns and to maintain satisfactory conduction.

Persons with serious heart block who require very frequent or continuous artificial stimulation may have an electrical pacemaker implanted internally. A soft flexible electrode catheter is passed into the right ventricle via the right jugular vein or a femoral vein. The electrical charge passes from the electrode through the blood to the ventricular wall. The catheter is connected to a small transistorized pacemaker which is implanted subcutaneously. In this way, no part of the unit is external, thus reducing the possibility of infection. This transvenous method of implantation also has the distinct advantage of not involving a thoracotomy (surgical incision into the thoracic cavity).

A more recent model does not provide continuous stimulation, but only discharges impulses when the heart fails to contract after a certain interval and is referred to as a demand-pacemaker.

Following the implantation of a pacemaker, close observation is required to determine its effectiveness and any reaction to its presence. The pulse, blood pressure and the patient's alertness are noted at 15-minute intervals. The latter are gradually increased if the condition is satisfactory. In some instances, a continuous monitoring of the heart action may be made and the monitor set to sound an alarm to alert the staff if there is a cessation of heartbeats or if they fall to a certain rate.

Previous to the implantation, the pacemaker and the procedure are explained to the patient and family. In preparation for discharge the family and patient must understand that the primary condition (heart block) still exists and that continuous functioning of the pacemaker is necessary. For this reason, frequent checking is necessary. The patient and a family member are taught the taking of pulse and are advised that it should be done twice daily for a full minute. Any increase or decrease in the rate is reported promptly to the doctor or clinic. Regularly scheduled visits to the clinic or doctor are stressed.

CAUSES AND TYPES OF HEART DISORDERS

Inflammatory Disease Involving Heart Structures

In any tissue, the inflammatory process may result in destruction of normal functional tissue followed by its replacement with scar tissue, which is fibrous in nature and less specialized.

Diseases which produce inflammatory heart lesions and impaired function include rheumatic fever, bacterial endocarditis, syphilis and pericarditis.

Rheumatic Fever. This is the most common cause of inflammation in the heart structures. Although any or all parts may be affected by rheumatic fever, the valves and the myocardium are the most frequent sites and tend to sustain greater permanent damage. The disease is a complication of a group A streptococcal infection which is usually respiratory. A period of 1 to 5 weeks may lapse between the infection and the onset of the rheumatic fever, during which time the patient may have recovered completely from the infection.

The inflammatory response, which may occur in the joints as well as in the heart, is thought to be due to a sensitivity of the affected persons to the antibodies that were formed in response to the invading bacteria. The antistreptococcal lysin titer is found to be high in these persons at the onset of rheumatic fever. This sensitivity is only present in certain individuals, since not all persons with streptococcal infection develop rheumatic fever. (Rammelkamp says only 2 to 3 per cent of patients with group A hemolytic streptococcal infections develop rheumatic fever.[9]) The symptoms of the acute stage vary in intensity and may be so mild that they go unrecognized. In some persons, joint involvement and fever may be predominant with no evident symptoms referable to the heart, and it is not until much later that it becomes known that cardiac tissue was involved and received permanent damage.

Rheumatic fever may cause acute myocarditis with subsequent scarred areas that reduce myocardial efficiency and impairment of the conduction system.

The valves are the most common area of the heart to be affected, and the mitral and aortic valves are the most susceptible. They frequently become scarred, distorted and functionally impaired. Both the valve ring at the opening and the valve cusps may be affected. Following the acute inflammation, scarring occurs, the orifice is diminished and the edges of the cusps may fuse. These changes result in resistance to the forward movement of the blood, thus increasing the work of the heart chamber behind the obstruction. Damage of this type is referred to as a stenosis. Normally, the mitral opening in an adult is large enough to admit three fingers; in severe stenosis it can become so restricted that only one finger may be introduced.

In some instances, the scarring of the valvular cusps produces a thickening and loss of tissue that prevents them from coming together to completely close off the opening. This incomplete closure allows a regurgitation or backflow of blood through the valve and is called valvular insufficiency. An added strain is placed on the heart chamber behind the insufficiency. Many patients with rheumatic heart disease have a combined stenosis and insufficiency in the affected valve. If the mitral valve is involved,

---

[9]C. H. Rammelkamp, Jr.: "Hemolytic Streptococcal Infections." *In* J. R. Harrison, et al. (Eds.): Principles of Internal Medicine, 4th ed. New York, The Blakiston Division, McGraw-Hill Book Co., 1962, p. 913.

the left atrium develops dilatation and hypertrophy to compensate for the resistance of stenosis and the backflow of insufficiency. In the case of aortic valvular damage, the left ventricle dilates and hypertrophies. Prolonged strain created by a damaged valve, increased demands on the already weakened heart, or further progress of the initial rheumatic disease process may result in decompensation or heart failure.

Bacterial Endocarditis. Inflammation of the endocardium, including the valves, may be caused by many different pathogenic organisms, but Streptococcus viridans accounts for the greatest number of cases.[10] Bacterial endocarditis has a higher incidence in those who have some valvular abnormality, either acquired or congenital in origin, or who have a history of rheumatic fever. Special precautions should be taken with such persons when they experience minor infections, tooth extraction, and surgery, all of which predispose to the entrance of organisms into the blood. In bacterial endocarditis the organisms, transient in the blood, implant on areas of the endocardium and clusters of vegetative structures form consisting of inflammatory exudate, fibrin, platelets and bacteria. These are quite friable and may break off to form an embolus which then may lodge in an artery, interrupting the blood supply to an area of tissue. Should the embolus derive from the right side of the heart, it is likely to obstruct a pulmonary artery, causing a pulmonary infarct.* If the embolus originates in the left side of the heart, it may enter any systemic artery, resulting in an infarction. For example, it may lodge in a cerebral artery, leading to a stroke, or in a femoral artery, interrupting the blood supply to the limb.

As the infection subsides in endocarditis, the affected areas become scarred; if a valve was involved, a stenosis or insufficiency is likely to develop, and the patient then has the same problems as cited in relation to the patient with rheumatic fever.

Syphilis. Another type of infection that may produce a valvular lesion is syphilis.

---

[10]Paul B. Beeson: Endocarditis. *In* P. B. Beeson and W. McDermott (Eds.): Cecil-Loeb Textbook of Medicine, 13th ed. Philadelphia, W. B. Saunders Co., 1971, pp. 1098–1099.

*An infarct is an area of tissue which undergoes necrosis because it is deprived of its blood supply.

Most frequently it is the aortic valve that is affected, and an insufficiency develops.

Pericarditis. Bacteria may invade the pericardium and an accumulation of fluid results as part of the inflammatory response. The pressure exerted on the heart by this fluid may prevent its normal filling, creating a condition referred to as cardiac tamponade. In some instances, extensive scarring of the visceral pericardium may prevent normal stretching of the heart chambers.

It can be seen that in the inflammatory conditions cited in the preceding paragraphs, permanent heart damage can occur from the formation of scar tissue. The patient may remain active as long as his heart compensates, but he may have limitations due to reduced cardiac efficiency.

Resistance to the Flow of Blood from the Heart

Any increase in the resistance to the flow of blood from the heart increases the work of the heart, which strives to maintain a normal cardiac output. Narrowing of the lumen of the vessels by atherosclerosis and arteriosclerosis, and the increased arteriolar resistance characteristic of hypertension, place an added strain on the left ventricle. Pulmonary conditions such as emphysema, in which the alveoli are overdistended, and fibrosis of the lungs resist the flow of blood through the pulmonary circulatory system and increase the work of the right ventricle. The ventricle involved will respond by dilatation and hypertrophy. The period of time that the heart can compensate for the continuous added strain will vary with such factors as the degree of resistance, the age of the patient and the adequacy of coronary circulation. Eventually, decompensation or hypertensive cardiac failure is likely to ensue.

Deficiency in the Blood Supply to the Myocardium

A narrowing or obstruction in the coronary arteries reduces the blood supply to the myocardium and causes what is called ischemic heart disease. It results in a deficiency of oxygen and nutrients to the muscle. The reduced oxygen supply is most significant and is quickly reflected in reduced myocardial efficiency. The heart muscle can incur only a very small oxygen debt, as it is much more susceptible to a reduced oxygen supply than skeletal muscle.

The commonest cause of reduced coronary blood supply is atherosclerosis, which progressively increases with age. Atherosclerosis involves a thickening of the intima and fatty deposits, which slow the flow of blood through the vessel and predispose to thrombosis. Hypertrophy of the heart in response to some other condition may produce a coronary insufficiency; as the muscle cells enlarge they demand more oxygen and nutrients but there is not a proportional increase in the blood supply.

Angina Pectoris. This is a condition in which there is a discrepancy between the oxygen being supplied to the myocardium and the energy expenditure. The work load of the heart creates a need for a greater blood supply than is being delivered by the coronary circulation. The condition is manifested by severe pain in the sternal region, radiating to the left shoulder and down the arm; the patient may describe it as a choking or compressing sensation or a tightness. The pain, arising from the heart muscle fibers which are deficient in oxygen, is usually precipitated by physical exertion or emotional responses which increase the work load of the heart. Progressive restriction of the coronary vessels may eventually result in the patient experiencing a continuous ischemia, necessitating a reduction in his activity to a minimum.

Myocardial Infarction (Coronary Occlusion or Thrombosis). When the flow of blood through a coronary artery is blocked, the portion of the heart muscle normally supplied by that vessel suffers serious oxygen and nutritional deprivation. The area is damaged or destroyed and ceases to contract, reducing the heart's efficiency as a pump. The cardiac output may be decreased and the arterial blood pressure will fall, which accounts for the patient's state of shock. The damaged cells leak enzymes, and necrosis follows. This area of necrotic tissue, known as an infarct, becomes soft and then eventually fills in with firm, fibrous scar tissue. Survival and the extent of subsequent restrictions depend on the size of the artery occluded, since this determines the size of the infarct and the amount of myocardial

damage. Death may occur immediately or within a few hours if a large artery is involved. Obviously, the remaining viable heart tissue must compensate for the loss of functional tissue. If the patient survives the acute stage, his future activities are determined by the amount of permanent damage and his heart's compensatory ability.

The blocking of the artery is most frequently due to a thrombus forming within the vessel as a result of atherosclerosis; occasionally, an embolus is the cause. It may occur in any part of the coronary system but most often develops in an artery supplying the left ventricle.[11] Occlusion may be preceded by some manifestations of coronary insufficiency (e.g., angina pectoris) or it may take place suddenly without any previous warning.

Systemic Disease

Cardiac insufficiency may be a secondary development in some disease in an area other than the heart. The primary disease may have placed an added strain on the circulation or may have produced toxins or deficiencies in essential materials. Examples of these are diphtheria, hyperthyroidism, leukemia and pneumonia. Diphtheria produces a toxin that may cause myocarditis or may damage the conduction system. Diseases in which there is a prolonged and marked increase in the metabolic rate, as in hyperthyroidism and leukemia, place an increased demand on the circulatory system to keep the overactive body cells supplied. Pulmonary conditions, such as pneumonia and emphysema, may produce a respiratory insufficiency that results in an inadequate oxygen supply to the heart muscle and a consequent cardiac inefficiency.

Congenital Cardiovascular Defects

Congenital cardiovascular defect implies a structural abnormality that was present at birth in the heart or the large proximal blood vessels. It is only within the last two to three decades that many of the congenital cardiovascular defects have been identified and

---

[11]William A. Sodeman and William A. Sodeman, Jr. Pathologic Physiology, 4th ed. Philadelphia, W. B. Saunders Co., 1967, pp. 436 and 547.

successfully treated by surgery. Many are recognized shortly after birth if the infant survives. Others may go undiscovered for months or years because the heart maintains an adequate circulation by compensation. As in so many congenital deformities, the cause remains obscure. In some instances, it is thought that a virus infection, such as German measles, occurring in the mother in the first trimester of her pregnancy may cause the defect. Not infrequently, cardiovascular malformations accompany other congenital defects such as cataract, mental retardation and deaf-mutism.

Many types of heart malformations occur. They may be classified into three main groups: those which produce a left-to-right shunt of blood; those which offer resistance to the blood flow; and those which cause a right-to-left shunt.

Anomalies Which Cause a Left-to-Right Shunt. Several malformations occur which produce an abnormal pathway that permits a direct flow of blood from the left side of the heart or aorta to the right heart or pulmonary artery, creating a bypass of the systemic circulation and an overloading of the pulmonary circulation. These anomalies include patent ductus arteriosus and septal defects.

PATENT DUCTUS ARTERIOSUS. Normally, after birth a gradual spontaneous constriction and atrophy of the ductus takes place. If it remains open, the blood in the aorta, under a pressure approximately 5 to 6 times that in the pulmonary artery, is shunted into the pulmonary artery. This increases the volume of blood entering the lungs, resulting in a high pulmonary blood pressure and dilatation of the pulmonary vessels. The patient experiences dyspnea, particularly on exertion. There is a corresponding increase in the venous flow into the left atrium and left ventricle, causing

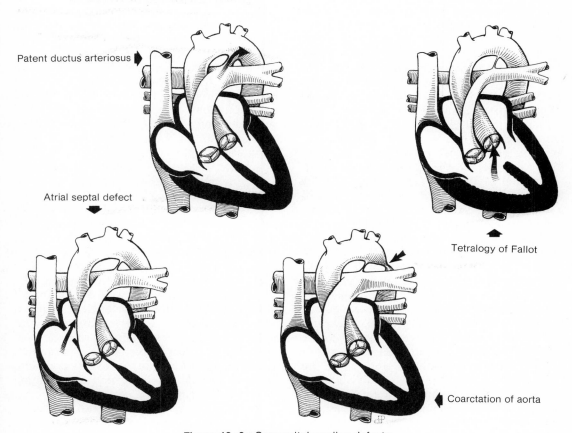

Patent ductus arteriosus

Atrial septal defect

Tetralogy of Fallot

Coarctation of aorta

Figure 13–6 Congenital cardiac defects.

dilatation and hypertrophy of the left side of the heart. The volume of blood in the systemic circulatory system is less than normal, and the resulting oxygen and nutritional deficiencies retard normal mental and physical development.

The patent ductus arteriosus is corrected by surgical division and suturing of the two ends of the vessel.

ATRIAL SEPTAL DEFECT. An opening between the two atria may be due to failure of the foramen ovale to close after birth or to a gap in the septum either above or below the foramen ovale. Blood in the left atrium, under higher pressure, will flow through the opening into the right atrium, increasing the volume of blood in the pulmonary system. The right atrium, right ventricle and pulmonary artery enlarge. Pulmonary hypertension develops and causes dyspnea, particularly on exertion. The reduced systemic circulatory volume retards physical and mental development and efficiency. The size of the opening may be so small that it goes undiscovered, and the patient may not experience any respiratory or circulatory difficulty.

Surgical repair of an atrial septal defect is usually done by open heart surgery. The heart is actually opened up; this necessitates diverting the blood in the venae cavae through an extracorporeal pump oxygenator to a femoral artery. Some defects may be closed simply by suturing others may require a patch of teflon, which is an inert material to which the tissues do not react.

VENTRICULAR SEPTAL DEFECT. An opening in the ventricular septum results in a left-to-right shunt, producing problems similar to those cited in atrial septal defect, namely, pulmonary hypertension, enlargement of the right ventricle and pulmonary arteries and a deficient systemic circulation.

Surgical repair of the septal defect is not undertaken in infants and very young children because they stand open heart surgery less well than those of five to six years and older. If the shunt involves a large volume of blood and severe pulmonary hypertension, a temporary artificial stenosis of the pulmonary artery may be established. A teflon band may be placed around the artery just beyond its origin. This reduces the volume of blood entering the pulmonary system and increases the pressure in the right ventricle; this in turn decreases the pressure differential between the two ventricles and reduces the volume of blood shunted from the left to the right ventricle. The primary defect may then be repaired by suturing or by the application of a teflon patch when the child is a few years older. At the same time, the restricting band is removed from the pulmonary artery. Occasionally, the defect closes spontaneously in the young child.

Anomalies Which Cause Resistance to Blood Flow Within the Circuit. The seriousness of the resistance is determined by the degree of constriction or stenosis which may be found in the pulmonary artery or the aorta.

PULMONARY STENOSIS. A stenosis of the pulmonary valve or artery offers resistance to the outflow of blood from the right side of the heart. The right ventricle enlarges and the pressure in both the right atrium and ventricle is above normal. Blood may be backed up in the venous system while the blood volume entering the pulmonary system is below normal. The latter creates an oxygen deficiency throughout the body which is manifested by cyanosis, shortness of breath and weakness.

This malformation may be treated by incision of the constricted ring. Depending on the information provided by cardiac catheterization and pressure studies, the approach may be through the artery below the stenosis or from above the stenosis through the right ventricle.

AORTIC STENOSIS. A defect comparable to pulmonary stenosis may occur in the aorta and offer resistance to left ventricular outflow. The left side of the heart enlarges and the pressure in both left chambers is above normal; this may be reflected in an increased pulmonary pressure if the restriction is severe. The cardiac output is lower and reduces arterial blood pressure and the systemic circulation as well as the blood supply into the coronary arteries. The defect may be treated by surgery, using an extracorporeal pump oxygenator during the procedure. In correcting the constriction, precautions are taken to avoid complete incision through the ring and the creating of an insufficient valve.

COARCTATION OF THORACIC AORTA. Coarctation is a stricture in a segment of the aorta. Postductal coarctation occurs just beyond the obliterated ductus arteriosus and distal to the origin of the left subclavian artery. The second type, preductal coarctation, develops in the segment of aorta before the entrance of the ductus arteriosus. With this latter type, the ductus usually remains patent.

Blood volume and pressure are increased behind the stricture, and the work of the left side of the heart is greatly increased. The blood volume and pressure are high in the upper extremities and head but are abnormally low in the body parts which derive their blood supply from below the stricture. A difference in growth and development may be seen between the areas supplied from behind the stricture and those supplied from the aortic flow distal to the stricture. The patient may experience headaches, epistaxis, dyspnea on exertion, leg cramps and fatigue.

Surgical treatment of the condition involves resection of the constricted area and an end-to-end anastomosis, or in some instances, the area is excised and a graft of inert material introduced.

Anomalies Which Cause a Right-to-Left Shunt.

A shunting of blood from the right side of the heart to the left involves a combination of two or more anomalies. Normally, the pressure is much higher in the left side of the heart than in the right side. A stenosis which offers resistance to flow from the right ventricle may increase the pressure in the right side to a level exceeding that in the left side. If a septal defect should coexist with this increased pressure, blood will be shunted from the right to the left side of the heart.

One of the most frequently seen combinations of anomalies which produces a right-to-left shunt is the tetralogy of Fallot. The term tetralogy denotes a set of four conditions: pulmonary stenosis; ventricular septal defect; dextroposition of the aorta, causing it to override the septal defect; and right ventricular hypertrophy. The pulmonic stenosis gives rise to an increased pressure in the right ventricle, causing a right-to-left shunt. The volume of blood flowing through the pulmonary system for oxygenation is reduced. Unoxygenated blood escapes into the aorta and a general systemic hypoxia occurs, manifested by cyanosis, especially on physical exertion. Compensatory responses to the oxygen deficiency develop in the form of polycythemia, high hemoglobin level and increased pulse and respiratory rates. In the very young, an increased collateral circulation causes a clubbing of the fingers.

Correction of these defects is possible by means of open heart surgery and the use of the pump oxygenator. The septal opening is patched, and the pulmonary stenosis is relieved. In some cases, the surgeon may decide not to do corrective surgery but will proceed with a palliative surgical procedure. This consists of an anastomosis between the subclavian and pulmonary arteries (Blalock operation) or between the aorta and pulmonary artery (Potts operation). The purpose of the anastomosis is to divert a larger volume of blood through the lungs for oxygenation.

Miscellaneous Congenital Cardiac Anomalies.

Only the more common anomalies that are recognized and treated have been presented here. A wide variety of anomalies can occur; many are not yet amenable to treatment, and others may be so severe that the infant cannot survive. Transposition of the great vessels is relatively common and attempts are now being made to find a successful surgical treatment. In this anomaly, the pulmonary artery originates from the left side of the heart and conducts the oxygenated blood back to the lungs; the aorta rises from the right ventricle, carrying unoxygenated blood into the systemic circulation.

Rarely, transposition of the pulmonary veins to the right of the heart is seen, and transplantation of the veins to the left atrium may be attempted.

Valvular atresia (absence of an opening) is another form of anomaly which occurs most frequently with the tricuspid valve but may also develop with the aortic valve. Tricuspid atresia raises the pressure within the right atrium to a level exceeding that in the left atrium, and blood flows through the foramen ovale. This anomaly frequently is accompanied by a ventricular septal defect which permits some blood to enter the right ventricle and pass into the pulmonary artery. Either the Blalock or Potts operation (see previous section), or an anastomosis between the superior vena cava and the pulmonary artery may be done for the purpose of increasing the volume of blood through the lungs.

Heart Compensation and Decompensation

Compensation. Heart compensation implies that the heart is maintaining circulation in the presence of some impairment. Many persons live a normal, active life with a heart condition that goes unrecognized for a long period. Others may have a known heart abnormality but, by respecting certain limitations, which in some cases may be very slight, are able to lead active, useful lives and live to a good age. In these latter persons, the heart condition may have been cured, but their cardiac reserve may be reduced, necessitating some adjustment in their activities. In still others, the heart condition is not cured and may even be progressive, but circulation is maintained by decreasing the demands on the heart and by compensating changes in the cardiovascular system. The adaptive changes that may occur are dilatation of the heart chambers, hypertrophy of the myocardium, increased pulse rate and peripheral vasoconstriction.

Dilatation occurs to accommodate an increase in the volume of blood returned to the heart or the blood that accumulates when the normal volume is not being forwarded. In accordance with the law of the heart, the increased stretching of the muscle fibers encourages an increase in the strength of the contraction of the heart muscle with a corresponding increase in the outflow.

Hypertrophy of the heart is due to an increase in the size of the individual muscle fibers in response to the persistent stretching of the fibers. This response is similar to that seen in skeletal muscles which enlarge when demands upon them are increased by exercise. In order to enlarge, the muscle fibers must have a good blood supply. If coronary circulation is deficient, hypertrophy may not be possible. Hypertrophy develops more readily in the young than in older persons. It requires time, and in sudden, severe heart damage when compensation cannot be supported by hypertrophy, heart failure may develop quickly. Both dilatation and hypertrophy are localized to the area of the heart involved; they may occur in relation to one chamber or one side of the heart only.

The autonomic reflexes that occur with cardiac insufficiency are principally those initiated by the pressoreceptors. The reduced cardiac output causes a corresponding fall in arterial blood pressure; impulses from the pressoreceptors are delivered to the cardiac and vasomotor centers in the medulla. As a result, general peripheral vasoconstriction and an increased pulse rate occur. The former increases the volume of venous return to the heart. The increased stretching of the muscle fibers may stimulate the pump, but if the heart is severely damaged it may be unable to respond and becomes further compromised by the overloading.

Decompensation. The ability of the heart to dilate and hypertrophy to compensate for an abnormal condition is limited. Excessive dilatation overstretches the muscle fibers to the point of injury; increasing hypertrophy creates a need for a corresponding increase in oxygen and nutrients, but there is not a proportional increase in the coronary blood supply.

Prolonged strain, progressive disease and demands exceeding the individual's cardiac compensation are likely to lead to a reduced cardiac output that will not meet the needs of the body. The heart is then said to be decompensated or in failure. Heart failure may be designated as left-sided or right-sided heart failure, as acute or chronic failure, or as congestive heart failure.

Failure of the heart to forward the volume of blood it receives is usually confined to one side of the heart, although the other side may fail later as a result of the primary failure. The side affected is determined by the site of the causative lesion. If the left side of the heart cannot forward the blood offered to it, blood is backed up in the pulmonary circulatory system. The vessels become engorged and fluid escapes into the alveoli, giving rise to dyspnea and cough. Right-sided failure may be secondary to that of the left side, or it may occur independently. If the right heart chambers cannot forward the blood being returned to the heart by the venae cavae, the systemic system becomes congested and edema develops in the tissues and organs.

Acute cardiac failure occurs suddenly and is considered a more serious threat to the patient's life. Chronic heart failure develops gradually and may only appear when the patient increases his activities and energy expenditure.

The term congestive is applied to cardiac

failure to describe the condition in the circulatory system behind the failure. It implies an excessive accumulation of blood in the system because the heart cannot accept and forward it.

Classification of Cardiac Patients

The required care is not the same for all cardiac patients since there are varying degrees of heart impairment and reduced efficiency as well as different pathological conditions.

There are those persons who have a slight abnormality or who have had a condition which has been cured. Their heart may carry some structural change or scar, but their cardiac efficiency and reserve are such that no restrictions on their activities are necessary. Some of these persons have unwarranted fears and restrict their activity unnecessarily even though they have been advised by their physician to live a normal, active life. The role of the nurse with these patients is to try to dispel their unsound fear and encourage them to be active. In some instances, overprotection by the family may be a problem.

A second group of persons whom the nurse may help are those who are not ill but have a reduced cardiac reserve. Their heart condition has resulted in adaptive changes (dilatation hypertrophy and/or acceleration) to compensate for the defect in order to maintain circulation. Energy expenditure must be restricted to correspond to the functional capacity of the heart in order to avoid failure. Obviously, the limitations vary with the extent of pathology and physiologic changes in the heart and its resulting capacity. For some, it may mean only the giving up of strenuous competitive sports; for others, greater restrictions are necessary. The aim of the care of these persons is to have each one live within his compensatory limits and, at the same time, live as useful and satisfying a life as possible. Continuous treatment may be necessary for some for

THE CLASSIFICATION OF PATIENTS WITH DISEASES OF THE HEART[12]

FUNCTIONAL CAPACITY

Class I. Patients with cardiac disease but without resulting limitations of physical activity. Ordinary physical activity does not cause undue fatigue, palpitation, dyspnea or anginal pain.

Class II. Patients with cardiac disease resulting in slight limitation of physical activity. They are comfortable at rest. Ordinary physical activity results in fatigue, palpitation, dyspnea or anginal pain.

Class III. Patients with cardiac disease resulting in marked limitation of physical activity. They are comfortable at rest. Less than ordinary activity causes fatigue, palpitation, dyspnea or anginal pain.

Class IV. Patients with cardiac disease resulting in inability to carry on any physical activity without discomfort. Symptoms of cardiac insufficiency or of the anginal syndrome are present even at rest. If any physical activity is undertaken discomfort is increased.

THERAPEUTIC CLASSIFICATION

Class A. Patients with a cardiac disease whose ordinary physical activity need not be restricted.

Class B. Patients with cardiac disease whose ordinary physical activity need not be restricted, but who should be advised against severe or competitive physical efforts.

Class C. Patients with cardiac disease whose ordinary physical activity should be moderately restricted and whose more strenuous efforts should be discontinued.

Class D. Patients with cardiac disease whose ordinary physical activity should be markedly restricted.

Class E. Patients with cardiac disease who should be at complete rest, confined to bed or chair.

[12]New York Heart Association: The Classification of Patients with Disease of the Heart. New York, American Heart Association. (Available in Canada through the Canadian Heart Foundation.)

them to remain asymptomatic. The physician assesses each patient's capacity, and the nurse helps the patient and family accept and adjust to the necessary restrictions. Emphasis is placed on the positive; suggestions are made as to what the patient can do, remembering that appropriate amounts of work, recreation and rest are more satisfying.

The functional capacity of some cardiac patients may be so limited that they cannot participate in any physical activity without experiencing symptoms of cardiac insufficiency. They may be restricted to self-care activities or may be confined to a chair or bed, completely dependent on others. The nurse's role with these patients is to provide the prescribed treatment and necessary care.

The physician may use the functional and therapeutic classifications developed by the New York Heart Association and published by the American Heart Association. This serves as a general guide to the type of care required and is useful in finding suitable employment for the patient (see p. 211).

NURSING IN HEART FAILURE

In heart failure, which may also be referred to as cardiac insufficiency or decompensation, care is directed toward (1) having the heart recover its ability to receive the normal venous return and forward the blood and (2) having the patient live within his cardiac capacity. Nursing responsibilities include the following considerations.

Observations

The patient's treatment and progress may be largely dependent upon the observations and recordings of the nurse.

Pulse. The strength, rate and rhythm of the pulse are noted at frequent intervals. The rate is determined on a count of a full minute. With some patients, the apical pulse as well as the radial is recorded, since a pulse deficit may be present. In some instances, there may be continuous electrocardiographic monitoring of the heart activity.

Respirations. It is important to know if the patient is experiencing shortness of breath and whether moist or abnormal sounds accompany respirations. These are indications of oxygen deficiency and pul-

monary congestion. The rate and depth of the respirations are significant, as well as the chest movement and use of accessory respiratory muscles. The position the person assumes may be helpful in denoting the amount of respiratory distress. Cheyne-Stokes respirations or alternating periods of apnea and hyperpnea frequently replace normal rhythm in cardiac patients.

Blood Pressure. Since the systolic pressure represents the cardiac output, it provides valuable information on heart action and the circulatory status. Frequent monitoring of the central venous pressure provides information about the heart's ability to receive and forward the blood (see p. 190).

Cough. Any cough is noted, since it is probably due to congestion and fluid in the alveoli and bronchial tubes. Its frequency and effect on the patient are recorded; the cough may be exhausting. The characteristics and amount of any sputum are noted. Frothy, colorless sputum occurs in pulmonary edema, and blood may appear if there is severe congestion from the rupture of capillaries and arterioles.

Color. The color of the lips, nail beds and skin is observed. Cyanosis (blueness) points to an oxygen deficiency, and the more pronounced, the more severe the circulatory failure. The blueness is produced by reduced (deoxygenated) hemoglobin. If the rate of blood flow through the tissues is slowed, the hemoglobin gives up more of its oxygen than it does normally. It must be remembered that serious heart conditions can exist without the patient exhibiting cyanosis. For example, this is seen in patients with left-to-right shunts in congenital defects. The person who suffers sudden cardiac arrest or myocardial infarction will probably show the extreme pallor characteristic of shock rather than cyanosis.

Orientation and Level of Consciousness. The degree to which the patient is oriented and his level of response provide some information about the circulation and oxygen supply to the brain.

Generalized Edema. The most accurate method of observing the patient for edema is by weighing him daily if his condition makes this possible. Ten to 15 pounds of water may be retained before edema becomes apparent. He should be weighed at the same time each day with the same weight of clothes. One looks for edema in the dependent areas of the body. If the person is ambulant, swelling first appears in the feet and ankles; but if he is confined to bed, edema may first become apparent in the back and sacral region. As it becomes more severe, all body tissues become affected and ascites and hydrothorax may develop. The latter further embarrasses the patient's breathing.

Fluid Balance. An accurate record is kept of the patient's fluid intake and output. A positive balance is brought to the attention of the physician, particularly if the urinary output is decreased to 20 to 25 ml. per hour.

Body Temperature. Many patients with cardiac insufficiency register a subnormal temperature, since their heat production is reduced because of the inadequate oxygen supply for cell metabolism.

With some patients, the temperature is recorded at least every 4 hours. In inflammatory disease and in myocardial infarction, the degree to which the temperature is elevated is significant in determining the severity of the disease process.

Anxiety. It is very important to observe the patient for fear and apprehension. Anxiety increases the demands on the heart and may indicate the need for information, explanations or sedation.

Care in Acute Pulmonary Edema

In failure of the left side of the heart, more blood is pumped into the pulmonary system than the left side of the heart can receive and forward. The vessels become congested and the alveoli gradually fill with serous fluid and blood. Unless this is checked, the respiratory exchange is cut off and the patient literally drowns. It can be seen that left cardiac failure precipitates an emergency which demands prompt action. Efforts are made to reduce the venous return to the heart and at the same time strengthen the heart in order to increase the output from the left side. A reduction in venous return may be achieved by the application of rotating tourniquets and by a phlebotomy.

Three tourniquets are necessary, and one is applied to the upper part of three extremities with just sufficient pressure to interfere with superficial venous circulation. One

tourniquet is moved to the free limb every 10 to 15 minutes and a definite pattern, either clockwise or counterclockwise, is established (see Fig. 13–7). The physician will indicate the period between moves and how long the tourniquet procedure is to be used. Too long a period of venous compression may produce the risk of phlebothrombosis and embolism.

The second emergency measure that may be used to reduce venous return is phlebotomy. The doctor withdraws 250 to 700 ml. of blood from a vein. Usually a blood donor set is quickly made available for this procedure, and the blood is donated to the blood bank.

The patient with severe pulmonary edema is naturally very fearful, which only further aggravates his primary condition. The physician will probably administer morphine intravenously, along with aminophylline to dilate the bronchial tree and digitalis to strengthen the myocardial contractions. Oxygen may also be used to support respirations.

To summarize briefly, pulmonary edema or sudden left-sided cardiac failure is an emergency. Quick action is necessary to save the patient's life. The nurse, advised that such a patient is to be admitted, quickly assembles the necessary equipment and medications for the treatments so there will be no delay.

Rest

Rest is important in the treatment of the cardiac patient since it reduces the demand on the heart by reducing body requirements for oxygen. For the patient threatened with failure or in failure, rest in bed is necessary. The doctor's order may read "complete (or absolute) bed rest" or simply "bed rest." These usually mean something different, and the nurse determines exactly what is meant by each in the particular situation. Generally, "complete bed rest" is interpreted as the absolute minimal activity on the patient's part, with the nurse doing everything possible for him. He is fed, bathed, turned and assisted on and off the bedpan; his teeth are cleaned and his hair combed. "Bed rest" usually means that the patient may participate to some degree in his personal care, and the nurse observes the effects of such

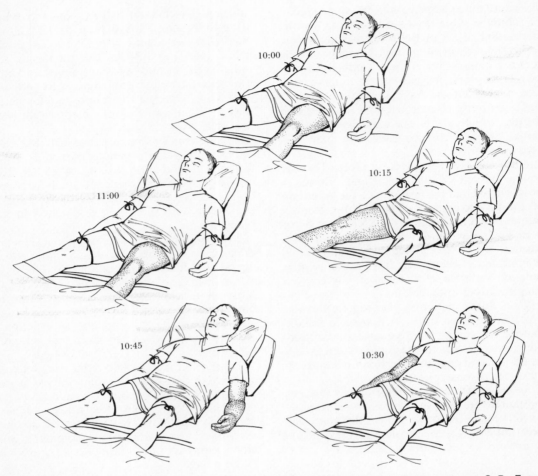

Figure 13–7 Rotation of tourniquets in pulmonary edema at 15-minute intervals. (From Keane, C. B.: Essentials of Nursing, 2nd ed. Philadelphia, W. B. Saunders Co., 1969, page 237.)

activities on the patient. If they produce shortness of breath, an increase in pulse rate and excessive fatigue, his activities are reduced.

Mental rest is as important as physical rest but often difficult to promote. The common knowledge that the heart is a most vital organ and that heart disease is a frequent cause of death makes for greater emotional reaction on the part of the person advised of a diagnosis of a heart ailment. He becomes fearful and apprehensive; his life, his job, his family's security and his whole future are threatened. Rarely does any other condition, even though it may be an equally severe threat, engender as much fear and concern. Frequently, the anxiety may be out of all proportion to the threat. Emotional

reactions increase respirations and the work load of the heart. A patient may appear to be at rest but is actually in a mental turmoil. The sensitive, observant nurse who understands the possible implications illness has for this patient is likely to detect this mental unrest and should endeavor to promote the peace of mind essential to optimum rest.

The nurse who understands the patient's condition, knows what to look for and knows what to do usually displays calm and composure, which contribute to a patient's confidence and security. A quiet, controlled atmosphere will do more toward allaying fear than verbal reassurance. The doctor will decide on how much the patient should know about his condition. This is a matter that must be dealt with on an individual basis. Withholding information and evading the patient's questions may produce more anxiety than knowledge of his condition. With another patient, the doctor may consider it unwise to tell him much about his condition. The nurse should know the doctor's decision on this matter and be willing to answer the patient's and his family's questions within the limits of the information deemed advisable.

It is helpful to have someone remain with the anxious patient; alone, he may panic, thinking he is cut off from help. If a nurse is not available, the presence of an auxiliary worker or a member of the family will provide some reassurance. Emotionally disturbed relatives should not be permitted to visit or remain with the patient unless they can conceal their feelings and control their reactions.

There may be a home problem that contributes to the patient's unrest. Some solution may be suggested or arrangements made for assistance from the social service. The nurse encourages the patient to express his anxieties and endeavors to identify his feelings and his problems as he sees them. Frequently, verbal expression of his concerns may reduce their proportions; having shared them, he now has the support of someone who knows his problems. It may be necessary, with some patients, to seek the assistance of the doctor or the patient's religious adviser to deal with questions or expressions of fear.

In the interest of providing optimum rest for the patient, consideration is given to his placement on the ward. He is not located next to disturbing persons and will most likely feel more secure if he is close to the nursing station. A light left burning at night may contribute to his security as well as making it easier for the nurse to make frequent, reassuring visits and the necessary observations. If his degree of activity permits, reading or listening to the radio may provide diversion and relaxation.

There is no specific formula for dealing with the cardiac patient's anxiety in order to provide the much needed rest. The nurse must be alert to the problem and work at it; that which proves successful with one patient will not be the answer for all.

Physical comfort will contribute to the patient's rest and may be promoted by change of position, back rub, bathing, warmth, etc. Anticipation of his needs and the planning and provision of undisturbed rest periods are important. Cooperation is sought from the laboratory, dietary and housekeeping staff to control the interruptions. Sedatives may be prescribed to reduce anxiety and restlessness, and the nurse provides the necessary attention to ensure maximum benefits from the drug.

Positioning

The position the cardiac patient finds most comfortable in bed is determined by his breathing. The patient who is experiencing dyspnea will be more comfortable with the head of the bed elevated, but the height of elevation should only be that at which his dyspnea is minimal. The horizontal position is less fatiguing if it can be tolerated.

Patients with congestive failure manifest orthopnea (i.e., less difficulty in breathing with the trunk in the upright position). The sitting position increases the vital capacity and tends to reduce the volume of blood returned to the heart and to the pulmonary system. Pressure of abdominal viscera on the diaphragm is reduced. Some patients may be still more comfortable in a true sitting position, that is, with the lower limbs down. A special cardiac bed on which the foot of the bed can be lowered to provide a chairlike support is available. The sitting position promotes the formation of peripheral edema in the dependent parts but relieves the pulmonary congestion to some extent; peripheral edema is much less serious than pulmonary edema.

In the sitting position, a pillow placed longitudinally at the patient's back may help provide some comfort. Pillows should be used at the sides to support the arms and relieve the fatiguing pull on the shoulders. A change may be made by arranging an overbed table and pillow in front of him on which he may rest his head and arms. Crib sides are kept up on the bed to safeguard the patient when he is in the upright position, since he may become drowsy and fall to the side or may experience cerebral hypoxia, which causes disorientation. The sides are also useful when a change of position is made, since they may be grasped by the patient and used for added support. Patients in the upright position are encouraged to assume the recumbent position for brief periods to help reduce the circulatory stasis and edema in the lower parts of the body. This should not be forced in severe dyspnea.

In the heart patient, as with all patients, the general principles of positioning apply. Good body alignment is respected to prevent contractures, hyperextension and circulatory stasis. Even a slight change in position every 1 to 2 hours is helpful. A footboard is used to prevent foot drop.

Activity

Rest has been emphasized as an important phase of the treatment of cardiac patients, but it is well known that there are certain disadvantages inherent in bed rest. The limbs should be put through passive movements to promote venous drainage and prevent phlebothrombosis. Gentle massage will also be helpful. If the patient's condition permits, the doctor will have him gradually commence foot, leg and arm exercises. The patient is also encouraged to take 5 to 10 deep breaths every 1 to 2 hours. As soon as possible, he is allowed to get out of bed to use a commode, since the use of a bedpan for defecation places considerable strain on the patient.

Observations should be made of the reactions to any activity so that undue stress on the heart may be avoided. This will also assist the doctor in defining the patient's future activities and the amount of rest and restriction that will be necessary.

Nutrition and Fluids

Adaptations in the diet for cardiac patients are based, first, on their retention of an excess of sodium, which causes the formation of edema, and, secondly, on the knowledge that overeating and overweight increase the work load of the heart.

Low sodium diets are prescribed to reduce edema and to prevent further accumulation of fluid in the tissues. The sodium restriction varies with patients, depending on their heart efficiency and amount of edema. Normally, the average daily salt intake is 10 to 12 grams. If no salt is added to food either at the table or in cooking and no salted foods are used, the intake may be reduced to approximately 3 grams. In congestive heart failure, more stringent restrictions are necessary and foods are selected that will provide still less sodium. Diets that contain as low as 0.25 gram can be prepared.

Low sodium diets are unpalatable, and the patient finds it difficult to adhere to the prescribed restriction. Frequently, the result is that he does not take sufficient food to meet his nutritional needs. The nurse explains the purpose of the diet and relates it to symptoms the patient is experiencing. There are many spices and allowable foods that help to make a low sodium diet more palatable. A list of such foods appeared in an issue of the American Journal of Nursing under the title of "Spicy Suggestions for Cardiacs."[13] In prolonged, severe restriction of sodium, the patient may develop a sodium deficiency. The doctor should be informed of any complaints of muscular cramps and weakness.

If the cardiac patient is overweight, his caloric intake is reduced in an effort to bring his weight to normal. A maintenance diet is then prescribed. The diet of lower calories should contain less fat but enough of the other food principles to meet nutritional requirements.

For patients with atherosclerosis, the doctor may suggest a change in the fat content of their diet. Atherosclerosis is a degenerative change in the wall of arteries due to fatty deposits which contain cholesterol. The intima of the vessel becomes scarred and thickened, resulting in a narrow lumen which restricts the flow of blood. The coronary arteries seems to be a particularly vulnerable site. Some patients may be advised to decrease their intake of saturated fats, which are mainly of animal origin (meat, butter, cream, whole milk and cheese). The foods containing saturated fats may be substituted for by the use of polyunsaturated fats, which are of vegetable origin (corn, soybean, and cottonseed oils). By reducing the animal fat and foods which contribute to the formation of cholesterol, it is thought the development of atherosclerosis may be prevented or arrested. Therapeutic diets for cardiac patients are

---

[13]Medical Highlights: "Spicy Suggestions for Cardiacs." Amer. J. Nurs., Vol. 58, No. 2 (Feb. 1958), p. 169.

available in booklet form from the Heart Foundation. These have been prepared according to the usual prescribed sodium restrictions (500 mg., 1000 mg., 2000 mg., 3000 mg.). The foundation also has booklets containing diet suggestions for restricted calories as well as those for controlled fat intake to produce lower blood cholesterol levels.

The food for heart patients should be easily digestible, and gas-forming foods should be avoided. Overeating should be avoided; smaller, frequent meals are more desirable than fewer large meals.

During the acute phase of a heart illness, the diet is usually fluid to start with and is graduated to soft foods and then light solid foods as the patient improves. The patient may have to be fed, and this is done by unhurried, willing personnel. If the patient feels that this is a burden on the ward staff, he may go without his food and may also resent the whole situation. This reaction creates an emotional response which negates the energy-sparing purpose of feeding the patient. When allowed to feed himself, his appetite generally improves, since it indicates to him that his condition is improving.

Restrictions are rarely placed on fluid intake, especially if sodium is restricted and diuresis is established. A record is kept of the intake and output, and if a positive balance occurs, the physician is consulted about the fluid intake. Harrison and Resnick suggest that "the intake of water should usually be regulated by the desire of the patient."[14] The general opinion would seem to be that there is no danger of overloading by fluid intake if the sodium is restricted and circulation and diuresis are improved, but there is danger if fluids are restricted, since intracellular water may shift and cause a disturbance in cell metabolism.

Elimination

Constipation and straining at defecation are to be avoided because of the undue strain placed on the heart. A mild laxative may have to be given to keep the stool soft. If constipation does occur, an oil enema may be given. Abdominal distention is also to be avoided, since it raises the diaphragm, further embarrassing the patient's breathing. It has been shown that the use of the bedpan requires more energy than getting out of bed and using a commode. For this reason the physican may prefer to have the patient use a bedside commode for defecation.

The cardiac patient who has edema is most likely receiving a diuretic. The intake and output are measured so that the effect of the drug may be noted. When a patient receives a diuretic it will mean frequent use of the bedpan or commode, which can be very exhausting. The nurse provides the necessary assistance, and the patient is allowed to rest undisturbed between voidings.

Care of the Mouth and Skin

The dyspnea and the retention of sodium experienced by the cardiac patient cause a decrease in the normal salivary secretions. The tongue is rough and dry, and a thick mucus accumulates and adheres to the teeth and mucous membrane, providing a medium for organisms. Under such conditions, older patients are especially predisposed to parotitis. The mouth is cleansed every 2 to 3 hours and is kept moist.

The poor circulation, edema, bed rest and restricted activity necessitate special skin care to prevent pressure sores. Bony prominences and pressure areas are kept clean and dry and are massaged gently but with sufficient pressure to promote circulation. Alcohol may help toughen the skin, but if found to be too drying, a small amount of oil may be applied occasionally. The alternating air pressure mattress is useful in protecting pressure areas; but if not available, a sponge rubber mattress may be used, or piece of sponge rubber or sheepskin may be placed under pressure areas such as the sacrum, buttocks and heels.

Medications

Several different groups of medicines are used in the treatment of heart disease. They comprise a large part of the treatment, and

[14]T. R. Harrison and W. H. Resnick: "Congestive Heart Failure." *In* T. R. Harrison, et al. (Eds.): Principles of Internal Medicine, 4th ed. New York, The Blakiston Division, McGraw-Hill Book Co., Inc., 1962, p. 1386.

the nurse is responsible for the administration of most of these drugs during hospitalization. Each drug may bear specific nursing responsibilities with its administration, and the nurse must be familiar with these.

The more commonly used drugs for cardiac patients are grouped and presented here according to their purpose.

1. To Relieve Hypoxia and Dyspnea

Oxygen may be administered by tent, mask or catheter to increase arterial oxygen concentration. It will only be effective, however, if the delivery to the tissues is improved.

The nurse briefly explains the procedure to the patient and remains with him until he is accustomed to the tent or mask. Observations are made of the patient's response to the oxygen. Its effectiveness will be indicated by reduced pulse rate, less dyspnea, improvement in color and less restlessness. (For details of administration of oxygen see p. 279.)

In severe pulmonary edema, the physician may administer oxygen under positive pressure to counteract the movement of fluid from the capillaries into the alveoli. A 50 to 100 per cent concentration of oxygen may be used at a pressure of 30 cm. of water for 10 to 15 minutes every few hours.

THEOPHYLLINE (AMINOPHYLLINE). This drug is frequently given intravenously at the onset of acute cardiac failure. Later it may be given orally or by rectal suppository. It dilates the bronchial tubes and bronchioles, contributing to the relief of cardiac dyspnea.

2. Drugs to Strengthen the Heart Muscle

DIGITALIS. This drug is used to strengthen and slow the myocardial contraction and thereby increase the cardiac output. It slows the pulse rate by depressing the A-V conduction and by increasing vagal nerve stimulation. The resulting fewer contractions give the heart muscle time to rest and recover.

A secondary action is diuresis. As it improves circulation, the urinary output increases and helps to reduce edema if present.

There are many preparations of digitalis: digitalis, digitalin, digitoxin, digoxin and digifolin are but a few. There are preparations for intravenous, intramuscular and oral administration. A large dose is prescribed for the first 2 to 3 days in order to achieve a therapeutic concentration of the drug in the blood. This is referred to as digitalization. The dosage is then reduced to a smaller maintenance dose.

Nursing responsibilities in administering digitalis preparations include taking the radial pulse before each dose. If it is 60 or less per minute, the apical pulse should be checked. If the apical pulse also is 60 or less per minute, the physician is consulted before giving the drug. Bradycardia, anorexia, nausea and vomiting, diarrhea, abdominal discomfort and visual disturbances are toxic signs for which the nurse must be alert.

3. Antiarrhythmic Drugs

QUINIDINE SULFATE. This drug is most frequently prescribed when the heart is fibrillating. It increases the refractory period of the myocardial cells and slows the rate and may re-establish the normal rhythm.

The drug is administered by mouth, and the radial and apical pulses are taken before each dose. Toxic symptoms which may develop are excessive cardiac acceleration, cardiac arrest, headache, tinnitus, visual disturbances, nausea, vomiting and diarrhea. A patient may have an idiosyncrasy to the drug, and the nurse is required to observe the patient closely following the first two or three doses for any toxic effects.

PROCAINAMIDE HYDROCHLORIDE (PRONESTYL). This drug is used in atrial fibrillation and tachycardia and has similar effects to quinidine. It may be given intravenously, intramuscularly or orally. The blood pressure is checked during intravenous administration, and the patient is observed closely for any indication of hypersensitivity, which may be manifested by a chill, joint and muscle pain, itching, weakness, dizziness or gastrointestinal disturbances. Norepinephrine and epinephrine should be quickly available in the event of a reaction.

LIDOCAINE HYDROCHLORIDE (XYLOCAINE). This preparation is commonly used to decrease premature ventricular contractions which frequently precede ventricular fibrillation. It depresses the rate of impulse discharge and conduction. Lidocaine is administered slowly by intravenous injection or by slow intravenous drip. It acts rapidly, within a matter of 2 to 4 minutes. The patient is observed closely for possible hypotension, and the heart action is checked by monitor. The drug is kept readily available for use following a myocardial infarction, during a cardiac catheterization and following cardiac surgery.

4. Drugs to Produce Diuresis

There are various groups of diuretics used to relieve cardiac edema, including preparations for parenteral and oral administration. The reader is referred to a clinical pharmacology text for a complete list and details of these drugs and their administration. Only a few are presented here.

MERCURIAL DIURETICS. Mercurial preparations such as Thiomerin and Mercuhydrin may be used. They induce diuresis by depressing the reabsorption of sodium chloride and water by the renal tubules.

BENZOTHIADIAZIDES. This group of drugs inhibits the reabsorption of sodium and chloride ions by the renal tubules. They have the distinct advantage of being available in preparations for oral administration. Preparations currently in frequent use include chlorothiazide (Diuril) and hydrochlorothiazide (Hydrodiuril).

AMMONIUM CHLORIDE. This is usually prescribed in conjunction with a mercurial diuretic. It is given orally and only for 2 to 3 days at a time, since it may reduce the pH of the body fluids.

SPIRONOLACTONE (ALDACTONE). This diuretic acts by inhibiting aldosterone. The latter is secreted by the cortex of the adrenal glands and promotes the absorption of sodium ions and water by the kidney tubules. The drug, unlike most other diuretics, does not inhibit the reabsorption of potassium ions by the kidneys. For this reason, it may be given in conjunction with another type of diuretic (e.g., Diuril).

FUROSEMIDE (LASIX). This sulfonamide derivative has been introduced more recently as a very effective diuretic. It acts quickly, producing diuresis in one-half to one hour following oral administration. It is used principally with patients in the hospital since a close check on potassium, sodium and chloride blood levels is necessary.

In order to judge the effectiveness of a diuretic, the nurse keeps an accurate record of the patient's fluid intake and output and, if possible, weighs the patient daily. Because the large and frequent urinary output may be very exhausting and distressing to the patient, the significance of the diuresis is explained, and the necesssary assistance is provided to avoid excessive fatigue. The diuretic is administered in the morning so the patient is not disturbed at night.

The nurse is always alert for untoward effects. Any complaint of gastrointestinal disturbance of sign of skin irritation should be brought to the physician's attention. Frequent and large urinary output may cause an excessive loss of potassium from the body fluids, further weakening the heart muscle.

5. Drugs to Produce Vasodilation of the Coronary Vessels

Dilation of the coronary arteries will improve the blood supply to the myocardium in ischemic heart disease (see section on Angina Pectoris and Myocardial Infarction).

NITROGLYCERIN (GLYCERYL TRINITRATE). This vasodilator is administered in tablet form, 0.1 mg. to 0.6 mg. The tablet is placed under the tongue where it is absorbed very quickly. It reduces vascular tone, allowing more blood through the vessels. The patient is started with a small dose which will most likely have to be increased as a tolerance is developed. Persons who suffer attacks of angina are advised to carry the drug at all times.

PENTAERYTHRITOL TETRANITRATE (PERITRATE). This is a slower acting vasodilator and is effective for a longer period. It is given orally and may significantly reduce the number of anginal attacks.

6. Drugs to Reduce Coagulation

Following a myocardial infarction, thrombi tend to form within the heart chamber involved and may cause pulmonary or cerebral embolism. The very restricted activity to which the coronary patient is subjected, coupled with impaired circulation, predisposes to phlebothrombosis. For these reasons, anticoagulants are frequently prescribed.

The two most widely used anticoagulants are heparin and dicoumarol. The former must be given parenterally, since it has no effect orally. Heparin is thought to block the effect of thrombin on fibrinogen, thereby preventing clot formation. It may be given for 24 to 48 hours and then gradually replaced by dicoumarol, which is given by mouth. Dicoumarol takes longer than heparin to take effect, so it is frequently started before the heparin is withdrawn.

The daily administration and dosage of either anticoagulant are dependent each day on the prothrombin time of that day. These drugs produce the risk of bleeding but their therapeutic value may be considered to outweigh this risk.

The nurse's responsibilities include close observation for signs of hemorrhage. Profuse bleeding from minor cuts, bleeding gums, hematuria, hematemesis, blood in the stool, petechiae and abnormal vaginal bleeding are reported promptly. In the event of bleeding the drug is discontinued, and vitamin K and a blood transfusion may be given to counteract the reduced coagulation.

Each day the nurse makes sure that the prothrombin time is determined before the anticoagulant drug is administered and that the physician is notified promptly if the prothrombin time is not within the desired range previously indicated by him. Patients outside the hospital on an anticoagulant are usually required to report to clinic weekly for a prothrombin time check.

7. Drugs to Treat and Prevent Infection and Inflammation

ANTIMICROBIALS. In the acute stage of rheumatic heart disease the patient may receive large doses of penicillin to destroy any hemolytic streptococci which may still be active in the body. Reactivation of the disease occurs very readily with any subsequent streptococcal infection. Rheumatic fever patients, particularly children, continue on prophylactic doses of oral penicillin or on a monthly intramuscular injection of a large dose which is slowly absorbed. For better absorption, the oral penicillin is given before food is taken in the morning and again at bedtime when the stomach is empty. Sulfadiazine may be used for prophylactic therapy in place of the penicillin, and the patient is advised to take a minimum of six to eight glasses of fluid each day to prevent precipitation of the drug in the renal tubules. Antibiotics are also used in the treatment of bacterial endocarditis.

With the initial administration of penicillin the nurse is alert for symptoms of allergic reactions. If the patient has not previously had the drug, a test dose may be given intracutaneously. Any information of previous reactions or of asthma or hay fever should be passed on to the doctor before the drug is given.

SALICYLATES. Sodium salicylate and acetylsalicylic acid (Aspirin) are preparations commonly used in rheumatic fever. These relieve the symptoms by suppressing tissue reaction. They are given orally and may produce gastric distress, so they should be given with meals or with a snack or a large volume of fluid. If the patient complains of dizziness, headache, tinnitus or dullness of hearing, the doctor is informed. Frequently, sodium bicarbonate tablets are administered with the salicylate to prevent the gastric symptoms, or enteric-coated acetylsalicylic acid tablets are used.

CORTICOIDS. Various preparations of cortisone are also used in the treatment of rheumatic heart disease. Their action is similar to that of salicylates in that they are anti-inflammatory and reduce tissue responses. While a patient is receiving a corticoid preparation his sodium intake may be restricted, since there tends to be an excessive reabsorption of sodium by the kidney tubules, leading to edema. The patient is weighed daily if possible and is observed for other indications of edema.

8. Drugs to Provide Rest and Relieve Pain

MORPHINE. This may be used to reduce anxiety and restlessness in cardiac insufficiency or to relieve the severe pain in myocardial infarction. The effect of the drug on the respirations should be carefully noted, since depression of the respiratory center may occur. If P.R.N. orders are left for morphine, very judicious use should be made of the drug.

MEPERIDINE HYDROCHLORIDE (DEMEROL). This drug may be used in place of morphine and for the same purposes.

BARBITURATES. The patient may be given small doses of a sedative, such as phenobarbital or amytal, three or four times a day to reduce his anxiety and promote rest.

Prevention of Complications

The impaired circulation and venous stasis, the vegetative clusters on the valve flaps in bacterial endocarditis and rheumatic heart disease, and the hemoconcentration found in some congenital heart conditions predispose to thrombus formation and possible embolism. Circulatory stasis may be prevented by passive movement of the lower limbs and by the encouragement of active exercise and activity as soon as the physician indicates that the patient's condition will permit these.

The patient should be protected from contact with infection since the heart patient's resistance is usually lowered. Any infection increases the work of the heart.

The need for bedsides was previously cited. These patients frequently display some confusion, particularly at night, and may attempt to get out of bed. This increases both the demands on their heart and the risk of injury by falling.

Rehabilitation

The philosophy and principles of rehabilitation are applicable to heart patients just as they are to patients with other conditions in which there is some residual damage or progressive disease. These persons may require help to learn to live within the limits of their cardiac capacity and at the same time achieve personal satisfaction and be able to function as productive members of society.

When a patient learns that he has a heart condition or recovers from an acute heart illness, he is advised as to whether he may resume his former activities or if it will be necessary for him to curtail some activities. The amount of activity and necessary restrictions are defined by the physician on the basis of the functional capacity of the heart. Many of these persons consider themselves doomed to complete invalidism and an early death. They may have an unjustified fear of another attack or of participating in any activity and may become helpless and dependent, creating unnecessary problems and hardships for themselves and their families.

Heart disease does not differ from many other diseases in that the patient may recover and take up his life where he left off. Some may find that a few simple adjustments in their pattern of living are necessary, while others are more restricted.

The physician has several ways of assessing the patient's capacity for activity and his limitations. He may observe the patient's responses to a gradual increase in energy expenditure. This will probably begin with self-care activities which are progressively extended to more strenuous efforts. The assessment program may go on over several weeks or months, and the patient may re-

quire considerable encouragement to persevere.

An evaluation by standardized tests may be made in a heart clinic. In some situations, work evaluation clinics are established and serve to determine how much activity the patient's heart will permit. Following an assessment, a functional and therapeutic classification may be made (see p. 211). This is particularly useful in placing the patient in employment.

The nurse may assist in the assessment of the patient by observing and recording his responses to various activities. Any complaint or shortness of breath, palpitation, fatigue or an undue increase in the pulse rate are reported, and the effort is discontinued until the patient is checked by the doctor.

It is sometimes helpful to have the patient list his accustomed pattern of activities. The doctor may then indicate what changes, if any, are necessary. This is useful in getting the patient to think and talk about how much he will be able to do. It encourages him to plan independently and to reach a compromise between activity and restrictions.

The patient should realize that he has some responsibility for his future. The length of time he will live, and with what degree of satisfaction, depends largely on his own efforts. Each person reacts differently to illness and to restrictions. One may refuse to take advice or accept limitations and decide to "live it up." Another may become depressed or may display hostility, and still others become overdependent. It is usually more difficult for the adult patient to accept and adjust to restrictions. Heart insufficiency so often occurs just when the patient has reached a high position in his job and when life has become easier. The adult required to change to a less strenuous occupation finds it difficult to face a retraining program. Often his age makes it difficult for him to get another job.

With emphasis on the positive aspects, the nurse helps the patient and his family understand and accept the decision of the doctor and to plan for the necessary adjustments. In the following paragraphs, consideration is given to the planning of assistance and guidance for these patients, remembering that every program must be planned in relation to each individual.

The nurse should have a copy of the many

useful pamphlets and booklets available from the Heart Foundation. Many of these deal with rehabilitation, and appropriate copies may be given to the patient to read with the doctor's approval.

Progressively increased activity is encouraged and directed by the nurse to condition the patient to the level of activity that corresponds to his heart's ability.

Changes may be necessary in the patient's home if he is not allowed to use stairs. It may be helpful to have a visiting nurse or social worker assess the home situation before the patient returns to it. Suggestions may be made in the interest of the patient and those who will be caring for him. For example, a bedroom and bathroom may have to be provided on the ground floor. Distance from public transportation and work may be factors that require consideration for some patients.

It should be pointed out to the patient and his family that moderation in everything is a good rule for persons who have had a heart illness. Some work, exercise, rest and recreation are important for everyone. Situations that are likely to add undue strain should be anticipated and avoided. Enough time should be allowed to prevent rushing. For example, rather than run the risk of running for a bus, the patient should plan to leave earlier. Climbing, walking against a strong wind, lifting, pushing and fatigue are to be avoided. Constipation, infections and emotional upsets also tend to increase the demands on the heart. The patient should strive for equanimity and develop the philosophy that what cannot be changed must be accepted. Suitable recreational activities, which meet both his interests and his cardiac functional capacity, may be suggested. Some exercise is beneficial and appropriate forms are discussed. Walking is considered a good exercise. Regular hours of rest at night and, if necessary, a rest period during the day are recommended.

Since smoking, particularly cigarettes, is found to be vasoconstricting, the heart patient is well advised to discontinue smoking.

Shortness of breath, palpitation, faintness, persisting fatigue, pain and edema are indications for the person to slow up and report to the clinic or his doctor.

The doctor, a social worker or the nurse may discuss necessary adjustments in the person's work situation with his employer or the industrial nurse. Assistance might be given to find suitable employment or to obtain retraining if a change in occupation is indicated.

Clarification of the prescribed diet is made. Many heart patients are advised to continue with a low sodium intake and a limited number of calories. Foods allowed, those restricted and meal planning are discussed. The importance of keeping the weight normal and avoiding large meals is explained. Preferably, the discussion of the diet should be with the homemaker as well as the patient. Directions and suggestions are given to the patient in writing, and an appropriate diet booklet is obtained from the Heart Foundation.

The medications that are to be continued are discussed, and written instructions are provided. Early signs of untoward reactions are cited and included with these are directions about what to do if they develop. For example, if an anticoagulant such as dicoumarol is to be continued, the patient and a family member are advised of the action of the drug and the necessary observations to recognize bleeding. They are told that bleeding from body orifices, discolored areas of the skin (bruises and petechiae), bleeding gums, and persistent bleeding from minor cuts or injuries are to be reported immediately to the doctor or clinic. If he is to have dental work done, the patient should advise his dentist that he is receiving dicoumarol. He is given an identification card to carry which states that he is receiving dicoumarol. A weekly visit to clinic for prothrombin time evaluation is usually requested by the physician.

Many heart patients are required to take digitalis continuously and should understand that loss of appetite, nausea or diarrhea may indicate the need for some adjustment in the dosage of the drug. If the patient is an elderly person who lives alone, he is advised to keep a calendar available with the days that he is to take a medication clearly marked. It is stressed that he adopt the habit of marking off the medication as soon as he takes it.

Some follow-up service is important. The patient and family are advised of the resources outside the hospital, and a referral may be made to the visiting nurse or public health agency. Home visits by a nurse can be very helpful; they provide an opportunity for the patient and family to ask questions and receive counseling on the various aspects of care. At the same time, the patient's condition and progress are noted.

If the patient's heart condition demands fairly stringent restrictions on his activity, it may be necessary to assist the family in planning how they will provide the required care. Some patients need provision made for their ordinary personal care. The family is advised about the amount of care needed, how to provide it and how to protect their own health. They are encouraged not to overprotect the patient or foster an over-dependent role. The family should plan together and all share in the necessary care. The nurse may recognize that the care of the patient will impose too heavy a burden on the family and help them to seek some other solution. A referral may be made for home care service or the patient may be transferred to a nursing home. Circumstances might necessitate the family receiving social welfare assistance. The nurse may have to help the patient accept this situation.

The importance of regular medical supervision is stressed. The severely handicapped person may have difficulty getting to the clinic or doctor's office; transportation may be requested of a voluntary organization such as the Red Cross Society or a service club.

Obviously, the child with heart disease will present different rehabilitative needs from those of an adult. While the child is still in the hospital, the nurse starts to plan with the parents for the child's home care. This can be greatly reinforced by counseling and demonstrations given by a visiting nurse in the home situation. For example, the nurse might suggest that if the child was in a room on the ground floor, with a bright interesting outlook and nearer to the center of activity, he would feel less isolated and more contented. This would also save steps for the mother.

The parents are given instructions on how to care for the child who is confined to bed, give medications, take temperature and pulse, plan the patient's meals and how to organize his and their day. Booklets such as "Home Care of the Child with Rheumatic

Fever" and other pamphlets may be appropriate and helpful.[15] It is of value, particularly for younger children, if a fairly rigid schedule from hour to hour is set up, and activities are included that are approved by the doctor. Definite hours of rest are respected to avoid overtaxing the heart.

If the patient is a school child, when he is well enough, plans are made for some school work to be continued. The department of education will arrange for a teacher to visit at regular intervals or send an outline of work which the parent or an older sibling can help the patient pursue.

Since it is difficult to keep children amused and contented while in bed, especially when they are alone in a room, the reader is referred to Dodds' booklet entitled "Have Fun . . . Get Well!"[16] which suggests crafts, hobbies and interests for the child and teen-ager.

Adolescents approaching the age when they must make a decision about a vocation or career may require aptitude and vocational tests. They are then helped to select on the basis of both these tests and the doctor's opinion of the individual's heart capacity.

Playmates, family friends and members of volunteer groups may be helpful by visiting and reading or playing games for a specified period. This may relieve the parents who frequently need some guidance as to how they may best protect their own health in such a situation. Occasionally, the observant nurse will recognize the need to tactfully discuss the adverse effects of their overprotection of the ill child and how this may be causing neglect of the other children.

The homemaker with a cardiac condition is given assistance in learning to continue her home functions within her heart capacity. Again, the reader is referred to the appropriate publications available through the Canadian Heart Foundation.[17] Much work

---

[15] Published by the American Heart Association, New York. Available in Canada through the Canadian Heart Foundation, Ottawa.

[16] Maryelle Dodds: "Have Fun . . . Get Well!" 8th ed. New York, American Heart Association, 1961. Available in Canada through the Canadian Heart Foundation, Ottawa.

[17] Example: "The Heart of the Home." Published by the American Heart Association, New York. Available in Canada through the Canadian Heart Foundation.

has been done on work simplification in the home, and there are many simple and inexpensive ways of making it possible to achieve more with less effort. In some communities, a consultant is available through the American Heart Association or a rehabilitation unit who will visit the home and make suggestions as to how the housekeeper's work can be made easier. Some physical changes, a reorganization in the placement of equipment, elimination of unnecessary chores, and the management of many tasks to economize on time and motion may be suggested and demonstrated. The success of rehabilitating the homemaker is largely dependent on how willing she is to change her ways of doing things. The nurse and rehabilitation worker may find that much time will have to be devoted to persuasion.

The patient's health and degree of satisfaction in living will depend to a large extent on his recognition and acceptance of the limitations imposed.

NURSING IN ISCHEMIC HEART DISEASE

Ischemic heart disease indicates an insufficiency in the coronary blood supply and includes the conditions angina pectoris, coronary insufficiency and myocardial infarction. In most instances, the decreased blood supply to the myocardium is due to degenerative changes in the arteries that produce a narrowing of the lumen of the vessels. Fatty substances which include cholesterol are deposited within the intima of the arteries, causing atherosclerosis. These fatty plaques interfere with the nutrition of the cells in the intima, leading to necrosis, scarring and calcification, which leave the surface rough and the lumen reduced. These roughened constricted areas allow less blood through and predispose to thrombus formation and occlusion of the vessel.

Atherosclerosis usually develops gradually. While the blood supply through the artery is being reduced, a collateral circulation develops in an effort to increase the supply to the myocardium, but this supplementary circulation is rarely sufficient to provide enough oxygen to the heart muscle during strenuous physical exertion.

The oxygen deficiency in the heart muscle is manifested by severe pain, giving rise to the condition known as angina pectoris or coronary insufficiency. The blocking of a coronary artery and sudden, complete withdrawal of oxygen from an area of heart muscle causes a myocardial infarction, also referred to as coronary occlusion or coronary thrombosis.

Angina Pectoris

The term angina pectoris describes the pain which the patient with ischemic heart disease experiences. Pectoris indicates the general location, and angina refers to the choking suffocating nature of the pain.

The patient suddenly develops pain in the chest which may radiate to one or both shoulders and arms and, occasionally, up the neck to the jaws. The pain is described as being crushing, constricting, suffocating or as a sensation of weight in the chest. The onset usually corresponds to some exertion on the part of the patient and is sufficiently severe to force him to stop. With the patient at rest, the pain usually subsides within a few minutes.

If rest does not promptly relieve the attack, nitroglycerine, 0.3 to 0.6 mg., taken under the tongue is usually effective. The angina patient is instructed to carry these nitroglycerine tablets with him at all times and is advised about the dosage and the sublingual administration. The doctor may recommend that he take a dose before doing anything likely to bring on an attack. Peritrate may be prescribed for a more prolonged effect.

Strenuous physical exertion and emotional conflicts should be avoided. The patient's occupation, ways of doing things, forms of recreation and social life may have to be changed. Smoking is discouraged, since it favors vasoconstriction. Overweight should be corrected and normal weight maintained.

The attacks may eventually become fewer and less severe as collateral circulation becomes established, but rarely does the patient escape some continued restrictions in his activities. Some patients gradually become seriously handicapped as their attacks increase in frequency and severity, and the term coronary insufficiency is then applied.

Acute Myocardial Infarction

Acute myocardial infarction (also known as coronary occlusion or thrombosis) is the most serious and acute form of ischemic heart disease. A coronary artery becomes blocked, and the myocardial area which it supplied suffers oxygen deficiency and necrosis. It occurs suddenly, and compensation through collateral channels is inadequate to maintain the myocardial cells. The resulting area of necrotic tissue is referred to as an infarct.

The patient suddenly becomes seriously ill and experiences excruciating pain, helplessness and a sense of impending death. The pain is similar to anginal pain except that it is not necessarily precipitated by exertion, is not relieved by rest or nitroglycerin and is more intense and prolonged. The patient may have been at complete rest when the attack struck.

Signs of shock appear quickly. The blood pressure falls; the skin is cool, moist and of a grayish pallor; and the pulse becomes rapid and weak or may be imperceptible because of the decrease in cardiac output. The patient may experience nausea and vomiting, dyspnea and extreme weakness. Characteristic electrocardiographic changes occur, indicating to the physician that myocardial damage has occurred and probably its location and extent.

The myocardial necrosis causes an elevation of body temperature ranging from 37.7° to 39° C. (100 to 103° F.), leukocytosis, an increased erythrocyte sedimentation rate and increased concentrations of specific intracellular enzymes (see p. 197). The presence of these clinical manifestations of myocardial damage and necrosis serve to confirm the diagnosis, and their intensity corresponds to the size of the infarct.

The pain and shock may subside within a few hours, but the situation remains critical. The impaired myocardium may not be able to sustain circulation and signs of failure may appear (dyspnea, hypoxia and edema). There is danger of the infarct rupturing in the soft, necrotic phase, particularly with sudden increased exertion. Arrhythmias may develop in the form of tachycardia, fibrillation or heart block.

Nursing Care of the Patient with an Acute Myocardial Infarction. The location, severity and incapacitating nature of the pain at the onset of the attack point to the possibility of a "heart attack." The patient may even be known to have had angina and to have taken nitroglycerin but without relief. Prompt action is necessary. The doctor is called immediately. The patient is kept at rest in the position he assumes. This will probably be semi-sitting, because of dyspnea. Tight clothing (collars, belts, etc.) should be loosened and the patient covered sufficiently to prevent chilling. Food and fluids are withheld since they may induce vomiting, which places undue strain on the heart.

Treatment and nursing care are directed toward the relief of pain and shock and minimizing the work of the heart until it recovers its ability to maintain normal circulation.

General nursing care of heart patients has been discussed (see p. 212). Some specific and pertinent factors applicable to the care of the person who has had a myocardial infarction are as follows.

OBSERVATIONS. Constant observation of this patient is necessary. The nurse must be alert to significant changes and must make decisions about the need for prompt reporting, the seeking of assistance and the use of emergency measures. Changes in heart rate and rhythm, a fall in blood pressure, increasing dyspnea and cyanosis, persisting cardiac pain and continuing restlessness and apprehension are reported. A continuous monitoring of heart action is usually established; electrodes are applied to the chest wall and are connected to an electrocardiograph with an oscilloscope. The purpose of the monitor is explained to the patient and his family. The patient should understand that he need not lie immobile because of the electrodes. The nurse responsible for the patient must become sufficiently familiar with the monitoring system and oscilloscope graphs so that she will be able to recognize changes and arrhythmias that demand prompt action.

RESPIRATORY SUPPORT. Oxygen is usually administered by tent, mask or catheter in order to increase the arterial oxygen tension which may help to relieve the myocardial pain caused by hypoxia. Mechanical assistance by the use of a respirator may be necessary in cases of severe insufficiency (see p. 286).

REST. This is of the utmost importance in the treatment and care of the patient with an acute myocardial infarction. Unless otherwise directed, the nurse places the patient on complete bed rest, which means that everything must be done for him. This necessary dependency should be discussed with the patient as to its purpose, importance and what it involves. He may rebel and resist this enforced dependency to the point that the doctor may think it is doing more harm than good. After 2 or 3 days, the strict inactivity may be modified somewhat and the patient is observed closely for his reactions. Mild activities such as cleaning his teeth, washing his face and hands and feeding himself are permitted first, as long as reaching is avoided. In most instances, exercising of the lower limbs to prevent venous stasis is commenced on the second day. Some patients are permitted to use a bedside commode once a day, since this demands less energy than using a bedpan for defecation.

Activities and exertion are restricted and carefully controlled until the infarct heals and scars firmly and a collateral circulation is established. This may take 2 or 3 weeks. The physician is guided in this by the body temperature, leukocyte count, sedimentation rate and enzyme concentrations. Their decrease coincides with healing of the infarct. During the necrotic stage when the infarct is soft and there is a risk of rupture of the heart wall, any activity that is permitted should be undertaken slowly.

The patient may be kept nonambulatory for approximately 10 days to 6 weeks. This will vary with the patient's response, the size and effect of the infarct and the doctor's philosophy. More recently, the tendency is to favor the shorter period, since many physicians believe fewer complications occur and the psychological effect of early ambulation is worth a great deal.

As cited previously, mental rest is a significant part of therapy for the heart patient. This patient's anxiety is usually great and frequently the direct question, "Am I going to die?" or "How serious is this?" is posed. The physician is advised of the patient's concern so he may provide him with information about his condition. Considerable help and peace of mind may be derived from the patient's spiritual adviser, but this visit should only be arranged on the patient's or his family's request.

The nurse remains with the patient until he becomes less apprehensive and then assures him someone is close by and will be in and out frequently. The presence of a close family member who will not disturb the patient may provide additional comfort. Bustling, noisy activity should be avoided.

Competent, quiet performance without apparent concern and hurry provides some reassurance for the patient. Anticipation of the treatment needs and preparedness contribute to more effective care. Undisturbed periods are planned in order to provide the therapeutic rest.

The patient's needs are anticipated so that he is neither tempted to get up nor reach for something rather than ask. Articles likely to be wanted are left within reach.

MEDICATIONS. The first consideration is usually the need for an analgesic to relieve the severe pain. Morphine may be given intravenously, intramuscularly or subcutaneously, or meperidine hydrochloride may be used. The analgesic will also help to reduce the patient's anxiety and restlessness. Later, sedation such as phenobarbital or amytal may be prescribed for rest.

The anticoagulants heparin and dicoumarol may be prescribed unless the patient has a history of peptic ulcer, a blood dyscrasia which predisposes to bleeding, or renal or liver disease. Administration of these drugs immediately poses some specific responsibilities for the nurse (see p. 219).

To combat shock, a vasopressor may be given. Levarterenol (Levophed), metaraminol (Aramine) and methoxamine hydrochloride (Vasoxyl-P) are examples of vasopressors that may be used. These drugs are given by slow intravenous infusion, and the rate of flow is very precisely regulated according to the patient's blood pressure, which must be taken every 15 to 30 minutes. An intravenous infusion of glucose 5 per cent in distilled water is started on admission so that there is a route readily available for the administration of antiarrhythmic drugs. The solution is run very slowly. In some situations, a solution of lidocaine (Xylocaine) or procainamide hydrochloride (Pronestyl) is prepared and attached to the intravenous by a Y connecting tube so that it is ready for prompt administration if the electrocardiographic tracing indicates premature ventricular contractions or fibrillation.

DIET. Nausea and vomiting are common in the first 24 hours. One need not be too concerned about the patient's intake for the first day or two. In most instances nutrition and hydration are optimum at the time of the attack, and the patient's need is also suddenly greatly reduced.

Liquids are given in small amounts at first and gradually increased to easily digested, nongas-forming solids as tolerated. Large meals are to be avoided. If necessary, the caloric intake is decreased to reduce the patient's weight to normal and to correspond to reduced energy output. Sodium is usually restricted to some degree.

The fat content of the diet may be controlled to reduce blood cholesterol levels, with a view to decreasing further atherosclerosis. Less animal fat is used, and the total amount of fat in the diet should comprise not more than 25 to 30 per cent of the total caloric intake.

When the patient is permitted to feed himself, it is advisable that he start by handling only a part of the meal. This is gradually increased to managing a complete meal, if he does not become excessively tired or manifest undue strain.

SMOKING. The patient is advised to refrain from smoking, since this is thought to contribute to the risk of further coronary disease.

ACTIVITY AND DIVERSION. The resumption of activities progresses gradually from self-care through sitting up in a chair to walking. The progression of increasing activities continues for weeks to months after the patient leaves the hospital. Limitations are applied to those activities which precipitate dyspnea or pain.

Once the patient is free of pain and recovers from shock, his fears and anxiety are somewhat reduced, and he feels fairly good but must still remain in bed. Time hangs heavy on his hands, so some effort should be made to provide suitable diversion in which the patient is interested. Reading and radio and television programs may occupy the patient but these should be selected to avoid overexcitement and fatigue. He may have some hobby which he can pursue without overtaxing his heart. Visitors are restricted at first but later they could help relieve the patient's boredom. Selection of the visitors should be made by the family to avoid persons who might excite or distress the patient.

Convalescence and Rehabilitation (see p. 221). The length of time the patient continues his convalescence before returning to work will depend on his freedom from dyspnea and pain as he progressively increases his activities. Many are advised to work only part time when they first return to work. Full time is resumed if there are no signs of distress. To be able to return to work boosts the patient's morale. It proves he is not relegated to complete invalidism and dependency.

Myocardial damage may have reduced the functional capacity of the person's heart. He may have to adjust to fewer hours of work and more hours of rest. Some persons may be restricted by progressive artherosclerosis and coronary insufficiency. A late complication that may develop following a coronary thrombosis is a weakening of the scarred area of the myocardium which balloons out to form an aneurysm. This complication usually leads to congestive heart failure. A few become incapacitated by their fear of another attack even though their functional heart capacity is such that they could do much more than they do.

Surgical Treatment in Ischemic Heart Disease. In severe coronary insufficiency, revascularization surgery may be undertaken to increase the supply of oxygenated blood to the myocardium. One procedure, referred to as the Vineberg operation, involves the transplantation of the internal mammary arteries into the myocardium. Anastomoses gradually develop between the transplants and the coronary vessels.

A more direct approach to the problem of coronary insufficiency is by coronary endarterectomy or by establishing a bypass graft from the ascending aorta to the coronary artery beyond the stenosed or occluded area. In the endarterectomy, the vessel is opened and the atheromatous plaque is removed. In the bypass procedure, a section of a saphenous vein is used as a graft.

For nursing care, see p. 230.

CARDIAC ARREST

Cardiac standstill or arrest means the sudden cessation of effective ventricular contraction. Possible causes are myocardial ischemia, respiratory insufficiency, ventricular fibrillation, heart block, electric shock and adverse reactions to an anesthetic or a drug.

The condition must be recognized as an

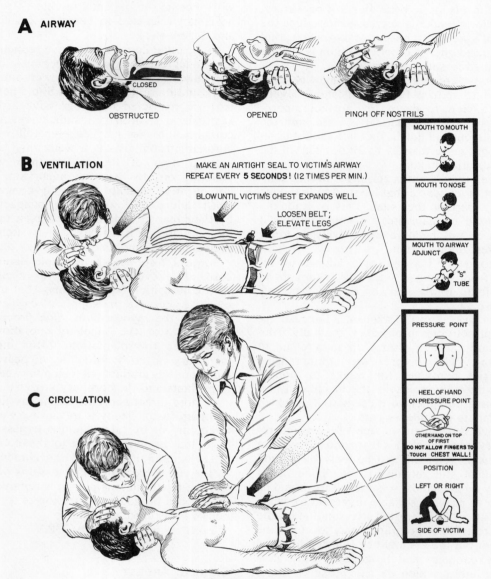

A AIRWAY

CLOSED

OBSTRUCTED   OPENED   PINCH OFF NOSTRILS

B VENTILATION

MAKE AN AIRTIGHT SEAL TO VICTIM'S AIRWAY
REPEAT EVERY **5 SECONDS!** (12 TIMES PER MIN.)

BLOW UNTIL VICTIM'S CHEST EXPANDS WELL

LOOSEN BELT;
ELEVATE LEGS

MOUTH TO MOUTH

MOUTH TO NOSE

MOUTH TO AIRWAY
ADJUNCT
"S" TUBE

C CIRCULATION

PRESSURE POINT

HEEL OF HAND
ON PRESSURE POINT

OTHER HAND ON TOP
OF FIRST
DO NOT ALLOW FINGERS TO
TOUCH CHEST WALL!

POSITION

LEFT OR RIGHT

SIDE OF VICTIM

Figure 13–8 Resuscitation in cardiac arrest.

STEPS IN EXTERNAL CARDIAC MASSAGE

1. Someone is dispatched for the necessary medical assistance.
2. The victim is placed on his back on a firm surface, such as the floor or ground. In the case of a bed patient, a board is placed under the patient. Each hospital ward is usually equipped with an "emergency board" that is easily handled and may be quickly placed under the upper half of the patient's trunk.
3. The operator places the heel of one hand over the lower third of the sternum and the other hand over the first hand. Pressure is applied vertically downward, depressing the sternum 1 to 2 inches about once each second. The pressure should be sufficient to produce a carotid and femoral pulse, which may be checked by a second person. Less pressure is required in cardiac massage for children up to 10 to 12 years, since the thoracic cage is very flexible. The pressure delivered by the heel of one hand is sufficient. In infants, the pressure is exerted by the fingers of one hand.
4. At the end of each pressure stroke, the hands are completely relaxed.
5. Mouth-to-mouth respirations are started as soon as possible if assistance is at hand. If the person doing the cardiac massage is alone, he interrupts the massage approximately every 30 pressure strokes (every 25 to 30 seconds) to give 3 or 4 artificial respirations.
6. The massage is continued until heart action resumes and is producing a strong peripheral pulse or until some other form of treatment is instituted. The operator pauses every 2 to 3 minutes to determine if heart action has resumed. As circulation is restored, spontaneous respirations and constriction of the pupils should occur.

STEPS IN MOUTH-TO-MOUTH ARTIFICIAL RESPIRATION

1. The mouth is cleared of any foreign matter.
2. The head is hyperextended, the lower jaw held forward and the nostrils are pinched.
3. The operator takes a large breath, places his mouth tightly over the patient's mouth and blows out his breath to inflate the patient's lungs. In the case of a small child, the operator's mouth is placed over the mouth and nose. If effective, the chest will rise with each blowing.
4. The operator removes his mouth and releases the nostrils. Air should be heard escaping from the patient's lungs, and the chest should fall.
5. The procedure is repeated approximately 12 to 15 times per minute.
6. If the patient's chest does not rise with the first respiration, the position of the head, neck, and lower jaw are checked again to ensure an open airway. If air still does not enter the patient's lungs, check the mouth for mucus and turn him to one side. Several sharp blows are then struck between the shoulder blades to dislodge a mucus plug or foreign substance which may be blocking the airway.
7. The artificial respirations and the pressure strokes of the cardiac massage must be coordinated. About 1 respiration to 4 pressure strokes is given, and the blowing in of air must occur during the release of sternal pressure.

emergency. It is urgent that circulation be sufficiently re-established to deliver oxygen to the brain within 4 minutes to prevent permanent cerebral damage. Cardiac arrest may be manifested by sudden collapse and loss of consciousness, an absence of pulse in the radial, carotid and femoral arteries, apnea and dilatation of the pupils.

External cardiac massage and artificial respirations should be commenced at once.

External Cardiac Massage

External cardiac massage consists of the intermittent application of vertical pressure over the lower third of the sternum. The pressure stroke compresses the heart between the sternum and the spine and empties the ventricles. To be effective, the compression must force a volume of blood into the arteries sufficient to produce pulsation in the carotid and femoral arteries. The pressure should depress the sternum 1 to 2 inches and is exerted about once a second. The thoracic cage is quite flexible in an unconscious person and the possibility of injury to the ribs is reduced. Relief of the pressure allows the heart to refill. This technique of resuscitation is simple, requires no special equipment and may be done anywhere.

Since cardiac arrest causes respiratory failure, artificial respirations must accompany cardiac massage; otherwise, the persisting oxygen deficiency to the cardiac muscle will prevent its response and increase the possibility of cerebral damage. The mouth-to-mouth method of artificial respirations is the one of choice unless the victim is in a situation where an intermittent positive pressure respirator, capable of delivering a higher concentration of oxygen, is available. If a second person is not available to perform the respiratory resuscitation efforts, cardiac massage is interrupted every 25 to 30 seconds to ventilate the victim's lungs 3 or 4 times.

In the hospital an external pacemaker may be used to stimulate heart action (see p. 203). If ventricular fibrillation has caused the arrest, an electric defibrillator may be used. An electric current of approximately 400 to 500 volts is delivered through electrodes into the chest wall.

Drugs may also be used as an adjunct to cardiac massage. Epinephrine hydrochloride (Adrenalin) 1:1000 may be injected directly into the myocardium by the physician. Preparations of sodium bicarbonate, calcium chloride and potassium should be readily available for intravenous injection or infusion.

Mouth-to-mouth respirations may be replaced by an intermittent positive pressure respirator which will deliver a higher concentration of oxygen.

Care Following Resuscitation. The patient who has been resuscitated requires constant observations of the vital signs. A continuous monitoring of heart action may be established and a pacemaker applied which will deliver a stimulus to the heart in the event of recurring arrest. Peripheral pulses are checked for quality and rate.

Respirations, temperature and blood pressure are noted and recorded at least hourly.

The defibrillator and respirator are kept close at hand and ready for immediate use.

The patient will be very apprehensive. He is advised of improvement in his condition and of the importance of rest and minimal emotional upset. He is assured that someone will either be with him or close by so that treatment may be quickly instituted should he need it.

NURSING THE CARDIAC SURGICAL PATIENT

Cardiac surgery is a relatively new and very specialized field of surgery. It deals with both congenital and acquired heart defects; the latter may be lesions resulting from organic disease or trauma. Most of the surgery undertaken at present is simply to close an abnormal opening or to remove an obstruction and enlarge an opening. Examples are the closing of septal defects and the correction of stenosed valves or an aortic coarctation. New surgical procedures are continuously evolving. Transplants, grafts and prostheses for reconstructive procedures are now being undertaken to correct more complex defects. The fact that the heart must function immediately after the surgery presents a problem different from that in many areas of the body. It must heal while continuing to maintain adequate circulation. This creates the need for greater support and for minimizing physiologic demands.

Progress in this area of surgery was delayed until the introduction of the pump oxygenator. This machine permits extracorporeal oxygenation of the blood and maintenance of circulation while the heart is arrested and opened to provide a direct approach to defects within the heart. Circulation bypasses the heart and lungs. The venae cavae are cannulated, and the blood passes from them into tubes leading to the mechanical oxygenator, which takes the place of the lungs. It is then pumped through a heat exchanger and filtered into a femoral or subclavian artery. The blood flows in a reverse direction in the aorta, keeping the aortic valve closed. Sufficient blood enters the coronary system to sustain the myocardial cells. The blood is heparinized in order to prevent coagulation and thrombus formation. On completion of the cardio-pulmonary bypass, the heparin is neutralized by the administration of protamine sulfate.

If surgery is to be performed on the aortic valve, the entrance of blood into the coronary system may have to be briefly curtailed. Hypothermia may be used to reduce the metabolic activity of the heart so the cells can survive interruption of the coronary circulation. Reducing the body temperature to within a range of 20 to 30° C. (hypothermia) may be used in heart surgery either alone or as an adjunct to the extracorporeal circulation. It reduces the metabolic activity of cells throughout the body and therefore their oxygen and nutritional needs. Hypothermia prevents damage to the brain and other vital organs when an interruption of circulation or a reduction in oxygenated blood to a dangerously low level is anticipated (see Section on Hypothermia, p. 71).

Preoperative Nursing Care

The preoperative preparation for cardiac surgery may extend through days to weeks, while the patient is thoroughly investigated and his physical and mental conditions are improved.

Psychological Preparation. In most instances, heart surgery carries more than the ordinary risk. The incision may be midsternal, which avoids entrance into the left pleural cavity and collapse of the left lung, or it may be through the left chest and may result in collapse of the left lung. Because of the tremendous emphasis placed on the heart by the average person, it is understandable that the patient and his family will be very apprehensive. The surgeon describes the patient's condition to the patient and his family and the likely prognosis if he continues untreated. An explanation is then made of what can be done surgically and the inherent risk.

It takes courage to face heart surgery; the patient or (in the case of a child) the parents may find it difficult to arrive at a decision. They require a great deal of emotional support. The nurse assesses the patient's anxiety and fears, and efforts are directed towards minimizing them, since they will affect the patient's reaction to surgery and his postoperative progress. He is encouraged to talk about his concerns and to ask questions. Worries may become less significant through verbalizing them and being able to share them. Socioeconomic problems may come to light which necessitate voluntary or welfare assistance for the patient and family. The patient may fear death and may wish to talk about this. A visit from the patient's spiritual adviser may provide him with considerable support.

Acquainting the patient with what to expect when he goes to the operating room and after the surgery will reduce some of his fear of the future. Preparation continues over several days, and as the patient talks more and more about the whole major event, he will begin to accept it with less stress. In all discussions with the patient and his family, what is said should be informative, in understandable terms, and judiciously selected to prevent inducing unnecessary anxiety. Sincere interest and understanding of their problems are frequently better expressed by feeling tones than by words.

To prevent unnecessary concern, the patient is advised of the multiple and complex equipment that will surround him after his operation. It may be helpful with some patients to actually let them see some of the equipment in this preoperative period. The patient is told that he will be receiving oxygen by a mask or probably by a respirator which will reduce the work of breathing, that his blood pressure and pulse will be taken at very frequent intervals to reveal information about his condition, and that there will be a tube in the chest as well as a nasogastric tube, intravenous tube and an indwelling catheter. He is advised that he will likely experience a sensation of heaviness and tightness as well as some pain in the chest and is reassured that the staff will do everything possible to provide relief.

Observations. During the preoperative period, vital signs, fluid intake and output, daily weight and reactions to any exertion are noted. The patient is also observed closely for indications of any condition, such as a cold or skin infection, which could cause serious postoperative complications. A detailed knowledge of the patient and his vital signs serves as a basis for comparison postoperatively.

Operative Consent. The patient, if responsible and of age, will sign his consent for operation. In some situations, the hospital and/or the surgeon may also require the signature of a close relative on the consent. The patient and his family should have had a description of the operation and its expected outcome before being asked to sign the operation permit. In the case of a minor, both parents may be required to give permission.

Functional Tests (see p. 196). Cardiac and respiratory functional tests, as well as complete blood studies, are done to further assess the patient's condition. The blood work will include typing and cross-matching so that compatible blood will be available at the time of operation. The nurse explains the tests to the patient and provides the required preparation and after-care applicable to each one. For 2 to 3 days following the more complex cardiac tests, such as catheterization, close observation is necessary for manifestations of reactions or complications. Bleeding or irritation at the site of entrance into the blood vessel, reaction to the radiopaque substance, fibrillation and cardiac arrest occur rarely.

Physical Preparation. Optimum nutritional status is important; attention is directed to having the patient take adequate meals. Protein and vitamin C are particularly important, for they contribute to tissue repair. If the patient has been on a low sodium diet previously, this will be continued. Optimum hydration is desirable; a daily intake of 2000 to 2500 ml. is encouraged as long as his output is adequate. A record is made of the fluid intake and output, and any indication of a positive balance is brought to the doctor's attention.

The patient is advised that he will be required to cough, take five to ten deep respirations, change position and do some simple leg and foot exercises frequently for several days after the operation. Arm exercises will also be necessary later. The purposes of these activities are explained. Instructions are given on how to cough and do the exercises, and the patient is encouraged to practice. To cough, he is instructed to take a deep breath, contract the abdominal muscles and then cough with the mouth and throat open. Postoperative coughing and deep breathing promote expansion of the lungs, the removal of secretions from the tract and the removal of air and fluid from the thoracic cavity. The foot and leg exercises are to prevent phlebothrombosis. The arm exercises promote a return to the full range of motion of the left arm, since the patient will tend to favor it following the operation.

Particular attention is paid to skin and oral hygiene during this period. Daily bathing with a mild antiseptic solution or soap minimizes the possibility of staphylococcal wound infection. Antiseptic mouthwash will help to prevent mouth and respiratory infection.

Immediate Preoperative Care. Extra precautions are taken with these patients in preparing the skin. Infection superimposed on their surgery could prove fatal. The day before operation, practically the whole trunk is shaved and cleansed including the axillae. Since a femoral artery may be cannulated, the upper thighs are also prepared. The surgeon will indicate what antiseptic, if any, is to be applied; following the shave, the patient may be given an antiseptic bath and placed in fresh bed linen. Care is taken during the shave to keep the skin intact. It is important that the fingernails are free of nail polish so that their true color may be detected.

Solid food is withheld for 10 to 12 hours previous to operation and the meal preceding this period should be light. Water may be given up to 4 to 6 hours prior to operation.

The doctor may or may not want the patient to have a small cleansing enema the afternoon before operation. A sedative is prescribed to ensure the patient a good sleep the night before operation. The nurse makes a final check to see that the required blood is available, the urinalysis report and vital signs are satisfactory, and that the operative consent has been signed.

The morning of operation, a nasogastric tube is inserted to prevent vomiting and abdominal distention later. An indwelling catheter may be placed in the bladder, but if not, the patient empties his bladder just before the sedative is given. An intravenous infusion will probably be started, or a venesection (cut-down) done and a cannula secured in the vein. All procedures are completed when the patient receives his preoperative medication so that he may be left undisturbed to derive the maximum benefit from the drug. A nurse accompanies the patient to the operating room and remains with him until the anesthetist or operating room staff takes over.

Consideration is given to the relatives during this stressful situation. A spouse, parent or someone close whom the patient wishes to have may be allowed to visit before the preoperative medication is administered. The family may wish to remain at the hospital during the operation, or may decide to return home to await word by telephone. If they remain, they are shown to a sitting room where an understanding hostess may be provided to help them through the difficult hours. If there is no hostess, the nurse should take a few moments at intervals to go and speak with them and to see that they have refreshments. Recognition on the part of the nurse or others that this is a difficult time will help. Many surgeons, knowing the family's stress, will forward a message from time to time to reassure them.

Postoperative Nursing Care

The patient who has had cardiac surgery is cared for in an intensive care unit where the necessary special equipment is assembled. Continuous observation and constant, expert nursing care are required. The patient becomes very anxious and fearful if left alone for even a very brief period the first day or two.

The care must be adapted to the patient's particular needs and the surgeon's directives. The following points of care may not be applicable nor complete in all situations but may serve as a guide to the nurse who is planning and providing care for the surgical cardiac patient.

Preparation to Receive the Patient. During the operation the necessary equipment is assembled in the patient's room and checked for normal functioning. Nonessential pieces of furniture should be removed from the room. Placement of the multiple pieces of equipment is important. Some will be in constant use; others will be used only occasionally or in an emergency, so they must be readily accessible but not in the way. Electrical cords and leads are kept untangled and out of the line of traffic.

A suggested list of necessary equipment follows:

Pharyngeal tube or airway
Sphygmomanometer and stethoscope
Respiratory and gastric suction equipment
Infusion poles

Equipment for oxygen administration (tent, mask or catheter)
I.P.P. respirator
Bottles for closed chest drainage
Two large hemostats
Cardiac monitoring equipment—with audible and visible signals
Respirometers
Defibrillator
Pacemaker
Emergency drug tray
Equipment for heart massage
Equipment for chest aspiration
Equipment for wound dressing
Equipment for tracheotomy
Equipment for measurement of central venous pressure
Equipment for measurement of arterial pressure
Electric thermometer
Drainage bottle for indwelling catheter

Reception of the Patient. On receiving the patient, a quick assessment is made of his pulse, blood pressure, respirations, color, skin temperature and moisture, and level of consciousness. The closed chest drainage and intravenous infusion are checked for function, the limb with the infusion is secured, nasogastric tube drainage is established and the indwelling catheter is connected to a urinary drainage bottle or bag. Oxygen administration is started by the method ordered.

Positioning. The patient is kept flat until the systolic blood pressure is 100 mm. Hg or more. He is raised gradually and his responses noted. Unless otherwise directed, his position is changed every 2 hours from back to left side to back and to right side, etc. If the patient manifests respiratory distress while on the right side, this position may have to be avoided for a day or two to allow full expansion of the right lung to compensate for the left lung which may not yet be fully re-expanded. Precautions are necessary to avoid dislodging any tubes when turning the patient.

Observations. A constant monitoring of the heart action may be used so that cardiac arrhythmias and change of rate may be quickly detected. Blood pressure, radial and apical pulses, respirations and color are checked and recorded every 15 minutes at first and the interval only increased as the vital signs become stabilized. Movement of both sides of the chest is noted in respiration; unequal expansion of the two sides, audible moist sounds and dyspnea should be reported. Continuous recording of the body temperature by the electric thermometer may be used for the first day or two; if not, the rectal temperature is taken every 2 hours for several days. The wound area is observed at frequent intervals for possible bleeding.

Orientation, level of consciousness, restlessness and anxiety are significant and should be noted. Stasis of circulation during the surgery may have resulted in the formation of a thrombus which later may move out as an embolus. Also, a small amount of air left in the heart on closing may cause an air embolism. For these reasons the patient's ability to move his limbs and his speech are tested every 1 to 2 hours. Any weakness or loss of function is promptly reported. Peripheral pulses in the limbs other than the radial pulse are also checked (dorsalis pedis, femoral and posterior tibial). The absence of one of these may point to a thrombosis or embolism.

Fluid intake and output are recorded. When his condition permits, the patient is weighed daily to detect possible retention of fluid.

Respiratory tests may be required at frequent intervals; the expiratory volume per minute may be estimated by the use of a respirometer. Arterial blood specimens are collected for determination of blood gases, electrolyte concentrations and the pH. Frequently, these patients have suffered some permanent alveolar changes before their surgery and normal gas exchanges do not take place. An excessive retention of carbon dioxide may cause acidosis.

Venous pressure is taken to detect congestion caused by heart failure and to determine intravascular volume. Roentgenograms of the lungs are frequently made to determine lung expansion and to detect the presence of fluid in the alveoli and thoracic cavity.

Assisting Respiratory Function. Oxygen may be administered by mask, catheter or, rarely, by tent.

Frequent suctioning is required; the catheter is introduced deep into the pharynx. The patient will gag or cough, which helps to raise the secretions.

Coughing every 1 to 2 hours is started as soon as the blood pressure is stabilized. The nurse assists the patient by elevating him to a sitting position and supporting the left chest, back and front. If the coughing is not productive, and it is evident that secretions are there, endotracheal suctioning may have to be done by the physician.

The patient may be placed on an intermittent positive pressure respirator if he is experiencing respiratory insufficiency. This ensures more efficient ventilation and lessens the work of breathing for the patient. A tracheostomy may be done and the respirator attached to the tracheostomy tube. This provides more efficient management of secretions because deeper suctioning is possible. (For nursing responsibilities associated with the I.P.P. respirator and tracheotomy the reader should consult Chapter 14.) If the patient is not on a respirator, he is encouraged to take 5 to 10 deep breaths every 1 to 2 hours.

Deep breathing, coughing, turning, and skin care should be done at one time in order to provide a longer undisturbed period for the patient.

Care of Drainage Tubes. The drainage tube in the thoracic cavity is connected to a tube which extends into the fluid in a drainage bottle. Keeping the end of the tube submerged in the water allows fluid and air to escape from the chest cavity but prevents air from entering the chest. (For details of closed, water-sealed drainage in chest surgery see p. 309). The system is observed at frequent intervals for functioning; the level of the fluid should fluctuate in the tube in the bottle with respirations and with coughing. If it does not, the tube is probably blocked by a clot and should be "milked" or stripped to remove the obstruction. If this is not successful, it is reported promptly, since an accumulation of fluid in the thoracic cavity could cause serious cardiac embarrassment. The drainage is examined frequently for possible bleeding, and the volume is measured at regular intervals. The tube must be clamped with two hemostats close to the chest wall when the bottle is changed or moved from one side of the bed to the other or in the event of any disruption of the seal.

The gastrointestinal drainage is measured and recorded as fluid output. When the condition improves and there is no abdominal distention or nausea, this tube is removed.

The urine drainage is checked hourly for the first 24 to 36 hours, particularly if the blood pressure is low. An hourly output of 25 ml. or less is brought to the doctor's attention since it may indicate the onset of a renal shut-down. The physician may require the bladder to be irrigated once or twice daily as long as the patient has an indwelling catheter.

The total 12-hour or 24-hour output is recorded and the fluid balance determined.

Nutrition and Fluids. For the first 24 to 48 hours the patient is maintained on intravenous infusion. The maximum amount to be given in an hour is specified and the rate of flow carefully controlled to prevent overloading the circulatory system and increasing the demand on the heart. The intravenous fluid is usually glucose in distilled water rather than saline.

Sips of water may be permitted to relieve the thirst sensation if there is gastrointestinal drainage. Frequent mouth care also helps and is necessary to prevent infection. When the gastrointestinal drainage tube is removed, clear fluids are given in small amounts and gradually increased. All fluid intake is measured and recorded. A positive balance may necessitate restricting the fluid intake to a prescribed volume.

The diet progresses from fluids to soft foods and then to light solid foods as tolerated. Frequent small amounts are more acceptable than larger amounts less often. Gas-forming foods are to be avoided, and sodium restriction may be indicated.

Rest. Uninterrupted periods of rest are important to reduce the demands on the heart. The various observations that must be made and the treatments, tests and doctors' visits sometimes make it difficult for the patient to get sufficient rest. The nurse should be alert to the problem and, if necessary, consult the physician.

Psychological Care. The patient who has had considerable preparation for what will follow the operation tends to accept the postoperative situation with less anxiety than patients who have not had a similar preparation. It is important that his questions are answered and that he receive some information as to his progress. Brief explanations of what is going to be done are

appreciated by the patient and a visit from a family member is also reassuring.

It is not uncommon for the patient's spirits to fluctuate; he may have brief periods of depression and may become very irritable. Patience and understanding on the part of the nurse are important. An expression that indicates to the patient that she knows how he feels may provide some support.

Medications. Analgesics and sedatives are used very sparingly with the cardiac surgical patient since they tend to depress respirations and the cough reflex.

A small dose of morphine or meperidine hydrochloride (Demerol) may be ordered for the relief of pain. Close observation of the patient's response to the drug is necessary; respirations are checked before the administration and for the period following. Very judicious use of these drugs is necessary; to withhold the drug unnecessarily may be harmful, since pain and the patient's response to it may increase the demands on the respiratory system and the heart. The narcotic ordered by the doctor should be used only for pain — not for restlessness. The latter condition indicates the need for increased observation to determine its cause; it may be due to hypoxia or hemorrhage and should be reported.

A prophylactic antibiotic may be administered for a period of 5 to 10 days. The number of days will depend on the patient's history; if he has had rheumatic fever and rheumatic heart disease he will probably receive the antibiotic for a longer period to prevent reactivation of the rheumatic disease.

Digitalis may be prescribed to strengthen the heart. Quinidine sulfate or another antiarrhythmic drug may be necessary to treat fibrillation.

Exercises and Mobility. To prevent circulatory stasis and thrombus formation some activity is desirable. Passive movements of the limbs are initiated first and are followed by active foot and leg exercises when indicated by the doctor. Later, active exercises are extended to include the arms. A pull cord by which the patient may pull himself up may be attached to the foot of the bed. His next move will be to the side of the bed, then to a chair, and finally to self-care activities and walking.

The patient tends to immobilize the left

shoulder and arm and may develop a "frozen shoulder." Gentle passive movement is all he may tolerate at first, but as soon as possible he is encouraged to use his arm and put it through a full range of motion as he was instructed preoperatively.

The start of exercises and the rate of progression and degree of mobility will be decided by the doctor for each patient. For example, the patient who has the surgical correction of a coarctation of the aorta must remain inactive for a much longer period than many other patients. The patient's responses will also be a factor in determining the amount of activity and when it should be started.

The Family. When the operation is completed, the surgeon sees the family, informs them as to what was done and advises them of the patient's condition. It is then helpful if they may see the patient without disturbing him. Before taking them to the patient's room, a brief description of some of the equipment in use may reduce their concern when they enter the room. A close family member may wish to remain in the hospital for most of the day and may be allowed to look in on the patient briefly at intervals. The nurse who stops to speak briefly with the family and inform them of the patient's condition conveys to them an understanding of their anxiety.

Convalescence and Rehabilitation. While the patient's physical activity is increased, his tolerance is noted. Any shortness of breath, cardiac pain, or edema is promptly reported and activity is stopped until the doctor has seen the patient.

Prescribed exercises are continued throughout convalescence and rehabilitation. The patient is encouraged to use his left arm and put it through a full range of motion. A member of the family and the patient are given instructions about his care after discharge. How long he must curtail his activities and to what extent will depend on the patient's condition before and after the operation and on his responses to activity.

Planning for his return home and his rehabilitation should include consideration of the factors suggested on page 221 under The Rehabilitation of the Cardiac Patient, recognizing of course that every program must be determined on an individual basis.

HEART DISEASE IN PREGNANCY

The woman with a heart disease who contemplates having a child should consult a cardiologist. Many such women are quite able to bear a child and come through safely if they are closely supervised throughout pregnancy and follow the doctor's instructions. For others, pregnancy may carry considerable risk, since it creates increased demands on the heart.

During pregnancy, the total blood volume is increased as much as 25 per cent by the seventh or eighth month. This increases the work load of the heart and persists 24 hours of the day, not just with physical activity. Some enlargement of the heart usually occurs in the normal pregnant woman. The changes in the concentration of certain hormones in pregnancy cause some retention of sodium. This varies in different women but does produce a hazard for the heart patient who, because of some cardiac insufficiency, may already be retaining an excess of sodium. The pregnant woman also experiences some shortness of breath as the enlarging uterus rises in the abdominal cavity, causing pressure on the diaphragm.

The nurse may be asked by the woman with a heart condition whether it is safe for her to become pregnant. She is advised to go to a heart clinic or to consult her doctor. If the woman confides in the nurse that she thinks she is already pregnant, she is urged to see her doctor or go to the clinic at once. A thorough history is taken, and her heart's functional capacity is assessed. The doctor may tell her he believes it would be safe for her to have a child, but that it will be necessary for her to follow his instructions closely. The fact that pregnancy imposes an increased work load on the heart and that she has a reduced cardiac reserve should be explained to her and to her husband. Pregnancy for her will necessitate reduced activity, longer and more frequent rest periods, avoidance of infection and emotional stresses, weight control and restricted salt intake.

The patient and her husband will be instructed to get in touch promptly with the doctor if she experiences shortness of breath, palpitation, vomiting, any infection or a gain in weight in excess of that suggested by the doctor. Frequent visits to the obstetrician and cardiologist are necessary. Weekly visits alternating between these two physicians may be requested.

If the woman develops any signs of cardiac failure, she is put to bed, and digitalis and a diuretic are prescribed. More stringent restrictions of sodium will be used. The visiting nurse can give this patient a great deal of help and support and should know that the strain on the heart reaches a peak in the seventh and eighth months. During these later months of pregnancy, closer observation of the patient and a strict regimen are very important.

The patient may be allowed to go to full term, or the doctor may think it advisable to induce labor a few weeks before term. In caring for the patient during labor, the nurse is alert for early signs of cardiac failure. The pulse, blood pressure and respirations are noted at frequent intervals. Every effort is made to prevent unnecessary exertion and to provide the patient with as much rest as possible. Fluid intake and output are measured and recorded. The equipment and supplies used in the treatment of any heart patient are kept at hand.

Following delivery, close observation for manifestations of cardiac insufficiency and precautions to reduce the work load of the heart are continued for 2 to 3 days. Davidson warns that the seventh and eighth months and the first few days following delivery are the most dangerous periods.[18]

THE SURGICAL PATIENT WITH IMPAIRED CARDIAC FUNCTION

The person with some cardiac insufficiency may require an operation. Unless it is an emergency, time is taken to assess carefully the functional capacity of the heart. Several tests are likely to be done which bear nursing responsibilities as discussed on page 196. The patient is closely observed during the period of preparation for any signs of failure; the recognition of such signs may influence his treatment and the risk which the surgery may carry.

This patient, knowing he has a heart condition, is likely to be more fearful than other surgical patients. The nurse encourages him to verbalize his concerns and takes time to help him work through them. He should be advised that there will be a nurse with him constantly until he is conscious, that when he regains consciousness one will remain close by and visit him at frequent intervals, and that a doctor will be notified promptly of any change in his condition.

Surgery carries less risk for these patients than it used to; recent knowledge and new and improved techniques, equipment and anesthetics have made surgery safer and provide more physiological support.

Postoperatively, the nurse provides even closer attention for this patient, since his condition could change suddenly. Frequent checking of vital signs, color, level of consciousness and accurate recording of the fluid intake and output are necessary for several days longer than for most surgical patients. Any dyspnea, cyanosis, abnormal pulse rate, rhythm or volume, positive fluid balance, apathy and loss of consciousness are reported to the physician promptly since they may indicate a reduced cardiac sufficiency. If the patient is to receive intravenous fluids, the rate of flow and volume must be carefully controlled to avoid a sudden increase in the intravascular volume and an overloading of the impaired heart. Any surgical complications, such as infection and phlebitis, are extremely hazardous because they may precipitate failure.

NURSING IN SHOCK

Shock is a circulatory failure in which there is a deficiency in the blood flow through all tissues, reduction in the venous return and a corresponding decrease in the cardiac output. The blood flow is below that necessary for normal cellular metabolism; cellular injury and destruction may occur, and tissue functions may deteriorate. It may be due to injury or stress which causes a reduced venous return or reduces the heart's ability to forward the blood it receives. The reduced venous return may result from a loss of intravascular fluid, a widespread vasodilatation or the trapping of blood in an area by a thrombosis or severe vasocon-

---

[18]Sir Stanley Davidson: *The Principles and Practice of Medicine,* 7th ed. London, E. & S. Livingstone Ltd., 1965, pp. 230–32.

striction. The failure of the heart as a pump may occur as a result of a number of conditions which have been cited in the preceding section on impaired cardiac function. The disturbance may begin in one portion of the circulatory system but will inevitably be reflected in other parts, since the system is a functional unit.

Classification of Shock

A multiplicity of descriptive and qualifying terms are used with the term shock. It may be described as medical, surgical or obstetrical, according to the clinical nature of the causative condition. Such adjectives as traumatic, hemorrhagic, toxemic, cardiac, anaphylactic or psychogenic may be used to denote the initiating factor of the shock.

Shock may be classified as hypovolemic or normovolemic. Hypovolemic shock implies a reduction in the intravascular fluid as may occur in hemorrhage, severe dehydration and tissue injury, such as burns, resulting in increased capillary permeability. Normovolemic shock indicates no reduction in the blood volume, but there is an increase in the capacity of the vascular system. The latter type of shock may be further qualified as vasogenic or neurogenic. In vasogenic shock there is a loss of vasomotor tone because of the direct effect on the vessel walls of some substance such as nitroglycerine, histamine or bacterial products. Pain, trauma, extreme fear or tragedy may produce neurogenic shock in which there is a reflex vasodilatation mediated through the central nervous system and vasomotor nerves.

The terms reversible and irreversible may also be used to classify shock according to the patient's progress. Shock is said to be reversible when the patient recovers independently or in response to treatment. It is labeled irreversible when the condition is not amenable to treatment and the patient's condition progressively deteriorates.

Stages of Shock

The process of shock goes through an initial phase, then through the compensatory (reversible) or progressive stage and then to the irreversible stage. In the initial phase, a disproportion occurs between the intra-vascular volume of fluid and the vascular compartment, reducing the venous return, cardiac output and arterial blood pressure. The latter falls below 100 mm. Hg. The hypotension and the reduced blood flow through the tissues and the accompanying hypoxia stimulate compensatory mechanisms. A reflex selective vasoconstriction and an increase in the pulse rate occur through stimulation of the aortic and carotid pressoreceptors. The adrenals discharge epinephrine, which augments these responses. The vasoconstriction is greater in the skin, kidneys, muscles and splanchnic area and is designed to increase the venous return to the heart and maintain the blood supply to more vital areas. An increase in the rate and depth of respirations may occur; this also promotes venous return and cardiac filling. The hypotension in the capillaries diminishes the hydrostatic pressure, and the colloidal osmotic pressure of the blood then becomes effective in attracting fluid into the vessels from the interstitial spaces, thus increasing the intravascular volume. The patient develops an increased thirst, leading to fluid intake if he is able to take it. These physiological responses may be sufficient to increase the cardiac output and restore adequate circulation. It may be necessary to assist in the recovery by blood or plasma infusion and other treatment. The shock is said to be reversible if circulation is re-established by effective compensatory mechanisms and treatment. If the initiating factor has not been too severe and the patient receives prompt treatment, recovery usually takes place in a few hours.

A prolonged hypotension of less than 90 mm. Hg is considered to be serious because of the severe oxygen deficiency in the tissues. The patient may be in the progressive stage, in which the circulatory structures suffer from the hypoxia, causing a still further decrease in the movement of blood through the tissues and a further reduction in the venous return and cardiac output. Cell metabolism becomes disrupted, and toxic substances may be released by the ischemic tissues to further complicate the situation. The tissues become less responsive and compensatory mechanisms fail, leading to further deterioration and more severe shock. There may be a brief period in the progressive phase when treatment restores the cardiac output and blood pressure to normal limits, but if this cannot be sustained, the patient's condition will reach a stage in which there is no response to any treatment. Shock has then progressed to the irreversible phase, and death ensues.

The degree of shock is not always the same for all persons following stress and injuries of equal intensity. There is considerable variation in response and also in the ease with which some persons progress to the irreversible stage. Elderly persons, the very young, those with chronic disease or infection and those of lesser emotional stability are more susceptible to shock.

Manifestations of Shock

Premonitory Signs. Unless the shock is very severe and develops very quickly, premonitory signs are restlessness, apprehension and thirst. Later, the restlessness and apprehension may be replaced by listlessness and apathy which may progress to loss of consciousness due to increasing cerebral hypoxia. A depression of reflex responses also occurs.

Color. The skin is pale or gray and cold because of superficial vasoconstriction. It may be moist because of the sympathetic nervous stimulation of the sweat glands. If the skin vessels are blanched by pressure, they refill slowly.

Vital Signs. Failing circulation is detected in the rapid, weak pulse and in the fall in both the systolic and diastolic blood pressures. Respirations may be rapid and deep because of the hypoxia, but in severe and progressive shock, depression of the respiratory center in the medulla causes slower, shallow and possibly irregular respirations. The body temperature is usually subnormal because cellular metabolism and heat production are reduced. The exception to this is a case in which the initial cause is infection, because there is likely to be a high fever.

Thirst. This is very distressing especially in hypovolemic shock. The mouth becomes parched as a result of the increased withdrawal of fluid from the interstitial spaces into the intravascular compartment.

Urinary Output. The volume of urine excreted by the kidneys may be seriously decreased because of the reduced renal blood supply and blood pressure.

Nursing Care

The treatment of shock is urgent and should be instituted as soon as possible to prevent progression of the condition to an irreversible phase. The nurse, who is with the patient for longer periods than the doctor, may recognize early changes and may be instrumental in the patient receiving early treatment. The aims in shock are (1) to improve the circulation in order to increase the oxygen supply to the tissues throughout the body and (2) to correct the specific cause. The care and treatment mentioned here relate only to the circulatory failure and not to the specific cause, although the one is somewhat conditioned by the other. For example, if the cause of the shock is hemorrhage, the treatment is directed toward arresting the loss of blood, and the infusion solution of choice will be whole blood to replace that which was lost. On recognition of early symptoms of shock, the nurse may prevent delay by anticipating the likely treatment and having the necessary equipment and drugs ready. These would include the equipment necessary for intravenous infusion, blood transfusion and oxygen therapy as well as vasopressor drugs. The sphygmomanometer cuff may be placed on the arm and left there for frequent readings. Other equipment may be necessary to deal with the initiating cause of the shock such as, for example, that necessary to check hemorrhage.

Observations. The patient in shock must be under constant observation. The pulse, blood pressure and respirations are recorded every 15 minutes and the interval is increased only as the patient's condition improves. Blood pressure and pulse are considered to be the best indexes of the degree of shock. A rapid, weak pulse and a systolic blood pressure below 90 mm. Hg signify danger. The lower the diastolic blood pressure, the more serious the shock, as this points to a lesser degree of compensation. The temperature is recorded, and the skin is checked for color and moisture. It is important to note the patient's level of response and to recognize possible fear and worry, which may aggravate his condition. The mouth and mucous membranes are observed for dryness. Accurate records are made of the fluid intake and output. The amount of urine excreted is an important indication of the degree of shock and the response to treatment. An indwelling catheter may be used, and the urine is measured hourly. The doctor is informed of an output of 25 ml. or less per hour.

Rest. The patient is kept at absolute rest. He is not to be moved, and his head must not be raised during hypotension. When the patient must be moved for a treatment or the use of a bedpan, sufficient assistance is given to avoid energy expenditure on his part. All handling must be gentle and kept to a minimum. The environment is kept as quiet and as free of stimuli as possible.

Positioning. The shock patient is kept in the recumbent position. Since gravity affects the blood flow, elevation of the lower limbs may be ordered to increase venous return. This position is not used in cases of embolism, head injury or with an obese person. Occasionally, elevation of foot of the bed causes respiratory embarrassment, and the flat position is preferable.

Warmth. Loss of body heat is prevented by the application of blankets, but sweating should be avoided. Heat applications are not used, since they produce vasodilatation (which directly opposes the compensatory reflex vasoconstriction) and cause perspiration, resulting in a loss of valuable body fluid. Heat also increases metabolism in the tissues, making a greater demand on the already depleted oxygen supply.

Pain. Pain may or may not be present, but if it is being experienced, it may aggravate the patient's shock. Morphine may be given subcutaneously, or it may be given intravenously by the doctor, in which case the dose is usually only one-half to two-thirds of that used hypodermically. Analgesics are used judiciously since they may depress respirations and may further increase the hypoxia, but the initial dose is not usually withheld if there is pain, since severe pain causes reflex vasodilatation, further increasing the shock. Sedatives and analgesics are not used when the shock is due to cerebral injury. The patient's pain may sometimes be relieved by immobilizing the injured part, as in the case of a fractured limb.

Fluids. One of the first considerations in the treatment of the shock patient is to restore an effective blood volume. Intravenous infusion of whole blood, plasma or a plasma volume expander is given just as soon as possible. Blood is usually the solution of choice, but the others may be used while compatible blood is being obtained. The plasma volume expander most commonly used is dextran 6 per cent and the amount used is generally restricted to 1200 to 2000 ml. Larger quantities tend to prolong the bleeding time.

The blood transfusion may be followed by an intravenous infusion of electrolyte and glucose solutions. Laboratory studies of relative volumes and concentrations of blood cells, hemoglobin, plasma proteins and electrolytes are made frequently to determine the physiological needs. Occasionally, impairment of the circulation is such that the blood will not run by gravity, and a pressure pump is used by the doctor. With any intravenous infusion, frequent observation is made to determine if the desired rate of flow and supply of solution are being maintained and to see that the solution is not leaking into the subcutaneous tissues. Veins collapse readily in shock, and it is frequently difficult to establish an intravenous infusion without a phlebotomy (cut-down). Since this is a possibility, the nurse prepares by having the necessary equipment readily available.

Fluids may be given by mouth to relieve the patient's thirst if they are tolerated, if no lesion of the gastrointestinal tract is known or suspected and if no surgery is anticipated. If fluids cannot be given orally, frequent rinsing of the mouth may provide some comfort and help to prevent possible parotitis.

No alcoholic beverage should be given to a person in shock because it counteracts the compensatory reactions and decreases the possibility of reversing the shock process. This is particularly applicable outside the hospital in emergency situations in which, frequently, lay persons consider this of benefit.

Oxygen. Since there is a severe oxygen deficiency throughout the tissues, oxygen may be ordered in high concentration. Some physicians think this of little value, inferring that with the impaired circulation it will not go farther than the lungs.

Vasopressor Drugs. The use of a drug that produces vasoconstriction may be considered by the physician. Some of the preparations used are levarterenol bitartrate (Levophed), metaraminol bitartrate (Aramine) and methoxamine hydrochloride (Vasoxyl-P). These drugs are usually given intravenously, although the latter two may also be given intramuscularly. The dosage and rate of intravenous flow are carefully regulated according to the blood pressure, which must be recorded every 10 to 15 minutes.

If a vasopressor drug is used, it is discontinued gradually and the patient is kept under close observation, since sudden severe hypotension may occur when the drug is withdrawn.

Recovery Period. When treatment has been instituted the nurse observes the patient closely for signs of its effectiveness. Criteria for effectiveness are: an increase in the blood pressure and pulse volume, a decrease in pulse rate, an increased urinary output, improved color and the recovery of normal responses. When the patient's condition has improved and he is permitted to move or be moved, any change in position should be assumed slowly. It may take some time for the circulatory system to recover its ability to adjust to postural changes. Renal ischemia incurred during the period of hypotension may result in residual damage to the tubular cells, reducing kidney efficiency. The urinary output should still be measured, and tests may be ordered to check the ability of the kidneys to concentrate solid wastes.

The skin may have suffered as a result of the period of immobility, impaired circulation and hypoxia. It is carefully examined, and the necessary care is taken to improve its general condition.

NURSING IN VASCULAR DISEASES

Disturbance of circulation within the vascular system may originate in the arterial system (arteries and arterioles) or in the veins. In the case of the former, a partial or complete occlusion reduces the volume of blood into the part which the vessel supplies, and the tissues suffer oxygen and nutritional deficiency. If the site of the vascular problem is the veins, there is interference with the normal outflow of venous blood, causing congestion and edema within the tissues. Vascular conditions may be chronic, developing slowly over a considerable period of time, or they may be sudden and acute.

Arterial Disorders

Chronic Arterial Occlusion

This most frequently develops as a result of gradual changes in the walls of the vessels, causing narrowing of the lumen. It may also be of functional origin due to a hyperactivity of the sympathetic nervous system, causing an excessive vasoconstriction. Gradual occlusion of the vessels allows for collateral circulation to be established, lessening the problem of deprivation in the tissues distal to the occlusion.

The most common causes of chronic occlusion are atherosclerosis and arteriosclerosis. The arteries in any area of the body may be affected, but the coronary, cerebral and renal arteries are frequent sites. The problems caused by their insufficiency are discussed under disorders of the relative structures. The arteries of the extremities are also a relatively frequent site of chronic occlusion that may be referred to as peripheral vascular disease. Two common forms of peripheral vascular disease are Raynaud's disease and thromboangiitis obliterans.

Raynaud's disease is a condition in which episodes of excessive vasoconstriction occur in the digits of the hands and/or feet. The cause is obscure, but the episodes are most frequently precipitated by cold or emotional stress. The disease is more common in females, usually develops before the age of 40 to 45 years and is bilateral.

Thromboangiitis obliterans (Buerger's disease) is a chronic occlusive disease in which there is an inflammation and thickening of the walls of limb arteries, predisposing to thrombosis. It has a higher incidence in young males and in Jewish persons. The parts are very tender and painful, and necrotic areas develop in the distal portions of the digits. The condition is seriously aggravated if the person smokes. The cause of this disease is unknown.

Acute Arterial Occlusion

Acute occlusion occurs suddenly as a result of external compression, thrombosis or embolism. It is serious because there is a lack of collateral circulation to the tissues supplied by the artery.

Arterial thrombosis occurs with the formation of an abnormal blood clot (thrombus) within an artery. It is usually the result of narrowing of the lumen of the artery by atherosclerotic changes. The stasis in the blood flow predisposes to the formation of the clot, partially or completely blocking the vessel. If the vessel is not completely blocked, treatment is directed toward preventing the clot from enlarging to occlude the vessel and toward keeping it at the site of formation to prevent an embolism.

Arterial embolism is the blocking of an artery by a foreign mass that has been carried by the blood stream until it reaches an artery too small for it to pass through. The foreign mass is referred to as an embolus.

It most frequently is a thrombus that breaks loose from its site of origin, but it may consist of air, fragments of vegetations from diseased cardiac valves, fat, atherosclerotic plaques or small masses of tissue or cancerous cells. The effects of an embolism are determined by the localization of the embolus. The vessel the embolus lodges in and obstructs depends upon the size of the embolus, its origin, and whether the artery blocked is an end-artery or one that anastomoses above the block with smaller vessels in the part supplied. Obviously, if it is an end-artery, the tissue entirely dependent on it becomes necrotic. An embolus originating in a vein or the right side of the heart is likely to cause a pulmonary embolism. One arising from the left side of the heart or a large systemic artery may produce a cerebral embolism or may plug a smaller arterial artery. Occasionally, the site of arterial occlusion by an embolus is a lower extremity.

Manifestations of Arterial Insufficiency in the Extremities

These manifestations are due to the deficiencies in oxygen and nutrients to the tissues resulting from the decreased blood supply into the limb. If there is a complete deprivation, the tissue cells die, and necrosis occurs in the form of ulceration or gangrene.

Pain. The patient may experience intermittent claudication. This is pain that occurs on exercise and is relieved by rest. The blood supply is sufficient to meet the tissue needs only when the part is at rest; on exercise, oxygen demands cannot be met. The pain may be constant even with the part at rest, indicating a decreased blood flow into the tissues or a complete obstruction. The patient may complain of a numbness or tingling in the extremity.

Pulse. A weakness or absence of peripheral pulses may be evident. In the arm, the radial, ulnar, brachial or axillary artery may be palpated with the fingertips, and in the leg the dorsalis pedis, popliteal or femoral artery may be felt. An oscillometer may be used to palpate the pulsation of arteries in an area where the vessels are deeper and cannot be palpated by the fingers. A comparison is made of the pulse in the different arteries and would reveal a partial block if one were present. Complete occlusion would be indicated by an absence of the pulse.

Color. A difference in the color of the two extremities or an abnormal change in both extremities, if both are involved, will most likely be present. The skin may become white and blanched, or it may become a dusky red or cyanosed, depending on the amount of blood in the capillaries and the amount of unsaturated hemoglobin in the blood. On being raised, the limb becomes even paler as the venous drainage increases, but on being lowered, it fails to increase its color as the normal limb would do quickly with the rush of arterial blood into it. The superficial veins are slow in filling when the limb is lowered; normally, they fill in approximately 5 seconds.

Skin Temperature. The skin temperature and moisture may be different in the two limbs. The affected one exhibits a coldness to the touch and may be unusually moist. The warmth of the skin is dependent on the heat brought to the part by the blood. The moisture may point to excessive sympathetic stimulation, causing vasospasm.

Atrophy of Tissues. Limb tissues may atrophy, causing the affected limb to become smaller than the other. The skin becomes dry and shiny and loses its hair. Nails thicken and become brittle and ridged.

Necrosis. Ulcerated or gangrenous areas may develop, denoting areas of tissue completely deprived of a blood supply. Ulceration is a superficial area of devitalized tissue; gangrene is a more massive area of dead tissue.

Diagnostic Procedures

Various tests may be used by the physician in diagnosing and assessing vascular disease.

Exercise Tolerance. The patient is required to walk or perform some form of exercise until intermittent claudication occurs. The length of time from the start of activity until pain occurs is noted.

Oscillometry. An inflatable cuff is applied to the limb at various levels and arterial pulsations and pressure are transmitted to the oscillometer. This examination will point to the approximate level of reduced flow through the artery.

Skin Temperature Determinations. This test is not considered very reliable, since the patient's emotions or activity may influence the vasomotor tone, thus affecting the skin temperature. The procedure comprises a comparison of temperature response in the two limbs. One limb is immersed in warm water at 42° to 44° C. (108° to 112° F.), and the temperature of the other limb is noted. Normally, there should be an increase of several degrees in the unimmersed limb up to a minimum skin temperature of 34° C. (93° F.) in 30 to 35 minutes. Another method is to place a hot water bottle or heating pad to the patient's abdomen and test the extremities for temperature change. Normally, there should be a reflex vasodilatation of the blood vessels, increasing the skin temperature in the limbs.

Angiography. A radiopaque dye is introduced into the arteries, and roentgenograms are made of the vessels. The site of narrowing or obstruction may be located in this way, and some information as to the amount of collateral circulation present may also be obtained.

Reactive Hyperemia. In this test, the flow of blood into the limb is reduced by the application of a tourniquet or blood pressure cuff for 2 to 3 minutes. On release, vasodilation normally follows and blood flows in very quickly to produce warmth and flushing of the skin. In arterial insufficiency the flow of blood into the part is delayed.

Radiography. If the problem is arteriosclerosis, calcified deposits may show up in x-ray pictures.

Sympathetic Ganglionic Block. The sympathetic vasomotor nerve fibers to the affected limb are temporarily blocked by procaine at the associated ganglia. Vasodilation in the affected limb with a subsequent increase in skin temperature should occur.

Treatment and Nursing Care of the Patient with Arterial Occlusive Disease

The aims in the care of the patient are: to prevent further progress of the condition causing the ischemia in the limbs; to prevent complications, such as dryness and cracking of the skin, infection and ulceration, since the resistance of the tissues is lower; to increase the blood supply to the extremities; and to keep the demands of the tissues within the limits of the existing blood supply into the limb.

Arterial occlusive disease (peripheral vascular disease) is a chronic condition, and the patient will most likely have to continue with the prescribed care and precautions indefinitely. It may create considerable hardship for the patient and his family, depending on the severity of the disease and the limitations it imposes. Adjustments may have to be made in his occupational and social life; he may become partially or completely dependent financially and for his personal care. The patient will certainly find it difficult to accept the situation and will react accordingly. The nurse will be alert to the possible implications for the patient and family and will provide the necessary assistance and guidance.

The patient and a family member are instructed in the necessary care. They should understand that adherence to the physician's suggestions and regular supervision are all important in preventing serious complications.

Diet. Obesity should be avoided, since excess tissue always increases the demands on the circulatory system. Overweight persons tend to be less active, which does not favor circulation. Protein and vitamin C are usually increased for maximum maintenance and support of the tissues suffering a degree of ischemia. An increase in B vitamins may be recommended, especially if there is peripheral nerve involvement and the patient is experiencing peripheral neuritis. The fat content of the diet will probably be reduced and vegetable fat substituted for most of the animal fat if the arterial insufficiency is due to atherosclerosis.

An optimum fluid intake is important in maintaining a normal vascular volume and in preventing possible hemoconcentration predisposing to thrombus formation.

Smoking. The use of tobacco is discontinued, since it promotes vasoconstriction and aggravates the disease.

Protection from Cold. Exposure to cold with lowering of normal body temperature incites undesirable responses, namely, peripheral vasoconstriction and increased metabolism. Special precautions are necessary in cold weather. Extra, warm clothing should be worn, and a change of residence to a warmer climate may be helpful. If exposure to cold precipitates an episode, the patient is advised to take a warm drink and seek a warm environment. A warm bath or a heating pad to the abdomen may be used to produce reflex vasodilation in the limbs. Local heat applications to the affected parts are discouraged because the tissue resistance is lowered, and frequently, there is a reduced nerve sensitivity.

Protection of the Affected Limbs. Extra precautions are necessary to protect the affected limbs from trauma and infection. Daily bathing in comfortably warm (not hot) water using a mild soap is recommended. Gentle and thorough drying is important, and special attention is given to the areas between the digits. If the skin is dry, the limbs may be gently massaged with lanolin or some light emollient. Nails are cut straight across but not right down to the soft tissue. A pumice stone may be used on calluses, but the physician's advice is sought as to the treatment of corns; the patient should not undertake to "pare" them with sharp instruments. The extremities, especially the terminal portions, are examined daily for changes; any discoloration, blister, broken area of skin, tenderness and swelling are to be promptly seen by the doctor.

The patient is advised of the importance of well-fitting shoes and socks or stockings. Socks should be loose and are changed daily. The patient is instructed to avoid walking about in bare feet; a cut, abrasion, sliver or infection could be quite serious, since the tissue resistance is lowered and healing is poor. Anything tight or restricting, such as round garters, must not be worn. The pressure of bedclothes can be prevented by using a footboard at the foot of the bed.

Positioning. The horizontal position is used when the patient rests unless the doctor suggests otherwise. Occasionally, raising the head of the bed may be used to encourage the flow of blood into the lower limbs by gravity. Position should be changed at frequent intervals throughout the day, and long periods of standing must be avoided. The patient is advised not to cross his legs and, when sitting, pressure on the popliteal region is avoided.

Rest and Activity. Some exercise and activity are encouraged to promote circulation. These should be stopped short of fatigue and if any pain occurs, since this would indicate oxygen deficiency in the muscles.

Measures to Increase the Blood Supply to the Extremities

1. EXERCISES. For arterial insufficiency in the lower limbs, Buerger-Allen exercises may be used. The leg is raised to approximately 45° above the horizontal and held until it blanches (1 to 2 minutes). It is then lowered to below the horizontal (over the side of the bed) until it becomes pink and then returned to the horizontal level for 1 to 2 minutes. This is repeated 5 to 10 times every 6 or 8 hours. A padded support at the required height is provided for the elevation part of the cycle. The timing is determined by the time it takes for the venous drainage and for the refilling of the vessels, so the color must be observed closely and timed at first.

Passive and active exercises may also be prescribed; flexion and extension of the legs, feet and toes may be used for lower limbs, and similar exercises may be employed for the arms and fingers if these are the site of the arterial insufficiency. Exercises promote emptying and filling of the vessels and stimulate the development of collateral circulation.

2. REFLEX DILATATION. Warm baths or increasing general body warmth by a higher environmental temperature may produce a reflex vasodilatation.

Occasionally, injections of typhoid vaccine may be given to the patient with Buerger's disease. The basis of such treatment is to produce a high fever, which should then cause vasodilatation.

3. CONTRAST BATHS. Immersion of the affected extremities alternately in warm and cold water may be prescribed. The limbs are placed first in a tub of warm water 37° to 47° C. (100° to 110° F.) for 1 minute. Then they are immersed in cold water for 1 minute. This is repeated for a period of 15 minutes approximately 2 to 3 times daily, always beginning and ending with the warm immersion. The limbs are gently and thoroughly dried and are lubricated with lanolin or some prescribed emollient to prevent excessive drying of the skin.

4. OSCILLATING BED. Alternate raising and lowering of the limbs to promote more efficient emptying and filling of the blood vessels may be achieved passively by placing the patient on an electric oscillating bed. A rocking motion is produced by a motor that can be set to tilt the bed longitudinally at a definite rate. The length of the period for operation may gradually be lengthened as the patient adjusts to the repeated tilting. It may be operated day and night and is helpful in relieving and preventing the pain which is associated with immobility. The patient is taught how to operate the motor, since the switch is readily available to him.

Drugs. Vasodilating and anticoagulant drugs may be used to treat patients with arterial occlusive disease. Examples of vasodilators used are: tolazoline hydrochloride (Priscoline), dibenzyl-β-chlorethylamine (Dibenamine), azapetine hydrochloride (Ilidar), phenoxybenzamine hydrochloride (Dibenzyline) and papaverine. Toxic effects of these drugs are manifested by nausea and vomiting, palpitation, skin irritation and hypotension. Alcohol is also a vasodilator, and the physician may suggest a dose at bedtime to promote relaxation of the vessels while the patient is at rest.

The anticoagulants heparin and a coumarin preparation (e.g., Dicoumarol) are prescribed to prevent and treat thrombosis. Implications for the nurse who is caring for a patient receiving an anticoagulant are presented on page 219.

Surgical Treatment and Care. If there is evidence of a decrease in vasomotor tone and improved circulation in the limbs in a diagnostic sympathetic block, a lumbar sympathectomy (removal of the second, third and fourth ganglia) may be performed. A direct surgical approach may be employed in which the surgeon chooses to do an endarterectomy, a bypass or a graft. An endarterectomy is the removal of the thickened intima and atheromatous plaques from the artery and is used when the disease is localized to a relatively small area. The establishment of a bypass channel in order to reduce the arterial insufficiency may be achieved by the transplanting of one end of another artery into the occluded artery below the site of obstruction or by an autogenous venous graft. The latter consists of the removal of a section of a vein (usually the saphenous), reversing it (because of the valves) to ensure flow in the right direction and attaching it to the affected artery above and below the occlusion. The surgeon may elect to resect the affected segment of the artery and replace it with an inert synthetic (teflon or dacron) graft. This type of graft is relatively porous and is eventually incorporated into host tissues. An intima develops within it fairly quickly as cells proliferate through the interstices and from the host intima of the artery at each end of the graft. A layer of fibrous tissue also develops on the exterior surface, reinforcing the tube.

The most frequent site of major vascular surgery for occlusive disease is the aorta and the iliac and femoral arteries.

Nursing responsibilities in the care of a patient having major vascular surgery include those applicable to most surgical patients as cited in Chapter 10 as well as the following considerations.

PREOPERATIVE PREPARATION. Local preparation involves the shaving and cleansing of the skin from the nipple line to the knees. The patient's blood is typed and cross-matched in readiness for transfusions during and after the operation.

The patient and his family are advised that he will be taken to the intensive care unit following surgery. To avoid unnecessary concern later, they are given some information about the nasogastric tube and the suction-siphonage decompression, intravenous infusion, urinary catheter drainage, cardiac monitoring and frequent checking of his pulse and blood pressure that will follow surgery.

POSTOPERATIVE CARE. It is very important that the nurse understand the patient's disease process and the corrective surgical procedure used.

OBSERVATIONS. The nurse is alerted to the possible complications of thrombosis in the graft, hemorrhage and embolism. Heart action is constantly monitored so that any adverse change is quickly detected. Arterial and central venous pressures are recorded at frequent intervals. The latter indicates the pressure under which the blood is returned to the heart and provides information about the blood volume and the ability of the heart to forward the blood. To determine central venous pressure, a catheter is placed in an antecubital vein and is attached to a manometer, or a three-way stopcock may be used on an intravenous infusion tube. The manometer is placed vertically and records the pressure in centimeters of water. For an accurate reading, the zero point on the manometer must be placed in line with the patient's midchest to coincide with the mid-atrial level, and the patient must be relaxed in the supine position with the bed flat. Coughing, holding of the breath or any activity that raises the intrathoracic pressure will result in an inaccurate recording. A venous pressure of 5 to 15 cm. of water is considered within normal limits. A decrease below the normal may indicate hemorrhage. An abnormal elevation of the venous pressure may be the result of cardiac insufficiency or of the overloading of the circulatory system with fluid or blood infusions.

Peripheral pulses in the lower limbs are checked frequently. Those in the feet are not usually detectable for 6 to 8 hours after surgery, but if they cannot be felt after this period, it is brought to the surgeon's attention. The pulses used are the femoral, popliteal, dorsalis pedis and posterior tibial. The femoral pulse may be felt in the middle of the groin, and the popliteal is located behind the knee. The dorsalis pedis pulse is found in the central region of the dorsum of the foot, and the posterior tibial behind the medial malleolus. With the latter two, it is helpful to mark the location on the skin so they can be readily checked. When only one limb has been affected, a comparison of the distal pulse is made with that of the unaffected limb.

Skin temperature and color are assessed and, where applicable, a comparison is made between the affected and unaffected limbs. Blanching or cyanosis and a lowering of the temperature in areas distal to the operative site must be reported.

Restlessness, general pallor, a rapid pulse of decreased volume, increased respirations and a fall in arterial and venous blood pressures are associated with bleeding and necessitate prompt medical attention.

The patient's level of consciousness, speech, strength of hand grip and ability to move his limbs are checked frequently. A disturbance in any one area may indicate a cerebral embolism.

POSITIONING. The revascularized area is usually elevated to a level above that of the heart to promote venous and lymphatic drainage and to prevent edema. The sudden increase in the blood supply may exceed the drainage capacity unless it is assisted by gravity.

When vascular grafts cross flexion lines, such as the groin and knee, precautions are taken to prevent flexion for 7 to 10 days. The patient is rolled to either side as though he were one straight rigid piece. It may be necessary to get him out of bed in a stiff-legged fashion to stand and walk. An explanation to the patient of the need to avoid flexion is necessary. Padded splints or restraints may be necessary to ensure non-flexion for the required length of time. When flexion is permitted, it is for very limited periods.

CARE OF AFFECTED LIMB. The skin breaks down very easily, necessitating special protective measures against pressure and trauma. A padded bed cradle is used to relieve the limb of the weight of bedclothes, and the foot rests on sheepskin. The toes are separated by loose absorbent cotton to prevent maceration. The skin is bathed and handled gently. A light application of lanolin may be used to relieve dryness and scaling.

COUGHING AND EXERCISES. The patient is required to breathe deeply and cough hourly to improve pulmonary ventilation. The ankles and toes are flexed 10 times hourly to prevent venous stasis. These flexion exercises may have to be passive until the patient is sufficiently responsive to carry them out himself.

FLUIDS AND NUTRITION. The patient is sustained by intravenous infusions of 5 to 8 per cent glucose in water. Saline solutions are avoided with most patients because of their tendency to retain the sodium.

The suction-siphonage decompression is discontinued and the nasogastric tube removed 2 or 3 days after surgery if there is no nausea or abdominal distention. The patient receives clear fluids at first, and if these are tolerated, the diet is gradually increased. High protein and vitamin C content contribute to the healing and resistance of affected tissues.

INSTRUCTION. In preparation for the patient's discharge from hospital, he is advised of his need to avoid sitting with his hips and knees flexed for long periods. If necessary, continued abstinence from smoking is stressed. He is made aware of ominous changes (pain, discoloration, cold, abrasions, edema) in his limbs that would necessitate prompt medical attention. The doctor gives him some idea of when he may expect to resume former activities and makes an appointment for a follow-up visit to him or the clinic.

Venous Disorders

As stated earlier, interference with the flow of blood through the veins reduces venous return from the part, inducing congestion and edema, which interfere with normal cell function and eventually prevent a normal arterial volume from reaching the tissue cells. Common venous conditions are varicose veins, thrombophlebitis and phlebothrombosis.

Varicose Veins

When venous blood meets with increased resistance to its forward flow, the walls of the veins become dilated and tortuous, the valves become damaged and incompetent and the blood tends to pool and stagnate. The condition may be referred to as varicosities, or as varicose veins. The superficial veins of the lower extremities are most susceptible. Because of our upright position, the venous pressure in the lower limbs is increased by gravity. Other common sites of varicosities are the veins of the anal canal (hemorrhoids), spermatic veins (varicocele), esophageal veins and the vulvar veins in the pregnant woman due to pressure from the enlarging uterus. Although resistance to the flow of blood is the main cause of varicosi-

ties, an inherited weakness of the valves of the veins is said to be a factor. Long periods of standing also predispose to the development of varicose veins in the lower extremities.

The over-full veins result in local edema of the tissues, crampy pains or aching, and a full, heavy feeling in the affected area. The congestion and edema in the tissues interfere with the normal supply of oxygen and nutrients reaching the cells, leading to fibrosing of subcutaneous tissues and, in some instances, necrosis of superficial tissue, producing what is referred to as a varicose ulcer. The affected area appears swollen and discolored, and the veins are seen as tortuous, bulbous protusions. These veins readily develop phlebitis, and occasionally the vessel wall ruptures, causing hemorrhage.

The test most frequently done for varicosities in the lower limbs is the Trendelenburg test. While the patient is in the horizontal position, the leg is elevated above the level of the pelvis until the superficial veins appear to be empty. The patient then stands, and the veins are observed as they fill. Normally they fill relatively slowly from below; in varicosities, the incompetent valves allow them to fill from above as well.

Treatment and Nursing Care of a Patient with Varicose Veins. Treatment may be conservative. The patient is instructed to avoid situations and factors that tend to increase the resistance to venous flow, to provide support to the veins and tissues by bandages or special hose, and to assist drainage by elevation of the limb at intervals.

If the varicosity is not extensive, the physician may inject a sclerosing agent (e.g., sodium morrhuate, sodium tetradecyl sulfate) into the veins. The varicosed segment becomes inflamed, scarred and thrombosed by the sclerosing agent. Antihistamines and the emergency drug tray are kept readily available in the event of a reaction.

With more severe varicosities in the lower limbs, surgical treatment in the form of ligation and stripping of the veins may be employed under local anesthesia. The affected vein is ligated above the varicosity, its connecting branches are severed and tied, and the vein removed. The venous blood then returns via the deep veins. The great saphenous vein is the one most frequently ligated and removed from the groin to the ankle. This necessitates several small horizontal incisions along the course of the vein. Elastic bandages are applied from the foot to the groin after the operation, and the foot of the bed is elevated. Beginning soon after operation the patient will be required to get up at regular intervals and walk about to prevent thrombosis. He may experience stiffness and some pain on movement and is given the necessary assistance and support. Early regular activity is very important and is explained to the patient in order to gain his cooperation.

In the postoperative period, the nurse observes the limb at regular, frequent intervals. The wound areas are checked for bleeding, and the distal parts and digits are examined for color, warmth and sensation so that any disturbance in the circulation will receive early recognition. If there is bleeding, if the distal parts are cold or cyanosed, or the patient experiences numbness, pain or "pins and needles," the surgeon is informed promptly.

The patient is usually only hospitalized for a brief period of 2 to 3 days. He is advised as to how long to continue the alternating periods of rest and walking and the bandaging and elevation of the limbs. He is taught how to apply and care for the elastic bandages and is told when to return to the doctor or clinic. Since the superficial tissue continues to be tender and has less resistance, he is instructed to use precautions against injuries and abrasions. Long periods of standing are still to be avoided.

All patients with leg varicosities should avoid constricting clothing, such as round garters and tight girdles. They are also advised not to sit with their legs crossed. As with all circulatory conditions, obesity is to be avoided.

Varicose ulcers develop very easily with the circulatory stasis but are very slow to heal. The patient may have to rest in bed with the affected leg elevated, or if he remains active, an elastic bandage or stocking is applied in an effort to reduce the edema and congestion.

Moist antiseptic dressings may be applied to the ulcer, and when it is free of infection and necrotic tissue, the physician may enclose the foot and leg in a "boot" of Unna's paste. A mixture of gelatin, zinc oxide, glycerine and water is prepared and applied along with bandages to the foot and leg. The ulcer is protected by a thin sterile dressing and a layer of paste is then applied with a brush directly to the skin. This is followed with a layer of bandage and the two are alternated until 3 or 4 layers of each are applied. The "boot" provides even pressure to the veins and protects the ulcer. It dries to a firm support in approximately one-half hour, but the patient remains where the nurse may check the exposed distal portions of the limb for circulation and sensitivity. The toes should be warm, a normal color, sensitive to touch and comfortable. The boot is usually changed every 12 to 14 days until the ulcer heals. Large ulcers that are difficult to keep uninfected and are resistant to healing may be treated by skin grafts.

Thrombophlebitis and Phlebothrombosis

Phlebitis is an inflammation of the walls of a vein and may be caused by injury, prolonged pressure or infection. The endothelial lining is damaged and a thrombus develops at the site of inflammation, producing a secondary condition known as thrombophlebitis.

Phlebothrombosis is the formation of a blood clot within a vein with no associated inflammation and for this reason may be referred to as a bland or silent thrombosis. It is nearly always due to slowness or stasis of the circulation, such as occurs with prolonged bed rest, inactivity or pressure, causing resistance to the venous blood flow. The serious factor in both phlebothrombosis and thrombophlebitis is the blood clot, which becomes a potential embolus. The silent thrombus or that associated with inflammation may be carried along in the blood stream and may eventually lodge in an artery to cause an embolism. Phlebitis and venous thrombosis may occur in any vein, but the most frequent site is the saphenous veins of the legs.

Manifestations. Thrombophlebitis in superficial veins produces local pain, tenderness and swelling. Systemic symptoms such as fever, headache, and general malaise develop. If the vein is superficial, the overlying skin becomes red and hot.

In phlebothrombosis, the process is silent and the clot is unattached. Usually, no symptoms present until the thrombus is swept along and causes an embolism. In either phlebothrombosis or thrombophlebitis, the thrombus may become large enough to block the vein, causing severe congestion, edema and pain.

Circulatory stasis in the lower limbs is the principal cause of phlebothrombosis, so efforts are directed toward avoiding prolonged inactivity and positions which favor its development. Passive movement and active exercises, especially of the lower limbs, and frequent change of position are used for patients who are inactive or confined to bed. Early ambulation is always to be encouraged when the condition permits. A dorsal recumbent position with the knees flexed and supported by a pillow or elevated gatch frame is always contraindicated, since it promotes a venous stasis in the legs. Sitting for hours is discouraged because the legs are dependent and there is a risk of pressure on the veins in the popliteal region. Sitting should be alternated with periods of walking around or lying down. The patient is instructed not to sit with his legs crossed, but to extend his legs, rotate his feet at the ankles, and flex and extend his toes 5 to 10 times hourly when sitting for an extended period. Persons with leg varicosities are predisposed to phlebothrombosis and thrombophlebitis. Bandaging their lower limbs up to the groin with elastic or crepe bandages provides support to the veins and promotes venous return when they are nonambulatory.

Treatment and Nursing Care of a Patient with Thrombophlebitis. When thrombophlebitis develops, care is directed toward preventing an embolism and relieving the congestion and edema of the tissues. The nurse obtains specific directives from the physician about the activity and positioning of the patient. The patient may be confined to bed, and the affected limb immobilized in an elevated position to promote venous and lymphatic drainage. Active exercise and massage of the limb are contraindicated to avoid possible dislodging of the thrombus and ensuing embolism. All strenuous activity, straining at stool, coughing and deep breathing are discouraged.

Local heat applications, moist or dry, may be prescribed. Precautions are taken to avoid burns since the skin is very susceptible to injury. A footboard or cradle is used to keep the weight of the bedclothes off the limbs. Anticoagulant therapy is started as soon

as the thrombosis is recognized. Rarely, if the patient is experiencing severe pain from vascular spasm, a sympathetic ganglionic block may be done to relax the veins. Analgesics are ordered for the relief of pain.

If the clot is dislodged, it will be carried along by the venous blood through the right side of the heart into the pulmonary circulation, where it is likely to cause a pulmonary embolism. Pain in the chest, dyspnea, coughing, hemoptysis, rapid weak pulse and pallor are reported promptly.

After 7 to 10 days, if the symptoms have subsided, ambulation is permitted. An elastic bandage or elastic stocking is applied before the patient gets out of bed. Activity is alternated with periods of rest. During the rest period the limb is elevated to the horizontal position or higher. The leg is examined for swelling and discoloration following ambulation and following a period of sitting. The patient may have to wear an elastic support indefinitely and must plan to avoid prolonged periods in which the limb is in the dependent position. The doctor may suggest that it is important for him to elevate the limb above heart level for several brief periods through the day. This is more often necessary following a thrombosis of the larger deep veins. Before going home, the nurse teaches the patient the application and care of the bandages or elastic stockings. He is helped to understand the importance of the prescribed periods of elevation of the limbs and that he must be in the dorsal recumbent position to do this. The patient is followed closely in the clinic or the doctor's office for some time following the phlebothrombosis.

NURSING IN HYPERTENSION

Hypertension is a condition in which there is a sustained elevation of the arterial blood pressure. The level at which the normal blood pressure becomes abnormally high is not firmly established, but hypertension may be said to occur if the systolic pressure exceeds 140 mm. Hg and the diastolic pressure exceeds 90 mm. Hg.[19, 20] The diastolic

---

[19] E. E. Selkurt (Ed.): Physiology. Boston, Little, Brown and Co., 1965, p. 376.
[20] P. B. Beeson and W. McDermott (Eds.): Cecil-Loeb Textbook of Medicine, 13th ed. Philadelphia, W. B. Saunders Co., 1971, p. 1050.

pressure is the more significant since it reflects the degree of peripheral resistance.

Hypertension is a serious condition; it is a common cause of heart failure and cerebral vascular hemorrhage. Guyton claims that "about 12 per cent of all persons die as a direct result of hypertension."[21] The sustained elevation in the arterial blood pressure seriously increases the work load of the heart and causes organic changes in the arteries. The myocardium hypertrophies in response to the increased demands, but there is not an adequate increase in the coronary blood supply and eventually some failure develops. The changes in the arterial walls involve thickening and sclerosis which alter the blood supply to tissues and ultimately may reduce their functional ability. The arteries may develop necrotic areas that weaken and tend to rupture under the high pressure of the blood, or they may thicken and narrow the lumen, predisposing to thrombosis. The areas of most serious damage are the heart, kidneys, brain and eyes, and these most often account for the symptoms seen in hypertensive patients. Cerebral hemorrhage (stroke) is a common sequela. Kidney function becomes impaired as the result of sclerosing hemorrhage or thrombosis of the renal arteries which destroys functional tissue. Retinal hemorrhages and edema of the optic disc occur frequently, resulting in degenerative changes in the eyes. Thickening and sclerosis of the coronary arteries may cause ischemic heart disease; the patient may experience angina pectoris or suffer a coronary occlusion in addition to developing the myocardial hypertrophy previously mentioned.

Hypertension may be classified as primary (essential) or secondary. Approximately 90 per cent of the persons with hypertensive disease are said to have essential hypertension; the remaining 10 per cent have secondary hypertension.[22]

Essential or Idiopathic Hypertension

Primary hypertension is most frequently referred to as essential or idiopathic hypertension. The cause of this type of hypertensive disease is not known; no initial disturbance in the areas commonly associated with secondary hypertension has been established. It may cause cardiac or kidney disease but is not preceded by either. Heredity is thought to play a role, since most persons with the condition have a history of a parent or grandparent having had it. There is a higher incidence in females, and the majority of hypertensive women are overweight.

Essential hypertension may be referred to as benign or malignant. The term benign, rarely used, is applied to essential hypertension that persists over 10 to 20 years without causing serious problems. Malignant indicates a rapidly progressive and serious condition. The patient develops kidney and heart complications and other sequelae very quickly and survives only a few months to 1 or 2 years at the most.

Essential hypertension may be classified according to the degree of severity of the disease. The numerical grading is based on changes in the ocular fundi, the response to treatment, the amount of cardiac hypertrophy and the effect on kidney function. Grades 3 and 4 are considered serious, and the patient with a Grade 4 hypertension as well as papilledema may be said to have a malignant hypertension.[23]

Secondary Hypertension

Causes of secondary hypertension include the following:

Coarctation of the Aorta. Obviously, a congenital stricture of an area of the aorta increases the resistance to the flow of blood through the vessel, causing an increase in the arterial pressure behind the coarctation. This may be corrected by surgery.

Disturbances Within the Central Nervous System. Interference with the vasomotor center or with pathways from the center may result in an increased vasoconstriction and peripheral resistance. Space-occupying lesions, such as a brain tumor, increased intracranial pressure, a cerebral thrombosis or poliomyelitis, are examples of conditions which may lead to the malfunctioning of the vasomotor center or pathway.

[21] A. C. Guyton: Textbook of Medical Physiology, 4th ed. Philadelphia, W. B. Saunders Co., 1971, p. 304.
[22] Ibid.

[23] G. C. Duncan, R. J. Gill, W. K. Jensen, and R. I. Fraser: "Office Management of Essential Hypertension." Med. Clin. North Amer., Vol. 5, No. 6 (Nov. 1961), pp. 1398–99.

Endocrine Disturbance. A pheochromocytoma is a tumor of the adrenal medulla. Just as the normal medullary cells do, the tumor cells secrete epinephrine, which produces vasoconstriction and an increased cardiac output with a corresponding elevation in arterial blood pressure. Removal of the tumor restores a normal blood pressure.

An increased output of aldosterone by the cortex of the adrenal glands may also be responsible for hypertension. The increased secretion may be idiopathic or may be due to a tumor. Aldosterone increases the reabsorption of sodium by the kidney, leading to water retention and an expansion of the intravascular volume, increasing the arterial blood pressure. It is suggested that aldosterone may also have a direct vasoconstricting effect. A general increase in the secretion of all of the adrenocorticoids causes Cushing's disease, which is also accompanied by hypertension.

Kidney Disturbance. Any condition which reduces the blood flow through the kidneys or destroys renal functional tissue causes hypertension. Examples of such conditions are sclerotic changes or stenosis of a renal artery, nephritis and polycystic disease. The ischemic kidney reacts by secreting a proteolytic enzyme called renin. In the blood stream, renin acts upon a plasma protein to produce angiotensin I which is then converted to angiotensin II by another enzyme. This angiotensin II causes widespread vasoconstriction of the arterioles and increased peripheral resistance, leading to an elevation in arterial blood pressure. Angiotensin II is also alleged to increase the secretion of aldosterone by the adrenal glands[24] which, as previously cited, increases the blood pressure through its influence on sodium and water retention.

Toxemia of Pregnancy. Hypertension is a feature of toxemia in pregnancy in which there is renal involvement.

Manifestations of Hypertension

A person may have an abnormally high arterial blood pressure for a long period without symptoms. The condition is often discovered on a routine physical examination. Some persons may exhibit a higher than

---

[24]Guyton, op. cit.

TABLE 13–2 SCHEMATIC OUTLINE OF THE RENIN-HYPERTENSION MECHANISM

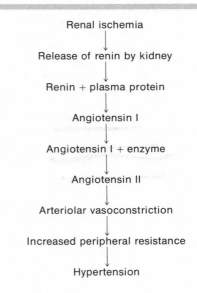

Renal ischemia

↓

Release of renin by kidney

↓

Renin + plasma protein

↓

Angiotensin I

↓

Angiotensin I + enzyme

↓

Angiotensin II

↓

Arteriolar vasoconstriction

↓

Increased peripheral resistance

↓

Hypertension

average normal blood pressure and on investigation may produce a higher than average response to stimuli that normally elicit an increase in blood pressure. The stimuli under which persons are observed are generally cold and exertion. Those who manifest an excessively high response are said to have vascular hyperactivity and are most likely headed for hypertension.

Those who do experience symptoms may complain of a throbbing occipital headache, especially on wakening in the morning, dizziness, visual disturbance, fatigue, irritability and restlessness, emotional instability or epistaxis. Later, more serious manifestations appear as the heart, kidneys, brain or eyes become damaged by the persisting hypertension. The person who manifests even a slight elevation above the normal in both systolic and diastolic blood pressures undergoes careful investigation to determine a possible primary cause.

Treatment and Nursing Care

If the hypertension is secondary, treatment is directed toward correcting the primary condition. In essential hypertension, treatment is directed at (1) lowering the blood pressure in an effort to prevent the serious complications and (2) having the patient adjust his life to reduce the demands on the cardiovascular system and kidneys. The treatment depends on the height and constancy of the blood pressure and the signs and symptoms of impaired function in vulnerable organs. The physician may decide to follow the mildly hypertensive who has no signs of complications without advising him of his hypertension. This is done on the basis that if told, the patient's concern and emotional response will only further aggravate his condition. This type of patient may simply be advised to reduce his weight to normal, avoid overwork and overexcitement, and decrease his salt intake to a prescribed level in order to prevent the development of hypertension.

Persons with more severe hypertension may receive a drug to lower the blood pressure and are likely to be more restricted in activities and diet. The patients seen in the hospital are usually those with Grade 3 or Grade 4 hypertension and those with cardiac, cerebral or renal complications.

Observations. The blood pressure is determined at regular intervals with the patient in the same position each time. The doctor may request several casual readings at times when the patient is not anticipating the recording. A record of the pressure each morning before the patient moves about may also be necessary, and in some instances there may be a request to obtain a reading while the patient is asleep. The nurse should know the patient's activities or experiences for the period preceding any reading. If frequent recordings cause anxiety, this is brought to the physician's attention. Fluid balance is noted, as a positive balance may point to either renal or cardiac failure. The patient's weight is recorded daily, either to indicate progress to his normal weight level or to indicate possible sodium and water retention. The pulse rate and volume are recorded at least twice daily, and the respirations are observed for any signs of dyspnea, particularly on exertion. Any complaint of headache or pain is reported.

Rest and Activity. The amount of rest needed, and whether it must be bed rest or not, will depend on the severity of the hypertension. Moderately severe hypertensive patients may require a period of bed rest. A sedative such as amytal or phenobarbital may be prescribed to encourage relaxation and rest. When activity is permitted, it is graduated and the patient's blood pressure response noted. Moderate exercise, such as walking and golfing, is encouraged once the blood pressure has been somewhat lowered and as long as there is no dyspnea nor undue fatigue.

Diet. The caloric intake is reduced to 1000 to 1200 calories daily until the weight is normal; then a maintenance diet is established. The sodium intake is usually reduced, and the degree of restriction depends upon the severity of the patient's disease. If the salt restriction is prolonged, one should be alert for sodium deficiency, which is manifested by muscular cramps, weakness, nausea and vomiting. The amount of coffee, tea and alcohol is usually limited with most hypertensive persons.

Elimination. Constipation is to be avoided since straining raises the blood pressure and could cause the rupture of a damaged sclerosed artery.

Medications. Drugs comprise the main treatment of essential hypertension at present. The patient may be receiving a hypotensive drug or a sympathetic blocking agent, a sedative and a diuretic.

1. HYPOTENSIVE DRUGS. A variety of drugs are used to produce vasodilatation and may achieve this through action upon the central nervous system or upon the peripheral nervous system. These include the following:

Rauwolfia alkaloid preparations (reserpine, Serpasil, Serpina, Rautensine, Raudixin, alseroxylon) act at midbrain level and produce a tranquilizing effect as well as vasodilatation. The preparations are given orally, and the patient is observed for possible side effects, such as nasal stuffiness, flushing of the skin, increased gastrointestinal motility, dizziness, drowsiness and mental depression.

Hydralazine hydrochloride (Apresoline) may be administered orally, intramuscularly or intravenously and acts at the midbrain level of the central nervous system. Toxic reactions are manifested by headache, dizziness, rapid pulse, palpitation, precordial pain, shortness of breath and postural hypotension.

Ganglionic Blocking Drugs. These drugs act by blocking the transmission of nerve impulses through the autonomic ganglia to the arterioles.

The hexamethonium salts pentolinium tartrate (Ansolysen) and trimethidinium methosulfate (Ostensin) are ammonium compounds that act as ganglionic blocking agents; i.e., they act by blocking the transmission of nerve impulses through the autonomic ganglia to the arterioles. The blocking of parasympathetic impulses may cause abdominal distention and constipation, dry mouth, gastric distress, disturbed visual accommodation, urinary retention, weakness and dizziness. Rarely, tremor and mental confusion may also occur.

Sympathetic Blocking Drugs. Guanethidine (Imelin) is an antihypertensive drug that acts by suppressing sympathetic nervous impulses but does not interfere with parasympathetic innervation. It is given orally and the side effect that may occur is diarrhea and, as with many hypotensive drugs, orthostatic hypotension.

When a patient is receiving a hypotensive drug, he must be observed for the particular side effects that are associated with the drug he is receiving. If they occur, the physician is informed promptly. Most of these drugs can cause orthostatic hypotension—a sudden fall of blood pressure to below the normal when a patient assumes the upright position. The nurse instructs the patient to move slowly and to assume the recumbent position on the first feeling of faintness. When getting up, he should sit on the side of the bed for a few minutes before standing.

The blood pressure is recorded at frequent intervals as indicated by the physician. The nurse may be requested to take the blood pressure with the patient standing, especially if the patient is on ganglionic blocking drugs. It may be necessary to take the blood pressure before each dose of the drug. The level frequently determines whether the drug should be given and in what dosage. The antihypertensive drug and the dosage are prescribed individually; one drug may be more effective than another with one patient, and the effective dosage will often vary from one patient to another.

If the patient develops a fever or a spell of hot weather occurs, the dosage of the antihypertensive drug may have to be reduced, since a higher temperature seems to intensify the effect of the drug.

2. SEDATIVES. Frequent small doses of amytal, phenobarbital or a tranquilizing drug are often ordered for the hypertensive patient to promote relaxation and rest.

3. DIURETICS. Chlorothiazide (Diuril) is frequently given to hypertensive patients to produce negative sodium and water balances. It is usually given in conjunction with a low sodium diet and a hypotensive drug. If administration is prolonged, the patient is observed for possible potassium deficiency and skin rash. As with the administration of any diuretic, the urinary output is measured, and the patient is weighed daily during hospitalization.

Surgical Treatment of Hypertension

Rarely, essential hypertension is treated by a sympathectomy which interrupts impulses to blood vessels in a large area of the body, causing their dilatation. Certain sections of the sympathetic chain of ganglia are resected, or the entire sympathetic chain may be removed. Surgical treatment by sympathectomy involves two operations, since only one chain (left or right) is resected at one time. Surgical treatment has been largely replaced by drug therapy.

The nurse required to care for a patient who has had a sympathectomy must be aware of certain responsibilities. The patient's hypertension with its possible effects on kidneys, heart and cerebral vessels necessitates close observation for possible complications in these areas. The disturbance of innervation to viscera may result in functional changes. The areas of the body deprived of sympathetic innervation do not perspire, so that the remaining areas may compensate by excessive perspiration. These factors are significant in relation to skin care. Since his vessels will not constrict to conserve body heat, the patient may suffer an excessive loss of heat unless protected by extra covers or clothing.

Orthostatic hypotension may present a problem as gravity causes pooling of blood in the large number of dilated vessels. Before the patient is allowed to sit up or assume the upright position, tensor bandages may have to be applied to the entire lower limbs. A tight abdominal binder may also help. These are gradually removed as the patient adjusts to changes of position.

More recently, surgical treatment is being done for hypertension that is secondary to renal artery stenosis or arteriosclerosis. A variety of operations may be performed to improve the blood flow into a kidney. The one of choice will depend on the findings revealed by renal arteriography. In this procedure, a radiopaque substance is introduced into the aorta, and roentgenograms are made of the renal blood vessels. Observation of the patient's pulse, respirations and blood pressure are checked at frequent intervals throughout this procedure and are continued until values become stabilized.

The site of entry into the artery must also be observed for bleeding.

Surgical intervention consists of a nephrectomy if only one kidney is involved. Resection of a stenosed area of the renal artery and an end-to-end anastomosis may be undertaken, or grafts may be implanted to channel the blood from the aorta to the renal artery beyond the affected area. A splenorenal anastomosis has also been used, attaching the splenic artery to the left renal artery to bypass a stenosed area.

References

PHYSIOLOGY

BOOKS

Guyton, A. C.: Function of the Human Body, 3rd ed. Philadelphia, W. B. Saunders Co., 1969. Chapters 11, 12, 13, 14, and 15.
Jacob, W. W., and Francone, C. A.: Structure and Function in Man, 2nd ed. Philadelphia, W. B. Saunders Co., 1970. Chapter 10.
Selkurt, E. E. (Ed.): Physiology. Boston, Little, Brown & Co., 1963. Chapters 13, 14, and 15.
Taylor, N. B., and McPhedran, M. G.: Basic Physiology and Anatomy. Toronto, The MacMillan Co. of Canada Ltd., 1965. Chapters 13 and 14.

IMPAIRED CARDIAC FUNCTION

BOOKS

Beeson, P. B., and McDermott, W. (Eds.): Cecil-Loeb Textbook of Medicine, 13th ed. Philadelphia, W. B. Saunders Co., 1971, pp. 947–1049, 1062–1106.
Beland, J. L.: Clinical Nursing. New York, The MacMillan Co., 1965, pp. 561–648.
Davidson, Sir Stanley (Ed.): The Principles and Practice of Medicine, 7th ed. Edinburgh, E & S Livingstone Ltd., 1965, pp. 88–238.
Fordham, M. E.: Cardiovascular Nursing. New York, The MacMillan Co., 1962.
Guyton, A. C.: Textbook of Medical Physiology, 4th ed. Philadelphia, W. B. Saunders Co., 1971, pp. 298–304, 337–347, and 362–366.
Harrison, T. R., et al. (Eds.): Principles of Internal Medicine, 4th ed. New York, Blakiston Division, McGraw-Hill Book Co., Inc., 1962, pp. 1377–1467.
Powers, M., and Storlie, F.: The Cardiac Surgical Patient. New York, The MacMillan Co., 1969.
Pitorak, E. F., Hudak, C., O'Gureck, J., and Hanusz, P. P.: Nurses' Guide to Cardiac Surgery and Nursing Care. New York, The Blakiston Division, McGraw-Hill Book Co., 1969.
Sodeman, W. A., and Sodeman, W. A., Jr.: Pathologic Physiology, 4th ed. Philadelphia, W. B. Saunders Co., 1967, pp. 386–500.

PERIODICALS AND PAMPHLETS

American Heart Association, New York, Books and Pamphlets. Available in Canada through the Canadian Heart Foundation, Ottawa.
Anderson, B. L.: "Nursing Care of the Patient with the Cardiac Pacemaker—Monitor." Technical Innovations in Health Care, A.N.A. Monograph No. 5, 1962, pp. 11–17.
Barnes, C. M.: "Working with Parents of Children Undergoing Heart Surgery." Nurs. Clin. North Amer., Vol. 4, No. 1 (March, 1969), pp. 11–18.
Belling, D. I.: "Complications After Open Heart Surgery." Nurs. Clin. North Amer., Vol. 4, No. 1 (March, 1969), pp. 123–129.
Carleton, R. A., Sessions, R. W., and Graettinger, J. S.: "Cardiac Pacemakers: Clinical and Physiological Studies." Med. Clin. North Amer., Vol. 50, No. 1 (Jan. 1966), pp. 325–340.

Cartier, P.: "Surgery of the Heart and Large Vessels." Canad. Nurse, Vol. 60, No. 3 (March 1964), pp. 270–276.

Huun, V. K.: "Cardiac Pacemakers." Amer. J. Nurs., Vol. 69, No. 4 (April 1969), pp. 749–754.

Kennedy, M. J.: "Coping with Emotional Stress in the Patient Awaiting Heart Surgery." Nurs. Clin. North Amer., Vol. 1, No. 1 (March 1966), pp. 3–13.

Killys, T.: "Management of the Patient with Acute Myocardial Infarction." Med. Clin. North Amer., Vol. 52, No. 5 (Sept. 1968), pp. 1061–1074.

Kory, R. C.: "Cardiac Catheterization and Related Procedures." Cardiov. Nurs. Vol. 4, No. 4 (July–Aug. 1968).

Levine, H. J.: "The Treatment of Congestive Heart Failure." Med. Clin. North Amer., Vol. 46, No. 5 (Sept. 1962), pp. 1261–1272.

Meltzer, L. E.: "Coronary Care, Electrocardiography, and the Nurse." Amer. J. Nurs., Vol. 65, No. 12 (Dec. 1965), pp. 63–67.

Moore, Sister Mary C.: "Nursing Care of a Patient with an Implanted Artificial Pacemaker." Cardiov. Nurs., Vol. 2, No. 1 (Winter 1966), pp. 19–22.

Pinneo, R.: "Nurses' Role in a Coronary Care Unit." Exploring Progress in Medical-Surgical Nursing, A.N.A. Monograph, 1966, pp. 26–30.

——————: "Nursing in a Coronary Care Unit." Cardiov. Nurs., Vol. 3, No. 1 (Jan.–Feb. 1967).

Ritchie, M.: "The Nurse's Responsibility in Cardiac Arrest." Emergency Intervention by the Nurse, A.N.A. Monograph, 1962, pp. 22–27.

Smith, B. C.: "Congestive Heart Failure." Amer. J. Nurs., Vol. 69, No. 2 (Feb. 1969), pp. 278–282.

Turell, D. J., "The Cardiac Patient Returns to Work." Amer. J. Nurs., Vol. 65, No. 8 (Aug. 1965), pp. 115–117.

Varvaro, F. F.: "Teaching the Patient about Open Heart Surgery." Amer. J. Nurs., Vol. 65, No. 10 (Oct. 1965), pp. 111–115.

Wass, J. R.: "Nursing the Patient After Heart Surgery." Canad. Nurse, Vol. 65, No. 1 (Jan. 1969), pp. 35–37.

SHOCK

BOOKS

Davis, L. (Ed.): Christopher's Textbook of Surgery, 9th ed. Philadelphia, W. B. Saunders Co., 1968. Chapter 8.

Guyton, A. C.: Textbook of Medical Physiology, 4th ed. Philadelphia, W. B. Saunders Co., 1971. Chapter 28.

PERIODICALS

Gurd, F. N.: "Pathogenesis and Treatment of Shock." Canad. Nurse, Vol. 62, No. 10 (Oct. 1966), pp. 33–37.

Simeone, F. A.: "The Nature of Shock." (Part I) and "The Treatment of Shock." (Part II) Amer. J. Nurs., Vol. 66, No. 6 (June 1966), pp. 1287–1294.

VASCULAR DISEASE

BOOKS

Davidson, Sir Stanley (Ed.): The Principles and Practice of Medicine, 7th ed. Edinburgh, E & S Livingstone Ltd., 1965, pp. 245–268.

Davis, L. (Ed.): Christopher's Textbook of Surgery, 9th ed. Philadelphia, W. B. Saunders Co., 1968, pp. 1249–1313.

Guyton, A. C.: Textbook of Medical Physiology, 4th ed. Philadelphia, W. B. Saunders Co., 1971, pp. 376–379.

PERIODICALS

Ajemian, S.: "Bypass Grafting for Femoral Artery Occlusion." Amer. J. Nurs., Vol. 67, No. 3 (March 1967), pp. 565–568.

Breslau, R.: "Intensive Care Following Vascular Surgery." Amer. J. Nurs., Vol. 68, No. 8 (Aug. 1968), pp. 1670–1676.

DeBakey, M. E. (Ed.): "Symposium on Vascular Surgery." Surg. Clin. North Amer., Vol. 46, No. 4 (Aug. 1966).

Fulcher, A.: "The Nurse and the Patient with Peripheral Vascular Disease." Nurs. Clin. North Amer., Vol. 1, No. 1 (March 1966), pp. 47–55.

Mary Elizabeth, Sister: "Occlusion of the Peripheral Arteries: Nursing Observations and Symptomatic Care." Amer. J. Nurs., Vol. 67, No. 3 (March 1967), pp. 562–564.

Roy, P.: "Angiography." Canad. Nurse, Vol. 60, No. 3 (March 1964), pp. 243–249.

HYPERTENSION

BOOKS

Beeson, P. B., and McDermott, W. (Eds.): Cecil-Loeb Textbook of Medicine, 13th ed. Philadelphia, W. B. Saunders Co., 1971, pp. 1050–1061.

Davidson, Sir Stanley (Ed.): The Principles and Practice of Medicine, 7th ed. Edinburgh, E & S Livingstone Ltd., 1965, pp. 194–212.

Guyton, A. C.: Textbook of Medical Physiology, 4th ed. Philadelphia, W. B. Saunders Co., 1971, pp. 304–310.

Harrison, T. R., et al. (Eds.): Principles of Internal Medicine, 4th ed. New York, Blakiston Division, McGraw-Hill Book Co., Inc., 1962, pp. 1346–1360.

PERIODICALS

Callow, A. D.: "A Surgeon Talks about Hypertension." Amer. J. Nurs., Vol. 64, No. 12 (Dec. 1964), pp. 74–78

Page, I. H. (Ed.): "Hypertension and Its Treatment." Med. Clin. North Amer., Vol. 45, No. 2 (March 1961).

Talso, P. J., and Remenchik, A. P.: "The Management of Office Patients with Hypertension." Med. Clin. North Amer., Vol. 50, No. 1 (Jan. 1966), pp. 287–289.

14
Nursing in Respiratory Disorders

RESPIRATION

A constant exchange of oxygen and carbon dioxide between the living organism and its environment is essential for survival. Respiration is the process which performs this function. The exchange takes place between the total organism and the external environment and between the tissue cells and the blood. The former involves pulmonary ventilation and diffusion of the gases through the alveolar membrane of the lungs. The exchange between the cells and the blood (sometimes called internal or tissue respiration) requires transportation of the gases by the blood and diffusion between the capillaries and tissue cells.

Pulmonary ventilation or breathing consists of the movement of air into and out of the lungs (inspiration and expiration). Diffusion involves the movement of gases between the air in the pulmonary air sacs (alveoli) and the blood in the pulmonary capillaries in the direction of the lower pressure.

As well as providing oxygen for cellular metabolism and removing the cellular metabolite carbon dioxide, respiration also functions in sound and speech production, the regulation of the pH of body fluids through adjusting the amount of carbon dioxide

eliminated, water and heat elimination and the return of venous blood to the right atrium through alternating intrathoracic pressures.

RESPIRATORY STRUCTURE AND FUNCTIONS

The structures concerned with ventilation are the upper and lower respiratory tracts, respiratory muscles and thorax.

Upper Respiratory Tract

The upper airway is formed by the nose, mouth and pharynx.

The nose has a highly vascularized and ciliated mucous membrane lining which serves to moisten, warm and filter inhaled air. The nasal cavities and their connecting sinuses act as resonating chambers in sound production. The posterior portion of the cavities contain olfactory receptors concerned with the sense of smell (olfactory sense). The external orifices are called the nostrils, or anterior nares.

The pharynx, a muscular tube lined with mucous membrane, provides a common passageway for air entering the larynx and food entering the esophagus. Air reaching

257

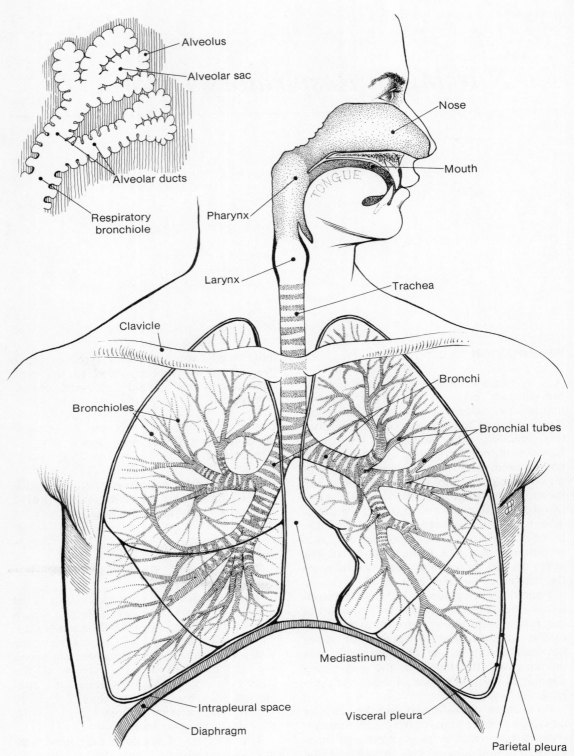

Figure 14–1 The respiratory system.

the pharynx passes readily into the larynx, but the presence of food or fluid stimulates a reflex contraction of the pharyngeal tube. The posterior nares (openings into the nasal cavities) are blocked off and the larynx is closed off by a lowering of the leaf-shaped structure, the epiglottis. These closures prevent the entrance of food or fluid into the nose and lower respiratory tract. As a result of the contraction, the pharyngeal content is directed into the esophagus.

Lower Respiratory Tract

The lower tract consists of the larynx, trachea, bronchi and two lungs.

The larynx is composed of muscle tissue and cartilages and is lined with mucous membrane. It functions as an air passage and contains the vocal cords, which are responsible for sound production. The laryngeal passageway is narrowed in one area by membranous folds reflected over the vocal cords. The slit-like space between these two folds is referred to as the glottis and is varied in size to produce different levels of pitch in voice production. In normal quiet inspiration and expiration the vocal cords are relaxed and the glottis is open.

The trachea is a continuation of the inferior end of the larynx and divides into two tubes—the right and left bronchi (singular, bronchus). The tracheal walls are composed of fibroelastic tissue in which incomplete cartilaginous rings are embedded to prevent collapse of the tube. The trachea simply serves as an air passageway.

Each bronchus enters a lung where it branches like a tree to form the bronchial tubes and, eventually, the very small tubes, the bronchioles. As the branches become more distal, the lumen of the tubes narrows and the walls change structure. The bronchi and bronchial tubes are similar in structure to the trachea except for the addition of plain muscle tissue in their walls. In the bronchioles, the cartilaginous tissue disappears and the smooth muscle tissue becomes more abundant.

The trachea and bronchial air passages are lined by a ciliated mucous membrane continuous with that of the upper air passages. The cilia are hair-like projections of protoplasm which alternately bend in one direction and straighten, providing a sweep-ing motion to remove mucus secretion and any foreign particles that may have been inhaled. Excessive secretions may initiate the cough reflex, which is a defense mechanism to rid the tract of such substances (see p. 268).

Each bronchiole terminates in clusters of microscopic sacs called alveoli (singular, alveolus). The walls of the alveoli consist mainly of thin elastic connective tissue and a network of capillaries. The air in the alveoli is separated from the blood in the capillaries by very thin semipermeable tissue which permits diffusion of the respiratory gases oxygen and carbon dioxide through it. The expanse of the alveolar surface is very great and is estimated to be approximately 30 to 40 times that of skin surface.

Each lung is made up mainly of bronchial tubes with their successive branches, alveoli and many blood vessels of the pulmonary circulatory system. The right lung is divided into 3 lobes, and the left is divided into 2 lobes only. The portion of lung derived from each main bronchial tube is referred to as a segment. Each lung is enclosed in an adherent serous membrane called the visceral pleura, which is continuous from the hilum of the lung with a similar layer that lines the thoracic wall and is known as the parietal pleura.

The lungs are well protected by the bony thoracic cage which is formed by the sternum, ribs and thoracic vertebrae. The thorax acts as an airtight box in which the lungs are suspended and in which pressure can be varied by the contraction of the respiratory muscles, altering the thoracic dimensions.

Blood Supply to the Lungs

Blood from two sources enters the lungs. The bronchial arteries convey blood from the aorta to nourish the respiratory structures. The pulmonary artery delivers the blood from the right side of the heart to be oxygenated. The blood from both sources is then collected from the capillaries around the alveoli into veins and is returned to the left side of the heart by the four pulmonary veins.

Secretions

The mucus which is secreted by the glandular cells of the mucous membrane lining of the respiratory tract serves to protect the organism in several ways. It provides a protective barrier against inhaled irritants and traps foreign particles, facilitating their removal by the cilia. It also waterproofs the surface, thus diminishing the loss of body water as well as setting up a barrier to inhaled organisms. Insufficient secretion of mucus or the production of a thick tenacious mucoid such as occurs in the congenital disorder mucoviscidosis (fibrocystic disease of the newborn) prevents the action of the cilia, predisposing to infection and partial or complete obstruction of bronchial tubes and bronchioles.

The alveolar epithelial cells secrete a lipoprotein substance onto the inner surface of the air sacs. Its action is similar to that of a detergent in that it reduces the surface tension of the fluid in the bronchioles and alveoli and prevents collapse of the latter. The alveoli and terminal bronchioles tend to collapse because of their elastic connective tissue and the surface tension of the contained fluid and mucus. A deficiency in the amount of surfactant produced increases surface tension, resulting in resistance to the inflow of air and reduced lung expansion. The condition is congenital and is known as hyaline membrane disease, or respiratory distress syndrome.

Chest Cavities and Their Pressures

The space between the visceral and parietal pleurae forms the intrapleural or pleural cavities. The space is normally only a potential space, since the surface of the lungs is in close apposition with the chest walls. The space between the lungs (interpleural space) is known as the mediastinum and contains large blood vessels, nerves, the heart, esophagus, trachea, bronchi and lymphatic ducts and nodes. The pressure within the pleural cavities is approximately 5 mm. Hg less than atmospheric pressure, which is 760 mm. Hg at sea level. It may also be expressed as a negative pressure equal to that exerted by a column of water 10 cm. in depth.

The intrapulmonic cavity is the space within the lungs, and since it communicates with the atmosphere, the intrapulmonary pressure varies above and below atmospheric pressure during expiration and in-

spiration respectively. Between expiration and inspiration, when there is no movement of air, the intrapulmonic pressure is that of the atmosphere.

Respiratory Muscles

The muscles used in normal breathing are principally the diaphragm and the intercostal muscles. The diaphragm is a dome-shaped muscular partition between the thoracic and abdominal cavities and is the most important respiratory muscle. When the diaphragm is relaxed, its thoracic surface is convex. On contraction, the convexity is reduced and the thoracic cavity is lengthened. The diaphragm also functions in coughing and sneezing and, in conjunction with the abdominal muscles, is used in defecation, vomiting and parturition. The external intercostal muscles increase the lateral and anteroposterior diameters of the thoracic cavity by elevating the sternum and moving the ribs into a more horizontal position.

Accessory muscles may be used to facilitate breathing. In labored and forced inspiration, the sternocleidomastoid, scalene and pectoralis muscles contract to raise the upper ribs. At the same time the nostrils dilate and the glottis widens. Forced or difficult expiration involves the abdominal and internal intercostal muscles. The abdominal muscles contract to raise the relaxed diaphragm higher in order to compress the lungs.

Mechanics of Pulmonary Ventilation

Each respiration involves inspiration and expiration. Inspiration is an active phase during which air moves into the lungs. Expiration, in normal breathing, is a passive phase during which air moves out of the lungs. Pulmonary ventilation is made possible by rhythmical variations in the dimensions of the thoracic and intrapulmonic spaces brought about by the alternate contraction and relaxation of the respiratory muscles.

Gases possess certain physical properties which explain the movement and exchange of respiratory gases. The molecules of a gas are in ceaseless movement and strike the walls of the container, creating a pressure. Within a given space, the greater the number of molecules of gas, the higher is the pressure produced. The pressure of a gas varies inversely with the space in which it is contained if the temperature remains constant; if the space in which the volume of gas is confined is reduced, more gas molecules strike a smaller area of the container, increasing the pressure. Conversely, if the space is increased, the pressure of the gas is decreased (Boyle's law). Gas molecules move from an area of higher pressure to one of lower pressure.

According to Dalton's law of partial pressure, each gas in a mixture of gases exerts the same pressure that it would exert if it were not in a mixture, and that pressure is proportional to its concentration. The pressure of the mixture is the sum of the pressures of the constituent gases. The pressure of each gas in the mixture is termed the partial pressure of that gas and is indicated by a "p" preceding the gas symbol. For example, the pressure of oxygen in a mixture of gases is recorded as pO_2.

The amount of a gas absorbed by a fluid is directly proportional to the partial pressure of the gas. The fluid will absorb the gas until the pressure of the gas is the same as that at the surface. This is referred to as Henry's law of the solution of gases.

Inspiration. The diaphragm and external intercostal muscles contract, increasing the closed, airtight thoracic space and resulting in a decrease of approximately 4 to 5 mm. Hg within the cavity. As the adherent moist parietal pleura moves out with the thoracic walls, the visceral pleura follows because of the cohesion between the two moist serous surfaces. The pressure in the intrapulmonic space is atmospheric and is greater than that of the expanded thoracic cavity. This pressure differential combined with the cohesion of the pleurae promotes a stretching of the elastic alveoli, resulting in the expansion of the lungs. The intrapulmonic space is now increased and the pressure of the contained air is reduced. A pressure gradient is produced between the atmospheric air and that in the lungs, so air moves into the respiratory tract, producing an inspiration.

Expiration. Relaxation of the respiratory muscles reverses the above process. As the intrathoracic space decreases, the pressure within the cavity increases. The elastic

alveoli which were stretched now recoil, diminishing the intrapulmonic space. The pressure of the air within the lungs is increased then to a level above that of the atmospheric air. This causes air to move out until the intrapulmonic pressure is equal to that of the atmosphere, thus producing an expiration. Normally, this mechanical cycle of inspiration and expiration is completed 14 to 18 times per minute in the adult.

Control of Ventilation. Breathing is under both nervous and chemical regulation. Muscular activities which perform ventilation are controlled by a respiratory center in the reticular formation of the medulla and pons. The center consists of inspiratory and expiratory neurons. Inspiratory neurons rhythmically discharge impulses which stimulate the respiratory muscles to contract, resulting in expansion of the thoracic and intrapulmonic cavities. The mechanism by which these neurons operate to produce rhythmical, alternating contraction and relaxation (inspiration and expiration) is not understood. It is suggested that the inspiratory neurons discharge impulses to the expiratory neurons as well as to the respiratory muscles. These impulses prompt the expiratory center to discharge impulses which inhibit the inspiratory neurons, allowing relaxation of the respiratory muscles and deflation of the lungs. Another explanation suggests that expansion of the lungs on inspiration gives rise to afferent impulses which are transmitted to the expiratory neurons which then discharge inhibitory impulses to the inspiratory center.

Impulses from the respiratory center descend into the spinal cord. Those carried to the diaphragm are transmitted by the phrenic nerves, which originate with the third, fourth and fifth cervical spinal nerves. The impulses to the intercostal muscles are delivered by the intercostal nerves that arise from the spinal cord with the third, fourth, fifth and sixth thoracic spinal nerves. The activity of the respiratory center is influenced by the level of activity of the reticular formation. Mental alertness and wakefulness normally have a stimulating effect on breathing, but sleep, sedatives and anesthesia tend to reduce the rate and volume of ventilation.

The major chemical factors that exert a control on ventilation are the pCO_2, pH and pO_2 of the blood.

The arterial carbon dioxide tension plays an important role in the regulation of breathing. An increase above the normal pCO_2 results in an increase in the volume and frequency of respirations. A decrease below the normal slows the respiratory rate. An increase in the hydrogen ion concentration (decrease in the pH) produces a similar response as that to an increase above normal in the pCO_2. The pO_2 influences respirations to a lesser extent than the carbon dioxide content. The cells which are sensitive to changes in these chemicals are not highly sensitive to slight variations in pO_2; the oxygen content may fall below 14 volumes per cent before there is a noticeable increase in respiratory activity.

It is not definite whether these chemicals exert their responses through a direct effect on the respiratory neurons or do so entirely through chemoreceptors, which are special sensory nerve endings that are sensitive to certain chemical changes. According to their location in relation to the nervous system, the chemoreceptors are of two types: peripheral and central.

The peripheral chemoreceptors are located in the carotid and aortic bodies* and are sensitive to changes in the pO_2 and hydrogen ion concentration of the blood. A decrease below the normal pO_2 and pH (increase in H^+ ion) initiates impulses in these receptors which are then transmitted to the respiratory neurons via the glossopharyngeal and vagus nerves, resulting in an increase in the rate and volume of respirations.

Central chemoreceptors which are located within the pia mater over the anterolateral surface of the medulla are sensitive to changes in the pH of the cerebrospinal fluid.[1] It is also suggested that these chemoreceptors may also react to changes in the arterial pCO_2.

When body metabolism increases, more oxygen is used by the tissues and more carbon dioxide and acid metabolites are pro-duced. Normally, this decreases the pO_2 and increases the pCO_2 and hydrogen ion concentration of the blood, and a corresponding increase in the rate and volume of respirations occurs.

Other factors which influence ventilatory activity include blood pressure changes, sensory stimuli, changes in body temperature, drugs, impulses from the higher brain centers and age.

Pressoreceptors in the aortic and carotid bodies are sensitive to changes in blood pressure. When they are stimulated, impulses are delivered to the respiratory center, which produce the appropriate response. A fall in blood pressure produces increased ventilation, and conversely, an elevated blood pressure generates impulses that give rise to a slower respiratory rate.

Certain sensory impulses may influence respirations. Severe pain produces faster and deeper respirations. Muscle activity increases respirations; this is attributed both to an increase in carbon dioxide production and to impulses originating in the stretch and pressure receptors of muscles, tendons and joints. A sudden cold application to the body produces a brief reflex apnea (cessation of breathing) followed by increased ventilation.

A high fever produces a noticeable increase in respiration which may be attributed principally to the increased oxygen consumption and carbon dioxide production by the accelerated cell metabolism. A decrease in temperature well below the normal, such as is produced in hypothermia, results in shallow, slow respirations.

Some drugs are known to depress the respiratory center, and overdosage may prove fatal for this reason. Narcotics such as morphine, barbiturates, anesthetics, alcohol and some tranquilizers are examples of drugs that reduce respiratory activity. Certain drugs have the reverse effect and in excess may cause hyperpnea (increased rate and volume of respiration). This could lead to exhaustion and respiratory alkalosis because of the excessive elimination of carbon dioxide. Salicylate preparations are perhaps the most common offenders in this area.

Impulses from the cerebral cortex may be delivered voluntarily or unconsciously to the respiratory center. Voluntary control is exerted on the respiratory center to facilitate

---

*The carotid bodies lie in the bifurcations of the carotid arteries; the aortic bodies are located on the wall of the aortic arch.

[1] J. Crofton, and A. Douglas: Respiratory Diseases. Edinburgh, Blackwell Scientific Publications, 1969, p. 25.

E. E. Chaffee, and E. M. Greisheimer: Basic Physiology and Anatomy, 2nd ed. Philadelphia, J. B. Lippincott Co., 1969, pp. 445–446.

such activities as speaking, singing and underwater swimming. One may arrest breathing for only a brief period before the center dominates. Hyperventilation may be voluntarily induced and, if prolonged, can produce a respiratory alkalosis due to the excessive reduction in the pCO_2 of the blood. Emotions can initiate impulses that may either increase or depress breathing.

Respiratory rate varies with age; it is more rapid in the young, decreasing with age. The rate at birth may be 40 to 70 respirations per minute; at 5 years of age it is approximately 25 to 30 per minute; at 10 years it is 20 to 22 per minute; and at 15 years of age and older it is 16 to 20 per minute.

The Work of Breathing. The inspiratory phase of breathing requires energy to overcome the elastic forces in the lungs and thorax and the flow-resistant forces within the air passages. Due to their elastic property, the lungs and chest wall tend to constantly maintain the position they occupy at the end of a normal expiration. When the respiratory muscles contract to expand the intrathoracic and intrapulmonic spaces to provide inhalation, they must overcome this elastic resistance. Compliance is a term used to indicate the distensibility of the lungs and the thorax. Pulmonary disease may produce changes in the lung tissue that make it "stiffer" and less elastic, causing a reduction in compliance. Similarly, the compliance of the thorax may be decreased by disorders affecting the chest wall.

Some energy is also necessary to overcome the frictional and viscous resistance offered by the surface tissues in the air passages. Any condition which reduces the caliber of the passages or causes an excessive production of mucus increases the flow-resistant forces. These forces create a demand for greater energy to move air in and out in ventilation.

Composition of Inspired, Expired and Alveolar Air

Inspired Air. Dry, inspired or atmospheric air at sea level is composed of nitrogen, oxygen and carbon dioxide in the following proportions:

oxygen	20.95 volumes per cent
carbon dioxide	0.04 volume per cent
nitrogen	78 volumes per cent.

Various quantities of water vapor, dust particles, and insignificant rare gases such as argon, neon and ozone may be present. Oxygen and carbon dioxide are the respiratory gases; nitrogen is not a concern since it is inert in the body. Some nitrogen does diffuse in and out of the blood, but under normal atmospheric pressures it has no physiological significance.

Expired Air. This shows a reduction in oxygen and an increase in the carbon dioxide as compared with atmospheric air. It is a mixture of alveolar air and atmospheric air from the passages above the alveoli. No exchange of gases is made in the air passages above the alveoli. This nonrespiratory area is called the anatomical dead space, and air contained in it may be referred to as dead air.

Alveolar Air. Since it is at this level that an exchange of the respiratory gases takes place with the capillary blood, the volume of oxygen in the contained air is reduced and that of carbon dioxide increases. Air that moves into the alveoli with each inspiration is a mixture of newly inspired air and air that moved into the dead space from the air sacs on previous expirations. In other words, as inspiration begins, alveolar air which had moved into the dead space on expiration is drawn back into the alveoli and mixed with a portion of newly inspired air. Thus, air entering the alveoli is not the exact composition of inspired atmospheric air.

A comparison of the approximate volumes of respiratory gases in inspired, expired and alveolar air may be made from Table 14–1.

Alveolar ventilation may be increased by increasing the inspiratory volume and the frequency of respirations per minute. The latter will only be effective if the inspiratory volume is increased at the same time. Rapid

TABLE 14–1 TENSIONS OF RESPIRATORY GASES IN INSPIRED, EXPIRED AND ALVEOLAR AIR

	VOLUMES PER CENT		PARTIAL PRESSURE MM. HG	
	Oxygen	Carbon Dioxide	Oxygen	Carbon Dioxide
Inspired (atmospheric) air	20.95	0.04	159	0.3
Expired air	16.3	4.5	116	28.0
Alveolar air	14.0	5.6	100	40.0

shallow respirations simply ventilate the dead space and expend considerable muscular energy to no avail. In exercise, when more oxygen is being used and more carbon dioxide is being produced, both the frequency of respirations and the inspired volume are automatically increased. These factors have a practical application in caring for inactive patients and point up the importance of having them take several deep breaths at regular intervals in order to adequately ventilate the alveoli.

Diffusion and Transportation of Respiratory Gases

Diffusion. The diffusion component of pulmonary respiration is the interchange of oxygen and carbon dioxide across the alveolar and capillary membranes. Gases move rapidly from areas of higher to lower pressure. A pressure differential occurs between the oxygen in the alveolar air and that in the blood in the pulmonary capillaries, and as a result, oxygen moves from the alveoli into the blood. Carbon dioxide moves in the opposite direction for the same reason.

Blood enters the vast number of pulmonary capillaries with the pO_2 at about 40 mm. Hg and the pCO_2 at approximately 46 mm. Hg. Alveolar air has a pO_2 of approximately 100 mm. Hg and a pCO_2 of about 35 to 40 mm. Hg. As a result of the diffusion exchange that quickly takes place as the blood flows through the pulmonary capillaries, blood enters the pulmonary veins with a pO_2 of 95 to 100 mm. Hg and a pCO_2 of approximately 40 mm. Hg (see Table 14-2).

Transportation of Respiratory Gases by the Blood. Oxygen is transported by the blood in solution in plasma and as a chemical compound in the red blood cells. The amount of gas that can be carried in solution is very limited; in order to carry sufficient oxygen through the body to meet the needs of the cells, most of the gas that enters the blood in the alveoli diffuses from the plasma into the red blood cells where it combines loosely with the hemoglobin to form the compound oxyhemoglobin. If the hemoglobin has its normal complement of iron, each gram can carry 1.34 ml. of oxygen. The chemical process that produces oxyhemoglobin is reversible so that as the oxygen in solution is used up by the tissues, more is made available by the dissociation of the unstable oxyhemoglobin ($Hb + O_2 \rightleftarrows HbO_2$). Of the 20 volumes per cent of oxygen in the arterial blood, only about 0.5 volume per cent remains in solution in plasma; the remaining 19.5 volumes per cent is carried as oxyhemoglobin.

The rate at which hemoglobin combines with oxygen and the rate of dissociation of oxyhemoglobin is influenced by the pO_2 and pCO_2 of the blood. An increase in the pO_2 and a decrease in the pCO_2 hasten the formation of oxyhemoglobin. Conversely, a decrease in the pO_2 and an increase in the pCO_2, as occurs in the systemic capillaries, promote the release of oxygen from hemoglobin. The pH of the blood has a significant effect on the dissociation of oxygen and hemoglobin. A decrease in the alkalinity below the normal (i.e., a decrease in the pH) promotes release of oxygen from the hemoglobin molecule. In the tissues this serves an important function; metabolites result in a decrease in the pH, and oxyhemoglobin dissociation is promoted in the capillary blood, allowing oxygen to diffuse into the tissues. Body temperature also influences oxygen-hemoglobin dissociation. An elevated temperature causes the release of oxygen from oxyhemoglobin.

Carbon dioxide is produced within the body by cellular metabolism and diffuses out of the cells through the tissue fluid into the blood where it is carried in several forms. Only a very limited amount remains in solution in plasma; the larger proportion is carried in the form of bicarbonate (HCO_3^-) and in combination with hemoglobin and plasma proteins (carbamins). About two-thirds of the total blood carbon dioxide is carried as sodium bicarbonate ($NaHCO_3$) in the plasma and serves to maintain the normal blood alkalinity (pH 7.4). A small,

TABLE 14-2 PARTIAL PRESSURES OF RESPIRATORY GASES

	PO_2 MM. HG	PCO_2 MM. HG
Alveolar air	100	40
Venous blood	40	46
Arterial blood	95	40

essential amount of potassium bicarbonate ($KHCO_3$) is found in the erythrocytes.

The chemical compounds are unstable and tend to dissociate with changes in the pressures of the gases in the blood. As the blood is circulated through the tissues, the increasing pCO_2 and decreasing pO_2 promote the formation of the compounds. A reverse of the pressure of these gases promotes dissociation of the compounds. In the pulmonary capillaries, where the pO_2 increases and pCO_2 decreases, a rapid dissociation takes place to release some of the CO_2.

Tissue Respiration. The exchange of carbon dioxide and oxygen which takes place between the cells and the blood in the systemic capillaries throughout the body comprises tissue or internal respiration. The basis of the gaseous exchange is the pressure gradient of each of the respiratory gases between the cells and the tissue fluid and between the tissue fluid and the blood. The pO_2 of the arterial blood when it enters the systemic capillaries is approximately 95 mm. Hg (20 volumes per cent) and is much higher than that of the interstitial fluid, so oxygen diffuses from the plasma into the tissue fluid. Continuous cell activity uses oxygen, so the higher pO_2 of the tissue fluid results in a movement of the oxygen into the cells. As the oxygen tension is reduced in the plasma, the loosely combined oxyhemoglobin dissociates to free oxygen. By the time the blood again reaches the pulmonary capillaries the oxyhemoglobin has given up considerable oxygen.

The chemical activities of the cells (metabolism) produce carbon dioxide. Its concentration in the cell produces a pressure gradient that results in its movement into the tissue fluid. From here, because of the difference in pressure, it moves into the capillary blood and gradually accumulates a higher concentration in the venous blood than that of the alveolar air. This promotes the diffusion of carbon dioxide from the pulmonary capillary blood into alveolar air.

The amount of gas exchanged in tissue respiration varies in different tissues and organs and with a decrease or increase in activity. The brain tissue, myocardium and skeletal muscles require a constant supply of oxygen. Any deficiency is quickly reflected in impaired function of these structures.

Chemical Reactions in Respiration

Several chemical reactions are involved in the transport and exchange of oxygen and carbon dioxide and go on continuously with great speed in the blood throughout all the tissues. A brief summary of the reactions follows, and since the reactions of oxygen and carbon dioxide are interrelated, they are considered together.

In the Tissues. Potassium oxyhemoglobin ($KHbO_2$) in red blood cells dissociates in the systemic capillaries to release O_2 which diffuses through the plasma into the interstitial fluid and on into the cells.

$$KHbO_2 \longrightarrow KHb + O_2$$

Carbon dioxide diffuses from the tissues into the plasma and on into red blood cells where an enzyme, carbonic anhydrase, promotes a reaction with water to form carbonic acid.

$$CO_2 + H_2O \xrightarrow{\text{carbonic anhydrase}} H_2CO_3$$

This is a very unstable acid and ionizes to hydrogen (H^+) and bicarbonate (HCO_3^-) ions. Some of the HCO_3^- ions move out into the plasma and form sodium bicarbonate ($NaHCO_3$). The H^+ ions unite with the hemoglobin (HHb).

$$H_2CO_3 \longrightarrow H^+ \cdot HCO_3^-$$
$$HCO_3^- + Na^+ \longrightarrow NaHCO_3$$
$$H^+ + Hb \longrightarrow HHb$$

Chloride (Cl^-) ions released by dissociation of $NaCl$ move into red blood cells from the plasma to replace the HCO_3^- ions to maintain ionic equilibrium. They react with potassium hemoglobin (KHb) and form potassium chloride (KCl) and hemoglobin (Hb).

$$Cl^- + KHb \longrightarrow KCl + Hb$$

Some bicarbonate (HCO_3^-) ions which remain within the red blood cells also react with KHb when it gives up O_2 to form potassium bicarbonate.

$$HCO_3^- + KHb \longrightarrow KHCO_3 + Hb$$

Some of the CO_2 entering the red blood cells unites with Hb, forming carbaminohemoglobin ($HbCO_2$).

$$CO_2 + Hb \longrightarrow HbCO_2$$

The above reactions at tissue level result in:

1. O_2 being released from Hb

2. The formation of $NaHCO_3$ and $KHCO_3$

3. The formation of $HbCO_2$

In the Lung Capillaries. The O_2 diffuses from the plasma into the red blood cells where it combines with HHb to form oxyhemoglobin ($HHbO_2$). The H^+ ion makes this compound acid, so it reacts with $KHCO_3$, yielding potassium hemoglobin ($KHbO_2$) and carbonic acid (H_2CO_3).

$$HHb + O_2 \longrightarrow HHbO_2$$
$$HHbO_2 + KHCO_3 \longrightarrow KHbO_2 + H_2CO_3$$

Dissociation of H_2CO_3 is promoted by carbonic anhydrase, and CO_2 and H_2O are produced. The CO_2 diffuses out of the red blood cell through the plasma into the alveolar air because of the pressure gradient.

$$H_2CO_3 \xrightarrow{\text{carbonic anhydrase}} H_2O + CO_2$$

With the loss of HCO_3^- ions in these reactions the ionic equilibrium is disturbed so dissociated Cl^- ions move out of the red blood cells into the plasma where they react with $NaHCO_3$ to form NaCl and bicarbonate (HCO_3^-).

$$Cl^- + NaHCO_3 \longrightarrow NaCl + HCO_3^-$$

Much of the HCO_3^- diffuses into the red blood cells and combines with the KHb to form $KHCO_3$.

As cited above, $KHCO_3$ reacts with the acidic oxyhemoglobin ($HHbO_2$) to yield carbonic acid (H_2CO_3).

The above reactions in lung capillaries result in:

1. Formation of oxyhemoglobin (HbO_2)
2. The formation of H_2CO_3
3. The dissociation of H_2CO_3 to H_2O and CO_2

Factors Which Influence Pulmonary Diffusion. The volumes of oxygen and carbon dioxide which diffuse across the pulmonary membrane depend on the pressure gradient of each gas between the alveolar air and capillary blood. Alveolar ventilation must be adequate to maintain an effective pO_2 to drive oxygen into the blood. Sufficient elimination of carbon dioxide in expiration to reduce the pCO_2 in the alveolar air is necessary to promote the movement of carbon dioxide out of the blood into the alveoli. Increased respiratory rate alone does not necessarily provide alveolar ventilation. If the respirations are shallow, it is mainly the dead space that is being ventilated.

Diffusion is greatly influenced by the ventilation-perfusion ratio. Normally, ventilation of the alveoli and perfusion (flow of blood) are relatively uniform. Any disparity that incurs underperfusion or underventilation results in reduced diffusion, which results in a decreased blood pO_2 and possibly an increased pCO_2.* A disturbance in the ventilation-perfusion ratio may be referred to as the mismatching or imbalance of ventilation and blood flow. Mismatching may be caused by such conditions as pulmonary embolism, which causes underperfusion, and emphysema, bronchial constriction or pneumonia, which result in a number of alveoli being underventilated.

Diffusion may be decreased by the presence of increased fluid in the alveoli or, rarely, by alveolar tissue changes resulting from chronic pulmonary disease (e.g., pulmonary fibrosis).

Any reduction in the alveolar surface area such as occurs with lobectomy, pneumonectomy or emphysema obviously greatly diminishes the diffusion of the respiratory gases.

Respiration and High Altitude

Atmospheric pressure decreases as the distance above sea level increases. The corresponding decreases in the partial pressure of oxygen at high altitudes reduces the pressure of oxygen in alveolar air, and less oxygen diffuses into the blood, causing a deficiency throughout the body. The height at which symptoms of hypoxia (deficiency of oxygen) are first experienced varies somewhat with different individuals and according to the speed with which they ascend. A rapid ascent to 10,000 feet where atmospheric pressure is approximately 523 mm. Hg and the pO_2 in alveolar air is 67 mm. Hg produces symptoms of oxygen deficiency in the brain. The person manifests reduced mental efficiency and a decrease in visual and auditory acuity. Greater heights produce further deterioration, and at 20,000 to 25,000 feet the person lapses into coma.

In a gradual ascent to a high altitude the

---

*Carbon dioxide is much more soluble than oxygen, so it diffuses more rapidly. Impaired diffusion is likely to cause hypoxia before hypercapnia.

person's physiology makes some adjustments to acclimatize. Respirations increase in rate and volume and the heart rate and output are increased. The number of red blood cells and the amount of hemoglobin are increased when one is exposed to a higher altitude for a period of one or more weeks. Since more carbon dioxide is lost at these heights, owing to the lower carbon dioxide pressure in the air and the increased respirations, blood alkalinity is increased. More base ions are excreted by the kidney in an effort to maintain a normal pH of the body fluids.

In aviation, the low atmospheric pressure of high altitudes is overcome by breathing pure oxygen to increase the oxygen concentration in the alveolar air or by pressurizing the cabin of the plane. Pressure within the plane is usually maintained at the pressure occurring at about 5000 feet above sea level.

Respiration and High Atmospheric Pressure

Atmospheric pressure increases as the distance below sea level increases. A depth of 33 feet below sea level doubles the atmospheric pressure. An abnormally high atmospheric pressure is experienced by deep sea divers and by workers in chambers or tunnels which are filled with compressed air to prevent cave-ins that might result from the increased pressure from without. The high pressure of the air causes greater amounts of oxygen and nitrogen to diffuse into the blood.

Excessive amounts of the gases are carried in solution in the body fluids. The high oxygen concentration may interfere with normal cellular activity; impaired brain function may be manifested by twitching, convulsions, confusion, stupor and coma. The excessive volume of nitrogen may also affect psychic behavior. Most frequently, it has a depressing or anesthetizing effect on the central nervous system and the person becomes very drowsy and inefficient. Nitrogen frequently causes more problems when the person ascends to normal atmospheric pressure. While exposed to the greater pressure the nitrogen remains in solution, but when he ascends to the surface, the decreased pressure on the body causes the nitrogen to expand and form bubbles in the

tissues or fluids. These may cause an embolism and tissue damage in any area of the body; severe pain, brain damage, paralysis or severe gastrointestinal distention may occur. To prevent bubble formation, the person is brought to sea level very slowly or is confined within a chamber in which the pressure is very gradually decreased while the excess nitrogen escapes.

Deep sea divers prevent the entry of excess gases into their blood by reducing the amount of oxygen in the gas they breathe, and in some instances they add helium. Disturbances due to extremely high atmospheric pressure may be referred to as caisson disease, decompression sickness or the bends.

Pulmonary Volumes and Capacities

The volume of air breathed in and out varies with the activity and demands of the body and with the age and size of each individual. The figure given with each of the following respiratory volumes is the average for normal male adults; for the normal average adult female the volumes are approximately 20 to 25 per cent less.

Tidal Volume (V_T). This represents the volume of air inspired or expired with each breath. During normal, quiet breathing the tidal volume measures about 500 ml. Approximately 150 ml. of this fills the anatomical dead space and does not exchange gases with the blood. The dead space gas is symbolized by V_D.

Minute Respiratory Volume (V min.). This is the total volume of air moved in or out of the lungs in one minute and is determined by multiplying the tidal volume by the respiratory rate per minute ($V_T \times f$).

Inspiratory Capacity (IC). This term indicates the maximum amount of air which can be inhaled in one breath. The normal is approximately 3500 ml.

Inspiratory Reserve Volume (IRV). This is the portion of the inspiratory capacity in excess of the tidal volume and is approximately 3000 ml.

Expiratory Reserve Volume (ERV). The maximum quantity of air that can be forcibly exhaled after an ordinary expiration is approximately 1000 to 1100 ml.

Forced Expiratory Volume (FEV). This is the maximum volume of air that can be rapidly exhaled following a maximum inspiration. It is usually recorded in liters per second.

Residual Volume (RV). The volume of air remaining in the lung after maximum expiration is referred to as residual air. The average normal volume is approximately 1200 ml. The lungs cannot be completely emptied of air if the chest cavity remains closed.

Vital Capacity (VC). This is the maximum volume of air that can be expired after an inspiration of maximum capacity. It equals the tidal volume plus the inspiratory and expiratory reserve volumes. The normal is approximately 4000 to 5000 ml.

Total Lung Capacity (TLC). The residual volume plus the vital capacity volume represents the total lung capacity. The normal amounts to approximately 5200 to 6000 ml.

RESPIRATORY DISORDERS

There are many different disorders which may adversely affect the movement of a normal volume of air in and out of the alveoli or the diffusion of the respiratory gases across the aveolar and capillary membranes. Acute and chronic respiratory disorders have a very high incidence and account for a large part of absenteeism at work and school as well as for permanent disability and dependence. The site of the problem may be within the upper or lower respiratory tract, or it may be extrinsic in areas such as the respiratory center (brain stem), respiratory muscles, chest wall and nonrespiratory structures within the mediastinum. The system is vulnerable to a wide variety of causative factors. A large proportion of the diseases are infectious and communicable; the infected person coughs or exhales contaminated droplets and air into the atmosphere which may then be inhaled by other persons in the environment. Other causes of respiratory disorders include allergic reaction, inhalation of irritating gas or dust, aspiration of foreign material or a foreign body, neoplasms and trauma. In many instances, the disorder is not of a serious nature but can be responsible for considerable discomfort for the affected person. Also, it must be remembered that the continuity and close relationship of the various respiratory structures

predispose to a minor disorder spreading to another part and becoming a more serious problem.

Regardless of the etiologic factor, the primary concern, especially when the lower tract is involved, is whether ventilation is adequate and whether the diffusion is sufficient to maintain normal blood gas levels (i.e., normal pO_2 and pCO_2).

Manifestations of Respiratory Disorders

Cough. A cough is a sudden, expulsive expiration for the purpose of removing an irritant from the air passages. It is a protective reflex that indicates there is some irritation in the tract.

The cough mechanism involves stimulation of receptors in the mucous membrane of the bronchial tubes, trachea, larynx or pharynx or stimulation at a point along the vagus nerve. The impulses travel via the vagus nerve or the glossopharyngeal nerve to the cough center formed by a group of neurons in the medulla of the brain. Responsive impulses are initiated in the center and travel to the respiratory muscles and the larynx, producing, in succession, a quick inhalation, closure of the glottis and contraction of the abdominal and internal intercostal muscles to increase the intrathoracic and intrapulmonic pressures. The latter is exerted against the closed glottis which opens suddenly, releasing a forceful gust-like expiration. A review of the sequence of activities shows three phases — namely, the inspiratory, compressive and expulsive phases. During the compressive phase, pressure is placed on the alveoli and their secretions are moved into the small bronchial tubes. The increased velocity of the airflow in the expiratory phase results in secretions being expelled from the air passages.

The cough is generally an involuntary response, although some voluntary control may be exerted to inhibit it or produce it. If a cough is unproductive, it may be helpful to instruct the patient to make an effort to inhibit the cough in order to conserve his energy and prevent exhaustion. In other instances, the patient may be required to initiate a series of coughs at regular intervals to prevent the accumulation of secretions in the air passages.

The origin of the cough stimulus may be within the respiratory tract or may be extrinsic to it. Intrinsic stimuli include inflammation, secretions, fluid, scar tissue which causes traction on the nerve endings, newgrowths, inhaled or aspirated particles of dust, irritating gases and foreign bodies and very cold or very hot air. Extrinsic stimuli are abnormal conditions in neighboring structures which exert pressure on some area of the tracheobronchial tree. Pleurisy, newgrowths of the esophagus, enlarged lymph nodes in the mediastinum and aortic aneurysm are examples of extrinsic causes. Rarely, a cough is psychogenic. Emotional tension may result in a failure of the epiglottis to close in swallowing, allowing saliva, fluid or food to enter the respiratory tract. Occasionally, a cough is used as an attention-seeking device.

IMPLICATIONS FOR NURSING. A persistent cough should always be considered as an indication of something abnormal that requires investigation. It is not unusual to find persons ignoring a cough until some more distressing sign or symptom appears, at which time the cause may have progressed to a serious or advanced stage.

Not all coughs should be suppressed; coughing is a reflex protective mechanism designed to remove foreign and irritating matter from the respiratory tract. It has been said that more deaths occur due to failure to cough than ever result from coughing. Efforts are directed toward making the cough less difficult and more effective. The patient may be instructed to extend the interval between paroxysms of coughing by exerting voluntary control and by remaining quiet and at rest for a period of 1 to 2 hours. He will then produce more forceful expiration and will raise more secretions than he could with frequent, shallow, hacking coughs. The fluid intake may be increased and medications prescribed to increase the secretions and make them less tenacious and easier to raise. If the cough is unproductive, frequent and exhausting, a drug may be ordered to depress the cough center.

Certain observations are made and recorded by the nurse. The frequency of the cough is noted as well as whether it is productive or nonproductive. Any sputum raised is observed as to the amount, character (mucus, watery, purulent, tenacious,

frothy, caseous or blood-streaked) and odor. The sound of the cough may be important; it may be hard and wracking, croupy, hacking, shallow, deep and rattling or may have a whooping sound. The cough may be worse at certain times of the day. Frequently, secretions accumulate during the night, and when the patient rouses and moves in the morning severe paroxysms of coughing are precipitated. If pain is experienced with coughing, its location and quality are ascertained. Finally, it is important to assess the effect of the cough on the patient. If the physical exertion and disturbance of rest are exhausting or if the cough is creating anxiety in the patient, the physician is informed. Its frequency may interrupt the patient's meal to the point that he gives up and does not take sufficient nourishment.

Some patients inhibit their cough because it causes pain; support may be given by the nurse who places a hand to the anterior and posterior chest walls in the painful area. If the pain is due to pleural irritation, the doctor may reduce the chest excursion by strapping the affected side with adhesive. Each strap is applied following an expiration when the lung is deflated.

Coughing and expectoration should always be considered potentially infectious. The mouth and nose should be covered by the patient with a tissue during a cough. Paper tissues are made available to receive the expectoration, and provision is made for the prompt disposal of used tissues in a paper bag kept within the patient's reach. If the sputum is profuse or is to be measured, a covered sputum container is used. Such containers have a disposable liner but the outer metal part requires daily cleansing and disinfection.

Drugs which may be used in treating a patient with a cough are:

EXPECTORANTS. These are drugs that increase and liquefy the secretions. Preparations of ammonium chloride or potassium iodide are examples of commonly used expectorants. Many persons do not tolerate potassium iodide and manifest toxic symptoms such as skin lesions, complaints of a metallic taste and burning irritation in the mouth or eyes.

MUCOLYTIC ENZYMES. A preparation of trypsin or pancreatic dornase may be used by aerosol administration to liquefy secretions, making it easier to raise them. Increased humidity of the atmosphere is also helpful.

ANTITUSSIVE DRUGS. These are drugs that depress the cough reflex. Examples are codeine and benzonatate (Tessalon).

Abnormal Breathing. Irregularities in breathing may relate to rate, volume, rhythm or to the ease with which the person breathes. The following terms are used to indicate characteristic breathing patterns.

Eupnea represents quiet normal breathing at the rate of about 16 to 20 times per minute in the adult.

Apnea is a temporary cessation of breathing.

Tachypnea is rapid breathing with the volume of the respirations below normal.

Hyperpnea is an increase in the volume of air breathed per minute due to either an increase in the rate or depth of respirations or to both.

Dyspnea refers to a subjective awareness of a disturbance in breathing. The patient experiences discomfort and/or the need for increased effort or work in ventilation.

Orthopnea is dyspnea which is present in the recumbent position but is relieved to some extent by elevation of the trunk.

Cheyne-Stokes respirations are characterized by a few seconds of apnea followed by respirations that gradually increase in frequency and volume to a peak intensity and then gradually subside to the period of apnea. This pattern is cyclic.

Abnormal Breath Sounds. Normal respirations present very little sound as the air enters the lungs. Absence of such sounds or the accompaniment of other sounds may indicate excessive secretions or fluid in an area or constriction or blockage of a section of the system. Abnormal sounds may be detected by the naked ear or by use of a stethoscope.

The following terms are used to describe abnormal breath sounds. Wheezing is a whistling sound heard mainly on expiration and is usually due to some narrowing of the bronchial tubes. Bubbling moist respirations heard with the naked ear indicate excessive secretions in the tract. Râles are bubbling sounds heard with a stethoscope and are produced by the movement of air through mucus. Rhonchi are coarse, loud râles produced by air moving through tenacious mucus in the bronchial tubes, bronchi or trachea. Crepitation may be used to describe the sound produced by air moving through fluid lying in the alveoli. Friction or pleural rub is a characteristic sound produced when an inflamed, roughened pleura rubs against the other pleura on inspiration. Stridor is a crowing-like or high-pitched sound that is emitted with each respiration as air passes through a constricted larynx or trachea.

Chest Pain. Pain associated with respiratory disorders originates mainly in the upper air passages or in the pleurae. Inflammation of the trachea or bronchial tubes causes a burning "raw" type of pain which is not affected by respirations but becomes worse on coughing. Pleural pain tends to be localized to one side of the chest and is due to the stretching of the affected pleura. It is sharp and stabbing on inspiration, causing the patient to take shallow breaths.

Abnormal Chest Movements. Unequal participation of the two sides of the chest in respiratory movements may be evident, or unusual retraction or ballooning of the intercostal spaces may occur. For example, in atelectasis or pneumothorax, in which a part or all of the lung is not being inflated, there is diminished movement of the chest wall on the affected side. Similarly, this may occur if a large section of alveoli is consolidated with fluid or secretions. Excessive retraction or ballooning is associated with extreme difficulty in getting air in or out of the air passages.

Secretions. Normally, the adult raises about 100 ml. of mucus daily. This may be increased when there is some irritation in the air passages and may change in color and consistency. The expectoration of blood occurs in many respiratory disorders and in varying degrees of severity. There may be only a slight streaking of the mucus with blood or there may be expectoration of frank blood. The latter is referred to as hemoptysis. Blood in the sputum is commonly associated with inflammatory conditions and lesions which cause erosion and necrosis of the tissues and blood vessels, such as bronchitis, pneumonia, tuberculosis, carcinoma and pulmonary infarction.

Clubbing of the Fingers and Toes. Occasionally, this unusual sign develops in chronic respiratory disease, and although its cause is not definitely known, it is thought to be due to increased vascularity in response to hypoxia.

Cyanosis. A dusky bluish color of the mucous membranes, skin and nail beds may be associated with respiratory disease due to excessive deoxygenation of the hemoglobin. When more than the usual amount of dissociation occurs, the hemoglobin presents a dark blue color. The absence of cyanosis is not always a reassuring sign unless the hemoglobin level is known. In a person with 50 per cent or less of the normal complement (13 to 15 Gm. per cent), the bluish hemoglobin may not be sufficiently concentrated to be reflected through superficial tissues.

Constitutional Symptoms in Respiratory Disorders. If the respiratory disturbance is due to infection or trauma, or if there is degeneration of tissue as in pulmonary infarction, the patient usually develops a fever and a corresponding increase in pulse rate. General debilitation occurs quickly in most respiratory disease; the patient complains of anorexia, weakness and fatigue and loses weight.

Abnormal Blood Gas Levels. Manifestations of disturbances in respiratory ventilation and/or diffusion may include changes in the arterial pO_2, pCO_2 and pH. For normal values see page 274.

Diagnostic Procedures and Respiratory Functional Tests

Investigation and assessment of the patient with a respiratory disorder includes observation of the rate and rhythm of the respirations and the associated chest movements, sounds and use of accessory muscles. A knowledge of familial incidence of respiratory disturbances and information about the patient's occupation, living customs and special concerns are an essential part of the investigation. The nutritional status and hydration are quite significant; the former influences his resistance and recuperative capacity. Dehydration may result in thick, tenacious secretions which are not readily raised and predispose to obstruction of the airway. On the other hand, overhydration and edema may increase the alveolar fluid content and interfere with ventilation and diffusion.

Examination includes percussion and auscultation. The former involves tapping of the chest and listening to the degree of resonance. Normally, the sounds are resonant, dull in consolidation of alveoli and hyperresonant in conditions such as emphysema, air-trapping and pneumothorax. Auscultation refers to listening to the breath sounds by means of a stethoscope.

The diagnostic procedures and respiratory functional tests used vary with each patient. In some instances, the diagnosis is made on the physical examination and the patient's history alone. In others, blood tests and special radiological, endoscopic, bacteriological and cytological investigative procedures are required. Similarly, respiratory function tests are necessary with some patients to determine to what extent, if any, they are experiencing respiratory insufficiency.

Roentgenogram of the Chest. Radiological examination of the chest is used to locate a lesion and obtain information about the size of the area involved and the nature of the lesion. The procedure is explained to the patient if it is unfamiliar to him. Clothing is removed to the waist to prevent the possibility of objects such as buttons restricting the entrance of the x-rays. The patient is protected from exposure by a hospital gown or drape.

Bacteriological and Cytological Examinations. Sputum is examined microscopically in a smear or by culture for disease organisms, bronchial casts, eosinophils and cancer cells. The physician may request that the sputum specimen be collected first thing in the morning, since the secretions that accumulate during the night may have a higher concentration of organisms. The mouth should be clean and free of residual food particles. The patient is given a wide-mouthed container, which is provided by the laboratory especially for a sputum specimen, and is instructed to cough deeply to raise the sputum from the lungs. A paper towel may be wrapped around the bottle to prevent contamination of the outside of the container. The specimen container is kept covered to prevent air contamination by the sputum and vice versa. When the specimen is obtained, the container is removed from the paper covering, labeled and delivered to the laboratory.

Pleural fluid obtained by aspiration that is

to be used for bacteriological or cytological examinations is placed in a sterile bottle or test tube and sealed with a sterile bottle cap or cork.

If the patient is unable to raise a satisfactory sputum specimen, a specimen of the gastric content may be requested, since some sputum may have been swallowed while sleeping. A gastric aspiration is done in the morning before anything is taken by mouth. A sterile gastric tube is passed and a syringe is used to withdraw a specimen. The fluid is placed in a sterile container. Sputum or aspiration specimens are examined microscopically and may also be used to inoculate a culture medium.

Endoscopic Investigation. An endoscope is a hollow instrument which is equipped with a light and is used for examining an area within the body. Each one is constructed as to size and shape for use in specific body areas; thus, there are the laryngoscope, bronchoscope, gastroscope, cystoscope, and so on. Investigation of a patient with a respiratory disorder may include a bronchoscopy and bronchogram.

In bronchoscopy, a rigid lighted tube is introduced through the mouth, pharynx, larynx and trachea into a bronchus. The air passages and the openings into the bronchial tree are viewed directly or by means of a telescopic lens passed through the bronchoscope. Special instruments may be passed through the bronchoscope to obtain a tissue specimen for biopsy, to remove a foreign body or to aspirate secretions or a mucus plug.

Preparation of a patient for a bronchoscopy includes an explanation of the procedure and what will be expected of him. He is advised that he will remain conscious since only topical anesthesia is used to introduce the instrument, relaxation during the examination will reduce the discomfort and breathing through the nose with the mouth open will be helpful. The patient is encouraged to practice these suggestions beforehand while lying flat on his back with his head extended. He should know that the room will be darkened and his eyes covered by a towel. Food and fluids are withheld 6 to 8 hours previous to the scheduled time for the examination to avoid vomiting and aspiration. Dentures are removed, atropine is generally administerd to reduce the secre-

tions and some sedation may be ordered to promote relaxation and reduce the patient's anxiety.

Following the examination the head of the bed is elevated, and the patient is encouraged to lie on either side to promote the drainage of secretions and prevent aspiration. An ice collar may be used to reduce soreness and possible edema. The swallowing and gag reflexes are usually absent for a few hours because of the local anesthesia used; fluids and food are withheld until they return. Restoration of the reflex may be determined by having the patient, after a minimum of 2 hours, try to swallow a small amount of water from a teaspoon or by gently touching the postpharyngeal wall with an absorbent-tipped applicator. When the normal reflexes are re-established, small amounts of fluids are given and are gradually increased if there is no vomiting. The patient is usually able to take a soft diet in 8 hours and his regular diet by the end of 24 hours. He is encouraged to rest quietly and not attempt to talk, cough or clear his throat.

Trauma of the larynx may produce hoarseness or loss of the voice; the patient needs reassurance that either is only temporary, and he is given a pencil and paper by which he can communicate.

The sputum may be streaked with blood if a biopsy was done but should clear in 24 to 48 hours. Any excessive amount of blood is reported promptly as it may manifest hemorrhage from the biopsy site.

A tracheostomy tray is kept close at hand following a bronchoscopy, for occasionally, some edema and difficulty in breathing develop. The patient is kept under close observation for several hours. Any indication of respiratory distress is brought to the physician's attention immediately.

In a bronchogram, a radiopaque liquid is injected into the tracheobronchial tree via a tube passed through the pharynx and larynx. The patient is then placed in various positions to distribute the fluid, and x-rays are taken on which the bronchial tubes are outlined.

Beforehand, the procedure is explained to the patient. No food or fluid is given for 6 to 8 hours preceding the bronchogram. Postural drainage (see p. 276) may be necessary before the procedure to clear the smaller distal tubes so the fluid can enter them. Dentures are removed, a mouthwash is given, and a sedative may be ordered.

Following the bronchogram, postural drainage is used to promote drainage of the fluid from the bronchial tree. Food and fluid are withheld and the same precautions used as cited above for after-care following a bronchoscopy.

Laryngoscopy may be used for direct viewing of the larynx. A laryngoscope is introduced using a local anesthesia. The care before and after the examination is similar to that necessary for the patient having a bronchoscopy.

Respiratory Function Tests. The more common ventilatory measurements are made with a spirometer and are particularly useful in assessing patients having obstructive pulmonary disease and reduced lung capacities.

VITAL CAPACITY (VC). This measures the maximum volume of air the patient can forcefully exhale into a spirometer after inhaling as deeply as possible. (Normal: 4000 to 5000 ml.) Less than 3000 ml. indicates some respiratory insufficiency.

TIMED VITAL CAPACITY (TVC). A timed vital capacity test records the percentage of vital capacity that can be expelled in 1, 2 and 3 seconds. The person is asked to take a maximum inspiration and then exhale as quickly as possible into the spirometer. Normally, about 80 per cent is expired in 1 second, 90 per cent in 2 seconds and 95 per cent within 3 seconds.

MINUTE VENTILATION (V MIN.). This represents the volume of ventilation per minute and is determined by measuring the tidal volume and multiplying that figure by the number of respirations per minute ($V_T \times f = V$ min.). The normal is about 6000 to 7500 ml.

FORCED EXPIRATORY VOLUME (FEV). This is the volume of air, recorded by a spirometer over a set period of time, that the person can exhale as rapidly as possible following a deep inspiration. This is used to determine if there is expiratory restriction.

BRONCHOSPIROMETRY. This is used to determine the capacity of each lung separately as well as the gas exchange between the alveoli of each lung and the blood. This is a more complex procedure than the measuring of the vital capacity. A double lumen tube is passed into the trachea and each bronchus is cannulated so that one lumen

connects with the right bronchus and the other with the left bronchus. One lumen is occluded in turn to measure the ventilatory capacity of the other lung; the proximal end of the tube is connected to the spirometer.

Care of the patient before and after bronchospirometry is the same as in bronchoscopy.

CARBON MONOXIDE (CO) TEST. This test provides information about the respiratory diffusion capacity and is based on the particular affinity of hemoglobin in the blood for carbon monoxide. The subject inhales a very low concentration of carbon monoxide (approximately 0.1 per cent), and the rate of uptake by the blood is determined. The latter is estimated by the difference between the concentrations in the inhaled and exhaled air. The patient is asked to hold his breath for a period of 10 seconds. Calculations may be made on a minute of regular breathing. The diffusing capacity is expressed as millimeters of CO diffused per minute per mm. Hg of the partial pressure of CO in the alveolar gas. The normal value for the person at rest is approximately 2.0 ml. per min. per mm. Hg.

Blood Tests. The following blood analyses may be made in investigating the patient with respiratory disturbances.

LEUKOCYTE COUNT. A total and differential may be ordered since this information may be useful in confirming infections and distinguishing between an acute disease, such as pneumonia, and a chronic one, such as tuberculosis. A leukocytosis with the increase being mainly in the polymorphonuclear granulocytes is generally associated with an acute infection. In chronic infection there is usually only a slight increase above the normal in the total number of leukocytes, and it is usually the lymphocytes that account for any increase. The eosinophils are increased in allergic asthma.

ERYTHROCYTE COUNT AND HEMOGLOBIN DETERMINATION. It is important to know if the erythrocyte count is normal since they contain the hemoglobin which carries the oxygen. Similarly, an assessment of the patient includes a determination of the hemoglobin concentration. Obviously, a deficiency of red blood cells or hemoglobin may produce an oxygen deficiency.

BLOOD GAS ANALYSIS. Determinations of the partial pressures of oxygen and carbon dioxide and of the hydrogen ion concentration of the arterial blood are valuable in diagnosis and progress assessment of patients with respiratory disorders.

Normal values:

pO_2	85 to 100 mm. Hg
pCO_2	35 to 40 mm. Hg
pH	7.35 to 7.45
CO_2	20 to 32 mEq./L.

LACTIC DEHYDROGENASE LEVEL (LDH). This is a cellular enzyme which promotes the conversion of lactic acid to pyruvic acid in metabolism. Injury or destruction of cells containing the enzyme results in its release into the plasma. Since this enzyme is characteristic of lung tissue cells, an elevation in its plasma concentration may confirm suspected cellular destruction such as occurs in pulmonary infarction.

Normal: 165 to 300 units

Hypoxia

Hypoxia may be defined as a deficiency of oxygen in the tissues. It may be due to external or internal factors and may be classified as arterial, anemic, circulatory or metabolic.

Arterial hypoxia indicates a lower than normal oxygen tension of the arterial blood due to a deficiency in oxygenation of the blood in the lungs. It may be caused by insufficient oxygen in the atmosphere; by hypoventilation of the alveoli due to interference with air entering the lungs, weak respirations or a reduction in functional alveoli; by reduced diffusion through the alveolar membrane; or by a mixing of venous and arterial blood via veno-arterial shunts as occurs in some congenital cardiac anomalies.

Anemic hypoxia is an oxygen deficiency in the blood due to a deficiency of hemoglobin to transport oxygen. Fewer than the normal number of erythrocytes or less than a normal complement of hemoglobin in the erythrocytes reduces the volume of oxygen uptake by the blood. This may also occur as a result of a chemical alteration of the hemoglobin to a form that reduces its oxygen-carrying function. An example of this is seen in carbon monoxide poisoning associated with prolonged inhalation of fuel gas or the gas from the exhaust of a motor car. The offending gas unites with hemoglobin even more readily than oxygen to form a more stable compound than oxyhemoglobin.

Circulatory hypoxia is due to inadequate delivery of sufficient oxygenated blood to the tissues. Cardiac failure or shock may account for a generalized hypoxia. Hypoxia may occur in just one area of the body as a result of a localized circulatory deficiency which could be caused by a thrombus or embolism or by interference with the venous return.

Metabolic hypoxia is an imbalance between the oxygen demands of the tissue cells and the quantity of oxygen available. The oxygen concentration of the arterial blood may be normal but the needs of the cells exceed the normal. Metabolic hypoxia may also occur because the tissues are unable to use the available oxygen. There may be some defect in the enzyme system that prevents the normal oxidative processes. This may occur in narcotic or cyanide poisoning and may also be referred to as histotoxic hypoxia.

Symptoms of Hypoxia. The symptoms presented depend on the severity of the condition and whether it is acute or chronic. If it is chronic, physiological adaptation by increasing the number of red blood cells may occur, such as is seen when a person resides at a high altitude. Acute hypoxia is manifested by rapid respirations interspersed with sighing and yawning and a rapid pulse which becomes weak as the myocardium suffers oxygen deficiency. If the hypoxia persists, respirations gradually fail as the respiratory center becomes depressed. Reduced mental activity and cellular metabolism produce a large range of symptoms. Early manifestations may be headache, restlessness, weakness and loss of visual acuity. As the oxygen supply to the brain diminishes, reduced mental efficiency may progress through confusion and stupor to coma. The patient may experience nausea and vomiting and may complain of precordial pain. Cyanosis is seen due to an excessive reduction of oxyhemoglobin. Since it is dependent on the presence of reduced hemoglobin, cyanosis is not present in those whose hemoglobin is reduced to 5 to 6 grams per cent or less.

Oxygen administration is used to increase the oxygen tension in the alveoli in conjunction with treatment directed toward the cause of the hypoxia. The patient is kept at rest to reduce his oxygen needs to a minimum.

Hypercapnia and Hypocapnia

Hypercapnia is an excessive retention of carbon dioxide in the body. It may occur as a result of insufficient pulmonary ventilation or impaired circulation. It develops more slowly than hypoxemia and does not necessarily occur when oxygen diffusion in the lungs is restricted, since CO_2 is more soluble and diffuses more readily and in greater amounts than O_2. A diminished movement of air in and out of the lungs decreases CO_2 elimination, and reduced circulation allows the gas to accumulate in the tissues. Hypercapnia may be reflected by changes in the activities of the pulmonary, central nervous and circulatory systems and the kidneys. The increase in CO_2 stimulates respirations and the rate and volume show a notable increase. The associated increased respiratory efforts cause the patient to experience severe dyspnea. If the hypercapnia becomes chronic, there is a decreased respiratory response as the respiratory chemoreceptors and center become accustomed to the higher pCO_2 of the blood. Respiration becomes more dependent on the hypoxic drive. Under such conditions, the administration of oxygen may depress respirations by removing the necessary hypoxic stimulus.

The central nervous system is depressed as a result of dilation of the cerebral blood vessels which causes edema and increased intracranial pressure. The patient experiences a headache and lethargy and may progress to a stuporous or comatose state. The retained CO_2 increases the hydrogen ion concentration (decreased pH) because of the increased formation of carbonic acid (H_2CO_3). The bicarbonate (HCO_3^-) becomes depleted, and respiratory acidosis develops.

Circulatory changes include dilation of peripheral vessels and vasoconstriction of the pulmonary vessels, which further aggravates the problem. The pulse rate and blood pressure rise; if the pCO_2 progressively increases, cardiac arrhythmias, myocardial depression and hypotension may develop. The urine becomes more acid as the kidneys form more HCO_3^- ions and reabsorb more sodium.

Hypocapnia is a decrease in the pCO_2 of the blood below normal. It is generally due to an excessive loss by hyperventilation, occurring as a result of hypermetabolism, overstimulation of the respiratory center by an intracranial disorder, salicylate poisoning or anxiety. Manifestations include slower deep respirations and disturbed cerebral function. The patient develops alkalosis as less carbon dioxide is available to form carbonic acid (H_2CO_3).

Respiratory Insufficiency

Respiratory insufficiency or failure is present when a person can no longer maintain normal arterial levels of oxygen and carbon dioxide.

The cause may be impaired ventilation, impaired diffusion, defective perfusion or transportation or a combination of these. The patient may manifest signs and symptoms of hypoxia and hypercapnia with a resultant decrease in the pH (acidosis) (see p. 63). In some instances, the PaO_2 may be below normal, and the $PaCO_2$ remains normal or below normal. This is accounted for by an increase in respirations in response to an increased CO_2 level and more is eliminated because of its greater solubility and dissociation. The conditions in which this occurs most often are those in which there is an imbalance in ventilation and perfusion. That is, areas of alveoli may be poorly ventilated but there is a normal flow of blood through the associated pulmonary capillaries, or the alveoli may be adequately ventilated but the pulmonary capillaries in areas may be underperfused. The adequately ventilated alveoli increase the total physiological dead space, for the air in the underperfused alveoli does not take part in gas exchange.

Ventilatory dysfunction may be due to obstructive or restrictive forces which impede the normal flow of air or to weakness or paralysis of the respiratory muscles. Obstructive and restrictive conditions in which the lumen of the air passages may be narrowed and/or there is reduced compliance include respiratory infection, retained secretions, hyperactive bronchial muscle tissue (e.g., asthma), aspirated foreign body, neoplasm, and deformity (e.g., kyphosis) or injury of the chest wall. Weakness or paralysis of the respiratory muscles may be associated with depression of the respiratory center by drug intoxication or excessive oxygen administration, pressure on the respiratory center as a result of an intracranial disease or injury, electric shock, poliomyelitis, myasthenia gravis, tetanus or polymyositis. Rarely, ventilatory insufficiency may be due to the lack of available air (suffocation) or to an abnormally low atmospheric pressure (high altitude).

Alveolar-capillary gas exchange may be impaired by pulmonary fibrosis, emphysema, edema or more often by ventilatory maldistribution such as occurs in atelectasis (collapse of a portion of a lung) or decreased pulmonary perfusion.

Conditions which may cause defective perfusion of the pulmonary blood vessels or impaired transportation of the respiratory gases include pulmonary thrombosis or embolism, a circulatory shunt resulting in blood bypassing the lung, anemia, circulatory failure (heart failure, shock) and carbon monoxide poisoning.

Certain factors are known to predispose to respiratory insufficiency. These include pre-existing pulmonary disease, immobility, coma, smoking, prolonged exposure to chemicals or air pollutants, pain or abdominal distention which tends to restrict the respiratory excursion, obesity, central nervous system depressants and the early and late years of life. In relation to age, in the infant and young child the lumen of the tracheobronchial tree is small and occludes more readily; in the elderly the cough is weak, the respirations are shallow and pulmonary edema develops more readily.

Treatment and Nursing Care. In caring for the patient with respiratory insufficiency, therapeutic measures are directed toward the correction of disorders in the blood gases, elimination of the primary cause, reduction of the demand for oxygen and the production of carbon dioxide to a minimum and control of infection.

Respiratory difficulty is a frightening experience for the patient; reassurance is given that his difficulty is recognized and that certain measures are being employed to provide relief. Mounting anxiety only increases the patient's demand for oxygen. Frequent determinations of the blood gas tensions, pH, and the tidal and minute volumes as well as the patient's general condition and primary disorder influence the therapeutic measures used. The patient requires constant attention. Nursing will be concerned with frequent assessment of the patient's respiratory rate, depth and sounds, his blood pressure, pulse, color and level of consciousness. It is also important to note his ability to cough and expectorate pulmonary secretions. Various procedures may be used to promote clearance of the airway and improve ventilation. These may include frequent change of position, postural drainage, physical therapy, medicinal preparations of expectorants and bronchodilators, suctioning, humidification of inspired air, oxygen inhalation, tracheal intubation, tracheostomy and mechanical ventilation.

POSTURAL DRAINAGE. To promote the elimination of pulmonary secretions, the patient may be placed in a position that initiates gravitational movement of the fluid and mucus to a level in the tracheobronchial tree that favors removal by coughing or suctioning. This may be carried out as part of a physical therapy program in which the special positioning is preceded by clapping of the chest to dislodge secretions. A bronchodilator may be administered just before each period of clapping and positioning. The position assumed depends on the area to be drained. An explanation is made to the patient before starting so that he will know what to expect and that he will be required to cough and attempt to raise the secretions.

The patient's condition and treatments being used (e.g., intravenous infusion) may necessitate modification of some positions, but the nurse should be familiar with the one appropriate to the drainage of various lung segments. To promote the movement of secretions out of upper lobes, the patient is placed in a sitting position and alternately leans forward and to each side to drain different segments. For drainage of middle and lower lobes, various side-lying, prone and supine positions are used. The patient may be horizontal or, to remove accumulations in lower segments, he may be tilted so that his head and chest are lower. An ambulatory patient may be positioned prone crosswise on the bed so that his head and thorax are dependent over one side. This position especially facilitates drainage of larger bronchial tubes, and if used, precautions are necessary to ensure safety and to prevent a fall and possible injury. The nurse remains with the patient each time until assured that he can safely handle the situation.

Each position is maintained for a minimum of 5 minutes if possible. The patient is then encouraged to cough, and suctioning may also be necessary to assist in eliminating the dislodged secretions.

BRONCHODILATORS AND EXPECTORANTS. Drugs which dilate the bronchial tubes may be used locally in the form of an aerosol preparation* or may be administered by the conventional routes. Examples of drugs used in aerosol form are isoproterenol (Isuprel), corticosteroid (dexamethasone) and epinephrine (Adrenalin). Bronchodilators given orally or parenterally include aminophylline, corticosteroid (Prednisone) and isoproterenol (Isuprel).

Similarly, preparations which promote the liquefaction and removal of pulmonary secretions may be used locally or given in internal systemic form. Those used locally in aerosol form are mucolytic agents. Examples of these include tyloxapol (Alevaire) and sodium ethasulfate (Tergemist), which are detergents mainly, acetylcysteine, and trypsin (Tryptar). Preparations of ammonium hydrochloride or potassium iodide may be given orally as expectorants.

A minimum fluid intake of 3000 ml., unless contraindicated by circulatory or renal insufficiency, and adequate humidification of the inspired gas are generally considered very effective expectorants.

CONTROL OF INFECTION. The patient with respiratory failure is very susceptible to infection. Frequently, it is the cause of the insufficiency, and a secondary invasion may readily be imposed on the primary infection. A minimum number of staff members should have contact with the patient, and obviously, no one with an infection, especially if it is respiratory, is permitted to care for the patient. Adequate facilities must be available for frequent hand washing. The nurse wears sterile gloves when handling the sterile catheter for deep suctioning and

a catheter is used only once for the procedure. Precautions are taken to prevent traumatizing the respiratory tract mucosa by gentle handling of the catheter and prompt release of the negative pressure should the mucosa be "drawn into" the opening of the tube. Placement on the ward receives consideration; the patient is not located next to someone with an infection of different cause. Visitors are restricted and screened.

A broad-spectrum, antimicrobial preparation is administered until the causative organism and its sensitivity are determined by culturing a specimen of the tract secretions.

As well as observing measures to protect the patient, if his problem is of infectious origin, the practice of strict medical asepsis is necessary to protect other patients.

SUCTIONING. This is a very important procedure that is used frequently to remove secretions in respiratory conditions. A catheter, connected to wall suction or a suction machine, may be passed gently into the oropharynx or through an endotracheal or tracheostomy tube into the trachea or proximal portion of either bronchus. An ordinary or whistle-tip catheter may be used for suctioning in the oropharynx. For deeper aspiration of secretions, a whistle-tip or, more often, a coude (bent) tip catheter is used. The size varies with the size of the patient or according to the size of the endotracheal or tracheostomy tube when either is used. An average size used with an adult is a number F. 14 or 16. When suctioning through a tube, the catheter should be smaller than the lumen of the tube to avoid too great a negative pressure that might cause atelectasis. If the suction catheter is too small, the procedure may be ineffective, especially if the secretions are thick and tenacious.

The introduction of the catheter through the mouth or nose into the oropharynx frequently initiates the cough reflex, resulting in the removal of deeper secretions as well as the aspiration of those in the pharynx.

When tracheal suctioning is done, the catheter is attached to one arm of a Y connecting tube which is connected to the source of the negative pressure. The free arm of the connecting tube acts as a vent. Precautions are observed to prevent the

---

*In an aerosol preparation, fine particles of a drug are suspended in a gas. It may be inhaled into the air passages or forced in by means of an intermittent positive-pressure respirator.

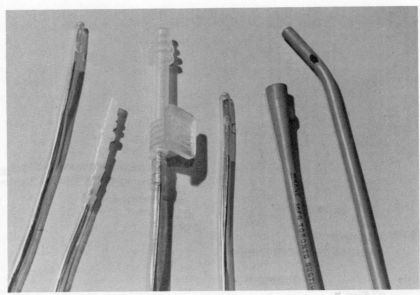

Figure 14–2 Three suction catheters, showing both ends. The center catheter has a special connecting tube which eliminates the need for a Y tube; the flat, square portion has an opening which serves as a vent. (Note: Wires have been inserted in these catheters to facilitate positioning them for photography.) (Courtesy of the New Mount Sinai Hospital, Toronto.)

introduction of infection. The hands are thoroughly washed and sterile gloves are worn to handle the catheter, which is also sterile. Before the catheter is passed into the trachea, it is moistened in sterile water or normal saline. While the catheter is being inserted, the vent on the **Y** tube is left open. When the tip of the catheter has reached the desired lower level, a finger is placed over the vent to establish suction. The aspiration must be brief, since it removes air as well as secretions, and the patient's respiratory insufficiency may be increased if the procedure is prolonged. Suctioning must not extend beyond 15 seconds. The catheter is slowly withdrawn while being gently rotated; suction is continued during the removal of the tube. If the aspiration was not sufficiently effective, allow ventilation for a few minutes before repeating the procedure. A fresh sterile catheter is used for each insertion.

Aspiration of the bronchi necessitates the use of a coude catheter and the introduction of its tip into the bronchus to be suctioned. Entry of the left bronchus is facilitated by having the patient turned partially on his left side with his head turned to the right and his chin up. To suction the opposite bronchus, the position is reversed.

The frequency of suctioning is determined according to the accumulation of secretions; unnecessary aspiration increases the risk of trauma to the mucosa by the tube. On the

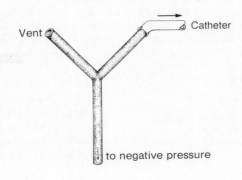

other hand, if the secretions are profuse, frequent suctioning must be done to promote adequate ventilation. When possible, the procedure is done when the cuff on the airway tube is deflated, the patient's position is changed, and regularly timed therapeutic activities are carried out. The patient may then have an undisturbed period.

Adequate humidification of the air or air-oxygen mixture that is inspired contributes to liquefaction of the pulmonary secretions, facilitating their elimination either by coughing or suctioning.

HUMIDIFICATION. Care of a patient with a respiratory disorder must give consideration to the need for humidification of the inspired air or oxygen. Normally, air is warmed and moistened as it passes through the upper air passages. This is necessary for normal functioning of the lower tract mucosa as it constantly produces a watery mucus that is continuously removed by the cilia. This sweeping out of the mucus is an important protective mechanism; it removes foreign particles, microorganisms and tissue debris. Lack of adequate humidification of the inspired gas promotes the drying of mucus and the retention of secretions which predisposes to infection, the plugging of bronchial tubes and the formation of crusts.

Various methods are used to humidify the air or gas to be inspired. The method de-

pends mainly on whether or not the upper airway is bypassed and the degree of dehydration of the secretions.

A steam kettle, vaporizer or room humidifier is probably the simplest means of increasing the moisture in the inspired air. Compressed oxygen is dry and always requires the addition of moisture. It is usually passed through warm water before reaching the patient. A more efficient means of providing the necessary moisture, especially if the secretions are thick and tenacious, is by forcing compressed air into water, thus forming an aerosol mist which is directed into the tube leading to the airway.

OXYGEN THERAPY. Oxygen may be administered by face mask, face tent, nasal catheter or cannulae, or regular oxygen tent. When using oxygen, it should be remembered that it is colorless, odorless, tasteless and heavier than air, and that it is hazardous because it supports combustion. Certain precautions must constantly be observed to avoid possible fire. Smoking is prohibited in the area and signs indicating the restriction are posted; cigarettes, pipe and matches are removed from the patient's bedside; the use of woollen blankets and other equipment which may produce static electricity is restricted; and inflammable solutions and electrical equipment (e.g., electric razor) may not be used in the room as long as the

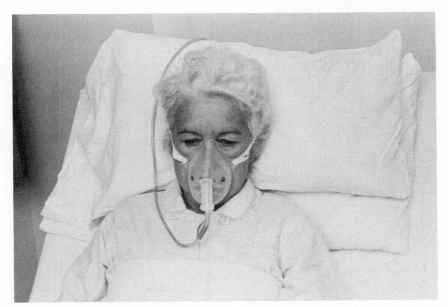

Figure 14-3 Oxygen may be administered by this type of mask. (Courtesy of the New Mount Sinai Hospital, Toronto.)

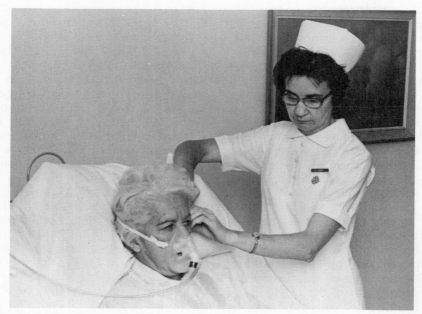

Figure 14–4 The oxygen mask with a rebreathing bag is being adjusted to fit snugly and comfortably. (Courtesy of the New Mount Sinai Hospital, Toronto.)

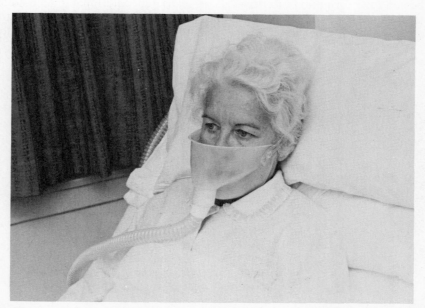

Figure 14–5 The face tent used for administering oxygen. (Courtesy of the New Mount Sinai Hospital, Toronto.)

oxygen is being given. Compressed oxygen is very dry and must be humidified before reaching the patient (see p. 279).

The face mask covers the nose and mouth and may be used to deliver relatively high concentrations of oxygen (50 to 100 per cent), depending on the type of mask used. Masks with no rebreathing bag usually have flutter valves and, if fitted snugly to the face, will provide an oxygen concentration of 60 to 80 per cent with the flow meter set at 8 to 10 liters. Masks with a reservoir bag, tightly fitted to the face, will deliver 100 per cent oxygen. The face tent is a transparent, firm, plastic mask that fits under the chin and to the sides of the face but is open at the top. Oxygen enters the lower part of the mask and, being heavier than air, does not readily escape. The flow meter on the oxygen source is usually set at 8 liters.

When a catheter is used, it is moistened and passed through a nostril into the nasopharynx. The length of tube to be inserted may be estimated by measuring the distance between the top of the nose and the ear lobe. The tip of the catheter should be visible just below the soft palate. The catheter is secured to the patient's face with adhesive, and the patient is advised to breathe through his nose if possible. Oxygen is lost if he breathes through his mouth. If the flow meter is set at 6 to 8 liters, an oxygen concentration of 30 to 40 per cent is provided. The catheter is changed every 8 to 10 hours; the nostrils are used alternately to minimize irritation.

Plastic nasal cannulae or nasoinhalors are available for the administration of an oxygen concentration up to approximately 35 per cent. Each of the two cannulae is inserted about one-half inch into a nostril. The two connect to a common tube that leads to the oxygen source.

The oxygen tent is used rarely for adults, since it is difficult to maintain a satisfactory concentration because of the repeated opening of the canopy and the fact that the oxygen, being heavier, settles to the bottom and tends to readily escape from the tent. With a high inflow of 10 to 12 liters per minute, the highest concentration inspired is about 50 per cent. However, the tent method of administration has some advantages. The patient is more comfortable and has more freedom than when a catheter

or mask is used, it is cool within the tent, and the air-oxygen mixture is adequately humidified. The clear, plastic canopy reduces the fear of being closed in that used to be experienced by patients.

ENDOTRACHEAL INTUBATION. This procedure involves the passage of a tube through the mouth or nose into the trachea to establish a free airway for the purpose of facilitating ventilation or the removal of secretions. The tube is equipped with an inflatable cuff which establishes a seal between the tube and the trachea. This prevents air from leaking out around the tube and the aspiration of secretions from the upper tract (Fig. 14–6). Inflation of the cuff is recognized by the lack of air escaping around the tube. A very slight air leak is permitted to prevent pressure necrosis of the tracheal wall by the cuff. Near the proximal end of the fine tube leading to the cuff there is a small balloon-like dilatation which remains inflated when the tube is clamped. It is observed frequently, and as long as it remains inflated, one knows the cuff is also inflated. An x-ray may be made to check the position of the tube; if the tube is too low, the inflated cuff could block off a bronchus completely. The endotracheal tube is generally used in conjunction with a respirator. It is very distressing and a source of discomfort to the conscious patient. If it is necessary for a period longer than 48 hours, a tracheostomy is done.

The cuff is deflated for 2 to 5 minutes every 1 to 2 hours to prevent ischemia and ensuing ulceration of the tracheal mucosa. Frequent mouth care is given, and suctioning of the oropharyngeal area may be necessary to remove secretions that may be a response to the presence of the tube. The removal of the secretions is especially important before deflating the cuff to prevent their entrance into the lower tract.

Frequent suctioning through the endotracheal tube is necessary. A sterile catheter is gently and quickly passed through the tube into the trachea.

TRACHEOSTOMY. The trachea is opened anteriorly, and a tube is inserted to establish an airway that bypasses the larynx and air passages above. A tracheostomy may be done because of an upper airway obstruction, prolonged, mechanically assisted ventilation, or the need for more efficient access

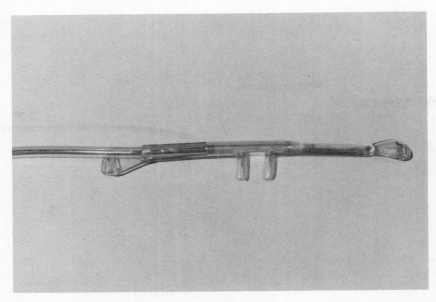

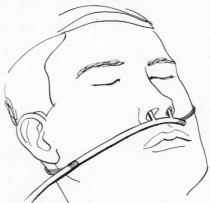

Figure 14–6 Plastic cannulae or prongs which are inserted into the nostrils to deliver oxygen. (Courtesy of the New Mount Sinai Hospital, Toronto.)

to retained tracheobronchial secretions which, unless removed, may cause serious respiratory problems, such as atelectasis and pneumonia.

It may be used in primary respiratory disorders, but it is frequently necessary with patients whose respiratory difficulty or insufficiency is secondary to trauma or disease elsewhere. For example, it may be necessary following cerebral injury or cardiac surgery or for the patient with myasthenia gravis who has developed dysfunction of the respiratory muscles. A tracheostomy reduces the work of breathing by eliminating the resistance offered by the upper airway. It also reduces the dead space by almost

50 per cent (the normal is approximately 150 ml.).

Since endotracheal intubation has been more commonly used, the incidence of emergency tracheostomy has been greatly reduced. The current procedure is generally elective and carried out under aseptic conditions in an operating room. The patient receives more careful preparation and has an airway already established through an endotracheal tube, which makes possible the administration of a general anesthetic if it is considered necessary.

With the neck well extended, a vertical or horizontal incision is made approximately 2 cm. above the suprasternal notch to

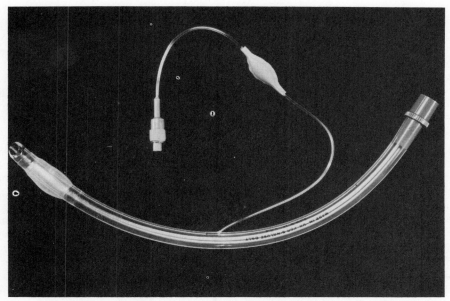

Figure 14–7 An endotracheal tube with an inflatable cuff which provides a seal between the trachea and tube. After the tube is inserted, the cuff is inflated by the introduction of a specified volume of air through the fine attached tube, which is then clamped. (Courtesy of the New Mount Sinai Hospital, Toronto.)

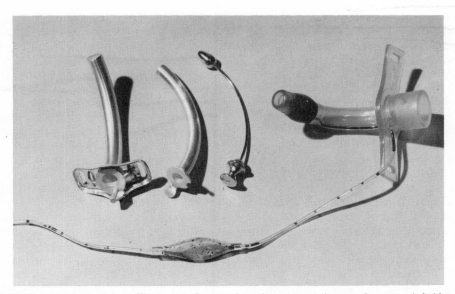

Figure 14–8 Tracheostomy tubes. The parts of a metal tracheostomy tube are shown on left (the outer and inner cannulae and the obturator, which is used during the insertion of the outer cannula into the trachea). The polyethylene tube on the right has an inflatable cuff at the distal end to provide a seal between the tube and the trachea. (Courtesy of the New Mount Sinai Hospital, Toronto.)

expose the upper part of the trachea. The latter is then opened usually at the level of the second or third cartilaginous ring, and a tracheostomy tube is introduced. The tube is held in position by laterally attached tapes which are tied securely around the patient's neck with his head flexed forward.

The tracheostomy tube may be made of silver or synthetic material, such as plastic and polyethylene, and may be single or may consist of 2 parts, an inner and outer cannula. When the metal one is used, the outer tube is fitted with an obturator that extends beyond the distal end of the tube. The end is blunt and smooth and facilitates the introduction of the tube. As soon as the tube is in position, the obturator is removed and the inner tube is inserted and secured. The latter can be removed and cleansed of secretions at frequent intervals while the outer cannula maintains a patent airway. The cannulae and obturators of the double tubes are not interchangeable.

Most of the synthetic tubes have a cuff which encircles the lower part of the outer tubes. After the tube is in position, the cuff is inflated by the introduction of a small amount of air via a fine tube that leads into it. The cuff creates a seal between the trachea and the tube and prevents air from entering or escaping around the tube as well as the aspiration of secretions or fluid into the tract below. This type of tube is used most frequently in patients who require mechanical assistance in breathing. A disadvantage of the cuff is possible ulceration of the tracheal mucosa due to pressure at the site. The cuff must be deflated at frequent, regular intervals and left deflated for a stated period of time. The amount of air required to produce a seal without unnecessary pressure varies from 2 to 10 cc. While introducing the air, the nurse listens and tests for the escape of air from around the tube. The tube may be blocked off momentarily while testing for leakage around the tube. On completing the inflation, the end of the fine tube is clamped with a small hemostat. The amount of air used in inflating the cuff is recorded each time; any significant change from one time to another is reported. A decreased amount may indicate swelling and edema of the air passage. Near the proximal end of the fine inflating tube is a small balloon-like dilatation. This is inflated and,

being visible, may be checked frequently to determine if the tube and the cuff below remain inflated. Obviously, if the small pilot balloon becomes deflated, a leak in the system is indicated, and the cuff will be deflated, thus losing the intratracheal seal.

Tracheostomy tubes are available in various sizes and number from 2 to 8 according to their internal diameter in millimeters. A No. 6 (internal diameter, 6 mm.) is commonly used for adults.

A small, dry dressing or a piece of gauze impregnated with petrolatum jelly is placed between the flanges of the tube and the wound. If the tube is open (i.e., no respirator is attached) a single layer of gauze (without any absorbent) may be placed over it to prevent the entrance of foreign particles.

Tracheostomy Care. If the patient is sufficiently alert and the delay does not invoke any risk, he is advised preferably by the physician about the need for a tracheostomy and what it involves. An explanation is made of his breathing through the tube and his temporary loss of voice. He is then reassured that provision will be made for him to communicate by writing if he wishes and that someone will be in frequent attendance. A similar explanation is given to the family.

Although a tracheostomy is frequently a life-saving measure, it does have certain significant disadvantages. These include loss of filtration and humidification of the inspired air, which is normally done by the upper air passages, and loss of the cough reflex as well as the verbal means of communication. The entry of unmoistened air predisposes to irritation of the lower tract mucosa and the drying of secretions, making them difficult to raise. Direct entrance of air into the trachea without filtration also permits ready inhalation of dust and microorganisms into the lungs.

Preparation to receive the patient following a tracheostomy includes assembling the following: suction equipment with sterile catheters of various sizes (Fr. 12, 14, 16 and 18); equipment for humidification of the air or air-oxygen mixture; respirator; Ambu bag; a sterile surgical tray with obturator of the tracheostomy tube, extra sterile tracheostomy tube in case the one inserted becomes dislodged, tape for securing the tube in place, gauze squares, forceps and tracheal dilator; syringe to inflate the cuff if a cuffed tube is used, and hemostats to clamp the tube leading to the cuff; equipment for frequent mouth cleansing; and a pencil and pad or slate.

Following the surgery, the head of the bed is elevated to approximately 45° when the patient regains consciousness and his blood pressure and pulse are stable. Constant nursing attention is necessary for at least the first 24 to 36 hours. The patient is likely to be fearful about his breathing and, being unable to speak, may panic if left alone.

Frequent observations are made of the patient's blood pressure, pulse, color, respiratory rate and sounds, movement of both sides of the chest, tidal and minute volumes and of the tracheal tube for patency. The wound around the tube is examined for possible bleeding and the characteristics of the tracheobronchial secretions are noted. The patient may still experience respiratory insufficiency due to obstruction in the tract below the tracheostomy. This could be evidenced by marked respiratory effort, unequal movement of the sides of the chest and retraction of the soft tissues in the intercostal and supraclavicular spaces. Cyanosis and distress not relieved by suctioning is reported promptly. Increasing restlessness, especially if accompanied by a rapid pulse rate, may indicate hypoxia or bleeding. Undue apprehension is reported to the physician as it may have an adverse effect on the patient's breathing and heart action. An x-ray may be done daily for 2 or 3 days to determine whether the tube is in the right position and to check the lungs for retained secretions, atelectasis and congestion.

Increased secretion occurs in response to the tracheal trauma and is usually colored by blood at first, but the blood content should gradually diminish and disappear. If frank blood appears or if bright blood-colored secretion persists beyond the first 6 to 8 hours, the surgeon is informed, as it may indicate bleeding into the tract. Suctioning through the tube is necessary to maintain a clear airway. It generally has to be done often the first 12 to 24 hours. Frequent introduction of the catheter into the trachea predisposes to irritation and trauma of the mucosa. As the secretions diminish, the interval between suctionings is gradually lengthened. If the secretion is thick and tenacious, the surgeon may recommend the instillation of approximately 2 to 3 ml. of saline into the trachea just before suctioning. For further details on the procedure see the section on Suctioning on page 277.

The wound is protected by a piece of sterile gauze placed under and around the tracheostomy tube. It is changed as often as necessary to keep the wound clean and dry; moisture predisposes to infection and maceration of the area. Using aseptic technique, the skin around the wound may be cleansed with sterile normal saline or a mild antiseptic as ordered. Precautions must be taken to prevent displacement of the tube; the tapes which secure it are checked frequently. It is necessary to remove and clean the inner cannula of the tracheostomy tube at frequent intervals to keep it free of mucus and encrustations. It is cleansed with a cold solution of hydrogen peroxide or sodium bicarbonate and then is washed with detergent, using a small tube-brush for the interior. The cannula is then sterilized, reinserted in the outer tube and locked in position. While the inner cannula is out, the outer tube is suctioned and cleansed. In some instances, a second sterile inner cannula of the same size as the one being removed is available for prompt replacement. The outer cannula is only changed by the doctor. If a cuffed tracheostomy tube is used, the cuff is deflated at regular intervals to prevent pressure necrosis of the trachea. Should the tube come out of the trachea because of vigorous coughing or carelessly tied tapes, the tracheal opening closes and the patient is threatened with asphyxia. Prompt action is necessary. The tracheal wound is quickly reopened with the sterile tracheal dilator or a hemostat which is always kept at the bedside in the event of such an emergency. The opening is held open until the doctor arrives and inserts the sterile tracheostomy tube, which must also always be available at the bedside.

If a mechanical ventilator is needed, a flexible swivel-connector is used to attach the ventilatory tube of the machine to the tracheostomy tube. This permits movement and turning of the patient with minimal risk of moving or dislodging the tracheostomy tube.

Oral hygiene is important to the patient's comfort and to reduce the possibility of infection. The mouth is cleansed and rinsed every 2 hours until the patient is taking normal meals, when regular cleansing of the teeth and rinsing of the mouth after each meal and at bedtime suffice.

The patient is encouraged to take extra fluids; a minimum of 3000 ml. is recommended to help liquefy the pulmonary secretions. An accurate record is kept of the intake and output. If he is unable to take sufficient fluids orally, intravenous solutions may be given. A soft diet is introduced a day or two after the surgery and is increased to a regular diet as soon as it can be tolerated. The patient is fed by the nurse at first as he is likely to have some apprehension about taking food for fear of choking.

A mild sedative or a tranquilizer may be ordered if the patient is fearful and emotionally disturbed. Morphine and narcotics, which depress the respiratory center and the cough reflex, are not generally used. His needs should be anticipated as much as possible, but he is also encouraged to use a slate or pad to communicate his "feelings" and needs.

When the tracheostomy is a temporary measure to improve ventilation, the patient is gradually returned to breathing through the upper tract. This may be done by the insertion of a special tube with a small opening into the tracheostomy tube. If this smaller opening is tolerated by the patient, the tube is removed and the wound closed. The patient may be fearful of not being able to breathe when the tube is removed; he is assured beforehand that his breathing is adequate via the normal route. A nurse remains with him following the removal to be certain that he experiences no difficulty. Blood specimens may be taken for a day or two to determine the PaO_2 and $PaCO_2$ levels. Following discharge, the patient who has had a tracheostomy is followed by his doctor or at clinic for at least a year. He is checked for possible scarring and tracheal stricture resulting from irritation and trauma.

If the tracheostomy is permanent, the patient is instructed about the care of the tube and the stoma (an artificial opening to the surface). This is done as soon as he is well enough to undertake the care in the hospital and develop confidence. A member of the family also receives the instruction about the necessary care and precautions.

A patient may continue to have excessive secretions and may require suction equipment at home. In this case, a family member is advised where such equipment may be obtained (e.g., the National Cancer Society) and, with the patient, is instructed in the use and care of the equipment. They are advised how to conceal the site of the tracheostomy. The shirt will cover the stoma in a man; a woman may wear a scarf or a high-necked blouse or dress.

An explanation is made of the danger of aspirating water through the tracheostomy tube; this precludes swimming or immersion in water to a high level. Precautions must also be used when taking a shower.

The patient is advised to return to the clinic or to his physician at regular intervals as directed for changing of the tube and examination of the stoma. Eventually, when the stoma is firmly healed and the tracheal opening remains patent, the doctor may permit the patient or a member of the family to change the outer cannula. Precautions should be used to avoid close contact with those in his environment with respiratory infection.

Mechanical Ventilation. When a patient is unable to adequately ventilate his lungs and maintain a satisfactory level of blood oxygenation and elimination of carbon dioxide, a mechanical respirator is used to inflate the lungs or assist the patient's inspiratory effort. The machine intermittently introduces air or a mixture of oxygen and air into the patient's airway by means of producing a positive pressure.* Expiration is passive when the inflow-regulating valve on the ventilator automatically closes. The respirator is connected to the patient's airway by means of a mask or an endotracheal or tracheostomy tube.

The machine may be designed to deliver a fixed volume of gas with each inspiratory phase (volume-cycled) or to deliver gas until a preset pressure (pressure-cycled) is achieved. In the second method the same pressure is reached in each inspiratory phase; with the volume-cycled machine, the preset volume of gas is delivered with what-

---

*Positive pressure implies a gas pressure greater than that of the atmosphere.

ever pressure is needed to deliver it. This may be elevated if the pulmonary resistance is increased. The respirator may be used to provide controlled ventilation or assisted ventilation. In controlled ventilation, the machine is set for automatic operation and produces a fixed number of cycles per minute, regardless of the patient's respiratory effort. It is important that the patient's spontaneous respirations be synchronized with the respirator. The patient is advised to relax and breathe with the machine. Occasionally, the patient "fights the respirator," finding it difficult to regulate his respirations to the machine. This reduces effective ventilation and should be brought to the physician's attention. In assisted ventilation, the inspiratory phase of the respirator's cycle is triggered by the patient's spontaneous inspiration, complementing his ventilatory volume. These machines are equipped with a safety control, so that if the patient fails to trigger an assistive cycle by a preset interval of time, controlled ventilation automatically takes over. All respirators have some means of humidifying the gas before it reaches the patient's airway.

When mechanical respiration is necessary, the physician indicates the machine settings which include controlled or assisted ventilation, the pressure, volume and mixture of gas to be delivered, and the number of cycles per minute. Many hospitals now have a staff of inhalation technicians who are available to assist with the operation of respirators. The nurse caring for a patient receiving mechanical ventilation must be familiar with the underlying principles, the operation of the particular machine being used, and the immediate indications of mechanical malfunction or untoward reactions in the patient and the appropriate action. It is essential that adequate instruction and supervision be given, reading references and visual aids be provided, and the specific directives prepared by the manufacturer are reviewed before the nurse assumes responsibility for the patient.

An Ambu bag, which is a self-inflating, manually operated bag with an expiratory valve, is kept at the bedside at all times. It is used to ventilate the patient in the event of mechanical failure of the respirator and when treatments or tests necessitate interruption.

Frequent determinations of the gas tensions of the arterial blood are made. The findings may indicate necessary corrective adjustments in the machine settings. For example, the flow rate of oxygen may have to be increased to provide a higher inhalation percentage. If the pCO_2 is below normal, the dead space may be increased by lengthening the tube between the patient and respirator or the number of cycles may be reduced. Lengthening the tube promotes rebreathing of some of the exhaled CO_2. Serum

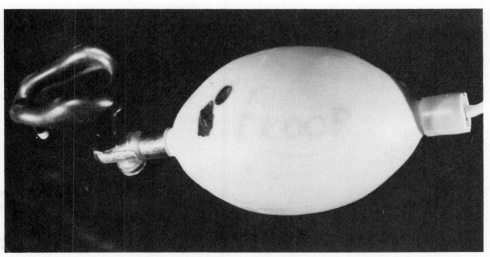

Figure 14–9 An Ambu bag which is manually operated to ventilate a patient in an emergency or when mechanical respiratory assistance is interrupted. (Courtesy of the New Mount Sinai Hospital, Toronto.)

electrolyte levels are determined frequently; changes may occur, especially in bicarbonate, sodium and potassium concentrations.

If the patient is sufficiently alert, an explanation of the respirator and its purpose is made. A nurse remains in constant attendance. Nursing responsibilities include frequent regular observation and recording (at least hourly) of the patient's blood pressure, radial and apical pulses, color, chest excursions (both sides), level of consciousness and reaction to the respirator. Underventilation may cause an increase in the blood pressure for a brief period, then a gradual fall. An increase in the rate and decrease in the volume of the pulse may indicate deterioration of the condition or may be the result of excessive intrathoracic pressure on inspiration. This excessive pressure reduces venous return, and subsequently, cardiac output is reduced. Reduced alertness or level of consciousness may be associated with insufficient blood oxygenation. The patient's tidal volume and minute ventilation are recorded hourly. The former may be measured by using a Wright respirometer or a built-in arrangement on the ventilator. A regular check is made of the peak inflationary pressure indicated on the pressure gauge. The pressure is rarely allowed to exceed 30 cm. of water; as cited previously, excessive pressure may diminish venous return to the heart.

The central venous pressure may be monitored hourly. A catheter is passed into the superior vena cava and is kept open between readings by maintaining an intravenous infusion. Abnormal intrathoracic pressures and venous return to the heart are reflected in central venous pressure. The physician generally indicates the range within which he wishes the pressure maintained; any deviation is promptly reported. The patient's fluid intake and output are accurately measured and the balance is noted.

The patient's airway must be kept as clear as possible. The nurse listens for breath sounds and notes increasing resistance to ventilation that indicate the need for suctioning. When the respirator is disconnected, the patient may be encouraged to cough. Regular turning and chest physical therapy are carried out to promote drainage. While the respirator is detached, 6 to 8 deep inflations with the Ambu bag may also be used. This may not be necessary if the respirator can be set to deliver deeper volume inflations ("sigh inspirations") at intervals to ensure greater alveolar ventilation. If an endotracheal tube or tracheostomy is used, hourly deflation of the cuff is necessary (see p. 281).

When caring for the patient who is being treated by a mechanical ventilator, the nurse must guard against becoming so occupied with the machines and technical procedures that the patient as a person is forgotten. Being unable to communicate verbally, he is dependent upon signs and facial and eye expressions to convey feelings and needs unless he is able to write and provision is made for him to do so. The family may be quite disturbed and fearful, especially on their initial visit. An explanation and reassurance should be provided.

If prolonged mechanical ventilation is necessary, the patient becomes very dependent on the respirator and is fearful of its discontinued use. Gradual weaning from the machine is introduced as soon as the tidal volume and blood gases reach satisfactory levels. It is important that use of the respiratory muscles be re-established as soon as possible in order to prevent loss of tone and slowness of response. The patient is taken off the machine for brief periods, which are progressively increased. A nurse remains with the patient during these periods and the patient's physiological responses, as well as the emotional reaction, are noted. The blood gas tensions, tidal volume, minute ventilation and vital capacity are assessed.

DISORDERS OF THE LARYNX

Disease of the larynx can present serious respiratory disturbance since the glottis narrows the air passageway. Children are particularly susceptible because their glottis and laryngeal space are much smaller. Any constriction or obstruction in the larynx is manifested quickly by dyspnea, stridor (high-pitched crowing breath sound), cyanosis, and increased but ineffective inspiratory effort which is evidenced by the retraction of the intercostal spaces. Prompt emergency treatment is necessary or death may ensue quickly as a result of asphyxia.

Laryngitis

Inflammation of the mucous membrane of the larynx may be acute or chronic. The acute form is usually caused by infection but may occur with the inhalation of irritant gases. Chronic laryngitis may develop as a result of excessive smoking, overuse of the voice, chronic alcoholism or repeated acute attacks. The mucous membrane is swollen and congested and the voice is hoarse or may be reduced to a whisper.

Laryngitis is treated by general rest and voice rest, the inhalation of warm moist air and restricted smoking. If the cause is infection, a specific antimicrobial drug will most likely be prescribed.

Obstruction of the Larynx

Edema, laryngeal spasm or aspiration of a foreign body may cause obstruction in the larynx. Severe edema and swelling of the larynx may develop rapidly and close off the glottis, completely obstructing the airway. It may occur as a result of serious inflammation, as in diphtheria and scarlet fever, or of an allergic response to a drug or foreign protein in hypersensitive individuals. Edema sometimes follows trauma that unavoidably may accompany examination by a laryngoscope or bronchoscope.

Laryngeal Spasm

A spasm of the muscle tissue within the walls of the larynx may occur occasionally following some types of general anesthesia and may seriously restrict the air passage; or it may be seen rarely in persons with a low calcium blood level. The latter is usually accompanied by other skeletal muscle hyperirritability and spasm, and the condition is known as tetany.

A foreign body that is aspirated may lodge above the narrow opening of the glottis, interfering with movement of air in and out of the tract and with vibration of the vocal cords. If a foreign body is known to be the cause, the patient should be slapped vigorously between the scapulae. If this does not dislodge the object, a laryngoscope may be quickly introduced by the physician through which the offending object may be retrieved.

For edema or spasm, intubation may be performed in which a firm tube is passed beyond the obstruction into the trachea to establish an airway or the physician may do a tracheostomy (see p. 281). If edema of the larynx is due to an allergic response, the patient is given epinephrine (Adrenalin) 1:1000 subcutaneously. An adrenal corticosteroid preparation such as prednisone may be prescribed for a brief period to reduce tissue sensitivity. Local applications of ice to the neck may also be suggested.

When laryngeal muscle spasm is the cause of the obstruction, calcium chloride or calcium gluconate is given intravenously.

Newgrowth

A benign papilloma or polyp may develop within the larynx, the most frequent source being the vocal cords. Hoarseness and coughing are generally the initial symptoms, but gradually, as the tumor enlarges, breathing may become difficult. The tumor may be removed through the laryngoscope or by open surgery. Rarely is there any permanent voice impairment with this type of neoplasm.

The more serious newgrowth, cancer, has a higher incidence in males in the later years of life. Symptoms include hoarseness, dyspnea, cough, expectoration of blood, pain and possibly dysphagia (difficulty in swallowing) as the mass encroaches on the esophagus.

Early recognition and treatment are important in the prevention of metastases. Diagnosis is confirmed by laryngoscopy and biopsy. A few cases may be treated by radiation alone, but the majority of patients undergo surgical treatment. A partial laryngectomy may be done if the newgrowth appears localized. Some residual impairment of voice is likely, necessitating speech therapy following recovery from the surgery. Many patients have a total laryngectomy, which means they will be left voiceless and with a permanent tracheostomy through which they will breathe. Following recovery from surgery the patient may be assisted to develop esophageal speech or to use an artificial larynx.

DISORDERS OF THE TRACHEA

Tracheitis

Inflammation of the trachea rarely occurs independently of laryngitis or bronchitis. Because of the size of the lumen of the trachea and its noncollapsible structure, it rarely causes any serious interference with breathing but does cause considerable discomfort and a burning, raw pain.

Compression of the Trachea

Pressure from an aortic aneurysm or new-growth of neighboring structures (e.g., esophagus, lymph nodes of the mediastinum) may narrow the tracheal lumen and offer resistance to the passage of air through the trachea.

BRONCHITIS

This is an inflammation of the bronchial tubes and may be acute or chronic. Acute bronchitis is frequently a sequela of an upper respiratory tract infection or influenza. The trachea is generally involved first and then the infection extends into the bronchial tubes.

Signs and Symptoms. The illness varies greatly from a mild indisposition, lasting 2 to 3 days, to severe symptoms and eventual pneumonia. At the onset, the patient may complain of substernal tightness and discomfort and may experience an unproductive, irritating cough. In a day or two, the cough becomes less distressing and the secretions more profuse and mucopurulent with flecks or streaks of blood. Fever, general malaise and wheezing respirations accompany the disorder. Dyspnea is common and is due to bronchospasm that develops as a reflex response to the irritation. In some instances bronchial constriction may be severe enough to result in hypoventilation and hypoxemia.

Treatment and Nursing Care. The patient is confined to bed in a room in which the temperature is kept relatively constant and the air humidified. An antimicrobial drug may be prescribed to shorten the course of the disease and prevent its extension to the bronchioles and alveoli. A sputum specimen may be required for identification of the causative organism and for determination of antibiotic sensitivity. Coughing is encouraged at regular intervals when the cough becomes productive. An expectorant such as an ammonium chloride or glycerol guaiacolate preparation is ordered. If signs of bronchospasm are present, the patient is given a bronchodilator, such as aminophylline, which may be administered orally or by rectal suppository, or he may be given isoproterenol (Isuprel), which may be inhaled in aerosol form.

An increased fluid intake up to 3000 to 4000 ml. daily is recommended to promote liquefaction of the bronchial secretions. A soft or light nutritious diet is encouraged to maintain the patient's resistance. The patient's position is changed frequently to promote the movement of secretions from distal portions of the bronchial tree to a level from which they may be more readily raised by coughing.

Bronchitis can be debilitating, and although it may clear up in a week to 10 days, the patient may find the need to resume his former activities gradually and to take extra rest. Older persons who develop the disorder recover more slowly and are more predisposed to extension of their disease to bronchial pneumonia. They may not have sufficient muscular strength to cough up the secretions, and if these are retained, they predispose to complications. A longer period of convalescence with plenty of rest, nutritious foods and the prevention of chilling is necessary for these elderly persons.

Chronic Bronchitis and Emphysema

These two disorders along with asthma are classified as chronic obstructive pulmonary diseases because they interfere with the normal flow of air in and out of the lungs. They are characterized by wheezing, dyspnea (especially on exertion), coughing and abnormal blood gas tensions. Chronic bronchitis and emphysema are considered together since the latter is frequently a sequela of chronic bronchitis.

Chronic bronchitis is a chronic inflammatory process of the bronchial mucosa in response to prolonged or frequently recurring irritation. The common irritants are infection, tobacco smoke and atmospheric pollutants such as dust, industrial fumes and smoke. Heredity is suggested as having a role. There is some evidence that members of the same family may show a predisposition to develop the disease.[2] The mucosa

---

[2]J. Crofton, and A. Douglas: Respiratory Diseases. Oxford, Blackwell Scientific Publications, 1969, p. 310.

becomes edematous, thickened and scarred, and the mucus glands hypertrophy and are overactive. The excessive mucus may plug bronchioles and reduce ventilation. There is an increased susceptibility of the tract to infection, particularly during cold weather. The disease progresses insidiously over years, interspersed with acute exacerbations. The edema, scarring and the frequently associated bronchial spasm reduce the lumen of the air passages. Obstruction to the flow of air is greater during expiration, resulting in air being trapped in the bronchioles and alveoli. Eventually the air sacs become permanently overdistended and may rupture. Infection may be imposed on this, causing still further tissue damage. The chronic bronchitis is now complicated by emphysema.

Pulmonary emphysema implies dilation of the alveoli with some loss of septal tissue, causing a coalescence of several air sacs into one larger space. Air is trapped in these spaces, and the loss of alveoli results in an imbalance in ventilation and perfusion generally reflected by an elevation in the pCO_2 and a decrease in the pO_2. The incidence of chronic bronchitis and emphysema is higher in middle-aged and older males and in cold, damp climates.

Signs and Symptoms. The respirations are continually wheezy, the patient becomes progressively more dyspneic and short of breath on exertion, and the increasing respiratory insufficiency leads to restricted physical activity. A persistent, hard, productive cough is troublesome, the sputum is tenacious, and there is white or mucopurulent mucus. Symptoms of hypoxia and hypercapnia appear with the reduction in alveolar ventilation and diffusion (see pp. 274–5). The patient with emphysema may gradually develop observable changes in the shape and dimensions of his chest as a result of the trapping of air in the alveoli and the overdistention of the lungs. The anteroposterior diameter of the chest increases, and the ribs assume a more horizontal position, giving the chest a barrel-shaped appearance. The normal rise and fall of the chest with inspiration and expiration are diminished. Right-sided heart failure may develop as a result of the increased pulmonary vascular resistance, and the cardiac output is diminished.

Treatment and Nursing Care. Care of the patient with chronic obstructive lung disease is directed toward preserving his existing lung function and preventing further irreversible tissue damage. Consideration is given to the prevention of acute exacerbations, improving the patient's ventilation, having him adapt his activities to his respiratory tolerance and, at the same time, providing as great a degree of independence and satisfaction as possible. An explanation of his condition is made to the patient and his family, indicating that certain preventive measures and adaptations in his activities will contribute to the control of his disease.

INFECTION CONTROL. The patient may receive an antimicrobial drug or a mixed bacterial vaccine as a preventive measure throughout the autumn and winter months. The avoidance of close contact with those who have infection is stressed. General debilitation and loss of weight are commonly associated with the disease. A well-balanced, nutritious diet which is high in vitamin C and plenty of rest help to maintain the patient's resistance.

The patient is advised to seek prompt medical treatment with the earliest symptoms of an acute infection or increasing respiratory insufficiency.

IMPROVING VENTILATION. Humidification of the room air, especially during the cold season, and a fluid intake of not less than 3000 ml. are important to keep the pulmonary secretions thin. The patient is helped to establish a regular routine or time for taking fluids to ensure a sufficient intake. Warm, normal saline may be used in a nebulizer to moisten the mucosa. Physical therapy may be used to promote dislodgement of mucus from distal areas of the tracheobronchial tree into larger bronchial tubes from which the mucus can be more readily raised by coughing. The treatment may include clapping over various lung segments, coughing and postural drainage (see p. 276). Respiratory insufficiency due to reduced lung compliance and restricted respiratory excursion may be helped by breathing exercises, improved posture and physical exercises to increase the patient's general muscular status.

When bronchospasm and air trapping are present, a bronchodilator preparation, such as aminophylline or isoproterenol (Isuprel), may be ordered. Aerosol or nebulizer administration is frequently prescribed when isoproterenol is used and involves the forcing of air or oxygen through a solution of the drug to produce a fine spray which is directed into the patient's mouth so it may be inhaled. Nebulization may be done by hand by squeezing a rubber bulb which directs air through the solution, or it may be done by a nebulizer attached to the equipment for oxygen administration. The patient is instructed to exhale to the maximum and then, just as he starts to take his next breath, the tube through which the aerosol or nebulized solution is being forced is placed in his mouth. The process is repeated until the required dose is given.

If the bronchospasm persists, a course of corticosteroid (prednisone) may be given.

OXYGEN THERAPY. The patient may require the administration of oxygen at frequent intervals or during any activity. The percentage to be administered and the rate of flow are based on the laboratory report of the blood gas tensions and the patient's response to activity. Some patients with chronic obstructive pulmonary disease constantly have a relatively high pCO_2. The respiratory center becomes accustomed to this higher pCO_2 and is less responsive to it. As a result, hypoxia becomes the principle respiratory drive. The administration of a high concentration of oxygen may depress respirations and cause increased retention of carbon dioxide.

Oxygen therapy may have to be continued after the patient leaves the hospital. He and his family are advised of the necessary equipment and source of supply. Specific instructions about the administration and the necessary precautions must be clearly given verbally and in writing. Supervision by frequent visits from a visiting nurse or inhalation technician is important, especially during the first 2 or 3 weeks. Portable, light-weight oxygen equipment is now available which permits greater freedom and more varied activities for the patient.

AVOIDANCE OF EXPOSURE TO TRACHEOBRONCHIAL IRRITANTS. The person with chronic bronchitis or emphysema should not smoke. Convincing him of the importance of this and providing necessary assistance in breaking the habit may present quite a challenge to the nurse. The patient and family are advised of the hazards of cigarette smoking. Pamphlets and booklets, published by the Tuberculosis and Respiratory Disease Association, citing the harmful effects of smoking may be made available. The nurse tries to be persuasive and supportive without being judgmental, and she should praise the patient for his success over set periods.

Bronchial irritation may be reduced by avoiding the inhalation of smoke, chemical fumes and dust. Very cold air frequently precipitates bronchospasm, coughing and dyspnea in the person with a chronic respiratory disorder. If he must go out when the temperature is low, a scarf worn over the nose and mouth may reduce the distress.

ACTIVITY AND REST. The restrictions on physical activity and degree of handicap vary with each patient. His ability to carry on his former occupation and social life frequently diminishes. In order to avoid bronchial irritants he may have to change his job. He may reject this recommendation. It may have to be emphasized that remaining in a situation which exposes him to an irritant promotes acute exacerbations and increasing respiratory insufficiency which, in all probability, will lead to an inability to work at all. A referral to a social worker or rehabilitation officer may be made to provide assistance in finding a suitable occupation.

The patient's usual total daily activities are reviewed; some may be simplified to reduce energy demands, others may have to be eliminated. Shorter work hours and more rest may be necessary. An effective physical therapy program, breathing exercises, chemoprophylaxis and improvement of his general condition may increase his tolerance and eventually permit the resumption of some former activities. In some cases, the patient may not be able to continue in any form of employment and may even require continuing care. The patient and his family may be faced with serious socioeconomic problems. The nurse, who is familiar with the resources, makes the appropriate referral so that prompt planning for the necessary assistance is initiated.

The living accommodations should be assessed and adjustments made to decrease the energy expenditure if necessary. Factors to be considered include stairs, distance to transportation and other facilities, means of humidifying the air in his room and who is available to provide assistance for the patient.

The wheezing, shortness of breath and fear of complete invalidism and dependence create anxiety and emotional reactions. These may aggravate his bronchospasm and dyspnea. A mild sedative (e.g., small doses of sodium amytal) or tranquilizer (e.g., valium) may be prescribed. These are used cautiously because of possible depression of the respiratory center and ensuing hypoxia and increased retention of carbon dioxide. The latter could lead to acidosis.

SUPERVISION. An important part of the nursing care plan for the patient with chronic bronchitis or emphysema is preparation for continuing care at home. Instruction begins with providing a simple, clear explanation of the disorder with emphasis on the role of continued care, much of which is the patient's responsibility. The points of care discussed in the foregoing paragraphs are presented to the patient and family. A referral is made to a visiting nurse agency early enough to allow a satisfactory assessment of the home situation and the necessary adjustments to be made. Regular visits are made when the patient is home in order to counsel and coordinate and assist with his care. Frequent visits and close surveillance are needed if the patient is receiving medications and oxygen therapy. Careful observations are made on each visit for signs of hypoxia, infection, impaired cardiac function and the patient's emotional reaction to his condition. Transportation may have to be arranged for visits to his doctor or the clinic. Arrangements may also have to be made for a physical therapist to continue treatment and exercises. Gradually the patient and his family may be able to follow the suggested program with a weekly supervisory visit by the therapist and visiting nurse. If the patient is permitted to return to his former employment, the occupational nurse in the health service there is informed of the patient's condition, therapeutic regimen, and necessary restrictions.

Bronchial Asthma

Asthma is an episodic obstructive pulmonary disorder in which there is a narrowing of the bronchial lumen. This narrowing is due to spasm of the bronchial muscle tissue, edema and swelling of the mucous membrane, and the secretion of viscid mucus that tends to plug some branches of the bronchial tree. Resistance is offered to airflow through the lower air passages and is greater during expiration; this results in air being trapped in the alveoli, leading to distention and weakening of the alveolar walls.

Etiology and Incidence. Three factors play an important etiologic role in asthma— namely, hypersensitivity, heredity and infection.

Asthma may be a manifestation of a bronchial hypersensitivity (allergy) to a food, drug or inhaled substance. Common antigenic inhalants are dust, pollen, feathers, animal dander and mold. Examples of foods to which some persons are frequently sensitive include eggs, milk, wheat, shellfish and chocolate. Acetylsalicylic acid (Aspirin), antibiotics, serum and iodide preparations are examples of common drug allergens (see p. 36).

Heredity is thought to play a significant role, since many asthmatic patients have some family history of an allergic condition, such as urticaria, eczema or hay fever. Hay fever is a hypersensitivity in the nasal mucosa manifested by sneezing, nasal congestion and excessive secretion.

Chronic infection or frequent acute episodes of infection in the respiratory tract may cause the bronchial tissues to develop the asthmatic response. This type of asthma may be referred to as infective asthma. It is thought that the person who develops this type of the disease may have had a mild sensitivity which in itself was not sufficient to produce asthma but, with an infection imposed upon it, bronchial spasm develops.

Allergic asthma begins most often in children or young adults; the infective type may have its onset at any age. Emotional stress, infection, air pollutants, strenuous physical exercise and smoking are considered to be exciting factors of episodic attacks.

Signs and Symptoms. Asthma usually has a sudden onset with the patient experiencing a sense of suffocation, tightness in the chest, wheezing and expiratory dyspnea. Inspiration is short, but expiration is a prolonged, conscious effort, using accessory muscles.

The patient appears distraught, assumes an upright sitting position, has a frequent hard cough and raises a thick, viscous mucus with difficulty. A microscopic examination of the sputum reveals numerous eosinophils and gelatinous-like casts of the smaller bronchial tubes (Laennec's pearls). In infective asthma, the sputum will be mucopurulent. A differential leukocyte count usually reveals a marked increase in the eosinophils in allergic asthma. The attacks are episodic and may end abruptly. In severe and prolonged spasm, the patient becomes cyanosed, and the developing respiratory insufficiency and hypoxia may threaten his life. This severe type of attack is known as status asthmaticus.

Treatment and Care of the Asthmatic Patient

PREVENTION OF ATTACKS. Skin tests are done when extrinsic asthma is suspected in an effort to identify the specific allergen(s) to which the patient is sensitive. This is done by the intracutaneous injection of various allergens on the back or arm. Sensitivity is indicated if an urticarial lesion (hive) develops at the site of an injection. If the allergen is identified, efforts are made to have the patient avoid it. A series of subcutaneous injections of a solution of the particular antigen may be used to desensitize the patient. The dosage is very small to start with and is gradually increased. The patient is observed for approximately one-half to one hour following each injection, and epinephrine (Adrenalin) 1:1000 solution should be readily available in case a reaction is precipitated. If the allergen is a particular food, it is eliminated from the patient's diet. In the case of a drug being the antigen, the patient and his family are told that any doctor treating the patient should be advised of the allergy. It may also be helpful if the patient indicates the drug allergy on his identification card or wears a Medic Alert bracelet or pendant. The use of tobacco should be discontinued and irritating inhalants (dust, smoke, extremes of temperature) avoided as much as possible.

When asthma develops because of infection, preventive measures are directed toward the avoidance of factors that predispose to it, such as fatigue, malnutrition, chilling and exposure to infected persons. Bacterial vaccine may also provide some protection for the patient; regular doses at prescribed intervals maintain a more protective concentration of antibodies. Prompt medical treatment is recommended when an infection develops; this may prevent or reduce the bronchial irritation before asthma develops.

Frequently, emotional stress is a precipitating factor in asthma. An attempt is made to determine whether the patient is worried or disturbed about something. Discussion and bringing the problem out into the open may lead to elimination of the stress. Small frequent doses of a sedative (such as phenobarbital or amytal) or tranquilizer (e.g., chlorpromazine) may be prescribed to reduce emotional strain and promote relaxation.

CARE DURING AN ATTACK. During an attack the aim is to relieve the bronchial spasm, encourage expectoration of secretions and improve the patient's respiratory function. Medicinal preparations which are commonly used to relax and dilate the bronchial tubes include: epinephrine, ephedrine sulfate preparations, aminophylline, antihistamine preparations and adrenal corticosteroids. Epinephrine (Adrenalin) 1:1000 may be administered subcutaneously to provide quick relief. The patient will most likely experience some tachycardia, palpitation and tremor, and may become pale as a result of the vasoconstricting effect of this drug.

Ephedrine sulfate may be given orally 3 or 4 times a day and is usually used in combination with small doses of a mild sedative (e.g., phenobarbital). The sedative reduces the stimulating effect of the ephedrine.

Aminophylline is frequently used and may be given orally (by tablet or solution) or by rectal suppository. Frequent use of the latter may cause anorectal irritation. In very severe attacks and in status asthmaticus, aminophylline may be administered slowly by the intravenous route.

Isoproterenol (Isuprel) may be inhaled in a nebulized form to provide relief. Many asthma victims find that if they use the spray when early symptoms are experienced it prevents an attack. In using the nebulizer, the spray should be released to coincide with an inspiration so that more efficient inhalation takes place. Isoproterenol is also available in tablets for sublingual administration.

If the bronchial spasm is not responding to the above bronchodilators, an adrenocorticoid preparation, such as prednisone, may be prescribed. Dramatic relief occurs in many patients who receive the corticoid, and there is a danger that they may develop a dependency on the drug. If it is used, the dosage is kept to a minimum, and it is administered for only a very limited period and then gradually withdrawn.

ENVIRONMENT AND POSITIONING. Possible irritants in the patient's environment are kept to a minimum. The room should be devoid of rugs, drapes, flowers and smoke. Pillows of sponge rubber or other non-allergenic material are recommended. The floors and furniture are dusted with a damp cloth. Although the bed is elevated, the patient may be reluctant to lie back against it because of the sensation that any pressure on his back interferes with his breathing. Since he tends to lean forward constantly, an over-bed table with pillows may be placed in front of him for support of his arms and head. This may provide some comfort and rest. Crib sides are advisable to prevent him from falling if he should become drowsy or lose his balance in the upright sitting position. Special care is given to the sacral and buttock regions, as the patient tends to remain constantly in the one position. Flannelette sheets are usually more comfortable and are softer to the skin.

OBSERVATIONS. Close observation is made of the patient's color and pulse during an attack. Cyanosis, a progressively rising pulse rate, restlessness and confusion may indicate hypoxia and are brought to the physician's attention. The amount and characteristics of the sputum are noted. The fluid intake and output are recorded, and the balance is calculated. The nurse is alert for emotional stresses that may be aggravating the condition. These may be revealed in conversation with the patient and his family or through observing their interactions.

REST. The increased work involved in breathing and coughing, the loss of sleep, and the fear and tension associated with respiratory distress exhaust the patient. Nursing care is organized so that he is disturbed as little as possible, and environmental stimuli are kept to a minimum. Everything should be done for the patient during an attack to conserve his energy (feeding, bathing, lifting, etc.).

CLEARING THE TRACT OF SECRETIONS. The thick, tenacious secretions that may collect can plug the small bronchial tubes and bronchioles and seriously threaten adequate ventilation. An expectorant, such as a preparation of ammonium chloride or potassium iodide, may be given to thin the secretions and facilitate expectoration. Alevaire (a detergent preparation) or trypsin (an enzymatic preparation) may be used by aerosol administration to assist in clearing the tubes of mucus. A fluid intake of 3000 to 4000 ml. daily for an adult is important in thinning the secretions and maintaining normal hydration. The patient with acute asthma usually perspires freely due to increased sympathetic innervation. A record is kept of the patient's intake and output. Intravenous fluids are frequently necessary the first few days in severe episodes, as the patient may find it difficult to take adequate fluid while experiencing such acute respiratory distress.

CONTROL OF COUGH. Frequent coughing is physically exhausting and aggravates bronchospasm. The patient is instructed to try to suppress the cough and prolong the intervals between paroxysms. Swallowing inhibits coughing, so taking a sip of fluid or keeping hard candy in his mouth may help. A humidifier or steam vaporizer in the room to moisten the inhaled air may help to reduce bronchial irritation and coughing.

A confident, reassuring nurse at the bedside lessens the fear that the patient has of suffocation. At the same time, his needs are anticipated and his efforts are spared.

OXYGEN THERAPY. In acute asthma, when the respiratory insufficiency produces hypoxia and cyanosis, oxygen may be given by nasal catheter, mask, nasal cannulae or, rarely, by tent. The patient may object to mask administration because it covers his nose and mouth, increasing his sense of suffocation. The tent has the distinct advantage here since it provides an air-conditioned, allergen-free atmosphere.

TREATMENT OF INFECTION. When infection is also involved, the patient generally receives an antibiotic. If penicillin is ordered, a sensitivity test is done before the first dose is administered, since many of these patients show a hypersensitivity to the drug. For this reason, the physician tends to prescribe an oral antibiotic. The sputum may be cultured for purposes of identifying the causative organism.

NUTRITION. Nourishing fluids and soft foods are encouraged during an acute attack. The patient is using considerable energy and requires nourishment to provide it as well as to maintain his resistance to infection. He may tire readily while eating, so he is given small amounts at a time and assistance is provided.

INSTRUCTION. When the acute attack has been abated, the necessary care to prevent another attack is discussed with the patient and his family. Appropriate instruction is given in relation to the following: the control of the environment to avoid irritants; medications and their administration; the prevention of respiratory infection; the importance of prompt medical treatment if an infection is imminent; keeping emotional strain to a minimum; and physical exercise within his limits of tolerance.

Pneumonia

Crofton and Douglas indicate that the term "pneumonia" is generally used to imply an inflammation in the lung tissue and that "pneumonitis" is synonymous but is most commonly used in reference to mild segmental pneumonia.[3] Guyton defines pneumonia as "any lung condition in which the alveoli become filled with a fluid and/or blood cells."[4] In the latter description, the fluid may be a transudate, as in pulmonary edema, or it may be an inflammatory exudate, as forms in infective pneumonia.

Classification and Causes. Pneumonia may be classified in several ways. If Guyton's definition is applied, it may be considered as being noninfective or infective; however, fluid in the alveoli rarely remains uninfected for long since it provides a warm, moist, culture medium for common airborne organisms. Infective pneumonia may be bacterial or viral, or it may be classified

according to the specific causative organism; for example, the disease may be referred to as pneumococcal, staphylococcal, streptococcal, Friedländer's bacillus or influenzal viral pneumonia. The classification by organism is now commonly used since identification of the specific microbe is considered important in determining the appropriate anti-infective drug to be used. Still another classification which may be applied is according to the structural distribution of the disease. The pneumonia is lobar if a complete lobe is affected, segmental if involving a segment, and bronchial or lobular if the disease is patchy throughout one or both lungs. Initial causes of inflammation of lung tissue also include irritating chemical gases and aspirated vomitus.

Incidence and Predisposing Factors. Pneumonia has a higher incidence in the colder seasons and is probably related to overcrowding, hot dry indoor air and increased air pollution by fuel smoke. Predisposing factors also include chronic respiratory infection (e.g., chronic bronchitis), smoking, alcoholism which depresses reflexes (e.g., cough) and the production of antibodies, and fibrocystic disease (muscoviscidosis). All ages are susceptible, but pneumonia is especially serious in the aged and debilitated.

Manifestations. The onset, symptoms and course vary with different types of pneumonia. Infection of the alveoli results in their filling with inflammatory exudate (plasma, blood cells, pathological organisms and cellular debris) which readily overflows into other alveoli, extending the infection. A large area of lung tissue may become consolidated; pulmonary ventilation and diffusion are impaired, and the oxygen tension of the blood is reduced to below normal. The pCO_2 level generally remains normal; the increased respiratory rate in response to the initial increase in the pCO_2 results in increased amounts of CO_2 being excreted by the normal areas of the lung. In a few days, the exudate becomes more liquid and may be gradually eliminated from the alveoli by expectoration and absorption. This process is referred to as resolution. The disease may clear up with dramatic rapidity when specific antibacterial drugs are administered. It may run a course of

[3] J. Crofton, and A. Douglas: Respiratory Diseases. Oxford, Blackwell Scientific Publications, 1969, p. 112.

[4] A. C. Guyton: Textbook of Medical Physiology, 4th ed. Philadelphia, W.B. Saunders Co., 1971, p. 510.

5 to 10 days; untreated, it may rapidly prove terminal.

The onset of infective pneumonia may be very sudden and is frequently ushered in by a chill followed by fever. The pulse rate and respirations increase. The latter may be shallow and accompanied by an audible grunt. The nostrils flare on inspiration and the face may be flushed. Cyanosis of the lips and nail beds may develop. The patient's cough may be hacking, painful and unproductive at first; later, it becomes less painful and is productive. The sputum is tenacious, blood-streaked and mucopurulent in bronchopneumonia. In pneumococcal pneumonia, the sputum is usually rust-colored, becoming purulent as resolution takes place. The patient experiences general malaise, weakness, headache and aching pains. The leukocyte count is elevated, especially in the pneumococcal type.

Herpes simplex (cold sore or fever blister) frequently appears on the lips or around the nose and mouth. These lesions are attributed to activation of a virus that may have been dormant in the tissues. They appear as blisters first, then rupture and become encrusted.

Treatment and Nursing Care in Infective Pneumonia. The pneumonia patient requires prompt anti-infective treatment and supportive care to combat his acute communicable infection and correct the interference with pulmonary ventilation and diffusion. Nursing care includes the following considerations:

OBSERVATIONS. The vital signs are recorded at frequent intervals. A sudden fall in the temperature while the pulse and respirations remain rapid is reported, especially if the blood pressure also falls. These unfavorable signs may indicate shock or a serious spread of the infection. Respiratory movements of both sides of the chest are noted, and the patient's color is checked for pallor or cyanosis. The characteristics and amount of sputum are recorded. The fluid intake and output are measured and the balance recorded. The abdomen is examined for possible distention, which is not uncommon in pneumonia. The distention may interfere with normal diaphragmatic excursions, further embarrassing the patient's respirations.

The physician is informed of marked restlessness, cyanosis, disorientation and rising pulse rate, as they may indicate increasing hypoxemia. A sputum specimen is generally requested for culture and identification of the offending organism. This is collected if possible before the patient receives antimicrobial drugs. A leukocyte count and differential are done, and blood specimens may be obtained for pO_2, pCO_2 and electrolyte determinations. The chest is x-rayed to identify the areas of involvement.

REST. Physical and mental rest are important to reduce the patient's oxygen demands to a minimum. Care and treatments are organized to provide undisturbed periods. The diagnosis of pneumonia is generally very ominous and threatening to the patient; he requires reassurance and explanations of what is being done. Persisting anxiety and apprehension which are interfering with the patient's relaxation and rest are brought to the physician's attention.

MEDICATIONS. If the patient is cyanosed, dyspneic or the pO_2 is reduced to 70 mm. Hg or less, oxygen inhalation may be prescribed. It is usually administered by nasal catheter or cannulae (prongs) since the frequent coughing and expectoration tends to preclude the use of a mask. The oxygen is moistened by bubbling it through water, and the rate of flow indicated by the doctor generally ranges from 5 to 8 liters per minute.

An antibiotic is prescribed immediately; a broad-spectrum preparation (e.g., tetracycline) may be given as soon as a sputum specimen is obtained for bacteriological study. When the causative organism is identified, the antibiotic may be changed to a specific preparation. Antimicrobial drugs must be given regularly and promptly as prescribed in order to maintain an effective blood concentration. Since some persons may be hypersensitive to penicillin, which may be ordered, and could develop a serious reaction, such as anaphylaxis, the patient is questioned about ever having had asthma, hay fever, eczema or hives and is asked if he has ever had penicillin. A sensitivity test is done before administering the first dose. A small test dose of penicillin is given intracutaneously; hypersensitivity is manifested by a wheal or urticaria developing at the site. If hypersensitivity is known or suspected, another antibiotic is substituted for penicillin.

A cough suppressant such as dihydrocodeinone (Hycodan or Mercodol) may be prescribed during the initial unproductive, painful phase. Later, this is likely to be replaced by an expectorant such as an ammonium chloride or potassium iodide preparation to facilitate elimination of the exudate and secretions.

Pleural pain may be very distressing and may interfere with the patient's rest. Acetylsalicylic acid (Aspirin) or dextropropoxyphene (Darvon) may provide relief, or a small dose of codeine may be prescribed if the pain is particularly severe. Repeated and prolonged use of any narcotic is avoided as it tends to depress the cough reflex and the respiratory center. Some sedation may be necessary if the patient is restless and confused. Chloral hydrate or a barbiturate (e.g., sodium amytal) may be ordered.

FLUIDS AND NUTRITION. The high fever, rapid respirations and increased pulmonary secretions necessitate a fluid intake of 3000 to 4000 ml. daily. This amount contributes to liquefaction of the secretions, facilitating their expectoration. The patient perspires freely and incurs a loss of sodium as well as water. The addition of salt to broth or soup may be suggested unless contraindicated by a positive fluid balance. Because cellular activity (metabolism) is accelerated to produce the elevated temperature and there is a loss of plasma and cells in the exudate, the patient should receive a minimum of 1200 to 1500 calories daily. If he cannot tolerate solid foods, nourishing fluids and soft foods such as eggnogs, milk, junkets and custards are encouraged. Food concentrates added to fluids are useful in providing the necessary calories. The diet is increased to a full complement as soon as it can be tolerated.

POSITIONING AND EXERCISE. The patient is generally more comfortable if his head and chest are elevated. His position is changed (side, to side, to back, to side) at least every 2 hours. The pain generally worsens with moving and coughing; the patient needs encouragement and support in these activities and is spared as much

effort as possible. The nurse may splint his chest during coughing by placing her hands over the painful area. Active exercises of the lower limbs are carried out every 2 hours to reduce the possibility of venous thrombosis. The patient is confined to bed until his temperature returns to normal. Depending on the severity of his disease, he may be allowed to use a commode at the bedside rather than expend the greater amount of energy in using a bedpan. When he is allowed up, activities are gradually increased. If spontaneous coughing does not occur at least hourly, the patient is prompted to initiate it. Physical therapy in the form of percussion and clapping may be necessary to dislodge tenacious, thick secretions.

MOUTH AND SKIN CARE. The fever and perspiration necessitate frequent changes of gown and bedding to prevent chilling and skin irritation and to provide comfort. Flannelette sheets are more satisfactory than cotton ones. Bathing at least once daily is necessary because of the fever and perspiration.

Frequent cleansing and moistening of the mouth are necessary because of the fever, mouth breathing and infected sputum. If herpes simplex develops, the doctor may suggest an application of spirits of camphor or tincture of benzoin in the vesicular stage, then an ointment may be applied when the lesion becomes encrusted.

ELIMINATION. A mild laxative or a low cleansing enema may be used if necessary for bowel elimination. As cited previously, abdominal distention may become a problem and should be relieved to prevent further respiratory difficulty. An enema may be effective, but a peristaltic stimulant such as neostigmine (Prostigmin) or Pitressin may have to be given intramuscularly with the enema to provide relief. The application of heat to the abdomen may also be suggested.

MEDICAL ASEPSIS. Bacterial and viral pneumonia are communicable diseases which may be transmitted to others by the dissemination of contaminated droplets when the patient coughs or by contact with the sputum. It may be necessary to instruct the patient to cover his mouth when he coughs, turn his head away from anyone at his bedside and promptly dispose of his used tissues into a paper bag kept within his reach. If a sputum cup is used, the disposable inner container is changed at least 3 times daily and the outer one is disinfected.

Visitors are restricted to the family during the acute phase and are advised of the necessary precautions for their protection. A gown is worn over the uniform while the nurse is caring for the patient and in contact with the bedding. A single room provides more rest for the patient and lessens the possibility of his disease being conveyed to others. If this is not possible, he should not be placed near very ill, elderly or debilitated patients.

DISORIENTATION. The combination of fever, toxins and hypoxemia may cause disorientation. Precautions are taken to prevent injury and overexertion. Crib sides are placed on the bed, and someone may have to remain with the patient. A sedative which is least likely to depress the respiratory center and cough reflex is generally ordered.

COMPLICATIONS. The nurse must be alert for possible complications even though these rarely occur if the pneumonia has been treated in the early stage with an antimicrobial preparation. This preparation usually arrests the pneumonic process in a few days, and resolution relieves the consolidation in a relatively short period. Lack of prompt treatment or infection by a very virulent or resistant organism may result in delayed resolution or one of the following complications.

Atelectasis, or collapse of a part or of a whole lobe of the lung, ensues with the obstruction of a bronchial tube by a mucus plug. The lung tissue distal to the obstruction collapses as its residual air is absorbed into the blood. This complication frequently may be prevented by encouraging the patient to cough deeply and effectively, giving copious fluids to thin the secretions and turning him regularly.

A patient with pneumonia caused by resistant or very virulent organisms or whose treatment has been delayed may develop a peripheral vascular collapse, leading to shock. The prognosis in this complication is grave. Early signs are a fall in temperature and blood pressure while the pulse remains rapid but of lesser volume. The skin becomes cold and clammy, and the patient is less responsive. Oxygen inhalation is given; a vasopressor drug such as isoproterenol (Isuprel) or levarterenol bitartrate (Levophed) may be given in normal saline or glucose 5 per cent by intravenous infusion. The rate of flow is indicated by the physician and adjusted to the blood pressure response.

A dread complication of pneumonia is septicemia, in which the causative organisms may enter the blood stream and may be deposited in other tissues or organs quite remote from the lungs. Pericarditis, endocarditis, meningitis and arthritis are examples of what may be incurred by septicemia.

Empyema is a collection of pus in the pleural cavity resulting from involvement of the pleurae in the pneumonic infection. Indications include persisting high fever, chest pain and increasing dyspnea as the lung becomes compressed by the accumulation of fluid. Surgical drainage of the cavity may have to be performed if the condition fails to respond to specific chemotherapy.

CONVALESCENCE. Pneumonia can be a very debilitating disease, especially in the elderly. The duration of bed rest and of convalescence varies from one patient to another, being influenced by the severity of his disease and complications as well as his age. Even if the acute illness is brief, the patient is advised to resume activities gradually. He may find that he tires quickly and that extra rest is necessary for several weeks. His resistance is lower for a period of time, so he is instructed to avoid contact with those with an infection as much as possible and to seek prompt treatment if he develops early symptoms. A high-calorie, high-protein, high-vitamin diet is recommended unless the patient is overweight. The nature of his occupation will largely determine how soon he may return to work.

It is recommended that the patient continue deep breathing exercises 4 times daily for 6 to 8 weeks to counteract the possible development of reduced compliance and vital capacity. These are commenced in the hospital when the temperature is normal.

Bronchiectasis

Bronchiectasis is a chronic tubular dilatation of bronchial tubes and bronchioles. It may involve any part of the lung, but the lower dependent segments are most often the areas affected.

Etiology and Disease Process. In the majority of patients, the causes of bronchiectasis are obstruction of a bronchial tube and infection. Obstruction of a bronchial tube by a mucus plug or a foreign body causes collapse of the bronchioles and alveoli beyond. The collapse increases the intrapleural negative pressure. The bronchial tubes above the block are subjected to this negative pressure and also communicate with the atmosphere. The increased differential between intrapleural and atmospheric pressures causes dilatation of the tubes above the block. If this is prolonged, the walls are weakened, and they may not return to their original size even with reexpansion of the collapsed segments. Bronchiectasis may also occur below an obstruction of a bronchus or bronchial tube. The retained secretions in the tubes and alveoli distal to the block readily become infected and may be the initiating cause. In this instance the infection is secondary to the obstruction.

Prolonged infection without obstruction may damage the walls, producing structural changes, weakening and dilation. Loss of cilia and normal muscle tone in the tubes results in the retention and pooling of the infective, purulent secretions which perpetuate and extend the infection.

The onset of bronchiectasis has a higher incidence in childhood which is probably due to the smaller lumen of the tracheobronchial tree. A congenital weakness in the bronchial walls and debilitation may be predisposing factors.

The degree of impairment of pulmonary ventilation and oxygen uptake depends on the amount of lung damage and chronic infection.

Symptoms. The symptoms of bronchiectasis include a persisting cough, profuse purulent sputum with an offensive odor, periodic hemoptysis due to erosion of a blood vessel by the infective process, shortness of breath on exertion, loss of weight and reduced work capacity. A severe paroxysm of coughing is common in the morning as a result of the overnight accumulation of secretions. A change of position may also precipitate coughing when the secretions flow from the dilated saccular area into healthier tubes which are capable of initiating the cough reflex. Clubbing of the fingers and toes may develop when the disease is of long standing. Episodes of acute respiratory infection (such as pneumonia) with chest pain, fever and dyspnea occur.

The diagnosis is confirmed, and the extent of the disease is determined by a bronchogram of both lungs (see p. 272).

Treatment and Care. The patient may be treated conservatively by the prolonged administration of an antibiotic. The choice of the anti-infective drug will depend on the organisms present in the sputum and their sensitivity. Postural drainage is used to empty the bronchiectatic cavities of their purulent secretions and reduce the frequent coughing (see p. 276). Bronchoscopic suctioning may be used if the cavity is readily accessible and the secretions are viscous and difficult to raise. Deep breathing exercises are encouraged to improve alveolar ventilation; the fuller inflation of the lungs also helps to move the secretions out. The avoidance of chilling, fatigue, and contact with those with acute respiratory infection is recommended. A high-calorie, high-vitamin, well-balanced diet and extra rest contribute to the patient's resistance and the prevention of pneumonia. The patient is not usually hospitalized except during bronchoscopic investigation and when an acute pulmonary infection develops. The extent of his disease determines if he is able to continue at school or in his employment.

The initial period in the hospital during diagnosis usually provides an opportunity for the nurse to instruct the patient and his family about the management regimen (postural drainage, coughing, breathing exercises). A referral to a clinic or to a visiting nurse agency is desirable so that the patient is supervised and teaching is reinforced at intervals.

Surgical excision of the affected segment or lobe is considered to be the most effective treatment if the bronchiectatic cavity or cavities persist. Occasionally, if more than one lobe of a lung is involved, an entire lung is removed. For nursing care, see p. 305.

Pleural Effusion

A pleural effusion is an accumulation of an abnormal quantity of fluid in the interpleural space and is a symptom associated with a variety of conditions. The fluid may be a transudate or an exudate. A transudate may collect in the pleural space as a result of increased venous pressure incurred by congestive heart failure or an intrathoracic tumor which interferes with venous drainage in the area. Cirrhosis of the liver may cause a pleural effusion as well as ascites. An accumulation of exudate in the pleural space indicates irritation and inflammation of the pleura.

The patient with an effusion may experience some pleuritic pain, which is stabbing and is worse on inspiration before the excess fluid collects. The condition may develop insidiously and may go unrecognized until the increasing volume of fluid commences to compress the lung, causing dyspnea and impaired pulmonary ventilation.

A chest aspiration (thoracentesis) is done to relieve the pressure on the lung and to obtain a specimen of fluid for examination. Treatment is directed toward the disease causing the effusion.

If the exudative fluid in the pleural space becomes purulent, the condition is referred to as thoracic empyema. Its occurrence is rare since the advent of the improved antimicrobial drugs, but it is generally a complication of pneumonia or, less often, of tuberculosis. A culture is made of the aspirated fluid for identification of the causative organisms and their antibiotic sensitivity. The patient receives antibiotics parenterally or orally, and the drug may also be injected into the thoracic cavity following aspiration. Surgical drainage may be necessary, especially if the pus is thick. Early breathing exercises to promote re-expansion of the lung are important, since the visceral pleura tends to become thick, fibrous and resistant to stretching.

Pulmonary Tuberculosis

Tuberculosis is a reportable infectious disease that is caused by the tubercle bacillus. The organism may attack other tissues in the body, but the lungs are most frequently the primary site of invasion. The incidence of pulmonary tuberculosis has diminished in many countries where the standard of living is relatively higher (e.g., North America and European countries), but it still remains a major health problem in countries which are less well developed economically and socially.

Up until the last 2 to 3 decades, the disease was seen more often in children, adolescents and young adults. In recent years, fewer younger persons become infected, but many of the older age group are infected. Most of them have controlled their disease throughout their life; with poorer health and lowered resistance in the later years, some of them develop active disease. This change in incidence in relation to age is attributed to the improved socioeconomic conditions and effective chemotherapy.

Two types of tubercle bacilli may cause disease in man; one is the bovine, which is most often found in cattle and may be transmitted to man by the ingestion of infected dairy products. Fortunately, this is relatively well controlled now by the inspection and testing of herds and the pasteurization of milk. The second type of tubercle bacillus is classified as the human variety and may invade any body tissue but has a predilection for lungs.

Small, rounded nodules with a tendency toward central necrosis develop at the site of tissue invasion by the bacilli. These are referred to as tubercles and are comprised of lung tissue cells, leukocytes, other phagocytic cells and fibroblasts. If the body defenses are strong enough to destroy the organisms, the lesion heals and may calcify. In some instances, the reproduction of the tubercle bacilli may be minimal; a few continue to survive within the tubercle but remain confined and the infection becomes dormant. This person, having been infected and still harboring live bacilli, will show a positive tuberculin test. At a later date, if his resistance is lowered, the reproduction of the tubercle bacilli may be accelerated and he develops active disease. When the bacilli continue to multiple, the tubercle necroses centrally, producing soft, caseous material that may eventually be discharged from the tubercle, leaving a cavity. This caseous discharge is highly infective and bacilli are readily spread to others who inhale contaminated air or droplets which may be expelled by coughing or sneezing.

Resistance and Susceptibility. Susceptibility to tuberculosis appears to vary somewhat from one race of people to another, which suggests that some may have a natural resistance. The North American Indians and African Negroes show a high incidence and increased susceptibility.

Davidson indicates that some persons who have been infected and who have controlled their primary lesion are more resistant to the disease on subsequent exposure; this suggests some protection comparable to acquired immunity.[5]

Factors which lower the resistance and the ability to control the primary infection include nutritional deficiency, debilitating disease, chronic respiratory disease (e.g., asthma), excessive fatigue, overcrowding and prolonged dust inhalation such as that to which miners are subjected.

Persons receiving adrenocorticoid preparations (e.g., asthmatic and arthritic patients) also run a greater risk of developing tuberculosis because of the depressing effect of the drug on inflammation and lymphocyte and antibody production.

Signs and Symptoms. The onset of pulmonary tuberculosis tends to be insidious. A person may be active and may be leading his usual pattern of life over a long period during which the disease may be slowly progressing with the very gradual appearance of symptoms. The symptoms include those produced by the systemic effects of the disease and those due to the local effects of the tubercles.

The constitutional symptoms are vague and nonspecific, including lassitude, easy fatigue, malaise, loss of appetite and weight, fever (usually low grade) in the latter part of the day, tachycardia and night sweats. Those produced by the local disease process

---

[5]Sir Stanley Davidson: The Principles and Practice of Medicine, 9th ed. Edinburgh, E. & S. Livingstone Ltd., 1970, p. 411.

at the site of the lesion in the lungs are cough, sputum, hemoptysis, dyspnea and chest pain if the pleura is involved.

Diagnostic Investigation. The investigation of a patient for pulmonary tuberculosis involves tuberculin testing, chest x-ray and bacteriologic examination of sputum.

In tuberculin testing, a small amount of tuberculin may be injected intradermally at one site (Mantoux test) or by multiple puncture (Heaf and Tine tests). One of two preparations of tuberculin may be used—namely, pure protein derivative (PPD) or old tuberculin (OT). The Mantoux test generally uses PPD, and the site is examined for induration or swelling in 48 to 72 hours. The exact size of the area of induration is recorded in millimeters. An area of 10 mm. or over is considered positive. The Heaf test uses PPD and the site is examined on the fourth to seventh day after administration. Palpable induration around at least 4 puncture points indicates a positive reaction. The Tine test uses a concentrated solution of old tuberculin and the four-puncture site is examined in 48 to 72 hours. Induration of 2 mm. or more is generally considered to be a positive reaction.

If the tuberculin test is positive, this is usually followed by roentgenograms of the chest and a sputum examination. Even very small lesions are likely to be detected in a chest x-ray because of the natural air contrast available in the lungs. Healed lesions may be recognized by the contracted scar tissue and deposits of calcium. A sputum specimen, which is obtained in the morning when the patient first awakens, is cultured and examined for gram-positive, acid-fast bacilli. At least 3 specimens are examined to confirm the diagnosis, but it must be remembered that a negative bacteriological report does not necessarily exclude the disease. If it is difficult to obtain a satisfactory sputum specimen, gastric contents or washings aspirated before breakfast or laryngeal swabs may be cultured. Rarely, a bronchoscopy may be done and a specimen of secretions obtained by suction.

Treatment and Nursing Care. The principle forms of treatment are chemotherapy and rest. The three drugs most commonly used are streptomycin, para-aminosalicylic acid (PAS) and isoniazid (INH). The patient may receive a regimen of all three for a period of time, and is then changed over to a combination of two. The two are generally PAS and INH. The tubercle bacilli found in the patient's sputum may be tested for their sensitivity to the various drugs. A combination of any two is considered necessary in preventing the development of drug-resistant bacilli. Drug therapy is generally continued for a minimum of 2 years. These patients are usually under the supervision of a visiting or clinic nurse who must impress upon them the importance of strict adherence to the prescribed drug therapy. The patients must also be alerted for side effects, which are to be reported promptly. Streptomycin may cause auditory nerve damage manifested by dizziness and/or impaired hearing and a skin rash. Not infrequently, PAS results in anorexia and gastrointestinal irritation which causes nausea, vomiting and diarrhea. Isoniazid may incur skin irritation and, rarely, some renal damage manifested by a low urinary output, headache and drowsiness.

A period of hospitalization may be necessary during sensitivity studies and initial chemotherapy and until the infectiousness of the patient is reversed. This provides an excellent opportunity to help the patient understand his disease and the required therapy and to assist him in planning his care regimen as an outpatient.

Bed rest may be recommended until acute symptoms subside and the local lesion(s) manifests a favorable response to the chemotherapy. Activity is gradually resumed, and its effect on the patient is carefully assessed. He is encouraged to take a well-balanced, nutritious diet.

An important part of the teaching provided by the nurse is that which is related to preventing the spread of the patient's infection to others. He and his family are advised of the modes of transmission and the significance of covering his nose and mouth with tissues when coughing, sneezing or raising sputum; the adequate, prompt disposal of the used tissues; washing of the hands; and the avoidance of close contact with people. An important nursing responsibility is the identification and follow-up of patient contacts. These are members of the patient's immediate household, those in relatively close contact at school or at his place of employment, and those who are known to have been closely or frequently associated with the patient socially.

The patient with pulmonary tuberculosis requires long-term care; he and his family need long-term guidance and the support of interested, informed nurses.

In a few instances, a patient may develop a cavity which is difficult to heal by chemotherapy because of the respiratory movements. Pneumothorax may be used to place the lung at rest and bring the surfaces of the cavity together to promote healing. Rarely, surgical excision of an affected lobe or lung is undertaken if the disease is localized to one lung.

Carcinoma of the Lung

Only a very small percentage of tumors of the lung are nonmalignant. The majority of newgrowths arise from the bronchial epithelium and prove to be bronchogenic carcinoma. The incidence is higher in males but is occurring with greater frequency in females. There has been an alarming progressive increase in lung cancer in the last 3 or 4 decades, and chronic irritation of the bronchial tissues is considered to be an important etiological factor in cancer. Irritating inhalants such as cigarette smoke, air pollutants, dust and chemical gases are thought to play a significant role. Statistical surveys indicate a much higher incidence in cigarette smokers.

Manifestations. The symptoms depend somewhat on the location of the lesion; they may result from encroachment of the tumor on the bronchial lumen and/or its pressure on structures in the mediastinum, base of the neck or chest wall. A persistent cough, wheezing and hemoptysis are common, and as the tumor encroaches on the bronchial lumen, increasing respiratory distress is experienced. Eventually, the tube may be obstructed, causing atelectasis of the segment distal to the lesion. Recurring attacks of bronchitis and/or pneumonia may develop as a result of retained secretions. If the carcinoma is in a small bronchial tube in a peripheral area of the lung, the patient may be asymptomatic in the early stage. His disease may progress to a relatively advanced stage before it is discovered which, in some instances, occurs on a routine physical examination or routine chest x-ray. Pain may be present if the disease invades the chest wall, causing pressure on intercostal and brachial nerve fibers. Systemic effects of the malignant disease, such as anemia, loss of weight and progressive fatigue and weakness, develop gradually.

Diagnosis is by chest roentgenograms, bronchoscopic examination (see p. 272) and cytological examination of bronchial secretions or a biopsy for cancerous cells. The bronchoscopy may provide a direct view of the lesion, a biopsy and the collection of secretions.

Treatment and Care. Early diagnosis and treatment of lung cancer, as with all cancer, produce more favorable results. Pulmonary resection is generally undertaken as soon as the patient's general condition and pulmonary and cardiac function are carefully investigated. The surgery may entail the excision of the affected lobe or the removal of the lung (pneumonectomy) and affected contiguous structures, such as the mediastinal nodes. Postoperative radiation therapy may be used if there is suspicion of metastases in adjacent structures, such as the large blood vessels or the chest wall. If the patient's disease has advanced to an inoperable stage when it is discovered, radiation therapy may be used in an effort to arrest the growth of the neoplasm and metastasization. See Chapter 8 for the nursing care of the patient with a malignant disease and page 305 for care of the patient having chest surgery.

The prognosis is more favorable in those who have no evidence of metastases or spreading to contiguous structures at the time of operation, in younger patients and in females, and if the lesion is epidermoid carcinoma rather than adenocarcinoma and is located in the central or upper lobe. Early recognition and resection play a significant role. The nurse has a responsibility to urge persons to seek investigation of a chronic cough or recurring infections, discourage smoking and recommend frequent check-ups and chest x-rays for those who have smoked for 15 to 20 years.

Diaphragmatic Hernia (Hiatus Hernia)

The openings in the diaphragm which accommodate the esophagus and aorta are potential sites for the herniation of an abdominal viscus into the thoracic cavity. The hiatus through which the esophagus passes is the most vulnerable area. The chief cause of the defect in the diaphragm is considered to be a congenital weakness, resulting probably from a defect in the fusion of the tissues around the opening. The weakness or gap that occurs results in imperfect closure of the hiatus around the esophagus. Rarely, the hernia may be caused by trauma such as a fractured rib or perforating foreign object (e.g., bullet) or prolonged, extreme intra-abdominal pressure.

There are two major factors of concern, especially in large hiatal defects; a loop of the intestine or a portion of the stomach may move into the thoracic cavity and become constricted at the hiatus. A bowel obstruction may ensue, or in the case of the protrusion of the abdominal esophagus or stomach, gastric distress, heartburn, belching, feeling of fullness, vomiting and/or dysphagia may develop. Ulceration in the distal portion of the esophagus or the proximal portion of the stomach is not uncommon. Respiratory distress occurs as the viscus compresses the lungs; cardiac function may be impaired by direct pressure on the heart.

The symptoms depend on the size of the hernia and the amount of displaced viscus. Intermittent mild digestive disturbances only may be experienced. Diagnosis is made by a barium ingestion with fluoroscopic and roentgenographic studies.

A slight hernia may be controlled, and the patient is kept relatively asymptomatic by loss of weight (if he is obese), the avoidance of heavy lifting, eating more slowly and lesser amounts at one time, the elimination of gas-forming foods from the diet and remaining in an upright position after a meal.

If a loop of the intestine or a portion of the stomach becomes confined in the thoracic cavity, surgical treatment is essential to return the viscus to the abdominal cavity. The surgical approach is usually made through the chest but occasionally may be made via the abdominal cavity. Following replacement of the viscus, the hiatus hernia is repaired. A nasogastric tube is likely to be introduced, and mild suction is applied to prevent vomiting and intestinal distention. Fluids are administered by intravenous infusion for the first day or two, then gradually introduced by mouth when the gastric suction is discontinued. For nursing care when a thoracotomy is used, see below.

Chest Injuries

The commonest form of chest injury is a fracture of the ribs but unless the fragments penetrate or injure the pleura and lung, it is not considered serious. However, the pain interferes with normal respiratory function, since the patient tends to immobilize the chest and take shallow respirations to minimize the pain. If there is no visceral damage, the affected side may be immobilized by adhesive strapping; and, rarely, with severe pain that cannot be controlled by analgesics, an intercostal nerve block may be done to provide relief. The patient is usually more comfortable in an elevated position and is encouraged to breathe deeply. Sudden sharp chest pain, dyspnea or blood-streaked sputum is promptly brought to the physician's attention. A crushing injury of the chest is frequently sustained by an automobile driver in an accident. His chest is crushed by the steering wheel, and several ribs may receive multiple fractures. A portion of the rib cage is detached and displaced inward, producing a flail chest, which is serious. On inspiration, the flail section of the chest wall is pulled in, and on expiration it moves out. This is referred to as paradoxical respiration. Obviously, the patient suffers respiratory insufficiency, leading to hypoxia and retention of carbon dioxide which further stimulate respirations. Treatment is aimed at immobilizing the chest wall to reduce the paradoxical respirations. Pressure dressings may be used, or some form of traction to the chest wall may be employed by means of the application of towel clips or wires to the affected area and their connection to weights suspended by ropes over pulleys. Injury to the pleura or lung frequently complicates the condition, causing pneumothorax (collapse of the lung) or hemothorax (collection of blood in the thoracic cavity). Chest aspiration will probably be necessary to remove serum and blood, and a catheter may be left in the pleural cavity to allow for a continuous escape of air and fluid. An effort may be made to reduce the patient's pain with an intercostal nerve block. Narcotics are used sparingly, since they depress respirations and the cough reflex. The condition is usually complicated by severe shock and probably by other injuries.

Penetrating chest wounds produce what is commonly referred to as a sucking wound. Air passes freely in and out of the pleural cavity, and the lung of the affected side collapses. The air may accumulate to displace the mediastinum to the unaffected side, interfering with the normal respiratory capacity of the lung on that side by compression.

An immediate effort to seal off the opening into the chest wall is mandatory. In the emergency situation, a towel, handkerchief or any clean material at hand is used until surgical treatment is available. A thoracotomy may be done to control the bleeding and repair damaged tissues. The intrapleural cavity has been entered and the nursing care of the patient following the surgery is similar to that of any patient who has chest surgery.

Nursing the Thoracic Surgical Patient

In pulmonary disorders, the thoracic operative procedures performed include pneumonectomy, lobectomy, segmental resection and decortication.

Pneumonectomy, in which an entire lung is removed, involves the ligation of a large pulmonary artery, two large pulmonary veins and a bronchus. The phrenic nerve on the operative side is crushed or severed to permit the diaphragm to rise to reduce the size of the cavity that remains. Pneumonectomy is used in cancer of the lung or for widespread unilateral bronchiectasis, tuberculosis or abscesses. A lobectomy is the removal of a lobe of a lung and is used when the disease is confined to that particular lobe. Disease may be localized to a segment of a lung, making it possible to conserve functional tissue and lessen the degree of overdistention in the other lung by removing only the affected segment. Decortication is a surgical procedure in which a thick fibrous membrane that has replaced the visceral pleura is removed. The resistive membrane may develop with empyema (a collection of pus in the pleural cavity), pleural effusion or prolonged hemothorax (blood in the pleural cavity).

Preoperative Nursing Care. The patient who is to have chest surgery usually undergoes a period in which evaluation studies are made and care is given to improve his general condition.

PSYCHOLOGICAL PREPARATION. The patient facing chest surgery is likely to be quite apprehensive. He needs emotional support and some understanding of what is being done and what is going to take place. The physician describes the condition and the proposed surgery to the patient and his family. Following this, the nurse is usually required to answer questions and reinforce what the doctor has said. The patient is encouraged to express his fears and concerns; questions should not be evaded but answered knowledgeably. Home problems may be revealed and should be referred to the appropriate sources for assistance (e.g., Social Service or Welfare Department or a visiting nurse agency), thus relieving the patient's concerns.

A brief description of what to expect when he arrives in the operating room and after the surgery proves helpful. Since the frequent monitoring and recording of his blood pressure, pulse and respirations might cause him some concern for his condition, he is advised before the operation that these observations are made to inform the attendant staff as to his progress.

OBSERVATIONS. During the preoperative period, vital signs, hydration and nutritional status are noted, and the patient is observed for indications of any condition, such as an acute respiratory or skin infection, that may predispose to postoperative complications.

NUTRITION. The general nutritional status and resistance may be improved by a high-calorie diet with an increase in the protein and vitamin content. If the patient's appetite is poor and increased intake poses a problem, the calorie and protein intake may be provided for in commercial concentrates that can be added to a glass of milk or fruit juice. The fluid intake is generally increased to provide optimum hydration and to promote effective removal of pulmonary secretions.

SECRETIONS. If the patient has bronchiectasis, lung abscess or retained secretions, postural drainage may be used to clear the lung of as much infective material as possible (see p. 276). The sputum is measured and recorded for each 8- or 24-hour period.

ANTIBIOTICS. If the condition is infective, a broad-spectrum antibiotic will probably be prescribed to reduce the pathogenic organisms. It may be administered in an aerosol spray, orally or parenterally.

MOUTH CARE. Frequent antiseptic mouthwashes contribute to reducing infective organisms as well as to the comfort of the patient. Frequent expectoration of purulent sputum and the objectionable taste which may develop tend to depress the appetite. Keeping the mouth clean may encourage the patient to take necessary food.

INSTRUCTION AS TO POSTOPERATIVE ROLE. Much attention is given to preparing the patient for what will take place after the operation. Oxygen administration, the use of a respirator to reduce the patient's work of breathing, the frequent use of the suction to remove secretions, the drainage tubes in his chest, the frequent turning and early ambulation are judiciously explained.

The patient is advised that he will be expected to cough at least every 1 to 2 hours to promote re-expansion of the lung in the case of partial resection and to promote drainage from the thoracic cavity and the removal of intrapulmonary secretions. He is taught to inhale deeply and cough with the mouth and throat open and is encouraged to practice this during the preoperative period. The importance of regular periods of deep breathing, which he will be expected to carry out when not on a respirator, is emphasized. The nurse or a physiotherapist explains and demonstrates the leg exercises, which he will be required to do to prevent circulatory stasis and thrombus formation, and the posture training and arm exercises to preserve good posture and normal range of motion. The patient is advised if he is to be transferred to an intensive care unit following surgery and should, if possible, have some contact with the nurse who will care for him.

EVALUATION TESTS. Pulmonary function tests and complete blood studies are done. The blood work will include typing and arrangements for compatible blood to be available at the time of surgery. The procedures and their purpose are explained to the patient.

IMMEDIATE PREOPERATIVE CARE. The immediate preparation beginning the day before operation is similar to that suggested for most major surgery in Chapter 10. A large skin area is shaved and cleaned, since the exact site of incision varies. The doctor may not consider an enema necessary if early ambulation is anticipated. Postural drainage may be required before the patient goes to operation. It atropine is ordered as preoperative medication, the postural drainage should be done before the atropine is administered. A final check is made to see that the operative consent has been signed, that the urinalysis and vital signs are normal and that the patient's urinary bladder is empty. A close relative may be allowed to visit briefly with the patient before the preoperative sedative is administered and then is shown to a sitting room where the family may wait during the operation.

Postoperative Nursing Care. During the operation certain pieces of equipment are assembled in the patient's unit and are checked for functioning. These include the following as well as those prepared for all patients having major surgery (see p. 115).

Respiratory suction equipment

Equipment for closed chest (water-seal) drainage

Two large hemostats

Equipment for oxygen administration: mask, catheter or cannulae, tubing and bottle for humidification

Equipment for measuring central venous pressure

Thoracentesis (chest aspiration) tray

POSITIONING. With the return of consciousness and stabilization of the blood pressure and pulse, the head of the bed is raised gradually to a 30° to 45° angle. This facilitates the patient's breathing by lowering the diaphragm. The patient is turned every 1 to 2 hours, and the doctor usually specifies whether he may be turned on either side or to one side only. In the case of a pneumonectomy, turning is from the back to the affected side only so that there is no restriction placed on the remaining lung, which is carrying the full respiratory load. With partial resection, the patient usually may be turned from back, to left side, to back, to right side, etc. If a sternum-splitting incision is used, the patient is generally least uncomfortable on his back but is encouraged to assume a lateral position for at least brief periods. During any moving or turning of the patient, precautions are necessary to prevent dislodging the chest drainage tube. As the patient turns, the tube is firmly clamped near the chest with a forceps, and is lifted to prevent dragging or pulling. When he is positioned, a final check is made to be sure that the closed drainage system is patent.

Frequent change of position promotes drainage from the pleural cavity, loosens secretions within the lungs, stimulates circulation, helps to prevent pressure sores and generally reduces the patient's discomfort.

OBSERVATIONS. The arterial blood pressure, pulse and respirations are noted every 15 minutes for the first 2 to 3 hours and then the interval is increased to one-half to 1 hour for the succeeding 8 to 10 hours if the vital signs are stabilized. Since venous return to the right atrium is influenced by respiratory movements and intrathoracic pressure changes, hourly recording of the central venous pressure may be required. This pressure also reflects the ability of the heart to forward the blood. The reduction in the pulmonary vascular bed following lung resection may offer resistance to the outflow of the right side of the heart, causing an elevation of venous blood pressure. The pressure is obtained by the installation of a fine venous catheter threaded through an antecubital vein (basilic or cephalic vein) into the superior vena cava. The surgeon usually indicates the level of elevation of venous pressure at which he is to be notified and at which the fluid intake is restricted.

The rise and fall of both sides of the chest in respiration should be noted. Dyspnea, decreased movement of one side of the chest on inspiration (except in pneumonectomy), cyanosis or chest pain may manifest a pneumothorax and should be reported promptly to the doctor. This may develop as a result of air or fluid collecting in the pleural cavity and compressing the lung. It must be treated quickly by chest aspiration (thoracentesis), or the patient may die of respiratory insufficiency. Respirations are also observed for audible moist sounds. A portable chest x-ray may be done daily for 2 to 3 days to determine lung expansion and detect the presence of fluid and air in the pleural cavity.

The wound area and chest drainage are examined frequently for any indications of bleeding. The sealed-drainage system is checked frequently for functioning (see p. 309), and the tubing connections are examined for security. The volume of drainage is measured at regular 8-hour intervals. The intake and output are recorded, and the fluid balance is estimated.

The nurse may also be required to measure the patient's tidal and minute volumes. Arterial blood specimens may be necessary for blood gas determinations which indicate possible respiratory insufficiency and the need for mechanical assistance and/or increased oxygen inhalation.

OXYGEN ADMINISTRATION. The patient usually receives oxygen by mask, catheter or cannulae for at least the first 24 to 36 hours. The administration is not prolonged unless the patient is experiencing some respiratory insufficiency. Most patients seem to adapt fairly quickly to the remaining lung capacity. Occasionally a patient becomes dependent on the oxygen therapy and is fearful of having it discontinued. In such instances a gradual withdrawal is necessary.

SUCTIONING AND COUGHING. As soon as the blood pressure is stabilized, the patient is asked to cough every 1 to 2 hours or oftener if there is evidence of retained secretions. Removal of secretions may prevent atelectasis and infection and will improve ventilation of the lung. It is sufficiently important that the patient is wakened to cough at the regular intervals throughout the night. Even with preoperative instruction and practice, the patient is usually fearful and may find the procedure difficult. Suctioning is used to clear the pharyngeal part of the tract and will also precipitate coughing. The latter loosens secretions in the lower tracheo-bronchial passages and raises them to the upper tract from which the patient may cough them up or they may be reached by suction. The nurse assists the patient to a sitting position for coughing and, standing at the side of the bed which is opposite to the patient's incision, supports the operative side of the chest, back and front, with her hands. The patient is asked to take several deep breaths and to cough with each expiration. If the cough and suctioning are not productive, it is brought to the doctor's attention. An expectorant or aerosol preparation may be prescribed to liquefy the secretions, making them easier to raise. A

humidifier or steam inhalation in the room may also be helpful. Endotracheal suctioning may have to be done by the physician if the secretions continue to be retained. For this a number Fr. 14 or 16 catheter is attached to the suction and, with the patient in an upright sitting position, his tongue is gently pulled forward, and the catheter is passed via the nose into the larynx. The patient is asked to inhale deeply or cough which opens the glottis and the doctor quickly forwards the catheter into the trachea. Violent coughing ensues, dislodging secretions to within reach of the suction.

DEEP BREATHING. The patient's respirations tend to be shallow, since deep breaths are likely to cause some discomfort. He is encouraged to take 5 to 10 deep breaths hourly and is given an explanation of the need to promote full expansion of the remaining lung tissue and the drainage of air and fluid from the thoracic cavity. As the lung expands to occupy more space, the pressure increases within the pleural cavity, forcing air and fluid through the drainage tube.

FLUIDS AND NUTRITION. The blood loss at operation is replaced by a blood transfusion and fluids are usually given intravenously for the first 24 to 48 hours. The rate at which the fluid is given must be carefully controlled to prevent too rapid filling of the reduced vascular compartment and subsequent pulmonary edema, which is manifested by dyspnea, bubbling sounds and frothy sputum. The doctor may indicate the rate at which the intravenous fluid may be administered, which usually does not exceed 40 drops per minute. The rate of flow is also regulated according to the central venous pressure.

Clear fluids may be given as soon as there is no nausea and vomiting and gradually are increased in volume as tolerated. The patient may have a soft diet the first postoperative day, if he can take it, and a regular diet the following day. Extra fluids are provided, if tolerated, to reduce the tenaciousness of the respiratory secretions.

RELIEF OF PAIN. When closing the chest wall, the surgeon may inject the intercostal nerves with a novocaine preparation to reduce the pain. Narcotic drugs are used sparingly since they generally depress respirations and the cough reflex. A small dose of morphine or meperidine hydrochloride (Demerol) may be prescribed for pain, but judgment must be used in administering it. The patient should not be allowed to suffer unnecessarily, but it is also important that he cough to remove secretions and breathe deeply to adequately ventilate the remaining lung tissue.

EXERCISE AND MOBILITY. Passive extension and flexion movements of the lower limbs are carried out by the nurse every 3 to 4 hours until the doctor indicates that the patient may begin active exercises. The latter may be limited or delayed by the chest drainage, but if his progress is satisfactory, postural and arm exercises will probably be started the third postoperative day. If his condition is satisfactory, he may be assisted out of bed on the second or third day. The exercises and early ambulation stimulate circulation and respirations, prevent venous stasis and thrombus formation and promote normal posture. They also tend to assure the patient of a favorable progress and bolster his morale.

CONVALESCENCE AND REHABILITATION. The convalescence and rehabilitation must be adapted to each individual patient. Generally, the patient requires a fairly long period of convalescence during which he is encouraged to continue his exercises and deep breathing. Activity is gradually increased, and the patient's reaction to it is noted. The doctor is informed if there is persisting dyspnea or shortness of breath, and the activity is restricted until a greater exercise tolerance is developed. The body has to adjust to a reduced respiratory capacity, and the patient who has had a pneumonectomy will require a greater period of adjustment. The patient may not be able to resume his former occupation and may need help to find lighter work within his respiratory capacity.

In preparation for going home, the patient receives instructions about the exercises, deep breathing and coughing which are to be continued. The recommended amounts of rest and activity are explained. If distance and travel do not present too great a problem, the patient may be requested to return to the physiotherapy department for exercise supervision once or twice weekly. Or arrangements may be made to have a physiotherapist or a nurse visit him at home to counsel and assess his progress. He may experience some numbness, pain or heaviness in the operative area due to interruption of the intercostal nerves but may be reassured that this is generally temporary.

CLOSED CHEST DRAINAGE. Following intrathoracic surgery, fluid and air may collect in the space between the lungs and chest wall. If allowed to remain, the accumulation may prevent re-expansion of the lung on the operative side and may also cause pressure on the large blood vessels, heart and unaffected lung, interfering with circulation and reducing ventilation. A collection of serosanguinous fluid predisposes to infection as it serves as a good culture medium. It may also cause pleural thickening that could reduce the ventilatory and diffusion capacity of the lung.

When the surgery is completed, a closed or water-seal drainage system is established to allow the escape of air and fluid from the pleural cavity but prevent any reflux. Two tubes are generally placed in the operative area and are secured by a suture to the chest wall. One tube is placed in the anterior upper part of the operative area and principally serves in the escape of air; the second tube is usually placed in the posterior base of the cavity for fluid drainage.

Various methods are used to achieve closed drainage, but the principle is the same in all—namely, to allow air and fluid to pass in one direction only. The difference in the methods is mainly in the number of bottles used, whether or not suction is applied and whether or not a flutter valve is introduced into the system.

In water-seal drainage without suction, the drainage tubes are connected to a fairly long tube leading to the drainage bottle where it is connected to a glass or plastic tube which has its distal end submerged at all times in sterile water or sterile normal saline to a designated depth (usually 3 to 5 cm.). The depth of tube submersion determines the pressure exerted by the water. The drainage tube is sealed off by the water, hence the term "water-seal drainage." A small, short glass tube, serving as an air vent, passes through the second hole of the tight fitting, two-holed rubber stopper.

With each expiration, the intrapleural space is diminished and the pressure is increased to exceed that exerted by the water on the end of the tube, so fluid and air are forced from the cavity into the water in the bottle. The air may be seen bubbling through the water, from which it passes, escaping from the bottle through the vent. On inspiration, the pleural space enlarges and the pressure within it decreases, causing water to rise a few inches in the distal end of the tube. The alternating changes in pressure in the pleural cavity result in repeated fluctuations in the water level in the distal end of the drainage tube; these fluctuations correspond to the patient's breathing in and out and indicate a patent system and serve as a guide to the nurse. If the level of the water does not oscillate, one may suspect that the tube is blocked by a blood clot or fibrin. If this occurs, the tube is "milked" toward the drainage bottle in an effort to relieve the blockage, and if this is not successful, the physician is notified at once. In order to prevent blocking, the tube is generally milked at least hourly. Fluctuation of the fluid level in the tube ceases when the lung has fully re-expanded. The doctor confirms this by an x-ray of the chest before removing the drainage tube.

Coughing and deep breathing alter the intrapleural space and pressure to a greater degree than normal respirations and, as a result, play an important role in promoting drainage of the cavity, removal of air and re-expansion of remaining lung tissue.

To prevent water from being sucked into the chest, the drainage bottle must be kept at floor level or well below the level of the bed (2 to 3 feet below the patient's chest). The negative chest pressure is equivalent to 10 to 20 cm. of water and sucks the water up into the tube only to that level. If the bottle must be lifted or moved, the drainage tube is securely clamped near the chest wall by two strong hemostats which must always be available at the bedside.

A safer method to prevent the possibility of water accidentally entering the chest cavity and which also keeps the drainage separated from the water is to use a second bottle for the water, leaving the drainage bottle dry. When only one bottle is used, fluid drainage from the chest raises the level of the fluid, increasing the pressure at the distal end of the tube. More pressure, then, is required to force the fluid down on expiration and allow the escape of air fluid. Blood and serum are more likely to collect and clot in the tube. In the two-bottle system, the first bottle is sealed and does not contain water; the shorter of the glass tubes is connected to the second bottle which also has two glass tubes. The first (drainage) bottle is connected to the longer tube in the second bottle. The distal end of this tube is submerged in sterile water to a designated depth (3 to 5 cm.). The second tube (in bottle 2) is short and acts as an air vent (see Fig. 14–10).

If there is a considerable amount of air leaking into the pleural cavity from the intrapulmonary space or if the patient's cough and respirations are not sufficiently strong to facilitate the clearance of fluid and air from the chest cavity, continuous gentle suction may be applied. This usually necessitates a two-bottle system; the first bottle serves as a drainage bottle and is sealed. The short, air-vent tube in bottle 1 is connected to the second bottle which has a three-holed stopper through which 2 short tubes and one longer one pass (see Fig. 14-10). The lower end of the longer tube is submerged in water to a designated depth; the upper end is open to the air. This tube serves to control the degree of suction applied to the pleural cavity. One short tube is connected to bottle 1; the second short tube is connected to a suction apparatus. The usual suction machine creates too strong a negative pressure to be applied directly to the pleural cavity. This may be reduced by a valve and meter inserted between the suction and the water-seal bottle as is used on "wall suction." If the portable suction machine is used, the negative pressure is controlled by the depth of submersion of the lower end of the open glass tube in bottle 2. A continuous bubbling in the control bottle (bottle 2) indicates that the suction is being maintained.

Recently, disposable closed drainage receptacles have become available. These are used with suction and have 2 compartments comparable to the two-bottle system. The receptacle is suspended from the side of the bed to eliminate the danger of bottles being knocked over and broken.

The water-seal system is cumbersome and also restricts patient mobility. The nurse and patient are continuously apprehensive

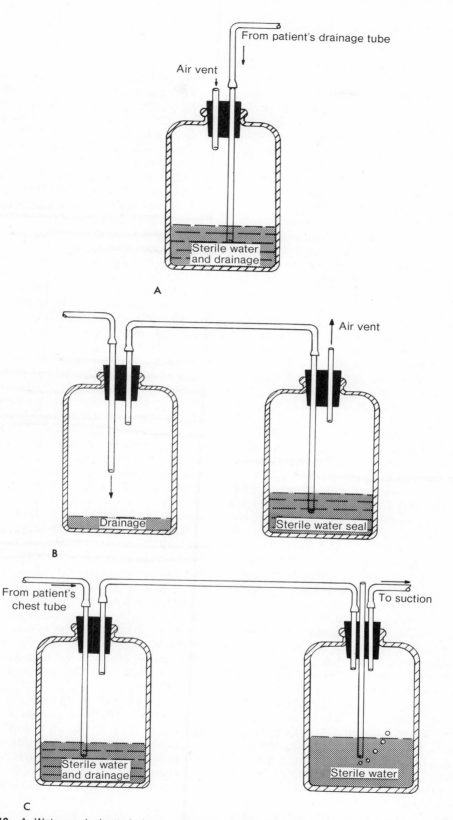

Figure 14–10 *A,* Water-seal chest drainage using one bottle. *B,* Water-seal chest drainage system using two bottles. *C,* Water-seal drainage system using two bottles and suction.

of tubes becoming disconnected, bottles being broken, and so on. As a safety measure and to permit greater freedom in turning and earlier ambulation, some surgeons prefer to introduce a plastic flutter valve into the system. It is placed between the chest drainage tube and the tube leading to the drainage bottle. Suction may still be applied.

When any method of water-seal drainage is used, nursing responsibilities include the following considerations:

It is important that the nurse understand the purpose and operating principles of the system as well as the precautions to be observed to prevent air and fluid from entering the chest cavity which could cause atelectasis and life-threatening respiratory insufficiency.

If the bottle system is used, a directive should be received from the physician as to the depth to which the underwater tube is to be submerged. The bottle should be calibrated so the volume of water used is known and so the drainage may be measured.

The system must be checked at frequent intervals for patency. This is determined by noting the oscillating water level in the submerged tube. It rises with inspiration and falls with expiration. When suction is employed, fluctuations of the water level do not occur because the continuous suction holds the water level in the tube at a fixed level. The suction may be interrupted briefly and the column of water observed for fluctuations. If the water level does not fluctuate in a closed system, the tube should be examined for possible kinks or compression caused by the patient lying on it. A clot may be obstructing the tube and may be dislodged by "milking" the tube toward the drainage bottle. If the system remains nonfunctional, the physician is informed at once.

As a precaution, all connections between the rubber and glass tubes are taped with adhesive to prevent their separation and to keep air from entering the system. The bottles are placed in a rack or taped to the floor to prevent accidental moving or knocking over. Visitors and ward personnel are warned not to disturb them and a warning sign placed by the bottles is helpful.

The drainage tube is supported and lies free in a trough formed by pinning a fold in the sheet. It should not be looped but should be long enough to avoid marked restriction of the patient's moving and turning.

The characteristics and volume of the drainage are noted and recorded frequently, especially during the first 24 to 48 hours. It is generally colored by blood at first but gradually clears and decreases in amount.

Changing the drainage bottle may be done by the doctor or is the responsibility of designated persons who fully understand closed drainage. Each drainage tube is clamped with 2 hemostats close to the chest wall, and the bottle is quickly replaced by a clean sterile bottle.

If an interruption or break in the closed system should occur as a result of the disconnection of a tube or a broken bottle, the drainage tube(s) should be clamped off close to the chest wall immediately to prevent air from entering the chest cavity. An accumulation of air in the pleural cavity could cause a collapse of the lung on the affected side and compression of the unaffected lung, heart and large blood vessels. Associated symptoms are a complaint by the patient of tightness or pressure in the chest, dyspnea, cyanosis and a rapid pulse. The surgeon is notified promptly of the break in the system, and arrangements are made to quickly reestablish drainage. As a precaution, an extra, sterile set of bottles and connections are always available. A thoracentesis may be necessary to remove air from the cavity.

Regular frequent coughing and deep breathing are important, since they increase the intrapulmonic and intrapleural pressure, forcing air and fluid out of the cavity and promoting lung expansion.

When turning the patient or when giving any care, precautions are taken not to dislodge or disconnect the drainage tubes. A check is made to make sure the patient is not lying on a portion of the tube and that there are no loops or kinks that would interfere with drainage.

Even if the system appears to be functioning satisfactorily, any patient complaint of pressure or pain in the chest, dyspnea, cyanosis or a rapid, weak pulse is promptly brought to the physician's attention.

When the lung is fully expanded and no fluid remains in the pleural cavity, the tubes are removed. The water in the closed drainage bottle will have stopped fluctuating, and the lung expansion is confirmed by the physician by percussion, auscultation and a chest x-ray.

When the tube is withdrawn from the chest cavity, the wound is sealed by the application of petroleum jelly gauze and adhesive. The patient is observed closely for the next 24 hours for possible leakage of air into the chest and ensuing pneumothorax.

References

BOOKS

Bates, D. V., Macklem, P. T., and Christie, R. V.: Respiratory Function in Disease, 2nd ed. Philadelphia, W. B. Saunders Co., 1971.

Bendixen, H. H., et al.: Respiratory Care. St. Louis, The C. V. Mosby Co., 1965.

Cherniak, R. M., Cherniak, L., and Naimark, A.: Respiration in Health and Disease, 2nd ed. Philadelphia, W. B. Saunders Co., 1972.

Crofton, J., and Douglas, A.: Respiratory Diseases. Oxford, Blackwell Scientific Publications, 1969.

Davidson, Sir Stanley: The Principles and Practices of Medicine, 9th ed. Edinburgh, E. & S. Livingstone Ltd., 1970, pp. 298–437.

Flitter, H. H.: An Introduction to Physics in Nursing, 5th ed. St. Louis, The C. V. Mosby Co., 1967, pp. 90–99.

Guyton, A. C.: Basic Human Physiology. Philadelphia, W. B. Saunders Co., 1971. Chapters 27, 28, 29 and 30.

Guyton, A. C.: Textbook of Medical Physiology, 4th ed. Philadelphia, W. B. Saunders Co., 1971. Chapters 39, 40, 41, 42, 43 and 44.

Jacob, S. W., and Francone, C. A.: Structure and Function in Man, 2nd ed. Philadelphia, W. B. Saunders Co., 1970, Chapter 12.

Langley, L. L.: Outline of Physiology, 2nd ed. New York, McGraw-Hill Book Co., 1965. Chapters 19, 20 and 21.

National Tuberculosis and Respiratory Disease Association: Introduction to Respiratory Diseases, 4th ed. New York, National Tuberculosis and Respiratory Disease Association, 1969.

Oswald, N. C., and Fry, J.: Diseases of the Respiratory System. Oxford, Blackwell Scientific Publications, 1962.

Secor, J.: Patient Care in Respiratory Problems. Philadelphia, W. B. Saunders Co., 1969.

South, J.: Tuberculosis Handbook for Public Health Nurses. New York, National Tuberculosis and Respiratory Disease Association, 1965.

Sutton, A. F.: Bedside Nursing Techniques in Medicine and Surgery, 2nd ed. Philadelphia, W. B. Saunders Co., 1969. Chapters 4, 5 and 13.

PERIODICALS

Betson, C.: "Blood Gases." Amer. J. Nurs., Vol. 68, No. 5 (May 1968), pp. 1010–1012.

Bradley, J.: "Emphysema: Are Nurses Prepared?" R.N., Jan. 1968, pp. 41–43.

Crowell, C. E. (Educational Designs Inc. of New York): "Respiratory Tract Aspiration, Programmed Instruction." Amer. J. Nurs., Vol. 66, No. 11 (Nov. 1966), pp. 2483–2510.

Dittbrenner, Sister Marilyn, and Hebert, W. M.: "Regimen for a Thoractomy Patient." Amer. J. Nurs. Vol. 67, No. 10 (October 1967), pp. 2072–2075.

Hadley, F., and Bordicks, K. J.: "When a Patient Has Respiratory Difficulty." Amer. J. Nurs., Vol. 62, No. 11 (October 1962), pp. 64–67.

Helming, M. G. (Ed.): Symposium on Nursing in Respiratory Diseases. Nurs. Clin. North Amer., Vol. 3, No. 3 (Sept. 1968).

Kearns, B.: "Tracheotomy Suctioning Technique." Canad. Nurse, Vol. 66, No. 2 (Feb. 1970), pp. 44–48.

Kirby, W. M. M. (Ed.): Symposium on Modern Management of Respiratory Disease. Med. Clin. North Amer., Vol. 51, No. 2. (Mar. 1967).

Kurihara, M.: "Postural Drainage, Clapping and Vibrating." Amer. J. Nurs., Vol. 65, No. 11 (Nov. 1965), pp. 76–79.

McArdle, K. H.: "The Patient on the Bennett." Nurs. Clin. North Amer., Vol. 1, No. 1. (Mar. 1966), pp. 143–152.

Nealon, T. F., Jr., and Sandler, S. C.: "The Treatment of Respiratory Failure with Continuous Ventilatory Support." Surg. Clin. North Amer., Vol. 47, No. 5 (Oct. 1967), pp. 1207–1222.

Nett, L. M., and Petty, T. L.: "Acute Respiratory Failure." Amer. J. Nurs., Vol. 67, No. 9 (Sept., 1967), pp. 1847–1853.

Nett, L. M., and Petty, T. L.: "Why Emphysema Patients Are the Way They Are." Amer. J. Nurs., Vol. 70, No. 6 (June 1970), pp. 1251–1253.

Ochsner, J. L., and Keller, C. H.: "Removing Bronchial Secretions." Nurs. Clin. North Amer., Vol. 2, No. 3 (Sept. 1967), pp. 521–527.

Oschner, A., and Oschner, A., Jr.: "Cancer of the Lung: Recognition and Management." Surg. Clin. North Amer., Vol. 46, No. 6 (Dec. 1966), pp. 1411–1425.

Rodman, T.: "Management of Tracheobronchial Secretions." Amer. J. Nurs., Vol. 66, No. 11 (Nov. 1966), pp. 2474–2477.

Schwaid, M. C.: "The Impact of Emphysema." Amer. J. Nurs., Vol. 70, No. 6 (June, 1970), pp. 1247–1250.

Sovie, M., and Israel, J. S.: "Use of the Cuffed Tracheostomy Tube." Amer. J. Nurs., Vol. 67, No. 9 (Sept. 1967), pp. 1854–1856.

Ujiki, G. T., and Shields, T. W.: "Newer Trends in the Diagnosis and Treatment of Bronchogenic Carcinoma." Surg. Clin. North Amer., Vol. 51, No. 1 (Feb. 1971), pp. 183–192.

Winter, P. M., and Lowenstein, E.: "Acute Respiratory Failure." Sci. Amer., Vol. 221, No. 5 (Nov. 1969), pp. 23–29.

PAMPHLETS

Living with Asthma, Chronic Bronchitis, and Emphysema — A Guide to Self-care, Prepared and distributed by Riker Laboratories, Northridge, California, 1968.

Asthma — A Practical Guide for Physicians. Prepared by a Joint Committee of the Allergy Foundation of America and American Thoracic Society, 1968.

15
Nursing in Disorders of the Alimentary Canal

DIGESTION

DIGESTIVE STRUCTURES AND FUNCTIONS

The Alimentary Canal

The alimentary canal is a long hollow tube extending from the lips to the anus. It is wider in some parts than in others and is divided into the mouth, pharynx, esophagus, stomach (Greek, *gaster*) and intestines (Greek, *enteron*). Its functions are digestion, absorption of food and fluid into the blood and elimination of residue and waste products. Modifications in the structure occur in the different parts of the canal and are correlated with the particular functions featured in the respective area.

The mouth or oral cavity, the initial part of the tract, is lined by a mucous membrane which secretes mucus to mix with the food, facilitating its movement through the pharynx and esophagus. Although the mouth is primarily concerned with the ingestion of food, it also plays an important role in speech.

The tongue, teeth and salivary glands are contained within the mouth. The tongue is comprised of muscular tissue enclosed in mucous membrane. The upper surface is studded with numerous papillae and contains taste buds. The tongue functions in swallowing and speech as well as in taste.

Early in life, the human organism develops 20 primary deciduous teeth—10 upper and 10 lower. Beginning in the fifth or sixth year and continuing over a period of several years, the deciduous teeth are replaced by a permanent set of 16 in the upper jaw and 16 in the lower jaw. The front teeth are shaped for biting and tearing, the remainder for grinding and masticating food. Hence, loss of teeth, or defects in them, can lead to indigestion or malnutrition.

Each tooth consists of a crown and root. The crown is the exposed portion which has a hard external covering of enamel and an internal substance called dentine. The root is the part buried in the jaw bone and has a covering of cementum, a substance less hard and less smooth than the enamel. A central cavity running the length of the tooth contains nerves and blood vessels.

There are three pairs of salivary glands whose ducts open onto the surface of the mouth. The parotid glands lie in front of and below the ear and produce a thin, watery secretion that includes an important digestive enzyme, ptyalin. The submaxillary and sublingual glands are located in the floor of the mouth. The sublingual glands secrete only mucus; the submaxillary glands produce both a watery and mucous secretion. The secretions of the salivary glands and the oral mucosa collectively form the saliva. For the composition and functions of saliva see page 319.

The second segment of the tract is the pharynx, which is a muscular tube lined with mucous membrane continuous with that of the mouth, respiratory tract and esophagus. It serves as a common pathway for food and air. When its muscular tissue contracts, it directs food and fluid into the esophagus, closing off the entrances to the larynx and nasal cavities at the same time.

The esophagus is a narrow muscular tube, approximately 10 inches long, that passes down behind the trachea and heart, through the mediastinum and diaphragm to the stomach. It is lined with mucous membrane and has an outer protective coat of fibrous tissue.

The stomach and the intestines, the remaining portions of the digestive tract, lie within the abdominal cavity. The stomach is located just below the diaphragm and is the widest part of the alimentary canal which makes possible its retention of a considerable amount of food while the food undergoes certain changes. It is divided into 3 segments: the fundus, body and pylorus (Fig. 15–1).

The gastric walls have 3 layers of muscle tissue; one in which the fibers run longitudinally, a second one in which they are circular, and a third in which they run obliquely to the others. The circular muscle layer is thickened at the opening of the esophagus into the stomach to form the cardiac sphincter. Similarly, the opening into the small intestine is guarded by the pyloric sphincter.

The mucous membrane lining is thick and lies in folds to allow for distensibility as the stomach fills. It contains numerous minute glands made up of 3 types of secreting cells: the chief, or zymogen, cells secrete the gastric enzymes; the parietal cells produce hydrochloric acid; and mucous glands provide mucus. The glandular secretions are poured out into the stomach to form collectively the gastric juice.

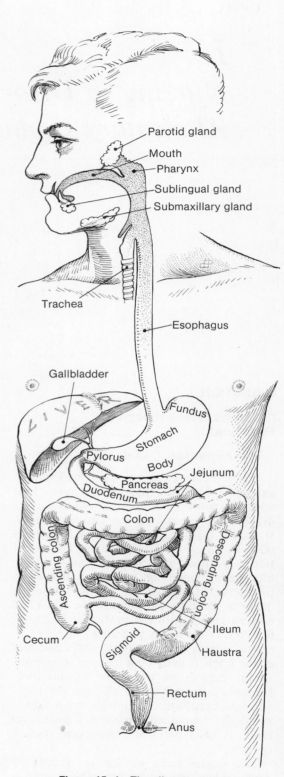

Figure 15–1 The alimentary tract.

The small intestine is the longest portion of the alimentary canal, being approximately 18 to 20 feet, and is divided into the duodenum, jejunum and ileum. The duodenum is the short, proximal portion which originates with the gastric pylorus. It receives the bile and the pancreatic enzymes through a sphincter (sphincter of Oddi) at the junction of the common bile duct and the duodenum. The long jejunum and ileum lie in loops and fill the greater part of the abdominal cavity.

The mucosal surface of the small intestine is covered with many finger-like processes called villi, each of which contains a central lymph channel, called a lacteal, and a network of capillaries. Most digestion and absorption take place in the small intestine where circular folds increase the surface area and somewhat retard the passage of the food, thus favoring absorption. The molecules of digested food are picked up by the blood in the capillaries or the lymph in the lacteals.

The small intestine contains many glands which secrete digestive enzymes (see p. 323) and mucus into the lumen of the tube. Lymph nodes appear in clusters throughout the small intestine and are referred to as Peyer's patches.

The large intestine has a greater diameter than that of the small intestine and is divided into the cecum, colon, rectum and anal canal. The ileum opens into a pouch-like structure, the cecum, in the right lower abdominal quadrant. The appendix, a slender blind tube, is attached to the cecum and is a frequent site of inflammation and infection (appendicitis). At the junction of the ileum and cecum, an ileocecal valve functions to allow contents to pass in one direction only— from the ileum to the cecum.

The large intestine ascends the right side of the abdominal cavity from the cecum as the ascending colon and flexes at the undersurface of the liver to form the transverse colon. The descending colon passes down the left side of the abdomen and, since it takes an S-shaped course through the pelvis, becomes the sigmoid colon.

The mucosa of the large intestine has no villi and its glands secrete only mucus. The longitudinal muscle tissue is arranged in 3 strips that are shorter than the other tissues, resulting in small sacs along the wall of the tube called haustra (Fig. 15–1).

The rectum is a continuation of the sigmoid along the anterior surface of the sacrum and coccyx. It is about 6 to 7 inches long and contains vertical folds referred to as rectal columns. Each column contains an artery and vein. The veins frequently become varicosed, forming hemorrhoids.

The short terminal portion of the alimentary tube, the anal canal, opens on to the body surface at the anus. The opening between the rectum and the anal canal is controlled by the internal anal sphincter, which is involuntary. The anus is controlled by the external anal sphincter which, after infancy, is under voluntary control.

Peritoneum. The outer protective coat of the stomach and intestines is serous membrane and is known as the visceral peritoneum. The abdominal cavity is lined with serous membrane called the parietal peritoneum. A fan-like expanse is reflected off the posterior abdominal wall and extends to the intestine where it become continuous with the visceral peritoneum. This portion of serous membrane is known as the mesentery; it supports the intestine and transmits blood vessels, lymphatics and nerves. A sheet of peritoneum, the great omentum, is reflected off the stomach to lie like an apron in front of the intestines. The great omentum protects the intestines, and when infection or inflammation of the peritoneum (peritonitis) occurs, it makes an effort to wall off the affected area by surrounding it to prevent a spread of the infection. The lesser omentum is a fold of peritoneum extending from the liver to the stomach.

Blood Supply to the Alimentary Canal. The mouth, tongue and pharynx derive their blood supply from the external carotid artery via the lingual and external maxillary arteries. The esophageal artery arises from the thoracic aorta. Three main arteries supply the stomach: the left, right and short gastric arteries. The left gastric is a branch of the celiac which is a large, short artery arising from the abdominal aorta. The other two gastrics originate from the other main branches of the celiac, the hepatic and splenic arteries.

The remainder of the tract is nourished by the superior and inferior mesenteric arteries, direct branches of the abdominal aorta.

The blood into which the digested food

products are absorbed is carried by the superior and inferior mesenteric veins into the portal vein, which transmits it to the liver. This makes the food products immediately available to the liver for its functions.

Nerve Supply to the Alimentary Canal. The glands that secrete enzymes and mucus in various parts of the digestive tract are innervated by parasympathetic and sympathetic nerve fibers. The muscle tissue of the mouth, pharynx and upper third of the esophagus is controlled by impulses transmitted by fibers of cranial nerves directly from the brain (trigeminal, glossopharyngeal and vagus nerves). The musculature of the remainder of the tract is innervated by sympathetic and parasympathetic fibers. The parasympathetic fibers increase activity, and the sympathetic impulses depress gastrointestinal activity.

Accessory Structures of Digestion

The Bile System and Pancreas. The bile system and pancreas are discussed in separate chapters. See Chapter 16 for the biliary system and Chapter 17 for the pancreas.

PHYSIOLOGY

Digestion consists of mechanical and chemical processes. The mechanical processes, involving the neuromuscular tissues of the alimentary tract, have as their purposes the movement of food through the tract, the mixing of it with digestive secretions, and the repeated breaking up of the food mass to bring more of it in contact with the absorptive surface. These processes include mastication, deglutition (swallowing), movements of the stomach and intestines, and defecation. The chemical processes are chemical reactions promoted by enzymes to reduce the food to simpler compounds.

The digestive enzymes are substances secreted by mucosal cells of the alimentary tract or by the associated digestive organs. Like all enzymes in the body, they act as catalysts (i.e., they promote and speed up chemical reactions without becoming a part of them). All enzymes are specific, and in the case of the digestive enzymes, each is

secreted only by cells in a certain area of the digestive system. They are classified according to the food they act upon. An enzyme which promotes the breakdown of protein is called a proteinase; one that acts upon starches is an amylase; and a fat-splitting enzyme is known as a lipase.

The principal reaction in chemical digestion is hydrolysis, which is the breaking up of a large molecule of a substance into smaller molecules by combining it with water. For example, in the digestion of cane sugar, 1 molecule of the sugar and 1 molecule of water yields 2 molecules of simple diffusable glucose that can be absorbed

$$(C_{12}H_{22}O_{11} + H_2O \xrightarrow{\text{enzyme}} 2(C_6H_{12}O_6)).$$

Most food undergoes several chemical reactions before it is reduced to a form that can be absorbed. The steps in the digestive breakdown of protein, carbohydrate and fat follow.

Protein → proteoses → peptones → polypeptides → amino acids

Carbohydrate
   a. Starch (polysaccharide) → maltose → glucose
   b. Disaccharides
      maltose → glucose
      sucrose → glucose and fructose
      lactose → glucose and galactose

Fat → glycerol and fatty acids

Digestion takes place entirely within the alimentary canal, and the mechanical and chemical processes vary from one area of the digestive tract to another. In the following section, digestion is discussed as it occurs in each of the different parts of the alimentary tract.

Movement, Secretion and Digestion in the Mouth, Pharynx and Esophagus

Movement in the Mouth, Pharynx and Esophagus. The mouth performs mastication and the initial part of swallowing. The pharynx and esophagus are concerned only with swallowing.

MASTICATION. Most of the food entering the mouth undergoes biting and grinding by the teeth and is mixed with the saliva to produce a moist pulpy mass, called a bolus, for swallowing. Mastication is achieved by contractions of the muscles of the jaws, lips, cheeks and tongue.

DEGLUTITION. Deglutition is the term applied to the transmission of food and fluid from the mouth to the stomach and is commonly referred to as swallowing. When mastication is completed, the food is moved to the posterior oral cavity by the tongue and cheeks and then forced into the pharynx. Certain reflexes then occur in rapid succession. Muscles in the walls of the pharynx contract, drawing the soft palate up and back and closing off the entrance to the nasal cavities. The larynx is raised, bringing its opening against the epiglottis and the base of the tongue, thus preventing the food from entering the respiratory tract. The food cannot re-enter the mouth, for the back of the tongue is raised to block the opening. The pressure exerted on the bolus by the pharyngeal constriction forces the food into the only open route, the esophagus.

The reflex responses of the pharynx to the entrance of food or fluid may be depressed by local anesthetic. To prevent aspiration following anesthetization of the pharynx, food and fluid are withheld until the swallowing reflexes have returned. This applies following laryngoscopy, bronchoscopy, esophagoscopy, gastroscopy and surgery on the mouth or throat.

When the bolus enters the esophagus, it stimulates the circular muscle of the section it is in and inhibits that of the portion immediately ahead. Thus, the food is squeezed out of the first section into the relaxed portion. The process is repeated, producing a wave of alternating contractions and relaxations along the esophagus. The wave of inhibition which precedes the bolus reaches the cardiac sphincter, causing it to open, and the bolus enters the stomach.

The more liquid the bolus, the more rapidly it travels through the esophagus.

Secretion and Digestion in the Mouth, Pharynx and Esophagus. Saliva is secreted by the salivary glands; added to it is a small amount of mucus produced by the mucous membrane of the oral cavity. The amount of saliva secreted varies from approximately 1 to 1.5 L. per day, depending on the quantity and quality of food taken. A greater volume of food requires an increased output of saliva and appetizing foods also stimulate the output. The saliva is swallowed and much of the fluid is reclaimed by absorption. Any interference with swallowing or any condition that provokes loss of saliva from the mouth results in a considerable loss of body fluid, contributing to dehydration.

Saliva is usually slightly acidic with a pH of 6.6 to 6.9 and consists of the following:

Water (97 to 99 per cent)

Mucin

Salts of sodium, potassium and calcium. (The bicarbonate salts of saliva are responsible for the formation of most of the tartar on the teeth. The salts, when exposed to air, release CO_2 and the bicarbonate is transformed to an insoluble carbonate.)

Organisms

Epithelial cells from the mucosa

FUNCTIONS OF SALIVA. One of the functions of saliva is to moisten the food and lubricate the oral cavity in order to facilitate swallowing. Dry food is put into solution by saliva, making possible the taste sensation, since only food in solution reaches the taste buds which are recessed in small pits in the tongue. Speech is made more articulate when the oral structures are moist.

The enzyme ptyalin acts on starches, reducing them to maltose. This is the only chemical digestive function performed by saliva. The action of ptyalin may be continued for a brief period in the stomach, as the saliva is swallowed with the food. Ptyalin is only effective in an alkaline medium or very mild acid; in the stomach it is inactivated by the presence of the hydrochloric acid.

Saliva has a cleansing effect; it washes away food particles and other debris. If these are allowed to accumulate, they could act as a culture medium for organisms. Patients who are not secreting the normal amount of saliva require frequent cleansing mouth care.

The salivary glands excrete certain substances from the blood into the saliva. Lead, sulfur and potassium iodide may be transferred to the saliva. Similarly, urea may be noticeable in the saliva of persons whose kidneys fail to excrete the normal amount of urea.

Finally, saliva has a role in relation to the water balance. The moisture of the mouth largely determines the sense of thirst. A reduction in salivary output occurs with dehydration and a sense of thirst accompanies the dry mouth. When the fluids are replenished, the mouth again becomes moistened by saliva and the sense of thirst is alleviated.

REGULATION OF SALIVARY SECRETION. Control of the salivary glands is by the autonomic nervous system; each gland has both a parasympathetic and sympathetic nerve supply which deliver impulses from a salivary center in the medulla of the brain stem. Sensory nerves conduct impulses from the mouth to the salivary center to influence its action. The sensory impulses arise from taste and from pressure created by the presence of food or some instrument in the mouth. One is familiar with the experience of increased salivation when the dentist is working in the mouth.

An increased output of saliva may be a conditioned response to the sight, smell or thought of food. It implies previous experience with food and impulses are transmitted from higher centers of the brain to the salivary center in the medulla.

Parasympathetic innervation results in an increased volume of a watery secretion containing the enzyme ptyalin; sympathetic innervation causes a scanty flow of a thick, viscous saliva. The generalized sympathetic innervation associated with fright or nervousness and stress frequently produces a dry, "sticky" mouth.

No enzymes are secreted by the pharynx and esophagus; therefore, no chemical digestion is attributed to these areas. The mucous membrane produces mucus that facilitates the movement of food in swallowing. The mucus also protects the mucosa from any abrasive effect the food might have upon it and from tissue digestion by gastric juice that might escape into the esophagus.

There is an esophagosalivary reflex that increases salivation. A mass or bolus pressing on the walls of the esophagus for any length of time gives rise to sensory impulses, resulting in stimulation of the salivary glands. The increased volume of saliva which is swallowed is an effort to "wash down" the mass. One sees this in the patient with cancer of the esophagus who experiences the problem of excessive salivation.

Movement, Secretion and Digestion in the Stomach

Gastric Movement. The stomach retains the food and churns it about for a period of time until it undergoes certain chemical and physical changes. It ejects its content in frequent small spurts into the duodenum. When the content has become mixed with the gastric secretions, its consistency changes to a thick fluid. This fluid is referred to as chyme.

When the stomach is empty it produces periodic contractions that give the sensation of hunger. The contractions may gradually increase in intensity and be referred to as hunger pains. With the entrance of food, the gastric muscle tissue relaxes and the stomach dilates to accommodate the food (receptive relaxation). Small waves of contraction are gradually resumed, beginning in the body of the stomach, and the food is delivered into the pylorus. When strong contractions occur, the pyloric sphincter relaxes and a portion of the gastric content moves into the duodenum.

Fluid substances pass through the stomach quickly; solid food may take three to five hours, depending on the type of food. Fat remains in the stomach longer than protein, and protein longer than carbohydrate.

Gastric motility and emptying are influenced by mechanical and chemical factors in the duodenum. A volume of chyme filling the duodenum initiates an enterogastric reflex; sensory impulses arise in the walls of the duodenum that result in inhibitory reflex responses by the gastric muscle. The fat content of chyme stimulates the duodenal mucosa to secrete a hormone, enterogastrone, into the blood. On reaching the stomach, enterogastrone depresses gastric contractions.

To summarize, gastric motility is increased as the stomach becomes empty and as the content becomes fluid. It decreases when the gastric content is semisolid, high in fat and when the duodenum is full.

Gastric Secretion and Digestion. The gastric glands secrete a clear, colorless, slimy fluid of high acidity (pH 0.9 to 1.5) that contributes to chemical digestion and changes the food to a more fluid consistency.

The constituents of gastric juice are:
Water (97 to 99 per cent)
Hydrochloric acid (0.2 to 0.5 per cent)
Enzymes:
    pepsinogen (inactive pepsin)
    rennin
    gastric lipase
Inorganic salts of sodium, potassium and calcium

Hematopoietic or intrinsic factor (promotes absorption of Vitamin B_{12})

Mucus

The hydrochloric acid and enzymes are the factors concerned with chemical digestion. Pepsinogen is activated to pepsin by the hydrochloric acid, and the initial breakdown of proteins occurs. Pepsin reduces proteins to proteoses and peptones. Rennin is a specific proteolytic enzyme that converts the soluble caseinogen of milk to insoluble paracasein. The paracasein with the calcium of the milk produces a curd, a more solid form that results in its retention in the stomach while it is digested by pepsin. Gastric lipase is produced in small amounts. Emulsified fats may undergo some reduction, but fat digestion in the stomach is relatively insignificant.

The hydrochloric acid of the gastric juice destroys many bacteria which are ingested with food. The acidity of chyme, due to the hydrochloric acid secretion, stimulates the secretion of the hormone secretin (prosecretin) by the duodenal mucosa. Secretin influences the pancreatic cells to release a fluid high in sodium bicarbonate.

REGULATION OF GASTRIC SECRETION. The amount of gastric juice produced varies somewhat with the types of food taken, but with average meals, it is about 2 L. per day. With fasting, the volume is reduced to a rate of approximately 8 to 15 ml. per hour, or approximately 300 ml. per day.

Secretion is influenced by both nervous and hormonal factors, and it is customary to describe gastric secretion as occurring in certain phases—the psychic, gastric and intestinal phases. The psychic phase of gastric secretion occurs before the food reaches the stomach. When food is tasted and chewed, sensory impulses from the mouth enter the central nervous system and result in parasympathetic innervation via vagus nerve fibers, stimulating the gastric glands to pour out their secretions. The more appetizing the food is, the greater will be the vagal innervation and the response of the gastric glands. Psychic stimulation by the thought, smell or sight of appetizing food may produce the same effect. Conversely, sympathetic innervation depresses the gastric glands and secretion is reduced. Emotional disturbances such as worry, fear and grief result in a decrease in gastric secretion.

Food reaching the stomach further stimulates its secretion, producing what is known as the gastric phase. The food causes a direct mechanical stimulation of the gastric glands and initiates sensory nerve impulses that are delivered via vagus nerve fibers to the medulla, resulting in return impulses via vagal motor fibers that increase the activity of the gastric glands. Chemical stimulation is by a hormone, gastrin, that is released by the gastric mucosa into the blood. Distention of the stomach, particularly in the pyloric region, and certain foods, referred to as secretogogues, evoke the release of gastrin. Proteins, particularly meats, are high in secretogogues, which are soluble in water. Meat soups and broths increase gastric secretion and therefore are used at the beginning of a meal in preparation for the food to follow. Such preparations are excluded from the diet of peptic ulcer patients, since an increased output of the highly acid juice further irritates and erodes their lesion.

Histamine has been found to stimulate the parietal cells of the gastric glands, resulting in an increased output of hydrochloric acid. If the physician finds it necessary to determine if the patient's cells are producing acid or if he is lacking hydrochloric acid (achlorhydric), histamine is injected and the gastric juice aspirated for analysis.

Movement, Secretions and Digestion in the Small Intestine

Movement of the Small Intestine. Food moves slowly through the small intestine so that digestion may be completed and the simpler molecules absorbed. The motor activities perform three functions: food is mixed with bile and with pancreatic and intestinal secretions; the mass is broken up to bring it in contact with the absorptive surfaces; and the unabsorbed content is moved into the large intestine.

Contractions of the longitudinal and circular layers of muscle tissue produce two major types of movement, namely, segmentation and peristalsis. Segmentation occurs with areas of the circular muscle contracting and dividing the intestine into a series of alternating constricted and relaxed areas, giving the tube the appearance of a string of sausages. The mass of food stimulates the circular muscle of the section it is in, while those areas behind and ahead remain relaxed.

The content in the contracted area is divided into two segments: one being squeezed into the relaxed portion of the intestine ahead and the other being forced back into the relaxed area behind the constriction. The area of contracted circular muscle relaxes and contraction occurs in the previously relaxed areas. Segmentation serves to break up the mass of content so more of it is brought into contact with the digestive juice and the absorptive surfaces.

Because the circular muscle tissue of the intestines has an inherent ability to initiate contractions without nerve impulses, segmentation contractions can originate independently of nervous control.

Mixing of the chyme and intestinal juice and absorption are facilitated by oscillations of the villi of the mucosa.

Peristalsis is a wave-like muscular activity consisting of a wave of inhibition followed by a wave of contraction. The advancing portion of the wave involves relaxation of an area of the circular muscle and contraction of the longitudinal muscle, producing a sac-like dilatation. The posterior part of the wave consists of contraction of the circular muscle, producing a constricted area in the tube. The wave is initiated by distention of the intestine or by irritation of the mucosa. As food is moved along slowly, with more food following, a series of these peristaltic waves may occur along a considerable length of the intestine, moving the content toward the large intestine.

The small intestine terminates with the ileocecal valve, which guards the opening into the cecum. The pressure in the small intestine forces open the valve and the fluid passes through into the large bowel.

Pancreatic Juice and Bile. The digestive juice in the small intestine includes external pancreatic secretions, bile and the secretions of the intestinal mucosal glands. Approximately 700 to 1200 ml. of pancreatic secretions enter the duodenum daily and consist of:

Water (97 to 98 per cent)
Enzymes:
  amylase
    amylopsin

proteinases
  trypsinogen (inactive trypsin)
  chymotrypsinogen (inactive chymotrypsin)
  procarboxypeptidase (inactive carboxypeptidase)
lipase
  steapsin

Salts: principal ones are sodium and potassium bicarbonate and sodium alkaline phosphate

Because of the salts, the pancreatic secretion is alkaline with a pH of 7.5 to 8.4 and neutralizes the acid chyme.

For the secretion and composition of bile, see page 393. Bile does not contain a digestive enzyme, but the bile salts do facilitate the digestion of fat by the pancreatic lipase.

REGULATION OF PANCREATIC ENZYME AND BILE SECRETION. Pancreatic secretion into the intestine is regulated mainly by hormones secreted by the intestinal mucosa. The entrance of the acid solution chyme into the duodenum causes the release of secretin (prosecretin) into the blood. When secretin reaches the pancreas, it activates the cells to secrete a fluid high in sodium bicarbonate. Failure to produce this alkaline solution may result in damage to the duodenum by the chyme, which is strongly acid and contains pepsin. The duodenal mucosa is not as well protected by mucus as the gastric mucosa.

A second hormone, pancreozymin, is also produced by the duodenal mucosa when food enters from the stomach. It is carried to the pancreas where it causes the cells to produce a thicker solution rich in enzymes.

Some control of pancreatic secretion is also exerted via the vagus nerve. It is suggested that this is part of the gastric reflex. Sensory impulses are initiated by food in the stomach and result in vagal stimulation of the pancreatic cells to produce enzymes.

The liver cells secrete bile continuously, but the amount is increased when food is taken, especially fat and protein. However, it is thought that the hormone secretin which excites the pancreas may also cause an increased output of bile. Probably the most effective mechanism is stimulation of the liver cells by bile salts. The bile salts are absorbed from the intestine and activate the liver cells to form bile. The sphincter of Oddi relaxes when food enters the duodenum (see p. 395) and bile that has been stored in the gallbladder enters the intestine. Bile salts are then available to be absorbed to stimulate the liver cells. In a fasting state, bile does not enter the duodenum and the secretion of bile is somewhat decreased.

Intestinal Juice (Succus Entericus). The mucosa of the small intestine produces 2 to 3 L. of fluid per day. The solution, called succus entericus, is alkaline, and the pH varies from 7.0 to 9.0, depending on the region of the intestine. The composition of succus entericus is:

Water
Salts
Mucin
Epithelial cells
Enzymes:
  enterokinase, which activates the trypsinogen and probably procarboxypeptidase
  erepsin
  lipase
  sucrase
  maltase
  lactase

REGULATION OF SMALL INTESTINAL SECRETION. Several factors are said to influence intestinal secretion. The pressure of its content produces a direct effect on the mucosa which results in an increased amount of intestinal juice. There is also a hormone, enterocrinin, which is released by the mucosa and excites the production of the succus entericus. Secretion may also be influenced by the autonomic nervous system; parasympathetic innervation increases secretions, and sympathetic innervation decreases the output.

Digestion in the Small Intestine. Most chemical digestion takes place and is completed in the small intestine.

Any polysaccharides which have not been reduced by ptyalin to maltose are acted upon by the pancreatic amylase (amylopsin). The intestinal enzyme maltase hydrolyzes maltose; lactase splits lactose; and sucrase breaks down sucrose resulting in the simple absorbable sugars glucose, galactose and fructose.

Protein digestion which is initiated in the stomach by pepsin is completed by several pancreatic and intestinal enzymes. Trypsinogen is activated in the intestine by enterokinase and is then known as trypsin.

Chymotrypsinogen is converted to the active form chymotrypsin by trypsin, and procarboxypeptidase becomes active carboxypeptidase by either trypsin or enterokinase. Trypsin, chymotrypsin, carboxypeptidase and intestinal erepsin reduce proteins to absorbable amino acids.

The breaking down of fats into glycerol and fatty acids is done mainly by the pancreatic lipase, steapsin. The intestinal lipase is less effective. Fat digestion is greatly facilitated by bile, which emulsifies the fat.

Movement, Secretion and Digestion in the Large Intestine

Movement of the Large Intestine. Peristalsis in the colon occurs as a mass movement 3 or 4 times a day, moving the content toward the rectum. When the content reaches the distal portion of the colon, it is then moved into the rectum. As the food proceeded through the mouth, stomach and small intestine, a large amount of water was added to it. Much of this water is reclaimed by absorption in the colon which changes the consistency of the remaining content. The latter becomes a soft, solid mass referred to as feces.*

Peristaltic movements in the large intestine are reflexly stimulated by the entrance of food into the stomach. This gastrocolic reflex, as it is termed, is usually most evident after breakfast, when the stomach has been empty for a longer period of time. It results in the feces being moved into the rectum, giving rise to the desire to defecate. Reflex stimulation originating with emotion, and distention or irritation of the colon will initiate movement.

Defecation is the term applied to the expulsion of feces from the rectum and has both an involuntary and voluntary phase. Normally, the rectum remains empty until just before defecation. When feces enter the rectum, the local distention and pressure give rise to sensory impulses that initiate reflex impulses to the internal anal sphincter and to the muscle tissue of the sigmoid colon and the rectum. The sphincter relaxes and the muscle tissue contracts. The external anal sphincter is under voluntary control and must also relax for evacuation of the rectum.

---

*_Feces_ is the Latin word for dregs.

Defecation may be assisted voluntarily by contracting the abdominal muscles and by forceful expiration with the glottis closed to increase the intra-abdominal pressure.

If the defecation reflex is ignored and the external sphincter is kept closed, the defecation desire soon wanes. Eventually, with repeated ignoring of the defecation reflex, local stimulation by distention and pressure is lost. Feces accumulate in the rectum and lower colon, causing constipation.

Eight to ten hours are required normally for the chyme to pass through the small intestine and to reach the distal portion of the colon, where it accumulates until defecation. The content of the alimentary canal that is not absorbed may take 24 hours or longer to pass through the entire canal.

Fecal matter consists of the unabsorbed food residue, mucus, digestive secretions (gastric, intestinal, pancreatic and liver), water and microorganisms. The water content is progressively reduced by absorption as the feces move through the large intestine so that, normally, on elimination the stool is a formed mass. If the feces are moved rapidly through the large intestine, less water is absorbed and the stool is unformed and liquid. If movement of the feces and elimination are delayed, an excessive amount of water is absorbed and the stool becomes hard and dry.

Secretion and Digestion in the Large Intestine. The large intestine has no role in digestion. It secretes a large amount of viscous alkaline mucus that lubricates the feces, facilitating their movement through the large bowel. The mucus also protects the mucosa from mechanical and chemical injury, and its alkalinity neutralizes acids formed by bacterial action, which is considerable in the colon.

Irritation of an area of the large intestine results in an increased output of mucus as well as an outpouring by the mucosa of large amounts of water and electrolytes in an effort to dilute and wash away the irritant. This causes the condition known as diarrhea (frequent liquid stools). The loss of fluid and electrolytes may cause dehydration and an electrolyte imbalance.

Many microorganisms inhabit the large intestine, and colon bacilli are present in large numbers. The tract is sterile at birth, but in a short time organisms which have been ingested with food are present in the intestine. These organisms are useful in that they synthesize vitamin K, which is essential to the production of prothrombin. A deficiency of vitamin K can result in uncontrollable hemorrhage. Other substances in which bacteria may play a role are B_{12}, thiamin and riboflavin.

Bacteria cause some fermentation and putrefaction of the intestinal content. The fermentation process breaks the content down into still simpler components and at the same time produces gas. The organisms may cause a breakdown of unabsorbed amino acids which may release poisonous substances such as histamine, indol, choline, ammonia, skatol and hydrogen sulfide. However, since this usually takes place in the large bowel, little of these toxic products are absorbed. If they are absorbed, the liver detoxifies them.

Absorption

Absorption is the movement of food, water, or drugs from the alimentary canal into the blood to make them available to the cells throughout the body. It is performed passively by the physicochemical processes of diffusion, osmosis and filtration or by active transport by the cells.

There are two channels by which food may be absorbed: the capillaries of the mucosa and the lacteals. Water, salts, glucose, amino acids and some fatty acids and glycerol are absorbed into the capillaries. The larger proportion of the products of fat digestion is absorbed into the lacteals.

Like digestion, most of the absorption takes place in the small intestine. Its surface is especially adapted by the many circular folds in the mucous membrane to increase the surface area. The whole surface is also studded with millions of villi which are the most important structures of absorption. The network of capillaries and the central lymph channel of each villus take up much of the digested food. Special epithelial cells of the villi are responsible for the active transport of materials across the membrane.

Absorption in the Mouth. No food is absorbed from the mouth, but a few drugs may be taken into the blood through the buccal mucosa. Examples of these are nitroglycerine and epinephrine.

Absorption in the Stomach. Absorption in the stomach is relatively negligible. The gastric mucosa does not actively transport food molecules across it, but if the concentration is high in the stomach (creating a considerable gradient between the blood and the stomach), glucose, water and electrolytes may be absorbed. Alcohol and some drugs are also absorbed from the stomach.

Absorption in the Small Intestine. Minerals, vitamins, water, drugs, amino acids, simple sugars, fatty acids and glycerol are freely absorbed from the small intestine. Most absorption takes place in the upper part of the small intestine.

Absorption in the Colon. Large amounts of water are absorbed in the colon. Approximately 500 ml. of fluid pass from the small intestine into the colon daily. About 400 ml. of water are absorbed from this, leaving 100 ml. to be excreted in the feces. Small amounts of glucose and salts are also absorbed by the large intestine, and a number of drugs may be administered by this channel.

Absorption of Vitamins. The water-soluble vitamins B complex and C are generally readily absorbed from the small intestine. The exception is vitamin B_{12}. For absorption of B_{12}, a substance called the intrinsic factor is necessary and is secreted by the mucosa of the stomach. A deficiency of the intrinsic factor or of vitamin B_{12} causes a deficiency in the production of mature red blood cells.

The fat-soluble vitamins A, D, E and K are absorbed from the small intestine if bile salts are present.

Fate of Foods in the Body

When food is absorbed it is taken from the blood by tissue cells. Some of it is used by the cells to meet the material requirements for the construction of tissue for growth and maintenance or for the production of substances such as hormones and enzymes. Much of the food is broken down to produce the energy required by the body to carry out its many functions. All cells require substances that furnish energy, but since those of different tissues vary in composition and function, the cells select materials to meet their special needs in respect to such differences. Glucose and fat are used mainly to supply energy, while requirements for cellular structure and chemical products are met principally by the amino acids and minerals.

When the foods are taken into the cells they undergo physical and chemical changes which comprise metabolism. When the cellular activity results in the synthesis of tissue substance, the process is referred to as anabolism, or anabolic metabolism. The processes that break down the materials into simpler forms and release energy are called catabolism, or catabolic metabolism.

Fate of Carbohydrates in the Body. Carbohydrates are absorbed as glucose, fructose and galactose and are the main energy source. Fructose and most of the galactose are converted to glucose by the liver. Some galactose remains as such and is one of the components of the myelin sheath, found around many nerve fibers. The sheath is a fatty, insulating membrane that prevents the loss of the nerve impulse.

Glucose may be oxidized by the cells to provide energy; it is temporarily stored as glycogen in the liver or muscles or converted to fat and stored as such. It is also used in small amounts in the synthesis of tissue substances and secretions and is circulated in the blood for a period of time, providing what is known as the blood sugar. If it is in excess, some may be excreted in the urine.

OXIDATION OF GLUCOSE. The oxidation of glucose by the cells to acquire energy is a complex process involving a series of many chemical reactions. Each reaction is catalyzed by a specific enzyme with the final end products being energy, water and carbon dioxide.

It is not the intent to give the details here of the biochemical reactions that take place in the oxidation of glucose. If such information is desired, the reader should consult a textbook of biochemistry or medical physiology. The catabolism of glucose involves two main processes: glycolysis and the citric acid cycle (Kreb's cycle or tricarboxylic acid cycle).

Glycolysis splits the glucose molecule into two pyruvic acid molecules, at the same time releasing some energy. Ten successive chemical reactions are necessary to achieve glycolysis. The pyruvic acid molecules then embark on a series of chemical reactions which comprise the citric acid cycle. Each of the ten chemical changes occurring in the citric acid cycle also requires a specific enzyme. The net result of the metabolism of one molecule of glucose is energy plus 6 molecules of carbon dioxide plus 6 molecules of water ($C_6H_{12}O_6 + 6O_2 \longrightarrow E + 6CO_2 + 6H_2O$). Some of the energy that is released by the chemical reactions forms heat energy, and the remainder is stored in the cell as adenosine triphosphate (ATP). ATP is a compound with three phosphoric acid radicals; two of these radicals are connected to the compound by high energy bonds which can be split off readily when energy is needed by the cell to promote other chemical changes. If one phosphate radical is released, the compound is changed to adenosine diphosphate (ADP). As energy is released by other chemical reactions, the energy is used to bond the free phosphate radical to ADP to regenerate ATP. These energy changes go on continually with the chemical processes that comprise metabolism.

The glucose that is not needed to maintain a normal concentration in the blood or for immediate oxidation is converted by several chemical reactions and enzymes to glycogen and stored as such. Most of the glycogen is found in the muscle and liver cells. The muscle cells store it for their own use for contraction. The liver stores it and as the blood concentration falls, converts the glycogen back to glucose and releases it into the blood. The process by which the glucose is converted to glycogen is known as glycogenesis; the reconversion of the glycogen to glucose is called glycogenolysis.

BLOOD SUGAR. The blood sugar concentration is relatively constant, the normal being 80 to 120 mg. per 100 ml. of blood. It may rise to 130 to 140 mg. per cent after a meal, but falls to normal within 2 or 3 hours. A concentration of at least 80 mg. per cent of glucose in the blood is necessary in order to meet the needs of the cells.

Maintenance of the blood sugar level within normal limits is especially important for the survival and normal functioning of the brain cells.

A deficiency in the blood sugar concentration is quickly manifested by certain central nervous system disturbances. The person may become confused and may lose muscle coordination and strength. If the deficiency is severe, loss of consciousness may occur and, unless it is corrected, death may ensue. If the brain cells are deprived of glucose for even a very few hours, they may be permanently damaged.

Hypoglycemia is the term given to a blood sugar concentration below the normal. If the concentration is above the normal, the condition is known as hyperglycemia.

Regulation of the Blood Sugar Concentration. Maintenance of the blood glucose within normal limits is done mainly by hormones. When the blood sugar concentration falls, the liver cells may be activated by two hormones, glucagon and epinephrine, to convert glycogen to glucose and release it into the blood. Glucagon is secreted by the pancreas when the blood sugar falls below the normal level. Epinephrine is secreted by the medulla of the adrenal glands. Sympathetic innervation to the adrenal glands is excited by a low blood sugar concentration, resulting in a release of epinephrine into the blood.

Insulin, a hormone secreted by cells in the islands of Langerhans of the pancreas, brings about a decrease in the blood sugar concentration by promoting the transport of glucose into the tissue cells. If the blood sugar level decreases toward or below the lower normal limits, there is a corresponding decrease in the secretion of insulin.

The adrenal cortex also secretes hormones—glucocorticoids—that increase the blood sugar concentration. A decrease in the blood sugar stimulates the adenohypophysis (anterior pituitary gland) to release the adrenocorticotrophic (ACTH) hormone which brings about the release of glucocorticoids. The increase in blood sugar is brought about by the glucocorticoids stimulating the liver cells to form glucose from noncarbohydrate substances. Proteins and fats may be broken down and glycogen or glucose formed. This process may be referred to as glyconeogenesis or, if glucose is produced, as gluconeogenesis.

Similarly, the lowered blood sugar may cause the release of the thyroid stimulating hormone (TSH) by the adenohypophysis and a resulting increase in the output of thyroxin, which promotes gluconeogenesis.

LIPOGENESIS. When the absorbed glucose exceeds what the cells use and what can be stored as glycogen, it may be converted to fat and stored in the fat depots of the body.

EXCRETION OF GLUCOSE BY THE KID-NEYS. As the blood flows through the kidney, much of the plasma and its solutes escape into the kidney tubules. Normally, all of the glucose that escapes is reabsorbed and the urine is sugar free. If the blood sugar becomes abnormally high, not all the glucose is reabsorbed from the kidney tubule back into the blood; that rejected by the renal cells passes out into the urine. The level of blood sugar at which glucose is excreted in the urine is referred to as the renal glucose threshold and is approximately 160 to 165 mg. per cent, but this may vary with individuals. This excretion of the sugar, rather than its usual reabsorption, does reduce the blood sugar to some extent and is considered as a mechanism active in the regulation of the blood sugar.

Fate of Fats in the Body. Fatty acids and glycerol are absorbed into the lacteals of the villi and are combined in the process to form neutral fat. The absorbed fat is carried into the major lymph channels and reaches the blood through the thoracic lymphatic duct. Fats may be used by the body cells to provide energy, synthesize fat compounds or be stored as fatty tissue.

In the use of fats to provide energy, the neutral fat is first broken down by the liver into glycerol and fatty acids. The glycerol is converted to glycogen which is then converted to glucose.

The fatty acids are split by a series of chemical changes mainly in the liver. In each reaction, 2 carbon atoms and energy are freed in an oxidation process, finally ending up with acetoacetic acid and smaller amounts of beta-hydroxybutyric acid and acetone. These acids, because of their chemical structure, may be referred to as ketone acids or ketone bodies and the process by which they were formed is called ketogenesis. The ketones move out of the liver into the blood and are transported to the cells in need of energy where they are metabolized via the citric acid cycle, releasing energy and ending up as carbon dioxide and water. Although 1 gram of fat has more than twice as much energy value (9.3 calories) as does 1 gram of glucose (4.1 calories), as long as glucose is available to the cells, it is used in preference to fats.

The amount of ketones in the blood normally is very low and depends on a balance between the production by the liver and the assimilation by the tissue cells. Occasionally the rate of ketogenesis may exceed the rate at which the cells complete the metabolism, resulting in an accumulation of ketone acids in the blood and ketonuria. The condition is called ketosis and may occur when there is an increased use of endogenous fat for energy, as in starvation, or if there is a deficiency of glucose or a disturbance in the metabolism of glucose, as in diabetes mellitus. Ketosis may also develop with a diet high in fats (ketogenic diet).

Fat is necessary in the body for the formation of some essential fatty compounds such as phospholipids, lecithin, steroids and cholesterol. These compounds are built into other tissues. For example, phospholipids and cholesterol are necessary components of cell membranes.

The fat that is not used for energy or for the synthesis of certain tissue substances is stored as fatty tissue in areas of the body called the fat depots. Most of the fat is deposited in the subcutaneous tissue in the abdomen, especially on the mesentery and omentum, around the kidneys and between the muscle fibers.

A certain amount of stored fat is of value. The subcutaneous fatty tissue insulates the body against an excessive heat loss and against the cold of the external environment. Fatty tissue also provides a protective cushion for the body against trauma.

Following a meal not all the absorbed fat may enter the liver. Some of it moves directly into the fat depots so that the concentration of fat in the blood is quickly lowered. The fat in the tissues is mobilized when it is needed for energy. Thus, there is a constant movement of fat in and out of the fatty tissue.

As with carbohydrate metabolism, certain hormones produced in the body may influence fat metabolism. Most of them increase fat mobilization and fat utilization by the cells. These hormones include the growth, or somatotrophic, hormone secreted by the adenohypophysis; thyroxine; cortisone secreted by the adrenal cortices; and epinephrine released by the medulla of the adrenals. Insulin increases lipid synthesis and utilization. Estrogen secreted by the ovaries increases the deposition of fats in the tissues.

Fate of Protein in the Body. The absorbed amino acids may be built into body tissue or used in the synthesis of cell products, such as enzymes and hormones, or the formation of protein compounds, such as plasma proteins. They may be converted to non-nitrogenous substances, such as carbohydrate or fat, which may be stored or oxidized to produce energy. Amino acids are constantly being taken into the cells where they are used to construct the various protein substances of the body. From the large number of different amino acids, the cells select only those that they need to produce their particular type of protoplasm and cell products. Amino acids are very important to the child, whose protein requirement is more than twice that of the adult, since he grows and amasses more tissue.

The amino acids that are not used by the cells for structure or cell products are taken into the liver where they may be stored or converted to a non-nitrogenous compound. By this means the liver prevents an excessive concentration of amino acids in the blood. Only a small amount can be stored, but when the blood concentration of amino acids falls, the liver releases the reserve.

Amino acids may be converted to glucose by the liver cells by a process called deamination. The amino radical is removed from the amino acid, forming ammonia. Since the ammonia would be toxic to tissue cells, it is combined with carbon dioxide to form urea. The urea is released from the liver into the general circulation and excreted by the kidneys.

The residual molecular elements of the amino acid are converted to glucose or fat and are oxidized to meet energy requirements. Normally, carbohydrate and fat provide the energy required by the cells. If these become deficient, protein is moved into the liver and is deaminized to meet the cells' energy needs. In starvation, this involves the use of blood proteins and tissue protein and deprives the cells of structural and functional amino acids. The cells' normal activities are disrupted and survival is threatened.

Some amino acids may be synthesized by the liver cells. The amino radical is removed from one amino acid and is attached to the molecule of a carbohydrate or a fatty acid. This process is called transamination.

Protein metabolism is influenced by certain hormones. The somatotrophic (growth) hormone, thyroxine, and testosterone (male hormone) stimulate the use of protein in the synthesis of tissue and cell products. The glucocorticoids promote mobilization of amino acids into the blood from the cells and their conversion to glucose.

NURSING IN DISORDERS OF THE DIGESTIVE SYSTEM

Disorders of the Digestive System

Disorders of the digestive system are many and varied; they may interfere with the ingestion, digestion or absorption of food and fluids or with the elimination of residue. Any dysfunction threatens the well-being, functional capacity, and perhaps the survival of the patient. The manifestations depend largely on the location of the disorder in the system as well as the nature of the etiologic factor. Different diseases may cause similar disorders of function.

Modern health education places much emphasis on nutrition, and any interference with the ability to take and retain food may create anxiety in the patient. The common knowledge of the high incidence of malignant disease in the gastrointestinal tract may cause considerable concern in anyone with any digestive upset. Fortunately, the digestive system has considerable reserve; parts of it may be removed and the patient, with some necessary adjustments in diet and living habits, may continue to live a useful life.

Frequently a disturbance of function in the alimentary canal is secondary to disease in another part of the body. For example, some disorders of the brain may be manifested first by vomiting or difficulty in swallowing. It may be a complaint of indigestion that brings the patient with primary anemia to the physician. Fatigue or emotional stress may be the basis of malfunctioning of the gastrointestinal tract and most of us at some time have experienced functional disturbance in the stomach or bowel during a period of anxiety or grief. Some persons have an autonomic nervous system that appears to be more sensitive than that of others and, as a result, readily experience some malfunctioning of the digestive system coincidental with some form of stress. The patient may worry about the symptoms, creating a nervous stress that contributes to perpetuating the dysfunction.

"There is certain experimental evidence which illustrates the working of emotion on the gut. . . . In humans observed under the x-ray screen the pyloric valve mechanism is inhibited by fear and the stomach will not empty. Changes of mucosal colour and mobility in response to emotion have been observed in the colon and stomach. Anxiety has been shown to produce strong non-propulsive contractions of the colon and constipation. Anxiety will make the mouth dry and the breath offensive."[1]

The patient whose medical investigation rules out organic and structural disease still requires the nurse's understanding sympathy and must be observed for emotional stress that may be the basis of his illness.

Manifestations of Disorders of the Digestive System

Pain. Pain caused by a digestive disorder may be due to strong contractions of muscle tissue, stretching of a viscus, chemical or mechanical irritation of the mucosa, inflammation of the peritoneum, or direct irritation or pressure on associated nerves. It may occur in any part of the abdomen or in some instances is referred to a site remote from its origin. For example, pain arising from a peptic ulcer or from the biliary tract may be referred to an area of the back.

Heartburn is a form of pain that is described as a burning sensation felt behind the sternum. It is usually attributed to irritation of the esophageal mucosa by regurgitation of gastric acid fluid into the esophagus and may be accompanied by regurgitation of some stomach content into the mouth.

A patient may complain of a sense of fullness, especially after eating. Normally, the stomach relaxes and distends to accommodate food without increasing the intragastric pressure. This accommodation may not occur if there is disease, such as carcinoma, or if the patient is in an anxious state.

[1] J. A. Naish and A. E. A. Reed: Basic Gastro-Enterology. Bristol, John Wright and Sons Ltd., 1965, p. 3.

Significant characteristics of the pain must be noted and recorded. Meaningful clues include the duration, location, and the nature and onset of the pain as described by the patient. Aggravating factors such as activity, the taking of food or medicine, or some specific experience or emotional stress may exist. Nausea, vomiting, flatulence and defecation associated with the pain are pertinent observations. The effect of pain on each individual varies. The patient is observed for such changes as restlessness, pallor, perspiration, weakness and changes in the vital signs.

Anorexia. Loss of appetite is a common complaint of patients with digestive disease but is also associated with disorders in practically all parts of the body. It may be functional in origin, resulting from an emotional upset. Persistent refusal of food due to psychological disturbance is referred to as anorexia nervosa.

Nausea and Vomiting. Nausea is a psychic experience in which one has a feeling of discomfort in the region of the stomach and the inclination to vomit.

Vomiting is the ejection of the gastric contents through the mouth and is usually preceded by nausea and hypersalivation. There may be nausea without vomiting, and vomiting may occasionally occur without being preceded by nausea. The muscular activity that precedes or accompanies vomiting is referred to as retching.

Nausea and vomiting are very common symptoms and are seen in a great variety of conditions. They can be manifestations of a digestive dysfunction or they may accompany practically any acute illness or stress situation. The nurse is frequently called upon to comfort and support a patient who is vomiting and to make pertinent observations which may prove significant to the physician in making a diagnosis and planning treatment.

The vomiting process in initiated by a vomiting or emetic center in the medulla oblongata. This center may be excited by sensory impulses originating in the stomach or intestines; by impulses of psychic origin when fright, unpleasant sights, odors or severe pain are experienced; or by impulses from a group of neurons referred to as the chemoreceptor trigger zone in the floor of the fourth ventricle. The cells in the trigger zone are sensitive to certain chemicals in the blood and to impulses from the portion of the internal ear concerned with equilibrium. Vomiting in motion sickness, radiation therapy, toxemia and with the taking of certain drugs such as apomorphine and digitalis results from impulses that arise from the chemoreceptor trigger zone. The sensitivity of the vomiting center varies in different individuals; some vomit very readily and with little effort while others are not affected even though the stimulus may be similar and of equal intensity.

The impulses discharged by the vomiting center result in a quick, deep inspiration followed by closure of the glottis and epiglottis, closure of the nasopharynx by elevation of the soft palate, and relaxation of the esophagus, cardiac sphincter and stomach. Vigorous contraction of the diaphragm and abdominal muscles increases intra-abdominal pressure which forces the gastric content up through the relaxed esophagus and the mouth. The stomach plays a passive role.

One should be alert to the possible effects of vomiting, regardless of its cause. Considerable muscular energy can be expended in frequent vomiting and may result in exhaustion.

Obviously, nausea and vomiting interfere with normal nutrition, and if prolonged, malnutrition and loss of weight and strength occur. The reduced intake and loss of fluid may rapidly lead to dehydration. Loss of gastric secretion may deplete the body electrolytes and cause acid-base imbalance. Acidosis may develop as the patient becomes dependent on his body fat as a source of energy. The patient may complain of abdominal soreness from the retching and muscular effort and may become extremely worried about his condition, which may further aggravate the disturbance.

The patient who is nauseated and is vomiting, regardless of the cause, requires the following nursing considerations.

Sympathetic attention and understanding can mean a great deal to the patient. Remaining with him to hold his head or a painful site, holding the basin, cleansing his mouth and lips, and making sincere efforts to relieve the discomfort provide some support. Positioning should facilitate drainage of the vomitus from the mouth to prevent possible aspiration.

The following factors should be noted: whether the vomiting was preceded by nausea; whether there was retching or the vomitus was regurgitated without effort; the quantity, consistency, color, content and frequency of the emesis; the time of day and any association with the ingestion of food or drugs; and the effect on the patient (e.g., fluid balance, exhaustion).

Food and fluid are usually withheld for a period of time and are resumed gradually in small amounts. If the vomiting is due to local irritation, it may be helpful to have the patient take a whole glass of water to "wash out" the stomach. The mouth is rinsed after each emesis and the basin emptied promptly. Soiled bedding and clothing should be changed and the room ventilated. The odor or sight of vomitus may contribute to the patient's discomfort and may cause repetitive vomiting. The patient may be reassured by having a clean basin always within reach, but it is less suggestive if covered with a clean towel.

Rest, quiet and a minimum of disturbance may reduce the incidence of vomiting. Nausea tends to increase with motion; any change of position should be made slowly. Subdued lighting may reduce external stimuli and be conducive to rest. Sometimes encouraging the patient to take several deep breaths reduces nausea and may offset vomiting.

Since worry or fear can perpetuate nausea and vomiting, the patient is encouraged to verbalize his concerns. Problems may come to light which may be explained or solved. For example, he may be anxious about a home situation that could be cared for by the social or welfare service. The care must be individualized; what may prove helpful with one person may not be tolerated by another. If the vomiting continues, gastric drainage by a tube may be established (see p. 336).

An antiemetic or a sedative may be prescribed. Sodium phenobarbital may be administered orally or parenterally for sedation. Dimenhydrinate (Dramamine or Gravol) or pipamazine (Mornidine) are examples of antiemetics which may be used.

Regurgitation. Ejection of small amounts of chyme or gastric secretion through the esophagus into the mouth without the vomiting mechanism being employed is referred to as regurgitation. It may occur due to some incompetency of the esophageal-gastric (cardiac) sphincter, as seen in infants, or it may be a symptom of organic disease.

Bleeding from the Gastrointestinal Tract. Bleeding in the alimentary canal may be manifested by the vomiting of blood (hematemesis); by melena, which is the passage of a black, tarry stool containing blood pigments; or by the passage of frank blood from the bowel. Hematemesis and melena occur as a result of bleeding in the upper digestive tract. The characteristic black tarry appearance of the stool is due to the effect of the digestive enzymes on the blood. Frank blood in the stool usually originates with bleeding in the colon, rectum or anal canal.

It may be necessary in some instances to examine the blood that has been ejected through the mouth to determine whether it has been coughed up (hemoptysis) or vomited. Blood from the respiratory tract is a brighter red and frothy because of the contained air; that from the stomach is usually darker and may contain small clots and food particles.

Melena may be so slight that it goes unrecognized unless a stool specimen is submitted for laboratory examination for occult blood.

The most frequent cause of hematemesis and melena is peptic ulcer, but esophageal varices, carcinoma, injuries or a blood dyscrasia may account for the bleeding in other cases. Any evidence of bleeding should be promptly reported to the physician. The patient who has hematemesis or tarry stool is put at rest and his blood pressure, pulse, respirations, color and general state (e.g., strength and consciousness) are checked.

Bleeding from the lower part of the tract may be due to a newgrowth, ulcerative colitis, hemorrhoids or an anorectal fissure. The patient is advised to see a physician immediately for early diagnosis and treatment.

Dysphagia. Dysphagia is defined as difficulty in swallowing. The patient may be able to swallow soft foods and liquids but may be unable to take firmer, more solid foods. Others may be able to swallow but complain of pain on doing so. Dysphagia may be due to mechanical obstruction, dysfunction in the neuromuscular structures involved in swallowing or to diseases of the mouth, pharynx or larynx.

Loss of Weight and Strength. Obviously, if food cannot be taken, digested or absorbed, body tissue cells are deprived of their requirements for normal functioning. Body stores and actual tissue are mobilized to meet the needs, but eventually these may be depleted. The patient manifests loss of weight, strength and efficiency. If the problem is related to a specific food, symptoms characteristic of a lack of that particular food will appear. For example, if there is a disturbance in the absorption of vitamin K due to a lack of bile salts in the intestine, the deficiency may be manifested by bleeding, since prothrombin, necessary for blood coagulation, will not be produced by the liver.

Changes in the Mouth. Changes in the mouth may be of local origin or may be associated with digestive or general disorders. Disturbances may take the form of a coated or furry tongue, dryness, soreness, small ulcers (aphthous ulcers) and halitosis. Changes due to local conditions may be caused by inflammation and infection of the tongue and buccal mucosa, neoplastic disease and injuries.

Flatulence. Flatulence is an excessive amount of gas in the gastrointestinal tract. The patient may complain of a "full, bloated feeling," pressure or actual pain. The abdomen may be distended and the patient may eructate gas from the stomach through the mouth or may expel gas (flatus) from the bowel. Excessive gas in the stomach or bowel is frequently due to swallowed air. Aerophagia, or the unconscious swallowing of air, may be seen in nervous persons and in patients who are nauseated or experiencing some digestive stress. It is sometimes helpful to advise patients to make a conscious effort to avoid the swallowing or to hold something such as a wooden or plastic applicator or a cigarette holder between their teeth.

Excessive gas in the intestines may result from the ingestion of excessive amounts of gas-forming foods (cabbage, turnips, onions, etc.) or from abnormal fermentation of the food due to bacterial action. Flatulence and distention occur with any obstruction in the tract and with paralysis of peristalsis.

Borborygmi (singular, borborygmus) is a

term applied to the sounds made by the movement of a gas and fluid mixture in the intestines that are loud enough to be heard by the patient and others close by. The sound can be a significant observation, especially where there is some question of obstruction. The sounds do occur in the normal alimentary tract on occasion.

Abdominal Rigidity. Rigidity of any area of the abdominal wall due to excessively tense muscle tone may be evident in patients with disease of the gastrointestinal tract. The muscle contraction is usually a response to irritation of an underlying structure. This symptom is usually noted by the physician when he palpates the abdomen in examining the patient.

Change in the Normal Pattern of Bowel Elimination. A disorder of the intestine may cause a retarded or an accelerated movement of contents through the intestine. Delayed movement may cause constipation characterized by infrequent, hard, dry stools or may result in a complete failure of the passage of feces. Acceleration of the content causes diarrhea, which is frequent liquid or unformed stools. The person who experiences any persistent change in his normal pattern of bowel elimination should consult a physician.

For a discussion on constipation and diarrhea see page 365.

Hiccup (Singultus). Persisting hiccups or frequent attacks of hiccups may be associated with organic disease of the digestive system. They are caused by intermittent spasms of the diaphragm due to some irritation of the phrenic nerve. The frequency of the attacks and the effect of the hiccups on the patient should be noted. Dehydration, acid-base imbalance and malnutrition may develop, since hiccups may interfere with the taking of fluids and food. Disturbed rest and the expenditure of muscular energy may cause exhaustion. In many instances, the patient becomes fearful because of the persistence of the condition.

Jaundice. An excessive concentration of bilirubin in the blood causes a yellow discoloration of the sclerae, skin and mucous membranes. It is commonly associated with liver disease (liver cell jaundice), obstruction to the flow of bile through the biliary ducts (obstructive jaundice), and with a rapid increase in the destruction of red blood cells which frees bilirubin more rapidly than the liver cells can excrete it in bile (hemolytic jaundice). In obstructive jaundice the flow of bile may be impeded in the intrahepatic ducts, as in hepatitis (inflammation of the liver) and liver cirrhosis, or the obstruction may be in the extrahepatic ducts. The latter is most frequently caused by gallstones in the duct or by a neoplasm which constricts the biliary tract.

DIAGNOSTIC PROCEDURES

Except for the mouth, which is readily accessible to viewing and palpation, diagnosis of disorders of the digestive system are rarely made without the assistance of various investigative procedures. These include the following.

Blood Cell Counts

Leukocyte Count. An increase in the number of white blood cells (leukocytosis), particularly neutrophils, may indicate infection and an acute inflammatory process. This test is of significance in conditions such as appendicitis, acute enteritis, colitis and acute gallbladder disease (cholecystitis).

Normal: 5000 to 10,000 per cu. mm.

Erythrocyte Count and Hemoglobin Concentration. A deficiency in the number of red blood cells and in the amount of hemoglobin may point to the loss of blood or nutritional deficiency and provide information as to the patient's condition.

Normal: Erythrocytes, $4\frac{1}{2}$ to 5 million per cu. mm.; hemoglobin, 12 to 16 Gm. per 100 ml.

Endoscopy

Visual examination by means of a lighted tube (endoscope) may be made of the esophagus, stomach, sigmoid colon, rectum and anal canal.

Esophagoscopy. The esophagus may be examined and a biopsy specimen obtained through the esophagoscope. The instrument may also be used to remove a foreign body or a bolus which has lodged in the esophagus.

Gastroscopy. The gastroscope permits direct viewing of the gastric mucosa and the taking of a biopsy.

Nursing Care in Esophagoscopy and Gastroscopy. Preparation for either of these diagnostic procedures should begin with an explanation to the patient of what to expect. The physician may have described the examination and its values, but the patient will most likely still have questions. The nurse should have sufficient understanding of the procedure to be able to answer the patient's questions judiciously.

The patient is advised that he will be taken to the special treatment room or to the operating room for the examination. A written consent for the procedure is obtained. No food or fluid is given for 6 to 8 hours before the procedure. In gastroscopy, the physician may request a gastric lavage to be done several hours before the examination in patients in whom some pyloric obstruction is suspected. Dentures and jewelry are removed and, in the case of the female, the hair is confined under a turban, or if it is long, it should be braided. Adults usually receive a sedative such as meperidine (Demerol), morphine or a barbiturate preparation 30 minutes to 1 hour before the scheduled time. The patient empties his bladder before leaving his room to avoid such need during the examination.

The pharyngeal area is sprayed with a local anesthetic before the gastroscope or esophagoscope is introduced. A general anesthetic may be given in the case of a child, or, rarely, it may be used for a nervous adult in order to get better relaxation. A nurse remains beside the patient to give reassurance and support during the procedure and to assist with positioning. In esophagoscopy, the patient's head and shoulders are extended over the head of the table. In gastroscopy, a lateral position is used.

Following the examination, the patient is allowed to rest. All food and fluids are withheld for 4 to 6 hours—until the effect of the local anesthetic has worn off and the gag reflex returns. Before giving any fluid, the reflex may be tested by gently touching the back of the throat with an applicator or spoon. The patient may complain of a sore throat or soreness in midchest. Warm fluids may be soothing and may provide some relief. Any expectoration or vomiting of blood and severe pain should be reported promptly to the physician.

Sigmoidoscopy. A direct examination of the anal canal, the rectum and the sigmoid colon may be made by means of a sigmoidoscope.

Proctoscopy. This is direct viewing of the rectum and anal canal by means of a proctoscope.

Nursing Care in Sigmoidoscopy and Proctoscopy. These examinations may be performed in the doctor's office or in the ward treatment room of the hospital. A tissue specimen (biopsy) may also be obtained at the same time.

An explanation of the procedure is given to the patient in which he is advised of the position that he will be required to assume. The knee-chest and the left lateral are the positions commonly used. The lower bowel should be empty; a cleansing enema is usually given 2 to 3 hours before the scheduled time. A low residue diet may be prescribed for the preceding day.

A nurse remains with the patient to assist with the positioning and provide support. Unnecessary exposure should be avoided by adequate drapes. In the knee-chest position the patient lies face down and draws his knees up so that his weight is borne by the chest and knees. The feet are extended over the end of the table, arms at the sides or at sides of the head, and the head is turned to one side. In the left lateral or Sim's position the lower limbs are flexed with the right one being drawn up further than the left. Suction is made available to remove any secretion or fluid feces that interfere with visualization of the bowel mucosa.

After the examination, the anal region is cleansed and the patient is allowed to rest. The nurse may be responsible for seeing that the tissue specimen is placed in the appropriate container, correctly labeled and delivered to the pathology laboratory.

Roentgenography and Fluoroscopy

Radiologic examination is a very valuable procedure in diagnosing disorders of the digestive system, particularly those of the alimentary canal. A radiopaque substance, barium sulfate, may be given by mouth (barium swallow or barium meal), and fluoroscopic studies and x-ray pictures are taken as it passes through the esophagus, stomach and intestines. The rate it moves through the tract and outlines of the various parts are studied. When the barium is followed by a series of x-rays taken at intervals of several hours the procedure may be referred to as a gastrointestinal x-ray series.

The patient who is to have a barium swallow usually has a light evening meal and then nothing but sips of water until several hours after he has received the barium the next morning. As soon as the radiologist indicates that the patient may have a meal, it should be served promptly. The patient may be very tired and may be experiencing weakness and discomfort because of the lack of food.

Following the taking of the barium and when the first studies of the series are completed, the patient should be offered a mouthwash, since the barium is chalky and clings to the oral mucosa. When the series is completed, which may be the day after the barium was administered, the physician should be consulted as to whether a cleansing enema or a laxative is to be given to clear the tract of the barium. Otherwise, it tends to cause constipation, fecal impaction and considerable discomfort.

X-ray examination of the large intestine and rectum is done by giving an enema of the barium solution. The lower bowel has been emptied previously by the administration of a laxative and a cleansing enema. Specific directions as to what laxative and enema solution are to be used and the time they are to be administered should be received from the x-ray department or the attending physician. Food will probably be withheld for 18 to 24 hours preceding the barium enema, but the patient is allowed fluids.

The patient should receive an explanation as to why the food is withheld. Also, he should be advised as to what will take place when he goes to the x-ray department and the importance of his retaining the barium until the necessary studies and films are made.

The barium enema is given in the x-ray room, and its progress through the rectum and colon are observed by fluoroscopy. X-ray films are also made to be studied later. Provision is made for the expelling of the enema, and then more films are made. A mild laxative is usually prescribed to ensure the elimination of residual barium.

Radiography is also used in the diagnosis of gallbladder disease and may be referred to as cholecystography. A radiopaque organic iodine compound (e.g., Telepaque or Cholografin) that is eliminated in the bile is given orally or intravenously. The patient is allowed a fat-free evening meal which is followed by the administration of the "dye" the night before the x-ray examination. Then, only water is allowed until after the first x-ray. The iodine compound is absorbed, secreted by the liver cells in the bile and, normally, concentrated in the gallbladder, since there was no fat in the meal to stimulate the emptying of the gallbladder.

An x-ray film is taken in the morning (approximately 12 hours after the "dye" was given) to determine if the gallbladder filled. Calculi may be observed if present.

Following this first film, the patient is given a meal containing fat. A rich eggnog or thickly buttered toast and an egg may be used. After 1 hour, a final roentgenogram is taken. Normally, after a fatty meal, the gallbladder contracts and empties bile into the small intestine via the common bile duct.

To summarize, cholecystography will provide information as to whether the gallbladder fills and empties and whether it contains gallstones.

Gastric Analysis

Examination of a specimen of vomitus or of aspirated gastric content may be made to detect the presence of blood, bile or organisms (e.g. tubercle bacillus); to determine the hydrochloric acid concentration; or to test the secretory function of the stomach.

In aspiration, a nasogastric tube, such as the Levin tube, is introduced and left until the required number of specimens are collected (see p. 336 for intubation). The procedure of testing for acidity and secretion may vary somewhat from one institution to another but in general is as follows. A fasting period of 8 to 10 hours precedes the test. A tube is passed into the stomach and the gastric content is aspirated by a syringe. Following this initial specimen, the gastric secretion is aspirated at stated intervals (usually every 15 minutes for 1½ to 2 hours) until the required number of specimens are obtained. Each specimen is placed in a separate tube and is numbered according to the order in which it is collected. The tube

TABLE 15–1 NORMAL VOLUME AND ACID CONCENTRATION OF GASTRIC
SECRETION IN ANALYSIS

	FASTING	BASAL	Alcohol or Broth	Histamine	Insulin
			RESPONSE IN 10 MINUTES FOLLOWING ADMINISTRATION OF		
Volume	10–25 ml.	0–10 ml.	10–25 ml.	15–30 ml.	10–30 ml.
Free acid	0–30 units	10–30 units	30–60 units	70–110 units	50–100 units
Total acid	5–40 units	15–35 units	40–80 units	80–120 units	60–110 units

is clamped between aspirations to prevent the entrance of air into the stomach. This procedure is known as fractional gastric analysis.

Usually, fractional analysis to evaluate secretory function includes the administration of a secretory stimulant such as alcohol, histamine, insulin or a small amount of food. If alcohol is prescribed, a measured amount of pure ethyl alcohol is given via the nasogastric tube after the initial aspiration. The alcohol stimulates the secretion of acid but not enzymes.

Histamine phosphate is more commonly used. It stimulates the parietal cells to secrete hydrochloric acid and is frequently used to determine whether the gastric secretions are achlorhydric or hyperchlorhydric. Achlorhydria means an absence of hydrochloric acid from the gastric juice. Hyperchlorhydria is used to describe an excessive secretion of hydrochloric acid in the stomach. A decrease in hydrochloric acid secretion may be associated with cancer of the stomach, chronic gastritis, gastric ulcer or pernicious anemia. An increase in acid secretion may be seen in duodenal ulcer.

If histamine phosphate is used in fractional gastric analysis, it is given subcutaneously after the initial aspiration of gastric content. The patient must be observed for possible toxic effects; the drug is not given if there is a history of allergy or asthma. If the patient complains of dizziness or weakness or manifests local irritation at the site of injection, flushing of the face or pallor, sweating or a rapid weak pulse, the physician should be notified at once. A severe drop in blood pressure may occur and the patient may develop signs of shock. Epinephrine should be readily available for prompt administration in the event of a reaction. The physician may order an antihistamine preparation to be given one-half hour before the histamine is given to offset the undesirable effects of the drug. Antihistamines do not affect the parietal cell secretion.

Occasionally, the giving of some food to stimulate gastric secretion may be used. The doctor usually specifies what food and the amount to be given. A cereal such as shredded wheat or gruel may be suggested.

Regular insulin may be ordered subcutaneously or may be administered intravenously by the physician. Insulin stimulates a secretion of the hydrochloric acid. The patient is observed closely for signs of hypoglycemia (insulin shock). Complaints of nervousness, hunger pains, weakness or faintness or signs of cold, clammy perspiration, tremors, pallor, weak pulse or disorientation should be reported promptly.

The physician may start an intravenous infusion of normal saline before the insulin is given in order that 50 per cent glucose may be given without delay should hypoglycemia develop. Also, this facilitates the collation of samples when each gastric specimen is obtained; the blood sugar level is determined and correlated with the findings in studies of gastric secretions.

When the required number of aspiration specimens are collected the nasogastric tube is removed, the patient's face is washed to refresh him and his regular meal is served.

Harrison et al. have recorded the information shown in Table 15–1 as the normal volume and acid concentration of gastric secretion in analysis.[2]

---

[2]J. R. Harrison, R. D. Adams, J. L. Bennet, W. H. Resnick, G. W. Thorn, and M. M. Wintrobe (Eds.): Principles of Internal Medicine, 4th ed. New York, The Blakiston Division, McGraw-Hill Book Co., Inc., 1962, p. 1944.

Recently, a simpler test has been introduced to provide information on gastric secretion of hydrochloric acid. This test is known as the diagnex blue test or tubeless gastric analysis and involves the following. After a fasting period of 8 to 10 hours, the patient receives caffeine sodium benzoate and carbacrylic resin with azure. A dye (Diagnex blue, Azuresin) and water. The patient voids just before the drugs are given and then again in 2 hours to provide a urine specimen to be examined for the azure dye.

The caffeine sodium benzoate stimulates the gastric parietal cells to secrete hydrochloric acid. The acid frees the dye from the resin, allowing it to be absorbed. It is then excreted from the blood in the urine. Unless there is acid to react with the carbacrylic resin compound, the dye remains bound to the resin which is nonabsorbable from the digestive tract. The presence of dye in the urine indicates the secretion of hydrochloric acid in the stomach. The concentration of the dye corresponds to the amount of acid released. If the urine is negative for the dye, it is attributed to achlorhydria.

Nightly Gastric Aspiration. When the patient has some pyloric obstruction, the doctor may order a nightly aspiration. The patient receives his prescribed diet during the day; then, at about 10 P.M. his stomach content is aspirated and measured. The amount of food residue and secretions in the stomach at this time gives the physician information as to the severity of the obstruction. It also relieves the patient of the sense of fullness, pain and discomfort resulting from the overdistended stomach and prevents vomiting.

Stool Examination

A stool specimen may be examined in the investigation of disorders of the digestive system for blood, urobilinogen, parasites, organisms or specific food residue. A small amount of stool is removed on a tongue depressor to the appropriate container (a waxed cardboard container with a lid). If the examination is for parasites, the specimen is kept warm and must be delivered to the laboratory promptly. If it is to determine the presence of occult blood, red meat is not included in the patient's diet for the 24 hours preceding the stool collection. If an enema is necessary to obtain a stool specimen, the solution used is clear water or normal saline.

When anything unusual is noted about a patient's stool, such as the presence of blood, excessive mucus or parasites, the stool should be kept until it is seen by the doctor.

GASTRIC AND INTESTINAL INTUBATION

The investigation or treatment of many medical and surgical patients may include the passage of a tube into the stomach or small intestine via the nose or mouth and the esophagus. The purpose may be to withdraw fluid from the stomach or intestine for analysis; to remove fluid and gas (decompression); to wash out the stomach (gastric lavage); to apply cold or pressure to the walls of the esophagus, stomach or small intestine; or to administer feedings or drugs.

Types of Tubes

Many different tubes are encountered and the type used varies with the purpose. The tube may have 1 or 2 lumens and may have a small inflatable bag attached at the distal end. Longer tubes are necessary for intestinal intubation. The following are commonly used.

Levin Tube. This tube has a single lumen with several openings at the distal end and is used for gastric intubation.

Rehfuss Tube. The Rehfuss tube has only one lumen which terminates in a small metal bulb with vertical slits. It is used for the aspiration of gastric or duodenal secretions.

Stomach Pump or Ewald Tube. This large tube has a bulb incorporated into the proximal portion for the purpose of producing suction. It is introduced through the mouth into the stomach and is used to quickly withdraw larger volumes of gastric content and to wash out the stomach.

Miller-Abbott Tube. The Miller-Abbott tube used for intestinal intubation is quite long and has two lumens. One lumen serves to aspirate intestinal fluid and gas, the other lumen opens into a small rubber bag which is inflated after the tube is passed. The balloon causes pressure which stimulates intestinal motility. In some instances, mercury is used in the balloon instead of air; its weight

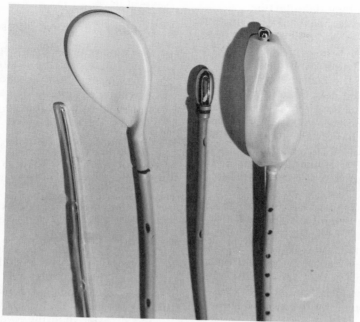

Figure 15–2 Tubes used in gastric and intestinal aspiration. From left to right: Levin tube; Cantor tube; Rehfuss tube; and Miller-Abbott tube. (Courtesy of the New Mount Sinai Hospital, Toronto.)

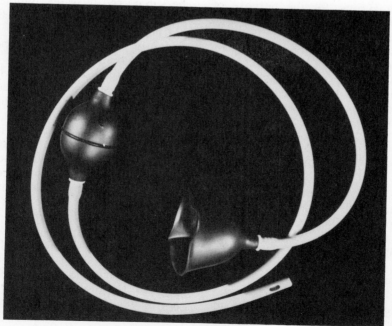

Figure 15–3 The Ewald tube, or stomach pump. (Courtesy of the New Mount Sinai Hospital, Toronto.)

facilitates the movement of the tube through the pylorus and along the intestine.

The inlets at the proximal end must be clearly marked as to which lumen is for drainage and which is kept clamped off to maintain the inflation of the balloon. The tube is marked off in centimeters so the distance it has passed may be determined.

Cantor Tube. The Cantor tube is used for intestinal aspiration. It has a small rubber bag at its distal end which contains 5 to 10 cc. of Hg. The lumen of the tube is sealed off at its junction with the bag, and the openings that permit aspiration are above the bag.

Harris Tube. This tube is smaller than the Cantor tube but resembles it in that it has a single lumen and a bag containing mercury attached below the holes. In both the Cantor and Harris tubes the mercury is introduced into the balloons before intubation by means of a syringe and needle. The mercury will not escape through the fine needle hole.

Gastric and Intestinal Aspiration

Suction may be applied intermittently or continuously for aspiration of gastric or intestinal contents. The suction may be provided by a syringe for the purpose of collecting specimens or for occasional aspiration of a small amount. More frequent or continuous suction may be provided by the Wangensteen set-up in which suction is created by water displacement or by a small electric pump at the patient's bedside. The electric suction apparatus may be set for intermittent or continuous suctioning. Piped suction from a central source may be available through a wall outlet with a valve and gauge by which the amount of suction is controlled.

Gastrointestinal suctioning must be gentle; the amount of suction or pull exerted is kept low to avoid drawing the soft tissue structures to the openings which would obstruct drainage and possibly damage the tissues.

Following gastric surgery, aspiration may be achieved by applying suction to a gastrostomy tube. A catheter with several side openings is inserted into the stomach through the abdominal incision and secured by sutures. This method of aspiration eliminates the discomfort and irritation associated with a nasogastric tube that is necessary for several days.

Nursing Responsibilities

Assisting With the Insertion of the Tube. An explanation of the treatment is made to the patient and he is advised that the insertion will be easier and quicker if he relaxes, breathes deeply through his mouth and swallows when instructed to do so to advance the tube.

The tube, if rubber, has been chilled in a bowl of ice chips so it is stiffer and less likely to curl up; it is lubricated with a water-soluble jelly.

The head of the bed is elevated, and the patient's head is hyperextended during the initial introduction of the tube through a naris or the mouth. When the patient is asked to swallow, the head is slightly flexed to the more natural position for swallowing. The tube is gently pushed downward as the patient swallows, but it should not be advanced faster than the swallowing or it will curl up in the pharynx and cause gagging. The patient may be allowed sips of water to make the swallowing easier.

To make sure the tube is in the esophagus and not in the trachea, the proximal end may be submerged in water; bubbles will appear as the patient exhales if the tube is in the trachea. Or the patient may be asked to speak or hum, which is not possible if the tube is in the larynx.

In intestinal intubation, when the tube reaches the stomach the patient is required to assume various positions to promote its passage through the pylorus and the duodenum. The usual procedure is to place the patient on his right side for 1 to 2 hours, then on his back with the head of the bed elevated for 1 to 2 hours. Advancement of the tube may be followed by fluoroscopy, and suggestions are made as to the desirable positioning of the patient. When the Miller-Abbott tube is used, the physician may inflate the balloon when it reaches the stomach on the basis that it simulates a food mass and stimulates motility to carry it through the pylorus. In other instances, the balloon may not be inflated until the tube has passed into the duodenum.

Securing the Tube. The tube is secured to the face with narrow strips of adhesive when it has been advanced to the desirable position if it is to be left in place for several hours or days. It must be checked several times daily for security, and the skin is examined for possible irritation from the adhesive.

If the tube is attached to a drainage bottle, it should be supported in a "trough" made in the bottom sheet or by a tape or towel pinned to the bedding to prevent tension on the nasogastric tube. The connecting tube should be long enough to prevent displacement of the gastrointestinal tube and to permit free movement of the patient in bed.

Mouth and Nose Care. The patient usually experiences considerable discomfort from the tube being in the nose and throat and from the dryness due to mouth breathing and restricted oral intake. The mouth should be cleansed and rinsed frequently. Normal cleansing of the teeth should be encouraged and need not interfere with the nasogastric tube. Vaseline, face cream or oil may be applied to the lips. Chewing gum may be permitted to stimulate salivary secretion and small sips of water may be allowed in some instances.

The nostril may become irritated and secretions accumulate and encrust. It should be gently cleansed with a swab moistened in water or normal saline and a light application of water-soluble jelly or mineral oil made.

Turning the patient hourly helps to shift the tube sufficiently to relieve constant pressure on one area of the throat. Throat lozenges may be ordered to lessen throat irritation.

Maintenance of Drainage. After the tube is in place and connected to the suction apparatus, it is necessary to check the system at frequent intervals for functioning. Mechanical failure of the apparatus might occur, or drainage may be interrupted by a blocking of the tube by mucus or a blood clot and could result in pain, vomiting, or serious distention of the stomach or intestine. The surgeon may order the tube to be irrigated by syringe at regular intervals or only if it is blocked. The solution and volume to be used for irrigating are specifically stated. After injection of the solution, some of the fluid may be aspirated using the syringe to determine if the tube is clear. The amounts of solution injected and aspirated are accurately measured and recorded on the fluid balance sheet.

The characteristics of the drainage fluid are noted and the total volume is recorded every 8 or 12 hours. The bottle is washed each time it is emptied as well as the connecting tubing.

Removal of the Tube. Before removal, the tube may be clamped and left in place while oral fluid is introduced. If the fluid is tolerated, an order may then be given to remove the tube. The gastric tube is withdrawn gently and quickly. The patient is instructed to hold his breath to avoid possible aspiration of fluid or mucus that may escape from the tube into the oropharynx.

The intestinal tube is removed slowly, a few inches at a time. The lumen into the air-inflated balloon is opened, and the air is allowed to escape. When slight resistance is encountered due to the intestinal peristalsis, the tube is left for a few minutes and then withdrawal is resumed. The physician should be notified if resistance to removal persists; force should not be used. If the tube has a mercury-filled bag at its distal end, the latter is brought out through the mouth and the bag removed. The remainder of the tube may then be pulled through the nostril. As with the removal of the gastric tube, the patient is asked to hold his breath as the terminal portion of the tube is drawn from the esophagus.

The mouth should be cleansed and rinsed immediately following the removal of the tube. The patient may complain of some soreness in the throat and nose which usually subsides in a day or two.

Gastric Gavage

When a patient is unable to take fluid and foods by mouth, a nasogastric tube (usually the Levin) may be passed through which a specially prepared solution of essential nutrients is introduced directly into the stomach. This method of feeding a patient may be referred to as gastric gavage or tube feeding. The nurse assists with the intubation as described on page 338. The tube may be left in place, but should be removed every 5 to 6 days, thoroughly cleaned and reinserted through the other naris. With infants and young children the tube is inserted prior to each feeding. When the tube is to be left in place, it is secured to the patient's face with narrow strips of adhesive.

The physician indicates the specific feeding to be used to meet the patient's nutritional needs. Various feedings are used. The foods of a normal diet may be liquefied in a blender and given, or a protein supplement and vitamins may be added to a mixture of eggs, milk and orange juice. For information as to the component, nutrients, amounts and the preparation of feedings, the reader is referred to recent publications on diet therapy.[3, 4]

The prescribed amount of solution is warmed (100 to 105° F.) in a water bath and brought to the bedside on a clean tray with a container of approximately 70 to 80 ml. of water and the barrel of an Asepto syringe. If this is the initial feeding, an explanation of the procedure is given to the patient. The head of the bed is elevated and 30 to 40 ml. of water is introduced into the tube to determine its patency.

The feeding is administered slowly and allowed to flow into the stomach by gravity. To avoid air entering the stomach, the funnel is not allowed to completely empty until all the fluid is given. When the feeding is completed, the tube is cleansed by rinsing it with 30 to 40 ml. of water and is then clamped. If regurgitation or vomiting occurs, it may be that the prescribed volume is too great. A smaller amount given more frequently may be tolerated.

Frequent mouth care is necessary and the nostril through which the tube passes requires attention.

For removal of the tube see page 339.

Gastrostomy

This is the surgical establishment of an opening into the stomach through the abdominal wall and the insertion of a tube through which fluids and liquefied food may be introduced directly into the stomach.

Before the gastrostomy, the procedure is discussed with the patient so he understands the purpose of the surgery and what is entailed postoperatively. The patient's written consent and the usual preoperative preparation for abdominal surgery are necessary. General or local anesthesia is used and a small incision made in the abdominal wall and stomach. A large catheter (No. 20 or 22F) is inserted into the stomach and secured by sutures put through the tissues and the tube. In some instances, a Foley catheter is used and a purse string suture used around it. The layers of tissue are then closed around the tube.

A gastrostomy may be a temporary procedure during a period of corrective surgery or it may be permanent when an obstructing esophageal condition is considered inoperable.

The patient generally finds it difficult to accept a gastrostomy. He is denied the natural process of eating and its associated pleasures, such as taste and sociability. Personnel caring for the patient, the family and friends should acknowledge to the patient that they understand his concern and tendency to withdraw. An effort should be made to find interests for the patient and to treat him as normally as possible.

For the first day or two postoperatively, water or a glucose solution in prescribed amounts is given through the tube; then, regular feedings, according to the doctor's orders, are given. The food preparations used in gastrostomy are similar to those cited above for gastric gavage. The required amount of feeding is warmed and given through a funnel or the barrel of a syringe attached to the gastric tube. The patient's head and shoulders should be elevated and he remains in this position for one-half hour after the feeding to prevent regurgitation into the esophagus and leakage around the tube. The tube is cleansed following the feeding by rinsing it with 30 to 40 ml. of water and is then clamped.

A gauze dressing is applied to the wound. The escape of even a small amount of gastric juice from around the tube may irritate the skin because of its acid-pepsin content. The dressing is changed whenever there is drainage, and the skin is cleansed thoroughly with soap and water and dried. A protective coating of vaseline or a prescribed ointment or powder is then applied.

The feedings may have to be adjusted from time to time. Too much fat or carbohydrate may cause diarrhea. Complaints of a full feeling or abdominal discomfort may necessitate a decrease in the amount of feed-

---

[3]L. F. Cooper, et al.: Nutrition in Health and Disease, 14th ed. Philadelphia, J. B. Lippincott Co., 1963, pp. 352–355.

[4]C. W. Shearman, Diets Are For People. New York, Appleton-Century-Crofts, 1963, pp. 22–23.

ing given. A record of the patient's weight is made which also serves as a guide in adjusting the caloric value of the feeding formula.

The tube is removed in approximately 1 to 2 weeks when the opening (stoma) and the channel through the layers of tissue are well established and healing has sealed off the peritoneal cavity. The tube is reinserted for each feeding and the stoma covered with a small dressing pad between feedings. Since the feedings correspond to the patient's meals, meticulous care should be used in relation to the equipment and to the preparation and administration. Such considerations as a clean, fresh towel covering the tray or clean equipment free of stains may lessen the patient's aversion to this unnatural method of taking his meal. When the patient receives blender feedings, he may feel more hopeful and "less different" if advised he is receiving foods included in a normal diet. Strict privacy should be provided during the feeding, as the patient is sensitive.

The patient's mouth will require special attention. Frequent cleansing and rinsing are essential. Some satisfaction may be derived from the taking of various fluids (e.g., fruit juice), retaining them in the mouth for a brief period and then expectorating them. The physician may encourage the patient to take foods which he desires, masticate them and then expectorate the bolus. These measures help to keep the mouth in better condition, stimulate gastric secretion and may provide some satisfaction through taste for the patient.

If the patient is to be fed by gastrostomy over a long period while various stages of treatment are carried out or if the gastrostomy is permanent, he is taught to feed himself. Instruction is given to the patient and a member of the family in the preparation of the feeding and the care of the stoma. Financial assistance may be necessary to provide a blender or prescribed commercial feeding preparations. The nurse may direct the family to the appropriate community resources for the necessary assistance or make the contact for them.

Gastric Hypothermia

A continuous internal application of cold may be used to treat gastric hemorrhage.

The stomach is first lavaged with ice-cold water or saline to remove the gastric content and blood clots in order that the cold may be brought in more direct contact with the stomach wall. This is also necessary to prevent overdistention of the stomach when the cooling bag is inflated. The large Ewald tube is then removed and replaced with a double-lumen tube with a large distensible bag resembling the shape of the stomach that is inflated with a cold solution. One lumen is used as an inflow tube to the bag, the other as an outflow.

A 50 per cent mixture of alcohol and water is cooled to 0° C. and approximately 600 ml. is introduced slowly into the bag. The inflow and outflow lumens are connected to a cooling reservoir in a refrigerating machine. The solution is continually circulated through the closed system by means of a pump. The inflated bag applies pressure as well as cold to the site of the bleeding.

A nasogastric tube may be inserted along with the cooling tube to maintain gastric decompression and provide information as to the bleeding.

The treatment may be continued up to 48 hours. The bag is gradually deflated and the tube left in place for a period of time in case bleeding starts again.

An electric warming blanket set on low is used to maintain body temperature and keep the patient comfortably warm. The rectal temperature is recorded at frequent intervals. The pulse and blood pressure will be observed closely because of the hemorrhage; pulse irregularity may develop as a result of the proximity of the cold tube to the heart and should be reported promptly.

MOUTH AND SALIVARY GLAND DISORDERS

Disorders of the mouth and contained structures are numerous and, as cited previously, may be of local origins or may be secondary to disease elsewhere in the digestive system or in some other system. Primary lesions may be due to bacterial, viral or fungal infection, chemical irritation, congenital malformation, injury or neoplastic disease. General diseases frequently accompanied by a mouth disorder include vitamin

B complex or C deficiency, blood dyscrasias, metallic medication intoxication, infectious disease and any condition that interferes with the normal fluid and food intake or salivary secretion.

Predisposing factors in mouth lesions are debilitation, poor dietary habits, poor oral and dental hygiene, dehydration, emotional stress and mouth breathing.

Only a few of the more common disorders are presented here.

Stomatitis

This is a term applied to inflammation of the oral mucosa. Its causes are numerous and include excessive smoking, dental sepsis, dehydration, vitamin deficiency, blood dyscrasia such as primary anemia and leukemia, systemic infection and a sensitivity to certain foods or drugs. The mucosa is very red and tender and ulcerative areas may develop.

Herpetic Stomatitis. This condition is thought to be caused by the herpes simplex virus and is also known as aphthous stomatitis. The lesion may occur singly or in crops on the mucosa of the mouth or on the tongue. It is commonly referred to as a canker sore and appears first as a small, sore inflamed area, followed by vesicle formation. The vesicle ruptures, leaving an ulcer which usually heals in a few days. The condition is painful and the patient complains of a burning sensation.

Frequent attacks of multiple lesions can be very distressing to the patient and may interfere with food intake. Treatment is usually on an empirical basis; what may be effective for one patient may not be so with another. Caustic agents such as silver nitrate should not be applied to the lesions as they only increase the erosion of tissue. A mild mouthwash such as sodium bicarbonate is used. Vitamin B complex and vitamin C may be prescribed. Local applications of cortisone in the form of an ointment or as a pellet may be used. A preparation commonly used is betamethasone disodium phosphate (Betnesol, Celestone) in pellet form; each tablet contains 0.1 to 0.2 mg. of cortisone. The pellet is held in the mouth as near the ulcers as possible. The doctor may also suggest some form of analgesic lozenge to relieve the

discomfort. Bland foods and fluids, not too hot, are taken.

In stubborn cases, typhoid and/or smallpox vaccine may be given to increase the patient's viral resistance.

Thrush (Moniliasis)

Thrush is caused by the fungus *Candida albicans*. It occurs most frequently in infants and children and in the very old but may also appear in debilitated persons. Occasionally, it follows the use of certain antibacterial drugs such as tetracycline (Achromycin) and chloramphenicol (Chloromycetin). Areas of superficial ulceration occur in the oral mucosa or gums, and the membrane over the lesion becomes white and is easily detached. The lesions respond to local application of 1 per cent gentian violet or to an antifungal antibiotic solution such as nystatin (Mycostatin). Attention is also directed to the patient's diet in an effort to improve his resistance and general condition.

Herpes Simplex

This condition is commonly called fever blisters or cold sores and occurs on the lips or skin surrounding the lips. It is due to a virus that is harbored by the cells in this region in a dormant state, the primary invasion having occurred early in life. Fever and a lowered resistance predispose the viral activity. The lesion appears as a small inflamed area which develops a vesicle that ruptures, leaving a superficial ulcer that forms a dry crust. There may be one or several lesions and they most frequently occur with acute infections. There is no specific treatment, but an ointment may be prescribed to soften the crust to prevent cracking and bleeding.

Vincent's Angina (Trench Mouth)

This is an inflammation of the gums (gingivitis) followed by ulceration and necrosis and is caused by specific fusiform bacilli and spirochetes. The gums are swollen, painful and bleed readily. Excessive salivary secretion and an offensive breath are usually present. There is a loss of marginal gum tissue and of the interdental papillae by the ulcerating process. Lesions may develop on the buccal and pharyngeal mucosa. A smear may be made from the affected area to confirm the diagnosis.

Predisposing factors are poor oral and dental hygiene, malnutrition and debilitation. Mouthwashes are given frequently; a solution of hydrogen peroxide, saline or sodium perborate may be used. An antibiotic by parenteral administration is prescribed and may be supplemented by topical administration. The patient will require instrumentative treatment by a dentist as soon as possible.

The condition is infectious and can be transmitted to other persons unless precautions are taken.

Leukoplakia

This condition is characterized by patchy, yellowish-white, firm, thickened areas of the oral mucous membrane or of the tongue. The increase in the surface epithelial tissue is referred to as keratinization. The lesions are painless and are considered serious since they may be precancerous. They occur most frequently in men after the fourth decade of life. The lesions usually develop in response to chronic irritation that may be mechanical, chemical, thermal or infective in origin. The lesions may disappear with elimination of the irritation.

Teeth are checked and defects corrected that may be causing irritation. Smoking should be discontinued and a high-vitamin diet is prescribed. If the area is fissured or ulcerated, a biopsy is done to determine if cancer has developed. If malignant changes have taken place, surgical excision and radiation therapy are used.

Cancer of the Mouth

Carcinoma may develop on the tongue and buccal mucosa, but the most frequent site is the lower lip. It usually appears first on the lip or mucosa as leukoplakia, as a roughened area or as a persisting ulcer. The lesion in cancer of the tongue usually appears as a small firm lump on the lateral margin. Later the area breaks down, leaving a painful ulcer. If the condition goes untreated, swallowing and speech become difficult, hypersalivation develops, the mucosa becomes infected and the malignant growth metastasizes to the jaw and to lymph nodes in the neck.

As with all malignant disease, early recognition and treatment are extremely important; any sore that resists treatment and persists for 3 weeks should receive prompt medical attention.

Treatment involves surgical excision of the cancerous tissue and radiation therapy. When metastasis to lymph nodes is suspected, more radical surgery is performed to include dissection of the cervical lymphatics. Extension of the malignant disease into the jaw may necessitate extirpation of the jaw.

Parotitis

Inflammation of a parotid gland is the most common disturbance of the salivary glands and may be due to infection by the specific virus that causes mumps, or it may develop as a result of any nonspecific bacterial invasion of the gland. Nonspecific parotitis may occur as a complication in febrile diseases or when dehydration is present and there is a lack of attention to oral hygiene. It tends to develop more readily in older and debilitated persons. The onset is sudden, the gland becomes swollen and painful and the patient develops a fever. It is treated by antibiotics and, if suppuration develops, surgical drainage is necessary. The fluid intake is increased and frequent mouth care is necessary. The local application of an ice bag to the area may be prescribed if pus has not formed.

Obstruction to the Flow of Saliva

Obstruction of any one of the salivary glands may be due to intrinsic or extrinsic causes. Disease within the gland or duct may be infection, newgrowth or a calculus. In conditions that cause inflammation, the duct may be occluded by swelling and edema or later by the resulting scar tissue. Extrinsic causes such as a tumor or infection in neighboring structures may compress the duct, or scar tissue resulting from stomatitis may close off the duct orifice.

The obstruction is manifested by swelling of the affected gland. The swelling is most pronounced during meals because of the salivary stimulation and may subside between meals. Pain and tenderness may be due to the pressure or to the condition causing the obstruction. Fever and general malaise may accompany infection.

Constriction of the duct is treated by probing and dilatation. A calculus may be removed via the duct, or if this approach should fail, surgical removal may have to be undertaken.

A tumor in a salivary gland causes a more gradual swelling unrelated to salivary stimulation. It is treated by prompt surgical excision of the gland. The parotid gland is the most frequent site of salivary tumors; the submaxillary gland is next in order of incidence. If the physician suspects the tumor is malignant because of its firmness, fixation and involvement of the facial nerve, a biopsy may be done to confirm the diagnosis. Carcinoma involves more radical surgery and radiation therapy. In the case of cancer of a parotid gland, removal of the mandible and dissection of the cervical lymphatics may be necessary. Surgical excision of the submaxillary gland for malignancy includes dissection of the cervical lymphatics and possibly resection of the mandible. Following such disfiguring surgery as the extirpation of the lower jaw, a prosthesis may be constructed of a synthetic material which is physically and chemically inert and is implanted in the area to restore a normal appearance.

Following any surgery on the parotid gland, the patient is observed for signs of facial paralysis because of the close proximity of the facial nerve to the operative site. In some instances, the facial nerve may be involved by a malignant tumor and is removed with the gland, leaving the patient with some permanent facial paralysis.

Nursing in Mouth Disorders

When caring for a patient with a mouth disorder, it should be remembered that the mouth and associated structures are concerned with the ingestion, mastication and swallowing of food, the sense of taste and with speech. Disease in the posterior part of the mouth may also cause respiratory difficulty.

Observations. An appreciation of the normal characteristics of the mouth and contained structures is necessary in order to recognize changes. A healthy oral mucosa is moist, intact and a dark pink color.

Healthy gums (gingivae) are a lighter pink, are firm and fit closely to the teeth, forming papillae to fill the interdental spaces.

The tongue, a light pink, is moist and has minute papillae on the superior surface. A slight white fur may be present, particularly in the morning.

Observation of the mouth may elicit significant information as to the patient's state of hydration and nutrition as well as manifestations of systemic disease and local disorders. The following should be noted: changes in color, degree of moisture, and coating of the tongue; prominence of the papillae; lesions; accumulation of secretions; bleeding; encrustations; odor of the breath; and general hygienic state. For example, the tongue and mouth are the first sites to reflect dehydration; the mouth and tongue become dry and the latter becomes furred. Bleeding of the gums may indicate a deficiency of vitamin C or an infection. Excessive salivation (sialorrhea) may be associated with a vitamin B deficiency, certain medications or a newgrowth in the mouth or esophagus.

Oral and Dental Care. Since the mouth is open to the environment, it is a normal habitat of organisms. A healthy, intact mucous membrane, a normal flow of saliva, good hygienic care and an adequate food and fluid intake maintain sufficient resistance to keep the organisms at a safe minimum. Also, the mouth is highly vascular, which contributes to its resistance and quick healing.

A patient may require encouragement and guidance in establishing better dental and mouth care. The importance of frequent brushing of the teeth, the technique of using an up-and-down movement and reaching all accessible areas, the avoidance of injury to soft tissues, regular visits to the dentist, and the role of nutrition and adequate fluids should be included in discussions with patients. Ill-fitting dentures may be a source of discomfort to a patient and may interfere with his taking an adequate diet or may cause actual mouth lesions. The person should be urged to have the problem corrected.

Frequently, ill persons are not able to perform their own dental and mouth care and the nurse accepts the responsibility. Care should be taken not to injure soft tissues and to reach the less accessible regions. Removable dentures are taken out frequently and cleaned, and the mouth is cared for before they are replaced.

If the tongue is coated, the mouth dry, and thick, tenacious secretions accumulate and encrust, special nursing attention is necessary. The mouth and teeth should be gently cleansed at least every 2 to 3 hours to reduce the patient's discomfort as well as the number of mouth organisms. A tongue depressor wrapped with gauze or cotton swabs moistened with an antiseptic mouthwash may be used. Saline or a solution of sodium bicarbonate or hydrogen peroxide may also be used. Following the cleansing, the mouth should be rinsed thoroughly. The rinsing may not be possible if the patient is unconscious or if there is danger of aspiration of the fluid, in which case moist applicators are used. A light application of mineral oil helps to protect the mucosa and prevent drying. A mixture of lemon juice and oil or glycerine may prove more palatable and refreshing to the patient; the lemon juice tends to increase salivation. Vaseline or cold cream may be applied to the lips.

If there are ulcers or infection and inflammation, the care and treatment are prescribed by the physician. Cleansing may be by mouthwashes or irrigations, since brushing or swabbing might injure the affected tissues or be too distressing to the patient. Local applications of drugs may be made directly by swabs to the affected areas, by mouthwash or by the dissolving of lozenges or pellets in the mouth. Systemic medications may also be prescribed to treat mouth conditions. Antibiotics and vitamins B complex and C are probably the most common.

Hypersalivation. Increased saliva may pose a problem in the care of some patients. It may result in very frequent expectorations or drooling, and the lips and skin around the mouth may become excoriated by the saliva. A coating of a protective substance such as vaseline should be applied to the lips and skin. A sputum cup or basin and soft tissues are supplied, and a paper bag for disposal of the wipes is placed within the patient's reach. Drainage may be cared for in some instances by the placing of one end of a gauze wick in the mouth and the other end in a basin. A lateral or semiprone position will facilitate drainage. The excessive saliva

may also be removed by a catheter attached to suction.

Nutrition and Fluids. The condition of the mouth is greatly influenced by the patient's nutrition and state of hydration. The ingestion of food and fluids stimulates salivary secretion and prevents an accumulation of secretions, cellular debris and organisms. Food and fluids should be encouraged, if permitted, when there are lesions and the mouth is sore; soft, nonirritating foods are served. Hot foods and fluids must be avoided. Fluids may have to be taken through a tube. Failure of the patient to take a sufficient quantity of food or fluid should be brought to the doctor's attention. Feedings via a nasogastric tube or parenteral fluids may be necessary.

Medical Asepsis. Strict medical asepsis should be observed in the care of patients with mouth disorders. The secretions are likely to contain organisms and precautions are necessary to prevent their spread to other persons. Equipment used for mouth care should be individualized and is disinfected at least once daily. Special attention should be given to thorough washing of the hands after any treatment or care given the patient. If the condition is infectious and the bedding possibly contaminated by oral secretions, a gown should be worn to avoid cross infection.

At the same time, in the interest of the patient, it is important that precautions are used to prevent introducing organisms into the mouth when there is any disorder and a lowered resistance. Also, for esthetic reasons, strict cleanliness should be observed; chipped mouthwash cups, basins and the like should be avoided and the nurse's hands should be washed just before giving mouth care.

Surgical Care. The patient facing surgery on the mouth or associated structures may be quite fearful and concerned about the results, particularly if radical surgery is to be performed. The surgery may be disfiguring or it may interfere with normal swallowing or speech. The patient is encouraged to verbalize his concerns and to ask questions. An explanation of what is entailed in the surgical treatment should be given to the patient and family. They are advised as to what they may expect after the operation. If the removal of a part of the jaw or other disfiguring surgery is involved, they may be advised of the reconstructive surgery and prosthesis that are now used to provide a normal appearance. Attention should be directed toward improving the patient's nutritional status and attaining optimal hydration during the preoperative period. Antiseptic mouthwashes or irrigations may be ordered so the mouth will be as clean as possible for the surgery.

Postoperative care depends on the extent of the surgery. The patient who has intra-oral or radical surgery will be more dependent and will require constant nursing attention.

To facilitate drainage and prevent aspiration, the patient is placed in a semiprone or lateral position. As soon as the vital signs are stable, the head of the bed is usually elevated. The patient will experience less difficulty with breathing in this position, and it also tends to reduce the edema in the operative area. Frequent gentle suctioning with a small catheter may be necessary.

The possibility of hemorrhage should be kept in mind, since the mouth is a very vascular area. After the first 24 hours, irrigations may be ordered to remove the secretions and old blood and to reduce the possibility of infection. Irrigation of the month generally contributes to the patient's comfort as well. Nutrition is provided by nasogastric tube for the first few days, and intravenous fluids are administered. When oral foods and fluids are permitted, a small amount of clear liquid is given to test the patient's ability to swallow. Any choking, coughing or difficulty in swallowing should be reported and the fluid withheld until further directions. If there is no problem, the fluids are gradually increased and soft, nonirritating foods are introduced. Extremes of temperature are avoided. The mouth is cleansed before each meal to improve the sense of taste and again following the meal.

Medications may include antibiotics to control infection and analgesics for the relief of pain.

Early ambulation is usually encouraged to prevent respiratory complications and improve the patient's morale.

The patient may be very sensitive about his appearance and may withdraw. Every effort should be made to have him feel accepted. The cooperation of family and friends is necessary in this; it may be helpful to discuss the problem with them and to advise them that it is important that the patient does not sense any revulsion on their part and that they treat him as normal. Cleanliness and tidiness of the patient and his immediate environment are important factors.

The surgery may have involved the tongue, interfering with communication.* Paper and a pencil or a slate should be kept within reach of the patient at all times. Anticipation of his needs by the thoughtful nurse will give him confidence and reduce his concern about his lack of ability to communicate.

In cases in which the external surface of the lips, face or neck is involved, care is taken to keep the area dry and free of contamination by vomitus and oral secretions in order to prevent infection and sloughing.

Nursing care should include consideration of the necessary care after the patient goes home from the hospital. His condition may be such that modifications in his diet and activities are needed and that continuing care is necessary.

Instructions concerning the patient's care should be given the patient and a member of his family. Before the patient leaves the hospital, he is provided with the opportunity for self-care in order to gain understanding and confidence. Appropriate referrals to a social service or a visiting nurse organization may be made by the nurse. A return to his former occupation may not be possible, and retraining for suitable work may be necessary.

DISORDERS OF SWALLOWING

The transmission of food and saliva from the mouth to the stomach — the only function of the esophagus — may be impaired by a disturbance in neuromuscular functioning, a decrease or obstruction in the lumen of the tube, or by inflammation and degeneration of tissue in the wall of the esophagus. Causes of these changes may be extrinsic or intrinsic.

---

*Surgical removal of the tongue (total glossectomy) or the excision of a portion of it (partial glossectomy).

Extrinsic Causes of Impaired Swallowing

Since the mouth, tongue and pharynx are involved in directing food into the esophagus, it is obvious that disease in any one of these structures may interfere with the initial phase of swallowing. This may be seen in severe stomatitis, pharyngitis, tonsillitis, cleft palate and neoplastic disease of the mouth or tongue. The condition may actually interfere with the swallowing process or cause so much pain that the patient avoids swallowing.

Compression of the esophagus by enlargement or newgrowths of neighboring structures occurs rarely. Examples are goiter (enlargement of the thyroid), aortic aneurysm and enlargement of the mediastinal lymph glands as in Hodgkin's disease.

Dysphagia (difficulty in swallowing) may result from nervous system disorders that affect innervation to the muscle tissue of the esophagus. Damage to the swallowing center in the medulla or to nerve fibers of the tenth cranial (vagus) nerve concerned with the swallowing mechanism may cause a partial or complete paralysis. Paralysis may occur in the pharyngeal area due to interference with the normal innervation via the ninth (glossopharyngeal) cranial nerve. Failure of the normal pharyngeal phase of swallowing may result in food passing into the trachea and the nasal cavities. The sphincter at the esophageal opening may remain relaxed, allowing air to be drawn into the esophagus during inspiration.

Conditions in which paralysis of swallowing is commonly seen include myasthenia gravis (failure of nerve impulse transmission at the neuromuscular junction), poliomyelitis that involves the motor neurons in the swallowing center, and cerebrovascular accident (stroke).

Intrinsic Causes of Impaired Swallowing

Congenital Anomalies. A congenital anomaly may occasionally be the cause of impaired swallowing in the newborn infant. The commonest malformations of the esophagus include atresia, stenosis and tracheo-esophageal fistula. In atresia, the esophagus is interrupted, ending in a blind pouch.

Stenosis is a constriction of the tube at one point that prevents the passage of food to the stomach. In a tracheo-esophageal fistula there is an opening between the trachea and the esophagus. This may be combined with atresia, in which case the esophagus opens into and ends in the trachea. In other instances, the esophagus may be complete, but a short tube exists between it and the trachea. Manifestations of an esophageal malformation in the newborn may be continuous drooling (since the normal amount of saliva cannot be swallowed), regurgitation of the feeding, choking and cyanosis. Prompt recognition and reporting of any indication of difficulty in swallowing may mean the infant's life. Early diagnosis and surgical treatment are necessary in the first few days of life if the infant is to survive. The infant's need for fluids and nourishment is paramount. A gastrostomy may be done in which an opening is made into the stomach through which a tube may be passed. Food is then introduced directly into the stomach. Later, surgery is undertaken to correct the anomaly.

Inflammation and Ulceration of the Esophagus. Inflammation and ulceration of the mucosa and underlying tissues of the esophagus may result from injury or irritation by a rough or sharp foreign body, corrosive substances (strong acids and alkalies), retained food that undergoes decomposition, or from regurgitated gastric juice. During the acute stage of the trauma and inflammation, the patient experiences pain and difficulty in swallowing. As the affected area heals, fibrous scar tissue forms, constricting the lumen of the tube, and resulting in dysphagia. The stricture is treated by gradual dilation by the introduction of bougies. Generally, repeated treatments at intervals for a year or longer are necessary to establish a satisfactory lumen.

Gastrostomy may be necessary in severe constriction in order to provide foods and fluids for the patient. The gastrostomy may also serve for retrograde bougienage in which a very fine bougie, usually a silk cord, is passed into the esophagus. It remains in place between dilation treatments, one end protruding from the nose, the other from the gastrostomy opening. The cord is secured by tying the two ends together. During dilations, the larger bougies are attached to the lower end of the cord and pulled up through the esophagus.

If bougie therapy is not successful, surgical resection of the constricted area with end-to-end anastomosis may be performed. When the area is extensive, surgical reconstruction of the esophagus may be undertaken. A plastic tube or a segment of intestine may be implanted to provide a patent passageway.

Achalasia (Cardiospasm). This condition is a failure of the esophagogastric (cardiac) sphincter to relax to allow the passage of food into the stomach accompanied by a lack of tone in the musculature and normal peristalsis, particularly in the lower part of the tube. The result is an accumulation and stagnation of food and fluids in the esophagus which may cause irritation and inflammation. The patient experiences regurgitation, discomfort and dysphagia. The weak peristalsis and failure of relaxation of the sphincter are attributed to degenerative changes or malfunctioning in the nerve plexus (Auerbach's plexus) that innervates the esophageal muscle tissue.

Treatment is by dilatation of the sphincter and is palliative, since the esophageal peristalsis remains ineffective. A bougie with an inflatable bag at the lower end is inserted under a fluoroscope. When the bag reaches the sphincter, it is filled with water. This stretches the muscle fibers of the sphincter, and many of them may be ruptured. The sphincter remains partially open and food enters by gravity. The dilatation procedure may have to be repeated, and if the results are still unsatisfactory, surgical division of the sphincter (cardiomyotomy) may be performed.

With the loss of sphincter control due to either bougie or surgical therapy, regurgitation of gastric content into the esophagus is likely to occur and may cause esophagitis. The patient is instructed to remain upright for 1 to 2 hours after a meal, to avoid activities that increase intra-abdominal pressure such as straining and stooping, and to sleep with the head of the bed elevated. These suggestions reduce the possibility of regurgitation of gastric contents into the esophagus.

Diverticulum of the Esophagus. An esophageal diverticulum is an outpouching of the wall and may be classified as a pulsion or a traction diverticulum. A pulsion diverticulum consists of mucosal and submucosal tissue protruding through a weakened area of the muscle tissue. The weakness of the muscle tissue is thought to be of congenital origin or due to aging in the older person. The most frequent site of this type of diverticulum is in the pharyngo-esophageal area and just above the diaphragm. A traction diverticulum develops most frequently in the midesophagus in the region of the bifurcation of the trachea. It usually involves all the layers of tissue and is less saccular than the pulsion diverticulum. The cause is inflammatory disease in adjacent structures, such as the mediastinal lymph nodes. The inflammation extends to the esophageal wall, and adhesions may form that put traction on the wall, causing the outpouching.

The symptoms depend on the size of the sacculation and the amount of food it retains. Regurgitation of stagnant food, dysphagia and pain in the chest may be experienced by the patient. Food collects in the diverticulum and may undergo decomposition and cause esophagitis. A traction diverticulum, being less saccular and having a wide-open neck, does not usually retain food and may actually go undiscovered until there is some x-ray examination.

When the symptoms of diverticulum are severe, surgical excision of the sac may be necessary. A pharyngo-esophageal diverticulum is approached through a cervical incision above the clavicular level. A transthoracic approach is used for the removal of diverticula located below the pharyngo-esophageal area.

Esophageal Varices. The flow of blood from the portal vein through the liver may meet with resistance due to disease and degenerative changes in the liver (cirrhosis of the liver). Since this resistance progresses over a period of time, collateral veins are developed by which some of the obstructed portal blood may reach the inferior vena cava. The major collateral channel is between the splenic vein and the esophageal veins. This increases the volume of blood and the pressure in the esophageal veins, causing dilatation and a weakening of the walls. These varicosed veins appear as large bulbous protrusions under the mucosa of the esophagus. Food passing over a protruded area may cause ulceration of the mucosa and wall of the vein, and severe hematemesis results. Some blood will enter the stomach and eventually the person passes tarry stools. Prompt emergency treatment is necessary and includes blood transfusion and the insertion of a nasogastric tube with balloons that are inflated to compress the area of bleeding and the cardiac portion of the stomach (balloon tamponade). The tube also has a lumen that opens into the stomach to permit gastric suction and is known as the Sengstaken-Blakemore tube.

A more recent form of treatment used to check the bleeding is the continuous application of cold to the esophagus and cardia of the stomach. A special double lumen tube is inserted. It permits a steady circulation, by a mechanical pump, of a cold mixture of alcohol and water through the balloons and a refrigeration unit.

Vitamin K may be ordered to increase the patient's clotting power. A drug such as methantheline bromide (Banthine) may be prescribed to depress gastric secretion. Antacids are used to neutralize the gastric acidity to prevent further irritation and erosion of the esophageal mucosa.

The patient requires constant observation and attention. The pressures in the balloons must be checked at frequent intervals and maintained. The blood pressure and respirations are checked, and the patient is kept at complete rest. Sedation may be necessary to allay the patient's fear and to provide rest. The head of the bed is usually elevated to reduce the flow of blood into the portal system. The patient is unable to swallow his saliva, so provision is made for suctioning or for expectoration into paper wipes or a basin.

Compression by the inflated balloons is not usually continued longer than 48 hours. Pressure for a longer period could cause edema, ulceration and perforation of the esophagus. The balloons are deflated and the tube left in place for continued gastric drainage and in case of recurrence of the bleeding.

Surgical treatment of esophageal varices may be done to relieve the hypertension of the portal venous system and to control esophageal bleeding. Different surgical procedures are used. A portocaval shunt in which an anastomosis is made between the portal vein and the inferior vena cava, a splenorenal venous shunt or a transesophageal ligation of the varices may be done.

Neoplasms of the Esophagus. Benign tumors occur rarely in the esophagus. The most common of these are leiomyomas which are tumors of nonstriated muscle tissue. Those encountered less frequently are polyps, cysts, fibromas, adenomas and fibrolipomas. As the tumor imposes itself on the lumen of the esophagus or interferes with normal muscle activity, dysphagia occurs. The patient first experiences difficulty in swallowing the more solid foods, such as meat and bread. The tumor is excised and whether the approach is transesophageal, cervical or thoracic will depend on the location and the nature of the tumor.

Cancer of the esophagus tends to develop more often in the older age group. Its incidence is mainly in males between 50 and 70 years of age, and the lower third of the esophagus is the most common site.

The majority of malignant tumors of the esophagus are squamous cell cancer. Adenocarcinoma may occur but is most frequently secondary to gastric carcinoma. The patient complains first of dysphagia with solid foods which gradually progresses to difficulty with liquids. Substernal discomfort and pain, regurgitation and loss of weight and strength are experienced with steadily increasing severity. In advanced stages, bleeding may occur.

Diagnosis is made by x-ray examination and an esophagoscopy. A biopsy is obtained and probably a smear from the lesion is taken for cytologic study during the endoscopic examination.

Various surgical procedures are employed; the surgeon's choice will depend on the location of the tumor and the stage to which the disease has advanced. The procedure may involve resection of the affected portion of the esophagus, removal of regional lymph nodes and the joining of the remaining portion of the esophagus to the stomach, which is drawn up into the thoracic cavity.

When a large portion of the esophagus is removed, a segment of the patient's intestine (jejunum or colon) may be implanted to replace the resected esophagus. More recently, a plastic tube has been used to re-establish a passageway between the remaining esophagus and the stomach. If the lesion is in the distal portion of the esophagus, most likely involving the esophagogastric junction, resection of both the esophagus and the stomach may be done (esophagogastrectomy).

Following diagnosis and investigation of the patient's general condition, the surgeon may conclude that radical surgery is inadvisable. Radiation therapy may be used with some benefit. A plastic nasogastric tube may be inserted through the constricted area and left in place so the patient can be given fluids and nourishment. Complications of ulceration and bleeding may develop with this latter palliative procedure. More often, a gastrostomy is employed by which nutrition is maintained for the remainder of the patient's life.

Nursing in Disorders of Swallowing

A disturbance in swallowing may interfere with the patient's ability to take food and fluid and to dispose of his saliva in the normal way. He may become very self-conscious about the latter problem and consider his life is really threatened by the former. Even slight dysphagia makes the patient very apprehensive; having experienced some difficulty, he may resort to fluids and soft foods that do not provide an adequate diet. He is nervous when eating with others because he fears the embarrassment of choking and regurgitation. Anxiety may only worsen his dysphagia. The patient requires sympathetic understanding and acknowledgement of his concerns.

Observations. An accurate recording should be made of the patient's fluid and food intake. Difficulty with any one type of food should be noted and that food avoided in future feedings. The physician may request a daily record of the patient's weight, but this may have to be omitted, since a loss of weight may only increase the patient's anxiety. The frequency of regurgitation should be noted and the amount and nature of the regurgitated material recorded.

Care of the Saliva. The patient may not be able to swallow his saliva. Soft paper wipes, a paper bag for their disposal and a sputum cup should be within his reach at all times. Hypersalivation is common in some esophageal conditions, such as tumors. A gauze wick placed in the side of the mouth with the other end in a basin may also be used. Frequent suctioning may be necessary with the very ill and weak patient.

Frequent expectoration and wiping of the mouth may cause irritation of the lips and the skin around the mouth. Gentle bathing, drying and an application of a protective cream at frequent intervals will prevent excoriation.

Some provision should be made at night for the salivary drainage. A thick towel folded over a plastic or rubber bed protector may be placed under the patient's face. He is encouraged to lie on either side to promote drainage and reduce the possibility of aspiration.

Mouth Hygiene. Frequent cleansing and rinsing of the mouth are necessary to decrease the number of organisms. Normally, many of these are swallowed and destroyed by the gastric juice. The patient with esophageal disease may experience an objectionable taste. Mouth care is refreshing, for the patient is constantly aware of the saliva that he cannot dispose of in the normal way.

Positioning. If the patient is still able to take some fluids and food by mouth, swallowing is less difficult if he is in the sitting position. The head of the bed may be raised, and the patient is given the necessary assistance to assume an upright position. The very ill and weak patient may have to be kept in a lateral or semiprone position to facilitate salivary drainage and prevent aspiration.

Hydration and Nutrition. The esophagus may not be completely obstructed, and the patient may be able to swallow liquids and semiliquids or even soft, solid food. He may, however, be very fearful of choking and regurgitation. Encouragement and reassurance from a nurse who remains with him during his meal may make the difference between his taking the essential nutrition and fluids and rejecting them. The more relaxed patient is more likely to have less difficulty in swallowing.

If swallowing is completely inhibited or obstructed, fluids and nourishment may have to be given by tube feedings. One method of tube feeding employs the use of a nasogastric tube which is usually left in place between feedings (see Gastric Gavage, p. 339). If the patient's esophagus is completely obstructed and a nasogastric tube cannot be passed, a gastrostomy may have to be done and feedings given via the tube that is inserted into the stomach through an abdominal incision (see Gastrostomy, p. 340).

Intravenous fluids may be necessary to maintain a normal fluid and electrolyte balance. The patient's fluid intake and output should be measured and recorded and observations made for any deficiency.

Preoperative Nursing Care. The care of the patient who is to have esophageal surgery is directed toward improving his nutritional status and establishing an optimal fluid and electrolyte balance. The patient is encouraged to take the maximum that he can manage orally. High-calorie, high-protein liquids or semiliquid foods may be used, but if the condition limits the oral intake and the patient is emaciated and dehydrated, tube feedings and parental fluids will most likely be ordered. Blood transfusions may be necessary to correct the anemia that has resulted from nutritional deficiency.

The patient and his family look for support and understanding from the nurse. They realize the seriousness of the surgery and are usually very apprehensive. The attentive nurse who gives consideration to the patient's needs and demonstrates understanding of his concern for his future may contribute much to lessening his fears and despair.

An explanation of what may be expected in the postoperative period should be made and the patient's and his family's questions answered willingly.

An explanation is given of the multiple pieces of equipment that will be necessary at his bedside after the operation and of the need for the nasogastric, chest and intravenous tubes and frequent suctioning. The importance of deep breathing, coughing, frequent turning and the simple foot and leg exercises is stressed, and instructions are given on how to cough and do the exercises (see Preparation of the Patient for Thoracic Surgery, p. 305). The discussion of the postoperative period should be extended over several periods, and as the patient talks about it and asks questions, his apprehension of the situation may be reduced. Any explanation should be discrete, in order to avoid arousing unnecessary anxiety, and should be in simple lay terms.

Particular attention is given to oral hygiene; rinsing frequently with antiseptic mouthwash will help to prevent mouth and respiratory infection.

The usual considerations are given to the immediate general preoperative care (see p. 107). Specific orders as to local preparation are received from the doctor, since the area of skin to be prepared will probably vary with the surgical approach planned.

If reconstructive surgery is anticipated that may involve the use of a segment of the patient's intestine (jejunum or colon) to replace the resected esophagus, an oral antibiotic or sulfonamide may be ordered to reduce the intestinal bacteria. If the patient is being tube-fed, the preparation is put into solution and given through the nasogastric or gastrostomy tube.

Postoperative Nursing Care. Preparation to receive the patient from the operating room includes the assembling of the following equipment:

Sphygmomanometer and stethoscope
Respiratory and gastric suctioning equipment
Infusion pole
Equipment for oxygen administration
Two large hemostats
Tray of equipment for chest aspiration
Tray of equipment for tracheotomy

Following operation, the principles of care include those applicable to the care of a patient having had chest and gastric surgery (see pp. 307 and 361).

If a nasogastric tube has been introduced in the operating room, this is usually attached to a suction apparatus for continuous removal of gastric secretions. This is observed for any sign of bleeding. The drainage may be colored with blood the first few hours but should gradually assume the characteristics of normal secretions. Directions will be given when nasogastric fluids and feedings are to be given and the suction discontinued. A temporary gastrostomy may be used for drainage and feedings; the nasogastric tube may simply be kept in position to maintain a patent esophagus.

The nasogastric tube may be removed in 4 to 5 days, and small amounts of water may then be given. Any difficulty in swallowing or regurgitation should be reported. The patient will find swallowing easier if he is sitting up. If he has no difficulty with water, the fluids are gradually varied and increased in volume. The diet gradually progresses to semiliquids, soft foods and a normal diet. Parenteral fluids and gastrostomy feedings are continued until the patient is able to swallow adequate amounts of fluids and food. If the surgical procedure entailed an esophagogastric anastomosis with the stomach being drawn up into the thoracic cavity, the patient may not be able to take the ordinary amount of food or fluid at one time without experiencing pressure in his chest and some dyspnea. In this event, the patient is fed smaller amounts at more frequent intervals and should remain upright in the sitting position for 1 to 2 hours after eating.

A frequent check is made of the patient's temperature and white blood cell count for any indication of infection. If either is increased to levels above the normal, parenteral administration of an antibiotic is ordered. In some instances the surgeon may prefer to start the antibiotic administration after the operation as a prophylactic measure against infection.

A record should be kept of the patient's intake and output until a normal intake by mouth is well established.

If the lesion was located in the proximal portion of the esophagus, a cervical approach may have been used in surgery without entry into the thoracic cavity. This eliminates the closed water seal drainage and reduces respiratory problems.

The convalescent period is usually prolonged, during which the patient will probably have to adjust to and learn to manage modifications in his diet and pattern of eating. Obviously, his condition will determine whether he returns to his former occupation. He and his family may be faced with socioeconomic problems that should be recognized by the nurse. Assistance may be sought from the social worker or an appropriate service or welfare organization. The visiting nurse may be contacted to assess the home situation and help the family plan for the patient's care.

GASTRIC DISORDERS

The gastric disorders seen most frequently are pyloric stenosis, gastritis, peptic ulcer and carcinoma.

Pyloric Stenosis

This condition may be congenital, or it may be secondary to peptic ulcer or carcinoma of the stomach. Secondary pyloric stenosis is discussed as a complication with the causative condition (see p. 359).

Gastritis

The term gastritis implies inflammation of the stomach. The condition may be acute or chronic and the pathological process is usually limited to the mucosa. The causes of acute inflammation may be the ingestion of large quantities of alcohol, contaminated foods, or foods to which the person is sensitive or allergic, such as seafood, mushrooms or salicylates (e.g., aspirin). Infective gastritis is most frequently due to the ingestion of foods bearing staphylococci or salmonella organisms.

The patient becomes ill suddenly and suffers severe epigastric pain, nausea, vomiting and fever. The attack may last a few hours to a few days. Dehydration develops rapidly and the patient becomes prostrate. The treatment includes nothing by mouth, bed rest and parenteral fluids. Clear fluids are given when the symptoms subside, and if tolerated, a bland diet of soft foods is introduced and progressively increased until a normal diet is resumed.

Chronic gastritis occurs with prolonged and repeated irritation of the mucosa and results in atrophic changes in the mucosa and glands. The cause may be evasive, since the condition may be associated with other diseases, such as pernicious anemia, and with the degenerative changes of aging. It may result from constant subjection of the stomach to an ingested irritant, such as alcohol, and frequently accompanies a gastric ulcer or gastric carcinoma.

The symptoms of chronic gastritis are usually ill-defined but may include anorexia, discomfort and a full feeling after meals, flatulence, nausea and occasionally hematemesis. A bland diet is recommended with abstinence from foods and fluids that seem to aggravate the condition. Spicy and raw foods, fats and very hot foods are poorly tolerated. The patient may lose considerable weight as he tends to restrict his food intake to avoid the distress it may precipitate. Attention is directed toward improving his general nutritional status by encouraging a well-balanced diet of nonirritating foods. Milk, buttermilk and eggnogs between meals may be tolerated and are nutritious.

Peptic Ulcer

A peptic ulcer is the erosion of a circumscribed area of tissue in the wall of the gastrointestinal tract resulting from the digestive action of hydrochloric acid and pepsin. The most frequent site of the ulcer is the stomach and proximal portion of the duodenum, as these areas are normally in contact with gastric juice. It occurs more frequently in the duodenum than the stomach, less often in the esophagus and rarely in the jejunum. The ulcer penetrates the mucosa and may invade the underlying submucosal and muscular tissues. Ulcers tend to recur; some heal promptly, others become chronic.

Etiology. There is no conclusion as to the initiating cause of peptic ulcer. The lesion develops when the mucosa is unable to resist the digestive action of the gastric juice.

Normally, the mucosa secretes sufficient mucus to provide a protective coating that prevents mucosal digestion by the acid-pepsin action. The duodenum has the additional protection of the strong alkalinity of the bile and pancreatic and intestinal secretions which neutralize the acidic chyme. Still another defense is a healthy resistant mucosa which has a good blood supply and is capable of continuous rapid regeneration of the mucosal epithelial cells.

A peptic ulcer may develop when the secretory output of hydrochloric acid and pepsin is in excess of the normal or when the protective mechanisms are inadequate in relation to the amount of acid and pepsin produced. Guyton states, "The usual cause of peptic ulceration is too much secretion of gastric juice in relation to the degree of protection afforded the mucosa by the mucus that is also secreted."[5] The problem is: what causes a hypersecretion of acid and pepsin or lowers mucosal resistance? The major factor is considered to be a disturbance in the autonomic nervous control of gastric secretion that results in increased vagal (parasympathetic) innervation, causing prolonged secretion of hydrochloric acid and pepsin.

There are several factors that may contribute to or predispose to the development of a peptic ulcer. Emotional tension, anxiety, frustration and stress may cause an imbalance in the autonomic nervous system, resulting in increased vagal stimulation of gastric secretion. Some drugs such as adrenal steroids (cortisone), acetylsalicylic acid (Aspirin) and phenylbutazone (Butazolidin) are ulcerogenic in some persons.

Poor dietary habits, particularly irregular meals, are thought to be an aggravating factor. Abnormally long periods between meals in persons with a prolonged hypersecretion of acid and pepsin leave the mucosa vulnerable. The protective mechanisms cannot withstand the acid-pepsin action without the diluting and neutralizing assistance of food. Smoking and excessive amounts of alcohol or coffee increase gastric secretion.

Incidence. Peptic ulcer is a common disease and has a higher incidence in males between the ages of 40 and 55 years. Approximately 10,000 deaths in Canada and the United States are attributed annually to the serious complications associated with peptic ulcer.[6]

A hereditary tendency is suggested, and those with type O blood appear to be more susceptible.

Manifestations. The prominent symptom of peptic ulcer is epigastric pain with definite characteristics. The pain is usually described by the patient as gnawing or burning and has had a rhythmicity in its development and relief in relation to the ingestion of food. The onset of pain may be 30 minutes to 4 hours after a meal and is relieved by taking food or an antacid. In the case of an esophageal ulcer, the pain develops within a half hour after the meal. Pain associated with a gastric ulcer usually occurs one-half to 1 hour after

---

[5]Arthur C. Guyton: Textbook of Medical Physiology, 4th ed. Philadelphia, W. B. Saunders Co., 1971, p. 776.

[6]Loyal Davis (Ed.): Christopher's Textbook of Surgery, 9th ed. Philadelphia, W. B. Saunders Co., 1968, p. 656.

the ingestion of food; that of duodenal ulcer is delayed for approximately 2 to 4 hours. The patient's rest is frequently disturbed by nocturnal pain, particularly with a duodenal ulcer. Although the ingestion of food generally provides relief, in a few instances it may be the initiating factor of the ulcer pain, particularly if the food is coarse or highly seasoned.

Vomiting is not a common incident in peptic ulcer but may occur if the ulcer pain is very severe or if the ulcer is in the pyloric region. In the case of the latter, inflammation and edema of the surrounding tissues, pyloric spasm or contracted scar tissue resulting from ulceration may narrow the lumen of the pylorus. This may delay the emptying of the stomach and may cause vomiting.

The ulcer patient usually maintains his weight, since he eats frequently to relieve his pain unless his condition is complicated by vomiting.

Investigation of the patient for peptic ulcer may include roentgenograms with a barium meal, gastric analysis to determine the hydrochloric acid secretion, gastroscopy and stool examination for occult blood (see p. 332).

Treatment and Nursing Care. Treatment of the peptic ulcer patient is directed toward the relief of symptoms, healing of the ulcer and the prevention of recurrence. A regime of rest, frequent bland feedings and various medications is designed to reduce gastric secretory and motor activity, dilute the gastric juice and to neutralize much of the hydrochloric acid that is secreted.

Hospitalization is not always necessary. It may be that the patient's home situation and his understanding and acceptance of the treatment are such that he may progress satisfactorily at home. If it is suspected that the patient will not adhere to the treatment regime or if his home situation is not conducive to the preparation of his diet or to relaxation, hospitalization is recommended until the symptoms are relieved and the patient and his family learn and plan for the necessary adjustments. A period in the hospital may be beneficial if the patient's usual environment is the source of incompatibilities, anxiety and frustration that aggravate his disease. Treatment and care should be individualized for all patients, but it is extremely important with the ulcer patient.

This means that those concerned with his care must get to know the patient and his pattern of living.

Nursing care includes the following considerations.

ADHERENCE TO TREATMENT REGIMEN. It is important that the nurse caring for the ulcer patient understands the treatment aims and the significance of strict adherence to the prescribed therapeutic regimen. The patient's response of annoyance to delayed or irregular feedings and medications can result in hypersecretion and hypermotility that further aggravate his condition and delay healing.

OBSERVATIONS. The patient's response to the treatment and his ability and willingness to cooperate in the prescribed schedule should be noted. He should be observed for evidence of mental conflicts, anxieties and emotional factors that may be influencing his disease.

Prompt recognition and reporting of early symptoms of complications which may develop are an important nursing responsibility.

REST. Mental and physical rest are necessary if reduced gastric activity is to be achieved. This is the basic principle of ulcer treatment. A brief period of bed rest may be recommended, or the patient may remain ambulatory with some restriction in activity and an increase in his hours of rest. A period away from his work situation is necessary if the symptoms are severe, but for some persons it may be considered better to let them carry on rather than impose the anxiety created by the loss of financial income or by the disorganization of their work. The need for a full "lunch hour," preferably away from the job, and for leaving the work behind when he leaves the work situation should be stressed with the patient who is continuing or resuming work. Other factors that contribute to rest should receive attention, such as a quiet pleasant environment, physical comfort, undisturbed rest periods, the avoidance of visitors who may arouse pent-up feelings, relaxing diversions of interest to the patient and the avoidance of delays in relation to his treatments and requests. The patient at home is encouraged to develop interests within his limitations.

The hospital or visiting nurse has an important role in recognizing and reducing underlying anxiety. Frequently, the ulcer patient tends to keep his concerns to himself, but if he recognizes the nurse as a sympathetic understanding person who is anxious to help and not to judge, he may confide his problems and emotional stress. The verbal expression of these in itself can be of value, for so often the problems tend to acquire inordinate proportions and therefore assume unrealistic importance. The nurse takes time to listen and encourages the patient to exhaust his pent-up tensions that tend to aggravate gastric hypersecretion and hypermotility. As an objective person, she may help the patient see the problems in normal perspective and may make constructive suggestions.

A sedative to promote rest and relaxation is usually administered at regular intervals in ulcer therapy.

DIET. Dietary measures are a major part of the treatment of the peptic ulcer patient. Frequent small feedings of foods that are chemically, mechanically and thermally nonirritating are used to minimize the gastric secretory and motor stimulation, dilute the gastric juice and neutralize much of the hydrochloric acid. All foods stimulate gastric secretion; proteins, particularly meat with the component secretagogue, cause greater stimulation than do carbohydrates and fats. Gastric contractions increase in intensity when the stomach is empty or when distended by a large volume of food. The ingestion of small frequent feedings keeps some food in the stomach most of the time and reduces gastric motor activity and acid-pepsin concentration.

The dietary modifications and restrictions will vary with the severity of the patient's symptoms and with the patient's response. Some physicians prescribe a very rigid dietary regimen, while others favor a more liberal diet. In the acute stage, the initial diet may consist only of 120 to 200 ml. of milk or milk and cream every waking hour. Milk is taken at night only if the patient wakens, or the doctor may want the patient wakened every 2 hours for feeding to neutralize the excess acid. In a few days, 3 small meals of soft, nonfibrous foods such as creamed soups, cooked cereals or gruel, custards, junkets, jello, milk puddings, melba toast, or soft boiled or poached egg are introduced with milk being continued every

1 or 2 hours between meals during the waking hours. If these additions are well tolerated and the patient's pain has subsided, the diet is gradually increased to include a greater variety of bland nonirritating light foods. A glass of milk and crackers, melba toast or arrowroot biscuits are taken midmorning, midafternoon and before retiring. Coarse and raw vegetables, fried food, pork products, spices, meat extracts, coffee and carbonated and alcoholic beverages should be avoided. If the patient is overweight or there is concern for hypercholesteremia or coronary artery disease, whole milk may be replaced by skimmed milk and the animal fat content of the diet reduced.

Later, the diet is liberalized in accord with the patient's symptoms and tolerance. Some raw fruits and vegetables, coffee once a day, a small amount of fried food and an alcoholic beverage before dinner, if desired, may be permitted. The continuance of regular unhurried meals with milk as a snack in between is very important. Coffee, tea and alcoholic beverages should be restricted to limited quantities. Meat, particularly beef, will be more readily tolerated if boiled or broiled. The importance of a well-balanced diet should be stressed to the patient in order to avoid nutritional deficiencies. Vitamin C and iron deficiencies may develop if the patient does not round out his diet sufficiently. Eventually the patient is encouraged to take as normal a diet as possible, eliminating only the foods that he finds give him discomfort.

The initial treatment of an acute peptic ulcer may consist of a continuous intragastric drip of milk or a solution of aluminum hydroxide passed through a nasogastric tube. The continuous drip provides more constant neutralization in the patient with a marked hypersecretion of acid. Its disadvantages are the discomfort of the tube to the patient and the restrictions it places on his mobility. Rarely, a gastrojejunal tube is passed, and frequent feedings are given through it which bypass the stomach and ulcer area; stimulation of gastric secretion and motility and irritation of the ulcer by direct contact with the food are eliminated.

MOUTH CARE. The patient should be encouraged to rinse his mouth after each milk feeding, since the residue in the mouth may tend to turn him against the feedings. A mild antiseptic mouthwash or just clear water may be used.

MEDICATIONS. An antacid is a drug used to increase the pH of the gastric juice. It is not always prescribed in the treatment of the patient with a peptic ulcer; many physicians claim that it is not actually necessary for the healing of the ulcer if adequate diet therapy is employed. Others consider it important in the relief of the patient's pain. Fairly large doses at frequent intervals over a period of weeks or months are necessary to keep the pH of gastric juice above 4.5; pepsin digestive activity increases as the pH decreases to below this figure.[7] There are several common antacids used. Calcium carbonate, which is given in hourly doses through the waking hours, is prone to cause constipation, and some physicians feel the patient ingests an excessive amount of calcium. Aluminum compounds in various liquid and tablet preparations may be used. These include aluminum hydroxide gel (Amphogel, Creamalin), aluminum phosphate gel (Phosphagel), and dihydroxy aluminum aminoacetate (Alglyn, Aspogen, Alzinox). Magnesium oxide and magnesium carbonate are effective antacids, but if given in sufficient dosage to neutralize the acid, they are likely to cause diarrhea. Magnesium trisilicate is frequently used as an antacid as it has a longer period of action and a milder laxative effect than the other magnesium compounds.

Various combinations of several antacids are prepared. Examples are aluminum hydroxide with magnesium trisilicate (Gelusil) and aluminum hydroxide with magnesium hydroxide (Maalox).

Magnesium hydroxide (Milk of Magnesia) is an alkali but is used mainly for its laxative effect. Sodium bicarbonate will neutralize gastric acidity and provide temporary relief of symptoms, but it is rarely used as medication for the ulcer patient since its effect lasts for a shorter period than that produced by the antacids cited above. Also, it is absorbed and may produce alkalosis.

In administering the antacids, those in powder form may be suspended in water; liquid preparations may be diluted. If the antacid is in tablet form, the tablets are chewed so they will disintegrate more readily in the stomach. The antacid is usually given midway between feedings. If the patient is on 3 regular meals with in-between feedings, the drug is usually given one-half hour before each meal.

Bowel action of the patient receiving an antacid should be noted, since some drugs may cause severe constipation and others may produce diarrhea.

Anticholinergic drugs that depress gastric secretion and motility may be used. Stimulation of parasympathetic nerve fibers results in the release of the chemical mediator acetylcholine at the junction of the fibers with the effector structures to initiate their responses. In the case of the stomach, parasympathetic innervation increases acid-pepsin secretion and muscular activity. Anticholinergic drugs may depress the release of acetylcholine or may block the nerve impulse before it reaches the neuro-effector junction, or they may block the action of acetylcholine even if it is released. These drugs do not inhibit total gastric acid-pepsin secretion, but they are considered of value in reducing the excessive secretion and hypermotility characteristic of peptic ulcer patients. The dosage of anticholinergic drugs is individualized since the reactions are variable from one person to another. Examples of such drugs are atropine sulfate; tincture of belladonna, which is more often used than atropine since its liquid form permits finer regulation of the dosage; synthetic anticholinergic drugs such as methantheline bromide (Banthine) given in tablet form, propantheline (Pro-Banthine) tablets, dicyclomine hydrochloride (Bentyl) capsules, and scopolamine methylbromide (Pamine) tablets may be administered. These drugs are given several times a day; the frequency may vary slightly with different physicians and with patients' responses.

Side effects are common to anticholinergic drugs and should be familiar to the nurse. The patient should be observed for dryness of the mouth, blurring of vision, urinary retention, constipation, tachycardia, palpitation and nervous excitation. Anticholinergic drugs are not given if the patient has glaucoma, prostatic hypertrophy or a rapid pulse rate. Older persons are more

---

[7]Franz Goldstein: "Newer Approaches to the Management of Peptic Ulcer." Med. Clin. North Amer., Volume 49, No. 5, Sept. 1965, p. 1265.

susceptible to the toxic effects of these drugs.

Tension and emotional stress are capable of increasing gastric secretion and motility. For this reason, sedatives are frequently a part of the treatment regimen of the ulcer patient. Small doses may be ordered throughout the day with a larger dose being given at bedtime. Elixir phenobarbital through the day and at bedtime may be ordered, or phenobarbital (Luminal) may be used. Amobarbital (Amytal) may be the preparation of choice.

SMOKING. Ulcer patients are advised to abstain from smoking, particularly cigarettes. It is considered to increase gastric motility and secretion and delay healing of the ulcer.

INSTRUCTIONS TO THE ULCER PATIENT. The nurse has an important role in helping the patient to understand and accept the treatment and adjustments recommended by the physician. His progress in the acute stage and the prevention of recurrence of the ulcer may be greatly influenced by the nurse's recognition of the patient's needs in this area and by careful planning to provide the necessary assistance. Obviously, some patients require more help than others, but generally the factors that should receive attention are as follows:

The patient should have some understanding of the nature of his disease and the principles of the suggested therapeutic measures. With such knowledge, he is more likely to cooperate. He is advised that ulcers are prone to recur and that his respect, or lack of it, for the prescribed regimen may play an important role in whether he remains symptom-free or has a recurrence.

An outline of the prescribed diet is given to the patient, and the necessary dietary modifications and their principles are discussed with him. The importance of regular unhurried meals in a relaxed environment, the continuance of the in-between feedings (usually a glass of milk) and the avoidance of excesses of roughage, coffee, tea, condiments, carbonated and alcoholic beverages and overeating are explained. Some directives relating to the selection and preparation of the patient's food may be necessary. For example, fried foods should be limited, and boiled or broiled meats are preferable in order to eliminate the stimulating extract (secretagogue). The process of puréeing or

sieving foods, if such is prescribed, and the usefulness of the commercially prepared baby foods may be suggested.

The patient is advised to continue the restrictions on smoking. If not completely prohibited, it should at least be limited. He is told of the inadvisability of taking aspirin or any medications that are not prescribed.

The need to avoid fatigue and emotional upsets and to forget his work when he leaves his work situation are discussed. The patient should understand the role of anxiety, worry and frustration in his disease. The importance of relaxation and some diversion should be stressed, and some practical suggestions made as to how these may be achieved.

Any pain, vomiting, abdominal distention or gastric distress should be reported promptly to his physician so early treatment may be instituted.

If possible, it is helpful to include a responsible family member in some of the discussions, which should be spread out over several days. The patient and family should be given sufficient opportunity to ask questions.

SURGICAL TREATMENT. If the ulcer fails to heal with medical treatment and the symptoms persist, surgical treatment may be considered necessary. Various operative procedures are used in the surgical treatment of an uncomplicated ulcer in order to reduce the gastric acid secretion.

Gastric resection (subtotal gastrectomy) is the removal of a portion of the stomach, including the ulcer-bearing area. An anastomosis is then made between the gastric stump and the duodenum or jejunum to restore gastrointestinal continuity.

Vagotomy is a resection of the vagus nerve to reduce the stimulation of gastric secretion. It also reduces the motility of the stomach and may interfere with gastric emptying. For this reason it is rarely performed alone but is combined with a gastric resection or with a gastroenterostomy to provide effective gastric emptying.

A combined vagotomy and resection of the antrum of the stomach (antrectomy) may be performed. The vagotomy reduces the innervation that increases the gastric secretion; removal of the antrum removes the source of the chemical stimulus—gastrin.

Complications of Peptic Ulceration. The

complications that commonly occur with peptic ulcer are serious and usually account for the deaths attributed to peptic ulcer. They are hemorrhage, perforation and pyloric obstruction.

HEMORRHAGE. Peptic ulceration is the commonest cause of hematemesis and melena. The loss of blood is due to erosion of a blood vessel at the ulcer site. Most of the patients who have a hemorrhage are known to have or to have had an ulcer, but in a few, it may be the first symptom that prompts them to seek treatment.

Vomiting of blood and the passing of black tarry stools are the prominent indications of serious ulcer bleeding. The patient experiences weakness, apprehension, dizziness and faintness which may progress rapidly to prostration and loss of consciousness. His skin becomes pale, cold and clammy, his pulse is rapid and thready and the blood pressure is abnormally low. Rapid respirations manifest an air hunger. If a large vessel is eroded, the signs and symptoms appear more rapidly and collapse occurs quickly.

Prompt hospital treatment is necessary and includes absolute rest, blood transfusions, parenteral fluids, oxygen administration and treatment of the ulcer.

The patient is restless and very apprehensive. Rest is promoted by the administration of a sedative, a quiet environment, a minimum of disturbance and reassurance. An effort must be made by those around the patient to avoid exhibiting apprehension. The patient may be less apprehensive if he is told something about his condition and is advised that treatment is well under control. He should not be left alone, and relatives are asked to control their emotions when in the patient's immediate environment.

The foot of the bed is usually elevated to encourage the maintenance of a blood supply to the more vital areas. A constant check is made of the patient's pulse, color and respirations, and the blood pressure is recorded every 15 minutes. This interval is lengthened as the patient shows improvement. Nothing is given by mouth at first. A nasogastric tube may be passed and gentle suction applied to remove the blood.

Frequent mouth care is necessary because of the hematemesis, dehydration and the discomfort of extreme thirst.

Small feedings of cold milk or milk and cream may be ordered within a few hours if the patient has recovered from the shock caused by the loss of blood and has stopped vomiting. The early feedings are considered to have several advantages; the milk reduces the acidity of the gastric juice and gives the ulcer a better chance to heal and check the bleeding; it provides nutrition and helps to maintain a normal fluid and electrolyte balance. If there is blood in the stomach, it is diluted by the milk and is less likely to cause nausea and vomiting. The patient's anxiety may be lessened and his general morale improved by the fact that he is receiving food again. Antacid medication may also be prescribed.

Local gastric hypothermia may be used to check the bleeding (see p. 341).

When the bleeding has ceased, a progressive ulcer diet is ordered as cited on page 355 in the care of the peptic ulcer patient. Bed rest is continued to promote ulcer healing and until the severe anemia is corrected. Bed exercises should be instituted, with the doctor's approval, to prevent vascular complications and weakness. It may be necessary to exclude the abdominal contractions that are usually a part of bed exercises.

A preparation of iron will probably be ordered for the development of hemoglobin. Parenteral injections may be used at first; then an oral preparation may be given with feedings.

Some blood may still remain in the intestine after bleeding is controlled, but laxatives and enemas are withheld for 3 to 4 days. The doctor may then order a small dose of a mild laxative, such as milk of magnesia, or a cleansing enema.

If the bleeding cannot be brought under control, emergency surgery may be undertaken. The ulcer area is resected, and the vessels leading to it are ligated.

PERFORATION. A peptic ulcer may progressively erode the submucosal, muscular and serous layers of the gastrointestinal wall. When the serous membranous layer is penetrated, some of the stomach or duodenal content escapes into the peritoneal cavity and causes a generalized peritonitis by chemical irritation and infection. Perforation has a higher incidence in duodenal ulceration and may occur in a few persons with no previous history of ulcer.

When perforation takes place, the patient immediately experiences sudden, incapacitating abdominal pain that begins in the epigastric region but spreads through the abdomen as more of the peritoneum becomes irritated by the intragastrointestinal content. The patient exhibits pallor, a cold clammy skin, rapid pulse, shallow grunting respirations and probably nausea and vomiting. The abdomen becomes rigid and board-like.

Perforation demands immediate treatment; the earlier the treatment is instituted, the greater is the patient's chance for recovery. The physician may consider emergency surgery advisable, or the patient's condition and history may be such that the perforation is treated by nonsurgical conservation methods. The surgical procedure may consist of gastric resection or simple closure of the perforation by suturing the serous layer and reinforcing the area with a patch of omentum. The peritoneal cavity is cleared of the intragastrointestinal fluid that seeped through the perforation. As well as the usual preoperative procedures for emergency surgery, preparation will include the insertion of a nasogastric tube and an intravenous infusion of electrolytes and fluids. An explanation of the need for surgery and what it entails will be made by the surgeon, and the nurse briefly explains the necessary preparatory procedures as she proceeds with them. For postoperative nursing care, see Nursing Care Following Gastric Surgery, page 362.

Nonoperative treatment usually includes an analgesic such as morphine or meperidine hydrochloride (Demerol) by parenteral administration, aspiration of the stomach content using a large tube followed by the insertion of a nasogastric tube and continuous gastric suctioning, and intravenous electrolytes and fluids (fluids may include whole blood) and antibiotic therapy. If the patient's condition is satisfactory, continuous gastric suctioning is replaced by intermittent aspiration after 30 to 48 hours. After 3 to 5 days, small amounts of fluid may be ordered by mouth at stated intervals, and if tolerated, the oral intake is progressively increased.

PYLORIC OBSTRUCTION. The third serious complication of peptic ulcer disease is contriction of the pylorus. This may be caused by inflammation and edema, spasm (when the ulcer is in the acute stage) or by scar tissue which is formed as the ulcer heals. The ulcer may be gastric in the region of the pylorus, or it may be in the duodenum. The constriction causes gastric retention and dilatation.

The patient complains of a full feeling which causes greater discomfort toward the end of the day. Pain may be experienced following eating as gastric contractions increase in intensity in an effort to overcome the obstruction. The contractions gradually decline and the stomach becomes atonic and dilates. Severe anorexia develops and the patient vomits large amounts irregularly. The loss of nutrients, water and electrolytes leads to loss of weight, weakness, dehydration and acid-base imbalance (alkalosis).

If the obstruction is due to the active ulceration process, it is treated medically by gastric aspiration and intravenous fluids. The stomach may be completely emptied of its contents and washed out with normal saline to begin with by means of a large stomach tube. Then a nasogastric tube is passed and continuous or intermittent suctioning is used for 2 to 3 days; withdrawal of gastric secretions reduces the acid-pepsin irritation of the ulcer, and the inflammation, edema and spasm that are responsible for the pyloric constriction gradually subside. The muscle tissue in the stomach walls gradually recover its tone and normal contractility.

Frequent small feedings are gradually introduced and the amount of gastric retention determined by a bedtime aspiration (4 hours after the last feeding). Normally, the volume of residue should not exceed 250 cc. When there is evidence of sufficient gastric outflow, aspirations are discontinued and the patient placed on the usual peptic ulcer dietary regimen.

The nursing care of the patient with a pyloric obstruction includes careful observations and recording of the exact amount and characteristics of all vomitus and aspirated material, the total fluid intake and output for each 12 or 24 hours, the time pain occurs in relation to food intake and the patient's weight and general condition. The upper abdomen should be examined for distention.

Obstruction due to contraction of fibrous

scar tissue is treated by surgery. A gastric resection or gastroenterostomy may be performed.

Cancer of the Stomach

Although cancer of the stomach still accounts for a large number of deaths each year, there has been a significant decline over the last 2 decades. The National Cancer Institute of Canada reports that from 1945 to 1963 the death rate from gastric cancer in males dropped 32.9 per cent and in females it dropped 43.8 per cent.[8] In the United States, deaths due to cancer of the stomach declined from 28.9 per 100,000 deaths in 1930 to 13 per 100,000 deaths in 1955.[9] The incidence is higher in males and in those persons 60 years of age and over.

As is the case with all cancers, the cause is unknown but certain factors are considered predisposing. Familial or hereditary tendency is thought to play a role. There is a higher incidence in persons belonging to blood group A and in persons with atrophy of the gastric mucosa, achlorhydria and chronic gastric ulceration.

Any region of the stomach may be involved, but the most frequent sites are the pylorus and antrum.

Symptoms. The manifestations are vague and insidious. At first, the patient may complain of some mild discomfort after he eats; but as the disease advances, belching, regurgitation, nausea and vomiting may be experienced, and there is a progressive loss of appetite, weight and strength. Blood may appear in the vomitus and stool when there is ulceration at the cancer site. Pain is usually a late symptom. Unfortunately, because the early symptoms are mild and vague, the person tends to delay seeing a physician, and the disease becomes well advanced before there is medical intervention. Nurses should be aware of this problem, and on learning that a patient is experiencing even mild "digestive" disturbances, should urge him to seek medical advice.

[8]The National Cancer Institute of Canada: Cancer Mortality Trends in Canada and the Provinces — 1944–1963. Toronto, The National Cancer Institute of Canada, 1965, pp. 5 and 10.

[9]Henry L. Bockus: Gastroenterology (Vol. I), 2nd ed. Philadelphia, W. B. Saunders Co., 1963, p. 745.

Investigation of the patient includes x-ray examinations, analysis of gastric content for acidity, cytologic studies of gastric fluid, gastroscopy and biopsy, examination of the stool for blood, hemoglobin estimation and blood cell counts. The gastric analysis is done to determine if there is a decrease in the secretion of hydrochloric acid, as the majority of patients with cancer of the stomach demonstrate a hypochlorhydria or an achlorhydria. The blood examinations will probably show some deficiency of hemoglobin and red blood cells as anemia is a characteristic of gastric cancer due to the chronic bleeding, reduced production of the intrinsic factor by the gastric mucosa, reduced absorption of iron because of the hypochlorhydria and to nutritional deficits.

Metastases. Gastric carcinoma develops and metastasizes rapidly; all too often there has been a spread to some other structure(s) by the time of diagnosis. There may be direct extension to neighboring organs (e.g., esophagus, duodenum) or an indirect spread via the lymph and venous blood. The spleen, abdominal lymph nodes, peritoneum, liver, pancreas and lungs are frequent sites of metastases. The left supraclavicular and axillary nodes may also be affected.

Treatment and Nursing Care. At present, surgery is considered to be the only therapeutic approach to gastric cancer. The surgical procedure used will depend on the site of the cancer and its extension or possible course of extension. A subtotal gastrectomy or total gastrectomy is performed and may include resection of the duodenum, excision of the areas of lymphatic spread (omentum, spleen), resection of the pancreas or resection of the lower esophagus. In subtotal gastrectomy the stomach is anastomosed to the jejunum (gastrojejunostomy) if it has been the lower part of the stomach that has been removed. In the case of removal of the proximal portion of the stomach the operation is completed by anastomosis of the esophagus to the remaining stomach (esophago-antrostomy). Total gastrectomy and a resection of the esophagus necessitate entrance into the thoracic cavity. Continuity of the alimentary tract is restored by an esophagojejunostomy.

The preoperative and postoperative nursing care of the gastric surgical patient is presented on the next page. Care of the patient following a complete gastrectomy will include the care necessary for any patient who has had chest surgery (p. 307). The patient who has had his stomach removed will require small frequent meals of easily digested bland foods and vitamin B_{12} injections throughout the remainder of his life.

NURSING THE PATIENT WHO HAS GASTRIC SURGERY

Preoperative Nursing Care

The patient is admitted to the hospital several days prior to surgery. A general assessment is made of his condition by the surgeon and anesthetist, and treatment is instituted according to their findings.

Psychological Preparation. Most patients who are to have elective gastric surgery have considerable anxiety and apprehension, particularly if the anticipated procedure is a gastrectomy. In addition to the fears and problems that any surgery may create for the patient and his family (see Chapter 10), this patient is probably concerned about how he can survive without a portion of his stomach, or he may fear malignancy. The surgeon, while recommending and explaining the operation, may mention the possible sequelae or changes in gastrointestinal function that a few patients may experience postoperatively.

The understanding nurse encourages the patient to express his feelings and ask questions. An explanation may be necessary to reassure him that the continuity of his gastrointestinal tract will be re-established, that he will be able to take food in the normal way, and that only a few dietary modifications may be necessary because of the diminished gastric capacity.

The postoperative care is discussed briefly so that the patient may have some idea as to what to expect and will not be alarmed by the frequent checking of his pulse and blood pressure, gastric suctioning, and intravenous and oxygen administration.

Physical Preparation. The patient's diet and fluid intake may have been inadequate for some time because of his disease. Nutritional, electrolyte and fluid deficits are determined, and efforts are made to correct them. When his condition permits, solid food, total calories and the protein and vitamin content are increased and given in frequent small feedings. Foods that are normally contraindicated for patients with peptic ulcer are avoided (fried foods, roughage, spices, etc.). Fluids are provided between meals, and if well diluted citrus fruit juices are tolerated, they are encouraged, since they provide vitamin C, potassium and calories. If solid food cannot be managed, semifluids, blender feeding or liquids containing commercial protein preparations may be ordered. The patient may not be able to take sufficient quantities by mouth and may receive various intravenous solutions (glucose, electrolytes, amino acids) to improve his fluid and nutritional status. Parenteral preparations of vitamins B complex, C and K may also be given.

Blood studies are done to determine the needs of the patient. The findings govern the medicinal preparations ordered, and if anemia is present, a blood transfusion is given.

An accurate record is made of the fluid intake and output, and the patient is weighed daily. The weight is significant in determining the patient's nutritional status and progress as well as establishing a comparative basis for the postoperative period.

Postoperatively, the patient who has had gastric surgery tends to take very shallow breaths. The normal excursion of the diaphragm and chest walls may cause pain in the operative area, which is in the upper part of the abdomen, so the patient restricts respiratory movements. Shallow respirations decrease the respiratory exchange of oxygen and carbon dioxide and promote the accumulation of respiratory secretions in the alveoli and bronchioles; this may lead to serious pulmonary complications. The importance of the deep breathing, coughing, exercises and the early ambulation that will be a part of his postoperative care is discussed with the patient. Demonstrations of these activities by the nurse and practice by the patient should accompany the explanation to make it easier for him after the operation and to ensure greater cooperation on his part. The patient is asked to stop smoking and is given the reasons.

Any indication of a respiratory disturbance or infection, such as a nasal discharge, expectoration of sputum, cough, shortness of breath and temperature elevation, should be brought to the physician's attention.

If the patient has been receiving oral feedings, these may be reduced to clear fluids the day before operation and nothing is given in the immediate 8 to 12 hours preceding operation. A nasogastric tube is inserted the night before operation, and suction is used to empty the stomach of secretions and any food residue. The tube is left in place when the patient goes to the operating room.

In addition to the foregoing considerations, preparation of the patient will include the general preoperative care cited in Chapter 10.

Postoperative Nursing Care

Special Equipment. Preparation to receive the patient from the operating room includes the assembling of equipment for gastric suctioning, intravenous infusion, mouth care and oxygen administration. The oxygen tent may be used, since the mask and catheter administration are not satisfactory because of the nasogastric tube.

Observations. When the patient returns, the nasogastric or gastrostomy tube is connected to the suction as ordered, and the intravenous infusion checked to make sure the movement has not displaced the needle.

Close observation is made of the patient for the first 24 to 48 hours for early signs of shock, hemorrhage and interference with the gastric drainage system. Blood pressure, pulse, respirations, color, the temperature and moisture of the skin, the gastric drainage, wound site and the patient's response are checked frequently.

An accurate record is made of the fluid intake and output. The latter will include any emesis and gastric drainage as well as the urinary output.

Oxygen Administration. Oxygen may be ordered but is not usually necessary for a prolonged period if the patient makes an uncomplicated progress.

Gastric Drainage (see p. 338). Gentle gastric suctioning and nothing by mouth are continued for the first few days to prevent the escape of gastric secretions and fluid through the stomach suture line into the peritoneal cavity and to minimize vomiting and distention. The number of days the nasogastric tube is left in and oral fluids withheld varies with each surgeon and will also depend on the patient's progress. The characteristics and exact volume of the drainage are noted. It will most likely be colored by blood at first but usually clears in a few hours. The doctor is notified if large amounts of blood appear or if the drainage continues to be blood-colored. The tube may become obstructed by mucus or a small blood clot. An order may be received to clear it with a syringe and a small amount of normal saline or water (25 to 30 cc.).

The surgeon's order may be for continuous suction, or the nasogastric tube may be attached to a pump which automatically applies intermittent suctioning. After 24 to 36 hours, the tube may be connected to the suctioning apparatus only for stated periods at intervals; the volume which is aspirated is noted each time.

Positioning. When the patient regains consciousness and his blood pressure and pulse are stabilized, the head of the bed may be gradually elevated to promote gastric drainage and deeper breathing. The patient is turned hourly from side, to side, to back to side.

Deep Breathing and Coughing. The patient is reminded hourly to take 5 to 10 deep breaths and to cough several times to prevent pulmonary complications. Necessary encouragement and support are provided by the nurse who places one hand lightly over the operative site and the other on the patient's back during the coughing. She acknowledges the patient's distress but at the same time emphasizes the importance of deep breathing and coughing in the prevention of other problems.

Exercises and Early Ambulation. Simple limb exercises to prevent venous stasis are started the morning after operation if the doctor approves. If the patient is too weak or too ill for active participation, the limbs are put through a range of passive movements by the nurse. The surgeon usually suggests that the patient be assisted to a sitting position on the side of the bed the day after operation and then to sit in a chair on the second day. Self-care activities should be gradually encouraged.

In addition to preventing pulmonary and vascular complications, early ambulation and patient activity help to re-establish normal gastrointestinal motility.

Nutrition and Fluids. Parenteral fluids are

used to sustain the patient over the first few days. Different procedures are used to introduce the first fluids; the surgeon may have the nasogastric tube removed and small stated amounts of water given every half hour or every hour. The amount is gradually increased if tolerated. The directive may be to introduce a specific amount of water at intervals through the nasogastric tube which is then clamped.

If the patient tolerates the increased amounts of water without experiencing vomiting, pain or distention, feeding of clear sweetened tea, equal parts of milk and water, whole milk, creamed soups, gruel and blender feedings are progressively added over 2 to 3 days but only on specific orders from the surgeon.

With normal progress, the patient is usually receiving a soft bland diet by the fifth to seventh day. The volume given at any one time should remain small because of the reduced capacity of the stomach. Foods high in calories are selected and served in frequent, small amounts. The patient's weight is recorded regularly, and the physician is advised if there is a loss or a failure to gain. Inability of the patient to take the prescribed diet and any regurgitation, vomiting, distention or complaint of pain should be reported.

By the time the patient is ready to leave the hospital he will most likely be taking a light bland diet of high-calorie foods divided into 6 meals. Fluids may be omitted from the meals and taken in-between so their volume will not curtail the patient taking sufficient solid food. The patient is advised that he may gradually increase the amount taken at regular meals, and if no discomfort is experienced, he may eventually need only 3 or 4 meals with milk and other fluids taken between them.

Mouth Care. Frequent cleansing and moistening of the mouth are necessary to lessen the patient's discomfort while the nasogastric tube is in place, and oral fluids are restricted. The tube may cause irritation that results in mucus secretion which, if allowed to collect, might be aspirated. The nostril through which the tube is passed should also receive attention.

Elimination. The urinary output should be recorded and totaled for each 24 hours. A small cleansing enema may be ordered on the third postoperative day to cleanse the lower bowel of blood that may be in the tract from the surgical procedure. The enema may be repeated every other day when oral intake is started. A mild laxative such as milk of magnesia may be prescribed after 4 or 5 days.

Medications. Considerable pain is experienced by the gastric surgery patient. An analgesic, such as morphine sulfate, or meperidine hydrochloride (Demerol) by parenteral administration, is usually ordered to relieve the patient's discomfort but judicious use is necessary. Oversedation makes it difficult to promote deep breathing and coughing; on the other hand, the patient should not be allowed to suffer unnecessarily, since pain may contribute to shock.

A parenteral antibiotic may be prescribed by some surgeons as a prophylactic measure; others believe antibiotic therapy is reserved for some indication of infection.

Vitamins B complex and C and iron may be ordered since the natural food sources of these will be restricted in the diet for a period of time.

Instructions. Preparation of the patient for leaving the hospital should include discussions with him and a member of his family of the necessary dietary and activity modifications. The importance of frequent small meals of nonirritating foods high in calories should be explained. Suggestions are made as to food selection and preparation. Written dietary instructions and outlines may be necessary for some patients. The patient is advised to weigh himself regularly, to report to the clinic or to his doctor at the scheduled dates and to get in touch with the doctor promptly if he has pain, vomiting or other distressing symptoms.

Considerable rest will be necessary for some time and he should lie down for at least one-half hour after each meal. Normal activities are resumed very gradually and should not be allowed to interfere with regularity of his meals.

The patient and family should be informed of the assistance available to them from the visiting nurse agencies. Economic problems may be a concern because of the prolonged illness and convalescence, and the family may have difficulty in providing the diet and care suggested for the patient. A social worker may be asked to see them to arrange for the necessary assistance, or the nurse may refer the problem to an appropriate source.

Problems Following Gastric Surgery

A few patients experience some gastrointestinal dysfunction after gastric surgery mainly because of the anatomical changes made by the surgery.

Dumping Syndrome. Following a gastric resection or a gastroenterostomy, the patient may experience a complex of symptoms referred to as the dumping syndrome. The symptoms are related to gastrointestinal and vasomotor disturbances and are precipitated by eating. The syndrome may appear before the meal is completed or immediately after and lasts only a few minutes to a half hour. It may not occur with every meal but is more likely to develop following a large meal or one that contained a high content of sweets or salt.

The patient may experience epigastric fullness, nausea, crampy abdominal pains, distention, diarrhea, muscular weakness, dizziness, fainting, palpitation and sweating. He is pale and his pulse is rapid.

Normally, the gastric content is delivered in small amounts into the intestine by the pylorus. Following a gastric resection or a gastroenterostomy, this pyloric control of the volume moving from the stomach into the small intestine is absent. The dumping syndrome is caused by the precipitous passage into the jejunum of a relatively large amount of gastric content that has not undergone the usual dilution and digestive changes. The exact mechanism by which the characteristic responses are initiated is not entirely clear but the syndrome is usually explained by the following facts. First, the sudden distention of the proximal portion of the jejunum initiates sympathetic reflexes. Secondly, the fluid that moved quickly out of the stomach is hypertonic, having a high concentration of sugar and/or electrolytes, and requires dilution for digestion and absorption. This results in the movement of fluid from the intravascular spaces into the jejunum. The complex of symptoms is attributed to the distention of the jejunum, the decreased intravascular volume and the reflex responses of the sympathetic nervous system.

It is also suggested that a substance, serotonin, is released into the blood by the jejunum in response to the distention and hypertonic solution. The serotonin influences intestinal and vasomotor activity, resulting in the syndrome.[10, 11]

Medical treatment of the dumping syndrome is by dietary modifications and the administration of anticholinergic drugs. The symptoms gradually subside in most patients, and eventually a more normal dietary pattern may be resumed. Rarely, if the condition cannot be controlled by dietary and drug management and is incapacitating, surgical treatment is employed. An operation is performed to delay gastric emptying and may consist of narrowing the anastomotic opening from the stomach into the small intestine or conversion of the gastrojejunostomy (established at the time of the gastric resection) to a gastroduodenostomy.

The necessary dietary modifications include the avoidance of large meals and a reduced intake of salty and sweet foods. No fluids are given with meals. Six small, dry meals consisting mainly of proteins, fats and starches are planned to meet the patient's calorie requirement. Liquids are taken between meals to maintain normal hydration but should be limited during the half hour preceding and following a meal. The patient is advised to eat slowly and to lie down for a half hour following each meal.

The symptoms cause considerable emotional reaction in the patient. He should be encouraged to persevere with the suggested dietary regimen and should be reassured that as time goes on the condition will gradually subside as the gastrointestinal tract adapts to the structural changes. To avoid the distressing symptoms, the patient may tend to reduce his food intake to dangerously low amounts that result in weight loss and nutritional deficiencies.

In addition to the dietary treatment, anticholinergic drugs may be prescribed to decrease gastrointestinal motility (see p. 356).

---

[10]Donald Silver, et al.: "The Mechanism of the Dumping Syndrome." Surg. Clin. North Amer., Vol. 46, No. 2 (April 1966), pp. 427–428.

[11]Loyal Davis (Ed.): Christopher's Textbook of Surgery, 9th ed. Philadelphia, W. B. Saunders Co., 1968, p. 696.

Nutritional Deficiency. The patient who has had a gastric resection may have a problem in maintaining his normal weight. The cause is usually a lack of sufficient food intake because the diminished gastric capacity results in quick satiety and an overfull feeling, or it may be as cited above—due to the distressing dumping syndrome precipitated by eating. Frequent high-calorie feedings that are acceptable to the patient are planned. Small amounts are given at first and are gradually increased with the patient's tolerance. Part of the problem may be the patient's psychological reaction to the need for continuing dietary modifications; he may have expected no problems or restrictions once he had surgical treatment. The need for a period of time for necessary adjustments by his digestive system should be discussed with the patient to obtain his cooperation.

Anemia. Iron deficiency may occur as a result of a decreased iron absorption. Normal absorption is facilitated by gastric acidity which has been reduced in the gastrectomy patient. The bypassing of the duodenum by a gastrojejunostomy may also reduce the amount of iron absorption in many of these patients. The deficiency may be due to a poor dietary intake of foods that provide iron (red meat, liver, leafy vegetables, whole milk, eggs and certain cereals). The diet may be corrected to contain the necessary sources and supplemented by an iron drug preparation, such as ferrous sulfate tablets.

Anemia may be present as a result of a deficiency in the secretion of the intrinsic factor (due to the loss of gastric mucosa by the gastric resection) which promotes the absorption of vitamin B_{12}. It may develop within a few months after the gastrectomy but is not common until 2 to 3 years have elapsed. The patient is given daily vitamin B_{12} by subcutaneous or intramuscular injections until a normal erythrocyte count is established. Then a maintenance dose is given monthly throughout the remainder of the patient's life.

Hypoglycemia. A few patients who have had a gastrectomy may exhibit the manifestations characteristic of hypoglycemia 2 to 3 hours after taking a meal. The condition is referred to as late postprandial or postcibal hypoglycemia. The patient's symptoms are weakness, tremulousness, faintness, sweating and palpitation due to a fall in the blood sugar level to 50 to 60 mg. per cent. It is explained on the basis of the rapid emptying of the stomach and the rapid absorption of glucose from the intestine, causing a sudden hyperglycemia. The latter stimulates an excessive output of insulin which rapidly lowers the blood sugar concentration to an abnormally low level.

The condition is controlled by the patient taking a high-protein diet, decreasing the carbohydrate intake, and by shortening the interval between meals. Some form of sugar (candy, honey, lump sugar or orange juice) should be quickly available to the patient as soon as the early symptoms of hypoglycemia are experienced.

DISORDERS OF THE INTESTINES

Disorders of the small intestine may cause disturbances in digestion, absorption and the movement of content along the gastrointestinal tract. A prolonged or serious dysfunction threatens the patient's nutritional status.

A disturbance in function of the large intestine interferes with the excretion of bowel waste, and if the right half of the colon is involved, the normal absorption of water and salts may be reduced and may cause dehydration.

Constipation and Diarrhea

Intestinal dysfunction may be manifested by a retarded or accelerated movement of contents through the intestine. Delayed movement causes constipation, which is characterized by infrequent, hard dry stools, or may result in a complete failure of the excretion of feces. The prolonged retention of the feces results in the absorption of increased amounts of water which accounts for the abnormal consistency of the stools. The symptom of dysfunction may be diarrhea, which is frequent liquid or unformed stools.

Constipation. The majority of persons normally defecate once every 24 hours, but there is considerable variance in the frequency among healthy persons. Some persons have more than one bowel movement daily, others may have an evacuation of a normally moist stool only once every 2 or 3 days. Such variances in frequency of bowel elimination may be compatible with health.

Constipation may be a delay in the passage of feces through the colon, which is referred to as colonic constipation, or it may be a prolonged retention of the feces in the rectum and is designated as rectal constipation or dyschezia.

CAUSES OF CONSTIPATION. The causes of constipation are many and varied. It may be associated with organic disease, or it may be a functional disturbance.

Disease within the colon or rectum may narrow the lumen of the bowel and offer resistance to the forward movement of content. Common examples are carcinoma of the intestine; inflammation which causes spasm, scarring and adhesions; and partial volvulus (twisting of the bowel). Severe ascites (accumulation of fluid in the peritoneal cavity) or a tumor, such as an ovarian cyst or uterine fibroid, may compress the colon and delay the movement of intestinal content.

Failure of the normal propulsive movement may occur due to some disturbance or imbalance in the innervation of the intestine. The derangement may result in an excessive tone and spasm in a segment of the bowel that retards the movement of the content. The spasm may be induced by a hypersensitivity of the colon or by anxiety. Constipation may be associated with injury or degeneration of the spinal cord or cauda equina, which affects the nerve supply to the colon and rectum.

Megacolon (large colon) may account for constipation in infants. It is a congenital anomaly in which there is an absence of certain nerve structures (parasympathetic ganglia) in a segment of the colon, resulting in failure of peristalsis in the affected portion of the bowel. The most frequent site is the sigmoid, and it is seen more often in males. The affected segment is constricted and does not participate in normal peristaltic activity. Fecal content accumulates in the adjacent preceding colon and dilation occurs. The condition is also known as Hirschsprung's disease. Surgical resection of the colon may be considered necessary and is done in two stages: a colostomy is done first, and then resection of the affected area.

Constipation may be associated with any illness in which there is a diminished intake of food and fluid or in cases in which the diet is modified and results in less residue. The lesser amount of food does not provide sufficient bulk to stimulate peristalsis. Dehydration causes a small, dry, hard stool that may irritate the colon, causing spasm, or may fail to stimulate the normal colon motility.

Occasionally, drugs used in treatment may depress peristalsis and cause a delay in the excretion of feces. Common examples of such drugs are opiates (e.g., codeine) and anticholinergic drugs (e.g., Pro-Banthine).

Expulsion of the feces is aided by increasing the intra-abdominal pressure to compress the colon and rectum. This involves contraction of the muscles of the abdominal wall and of the diaphragm. Weakness of these muscles due to disease, senility, malnutrition or inactivity may contribute to constipation. Similarly, lack of tone in the intestinal musculature or weakness of the levator ani muscles may impair peristalsis and the expulsive power.

Frequent causes of constipation in persons who are not ill are faulty defecation habits, faulty diet and the habitual use of laxatives. If the urge to defecate is ignored and evacuation delayed, the reflex becomes weak as the rectal mucosa adapts to the pressure of the content. Repeated failure to respond to the defecation reflex may eventually result in the rectum becoming insensitive to the presence of a fecal mass and the reflex is not initiated. The person may delay response to the defecation urge because he does not find it convenient to interrupt what he is doing or because toilet facilities may not be available.

A deficiency of foods with cellulose and fibrous content in the diet may be the cause of constipation. Refined foods and those that leave little residue after absorption fail to produce sufficient bulk to stimulate colonic motility.

Many persons have an inordinate concern about bowel elimination and think they must have a daily bowel movement or a frequent purge and resort to the unnecessary repeated use of a laxative. Loss of intestinal tone and reduced peristaltic response to normal food residue follow the use of a laxative, and too often the laxative is then repeated. The colon is not allowed to regain its natural rhythmic response to the normal fecal mass.

Constipation may cause considerable discomfort; the person may experience abdominal pain, a full feeling and abdominal distention. There is a loss of appetite accompanied by headache and probably nausea and vomiting. The hard dry masses of fecal matter may damage the intestinal mucosa and lead to a fissure. Hemorrhoids are frequently the result of chronic constipation.

MANAGEMENT OF CONSTIPATION. The person who experiences a change in his normal pattern of bowel elimination that persists beyond a few days or that recurs at frequent intervals is urged to consult a physician. The underlying cause of the constipation is then identified, and treatment may be initiated.

Dietary modifications may be necessary; each meal should include 1 or 2 foods that will provide a liberal amount of fiber (roughage). Emphasis is placed on whole grain cereals and bread, fresh fruits and vegetables, and fruit juices. A minimum of 8 glasses or approximately 2 liters of liquid should be taken each day.

If the constipation is due to spastic response of an irritable or hypersensitive colon, a bland diet with a minimum of roughage is recommended. Raw fruits and vegetables and those high in fiber content are avoided as well as whole grain cereals and tough meat fiber. Spiced and fried foods and iced food and fluids should be restricted. For more details as to the diet for constipation, the reader is referred to a diet therapy text.

It may be helpful to explain to the person in simple terms the physiological mechanism of defecation so he may grasp the significance of responding to the initial urge for defecation. The importance of establishing a regular time for bowel elimination preferably after breakfast, should be stressed. This may necessitate an increase in the amount of breakfast taken to provide sufficient food to stimulate the necessary wave of intestinal peristalsis.

Flexion of the thighs on the abdomen helps to promote bowel evacuation. A footstool placed in front of the toilet raises and supports the feet and assists in assuming the suggested flexion position.

Exercises may be suggested by the physi-cian to increase the strength of the abdominal muscles. Examples of the exercises prescribed are as follows: The patient lies on his back on the floor or bed with his arms folded across his chest and raises himself to the sitting position, keeping his heels on the floor. From the supine position, the patient raises his lower limbs without bending his knees. These exercises are done 2 or 3 times daily, and the patient is also encouraged to contract his abdominal muscles several times at frequent intervals through the day.

Laxatives, enemas and suppositories that the patient may be accustomed to using are discontinued. If the diet and exercises are not sufficient at the beginning to establish normal bowel elimination, special medication may be necessary until the defecation reflex is restored and bowel irritability and spasm are reduced. The physician may suggest the use of a preparation that swells when it combines with fluid in the gastrointestinal tract and provides a stimulating bulk. Examples of the bulking laxatives are agar and psyllium mucilloid (Metamucil).

A stool softener may be ordered to prevent severe straining at stool and injury to the rectal and anal tissues. The stool softeners in use are preparations of dioctyl sodium sulfosuccinate (Colace, Doxinate). These preparations act as wetting agents, allowing water to penetrate and mix with the fecal mass.

Some persons who have been addicted to the use of laxatives may require the use of a stronger laxative at first. The dosage should be gradually decreased and the drug withdrawn completely as soon as possible.

FECAL IMPACTION. Occasionally, feces accumulate in the rectum, producing a hard dry mass that forms a partial or complete obstruction. It occurs most often in older persons and in those with central nervous system disorders. Crampy pain is experienced in the lower abdomen and liquid stools may be passed without expelling the impacted mass.

A retention enema of warm oil or a solution of dioctyl sodium sulfosuccinate (strength of solution to be ordered by the physician) may be given. This is followed in a few hours by digital breaking up and removal of the mass. A cleansing enema of saline or tap water is then given; the patient is made comfortable and is allowed to rest.

Diarrhea. This term implies an accelerated movement of content through the intestine, resulting in frequent liquid or unformed stools. The feces pass through the colon before the normal amount of water is absorbed. Diarrhea is a symptom of many different disorders which may be within the bowel or may be extrinsic to the intestine. Changes characteristic of organic disease may occur in the intestine and result in diarrhea, or the bowel may be structurally normal with the hypermotility being functional. The more common causes of diarrhea are presented here as intrinsic or extrinsic, although one finds many different etiological classifications in medical literature.

INTRINSIC CAUSES OF DIARRHEA. Normally the stimulus for peristalsis arises within the intestine. It may cause direct stimulation of the muscle tissue, or it may initiate sensory nerve impulses that are transmitted into the central nervous system, resulting in parasympathetic nerve impulses being carried out to the intestine that then stimulate its motility. Disease or irritations within the bowel which may increase either direct stimulation or reflex hypermotility include the following:

Infection. Food or fluid contaminated by salmonella, shigella or staphylococcal organisms is the most common cause of intestinal infection and may be referred to as bacterial food poisoning.

The shigella bacilli cause bacillary dysentery, and the primary source is usually the excreta of an infected person. This disease is rare, except under crowded and poor sanitary conditions.

The salmonella bacilli may inhabit the intestine of both man and animals and may be the source of infection to others. It may be transmitted by the meat of infected animals and by food or water contaminated by the excreta of infected humans or animals. Sporadic outbreaks occur and may be due to a human carrier employed in the handling of food. Ingested salmonella or shigella organisms multiply, causing irritation and inflammation of the intestine, resulting in diarrhea accompanied by crampy abdominal pain, fever, nausea and vomiting.

If the infection is by staphylococci, the irritation and inflammation of the intestine are due to the toxin produced by the organisms. Food may become contaminated by a handler who has an infected lesion on his body or who is carrying the organisms in his nose or throat. Meat, custard and cream-filled desserts allowed to remain at ordinary room temperature are common offenders and may contain considerable toxin when ingested. As a result, the manifestations of food poisoning—nausea, vomiting, fever, and diarrhea—occur within a few hours of ingestion of the contaminated food. The patient becomes very ill and quickly prostrated.

Neoplasms. Diarrhea may be a symptom of a malignant newgrowth of the colon and may be alternated with periods of constipation.

Dietary Factors. An excessive amount of coarse foods or highly seasoned irritating foods may produce hypermotility of the bowel. Occasionally, allergy to a certain food may account for diarrhea; if the intestinal mucosa is sensitive to the food, it becomes hyperemic and edematous and causes increased reflex hypermotility.

Malabsorption. Impaired absorption of foods may be due to incomplete digestion or to a defect in the absorptive process of the small intestine. Obviously, with reduced digestion and absorption, an increase in the bulk of the colon content results which is a stimulus to intestinal motility. The stools are bulky, have an offensive odor and usually contain large amounts of fats which are irritating to the bowel mucosa and initiate reflex peristalsis. General malnutrition is also evident.

Diverticulitis. A pouch or sac may occur in the wall of the intestine and is known as a diverticulum. It may be congenital or may develop as a result of a weakening of an area of the muscle tissue in the wall. There may be several diverticula, or the defect may occur singly.

Diverticula of the large intestine are more likely to give rise to trouble, as the more solid fecal content tends to collect and be retained in the sac, setting up an inflammation that causes increased reflex peristalsis and diarrhea.

Laxatives. Many laxatives act by direct irritation of the intestinal mucosa, resulting in the content being hurried through the colon before the normal amount of water is absorbed.

Antibiotics. Diarrhea sometimes accompanies the oral administration of antibiotics. They may irritate the mucosa or alter the normal bacterial flora of the intestinal tract. The most frequent offenders are the tetracycline preparations (Aureomycin, Terramycin, Achromycin) and polymixin.

Idiopathic Inflammation. Patients with ulcerative colitis or regional enteritis experience severe diarrhea. No specific cause has been recognized for either condition (see p. 382).

EXTRINSIC CAUSES OF DIARRHEA. Diarrhea accompanies a variety of disorders in which the stimulus that results in increased parasympathetic innervation to the bowel originates outside the intestine.

Emotional Stress. Anxiety or underlying tension is frequently the basis of diarrhea. On investigation, disturbances may be revealed that are secondary to the diarrhea, but there is no organic disease in the intestine or elsewhere. The intestinal hypermotility is entirely functional and is considered psychogenic. The patient is usually sensitive and has a nervous temperament; a study of the patient's total life situation may reveal a specific emotional conflict that will probably account for his diarrhea.

General or Systemic Disorders. Frequently, diarrhea is associated with general diseases, particularly if they cause toxemia. Examples of such conditions are acute infectious disease, hyperthyroidism and uremia.

EFFECTS OF DIARRHEA. Depending on the cause, diarrhea may be self-limiting by ridding the intestine of the irritating causative factor, it may be persistent or there may be remissions and exacerbations. Severe diarrhea may produce serious changes in the body which in some instances may become irreversible and fatal. Infants, young children, and seriously ill and elderly persons stand diarrhea less well, and serious effects may develop rapidly; prompt action is necessary at the onset with these persons.

Body fluids, electrolytes and nutrients are lost in the frequent liquid stools; the patient becomes dehydrated, develops nutritional deficiencies and loses weight and strength. Acidosis may develop because of the depleted sodium and bicarbonate ions. Severe crampy abdominal pain and tenesmus (painful spasm of the anus) frequently accompany the diarrhea. The patient may become emotionally disturbed because he is embarrassed by the frequency and urgency of the diarrheal stools and perhaps is fearful of the cause.

NURSING THE PATIENT WITH DIARRHEA. Any person who experiences diarrhea for more than a day or two or who has recurring attacks is urged to seek medical advice. The symptom should not be ignored, since it may be an early manifestation of a serious condition.

Investigation by the physician to determine the cause of the diarrhea may require several days during which symptomatic and supportive treatment are necessary. Diagnostic procedures may include a sigmoidoscopy, stool cultures, x-rays of the bowel and blood chemistry studies to determine potassium, sodium, chloride and bicarbonate concentrations (see p. 56).

Bed rest, with the patient remaining flat, is recommended for acute diarrhea; this may help to reduce peristalsis and decreases the energy demands. The weak patient should be given the necessary assistance on and off the bedpan. Some patients are unable to relax and rest because of a constant fear of not receiving the bedpan in time; in such instances it may be helpful to make an exception and leave a clean covered bedpan at the bedside within the patient's reach.

Fluids and electrolytes are replaced by intravenous infusions. If oral fluids are tolerated, water, sweetened clear tea, fat-free broth and gruel may be given. Skim milk and strained fruit juices may also be allowed by some doctors. Carbonated drinks, whole milk and iced fluids are usually avoided.

The diet is expanded as soon as possible to reduce the possibility of nutritional deficiencies. A high-calorie, high-vitamin and high-protein bland diet is gradually introduced, and the patient is observed as to the intestinal response. Rough and gas-producing foods are eliminated; whole grain bread and cereals, raw fruits and vegetables and highly seasoned and fried foods are not used. Cooked vegetables and fruits may have to be puréed to remove the fiber content. Concentrated sweets and fats are likely to be poorly tolerated. If the diarrhea is due to malabsorption, a gluten-free diet may be ordered in which foods are avoided that contain any wheat, rye, and barley grains or flour.

The first few mouthfuls of a meal may initiate a mass peristaltic wave, and the meal is interrupted. The patient's tray should be removed from the room and the hot foods kept warm. Following the necessary post-defecation care, the tray is returned. The patient may require some persuasion to complete his meal, as he is discouraged and is afraid that if he eats it will just precipitate another stool.

Placement of the patient on the ward should receive consideration; if ambulatory, he should be near toilet facilities; if confined to bed, privacy should be provided so the patient is less embarrassed by his frequent use of the bedpan. The anal region should be left clean after each defecation, and if the skin around the anus is irritated, it should be washed and a protective cream applied. Soiled bedding or clothing should be changed promptly.

Cases of acute diarrhea should be considered potentially infectious until it is indicated otherwise. Precautions should be used to prevent the possible spread of infection to others. A gown is worn by all personnel when giving care, and the hands are scrubbed with soap and running water after each contact. The patient's linen should be disinfected before laundering. Treatment equipment and the bedpan should be disinfected after each use. It may be considered necessary to disinfect the feces before the usual disposal by covering the stool with a 10 per cent formalin or 5 per cent cresol (Lysol) solution for 60 minutes. Visitors should be restricted to members of the family who may be asked to wear a gown and to avoid any contact with the patient and his bed.

Something to occupy the patient and divert his attention may prove beneficial. If the diarrhea is a reaction to stress, efforts are directed toward identifying the source of the emotional disturbance. The patient is encouraged to express his feelings and is reassured that there is no serious disease. New interests and activity in hobbies or sports may be suggested. Sedatives or tranquilizers may be ordered to relieve the emotional tension.

Various drugs may be used in the treatment of diarrhea. Drugs to reduce intestinal spasm and peristalsis may be ordered. Examples are camphorated tincture of opium (paregoric), diphenoxylate hydrochloride (Lomotil) and tincture of belladonna. Drugs to provide a protective coating on intestinal mucosa or to provide an adsorbent which condenses and holds irritating substances are used. Examples are aluminum silicate (Kaolin, Kaopectate), aluminum hydroxide gel (Amphojel) and bismuth subcarbonate. An anti-infective drug may be ordered if the diarrhea is of microbial origin. Sulfonamide preparations that are poorly absorbed but have a local effect are frequently used orally. Examples are succinylsulfathiazole (Sulfasuxidine) and phthalylsulfacetamide (Thalamyd).

Acute infectious diarrhea may readily spread through a family, a school or a neighborhood because of a common source of infected food or water or by the spread from an infected person. The nurse may play an important role in the prevention of diarrhea by alerting people to the hazards of exposed and unrefrigerated foods, particularly meat and those with cream filling or topping. Opportunities may arise to emphasize the hygienic handling of food and the importance of thorough hand washing after going to the toilet and the handling of soiled clothing.

The family in which a member develops acute diarrhea should be advised of the necessary precautions in caring for him to prevent the spread to others. If several members of a family become ill at one time, questions should be raised as to recently ingested food and its source.

If a large number of cases are found in a school or community, the local health authorities should be notified so that a systematic investigation as to the possible source may be instituted. Occasionally, acute diarrhea may spread through the patients on one ward of a hospital. The primary source of such an outbreak should be sought. Ward personnel are urged to practice rigid medical asepsis, for infection may be carried from one patient to another or from a ward worker to patients through failure to thoroughly wash the hands between patients, after handling bedpans or linen, or after going to the toilet.

Intestinal Obstruction

Obstruction to the passage of intestinal content may occur in the small or large bowel.

Causes. The cause of the obstruction may be within the wall or lumen of the intestine itself, or it may be extrinsic; it may be classified as mechanical, neurogenic or vascular and may be acquired or congenital.

Causes of mechanical obstruction include inflammation, edema and scarring of the intestinal wall; tumors of the bowel or of a neighboring structure; adhesions, which are bands of fibrous scar tissue, formed by the peritoneal tissue following inflammation and which may cause kinking and constriction of the intestine; occlusion by a mass, such as a hard, dry fecal accumulation, a large bolus of unchewed and undigested food, a gallstone or a foreign body; and intra-abdominal abscess.

Strangulated hernia, in which a loop of the intestine escapes from the peritoneal cavity through the defect in the abdominal wall, results in constriction of the lumen of the bowel and compression of the blood vessels, causing a blockage. The blockage may lead to gangrene of the protruding segment of the intestine. Obstruction may result from intussusception, a condition in which a segment of the intestine is invaginated into the segment immediately below. This telescoping results in the attached mesentery being compressed between the layers of intestine in the intussusception and interference with the blood supply to the bowel. Intussusception occurs mainly in infants and young children. Volvulus, which is a twisting of a loop of bowel on itself, interrupts the passage of intestinal contents and the blood supply to the involved segment. Older persons are more often affected, and the twisted section of bowel is usually the sigmoid colon. Congenital malformations may be responsible for intestinal obstruction in the newborn. The anomaly may be a stenosis or atresia in an area of the small or large intestine, or it may be an imperforate anus. The infant fails to pass meconium.

In neurogenic obstruction, peristalsis is inhibited by a disturbance in the normal nerve supply to the intestine. Often this is an imbalance in the autonomic innervation which inhibits peristalsis. It may develop with peritonitis, pancreatitis, severe toxemia as in pneumonia and uremia, spinal cord lesions, or occasionally after extensive abdominal surgery. An electrolyte imbalance in which the blood potassium is below normal also predisposes to intestinal immobility. The inhibition of peristalsis due to disturbed innervation causes the condition known as paralytic or adynamic ileus.

Obstruction of vascular origin is due to interference with the blood supply to a segment of the intestine and may be secondary to mechanical obstruction, or it may be primary and itself cause failure of bowel activity. Thrombosis and occlusion of a mesenteric artery may occur, blocking the blood source to a large portion of the bowel and arresting peristalsis. When the interruption in the blood supply is secondary, the obstruction is referred to as being strangulated.

Symptoms and Effects. The symptoms and effects of obstruction depend on whether it is in the small or large bowel and whether or not the blood supply to the intestine is maintained.

The first symptom of mechanical obstruction is colicky abdominal pain due to the bowel spasms. In paralytic ileus, the pain is steady and is due mainly to the distention. No fecal matter or gas is passed after that which was below the obstruction is evacuated.

In small bowel obstruction, vomiting begins earlier, is frequent, and the vomitus at first consists of stomach content, then of fluid containing bile. Eventually it becomes dark brown and fecal in character as the intestine becomes distended with excessive fluids and gas which overflow into the stomach.

The abdomen becomes distended because of the accumulation of gas and fluids in the bowel. Intestinal secretions are increased and the loss of fluid and electrolytes in the emesis leads to severe dehydration and electrolyte imbalance. Extravasation of plasma from the capillaries adds to the accumulation of fluid in the intestine as the veins are compressed by distention. This depletes the circulating blood volume and causes shock.

The patient's general condition may deteriorate rapidly. Unless the bowel is decompressed and fluid and electrolytes are replaced, a serious state of shock develops, manifested by restlessness, anxiety, a rapid weak pulse, low blood pressure, subnormal temperature, grayish pallor and cold clammy skin.

The colicky pain changes to a continuous

one as peristalsis diminishes, and the intestine loses its tone because of the marked distention and strangulation. Bowel sounds are absent. The vomiting changes character; it is no longer preceded by nausea and retching—the vomitus comes up without effort.

Peritonitis may develop as the weakened intestinal wall becomes permeable to organisms. Generalized abdominal tenderness and rigidity become evident.

Large intestinal obstruction is less acute, and the symptoms develop over a longer period of time. Complete constipation and crampy abdominal pain are the patient's first complaints. Distention of the bowel develops more slowly since it absorbs fluid, but eventually the distention may be very marked since the segment of the bowel is closed off by the obstruction at one end and the ileocecal valve at the other. The ileocecal valve will permit the entrance of content from the ileum but not until the later stage does the content of the colon and cecum back up into the ileum. Vomiting and the attendant dehydration and electrolyte imbalance occur in this later stage.

Diagnostic investigation in intestinal obstruction may include an x-ray examination of the abdomen in which gas and fluid levels may be apparent without a contrast medium. Blood studies are made to determine the leukocyte and differential counts, since a leukocytosis may develop with certain causes of obstruction. Hemoglobin and hematocrit estimations are made since they rise as dehydration and hemoconcentration develop. Electrolyte deficiencies may also be determined.

Bowel content eliminated from below the obstruction may be examined for blood which may be present if the obstruction is due to intussusception or to cancer of the large intestine.

Intestinal obstruction other than that due to paralytic ileus is treated surgically. In simple mechanical obstruction without strangulation, the operation may be delayed for a period in which medical treatment is used to improve the patient's condition. This treatment usually includes intestinal intubation and suctioning to remove the accumulation of gas and fluid and to relieve the vomiting, pain and distention (see p.

338). Fluid and electrolytes are given intravenously to replace the losses; as much as 5 to 6 L. of fluid may be ordered daily as long as there is intestinal suctioning. An accurate record of all fluid output and intake is necessary. The physician bases the electrolyte replacement as well as the amount of intravenous fluid on the volume of intestinal fluid lost in vomiting and aspiration. Glucose is included in the intravenous solution to provide calories. A blood transfusion may be used to increase the circulating blood volume and relieve shock.

If there is evidence of interference with the blood supply to the obstructed intestine, emergency surgery is undertaken.

The operation for intestinal obstruction involves relief of the obstruction and examination of the intestine for viability. If the blood supply has been deficient for some time, a segment of the bowel may be gangrenous, necessitating resection and anastomosis. In some instances, the surgeon may consider it advisable to simply establish drainage above the obstruction by performing an ileostomy or colostomy, delaying more extensive surgery until the patient's condition improves.

For nursing care, see page 373.

Cancer of the Intestine

Cancer is rare in the small intestine, but its incidence in the colon and rectum is higher than that of any other cancer in the human.[12] The most common site is the rectum; the sigmoid, cecum and ascending colon are next in order of frequency. Cancer of the colon or rectum may occur at any age but has its highest incidence in the fifth and sixth decades.

Conditions that frequently precede cancer of the bowel are ulcerative colitis that has been active for several years and multiple polyps (polyposis) in the bowel.

The malignant growth may be papillary, soft and friable, or a firm nodular mass projecting into the lumen; it may be a ring-shaped (annular) mass of firm fibrous tissue,

---

[12]J. E. Rhoads, S. J. Dudrick, and L. D. Miller: "Colectomy for Cancer—Techniques and Pitfalls." Surg. Clin. North Amer., Vol. 46, No. 5 (Oct. 1966), p. 1163.

causing a constriction of the bowel, or it may be ulcerative and necrotic, leading to bleeding and perforation.

The commonest earliest signs are a change in bowel habit and blood in the stool. Any person manifesting either of these signs should be urged to seek prompt medical attention.

There may be increasing constipation or perhaps alternating bouts of constipation and diarrhea. The stool may gradually become smaller and ribbon-like in form and may be streaked with blood, mucus and pus. A continuous defecation urge and the feeling that evacuation is incomplete after passing a stool may be experienced. If the cancer is in the cecum or ascending colon, the early symptoms are more insidious and difficult to detect. The patient presents a more general picture of ill health with a loss of weight and a progressive anemia. Laboratory examination of the stool will probably reveal occult blood. In cancer of the large bowel, abdominal pain is usually a late symptom; at first the patient may have a vague discomfort, and later he may experience a colicky pain which gradually becomes more persisting. Occasionally, the first symptoms recognized are those associated with complications, such as obstruction or perforation of the bowel.

Diagnostic procedures used are sigmoidoscopy, x-ray with barium enema, and the examination of stool specimens for blood and pus (see pp. 333 and 336).

Cancer of the colon is treated by resection of the bowel and anastomosis. This operation may have to be preceded by an emergency colostomy or cecostomy (see p. 376) for the relief of bowel obstruction. The resection is performed and the colostomy closed when the patient has recovered from the acute bowel obstruction. If the cancer involves the sigmoid colon and rectum, an abdominoperineal resection is done in which the entire anus, rectum and sigmoid are removed, leaving the patient with a permanent colostomy.

When the malignant disease is advanced and has metastasized to other structures, it may be considered inoperable. Treatment is then directed toward relieving the obstruction by a cecostomy or colostomy, correcting the anemia, providing relief of pain and keeping the patient as comfortable as pos-

sible (see Nursing Care of Patients with Cancer, Chapter 8).

For nursing care of the patient who has bowel resection, see below. For colostomy care, see page 376.

NURSING THE PATIENT WHO HAS INTESTINAL SURGERY

Preoperative Nursing Care

The preoperative care for a patient undergoing intestinal surgery is the same as that for any patient undergoing abdominal surgery (see p. 107) plus the following special considerations because the actual intestinal tract is to be entered.

The patient is hospitalized several days before operation for assessment of his general condition and for correction of disorders secondary to his disease, such as anemia, nutritional and fluid deficiencies and infection. This may not be possible if there is an acute bowel obstruction or strangulation.

Psychological Preparation. Since the patient is facing major surgery, he and his family are likely to be very anxious. There is probably fear of malignancy as well as concern for the patient's survival. The doctor may have advised the patient that it might be necessary to divert his bowel content through an abdominal opening (colostomy or ileostomy), depending on his findings at operation. (See page 376 for information concerning an ileostomy.)

The patient is encouraged to talk about his fears and ask questions. The nurse helps by being a willing listener and by indicating understanding and acceptance of his concerns. His questions are discreetly answered if possible without adding to his anxiety. Frequent visits to the patient and appropriate forms of diversion reduce his concentration on his condition. In talking with the patient and his family, socioeconomic or home problems may come to light for which the nurse may be able to suggest a solution or arrange for assistance from suitable sources.

The equipment and procedures that will be used postoperatively are briefly described, and their purpose and the patient's role are explained. These procedures most likely include intestinal suctioning, intravenous therapy, frequent checking of vital signs, the withholding of oral fluids and food, frequent coughing and deep breathing, and early ambulation. Knowing something of what to expect prevents unnecessary concern for his condition when these procedures are put into use postoperatively.

Physical Preparation. Observations are made for signs of possible dehydration. Extra fluids are given for optimal hydration; parenteral fluids may be ordered if the patient is unable to take sufficient quantities by mouth or to correct electrolyte deficiencies. A high-calorie, low-residue diet that includes extra protein and vitamins is desirable if it can be taken. If sufficient solid foods cannot be taken, a protein concentrate (e.g., Sustagen) may be given in solution, and the necessary vitamins may be ordered in medicinal form.

Usually only clear fluids are allowed during the 24 hours preceding the operation so the intestine will be empty. The sudden change in diet is explained to the patient.

During the preoperative period, the patient generally receives an oral antimicrobial drug to destroy intestinal organisms ("sterilization" of the bowel). Examples of drugs used for this purpose are succinylsulfathiazole (Sulfasuxidine), phthalylsulfathiazole (Sulfathalidine), and neomycin sulfate. Very little, if any, of these drugs is absorbed. If the drug used causes diarrhea, it should be reported promptly, as the patient cannot afford loss of fluid and nutrients.

Some sedation may be necessary to reduce the patient's anxiety and to promote rest. A small dose, 3 or 4 times daily, may be ordered.

Blood transfusions may be given to correct existing anemia and to improve the patient's general condition.

Immediate Preoperative Care. A laxative may be ordered 2 nights before operation and a cleansing enema given the night before so that there will be as little intestinal content as possible at the time of operation. The surgeon may also request intestinal intubation and suctioning for the same purpose. The passage of the tube may be done 24 hours or more before operation, since it takes several hours for the tube to advance the desired distance in the intestine (see p. 338). The intestinal tube is left in place, and suctioning is resumed after surgery to remove blood, secretions and gas so that distention and leakage through the suture line may be prevented.

In some instances, only nasogastric intubation may be required, in which case the tube is passed a few hours before the operation.

Postoperative Nursing Care

See Section on General Postoperative Care also, page 116.

The postoperative care will vary somewhat with the different surgical procedures that may be done on the intestine and with the level of the intestine involved. The patient may have had a resection of a segment of the bowel and an end-to-end anastomosis to restore the continuity of the tract; or the bowel may be retained, but an opening is made into the bowel through which the content is discharged onto the surface of the abdomen (colostomy or ileostomy). In cancer of the rectum or sigmoid colon or in ulcerative colitis, the patient may have had and abdominoperineal resection in which the lower segment of the colon, the rectum and the anus are removed, and the remaining terminal part of the intestine is brought to the abdominal surface to establish a permanent colostomy.

Special Equipment. The following equipment may be necessary and should be assembled and ready for immediate use when the patient returns from operation: intestinal suctioning apparatus; equipment for intravenous infusion and blood transfusion; equipment for the administration of oxygen; urinary drainage bottle or bag and tubing to connect to the retention catheter; and equipment for mouth care.

Observations. A frequent check is made of the patient's vital signs, response, and wound areas for early signs of shock or hemorrhage. Frequent observation of the intestinal suction and drainage is necessary to make sure there is no blockage of the tube or mechanical failure of the suction apparatus.

An accurate record is made of the fluid intake and output which includes the intestinal drainage. The amount and types of solutions to be given intravenously may be estimated by the physician on such records.

The abdomen should be examined for distention and rigidity; the development of either condition should be brought to the surgeon's attention promptly.

Intestinal Drainage. When a resection of the bowel has been done, decompression is continued until the anastomosis is partially healed and peristalsis is re-established.

The characteristics, as well as the exact amount, of the drainage are noted. It may be slightly colored by blood at first but should clear in a few hours. Persistence of blood-colored drainage or the appearance of large amounts of blood should be reported.

The intestinal suction tube may become obstructed by a small clot or by mucus and may require irrigation; a specific order as to the solution and the amount to be used is necessary. The suctioning may be discontinued for stated intervals the second or third postoperative day, and the patient's reaction is noted. The volume aspirated following each period of nonsuctioning should be carefully noted and recorded.

Positioning. With the patient's return to consciousness and stabilization of his vital signs, the head of the bed may be slightly elevated. He is encouraged to change his position hourly and is given the necessary assistance.

The patient who has had an abdomino-perineal resection usually lies on either side; moving is very difficult and painful for him at first because of the perineal wound, so the nurse helps him to change sides every hour or two. A pillow used to support the lower limb that is uppermost may help to lessen the discomfort.

Deep Breathing and Coughing. Pain and weakness may result in shallow breathing and may predispose to pulmonary complications. The patient is required hourly to take 5 to 10 deep breaths to fully ventilate his alveoli and to cough several times to dislodge any mucus that may collect. The nurse supports the patient and may ease some distress by placing one hand lightly over the abdominal incision.

Mouth and Nasal Care. Frequent cleansing and moistening of the mouth are necessary to lessen the patient's discomfort and prevent parotitis during the restriction of oral fluids. The nostril through which the intestinal tube is passed requires cleansing of the mucus secreted in response to the irritation. A light application of a water-soluble lubricant may be made after swabbing with water or saline.

Nutrition and Hydration. Nothing is given orally the first few days; intravenous fluids are used to sustain the patient. Oral intake is started with specific small amounts of water. If there is no untoward response, the amount is gradually increased and other fluids are introduced.

During the initial introduction of oral fluids, the intestinal suctioning may be discontinued and the tube clamped and left in place until the patient's response is determined. If the fluids are tolerated, the tube is removed, and the diet progresses through fluids to soft foods and then to a light, bland diet.

Elimination. The patient who has an abdominoperineal resection will have a retention catheter inserted into the bladder either preoperatively or immediately on completion of the operation. This is to prevent urinary retention, since most patients have difficulty in voiding. In the case of the female, it protects the perineal wound from urine contamination. The catheter may have to be irrigated at regular intervals with an antiseptic solution.

In bowel resection and anastomosis, the passage of any gas by rectum should be recorded; this probably indicates the re-establishment of peristalsis. A small cleansing enema may be ordered on the fourth or fifth day, and a mild laxative may be prescribed when food is being taken by mouth.

Elimination via an ileostomy or colostomy and the necessary care involved are discussed on page 376.

Exercises and Ambulation. The patient who has had a resection with anastomosis is out of bed a day or two after operation. If an abdominoperineal resection has been done, the patient usually remains in bed for several days. Lower limb exercises are important to prevent circulatory stasis and thrombosis. The patient tends to lie with the thighs and knees flexed; they should be straightened out several times daily and dorsiflexion of the feet, flexion and extension of the toes and tensing of the thigh muscles carried out.

Care of Wounds. The patient who has an abdominoperineal resection has 3 wounds.

There is a large abdominal incision through which the colon is severed above the affected segment of the colon and the distal portion is dissected and placed in the pelvic cavity outside the peritoneal cavity. A second smaller incision lies in the left abdomen through which the end of the proximal colon is brought and secured to form a permanent colostomy. The colon is kept clamped until the operation is completed to prevent possible contamination by intestinal content. The third incision is in the perineum through which the lower severed portion of the colon, the rectum and anal canal are removed.

The larger abdominal wound should be protected from contamination from the colostomy drainage. A sheet of plastic or thin rubber may be used over the dressing.

The perineal wound may be packed with vaseline gauze or it may have a soft rubber tissue drain. There is likely to be free sero-sanguineous drainage from this area, and the dressing requires frequent reinforcing during the first 24 hours. The doctor changes the dressing the first few times, and if packing has been used, it is gradually removed and the wound cavity allowed to heal by granulation. The T binder should be kept snug to avoid dressings rubbing on the wound or becoming displaced. Irrigations with a solution, such as normal saline or hydrogen peroxide, by means of a small catheter inserted into the wound are used to remove tissue debris. As soon as the patient is able to be out of bed, a sitz bath at a temperature of 37.8 to 40.6° C. (100 to 105° F) is used once or twice daily to stimulate circulation in the perineal area and promote healing. A rubber air ring is placed under the patient so the water can readily reach the wound and to reduce the discomfort of direct pressure on the area. Someone remains with the patient during the baths in case he becomes weak or faint.

The perineal wound may not be completely healed when the patient leaves the hospital. He should be taught the management of the sitz baths and the dressings at home. A referral may be made to the visiting nurse organization in his district so that he will receive the necessary assistance and reassurance when on his own. If the required dressings pose an economic problem, they can probably be obtained from the local chapter of the National Cancer Society. If necessary, this agency may also provide a means of transportation for the patient to go to the clinic or the doctor's office.

Care of the colostomy is discussed in the following section.

Ileostomy and Colostomy Care

The treatment of some intestinal disorders may necessitate surgery that establishes an opening into the bowel through which the intestinal content is discharged on to the surface of the abdomen. The opening may be temporary or permanent. A temporary diversion of the bowel content may be necessary while some abnormal condition below the level of the stoma is corrected or for quick decompression and drainage in obstruction. Later, the normal continuity of the tract is restored and the stoma is eliminated. If the opening is permanent, the portion of the bowel below is generally removed.

The operations performed are ileostomy, cecostomy and colostomy.

Ileostomy. An ileostomy involves transection of the ileum and bringing the proximal end out to the abdominal surface to form a stoma. The removal of the distal severed portion of the bowel may be done at the same operation or may be postponed until the patient's condition is improved. If the lower part of the intestine is to be retained for a period of time, it is closed; in some instances, the severed end may also be brought out to the abdominal surface. The colectomy usually includes removal of the rectum and anal canal. The ileostomy is most frequently performed for ulcerative colitis that does not respond to medical treatment and is incapacitating. It may also be necessary for patients with multiple polyposis of the colon or an intestinal obstruction in the upper portion of the bowel.

Colostomy. A colostomy is an opening of the colon on to the surface of the abdomen. It may be in the transverse or descending colon. If the colostomy is a temporary measure, the transverse colon is usually the site used. A loop of the colon is brought to the abdominal surface, secured and left unopened until the peritoneum heals sufficiently to prevent fecal matter from escaping into the peritoneal cavity. The bowel becomes adherent to the wound edges and an incision is made into it in 2 to 4 days. When the sigmoid colon, rectum and anal canal have to be removed, as in cancer of the sigmoid and rectum, the terminal end of the descending colon is brought to the abdominal surface to form a permanent colostomy.

Cecostomy. Rarely, in large bowel obstruction, decompression of the distended bowel is achieved by a cecostomy. A small opening is made in the cecum through a small lower right abdominal incision and a fairly large tube is inserted through which the bowel content escapes to the exterior. The tube is attached to a drainage receptacle and remains in place until the patient's condition is such that he can withstand the more extensive surgery necessary to relieve the obstruction.

Nursing Considerations in Ileostomy and Colostomy

PSYCHOLOGICAL PREOPERATIVE PREPARATION. When the physician advises the patient preoperatively that a colostomy or ileostomy may be, or will be, necessary, the patient is likely to be emotionally disturbed. Obviously, if the colostomy is a temporary measure it will be more readily accepted, but if it is likely to be permanent, the patient may be more concerned about this than about the operation or his basic condition. His immediate response may be "it would be better to die than have that." He may become resentful or show marked depression and despair and may see this change in his body as making him unclean and unacceptable to society. There are fears because of odor and soiling. It is best to let the patient and his family vent their feelings before attempting explanations. The nurse can help by being a willing listener, answering their questions and using every available opportunity to assure the patient that the "ostomy" can be cared for without interfering with his work and social life. When the patient recovers from the initial blow, discussions may then be held as to how he will care for his ileostomy or colostomy.

It is very helpful if he is visited by a person who has an ileostomy or colostomy and who has learned to manage his care and live an active, independent life. The request for such a person to visit may be made to the local Ileostomy Association; the members of the association consider this service to be one of their functions. If there is no local association, the physician or the visiting nurse organization may know of some-

one. To see this person, who is cheerful and appears quite normal, makes a tremendous impression on the patient; his whole attitude may change and result in his acceptance of the situation. Following this, the patient is likely to manifest an interest in learning about the postoperative management. The nurse capitalizes on this and plans the appropriate instruction. He is advised that for the first few postoperative days the drainage may be fairly free and erratic but will gradually become more regular. This may offset some of the discouragement experienced when the patient is actually faced with the discharge of his bowel content on to the surface of the abdomen.

DIFFERENCES BETWEEN ILEOSTOMY AND COLOSTOMY. Certain differences exist between an ileostomy and colostomy that result in different problems and types of care. For example, the control of the discharge is determined by the location of the stoma; drainage from the ileum is of liquid consistency, is rich in enzymes that may cause excoriation and erosion of the skin, and flows almost continuously, necessitating the constant wearing of a receptive appliance. There may be quiescent periods but they are not predictable and cannot be controlled. Complications are a more common occurrence with an ileostomy than with a colostomy and odor presents a greater problem because of the continuous drainage. Irrigations are not used in ileostomy; the introduction of anything into the ileal stoma is discouraged for fear of injury to the intestine.

Colostomy drainage is more manageable and is less irritating to the skin. Since the opening is usually in the terminal transverse or the descending colon, much of the fluid and electrolytes have been absorbed from the fecal content, leaving it semisolid or solid by the time it reaches the stoma. Irrigations may be necessary, but in some instances, the sigmoid colostomy may be so well controlled that it resembles normal bowel movement, and the patient does not have to wear a receptive bag continuously.

Intestinal activity in a person with a colostomy or ileostomy may be influenced by diet, fluid intake and emotions just as it is in the normal person.

EQUIPMENT. On completing an ileostomy, the surgeon usually applies a disposable polyethylene or plastic bag to receive the drainage. It is attached to a square of double-faced adhesive which secures the bag to the abdomen. A hole is cut in the adhesive to fit the stoma, leaving a margin of approximately one-eighth of an inch; too large an opening exposes a larger area of skin to the irritating drainage. The stoma shrinks during the first week or two, necessitating readjustment of the size of the opening. The lower end of the bag is folded in and secured with elastic bands. This arrangement permits the emptying of the bag without removing the adhesive. The bag is changed once daily.

The surgeon may prefer dressings to be used for the first few days postoperatively. Gauze dressings are loosened and fitted closely around the stoma, and the area is completely covered with adequate gauze and pads to absorb the drainage. The dressings are held in place by a binder or by adhesive with cotton tapes that may be tied. The dressings are changed as often as necessary to keep the patient clean and to prevent excoriation of the skin.

The ileostomy patient is fitted for a permanent appliance as soon as possible so he can become familiar with its use and care before leaving the hospital. A well-fitting comfortable appliance means a great deal to the patient's future; it should fit closely enough to the skin to prevent any leakage but without causing injury to the skin and stoma. It should be inconspicuous, allow freedom of activity and be odor-proof. Several types of appliances are available from surgical supply companies, but the essential parts are a disc which fits over the stoma and adheres closely to the body to prevent leakage, a rubber or plastic bag which may or may not be detachable from the disc, and a lightweight elasticized belt which attaches to the disc. The lower end of the bag is tapered and open. It is closed by folding and secured with elastic bands. A latex cement is available for application to the skin and disc to provide a secure adherence and prevent leakage. A special solvent is necessary to remove the cement or adhesive from the skin and disc when there is a change of the complete appliance. The surgeon recommends the appliance most suited to meet the requirements of the patient. Advice in the selection of equipment may also be obtained

from the Ileostomy Association. The location and size of the stoma and the contour and firmness of the abdomen are factors that have to be taken into consideration in the selection and fitting of a permanent appliance.

The temporary plastic bag may be used initially for the colostomy patient, or dressings may be applied as described above for the ileostomy patient. Whether it is necessary for the patient with a colostomy to wear a bag continuously depends on the degree of regularity and control established. Since part of the colon remains, the feces tend to be retained, and sufficient water is absorbed so that the stool is formed and discharged once or twice daily, corresponding to normal defecation. If the colostomy drainage is well controlled, the patient may simply wear a small dressing over the stoma and cover the area with a square of plastic material or oil silk. These are held in place by an elasticized belt or girdle. If the colostomy is in the transverse colon, is not regulated, or if the patient feels insecure, a colostomy bag may be worn. The colostomy appliance is similar to that for the ileostomy, consisting of a disc or ring that fits over the stoma to which a rubber or plastic bag may be attached.

CARE OF AN ILEOSTOMY AND A COLOSTOMY. The ileostomy bag is usually emptied several times daily as necessary. The lower end of the bag is opened and the contents allowed to drain directly into the toilet or a basin. The lower part of the bag is then rinsed with lukewarm or cool water; care is taken not to let the water reach the stoma and disc. The complete appliance is removed every 2 days at first. Gradually the interval is increased to regular changing twice weekly if the condition of the skin and stoma is satisfactory. The equipment includes 2 bags so that the one removed can be thoroughly washed with a detergent, filled with a weak solution of chloride bleach or commercial appliance cleaner and left to soak for several hours. It is then rinsed thoroughly and is hung to dry and air.

If a colostomy bag is worn, it is removed daily and cleansed in the same manner as the ileostomy bag. The tight adherence and seal of the disc, essential for the ileostomy, is not usually necessary in a colostomy, since the fecal drainage is less liquid. The disc can be removed daily if cement or adhesive is not used. If the colostomy is well regulated and elimination occurs regularly once or twice a day, the patient is encouraged to wear a light dressing rather than the bag.

The skin around the stoma of an ileostomy must receive constant attention and is kept free of direct contact with the drainage. The skin is cleansed and a protective substance such as karaya gum powder (Protex powder, Derma-Guard) or neo-karaya (a combination of aluminum hydroxide gel and karaya) is applied. These preparations, being non-greasy, permit the cement or adhesive to adhere. The skin may also be protected by the insertion of a thin, closed-pore, foam rubber pad between the skin and the appliance disc. To prevent damage to the skin, a solvent should be used to dissolve the cement or adhesive when removing the appliance and cleansing the skin. The skin should be wiped gently and cleansed, not scrubbed, and the solvent washed away quickly. The appliance is changed daily if the skin becomes even slightly irritated. A break in the skin should be brought to the doctor's attention. A small dressing may be ordered to the area and the disc applied over it.

Fewer skin problems are encountered by the colostomy patient. The skin should be thoroughly cleansed and examined after each elimination. A light application of petrolatum, zinc oxide ointment or karaya gum powder may be used to protect the skin or treat excoriation.

Odor is a constant source of concern to the ileostomy or colostomy patient and his family. It may be controlled by a clean, odor-free, well-fitting appliance; efficient emptying and flushing of the bag; and by the use of commercial deodorant tablets. The deodorant tablets are placed in the pouch while it is worn. Deodorant tablets of bismuth sub-gallate or chlorophyll are also available for oral administration but should only be taken if prescribed by the physician. Bags should not be kept in use too long; eventually they absorb odors that are impossible to remove entirely.

DIET. The ileostomy or colostomy patient usually starts out on a light, low-residue diet to which foods of a regular normal diet are gradually added. Raw fruits and some vegetables may have to be limited. Cabbage, turnips, celery, corn, onions, nuts,

prunes and pineapple tend to increase the bulk and gas content in the intestine and cause excessive drainage. Tolerance varies with patients but by careful personal experimentation with foods the patient will recognize what he can and cannot take.

Considerable water and salts are lost in ileostomy drainage, especially during the first 2 or 3 months. Gradually, the small intestine adapts to the lack of the colon function and absorbs more water and salts. Until then, extra water and foods rich in sodium and potassium should be taken. The patient may erroneously think that limiting his fluid intake will cause the intestinal drainage to be less fluid.

COLOSTOMY IRRIGATION. A colostomy may be controlled entirely by diet in some persons; others may require an irrigation daily or every second day. The following equipment is necessary:

1. Two-quart enema can or bag with tubing (approximately 40 to 44 inches), connecting tube and clamp
2. Catheter, number 18 or 20 French
3. Lubricating jelly
4. Toilet tissue or cellucotton for cleaning and absorbing any leakage around the stoma
5. Basin and small rubber sheet to receive the drainage or an irrigating cup that is fitted over the stoma and held in place by a belt. The catheter is inserted through the cup and a large tube is also attached to it for drainage
6. Basin of water for cleansing
7. Paper bag or newspaper for discard
8. Dressings or clean colostomy bag

Five hundred to 2000 ml. of tap water at 105° F. may be used and the can or bag is elevated 18 to 24 inches above the colostomy. The head of the bed may be raised, or if the patient is ambulatory, he may sit on a chair or on the toilet. The toilet should be used as soon as the patient is able; it has a beneficial psychological effect because of the association with normal defecation. If the rubber irrigating cup and drainage tube are not available, a trough leading into the basin or toilet may be formed with a rubber sheet to receive the discharge. The catheter is lubricated and, after the air is expelled from the tubing, is inserted gently 4 to 8 inches. The rate of flow and pressure should be regulated according to the patient's reaction.

If he experiences cramps, the can should be lowered and the rate of flow decreased. Cramping indicates excessive contraction of the bowel which may actually retard the elimination of the bowel content. Five hundred ml. of fluid is given at first, and this is increased as the need is determined. The amount required to stimulate peristalsis and satisfactory elimination varies with patients; some may require 1500 to 2000 ml. The actual irrigation and elimination process takes approximately 30 to 40 minutes. Some form of diversion for the patient such as reading or listening to the radio is helpful.

When evacuation is complete, the patient is left clean and dry, the skin is protected with powder or petrolatum, and a clean dressing or colostomy bag is applied. Drainage between irrigations may indicate that insufficient irrigating fluid was given or the fluid was given too quickly, or may be the result of constipation. If there is evidence of the latter, diet adjustment and increased fluid intake may be necessary.

REGULARITY. A regular schedule should be set up for colostomy irrigation and for changing the ileostomy appliance. The irrigation is most effective early in the morning, since this approximates the normal time of defecation. The ileostomy appliance should be changed at a time of day when the drainage is at a minimum. This may be determined by observation and is usually an hour or so before mealtime.

COMPLICATIONS. Prolapse of the intestine through the ileal or colonic stoma occurs rarely and should be brought to the physician's attention. A truss may be applied, or surgical correction may be necessary. An excessive watery discharge with less fecal content from an ileostomy may be due to a narrowing of the stoma or an enteritis and should be reported if it persists longer than 24 hours. Extra fluids will be necessary to relieve the resulting dehydration, and dilation of the stoma may be necessary. A low-residue diet may be necessary until normal function is re-established.

Obstruction, indicated by lack of ileostomy or colostomy drainage, may develop. It is usually accompanied by crampy pain, distention and vomiting and may be due to adhesions or recurrence of the primary disease.

Herniation due to a weakening of the muscles at the site of the stoma may occur. It is recognized as a bulging area and is usually controlled by a supporting belt or by the disc of the ileostomy appliance.

INSTRUCTION. As soon as the patient has recovered sufficiently from the operation, the nurse concentrates on helping him accept his "ostomy" and on teaching him the necessary care and management of it. Although there may have been considerable discussion of the modified method of elimination preoperatively, when the patient is actually faced with it he is filled with revulsion and becomes discouraged and depressed. The patient is again concerned about his social acceptance in the future. Acceptance comes first from the nurse who willingly makes every effort to keep the patient clean and comfortable without any hesitancy or aversion and gradually introduces self-care with an understanding of the patient's reactions to the adjustments he must make.

A plan of instruction is developed to prepare the patient for assuming care of his "ostomy." Explanations and demonstrations are given as to the following: The necessary equipment, and the application, emptying and changing of the appliance if one is to be worn; the care of the skin; the necessary observations; colonic irrigation, if it is to be used; the establishment of a plan and schedule for care; the cleaning and care of the equipment; the prevention of odor; diet and fluids; and activities. He is made aware of the necessity for periodic visits to a clinic or his physician and of the assistance which is available from visiting nurses and the Ileostomy Association.

At first, as the nurse cares for the ileostomy or colostomy, each step of the procedure may be explained. Then gradually the patient is given the opportunity to perform a part of the care. His participation is increased from day to day until eventually he is prepared to undertake complete care. This progressive, step-by-step approach takes time and patience but is less frustrating and discouraging for the patient. As he learns to assume self-care in the hospital, the nurse offers suggestions as to how he may manage the same procedure at home. It is helpful to include a member of the family in the discussions.

Directions for care and use usually accompany the various appliances and should be read carefully by the patient. Several very useful booklets on ileostomy and colostomy care are published which are helpful to the patient when he is assuming his own care.[13, 14, 15, 16] These should be available within the hospital and given to the patient to read.

Visits from members of the Ileostomy Association are extremely valuable during this period of adjustment. The patient often will ask them questions that he hesitates to present to the doctor or nurse. He receives the ileostomist's personal assistance and is advised of the advantages of membership in their organization. Association meetings and bulletins will provide additional assistance, information and reassurance. The patient may feel insecure when removed from the protective hospital environment where help was readily available. A referral may be made to have a nurse visit the patient at home.

The expense of dressings or appliance equipment may pose a problem; the social worker may be asked to see the patient to suggest possible sources of assistance. If the colostomy was performed because of cancer of the bowel, the local chapter of the National Cancer Society will frequently help by providing dressings or other forms of assistance.

Appendicitis

The appendix, a narrow blind tube extending from the inferior part of the cecum, is a common site of inflammation and accounts for a large number of acute abdominal operations. The appendix has no essential function in the human, and there is no change in body function with its removal.

The commonest cause of appendicitis is obstruction of the lumen by a fecolith (a small, hard mass of accumulated feces), a solid foreign body, or by disease or scar tissue in the walls of the appendix. Secretion collects in the tube, causing distention that results in pressure on the intramural blood vessels. The mucosa ulcerates and readily becomes infected; the walls may become gangrenous because of the interference with the blood supply, and perforation is likely to occur. A ruptured appendix is serious; it allows the escape of organisms into the peritoneal cavity and may cause an abscess in the appendiceal region or a generalized peritonitis.

The disease may occur at any age but is more common in children over 4 years of age, adolescents and young adults.

Manifestations of appendicitis are abdominal pain, nausea and vomiting, a moderate elevation in temperature and a leukocytosis with the increase being in the polymorphonuclear cells. At the onset, the pain is usually referred to the central portion of the abdomen or the lower epigastric region and is described as crampy. As the inflammation involves the walls of the appendix, the pain becomes localized to the lower right quadrant. The area is tender on palpation and gradually develops rigidity in the muscles. The patient moves slowly and carefully to avoid jolting and movement that increase the pain and tends to keep his right thigh flexed.

The omentum and adjacent bowel may become adherent to the inflamed appendix, walling off the area. If the appendix ruptures, an abscess will most likely form in the walled-off cavity. But if perforation occurs before the area is walled off, a generalized peritonitis usually develops; the patient complains of pain and tenderness over the whole abdomen which becomes rigid (board-like) and distended. The distention is due to inhibited bowel motility, which may be referred to as paralytic or adynamic ileus.

The treatment of appendicitis depends on the stage to which the disease has advanced. If it is still localized to the appendix, an appendectomy is done as soon as the diagnosis is established. If the appendix has ruptured and there is an abscess or peritonitis, the patient may be treated conservatively with antibiotics and parenteral fluids and given very little or nothing by mouth to reduce gastrointestinal activity. Gastrointestinal decompression is used if

[13]QT Inc. Boston: Manual for Ileostomy Patients, 4th ed. QT Inc. Boston, c/o The Medical Foundation, 227 Commonwealth Ave., Boston, Mass. 02216.

[14]Reina Siegel: The A.B.C. of Ileostomy. Custom Service, 1170 Andrews Ave., Bronx, New York 10453.

[15]QT Inc. Boston: Your Ileostomy. A Guide for New Patients. QT Inc. Boston, c/o The Medical Foundation, 227 Commonwealth Ave., Boston, Mass. 02216.

[16]National Cancer Society: Living with Your Colostomy.

there is generalized peritonitis and a paralytic ileus.

Nursing in Appendicitis. The person with abdominal pain is urged to seek medical advice, and self-treatment is discouraged, particularly the taking of a laxative or an enema which could be serious, since either could cause perforation of the appendix through stimulation of peristalsis. The patient is also advised not to take food or fluid until seen by the doctor. This is in case immediate surgery is necessary. In most instances, surgery is performed as soon as the diagnosis is established unless perforation is suspected. For preparation for emergency surgery, see page 114. If the appendix was intact at the time of removal, the patient usually makes a rapid uneventful recovery with a short period of hospitalization (5 to 7 days). For postoperative nursing care, see page 116.

If an abscess is present, a drainage tube is placed in the abscess cavity at operation. This necessitates cleansing of the wound and changing of the dressing at intervals. The patient's head and shoulders are elevated; this may help to keep the infection localized to the appendiceal region. Large doses of an antibiotic are ordered, and the patient should receive plenty of fluids. An accurate record of the intake should be kept, and if the patient cannot take sufficient quantities by mouth, parenteral supplements may be ordered. Close observations are made for possible extension of the infection and generalized peritonitis. Abdominal distention, nausea and vomiting, lack of bowel activity, an elevated temperature and rapid pulse should be brought promptly to the surgeon's attention.

Regional Enteritis (Regional Ileitis, Crohn's Disease)

This is an inflammatory disease of unknown cause that may develop in any part of the intestine but has a predilection for the terminal portion of the ileum. The regional lymph nodes and mesentery are involved, and it is suggested that the disease originates in the lymphatics and spreads to the walls of the intestine.[17] The intestinal walls in the affected area are swollen and edematous, and the lumen is narrowed. Ulceration and infection occur, and the bowel may perforate and form an internal or external fistula (an abnormal passage) into another loop of the intestine or onto the skin. As the inflammation subsides, there is scarring and stenosis, which may lead to a partial obstruction of the bowel. More than one area of the intestine may be involved, while the intervening segments remain unaffected.

The primary symptoms are crampy abdominal pain, tenderness in the lower right quadrant, diarrhea, nausea and vomiting, and a low-grade fever. The diarrheal stools will probably contain mucus, pus and undigested food particles. Some abdominal rigidity, due to peritoneal irritation, may be seen, and there is usually a slight leukocytosis. As the disease progresses, malnutrition, loss of weight and strength, dehydration, and anemia develop because of loss of appetite and interference with the normal intestinal absorption.

The condition may persist, or there may be remissions and exacerbations. Treatment and care are supportive and symptomatic. Efforts are directed toward relief of the pain and diarrhea; correction of fluid, electrolyte and nutritional deficiencies; treatment of secondary infection; and reducing the patient's emotional distress. The physical condition and emotional state of the patient have important roles in arresting the progress of the disease and in preventing an exacerbation. Restriction of activity depends on the severity of the disease and on the patient's strength and nutritional status. In severe attacks, bed rest is recommended. Reduced energy expenditure and extra hours of rest during the day may be suggested for less debilitated patients whose disease is less active. A high-calorie, high-protein, low-residue diet free of all roughage and irritating foods is used. Coffee, iced fluids, fruit juices and alcohol are avoided, and milk is usually poorly tolerated. The fat content is limited; some is usually allowed in order to make the food more palatable since anorexia is a problem. Intravenous infusions may be necessary to replace fluid and electrolyte losses, and blood transfusions may be given to treat the anemia. Medications may include vitamin supplements, drugs that reduce intestinal spasm and peristalsis, and antimicrobial drugs to treat secondary infection. Mild

[17]P. Bentley, and M. D. Colcock: "Regional Enteritis: A Surgical Enigma." Surg. Clin. North Amer., Vol. 44, No. 3 (June 1964), p. 779.

sedatives such as amobarbital (Amytal) may be ordered to relieve the patient's anxiety and emotional stress.

In severe persisting cases, the physician may prescribe a brief course of a corticoid preparation such as prednisone, hydrocortisone, or adrenocorticotropin (ACTH, corticotropin) to be administered intravenously very slowly over 8 to 10 hours. The cortisone and ACTH preparations are not curative but are considered useful to induce a remission. They also improve the patient's appetite and create a sense of well-being. The physician is usually reluctant to use either of these latter preparations since there is the tendency for an exacerbation to occur on withdrawal and because there is a greater possibility of infection and perforation. The salt intake of the patient who is receiving ACTH or a corticoid may be restricted because of the proneness to sodium retention and ensuing edema. The fluid intake and output are measured, and the blood pressure and weight are recorded daily; these serve to determine the possible sodium and water retention.

Psychological support is important; the patient should receive some explanation as to the nature of his disease, and fear of malignancy should be dispelled. He should be encouraged to plan to return to his occupation. Some type of diversion should be provided, since worry may increase the intestinal motility.

Much of the nursing care discussed under Diarrhea (p. 369) is applicable to this patient.

When intestinal obstruction, perforation or a fistula occurs, surgery is necessary. If the patient has experienced frequent severe relapses or the disease is intractable and incapacitating, surgery may be recommended. This involves resection of the diseased portion of the bowel and an end-to-end anastomosis to restore intestinal continuity. In some instances the resection will include the terminal ileum, cecum and the proximal section of the colon. The terminal end of the small intestine is then anastomosed with the transverse colon (enterocolostomy). Unfortunately, even following resection the disease may recur.

Idiopathic Ulcerative Colitis

Ulcerative colitis is characterized by severe inflammation and ulceration of the mucosa of a part or all of the colon. The process usually begins in the rectosigmoid area and spreads up the descending colon. There is marked hyperemia and edema in the affected area followed by ulceration. The denuded areas result in infection and a loss of fluid, electrolytes and blood.

The patient has frequent diarrhea stools containing blood, mucus and pus, accompanied by colicky abdominal pain. Dehydration, anemia and a loss of weight and strength develop, and the patient usually has a low-grade fever. The prolonged and distressing symptoms and incapacitation cause emotional stress, and the patient may become very discouraged and depressed.

The cause of this disease remains obscure. Infection and allergy have been proposed as possible etiologic factors. There is at present support for the theory that it is due to an auto-immune reaction in which the body forms antibodies that destroy the normal protective mucus which coats the bowel. It has also been suggested that the condition is a manifestation of concealed emotional stress, since many of the affected persons tend to be very sensitive, easily hurt, immature and dependent. Frequently arthritis, skin lesions or iritis is associated with ulcerative colitis and is considered to be a response to the same causative factor responsible for the disease in the colon.

Ulcerative colitis affects both sexes equally, and although it may occur at any age, the onset occurs most frequently during the second and third decades. Its course is unpredictable. The onset is usually insidious; however, rarely, it may develop suddenly with intense severity. The patient may have a complete recovery, but more often, there are relapses in subsequent months or years. An acute exacerbation may be precipitated by nervous or physical strain. The patient's history may reveal a recent bereavement, a home or job conflict, an acute infection or probably dietary indiscretions or bowel irritation by laxatives.

Persisting and frequent recurrences are likely to cause serious complications. Severe hemorrhage may occur if a large vessel is eroded, necessitating emergency surgical treatment in which a colectomy is usually done. Perforation of an ulcerated area of the bowel, leading to generalized peritonitis, is a less common complication but very serious. Perforation of the rectum frequently causes an abscess and fistula in the perirectal or perianal regions. When the disease is prolonged, the affected colon tends to become a smooth, narrow, inflexible tube. The mucosa becomes thin and the walls are infiltrated by scar tissue that causes a stenosis that may result in obstruction. Occasionally, polyps develop in the ulcerated colon and may give rise to bleeding. The incidence of cancer of the colon is 20 to 30 times greater in persons who have had ulcerative colitis for several years than in the general population.[18]

Treatment and Nursing Care. The patient is usually hospitalized during an acute attack of ulcerative colitis so that a more intensive therapeutic and supportive program may be provided. Also, hospitalization may remove the patient from an environment that has stress factors which aggravate his disease. Treatment and care are directed toward reducing colonic activity, combating secondary infection, improving the patient's general condition by correcting the malnutrition and anemia, and alleviating emotional stress.

Emotional Support. It should be understood by all those caring for the ulcerative colitis patient that sensitivity, dependency and insecurity are common characteristics of these patients and that they tend to have inner tensions and bottled-up feelings which are not expressed. Imposed on these basic personality traits now are the distressing symptoms of his disease, which he most likely finds rather humiliating, and the problems created by prolonged incapacity. Every appropriate means possible should be considered to make the patient mentally and physically comfortable. It is important that the nurse convey to the patient by thoughtful attention and words that she knows and cares about what he is experiencing and how he feels about his total situation.

Understanding sympathetic care is extremely important in gradually establishing confidence and a relationship that is conducive to more effective treatment. The patient should tactfully be encouraged to talk about himself and his life activities while the nurse listens carefully for problems that may be responsible for aggravating

his disorder. He may actually feel better after talking to the nurse because someone has been interested enough to listen.

Orientation to the environment and an explanation of care and treatments are necessary. The best timing for certain activities and the beneficial effects of such may be discussed; for example, it may be advisable to leave the patient undisturbed following a meal and to delay the bath or other care procedures to avoid movement and activities that may stimulate bowel activity. However, if the sensitive patient who is easily hurt is not advised of the purpose of the delay, he may feel neglected.

Some form of appropriate diversion should be provided to reduce the patient's preoccupation with his disease. Visitors are screened to avoid those who may worry the patient or stir up inner conflicts.

OBSERVATIONS. The number, volume, consistency and content of the stools should be noted and recorded accurately. A close check should be made of the patient's hydration and nutritional state from day to day. His weight is recorded daily unless it proves a source of concern to the patient, in which case it will be discontinued and only noted once or twice weekly.

The nurse should be alert to the possibility of perforation and hemorrhage and should promptly report any changes in the patient that might be early indications of these complications.

The foods taken by the patient are determined and observations are made as to whether the patient's diarrhea increases after any one particular food is taken.

REST. Bed rest, quiet and relaxation tend to reduce intestinal motility and are recommended during the acute phase. Activity is gradually resumed as the severe diarrhea and fever subside. Nursing care is planned to permit undisturbed periods of rest. Assistance should be given the weak and debilitated patient in turning and in getting on and off the bedpan, which can be exhausting to him.

POSITIONING AND SKIN CARE. The patient with ulcerative colitis may become emaciated, which necessitates special attention to the bony prominences to prevent decubitus ulcers. The areas are kept clean and dry and are gently and frequently massaged. Pressure on the bony prominences may be relieved by using an alternating air mattress or pieces of sponge rubber or sheep-

---

[18]Sir Ronald Badley Scott (Ed.): Price's Textbook of the Practice of Medicine, 10th ed. New York, Oxford University Press, 1966, p. 529.

skin. The rim of the bedpan or the commode should be padded to protect the skin. The anal region should be washed after each defecation, and a protective ointment or cream such as petrolatum or zinc oxide is applied. If severe tenesmus is experienced, warm compresses or an ointment such as Nupercaine may be applied to the anus.

The patient tends to lie curled up in one position with the legs and thighs continuously flexed, which predisposes to contractures. There is a reluctance to move about in bed or turn for fear of stimulating peristalsis and another bowel movement. He must be encouraged to turn and change his position every 1 to 2 hours. Full extension of the lower limbs should be required at frequent intervals, and if possible, the prone position should be assumed for a few minutes 2 or 3 times daily.

NUTRITION AND HYDRATION. In serious acute attacks, oral food and fluids may be withdrawn for a brief period in an effort to reduce intestinal activity to a minimum while the patient is maintained on parenteral fluids.

When food is permitted, a high-calorie, high-protein, nonirritating low-residue diet is given. Milk is usually poorly tolerated. Iced fluids, carbonated drinks, raw fruits and vegetables and all foods suspected of stimulating bowel activity are avoided. Recently, some physicians have suggested a more liberal diet with elimination of only those foods that the patient recognizes as increasing the diarrhea.

Nutrition of the patient requires a great deal of attention. Anorexia presents a problem, and there are serious losses of essential nutrients, fluid and electrolytes in the frequent stools. In many instances, the nurse must work at getting the patient to take sufficient nourishment; it may be necessary to provide frequent small meals. An effort should be made to serve foods the patient likes, to provide variety, and to have the tray attractively arranged. A discouraging factor commonly encountered is that as soon as the patient starts to eat, peristalsis is stimulated and he must have the bedpan. When this happens the tray should be removed from the room and returned after the patient has used the pan, received the necessary hygienic care and the room is ventilated. Hot foods should have been kept warm or are reheated. Encouragement and praise are given as the patient manages to take larger amounts of food.

Even though a fair amount may be taken orally, fluid and electrolyte losses may have to be replaced by intravenous infusions. Blood transfusions may be given to correct anemia and to restore a normal blood volume. Impaired absorption of the foods and vitamins, as well as restriction of certain foods, contributes to the need for vitamin supplements, particularly ascorbic acid and the vitamin B complex.

ENVIRONMENT. Preferably, the ulcerative colitis patient should be in a room by himself so he will be less embarrassed by his frequent use of the bedpan and the odor involved. If this is not possible, he should be placed in an area that can be screened to provide privacy and can be readily ventilated. If he has bathroom privileges, he should be placed near the bathroom.

It may be necessary to keep a clean, covered bedpan at the bedside because of the patient's urgency and to prevent concern about getting it in time. The bed linen should be kept clean and fresh. Extra covers may be needed for the patient for warmth; chilling should be avoided because of his lowered resistance.

MEDICATIONS. Various drugs are used in treating the patient with colitis. Nearly all patients receive small, regular doses of a sedative to promote rest and relaxation and to alleviate some of the emotional stress so common to this disorder. Examples of sedatives that may be prescribed are phenobarbital (Luminal) and amobarbital (Amytal). If the patient is very emotionally disturbed, a tranquilizer such as chlordiazepoxide hydrochloride (Librium) orally or diazepam (Valium) orally or intramuscularly may be ordered.

Secondary infection of the raw ulcerated areas of the bowel is treated by the oral administration of an antibiotic (e.g., neomycin) or a sulfonamide such as succinylsulfathiazole. A compound of sulfapyridine and acetylsalicylic acid (salicylazosulfapyridine, Azulfidine) may be used. The patient receiving sulfonamide preparations is observed for side effects such as skin rash, nausea, vomiting and headache. If the infection extends deeply into the colonic wall, a parenteral antibiotic may be prescribed.

Anticholinergic drugs to reduce peristalsis

and a drug to coat the mucosa and adsorb irritating substances may also be used. Examples are propantheline (Pro-Banthine) and aluminum hydroxide (Amphojel).

Either adrenocorticotropin or adrenocorticosteroid is used to bring about a remission of the disease. It reduces tissue sensitivity and responses. Prednisone is a commonly used corticosteroid preparation given orally. The initial dosage is gradually decreased as the patient's symptoms subside. Prednisone or hydrocortisone dissolved in a small amount of water may be ordered to be given rectally. The patient is encouraged to retain the rectal injection as long as possible. This method of administration produces fewer side effects, since little of the drug is absorbed. The patient may find it too difficult to retain the solution long enough for it to be effective, making it necessary for an oral preparation to be prescribed.

Adrenocorticotropin (ACTH, corticotropin) may be given intravenously very slowly over 8 to 10 hours, or corticotropin gel (Acthar) may be administered intramuscularly. The gel delays absorption and prolongs the action.

The patient who is receiving any adrenocorticotropin or corticoid preparation, particularly over a long period, must be observed for possible undesirable effects. He may develop sodium and fluid retention and ensuing edema, a false sense of well-being, lowered resistance to infection, a moon face and hirsutism.

Hematinics such as iron may be prescribed to aid in correcting the anemia.

INSTRUCTIONS. The possibility of a recurrence of the ulcerative colitis is reduced if the patient understands and respects certain care and precautions. The patient is encouraged to return to his occupation and to live as normal and useful a life as possible. A balance between rest, work and recreation is advisable. Assistance is given the patient in solving home or socioeconomic problems, since a relapse can frequently be attributed to a psychological disturbance. A social worker may be asked to see the patient or family to help solve existing problems, or a referral may be made to a welfare department or service organization from which help may be obtained. The family should be advised as to their role in supporting the patient.

Emphasis is placed on the importance of a nourishing diet with the elimination of certain foods that are coarse and irritating to the colon. Chilling, exhaustion and contact with persons having a cold or infection are to be avoided, since a relapse may follow.

SURGICAL TREATMENT. A colectomy with a permanent ileostomy may be considered advisable in persisting colitis that fails to respond to medical treatment or when there are frequent severe exacerbations which cause physical and psychological disability to the extent that the patient cannot lead a useful and independent life. Longstanding ulcerative colitis predisposes malignant changes in the bowel. Several authors claim that approximately 3 to 10 per cent of the patients with colitis of 10 to 15 years' duration develop cancer.[19, 20]

Complications, such as hemorrhage and perforation of the bowel, are usually indications for emergency surgery.

For nursing care of the patient who has a colectomy and ileostomy, see page 374.

Anorectal complications are common in patients with ulcerative colitis. Infection passes through the wall of the rectum and causes perirectal or perianal abscesses and fistulas that open onto the perineal area, discharging blood and pus. These complications require surgical treatment; the abscesses are drained, the fistula is excised and the area is left open to heal by granulation from within out to the surface.

RECTAL AND ANAL DISORDERS

Hemorrhoids

Hemorrhoids are varicose dilatations of the veins lying under the membranous lining of the anal canal. They are a very common distressing condition and may be classified as internal or external. Internal hemorrhoids underlie the upper portion of the anal canal which is lined by mucous membrane similar to that of the intestine. External hemorrhoids occur in veins in the lower portion of the

[19]T. F. Nealon (Ed.): Management of the Patient With Cancer. Philadelphia, W. B. Saunders Co., 1965, p. 658.
[20]J. M. Naish, and A. E. A. Read: Basic Gastroenterology. Bristol, John Wright and Sons Ltd., 1965, p. 463.

canal, which is lined by smooth skin. The external hemorrhoids cause more pain and pruritus because the skin in that area contains pain receptors.

The cause of hemorrhoids is basically an increased back-pressure of the blood in the rectal and anal veins, leading to dilatation. In many instances no cause of the increased pressure and dilatation is identified. They have a high incidence in persons with varicosities in the legs and seem to be hereditary, for several members of the same family may be affected. Predisposing factors are chronic constipation, pregnancy, intra-abdominal tumors, portal hypertension and long periods of standing.

Manifestations of hemorrhoids are bleeding with defecation, protrusion of a small mass through the anus, pain (especially with and following defecation), itching, and a feeling of a mass or pressure in the anal canal. Protrusion of hemorrhoids usually occurs with defecation, and for a period of time, the person is able to manually replace them within the canal. The hemorrhoid may become thrombosed or strangulated because of prolapse and constriction by the anal sphincter. Edema, inflammation and swelling ensue and the person experiences severe pain.

Any person who has pain or bleeding in the anorectal area is urged to see a physician promptly, for these may be indications of a more ominous condition. Temporary relief in hemorrhoids may be obtained by the application of an analgesic ointment such as Nupercaine or the insertion of a suppository containing cortisone or an analgesic and astringent. A sitz bath or the application of warm moist compresses may also be used. Constipation should be avoided; mineral oil may be prescribed to keep the stool soft.

Hemorrhoids may be treated by surgical excision (hemorrhoidectomy) or by injection with a sclerosing agent such as sodium morrhuate. Injection treatment is not used if there is an infection, severe prolapse or thrombosis of the hemorrhoids.

Preparation for surgery includes cleansing of the lower bowel by enemas and cleansing and shaving of the anal and perianal area. At the completion of the excision of the hemorrhoids, a small rubber tube or vaseline gauze packing may be inserted into the rectum to permit the escape of flatus and the drainage of blood should bleeding occur. Hemorrhage is the most common complication following hemorrhoidectomy; therefore, the dressing, vital signs and the patient's reaction should be checked frequently during the first 12 hours. Considerable pain and discomfort are experienced and an analgesic is usually necessary to provide relief and ensure rest. The patient may find the prone position more comfortable. When on his back, pressure on the operative area may be relieved by a sponge rubber cushion.

If a tube or packing has been used, it is usually removed the first or second postoperative day, and a sitz bath is ordered twice daily which generally provides considerable comfort. A rubber air ring should be provided for the patient during the bath and someone should remain with him in case of weakness and fainting. The patient is encouraged to be active and may be out of bed and walking the day after operation.

Urinary retention is a common problem especially during the first 24 hours and catheterization may be necessary.

A light diet is usually permitted as soon as the patient can tolerate it. In some instances, a low-residue diet is ordered until the patient's bowels move.

A mild, stool-softening laxative, such as mineral oil or petrolagar, is usually given once or twice daily, starting on the second postoperative day. If there is no bowel action on the third day, an oil retention enema followed by a gentle cleansing water or saline enema may be ordered.

The patient may be permitted to leave the hospital once defecation is established and there is no abnormal rectal discharge. He is advised to continue the sitz baths, avoid constipation by taking plenty of fluids and including fresh fruits and roughage in his diet, and to resume a moderate amount of activity. The doctor may suggest that the laxative should be continued with a gradual decrease in the dosage until it can be omitted. The patient is given an appointment to see his surgeon or visit the clinic in 2 or 3 weeks for an examination. Occasionally anal stricture develops, and dilatation at regular intervals may be necessary.

Perianal Abscess

Infection and abscess formation may occur in the tissues around the rectum and anus.

The most frequent site is the fatty tissue in the space between the rectum and the ischial tuberosity. The infection may originate in the anal glands, which normally drain into the canal. A gland may become blocked and infected and may rupture into the ischiorectal tissue, causing infection and abscess formation. It may also be caused by organisms escaping from the anal canal through a fissure into the surrounding tissue. A fissure is an ulcerated linear area in the lining of the anal canal.

The patient complains of pain in and around the rectum and anus and develops a fever, leukocytosis and local tenderness and swelling near the anus.

The affected area is incised and drained as soon as possible to prevent rupture into the intestine. The incision is packed with vaseline gauze, and the area is allowed to heal and fill in by granulation. The packing is changed daily and moist hot compresses or vaseline gauze dressings are used over the area. Sitz baths may be ordered twice daily. Precautions are taken to prevent soiling of the dressing during voiding and defecation; a square of plastic material or oiled silk may be placed over the dressing. The female bed patient may lie in the prone position while voiding into a basin. A low-residue diet is given for several days, and laxatives that produce liquid stools are avoided.

The wound may still be open when the patient leaves hospital; instruction is necessary as to the wound care, the taking of sitz baths, the need for thorough cleansing after voiding and defecation, and the importance of follow-up visits to the clinic or the surgeon.

Fistula in Ano

This is an abnormal tract extending from the lumen of the anal canal through the peri-anal tissue to the skin surface beside the anus. It is usually the result of a perianal or ischiorectal abscess and may be associated with ulcerative colitis or a tubercular infection. There is a persistent blood-stained purulent discharge.

Surgical treatment may consist of dissection of the tract or of simply opening it up widely for adequate drainage. Gauze packing is inserted, and the wound is left to heal by granulation. This usually requires several weeks, and the patient is taught to care for

the wound so that he may convalesce at home.

Pilonidal Sinus

A pilonidal (hair-bearing) sinus is a small tract underneath the skin that develops in the cleft between the buttocks in the sacro-coccygeal region. It may have several openings onto the surface and occurs most frequently in persons with a deep cleft and a generous growth of hair on the skin. The moist, soft skin of the area and the movement of the buttocks contribute to the penetration of the skin by short stiff hairs. The area is constantly irritated and readily becomes infected, forming a pilonidal abscess. The person may not know of the sinus until infection becomes manifested by local pain, redness, swelling and purulent drainage.

The condition is treated by incision and drainage. The sinus is laid open and cleansed of hair and pus. A soft rubber drain or gauze packing is inserted and the wound heals by granulation. If there is no infection, the sinus tract is excised and the wound is closed.

Precautions are necessary to avoid contamination of the dressings and wound when the patient voids or defecates. Bowel movements are delayed for the first few days, and straining at stool is avoided. A stool-softening laxative may be used and an oil retention enema given before the first bowel movement.

The patient may be confined to bed for several days and is required to lie in the prone or lateral position. When moving or when allowed up, strain on the incision is avoided, and when walking is permitted, short steps should be taken.

HERNIA

A hernia is a defect in the normal continuity of the wall of a cavity through which a structure contained in the cavity may protrude. It applies most frequently to a defect in the abdominal wall, the respiratory diaphragm or the pelvic floor. A pelvic hernia, or weakness of the muscle and fascia that support the pelvic structures, may result in prolapse of the pelvic organs—the bladder, rectum and uterus. Pelvic herniation frequently occurs in the female following delivery of a child. Prolapse of the bladder is referred to as a cystocele, prolapse of the rectum as rectocele and that of the uterus is known simply as uterine prolapse.

Herniation of the diaphragm is discussed under Disorders of Respiration (see p. 304).

Abdominal Hernia

Unless qualified by diaphragmatic or pelvic, the term hernia refers to abdominal hernia. Various classifications and descriptive terms are used in relation to abdominal hernias.

Congenital or Acquired Hernias. A hernia may be congenital, which implies that the defect in the abdominal wall was present at birth. The acquired hernia develops later in life and is most often due to heavy lifting and excessive strain on the abdominal wall or to a weakening due to surgery.

Inguinal, Femoral and Umbilical Hernias. These terms denote the location of the hernia. The inguinal hernia may occur at the site at which either the left or right spermatic cord or the round ligament emerges from the abdominal cavity and enters the respective inguinal canal. Each canal proceeds obliquely through the abdominal muscles and terminates in the aponeurosis of the external oblique muscle. The spermatic cord passes from the canal and descends into the scrotum; the round ligament of the female emerges and inserts in the labium majus. The opening through which the cord or ligament enters the canal is referred to as the internal or deep inguinal ring; the point of exit is called the external or superficial inguinal ring. These inguinal rings are weak areas and may become the site of a hernia when intra-abdominal pressure is increased. During fetal development, when the cord or ligament enters the canal, it pushes ahead of it a portion of the peritoneum (processus vaginalis) that normally becomes obliterated. In some instances it may persist and predisposes to the protrusion of a segment of intestine or omentum into the canal.

An inguinal hernia may be classified as indirect or direct. The term indirect is applied when there is a herniation of a portion of the peritoneum and a segment of bowel through the internal ring and inguinal canal. The hernia contents may continue into the scrotum or labium. The indirect hernia is considered to be basically congenital.

A direct inguinal hernia is usually acquired and is a herniation of peritoneum and bowel through a weakened area in the abdominal wall in the inguinal region. It develops as a result of continuous or frequent increased intra-abdominal pressure.

A femoral hernia occurs in the area of the abdominal wall through which the femoral artery passes from the abdominal cavity into the thigh. The femoral ring of each side is located in the groin. A portion of bowel or omentum may escape through the femoral ring, producing a swelling and mass in the groin.

An umbilical hernia is due to a failure of the fascia in the area of the umbilicus to completely close or heal firmly. It is usually recognized with the increased intra-abdominal pressure associated with crying, straining and coughing.

Reducible or Irreducible (Incarcerated) Hernia. A reducible hernia is one in which the contents of the hernia can be manually replaced in the abdominal cavity. If the bowel or omentum cannot be returned to the cavity, it is referred to as an irreducible or incarcerated hernia. The irreducibility is determined by the size of the inguinal ring through which the viscera escaped and the amount of intra-abdominal pressure.

Strangulated Hernia. When a hernia is irreducible there may be compression at the internal ring of the blood vessels supplying the viscus within the hernia. Unless relieved promptly, the strangulated viscus becomes gangrenous.

Incisional or Ventral Hernia. Protrusion of a segment of intestine or omentum through an old incision may occur if there is incomplete or poor healing of the abdominal muscle and fascia.

Double Hernia. If herniation occurs in both inguinal canals or both femoral rings it is said to be double, or bilateral.

Causes and Incidence of Hernia. Most abdominal hernias other than incisional are thought to occur primarily as the result of a congenital weakness at the site. The hernia may be evident early in life, or it may not develop until later when the weakened area is subjected to increased intra-abdominal pressure or to an increased relaxation or weakening of the abdominal muscles and fascial tissues. The increased intra-abdominal pressure may be due to severe coughing, straining at stool, vomiting, heavy lifting, obesity, pregnancy or a tumor. Loss of muscular tone and weakening of the fascial tissues may develop as the result of sedentary habits, prolonged illness or malnutrition.

Incisional hernia occurs most frequently following wound infection and drainage and has occurred in patients who were very debilitated at the time of operation.

Inguinal hernia has a much higher incidence in males, and femoral hernia is more common in females. Umbilical hernia that becomes manifest after infancy is seen more often in females.

An abdominal hernia is usually recognized first as a swelling at the site involved when the patient is upright or when he coughs. The swelling disappears when the person lies down and the hernia contents return to the abdominal cavity. Pain may be present due to traction on the viscus or local irritation of the peritoneum and is relieved when the hernia is reduced. If the hernia cannot be reduced, impairment of the blood supply to the herniated bowel is likely to develop, causing strangulation, increasingly severe pain and symptoms of bowel obstruction. A strangulated hernia presents an acute surgical emergency.

Treatment and Nursing Care. The desirable and most effective treatment of hernia is surgical repair (herniorrhaphy). The hernia contents are replaced into the peritoneal cavity, the hernial sac is removed, and the weakened defective area in the abdominal wall is repaired by firm suturing of the muscular and fascial tissues over or around the openings. Precautions are taken in the inguinal hernia to avoid trauma of the spermatic cord or round ligament.

More conservative treatment may be necessary in some instances in which surgery would be too great a risk or the patient simply refuses operation. The hernia is reduced, and the patient is fitted for a truss, which is a firm pad that is placed directly to the skin against the hernia opening and held in place by a belt. It is fitted and applied while the patient is in the dorsal recumbent position. The truss is only worn during the day unless there is frequent coughing or vomiting that increases intra-abdominal pressure. The skin under the truss and belt should be bathed daily and lightly powdered to prevent irritation.

The truss is only applied if the hernia is reduced; otherwise serious damage could be done to the hernia contents. The physician advises the patient that he can probably reduce the hernia by lying flat with feet elevated and gently pushing the contents through the hernia orifice. If at any time he cannot readily reduce the hernia, prompt medical assistance should be sought. Overmanipulation in attempting reduction traumatizes the herniated viscera, causing swelling and edema that further predispose to strangulation.

The nurse has an important role in encouraging persons with a hernia to accept the physician's advice of surgical repair. The patient may find it difficult to submit to surgery when not experiencing any discomfort or disability. Left unrepaired, the hernia may become larger and may restrict certain activities which could condition his employment. The repair becomes more difficult as the defect in the abdominal wall becomes larger, and there is an increasing risk of the hernia becoming irreducible and strangulated, which would necessitate emergency surgery.

Preparation for herniorrhaphy includes the usual considerations cited in Preoperative Nursing Care on page 107. Close observation should be made to detect any signs of respiratory infection, since the increased intra-abdominal pressure associated with coughing could weaken or break down the repair postoperatively. Local skin preparation includes the abdomen, the pubis and the upper part of the thigh on the affected side.

If the hernia is irreducible and strangulated, demanding surgical intervention as quickly as possible, the preparation is the same as that for any emergency surgery (see p. 114) and will most likely include gastric or intestinal intubation and suctioning to relieve the vomiting and distention. Intravenous fluids may be given during the brief preparation and continued during the operation, as the patient may have lost much fluid. If signs of shock are present, a blood transfusion may be given to increase the circulating volume.

Postoperatively, the patient usually makes a rapid, uneventful recovery if the hernia was uncomplicated by strangulation at the time of repair. The male patient who has an inguinal herniorrhaphy may require a scrotal support in the form of a suspensory or elastic athletic support to reduce tension on the spermatic cord and the possible edema and swelling. The scrotum should be examined frequently during the first 2 or 3 postoperative days. Rarely, bleeding into the scrotum and the formation of a hematoma may occur, and swelling or discoloration should be reported. Application of ice bags to the scrotum may be suggested to relieve swelling and pain.

Urinary retention is a common postoperative problem and may necessitate catheterization. Excessive distention of the bladder is to be avoided because of pressure on the repair. If the patient's condition permits and the surgeon approves, he may be able to void more easily if he stands.

The patient who has had an inguinal or femoral herniorrhaphy is usually allowed out of bed the day after operation unless there is swelling of the scrotum, and is encouraged to move about. Before leaving the hospital, the patient is advised of the needed restriction on strenuous activities, such as lifting or pushing, and the importance of avoiding constipation and straining at stool. The physician discusses the patient's return to his occupation; the length of time needed before he returns to work is influenced by the type of work he does, his age and the size of the hernia that was repaired. If his job involves heavy lifting and straining that might predispose a recurrence of the hernia, the surgeon may recommend a change of job. This may be a problem for the patient, and the assistance of a social or rehabilitation worker may be necessary to place the patient in lighter work. There could be a period of unemployment that creates hardships for his family; it may be necessary to arrange for financial assistance or welfare service.

The surgical treatment of the irreducible hernia involves the release of the hernial contents and re-establishment of the blood supply to the bowel segment; the latter is encouraged by the application of warm moist towels. If the released bowel remains devoid of circulation and is gangrenous, it is resected and an end-to-end anastomosis is done. The hernia is repaired as quickly as possible. The nursing care involves the same considerations as for a regular herniorrhaphy as well as those necessary because of the bowel resection. For a discussion of care involved with a bowel resection, see page 374.

The repair of an incisional hernia involves the excision of the old scar, opening of the peritoneal sac, replacement of the protruding viscus into the abdominal cavity and firm closure of the peritoneum and fascia. Preparation of the patient for surgery may include the insertion of a nasogastric tube, which is left in place for 1 to 2 days postoperatively to prevent vomiting and distention, which would put a strain on the repaired area.

Treatment of an umbilical hernia in an infant will depend on the size of the fascial defect. The hernia may be treated by the continuous application of gentle pressure by means of elastic tape or a girdle-type of band made of crepe or elastic bandage. The mother should be instructed as to its purpose, and she is told to examine the area frequently to note any change. If the protruded area appears to be enlarging, the infant should be seen by the physician. The child's increasing activity, sitting up, standing and walking strengthen the abdominal wall and a small hernia may close without surgical intervention. If the defect is relatively large and protrusion of the intestine is readily apparent under the skin, the surgeon may consider early surgical repair necessary to prevent the possibility of rupture of the hernial sac (peritoneum) and ensuing peritonitis.

References

BOOKS

Beeson, P. B., and McDermott, W. (Eds.): Cecil-Loeb Textbook of Medicine, 13th ed. Philadelphia, W. B. Saunders Co., 1971, pp. 1233–1376 and 1420–1458.

Bockus, H. L.: Gastroenterology, 2nd ed. Volume I. Philadelphia, W. B. Saunders Co., 1963.

Davis, L. (Ed.): Christopher's Textbook of Surgery, 9th ed. Philadelphia, W. B. Saunders Co., 1968. Chapters 22 and 23.

Gius, J. A.: Fundamentals of General Surgery, 3rd ed. Chicago. Year Book Medical Publichers Inc., 1966, Chapters 13, 14, 15, 16 and 22.

Green, J. H.: An Introduction To Human Physiology, 2nd ed. London, Oxford University Press, 1968, Chapters 83 and 89.

Harrison, T. R., et al. (Eds.): Principles of Internal Medicine, 4th ed. New York, The Blakiston Division, McGraw-Hill Book Co., Inc., pp 1577–1669.

Jacob, S. W., and Francone, C. A.: Structure and Function in Man, 2nd ed. Philadelphia, W. B. Saunders Co., 1970. Chapter 13.

Jones, F. A., and Gummer, J. W. P.: Clinical Gastroenterology, Oxford, Blackwell Scientific Publications Ltd., 1960.

Naish, J. M., and Read, A. E. A.: Basic Gastro-Enterology, Bristol, John Wright and Sons Ltd., 1965.

Sodeman, W. A., and Sodeman, W. A., Jr.: Pathologic Physiology, Mechanisms of Disease, 4th ed. Philadelphia, W. B. Saunders Co., 1967, Chapters 23, 24, 25 and 26.

Sutton, A. L.: Bedside Nursing Techniques in Medicine and Surgery, 2nd ed. Philadelphia, W. B. Saunders Co., 1969, pp 309–311.

PERIODICALS

Dericks, V. C.: "Rehabilitation of Patients with Ileostomy." Amer. J. Nurs., Vol. 61, No. 5. (May 1961), pp. 48–51.

Drummond, E. E., and Anderson, M. L.: "Gastrointestinal Suction." Amer. J. Nurs., Vol. 63., No 12 (Dec. 1963), pp. 109–113.

Hallburg, J. C.: "The Patient with Surgery of the Colon." Amer. J. Nurs., Vol. 61., No. 3 (Mar. 1961), pp. 64–66.

Hansen, D. E.: "Abdominal Hernias." Amer. J. Nurs., Vol. 61, No. 3 (Mar. 1961), pp. 102–104.

Klug, T., Ellensohn, J. A., and Zollinger, R. M.: "Gastric Resection. Medical and Surgical Care." Amer. J. Nurs., Vol. 61, No. 12 (Dec. 1961), pp. 73–76.

Magruder, L., Ranch, M. K., and May, C.: "Gastric Resection. Nursing Care." Amer. J. Nurs., Vol. 61, No. 12 (Dec. 1961), pp. 76–77.

McKittrick, J. B., and Shotken, J. M.: "Ulcerative Colitis." Amer. J. Nurs., Vol. 62., No. 8. (Aug. 1962), pp. 60–64.

Parks, A. G.: "Hemorrhoidectomy." Surg. Clin. North Amer., Vol. 45., No. 5 (Oct. 1965), pp. 1305–1315.

Secor, S. M.: "Colostomy Care." Amer. J. Nurs., Vol. 64, No. 9 (Sept. 1964), p. 127.

Snively, W. D.: "Peptic Ulcer—An Industrial Health Problem." Amer. Ass. Industrial Nurses J., Sept. 1964, pp. 19–21.

Taylor, S. G., et al.: "Colon Cancer." Med. Clin. North Amer., Vol. 48, No. 1. (Jan. 1964), pp. 215–226.

Thomas, B.: "Nursing in Rectal Disorders." Canad. Nurse, Vol. 62, No. 3 (Mar. 1966), pp. 38–39.

White, D. R.: "I Have an Ileostomy." Amer. J. Nurs., Vol. 61, No 5. (May 1961), pp. 51–52.

Wolfman, E. F., and Fotte, C. T.: "Carcinoma of the Colon and Rectum." Amer. J. Nurs., Vol. 61., No. 3 (Mar. 1961), pp. 60–63.

Usher, F. C., and Matthews, J.: "Surgery: Treatment of Choice for Hernia." Amer. J. Nurs., Vol. 64., No. 9 (Sept. 1964), pp. 85–87.

16
Nursing in Disorders of the Liver and Biliary Tract

PHYSIOLOGY OF THE BILIARY SYSTEM

The biliary system consists of the liver, gallbladder and bile ducts.

LIVER

The liver is the largest organ of the body and is situated in the upper abdominal cavity immediately below the diaphragm. It is divided into 4 lobes and is highly vascular, receiving its blood supply from two sources. The portal vein carries blood from the stomach, intestines, spleen and pancreas into the liver. The hepatic* artery delivers blood from the aorta. The blood from both sources leaves the liver by a common pathway, the hepatic vein, which joins the inferior vena cava.

The liver tissue is organized in functional units called lobules. Each lobule consists of rows of cells radiating out from a central vein. Subdivisions of the hepatic artery and portal vein deliver blood into small spaces (called sinusoids) between the rows of cells,

bringing the blood in direct contact with the hepatic cells. From the sinusoids it enters the central vein. Large phagocytic, reticulo-endothelial cells called Kupffer cells lie scattered within the sinusoids to ingest and destroy organisms and other foreign material. The central veins from the lobules empty into the sublobular collecting veins, which unite to form the hepatic vein. Minute ducts into which bile is discharged are also formed between the rows of hepatic cells. The small lobular bile ducts are directed toward the surface of the lobules where they unite to form larger ducts. Eventually, the bile from the lobules is transmitted in one main channel, the hepatic duct, which joins the bile duct from the gallbladder (cystic duct) to form the common bile duct.

Functions of the Liver

The liver performs a variety of very important functions.

Production of Bile. The liver cells secrete 500 to 1000 cc. of bile daily. It is a yellow-green or brownish fluid that is strongly alkaline and bitter to taste. The constituents of bile are:

1. Water (90 to 97 per cent). The water

---

*From *hepar,* the Latin word meaning liver.

content is reduced when the bile is stored in the gallbladder where it is concentrated 6 to 10 times.

2. Bile pigments. The pigments resulting from the breakdown of red blood cells and from foods are excreted as the bile pigments bilirubin and biliverdin. Bilirubin is orange-red and is in greater concentration in man; the biliverdin is green and predominates in persons or species whose diet is predominantly vegetable.

In the intestine, bile pigments are acted upon by bacteria and are reduced to urobilinogen. Part of the urobilinogen is excreted in the feces, giving them the normal brown color. The remainder is absorbed into the blood and carried to the liver where it is reconverted to bilirubin and again is secreted in the bile.

3. Bile salts (sodium glycocholate and sodium taurocholate). These are sodium salts of certain amino acids,* and they function in digestion and absorption. The bile salts emulsify fats, increasing the digestive action of the fat-splitting enzyme, and promote absorption of fats, fat-soluble vitamins and calcium salts. The bile salts are reclaimed from the intestine and returned to the liver by the portal circulation where they stimulate the hepatic cells to secrete bile. They are reused in the secretion.

4. Other constituents. Sodium and calcium salts, cholesterol, fatty acids and mucin.

The functions of bile may be summarized as follows:

Bile aids the digestion and absorption of fats in the small intestine. Being alkaline, it neutralizes the acidic chyme when it moves into the small duodenum. It stimulates peristalsis of the large intestine which is the basis of the use of bile salts in preparations of laxatives. The reabsorbed bile salts stimulate hepatic cells to secrete bile. Bile is an excretory medium for some drugs (e.g., phenol), toxins, excess minerals (e.g., copper and zinc), pigments and cholesterol.

Metabolic Functions. The liver has a role in the metabolism of carbohydrates, proteins and fats. Briefly, it converts glucose to glycogen and stores it (glycogenesis), re-

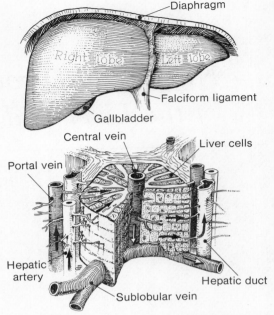

Figure 16-1 The liver and an enlarged section of its lobule.

converting it to glucose and releasing it into the blood when it is required in order to maintain an adequate blood sugar concentration. Glucose in excess of what can be converted to glycogen is changed to fat (lipogenesis) in the liver. The simple sugars, or monosaccharides, fructose and galactose cannot be utilized by the cells, so the liver changes the molecules to glucose.

Fats are desaturated; fatty compounds such as phospholipids, cholesterol and lecithin are formed; and fats are broken down, producing ketone acids.

Protein may be deaminized, a process in which the amine radical is removed and the remaining elements are used to form glycogen or other compounds to meet tissue needs. The amine radical is converted to urea and released into the blood for elimination by the kidneys. Amino acids are also used in the liver to form blood proteins.

Storage. The liver stores glycogen; vitamins A, D, and B_{12}; iron; phospholipids; cholesterol; and a small amount of protein and fat.

Formation of Certain Blood Components. In the fetus, the liver produces the erythrocytes. This activity gradually diminishes after midterm when erythropoiesis in the bone marrow increases. After birth, the

---

*Sodium glycocholate. Glycine + cholic acid → glycocholic acid + sodium → sodium glycocholate.

Sodium taurocholate. Taurine + cholic acid → taurocholic acid + sodium → sodium taurocholate.

liver stores vitamin B_{12} and releases it as necessary to promote the production of erythrocytes.

Prothrombin, heparin and the blood proteins serum albumin, fibrinogen and alpha and beta globulins are formed by the hepatic cells.

Destruction of Erythrocytes. The Kupffer cells break down the worn-out erythrocytes. The hemoglobin is released, the iron and globin are split off, and bilirubin is formed from the waste products and is excreted in bile. The iron is reclaimed, combined with a protein to form ferritin and stored until it is necessary for the formation of hemoglobin.

Detoxification of Poisonous Substances. Certain drugs and chemicals that could be harmful to tissue cells are changed by the liver and rendered harmless before being circulated and excreted by the kidneys. The liver detoxifies by conjugation, oxidation or hydrolysis. In conjugation, it combines the toxic substance with some other material to produce an inoffensive compound (e.g., benzoic acid is changed to hippuric acid). Barbiturates, nicotine and strychnine are drugs that are oxidized and completely destroyed by the liver.

The body itself produces certain chemicals (hormones) that, unless destroyed, would reach too high a concentration. Examples of physiological products that are destroyed in the liver are the antidiuretic hormone (ADH), progesterone and adrenocorticoid secretions.

The Kupffer cells also protect the body by their destruction of organisms that may have been absorbed from the intestine.

Heat Production. The liver is second only to muscle tissue in the production of heat by continuous cell activity. Under basal (resting) conditions, the liver is responsible for most of the body heat.

GALLBLADDER AND BILE DUCTS

The gallbladder is a sac on the undersurface of the liver with an average capacity of 40 to 50 ml. The cystic duct leading from the gallbladder merges with the hepatic duct to form the common bile duct. The latter unites with the pancreatic duct to form the ampulla of Vater which opens into the duodenum. This opening is controlled by the sphincter of Oddi.

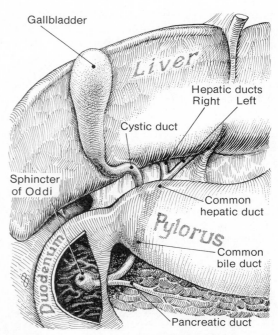

Figure 16–2 The gallbladder and the hepatic, cystic, pancreatic and common bile ducts.

Smooth muscle, connective tissue and a mucous membranous lining compose the walls of the gallbladder and ducts.

The functions of the gallbladder are to concentrate and store the bile. When the stomach and duodenum are empty of food, the opening from the ampulla of Vater remains closed. During this period, the bile that is continuously secreted accumulates in the gallbladder. Contraction of the sac to eject the bile is dependent upon hormonal stimulation. When food enters the duodenum, a hormone called cholecystokinin is secreted by cells of the duodenal mucosa. It is carried in the blood and, on reaching the gallbladder, stimulates the smooth muscle tissue to contract and eject bile. Movement of food through the duodenum causes a relaxation of the sphincter of Oddi, and bile flows into the duodenum.

LIVER DISORDERS

Liver function is essential to life, and fortunately, this large organ has exceptional functional ability and regenerative capacity. If liver disease is limited and tissue damage is localized to one area of the organ, the body is not likely to suffer serious impairment of function. If there is diffuse disease and parenchymal damage, dysfunction is more marked. Liver disease may be acute or chronic, and disturbed function may be reversible or irreversible, depending on the amount of tissue involved and the nature of the cause.

Manifestations of Impaired Liver Function

Jaundice (Icterus). This is an indication of an excess of bilirubin in the blood, resulting in a yellowish staining of the tissues that may be seen in the sclerae, mucous membranes and skin. The cause may be intrahepatic or extrahepatic disease, and according to the cause, the jaundice may be classified as hepatocellular, obstructive or hemolytic.

The hepatocellular type of jaundice is associated with intrinsic liver disease and is due to failure of the hepatic cells to take up the bilirubin resulting from the breakdown of red blood cells and excrete it as bile. Jaundice may not be present in chronic liver disease (e.g., cirrhosis), especially in the early stages, since regeneration of the hepatic cells may parallel the damage.

Obstructive jaundice is caused by an interference with the flow of bile in the extrahepatic ducts. It is most often due to the impaction of gallstones in the common bile duct but may occur as the result of a stricture in the duct or neoplastic disease in neighboring structures (e.g., pancreas). Hemolytic jaundice occurs when there is an inordinate destruction of red blood cells, resulting in excessive bilirubin formation.

The jaundiced patient's urine is likely to be dark because of the bilirubin or urobilinogen content. Urobilinogen is not present in obstructive jaundice, since it is formed in the intestine. The stools are pale gray in obstructive and severe hepatocellular jaundice.

The pruritus experienced by many patients with jaundice is attributed to irritation of the cutaneous sensory nerves by the retained bile salts.

General Constitutional Symptoms. The patient complains of a poor appetite, vague digestive discomfort and flatulence, and loses weight. Lassitude, weakness and muscle wasting develop as a result of the impaired storage of carbohydrates and protein metabolism. A low-grade fever may be present.

Pain. Dull, aching pain in the right upper abdominal quadrant is a common complaint, especially in acute liver disease, and tenderness is manifested on palpation.

Bleeding Tendency. Inadequate production of prothrombin and the accessory Factors V and VII result in failure of the normal clotting process. Spontaneous bleeding may occur, manifested by purpura, epistaxis, bleeding of the oral mucous membrane, and melena.

Ascites and Edema. An accumulation of fluid in the peritoneal cavity develops with progressive liver disease, such as cirrhosis. The hepatic tissue damage, obliteration of blood vessels, and compression by the fibrous tissue (scar) replacement produce a resistance to the outflow of blood from the portal vein. The resulting increase in the blood pressure within the portal vein and its contributaries promotes the escape of fluid into the peritoneal cavity.

Some patients also develop a generalized edema because of the failure of the liver to produce sufficient serum albumin to maintain the normal colloidal osmotic pressure of the blood (see p. 54). Reduced liver activity results in increased concentrations of antidiuretic hormone and aldosterone (an adrenocorticoid secretion), further contributing to edema. These secretions, normally destroyed by the liver, promote reabsorption of water and sodium by the kidneys.

Dilated Veins and Varicosities. The portal hypertension associated with liver disease is reflected in changes within the veins that drain into the portal vein. They become dilated and varicosities develop. The esophageal and gastric veins are commonly affected, and because they are close to the surface, one may rupture, resulting in massive hemorrhage manifested by hematemesis or melena or both. Hemorrhoids develop because of the pressure and resistance to blood flow within the rectal veins.

Splenomegaly. The spleen enlarges because of the hyperplasia of the reticuloendothelial tissue and congestion, causing considerable discomfort for the patient.

Skin Changes. In progressive chronic liver failure, several changes are likely to appear in the skin. Arterial spiders (spider angiomas or nevi) may develop in which a superficial arteriole gives rise to a series of fine, radiating branches readily visible on the surface. These lesions are seen predominantly on the face, neck, arms and chest.

The palms of the hands are frequently mottled, bright red and warm because of capillary dilatation (palmar erythema). There is a loss of axillary and pubic hair in both sexes, and facial hair grows more slowly than usual in the male.

Neurological Disturbances. Severe hepatic insufficiency leads to various mental changes. The patient may manifest irritability and behavior not previously characteristic. He may become inactive, apathetic, and forgetful. These symptoms may progress to confusion, lack of cooperation, stupor and eventually coma.

Twitching and a peculiar coarse tremor, referred to as the flapping tremor, develop. The flapping tremor consists of a series of rapid irregular alternating flexion, and extension movements at the wrist and finger joints occur when the arms and hands are extended.

Ammonia toxicity is considered to be an important factor in producing the mental changes, coma and other abnormal central nervous system responses. The liver is unable to convert the ammonia that results from a breakdown of amino acids to urea.

Fetor Hepaticus. In advanced liver disease, the breath has a fecal odor and the patient complains of a bad taste in the mouth. It is attributed to disturbed amino acid metabolism and abnormal bacterial action in the intestine.

Diagnostic and Liver Function Tests

Plasma Proteins (Serum Albumin and Globulin Concentrations). Serum albumin is produced by the liver and normally is of greater concentration than globulin, most of which is produced by the lymphoid tissues. In disease of the liver cells, the amount of albumin decreases, and the ratio of albumin to globulin is reversed.

Normal: Total serum proteins, 6 to 8 Gm. per 100 ml. Albumin, 3.5 to 5.5 Gm. per 100 ml. Globulin, 1.5 to 3 Gm. per 100 ml. A/G ratio, 3:1.

Serum Bilirubin (van den Bergh's Test). This test gives an estimation of the concentration of bilirubin in the blood and indicates whether it is conjugated or unconjugated. Normally, the liver cells extract the pigment from the blood and convert it to a water-soluble compound (bilirubin diglucuronide) before excreting it in bile. Unconjugated bilirubin is usually reported as "indirect bilirubin" and the conjugated form as "direct bilirubin." In obstructive jaundice, the conjugate (direct) bilirubin level is increased. In hemolytic jaundice, unconjugated (indirect) bilirubin is the predominant pigment in the blood.

Normal: Conjugated (direct) bilirubin, 0.2 mg. or less per cent. Unconjugated (indirect) bilirubin, 0.2 mg. to 0.7 mg. per cent. Total serum bilirubin, 0.4 to 1.1 mg. per cent.

Icterus Index. This test is a rough estimate of the concentration of bilirubin in the blood. The intensity of the yellowness of the serum is observed. It may be used to determine the decrease or increase of jaundice.

Normal: 4 to 6 units.

Serum Alkaline Phosphatase. Normally this enzyme is excreted in the bile by the hepatic cells. The blood concentration may be increased when there is liver disease or obstruction in the bile ducts.

Normal: 2.0 to 4.5 Bodansky units; 5.0 to 13.0 King-Armstrong units.

Serum Transaminases. The liver cells contain the enzymes serum glutamic oxalacetic transaminase (SGOT) and serum glutamic pyruvic transaminase (SGPT). Since they are released into the blood when the cells are damaged, their concentration may be used to estimate liver damage.

Normal: SGOT, 5 to 40 units; SGPT, 5 to 35 units.

Prothrombin Time. A decrease in the blood content of prothrombin may result from the failure of diseased liver cells to produce it or from a vitamin K deficiency. A vitamin K deficiency may result from the absence of bile salts in the small intestine, since they are necessary for the absorption of the fat-soluble vitamin.

Normal: 11 to 12 seconds.

Galactose Tolerance Test. Normally, most of the galactose is quickly taken from the blood and converted to glycogen by the liver cells. An abnormal concentration in the blood 1 to 2 hours following the administration of 100 ml. of a 25 per cent solution of galactose indicates impaired function of the liver. The galactose is given after an 8- to 10-hour fast, and a blood sample is collected in 1, 1½ and 2 hours following the administration.

Bromsulphalein (BSP) Test. Bromsulphalein is a dye normally excreted by the liver cells in the bile. The test is used to detect liver cell damage and impaired function. It is not used if obstruction in the bile ducts is suspected because the dye would be retained in the body. Five mg. of bromsulphalein for each kilogram of the patient's body weight is given intravenously, and a venous blood specimen is collected in 45 minutes. Normally, only 5 per cent or less of the dye given remains in the blood.

Hippuric Acid Test. Benzoic acid is detoxified by the liver cells by combining it with glycine to form hippuric acid, which is then circulated in the blood and eliminated in the urine. To test hepatic function, sodium benzoate is given either by mouth or by intravenous injection. Urine is then collected and examined for the hippuric acid concentration.

The procedure is as follows: 6 Gm. of sodium benzoate is dissolved in 250 ml. of water and given orally. The urine is collected over the next 1 to 4 hours. Intravenously, 1.77 Gm. of sodium benzoate is given slowly, and a urine specimen is collected in 1 hour.

Normally, with the oral administration of the sodium benzoate, 2 to 3.5 Gm. of hippuric acid will be excreted in the urine in 4 hours. Following the intravenous administration, 0.7 Gm. of hippuric acid should appear in the urine in 1 hour.

Serum Cholesterol. The concentration of cholesterol in the blood falls in liver disease when cell function is impaired and rises in obstructive jaundice.

Normal: 150 to 250 mg. per cent.

Urinary Bilirubin. A urine analysis may be requested for bilirubin. The pigment is present in the urine in obstructive jaundice and hepatocellular jaundice but is absent in hemolytic jaundice.

Urinary Urobilinogen. Conjugated bilirubin is changed to urobilinogen by bacterial action when the bile reaches the small intestine. Most of the urobilinogen is then excreted in the feces, and the remainder is absorbed. A small amount of the absorbed urobilinogen is excreted in the urine, but the larger portion is claimed by the liver to be excreted in the bile. If the liver cells are damaged, they may not perform this latter function, and the amount of urobilinogen excreted by the kidneys is increased. The amount of the pigment in the urine may be decreased below the normal amount in obstructive jaundice when bile is not reaching the intestine or if the bacterial content of the intestine is reduced, as it is in oral administration of antibiotics.

Normal: Less than 4 mg. in the urine per 24 hours or less than 1.0 Ehrlich units in 2 hours.

Blood Ammonia. In severe impairment of liver function, the ammonia concentration in the blood is elevated and may lead to hepatic coma.

Normal: 20 to 50 mg per cent.

Liver Biopsy. A small specimen of liver tissue may be examined microscopically to assist in the diagnosis of liver disease. The specimen is obtained by aspiration with a special liver biopsy needle. Using a lateral approach, the needle is passed through the ninth or tenth intercostal space or may be introduced below the costal margin if the liver is enlarged.

Previous to the procedure, the patient's bleeding, coagulation and prothrombin times are checked. The biopsy is not done if there is a prolongation of these. An explanation is made to the patient of the purpose of the biopsy and what will be expected of him during and after the procedure. He is required to sign a consent. His pulse, respirations and blood pressure are noted by the nurse for comparison following the biopsy.

The patient is placed in the supine position close to the right side of the bed. The area is cleansed, and an antiseptic and sterile drape are applied. A local anesthetic is then injected at the puncture site. The patient is instructed to take 2 or 3 deep breaths, then to stop breathing following exhalation. The physician quickly introduces the biopsy needle, aspirates and withdraws, taking only a few seconds.

Following the biopsy, absolute bed rest is necessary for 24 hours, The patient is required to lie on his right side with a small pillow under the costal margin. This position places pressure against the biopsy site, preventing the escape of blood and bile. Close observation is made of the patient for hemorrhage for 24 hours. The pulse, respirations, blood pressure, color and general condition are noted and recorded every 15 minutes for 2 to 3 hours. The interval is then gradually increased if there are no significant changes. Abdominal pain, tenderness and any rigidity are reported, since they may indicate irritation and inflammation of the peritoneum due to the leakage of bile from the liver.

Radioisotope Liver Scan. A radioactive isotope known to be taken up normally by the liver may be given intravenously, and an estimation is then made of the uptake by means of a special external detector of radioactivity. Rose bengal tagged with radioactive iodine (I^{131}), gold (Au^{198}) or vitamin B_{12} tagged with radioactive cobalt (Co^{60}) may be used. The photoscan made by the detector indicates nonfunctioning and functioning areas of the liver tissue. Areas or lesions which do not take up the radioactive material appear as blanks or as much lighter areas in the recording of the scan.

Other Studies. A barium swallow under fluoroscopic examination (see p. 333) or an esophagoscopy (see p. 333) may be done to detect venous dilation and varicosities in the esophagus resulting from portal hypertension. A splenoportogram may be undertaken in which an opaque dye is injected into the spleen and an x-ray taken of the upper abdomen and lower chest. The dilated portal vein and its branches show up, and gastroesophageal varices may be recognized.

Viral Hepatitis

The commonest inflammatory disease of the liver is due to viruses. Two types of these are currently recognized: one is referred to as the IH or A virus; the other is known as the SH or B virus. Hepatitis due to the former organism is classified as infectious hepatitis; that caused by the SH virus is known as homologous serum hepatitis.

Infectious hepatitis accounts for the greater number of cases of hepatitis. The disease can be epidemic and has a higher incidence in children and young adults. It has an incubation period of 10 to 40 days and is included in the reportable diseases.

The IH virus is present in the blood and feces and may be transmitted by contaminated food or water, parenteral injections of infected plasma or blood, or parenteral injections with contaminated syringes or needles.

Serum homologous hepatitis has a longer incubation period (2 to 6 months) and has no age preference. Transmission of the SH virus is via the parenteral route only by contaminated needles or syringes or infected blood, serum or plasma.

Manifestations. The virus attacks the hepatic cells, and inflammation and necrosis follow. The swelling and congestion interfere with normal bile formation and flow, resulting in jaundice and elevated blood bilirubin levels. Transaminase levels (SGOT and SGPT) rise sharply because of the necrosis, and the serum albumin-globulin ratio may indicate a reduced formation of albumin. Fortunately, in most cases complete regeneration of the liver cells occurs on recovery with a minimum of fibrous tissue formation and scarring. Very few patients experience residual impairment of liver function.

The signs and symptoms of the two infections are similar and may vary in intensity from one individual to another. The onset is usually manifested by vague symptoms such as fatigue, loss of appetite, nausea, vomiting, headache, fleeting abdominal and joint pains, and fever. After several days, abdominal discomfort and tenderness in the right upper quadrant are more predominant, the urine becomes dark, either constipation or diarrhea may be troublesome, the stools may be abnormally light in color and jaundice becomes evident.

Treatment and Nursing Care. Since there is no specific treatment for viral hepatitis, supportive therapy and attention to the patient's discomforts comprise the principal care.

REST. The patient is kept on bed rest during the active stage of the disease. With subsidence of fever, there is a decrease in the tenderness of the liver and a lowering of the serum bilirubin and transaminase levels. Activity is resumed slowly, and the patient is observed for reactions. Some persons regain their strength slowly and should not be encouraged to resume full activity until they feel equal to it.

Drugs (such as barbiturates and morphine) normally inactivated by the liver are not usually prescribed.

NUTRITION AND FLUIDS. In the acute stage, it is difficult for the patient to take sufficient fluids and food because of the nausea, vomiting and aversion to food. An increased fluid intake of at least 3000 ml. is necessary because of the fever and to promote urinary elimination of the serum bilirubin. If the patient cannot tolerate fluids orally, glucose 5 or 10 per cent is given intravenously to sustain the patient.

A high-calorie diet of 3000 calories is recommended; nutritional deficiency retards the liver's ability to overcome the infection and regenerate functional tissue. As soon as the nausea and vomiting are controlled, the patient is offered small amounts of high-calorie foods frequently. These are gradually increased until the ultimate goal of 3000 calories is achieved. The diet consists principally of protein and carbohydrate. The fat content may be restricted while there is jaundice but is increased, as tolerated, by the addition of whole milk, eggs and butter, which make the diet more palatable. Fried foods, fat meat and rich foods, such as pastries, usually are avoided for several weeks or months after recovery.

The patient's weight is checked at regular intervals, since there may have been a considerable loss in the early phase of the disease.

SKIN AND MOUTH CARE. Frequent bathing and changes of linen during the period of fever are necessary. The use of soap is avoided if the patient is jaundiced, and the water should be warm but not hot. The heat and the alkali in the soap tend to increase the pruritus frequently associated with jaundice. Starch or sodium bicarbonate added to the bath water or oatmeal tied in a bag and squeezed through the water may provide some relief from the itching. Caladryl lotion or cream, or calamine lotion with phenol 1 per cent applied following the bath may also be used. The fingernails are kept short and clean to prevent injury and infection of the skin in case of scratching.

PREVENTION OF THE SPREAD OF INFECTION. Unless the causative agent of the patient's hepatitis is definitely known to be the SH virus, all patients with viral hepatitis are treated as potentially infectious and are isolated. Personnel caring for the patient are informed of the sources of the infective organisms (feces and blood) and of the fact that they are unusually resistant to heat, disinfectants and prolonged exposure to cold and freezing.

The patient occupies a single room, and a gown is worn by those giving care. The hands are scrubbed under running water with hexachlorophene (pHisohex) after each contact. The bed linen is placed in a clean bag at the bedside and is disinfected before being laundered. Treatment equipment is disinfected after each use and is used only for the infected patient. Equipment used in procedures involving penetration of the skin (e.g., needles and syringes) is sterilized by high dry heat (oven) or autoclave (steam under pressure). If such facilities are not available, the equipment is boiled for at least 30 minutes. The use of disposable syringes and needles is recommended for all parenteral administrations.

If it is necessary to take the temperature by rectum, the nurse wears gloves while handling the thermometer, which is kept immersed in a strong disinfectant and thoroughly rinsed before use. Some institutions recommend discarding the thermometer when the patient is discharged since it cannot be sterilized by heat. The patient is advised of the importance of thorough hand washing after going to the toilet. The patient's bedpan is disinfected after each use. Stools are disinfected before the usual disposal by covering the feces with a disinfectant such as formalin 10 per cent or cresol (Lysol) 5 per cent for at least 1 hour.

The period of isolation is determined by the physician according to the patient's progress.

CONTACTS. Known contacts of infectious hepatitis are advised to consult a physician as soon as possible. An intramuscular injection of human serum gamma globulin may be given to provide protection. It is effective against the IH virus but not against the SH organism. The gamma globulin may not always provide immunity but is found to lessen the severity of the disease should the person develop it.

Toxic Hepatitis

Rarely, inflammation and degenerative changes in the liver occur as a result of a chemical. Carbon tetrachloride, phosphorous, sulfonamides, arsenical preparations and chloroform are examples of suggested offenders. The patient is treated by prompt withdrawal of the causative chemical, rest and supportive care.

Cirrhosis of the Liver

The term cirrhosis denotes chronic degenerative tissue changes in which there is destruction of parenchymal cells and formation of excessive dense fibrous scar tissue. Blood, lymph and bile channels within the liver become distorted, compressed and effaced with subsequent intrahepatic congestion, portal hypertension and impaired liver function. The fibrous tissue changes result in the liver becoming smaller and firmer. The surface is usually rough because of small projecting nodules of regenerated hepatic cells.

Etiological Factors and Classification

DIETARY DEFICIENCY. Many cases of cirrhosis of the liver are thought to be the result of malnutrition and a deficiency of protein. An accumulation of fat in the liver has been experimentally produced in animals by the restriction of protein. This dietary constituent is necessary for the provision of substances essential for normal fat metabolism in the liver, one of which is choline. Methionine, an amino acid, is necessary for the synthesis of choline by the body.

ALCOHOLISM. Cirrhosis of the liver is a common sequel to chronic alcoholism. It is suggested that the degenerative liver changes develop as a result of interference with normal nutrition over a relatively long period. Persons who become dependent on alcohol are often indifferent to food and consume less. The calories provided by the alcoholic beverages* suppress the appetite for food, resulting in a lack of essential food factors. Many persons show a marked improvement in the earlier stages of cirrhosis when alcohol ingestion is discontinued and a high-protein, high-vitamin diet is taken. Such evidence supports the theory that the liver changes in the alcoholic are secondary to the associated malnutrition.

It is also thought that liver damage in

---

*One ounce of alcohol provides approximately 75 to 90 calories.

the alcoholic may be related to an increased choline requirement incurred by the alcohol.

HEPATITIS. Severe hepatitis in which there has been extensive necrosis followed by considerable scarring may lead to cirrhosis.

CHRONIC CHOLESTASIS. Degenerative changes characteristic of cirrhosis may also occur with prolonged cholestasis (obstruction to the flow of bile). The cause is usually partial obstruction by a stone or stricture within the extrahepatic bile ducts but may be intrahepatic as a result of infection or inflammation and subsequent stricture of the small ducts within the liver.

Certain terms may be used to classify cirrhosis according to the cause. Cirrhosis due to nutritional deficiency and alcoholism may be referred to as Laennec's, portal or atrophic cirrhosis. When cirrhotic changes are a result of hepatic necrosis and subsequent fibrous scarring, the condition is known as postnecrotic cirrhosis. The term biliary cirrhosis is used to denote cirrhosis associated with cholestasis.

Signs and Symptoms. The liver has considerable reserve; early cirrhotic changes generally go unrecognized without apparent manifestations. With the characteristic insidious progress, signs and symptoms of impaired liver function appear gradually over a period of years. See page 396 for manifestations.

Treatment and Nursing Care. The care required by the patient with cirrhosis depends on the extent of the liver damage.

Since the progress of the disease is influenced by nutritional deficiency, a diet of 2500 to 3000 calories, high in protein (110 to 150 Gm.), carbohydrate and vitamins is recommended. Sufficient fat to make it palatable is added if the patient can tolerate it and is not jaundiced. Three small meals with in-between snacks will probably be more acceptable to the person than 3 large meals. The sodium intake is restricted because of the tendency to develop edema and ascites. Low sodium protein concentrate and low sodium milk are available and may be used to assist with the protein intake. Total abstinence from alcohol is very important.

Potentially toxic drugs normally inactivated by the liver are avoided. Examples of these are barbiturates, chlorpromazine and opiates. The patient's resistance to infection is lower and precautions are taken to avoid possible contacts.

If there is no ascites or signs of impending hepatic coma, the patient remains ambulatory, and a limited amount of activity that does not produce excessive fatigue is encouraged to promote appetite as well as circulation. In more advanced liver impairment, bed rest is recommended. The patient's lassitude necessitates thoughtful nursing measures such as frequent change of position, special skin care and passive exercises to combat the effects of prolonged inactivity.

The patient is weighed at the same time each day with the same amount of clothing and is observed for signs of edema. The daily fluid intake and output are measured and recorded. A diuretic such as chlorothiazide (Diuril), mercaptomerin sodium (Thiomerin) or spironolactone (Aldactone) is ordered if there is retention of fluid. The diuretic is given in the morning so the patient is not disturbed at night by frequent voiding. The total urinary output is noted to determine the effectiveness of the drug. The blood is checked for potassium and sodium levels, since the diuretic may cause hypokalemia and hyponatremia.

The abdomen is examined daily for evidence of developing ascites, and the girth is measured and recorded. An abdominal paracentesis may be necessary if the fluid in the peritoneal cavity reaches a volume that is causing respiratory distress, compression of abdominal viscera and blood vessels, and considerable pain and discomfort. The nurse explains the paracentesis procedure to the patient, and makes sure his bladder is empty. The head of the bed is elevated and the patient is supported with pillows. The physician may wish to have the patient sitting on the side of the bed with a support to his back and feet. A sphygmomanometer is placed in readiness on one arm. The necessary sterile equipment and fluid receptacle are brought to the bedside. Following the application of an antiseptic and sterile drapes, the physician injects the site with a local anesthetic before introducing the trocar and cannula. A tube is attached to the cannula to drain the fluid into the receptacle.

During the procedure, the nurse checks the patient's pulse, color and blood pressure

and provides necessary support. The physician is promptly alerted if the pulse becomes rapid and weak, pallor is noted, or there is a fall in blood pressure. Not more than 1 or 2 liters is withdrawn at one time. Removal of the fluid results in the loss of considerable plasma protein, especially serum albumin. Also, the sudden reduction of intra-abdominal pressure results in a dilatation of the abdominal blood vessels and a pooling of a large volume of blood that may lead to circulatory collapse and shock.

A sterile dressing is applied to the site of the paracentesis when the cannula is withdrawn, and an abdominal binder is applied snugly. The patient is returned to the dorsal recumbent position, and the head of the bed is lowered. The amount and character of the fluid are recorded. The abdominal site is kept clean and dry to prevent infection and discomfort. The pulse, color and blood pressure are checked at frequent intervals for several hours. A plasma or whole blood infusion may follow the paracentesis to replace the lost protein. Increased diuresis may be observed with the decreased pressure on the renal blood vessels.

The patient with cirrhosis is closely observed for signs of jaundice. If jaundice is present, the skin receives attention similar to that cited on page 400.

If liver insufficiency is serious and the patient is exhibiting neurological disturbances and an elevation in blood ammonia, protein is eliminated from the diet. The patient is sustained on carbohydrates, and if he is comatose, they are administered by nasogastric feedings or intravenous infusions. Crib sides are used to protect the confused, comatose patient. Nursing measures used in the care of any unconscious person are applicable to the patient in hepatic coma (see p. 103).

The patient who improves sufficiently to go home is advised as to what extent he must restrict his usual activity. Strict adherence to his diet, total abstinence from alcohol, and the avoidance of infection and physical strain are stressed when interpreting the regimen prescribed by the physician to the patient and family. He will be required to visit his doctor or a clinic at regular intervals. A referral to a visiting nursing agency may be necessary so that consistent supervision is ensured. The agency is advised of the recommended regimen and of the changes that may indicate regression, necessitating prompt medical care.

The prognosis for patients with cirrhosis depends on the degree of liver insufficiency. If treatment is instituted in the early stages and the patient is sufficiently motivated to adhere to the suggested care, he is likely to live a normal life span. If portal hypertension has developed with resultant ascites and esophageal varices, the prognosis is grave.

Esophageal Varices

As cited previously, the flow of blood from the portal vein through the liver may meet with resistance because of the degenerative changes in the liver. The volume of blood and the pressure in the esophageal veins cause dilatation and a weakening of the wall. These varicosed veins appear as large bulbous protrusions under the mucosa of the esophagus. Food passing over a protruded area may cause ulceration of the mucosa and wall of the vein, and severe hematemesis results. Some blood will enter the stomach and eventually the patient passes tarry stools. Prompt emergency treatment is necessary and includes blood transfusion and the insertion of a nasogastric tube with balloons that are inflated to compress the area of bleeding and the cardiac portion of the stomach (balloon tamponade). The tube also has a lumen that opens into the stomach to permit gastric drainage and is known as the Sengstaken-Blakemore tube.

A more recent form of treatment used to check the bleeding is the continuous application of cold to the esophagus and cardia of the stomach. A special double lumen tube is inserted that permits a continuous circulation of a mixture of alcohol and water through the balloons and a refrigeration unit.

Fresh blood is used in the transfusions to provide thrombocytes and prothrombin to promote clotting. Neither of these blood factors withstands prolonged refrigeration. Parenteral injections of vitamin K may be administered in an effort to increase the prothrombin level.

Bacterial action on the blood that reaches the intestine produces ammonia which is absorbed into the blood. An antibiotic such as neomycin is given to destroy intestinal organisms and prevent this reaction, since the ability of the liver to convert ammonia to urea is impaired.

The patient is critically ill and requires constant observation and attention. The pressure in the balloons must be maintained and is checked at frequent intervals. The blood pressure, pulse, and respirations are re-

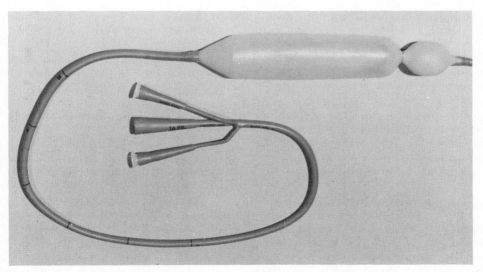

Figure 16–3 A Sengstaken-Blakemore tube which is used in the treatment of bleeding esophageal varices. The tube has three lumens. One leads to the longer inflatable balloon that is positioned in the esophagus to provide pressure. A second lumen ends in the smaller balloon that lies just within the stomach. The third lumen opens into the stomach to permit gastric drainage. (Courtesy of the New Mount Sinai Hospital, Toronto.)

corded frequently, and the patient is kept at complete rest. Narcotics may be necessary to allay the patient's fear and to provide rest. The head of the bed is usually elevated to reduce the flow of blood into the portal system. Since the patient is unable to swallow his saliva, provision is made for suctioning or for expectoration into paper wipes or a basin. Frequent mouth care is necessary, and the nostrils are cleansed and lubricated because of the irritation from the tube. Compression by the inflated balloons is not usually continued longer than 48 hours. Pressure for a longer period could cause edema, ulceration and perforation of the esophagus. The balloons are deflated gradually, and the tube is left in place for continued gastric drainage and in case of recurrence of the bleeding.

Surgical treatment of esophageal varices may be done to relieve the hypertension of the portal venous system and control esophageal bleeding. Various procedures are used. A portocaval shunt in which an anastomosis is made between the portal vein and the inferior vena cava or a splenorenal venous shunt may be done. Rarely, a transesophageal ligation of the veins is undertaken.

Care following a surgical shunt is similar to that of patients undergoing any abdominal surgery. Close observation for hemorrhage and abdominal distention is important. If a nasogastric tube is passed to control vomiting and distention, a soft rubber tube is selected and is introduced very gently to avoid precipitating variceal hemorrhage. Specific orders are received from the surgeon as to the amount of movement of the patient permitted and whether deep breathing, coughing, and leg exercises are to be carried out. Similarly, the patient receives nothing by mouth until specifically ordered.

In the case of a splenorenal shunt, a retention catheter is inserted, and a close check is kept on the urinary output.

Accidental Injury

Rupture of the liver in accidents is not uncommon. Any interruption of the capsule enclosing the hepatic tissue carries the risk of severe internal hemorrhage that may prove fatal before surgical intervention is possible. A blood transfusion is given, and surgical repair undertaken. Control of the bleeding is of prime importance. The area may be sutured or packed, or oxycel gauze (Gelfoam) may be applied. The latter supplies fibers on which the clot may form more easily. In addition to the loss of blood incurred in injury, peritonitis may develop as a result of the chemical irritation caused by the bile that may escape from the liver. Destruction of liver cells may also follow the injury, resulting in impaired liver function.

Neoplastic Disease

Benign and primary malignant newgrowths are rare in the liver, but it is a frequent site of metastasis, especially if the primary malignant neoplasm is in the abdominal cavity. The malignant cells may be transported to the liver via the portal venous or hepatic arterial blood or via the lymph. In many instances, secondaries in the liver are discovered before the primary sources. The liver enlarges and signs of liver insufficiency develop. The patient experiences pain, food intolerance, anemia, emaciation and ascites.

If a primary newgrowth is confined to one lobe of the liver, a hepatic lobectomy may be done. Following the operation, the patient is observed closely for possible hemorrhage and biliary peritonitis.

Liver Abscess

Infection with subsequent abscess formation occurs rarely and is most often associated with amebic dysentery. The causative organisms (*Entamoeba histolytica*) are carried by the portal blood stream from the bowel. The pyogenic infection may also be caused by staphylococcus, streptococcus or *Escherichia coli*. Along with manifestations of impaired liver function, the patient has chills and a high fever. There may be one or multiple small abscesses which frequently coalesce, forming one large cavity.

The patient is treated with antibiotics and also receives chloroquine or emetine hydrochloride (antiamebic drugs) if the abscess is a complication of amebiasis. The abscess is drained by aspiration followed by the injection of an antibiotic into the cavity. Open surgical drainage is avoided if possible because of the danger of dissemination of the infection within the peritoneal cavity and resultant peritonitis.

DISORDERS OF THE GALLBLADDER AND BILE DUCTS

Gallstone formation, inflammation or neoplastic disease may occur in the extrahepatic biliary system (gallbladder and ducts). These disease processes interfere with the normal flow of bile into the duodenum.

Manifestations

Disease of the extrahepatic biliary system may be acute or chronic, and the intensity of the signs and symptoms parallels the severity of the condition.

Pain. The pain associated with gallbladder or biliary duct disease may be felt in the right upper abdomen or mid-epigastric region or is referred to the right scapular area. It may be a persistent, dull ache or very severe and disabling. The onset may follow a meal containing fatty foods. When it is very severe and prostrating, the pain is described as biliary colic.

Digestive Disturbances. The patient may experience flatulence and an uncomfortable full feeling or nausea, especially after the ingestion of fatty or fried foods. Vomiting is usual if the patient has biliary colic or develops obstructive jaundice.

Jaundice. Obstruction of the hepatic or common bile duct as a result of a calculus, stricture or neoplasm causes regurgitation of bile into the blood, and the patient develops obstructive jaundice.

Fever. Chills and an elevation of temperature frequently accompany infection and inflammation within the gallbladder or bile ducts.

Bleeding Tendency. An obstruction to the flow of bile into the intestine decreases the absorption of vitamin K, resulting in a reduced prothrombin level and failure of the normal blood clotting process.

Cholelithiasis

This is the term used for stones in the gallbladder. Their formation is not understood. They vary in shape and size and consist mainly of cholesterol and bile pigments. There may be one stone or many, and although they may develop in both sexes, they occur more often in middle-aged females. Cholelithiasis may not give rise to any disturbance in many persons; in others, the stones cause signs and symptoms ranging from mild digestive disturbances following fat ingestion to all those previously cited under manifestations. Gallstones may cause acute or chronic inflammation of the gallbladder (cholecystitis) or cholestasis (stasis of the bile) within the liver, leading to impaired function of that organ. Small stones tend to cause more acute problems, since they may escape into the ducts. If this happens, the patient suffers intense, incapacitating pain (biliary colic). The stone may be passed into the duodenum, or it may lodge in the cystic or common bile duct or the ampulla of Vater. Impaction of a stone in the common bile duct leads to obstructive jaundice.

Cholelithiasis is treated surgically by removal of the gallbladder and exploration of the common bile duct for a stone or stricture. The surgery is not usually done during an acute attack unless obstruction of the common bile duct persists.

During an episode of biliary colic, the patient remains in bed. An antispasmodic drug such as atropine, propantheline (Pro-Banthine) or nitroglycerine may be ordered to relieve the painful reflex spasm that occurs in response to the stone in a duct. Morphine or meperidine hydrochloride (Demerol) may also be prescribed in conjunction with one of the above drugs, but some physicians avoid their use because they oppose relaxation of the sphincter of Oddi.

Food and fluids by mouth are withheld, and the patient is given intravenous fluids. If vomiting and abdominal distention occur, a nasogastric tube is passed and suction drainage established. Local applications of heat to the upper abdomen may be ordered; precautions to guard against burning are necessary, since the excruciating colic pain and the analgesics may dull the patient's awareness of the heat.

Following the acute episode and removal of the nasogastric tube, clear fluids are given and gradually increased to a light, low-fat diet as tolerated.

The patient is observed for signs of jaundice, and the color of all stools is noted. The nurse may be requested to save the stools for examination for the presence of the stone that has passed from the biliary tract into the intestine.

If the patient is jaundiced, and the stools are a pale gray, indicating an absence of bile in the intestine, a daily dose of vitamin K (Synkayvite, Mephyton, Hykinone) is given parenterally to maintain prothrombin formation and prevent bleeding.

Cholecystitis

Inflammation of the gallbladder may be acute or chronic. Acute cholecystitis is most often associated with gallstones but may occur without them due to infection. The patient manifests pain and tenderness in the right upper abdominal quadrant or mid-epigastrium, fever, nausea and vomiting and leukocytosis. The severity of the symptoms varies with the degree of inflammation. Jaundice may develop if the inflammation involves the biliary ducts.

The treatment includes bed rest, intravenous fluids, analgesics and antibiotics. If the condition persists or worsens, it may indicate suppuration (empyema of the gallbladder), necessitating surgery. A cholecystostomy (drainage of the gallbladder) or a cholecystectomy (removal of the gallbladder) may be done.

Chronic cholecystitis is characterized by a long history of vague digestive complaints. The patient experiences abdominal discomfort, and flatulence after a large rich meal or one high in fats. A dull, aching pain and nausea and vomiting may occur at times. The intensity and probably the frequency of the symptoms insidiously increase over months or years.

The chronic inflammation results in scarring and thickening of the wall of the gallbladder and cholestasis. If calculi are present, they progressively increase in size or number. The patient may have subacute or acute exacerbations in which he becomes incapacitated by nausea and vomiting, moderate fever and probably mild colic. The condition is usually treated surgically by removal of the gallbladder.

Carcinoma of Gallbladder

Cancer of the gallbladder is rare and is usually associated with calculi. It is usually recognized when a cholecystectomy is done because of stones. The symptoms may be similar to those of chronic cholecystitis,

gradually increasing in severity with persisting pain. Obstructive jaundice frequently develops with compression of the biliary ducts by the enlarging gallbladder. Obstructive jaundice may also result from extension of the malignant disease to the common bile duct.

Bile Duct Disorders

Obstruction of the common bile duct may occur as a result of a gallstone that has escaped from the gallbladder (choledocholithiasis), inflammation (choledochitis or cholangitis), neoplasm or a stricture formed by scar tissue following trauma and inflammation. The duct above the obstruction dilates and obstructive jaundice develops.

In the case of an impacted stone, the duct is opened and the calculus is removed. When a stricture is present and the area is sufficiently small, it is resected and an end-to-end anastomosis performed. If the obstruction is due to primary carcinoma, excision may be undertaken and the duct stump anastomosed to the duodenum (choledochoduodenostomy) or the jejunum (choledochojejunostomy).

Extrinsic pressure on the bile ducts obstructing the flow of bile may occur with cancer of the pancreas or duodenum.

When surgery involves an extrahepatic bile duct, a T-tube is inserted at the site of entry into the duct to maintain bile drainage during recovery of the tissues. The stem portion of the tube is brought out on the abdominal surface through a stab wound or the incision and is attached to a drainage bottle. Surgery on a bile duct is usually accompanied by a cholecystectomy, since the gallbladder is frequently the origin of the problem.

Nursing Care of Patients with Extrahepatic Disorders

Surgery is not usually done during an acute attack of cholecystitis or cholelithiasis unless the signs and symptoms are unremitting or progressive. The patient is kept at rest, and food is withheld. If there is vomiting, a nasogastric tube is passed and suction-siphonage is established (see p. 338). The temperature, pulse and respirations are recorded every 3 or 4 hours; a sudden elevation is reported promptly. The patient is checked for signs of obstructive jaundice and abdominal distention.

When the vomiting is controlled and the nasogastric tube removed, oral fluids are given and graduated, as tolerated, to a light, bland, low-fat diet. If the patient is obese, the caloric intake is limited to approximately 1000 calories daily.

Preoperative Care. Preoperative preparation (see p. 107) for surgery on the extrahepatic biliary system includes close observation for jaundice and the administration of vitamin K to raise the prothrombin level. Special attention is given to having the patient understand the importance of the frequent coughing and deep breathing that he will be required to carry out after the operation. Because of the site of the surgery, the patient tends to take very shallow breaths to prevent pain and discomfort, predisposing to respiratory complications. A nasogastric tube is usually passed before the patient is taken to the operating room.

Postoperative Care. General postoperative care as outlined in Chapter 10 is applicable. Close observation for bleeding is necessary, since low prothrombin levels may still exist. The drainage tube that is inserted in a cholecystostomy or choledochostomy is generally clamped during the transfer from the operating room; after the patient is transferred, it is immediately attached to a drainage receptacle which is placed at the level specified by the surgeon. The tubing leading to the receptacle is secured to the dressing and lower bed linen and should have sufficient slack to prevent traction and dislodgment. The patient is advised as to how to turn to avoid a pull on the tube and of the need to be sure that it is not kinked or compressed. The drainage is observed frequently during the first 24 hours in case of hemorrhage. There may be a small amount of blood mixed with bile in the first

few hours, but persistent bleeding is reported to the surgeon. The character and daily amount of bile drainage are recorded. If there is a prolonged loss of bile, it may be given back to the patient through a nasogastric tube for the purpose of promoting more normal digestion and absorption in the intestine. For esthetic reasons, the patient is not usually told of this procedure. The dressing is checked frequently for possible bleeding or bile leakage. After a few days, the drainage tube is clamped for stated intervals and is removed when the surgeon considers the common bile duct is patent. Following removal of the tube, the dressing is observed for bile seepage. If the dressing is soiled with bile, it is changed frequently, the skin and wound are cleansed, and vaseline gauze, an ointment or powder is applied to prevent excoriation and maceration. The patient is also observed for signs of peritonitis; an elevation of the temperature, abdominal pain, distention and rigidity are reported at once.

Until the procedures become less painful and the patient is less fearful, the nurse's assistance and support are required during the frequent, regular coughing, deep breathing and change of position. Early ambulation is generally urged, and provision is made for a small drainage receptacle that may be attached to the patient's dressing gown.

The urine, stools, sclerae and skin are checked for any indication of obstructive jaundice.

The patient receives intravenous solutions of glucose and electrolytes until the nasogastric tube is removed and oral fluids and food are tolerated. The fat content of the diet is limited.

In preparation for discharge, the patient's diet is discussed. Generally, the surgeon will suggest that the patient gradually increase the fat intake over a period of 4 to 6 months and find his own level of tolerance.

References

BOOKS

Beeson, P. B., and McDermott, W. (Eds.): Cecil-Loeb Textbook of Medicine, 13th ed. Philadelphia, W. B. Saunders Co., 1971, pp. 1377–1419.

Davidson, Sir Stanley: The Principles and Practice of Medicine, 7th ed. London, E. & S. Livingstone Ltd., 1965, pp. 963–1022.

Davis, L. (Ed.): Christopher's Textbook of Surgery, 9th ed. Philadelphia, W. B. Saunders Co., 1968. Chapter 24.

Harrison, T. R., et al. (Eds.): Principles of Internal Medicine, 4th ed. New York, Blakiston Division, McGraw-Hill Book Co., Inc., 1962, pp. 146–166 and 1670–1718.

Sherlock, S.: Diseases of the Liver and Biliary System, 3rd ed. Oxford, Blackwell Scientific Publications, 1963.

Sodeman, W. A., and Sodeman, W. A., Jr.: Pathologic Physiology, 4th ed. Philadelphia, W. B. Saunders Co., 1967. Chapters 27 and 28.

PERIODICALS

Bielski, M. T., and Molander, D. W.: "Laennec's Cirrhosis." Amer. J. Nurs., Vol. 65, No. 8 (Aug. 1965), pp. 82–86.

Bradley, S. E. (Ed.): Symposium on "The Liver and Its Diseases." Med. Clin. North Amer., Vol. 47, No. 3 (May 1963).

Conn, H. O., and Simpson, J. A.: "A Rational Program for the Diagnosis and Treatment of Bleeding Esophageal Varices." Med. Clin. North Amer., Vol. 52, No. 6 (Nov. 1968), pp. 1457–1472.

Hayter, J.: "Impaired Liver Function and Related Nursing Care." Amer. J. Nurs., Vol. 68, No. 11 (Nov. 1968), pp. 2374–2379.

Leevy, C. M.: "Cirrhosis in Alcoholics." Med. Clin. North Amer., Vol. 52, No. 6 (Nov. 1968), pp. 1445–1454.

Schimmel, E. M.: "Diagnostic Procedures in Liver Disease." Med. Clin. North Amer., Vol. 52, No. 6 (Nov. 1968), pp. 1407–1416.

17
Nursing in Disorders of the Pancreas

PHYSIOLOGY OF THE PANCREAS

The pancreas is a fish-shaped gland; the thicker portion, referred to as the head, lies in the curve of the duodenum, and the remainder extends to the left directly behind the stomach. It has two distinct types of essential functional cells. Groups of one type secrete into small ducts which drain into a main channel running the length of the gland. This collecting channel is called the pancreatic duct or the duct of Wirsung and passes out of the head of the pancreas to unite with the common bile duct to form the ampulla of Vater. In a few persons, the duct may have a direct entrance to the duodenum. Because the secretion of this type of cell flows through ducts, it is classified as an external, or exocrine, secretion.

The other type of parenchymal cell is scattered in insular groups, forming what are known as the islands of Langerhans. These cells produce secretions which are classified as internal, or endocrine, secretions because they are absorbed into the blood and are not secreted into ducts.

The external secretion passes through the ampulla of Vater and sphincter of Oddi into the duodenum. It contains several digestive enzymes (trypsinogen, chymotrypsin, procarboxypeptidase, amylopsin and lipase) concerned with the breakdown of proteins, carbohydrates and fats. Regulation of the secretion of these enzymes and their role in digestion is discussed under Digestion in the Small Intestine on page 322.

The endocrine functions of the pancreas are the production of insulin and glucagon,

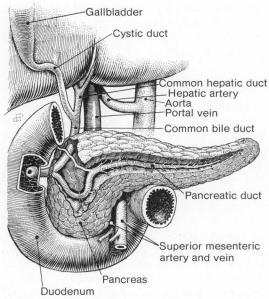

Figure 17–1 Diagram of the pancreas and central pancreatic duct in relationship to the duodenum and the common bile duct.

Labels (clockwise): Gallbladder, Cystic duct, Common hepatic duct, Hepatic artery, Aorta, Portal vein, Common bile duct, Pancreatic duct, Superior mesenteric artery and vein, Pancreas, Duodenum

409

which are concerned with the metabolism of glucose and the regulation of the blood sugar level. Insulin is secreted by the beta cells of the islands of Langerhans and produces a decrease in the blood sugar concentration. It promotes the utilization of glucose by tissue cells and the storage of glucose as glycogen in the liver (see p. 326). Glucagon is formed by the alpha cells of the islands of Langerhans and increases the blood sugar level by stimulating the conversion of liver glycogen to glucose and its release into the blood.

DISORDERS OF THE PANCREAS

Inflammation and neoplastic disease are the pathological conditions seen most frequently in the pancreas.

PANCREATITIS

Inflammation of the pancreas may be acute or chronic with recurrent acute episodes. The organ becomes edematous, and if the inflammatory process subsides in this stage, permanent damage usually results. If the process persists, necrosis and hemorrhage are likely to occur. Necrosis results from activation of the proteinases and lipase, initiating autodigestion of the pancreatic tissue and blood vessels. Enzymes and blood escape into surrounding tissue and the peritoneal cavity.

Etiology

Pancreatitis is considered to be the result of some factor or change within the pancreas that brings about activation of the proteinases and lipase of the exocrine secretion with subsequent breaking down of the ducts, parenchymal tissue and blood vessels. The causative factor may be an obstruction to the flow of the pancreatic secretion within the ducts. Continued secretion produces dilatation and back pressure, resulting in their disruption and the escape of enzymes into the parenchyma. A gallstone or newgrowth in the ampulla of Vater or spasm or edema of the sphincter of Oddi may be the initiating factor. It is suggested that such an obstruction promotes a reflux of bile into the pancreas, promoting activation of the enzymes and the ensuing autodigestion. The source of the obstruction may be a calculus, newgrowth or fibrosis following some irritation within the pancreas. Other possible etiologic factors are considered to be infection and injury of the pancreas. Pancreatitis is most frequently associated with biliary tract disease and alcoholism and has a higher incidence in middle-aged persons.

Manifestations

Acute pancreatitis has a sudden onset, being preceded usually by only mild, vague digestive disturbances. The principal signs and symptoms are pain, gastrointestinal disturbances, obstructive jaundice, shock and hypoglycemia.

Pain. At first, severe incapacitating pain occurs in the upper abdomen, radiating through to the back. It may be described as burning or boring. Later, with progression of the disease, the pain becomes more generalized in the abdomen.

Gastrointestinal Disturbances. Nausea and vomiting occur and persist. Food in the intestine remains undigested because of the lack of pancreatic enzymes and may cause diarrhea. The stools are bulky, greasy and foul-smelling as a result of the undigested fat and protein residue.

Abdominal distention and rigidity appear as a result of the development of peritonitis. The latter is caused by the chemical irritation of the viscera and peritoneum by the enzymes that escape from the pancreas. Peristalsis diminishes, and eventually paralytic ileus and intestinal obstruction may further complicate the patient's condition.

Shock. The patient may manifest severe shock when the pathological process includes necrosis and hemorrhage within the pancreas. This is attributed to the exudation of plasma into the peritoneal cavity that occurs with the peritonitis and also to the loss of blood resulting from the erosion of vessels within the pancreas.

Vital Signs. The temperature is elevated in the early stage but may become subnormal if peritonitis and shock develop. The pulse is rapid, and the blood pressure falls with the decrease in the intravascular volume and the concomitant shock. The patient is flushed at first, then usually becomes pale. If peritonitis develops, he is likely to become a dusky or cyanotic color.

Obstructive Jaundice. If the head of the pancreas is involved, it may compress the common bile duct and cause obstructive jaundice.

Blood Changes. With the escape of enzymes into the pancreatic parenchyma and peritoneal cavity, fatty tissue is broken down into glycerol and fatty acids. The latter combine with calcium to form insoluble calcium soaps. The serum calcium level falls and may be severe enough to produce tetany and affect heart action (prolonged diastole).

Hemoconcentration develops as a result of the loss of plasma. The prothrombin level falls because of the absence of absorption of vitamin K. Serum amylase and lipase levels are elevated.

Disturbance in Glucose Metabolism. A deficiency of insulin may develop when the islands of Langerhans are involved in the pathological process, and hyperglycemia and glycosuria (sugar in the urine) may be reported.

Diagnostic Procedures

The following diagnostic tests may be carried out on the patient suspected of having pancreatitis.

Blood Enzyme Concentrations. Some of the enzymes secreted by the pancreas are normally absorbed into the blood and eventually are excreted in the urine. An elevation of the serum amylase and lipase levels occurs when there is an obstruction of the pancreatic ducts and necrosis of the cells.

Normal: Serum amylase, 60 to 180 units per cent (Somogyi method). Serum lipase, 1.5 units or less or 450 to 850 mg. per cent.

Urinary Amylase Excretion. Urinalysis may indicate an increased excretion of the enzyme amylase in pancreatitis.

Normal: 260 to 950 units in a 24-hour specimen.

Blood Calcium Level. As cited in manifestations of pancreatitis, the disease causes a decrease in the blood calcium level.

Normal: 4.5 to 6.0 mEq. per L. or 9 to 11 mg. per cent.

Stool Examination. Analysis of a stool collection made over a specified number of hours is done to determine the quantitative fat content. With failure of the pancreatic lipase to reach the intestine, fat remains undigested and unabsorbed.

Normal: Less than 5 Gm. per 24 hours or up to 30 per cent of dry weight.

Blood Sugar Concentration. Damage to the islands of Langerhans may cause hyperglycemia and a reduction in insulin secretion.

Normal: Fasting, 80 to 120 mg. per cent.

Secretin-Pancreozymin Test. An evaluation of pancreatic exocrine function may be made by the analysis of aspirated duodenal content following stimulation by an intravenous injection of secretin followed by an injection of pancreozymin.

The dosage of the hormones is calculated by the physician on the basis of the patient's weight. A double lumen duodenal tube is passed; one lumen permits aspiration of the gastric content and the duodenal content is withdrawn through the other at stated intervals over a period of 80 minutes. The total volume is estimated, and the bicarbonate and amylase concentrations are determined.

Normal: Total secretion—at least 2.0 ml. per kg. of body weight. Bicarbonate concentration, 90 mEq. per L. Amylase, 6.0 units per kg. of body weight.

Lundh Test.[1] In chronic pancreatitis, exocrine function of the pancreas may be assessed by analyzing the duodenal content for the enzyme trypsin following a test meal of food that causes the release of the hormones secretin and pancreozymin, which stimulate pancreatic exocrine function. A single lumen duodenal tube (Rehfuss tube) is passed and the test meal consisting of skim milk powder and dextrose dissolved in water is given. Aspirations are made at stated intervals over 2 hours, and the specimens are analyzed for trypsin content.

Treatment and Nursing Care

The patient with acute pancreatitis is critically ill. Care is directed toward the reduction of pancreatic secretion to a minimum, the relief of pain, the prevention of shock or correction if it has developed and

[1]D. H. Hanscom: "Diagnostic Tests in Pancreatic Disease." Med. Clin. North Amer., Vol. 52, No. 6 (Nov. 1968), pp. 1483–1492.

the prevention of infection. Nursing responsibilities involve the following considerations.

Relief of Pain. Meperidine hydrochloride (Demerol) is used parenterally to relieve the patient's pain in preference to opiate preparations (morphine, codeine), since the latter tend to stimulate the contraction of the sphincter of Oddi. The patient is assisted in turning and moving and in finding the least painful position. Frequent attendance and verbal and nonverbal conveyance of an appreciation of the patient's suffering may contribute to making the pain less intolerable.

Observations. The patient's condition may change rapidly with progressive necrosis and resulting hemorrhage. The vital signs and the general response and appearance of the patient are observed frequently. A rapid weak pulse, a fall in blood pressure, pallor and increasing weakness may manifest hemorrhage or shock and are immediately brought to the physician's attention. Frequent hemoglobin and hematocrit estimations may be requested to detect hemoconcentration which would indicate the loss of plasma into the peritoneal cavity. An accurate record is kept of the fluid intake and output.

The intensity and location of the pain are noted, and the abdomen is examined for distention and rigidity. All stools are examined, and if they are bulky, greasy and foul-smelling or show other abnormalities, they are saved until seen by the doctor.

The sclerae and skin are observed for any yellow tinge that would indicate the development of jaundice.

Fluids. The patient receives nothing by mouth to avoid stimulation of the pancreatic secretion. The restoration and maintenance of normal blood volume is very important to prevent or correct shock. Plasma or whole blood may be given as well as electrolyte and glucose solutions intravenously. A close check is kept on the blood chemistry (potassium, sodium, chloride and calcium), gastric drainage volume, urinary output and amount of perspiration to determine the specific electrolyte and fluid needs.

Gastric Drainage. A nasogastric tube is passed and continuous suction drainage established. This relieves vomiting and distention and prevents the acid gastric secretion from entering the duodenum and stimulating the release of the hormones secretin and pancreozymin. The color, consistency and 24-hour volume of the drainage are recorded.

Mouth and Nasal Care. Frequent cleansing and rinsing of the mouth are necessary during the period in which oral intake is restricted because the anticholinergic drug which the patient may be receiving suppresses salivary secretion. Oil, vaseline or a cream is used on the lips to prevent cracking. The nostrils are cleansed with an applicator which has been slightly moistened with normal saline, and a light application of vaseline or water-soluble lubricant is made to the nostril through which the tube passes to prevent irritation and excoriation.

Medications. As well as analgesics, the patient usually receives an anticholinergic drug such as propantheline bromide (Pro-Banthine) and atropine sulfate by intramuscular or subcutaneous injection. These drugs inhibit vagal nerve stimulation of the pancreatic enzymes. Acetazolamide (Diamox) may also be used to suppress secretion through its effect at pancreatic cellular level.

An antibiotic is usually ordered as a prophylactic measure since the inflammation and necrosis make the pancreas very vulnerable to infection. When the gastric drainage is discontinued, an antacid such as aluminum hydroxide gel (Amphojel) may be given orally at frequent intervals to reduce the acidity of the chyme entering the duodenum. Parenteral administration of vitamin K may be necessary to maintain normal prothrombin production and prevent bleeding.

Nutrition. When oral intake is permitted, fluids are introduced in small amounts. The principal nutrient given at first is carbohydrate; protein is added gradually, according to the patient's tolerance. Fats are avoided. The diet is progressively increased to a high-protein, high-carbohydrate, low-fat, light diet. Four or five small meals are recommended. Extract of pancreas (pancreatin) may be given orally with meals to assist with digestion. Large meals are avoided, and total abstinence from alcohol is stressed.

Complications. If paralytic ileus and intestinal obstruction develop, a Miller-Abbott tube may be passed into the intestine and decompression suction established (see p. 338).

Chronic pancreatitis may develop following the initial episode, and acute exacerbations are likely to occur. The chronic form of the disease is associated with the fibrosing and calcification of areas in the pancreas following inflammation and necrosis. The degree of impaired function and the intensity of its signs and symptoms are proportionate to the amount of continuing inflammation or frequency of acute episodes and the ensuing tissue damage. In some instances, slight impairment may be controlled by dietary adjustments and the avoidance of emotional stress, fatigue and infection. In others, the patient may experience almost constant pain, requiring frequent doses of analgesics. Not infrequently, this becomes complicated by the patient's development of a tolerance for the drugs, necessitating progressively larger doses; actual addiction may become a problem. The patient's fear of precipitating more severe pain may lead to a reluctance to eat and a marked loss of weight. Impaired digestion due to the insufficient quantities of enzymes in the intestine and the ensuing steatorrhea also contribute to the loss of weight. Diabetes mellitus may develop, necessitating regular insulin administration to control glucose metabolism.

Another complication that rarely develops in pancreatitis is the formation of one or more pseudocysts. Accumulations of inflammatory exudate, liquefied necrotic tissue and secretions become walled off by a capsule of fibrous tissue. The cyst is atypical in that there is no epithelial lining characteristic of true cysts. This accounts for the term pseudocyst. A cyst may form within or on the surface of the pancreas or in a neighboring area into which pancreatic secretions have escaped. It may enlarge and impose on surrounding structures. The common bile duct may be blocked, the duodenum or stomach may be displaced, or the diaphragm may be elevated. The deviation and location are usually recognized in an x-ray.

The symptoms depend on the size and location of the cyst(s). In some instances resolution takes place spontaneously, or the cysts may produce persisting pain, digestive disturbances, anorexia, loss of weight and mechanical interference with other organs. Surgical drainage may be necessary and may be internal or external, depending on the location of the cyst. Internal drainage is achieved by anastomosing the cyst to the small intestine. If drainage is established through the skin, vaseline gauze or a protective ointment or powder is essential to prevent excoriation of the skin by the enzyme content of the drainage.

Preparation for Leaving Hospital. A long convalescence follows recovery from an acute episode of pancreatitis. The necessary care to avert an exacerbation is discussed with the patient and his family. The importance of strict adherence to the prescribed diet, total abstinence from alcohol and the avoidance of large meals are explained. Verbal and written instructions are given about the content and preparation of the recommended low-fat, high-protein, high-carbohydrate diet. If anticholinergic drugs or antacids are to be continued, verbal and written directions are given which include advice as to early side effects that should be reported to the doctor. To assist with digestion, the patient with chronic pancreatitis may need to continue to take extract of pancreas (pancreatin) orally with each meal.

The patient is encouraged to develop a special interest or hobby within his activity tolerance to help him through the convalescent period. A referral to a visiting nurse agency may be advisable to provide necessary supervision.

Surgical Treatment. Surgery is not usually undertaken during an acute attack of pancreatitis unless there is increasing obstructive jaundice due to an impacted stone. The various operative procedures that may be used to treat the patient may be performed on the biliary tract or directly on the pancreas. They include exploration of the common bile duct and ampulla of Vater and the insertion of a T-tube for drainage, cholecystostomy, cholecystectomy, sphincterotomy to relieve obstruction caused by spasm of the sphincter of Oddi, anastomosis between the common bile duct and duodenum, or anastomosis between the gallbladder and the jejunum. Surgery on the pancreas may be removal of the calculi in the pancreatic duct, drainage of a pseudocyst, or partial or complete pancreatectomy. Occasionally, in severe chronic pancreatitis, a sympathectomy may be done to relieve intractable pain.

The nursing care of patients having surgical treatment is similar to that required by patients having biliary tract surgery (see p. 407).

NEOPLASMS OF THE PANCREAS

Carcinoma

Cancer of the pancreas usually arises from the ducts, and although it may occur in any part of the organ, it is most commonly seen in the head. The patient experiences pain, progressive weakness and loss of weight. Jaundice develops as the newgrowth encroaches on the ampulla of Vater and common bile duct. The cancer may spread by direct invasion to adjacent structures and by metastasis to the liver.

The condition is treated surgically if recognized sufficiently early. A pancreato-duodenal resection may be done which involves resection of the head of the pancreas, ampulla of Vater, duodenum and pylorus with anastomosis between the common bile duct and jejunum, anastomosis between the pancreas and jejunum, and a gastrojejunostomy. This radical surgery is not usually undertaken if the cancer has spread beyond the pancreas. Palliative operations that may be used include a cholecystojejunostomy to relieve obstructive jaundice and a side-to-side anastomosis of the main pancreatic duct (duct of Wirsung) to the jejunum.

Preparation for surgery includes a high-calorie, low-fat diet if tolerated by the patient, intravenous infusion of glucose and electrolyte solutions, blood transfusions and parenteral vitamin K if there is jaundice. Postoperative care includes gastric suction to prevent distention of the jejunum and pressure on the sites of the anastomoses. The patient is supported by blood transfusions and intravenous electrolytes and glucose. Vitamin K administration may be continued.

Adenoma of the Islands of Langerhans

Occasionally an adenoma develops from beta cells of the islands of Langerhans, causing an excessive secretion of insulin (hyperinsulinism) and hypoglycemia. The adenoma is usually benign but, rarely, may be adenocarcinoma.

The symptoms presented by the patient are mainly due to the effect of the abnormally low blood sugar (50 mg. or less per cent) on the brain cells. Brain cells are more sensitive to glucose deficiency than other body cells. The initial symptoms are hunger, restlessness and apprehension. These progress to weakness, loss of coordination, tremors, diaphoresis, disorientation, convulsions and coma. The manifestations appear during a fasting period (early morning) or following extreme exertion. Prompt administration of some form of glucose is necessary to raise the blood sugar. If the hypoglycemia remains untreated, the glucose deficiency may result in permanent brain cell damage or death. When early signs are recognized, the patient is given sugar or orange juice with sugar. In the more advanced stage of hypoglycemia, glucose 50 per cent is given intravenously.

Surgical treatment may consist of excision of the adenoma or subtotal or total pancreatectomy. Preparation for the surgery includes a high-carbohydrate, high-protein diet and intravenous infusions of glucose solution to restore glycogen reserves. The glucose infusion is continued during the operation. Following surgery, close observation is made for a recurrence of hypoglycemia. If a total pancreatectomy is done, the patient will receive supplemental insulin and pancreatic extract for the remainder of his life.

CYSTIC FIBROSIS

Cystic fibrosis is a congenital disease characterized by impaired functioning of the exocrine and mucus-secreting glands throughout the body. The secretions, especially those of the respiratory tract, are abnormally viscous. The sweat and saliva of affected persons have inordinate concentrations of sodium and chloride.

This disease is usually recognized in infancy because of the serious respiratory problems incurred by the thick, tenacious mucus. The secretions are retained, blocking bronchioles and alveoli, and the patient's vital capacity is reduced. As a result, he is very vulnerable to infection. The viscous nature of the exocrine secretions of the pancreas causes a stasis and obstruction in ducts, which may result in cyst-like dilatations and degeneration of tissue and ensuing fibrosis. A deficiency of pancreatic enzymes in the intestine produces incomplete digestion and absorption as well as steatorrhea. The islands of Langerhans are not usually affected. In severe disease, the newborn may fail to pass meconium because of intestinal obstruction, and an ileostomy may have to be done.

Cystic fibrosis is currently considered to be a hereditary disease that is transmitted by a defective gene received from each parent. It is thought that the defect may result in the lack of a specific enzyme, causing interference with the cells' production of their secretions.

The child requires constant, intensive care and supervision. Special measures such as humidifiers and mist tents are used to keep the air in the patient's environment moist to help liquefy the respiratory secretions. Postural drainage, chest physical therapy, regular coughing and breathing exercises are also employed. Antimicrobial preparations may be prescribed to prevent infection. Obviously, any contact with persons who have an infection must be avoided.

The patient receives a high-calorie, high-carbohydrate, high-protein, low-fat diet. Pancreatic extract (pancreatin) is given to promote digestion and absorption. In warm weather, sodium and chloride depletion may occur as a result of increased sweating and may necessitate an increased intake of these electrolytes either orally or by intravenous infusion.

The family is referred to a visiting nursing organization and to a branch of the National Cystic Fibrosis Foundation. The parents generally need considerable assistance in establishing a plan of care for the patient. The socioeconomic demands are great. The medications and therapeutic equipment are expensive, and there is a continuous demand on the parents' time in providing the necessary observation and care. Frequent visits to the clinic or doctor's office are necessary.

References

BOOKS

Beeson, P. B., and McDermott, W. (Eds.): Cecil-Loeb Textbook of Medicine, 13th ed. Philadelphia, W. B. Saunders Co., 1971, pp. 1312–1327.

Cattell, R. B., and Warren, K. W.: Surgery of the Pancreas. Philadelphia, W. B. Saunders Co., 1953.

Davis, L. (Ed.): Christopher's Textbook of Surgery, 9th ed. Philadelphia, W. B. Saunders Co., 1968. Chapter 25.

Harrison, T. R., et al. (Eds.): Principles of Internal Medicine, 4th ed. New York, The Blakiston Division, McGraw-Hill Book Co., Inc., 1962, pp. 1660–1669.

Hess, W.: Surgery of the Biliary Passages and the Pancreas. New Jersey, Van Nostrand Co., Inc., 1965.

Sodeman, W. A., and Sodeman, W. A., Jr.: Pathologic Physiology, 4th ed. Philadelphia, W. B. Saunders Co., 1967, pp. 702–708.

PERIODICALS

Hanscom, D. H.: "Diagnostic Tests in Pancreatic Disease." Med. Clin. North Amer., Vol. 52, No. 6 (Nov. 1968), pp. 1483–1492.

Spencer, J. A., and Palmer, W. L.: "The Diagnosis and Management of Chronic Pancreatitis." Med. Clin. North Amer., Vol. 48, No. 1 (Jan. 1964), pp. 231–238.

18
Nursing in Disorders of the Urinary System

THE URINARY SYSTEM

The urinary system consists of 2 kidneys, 2 ureters, the bladder and urethra. The kidneys are the primary functional structures in which urine is formed. The ureters are drainage tubes which transmit the urine from the kidneys to the bladder where it is temporarily stored. The urethra is a duct that carries the urine to the exterior surface of the body.

Structure of the Kidneys

The kidneys are paired, bean-shaped organs that lie retroperitoneally against the dorsal abdominal wall. Each kidney is enclosed in a fibrous capsule and consists of approximately 1,000,000 nephrons, many collecting tubules and a pelvis. The blood vessels, nerves and ureter enter or leave the kidney at the hilum—the indentation on the medial surface.

Nephron. The nephron is the functional unit of the kidney. It consists of a narrow, convoluted tubule and a tuft of capillaries which is referred to as a glomerulus. The upper end of the tubule is dilated to envelop the glomerulus and is called Bowman's capsule. The remainder of the tubule is divided into three segments—the proximal convoluted tubule, the hairpin-like loop of Henle and the distal convoluted tubule (see Fig. 18-2). The thickness and structure of the walls differ from one segment to another;

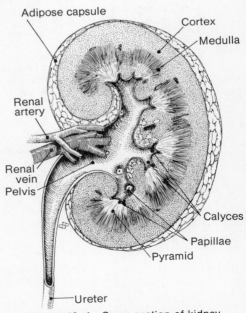

Figure 18-1 Cross section of kidney.

this arrangement accounts for different substances being reabsorbed in different sections of the tubule. The distal tubule terminates in a straight collecting tubule.

Collecting Tubules. The collecting tubules of the nephrons coalesce to form larger collecting tubules. Groups of the large tubes come together to form a pyramid-like structure. The apex of each pyramid is known as the papilla and contains the terminations of collecting tubules through which the urine passes into a cup-like pouch (calyx) of the renal pelvis.

Kidney Pelvis. When the ureter joins the kidney, it expands to form a funnel-shaped receiving basin for the urine delivered by the collecting tubules. It has numerous projecting pouches (calyces), each of which encases a renal papilla and is called a calyx.

Blood Supply. The renal artery to each kidney arises from the abdominal aorta. When the artery enters the kidney, it progressively subdivides to become afferent arterioles. Each afferent arteriole enters a nephron to form a glomerulus. The glomerular capillaries unite to form the efferent arteriole, which terminates in a second capillary network that surrounds the tubule. The blood pressure in this second set of capillaries is much lower than that in the glomerulus. The blood is then collected into venules and eventually into a renal vein that carries it to the inferior vena cava.

A large volume of blood is continuously circulated through the kidneys. It is estimated that the renal blood flow averages about 1000 to 1200 ml. per minute in an adult.

Just before the afferent arteriole becomes the glomerulus, there is an increase in the number of cells in the middle tissue layer of the walls. These cells are known as juxtaglomerular cells. It is suggested that they are responsible for the production of the chemical renin which, when released into the blood, combines with a blood protein (globulin) to form angiotensin. Angiotensin brings about an elevation in the blood pressure through vasoconstriction and stimulates the adrenal cortices to produce aldosterone, which promotes the reabsorption of sodium and water by the kidney tubules. The increased reabsorption leads to an increased intravascular volume, raising the blood pressure.

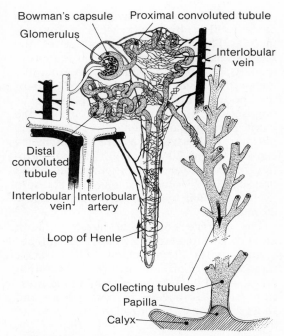

Figure 18–2 A renal unit or nephron of the cortex of the kidney is shown with its blood supply and a collecting tubule.

Innervation. Sympathetic nerve fibers from the thoracolumbar autonomic nervous system transmit impulses to the afferent and efferent arterioles, causing vasoconstriction.

Renal Function

Normal functioning of the body cells is greatly dependent upon a relative constancy of the internal environment. The kidneys play a major role in maintaining this constancy by regulating the water and electrolyte content and the acid-base balance of the body; they conserve appropriate amounts of essential substances vital to normal cellular function (e.g., glucose) and excrete the waste products of metabolism, toxic substances and drugs in the urine. The processes involved in these functions performed by the kidneys are filtration, selective reabsorption and secretion. What remains after these processes occur forms the urine to be excreted.

Filtration. The permeability of the glomerular capillaries is comparable to that of the capillaries elsewhere in the body, and the same principles that govern the movement of fluid out of the arterial ends of the capillaries throughout the body are applicable to the filtration process in the glomeruli. The hydrostatic pressure of the blood in the glomerular capillaries is approximately 70 mm. Hg, which is considerably higher than that in the other capillaries of the body. This hydrostatic pressure is opposed by the osmotic pressure of the blood proteins (approximately 30 mm. Hg) plus the hydrostatic pressure in Bowman's capsule (about 20 mm. Hg). The net filtration force is 20 mm. Hg (hydrostatic blood pressure (70) − colloidal osmotic pressure (30) − capsular hydrostatic pressure (20) = 20 mm. Hg).

The average volume of filtrate in both kidneys is estimated to be about 125 ml. per minute, or 180 liters each day. The filtration rate is directly proportional to the filtration force. A fall in systemic arterial blood pressure, such as occurs in hemorrhage and shock, reduces the filtration pressure and the volume of filtrate. Constriction of the afferent arterioles due to increased sympathetic innervation or obstruction of a renal artery causes a decrease in the quantity of blood reaching the glomeruli and in turn reduces the volume of filtrate. Conversely, dilatation of the afferent vessels increases filtration pressure and volume. Vasoconstriction of the efferent arteriole causes increased glomerular pressure and filtration at first, but if the vasoconstriction is prolonged, filtration is decreased as a result of the blood stasis in the glomerular capillaries.

The concentration of plasma proteins influences the effective filtration pressure; a deficiency lowers the osmotic pressure slightly, raising the net filtration force. Another factor that may reduce filtration is increased pressure within the capsule due to an inflammatory process or obstruction in the tubules or urinary tract. Normally, the formed elements (blood cells) and plasma proteins of the blood do not pass through the glomeruli; the composition of the filtrate is the same as plasma minus the plasma proteins.

Tubular Reabsorption. The composition and volume of the filtrate which enters Bowman's capsule differ markedly from those of urine. Of the 180 liters of filtrate produced in 24 hours, only about 1.5 liters are excreted as urine. Most of the water and many of the solid constituents of the filtrate are needed by the body to maintain homeostasis and normal cell metabolism. Other substances, such as urea, creatinine, uric acid, sulfates and phosphates are waste products of metabolism and are excreted in the urine. The tubule cells selectively reabsorb according to the body's needs. Certain substances, such as glucose and amino acids, are completely reabsorbed when their plasma concentrations are within normal range but appear in the urine when the normal is exceeded. About 99 per cent of the water in the filtrate is reclaimed. Reabsorption of the inorganic salts (e.g., sodium, chloride, calcium, potassium, bicarbonate) is variable, depending mainly on their plasma levels.

Some constituents of the filtrate are passively reabsorbed by diffusion and osmosis through the tubular membrane. Others are reabsorbed by active cellular transport, which entails energy expenditure on the part of the tubular cells and the presence of certain enzymes. The location of reabsorption in the tubules varies with different filtrate constituents. The proximal convoluted tubule is responsible for the greatest amount of reabsorption. All of the glucose and amino acids and a large proportion of the water and other essential substances are reabsorbed here. Only about 20 per cent of the total volume of filtrate enters the loop of Henle.

The maintenance of the volume and concentration of body fluids within a narrow normal range is largely controlled by the ability of the kidney tubules to concentrate or dilute the urine. When body fluids are diluted by an excess of water or diminished solute intake (especially sodium), the urine becomes dilute and the volume is increased. Conversely, if the concentration of body fluids is raised to above the normal level by an excessive intake of solutes or an extra renal loss of water, water reabsorption from the filtrate is increased, concentrating the urine and decreasing the output volume.

The dilution and concentration of urine depends principally on 2 factors: first, the osmotic pressure of the peritubular fluid, which in turn is mainly dependent on the normal functioning of the Henle's loop and the distal convoluted tubules; and secondly, on the concentration of the antidiuretic hormone in the blood.

The filtrate is made isotonic to the extracellular fluid and plasma in the proximal tube but is hypotonic when it flows out of the Henle's loop into the distal portion of the tubule. This change is attributed to the ascending limb of the loop; it is thicker and impermeable to water, and its cells actively transfer sodium chloride from the filtrate into the peritubular (interstitial) fluid. The tubular fluid thus becomes hypotonic, and by the addition of the sodium, the peritubular fluid is made hypertonic.

Reabsorption of water from the hypotonic filtrate in the distal convoluted and collecting tubules is regulated by the antidiuretic hormone (ADH), which increases the permeability of their membranous walls. It is produced by the hypothalamus in the brain and is stored and released into the blood by the neurohypophysis (posterior pituitary gland). Receptors in the hypothalamus are sensitive to changes in the osmotic pressure of the blood. When the pressure is increased to above normal (for example, by additional sodium), impulses are delivered to the neurohypophysis, resulting in the release of ADH and increasing water reabsorption in the tubules. Conversely, if the osmotic pressure falls below the homeostatic level, the release of ADH is inhibited. The tubular membrane becomes relatively impermeable, restricting the reabsorption of water and diluting the urine.

The reabsorption of sodium is by active cellular transport and its transfer is accompanied by chloride and bicarbonate ions. Eighty per cent of this occurs in the proximal tubule. As indicated previously, much of the 20 per cent is reabsorbed in the Henle's loop, but still more may be transferred in the distal tube. The latter amount is influenced by aldosterone, a hormone secreted by the cortex of the adrenal glands. A high concentration of aldosterone stimulates the distal tubular cells to reabsorb increasing amounts of sodium. A deficiency of the hormone, such as occurs in Addison's disease, reduces the amount of sodium reclaimed, resulting in an excessive loss in urine. Aldosterone also affects the amount of potassium reclaimed and excreted. Increased concentrations of the hormone promote excretion of the electrolyte, and a deficient amount of aldosterone produces excessive retention of potassium.

Tubular Secretion and Excretion. Tubular cells are capable of actively transporting some substances from the blood into the filtrate—a reverse process to that of reabsorption. The potassium concentration of plasma is regulated by this process. Practically all of the potassium that escapes from the plasma into the filtrate is reabsorbed in the proximal tubule. Any excess in the blood is then actively secreted by the distal tubules and is excreted in exchange for sodium ions.

Cells of the distal tubules play an important role in maintaining a normal acid-base balance. They do this by secreting hydrogen ions into the lumen of the tubules in exchange for sodium ions and by forming ammonium radicles that combine with chlorine ions to form ammonium chloride, which is excreted in the urine (see p. 61).

Some drugs are also excreted by active tubular removal from the blood into the tubules. These include diodrast, para-aminohippuric acid and phenosulfonphthalein which are used to investigate renal function.

Characteristics and Composition of Urine

When the filtrate flows into the main collecting tubules and renal pelvis, it becomes urine. The average volume excreted in 24 hours is approximately 1.5 liters but varies with fluid losses through other channels (e.g., perspiration) and the fluid intake. The reaction of urine is usually acid with a pH of about 6.0 but may range from 4.8 to 8.0 with a varied dietary intake. The acidity increases with high protein ingestion and tissue catabolism, while a vegetable diet produces an alkaline urine.

The specific gravity, which gives a rough estimate of the concentration of solids, ranges from 1.003 to 1.040. The composition of urine varies with the dietary intake and metabolic wastes produced. Normally, about 90 to 95 per cent of urine is water. An average of 60 Gm. of organic and inorganic solid wastes are eliminated daily. The chief solutes are urea, creatinine, uric acid and the chlorides, phosphates and sulfates of sodium, potassium, calcium, magnesium and ammonia.

Ureters, Bladder and Urethra

Each of the two ureters is a tube 10 to 12 inches in length, extending from a kidney to the bladder. They are situated behind the parietal peritoneum and enter the posterior wall of the lower half of the bladder obliquely. The slanted entrance forms a flap in the bladder wall that serves as a valve to prevent a reflux of urine as the bladder fills or contracts. Each ureter consists of an outer fibrous covering, a middle layer of muscle tissue, and a mucous membrane lining which is continuous with that of the bladder and the renal pelvis.

The function of these tubes is simply to convey urine from the kidneys to the bladder. Contraction of the ureteral muscular tissue produces peristaltic waves which move the urine along the tube and into the bladder in spurts.

The urinary bladder serves as a temporary reservoir for the urine, which it expels at intervals from the body. It is a collapsible muscular sac that lies behind the symphysis pubis. Three layers of plain muscle tissue form the bladder walls. The fibers are longitudinal in the inner and outer layers and are circular in the middle layer. Collectively, these layers are referred to as the detrusor muscle. The ureteral orifices in the posterior wall and the urethral opening outline a triangular area called the trigone. When the bladder is empty, the mucous membrane lining falls into folds (rugae) except in the area of the trigone.

The urethra is a slender tube that conveys urine from the bladder to the exterior. It has a thin layer of plain muscle tissue and is lined with a mucous membrane which is continuous with that of the bladder. The opening from the bladder is controlled by 2 sphincters: an internal one is under autonomic (involuntary) nervous system control, and an external one is voluntarily controlled by the cerebral cortex. The external urethral orifice is known as the urinary meatus.

In the female, the urethra is about 1.5 inches long and lies anterior to the vagina. The male urethra is approximately 8 inches in length and, on leaving the bladder, passes through the prostate gland. As well as conveying the urine, the male urethra receives the semen from the ejaculatory ducts of the reproductive system, transmitting it through the meatus.

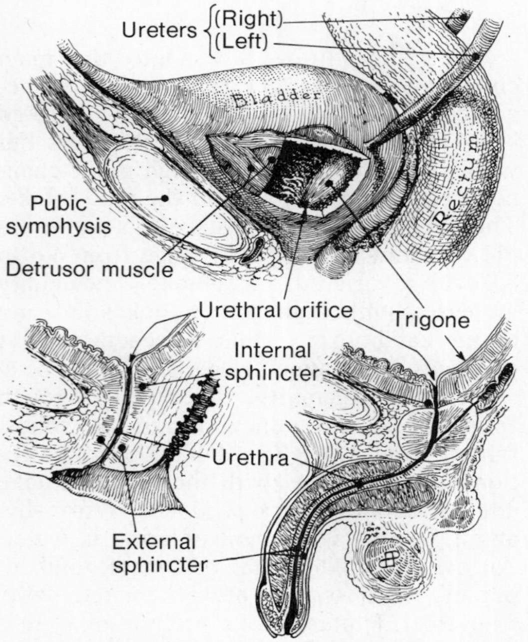

Micturition

This is a term used for the elimination of urine from the bladder. The process involves both autonomic (involuntary) and voluntary nervous impulses. When 300 to 400 ml. of urine collect in the bladder, receptors that are sensitive to stretching initiate impulses which are transmitted by afferent nerve fibers into the lower part of the spinal cord. A reflex response via parasympathetic nerves to the bladder results in contractions of the detrusor muscle and relaxation of the internal sphincter. The initial impulses from the stretch receptors are also relayed via a spinocortical tract to the cerebral cortex, producing an awareness of the need to void. When a person is prepared to empty the bladder, voluntary impulses are initiated which descend the cord and are carried out to the external sphincter, causing it to relax. With both sphincters relaxed, urine drains from the bladder through the urethra. Infants and very young children empty their bladder whenever the micturition reflex is

Figure 18–3 The bladder, ureters and urethra. Internal and external sphincters are shown in male and female.

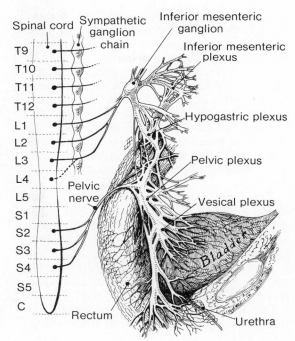

Figure 18–4 A diagram showing innervation of the bladder.

initiated as they have not yet developed voluntary control over the external sphincter. Obviously, any interruption of the spinocortical impulse pathway interferes with control of the external sphincter, resulting in involuntary voiding.

IMPAIRED RENAL FUNCTION

Impaired renal function may be due to primary disease in the kidneys, prerenal circulatory failure, involvement of the kidneys by a systemic disease or obstruction of the urinary tract. Renal dysfunction may be acute with a sudden onset, or it may be chronic, developing insidiously over a long period.

Manifestations

In impaired kidney function, the constancy of the internal environment (homeostasis), which is essential for the normal functioning of all body cells, is disrupted. The normal volume, composition and reaction of the body fluids may be altered by the inability of the kidneys to conserve essential substances and excrete excesses and meta-

bolic wastes. As a result, disturbances in the functioning of other organs readily develop. Consequently, the signs and symptoms of renal insufficiency are varied, and many are not directly referable to the urinary system. Whether the disease is acute or chronic and whether it affects the glomeruli or the tubules will also vary the manifestations.

Abnormal Urinary Volume. Oliguria or anuria may develop, especially in acute and advanced renal failure. Oliguria means that less than 500 ml. of urine is formed in 24 hours. Anuria implies a urinary output of less than 250 ml. in 24 hours and is sometimes referred to as a renal shutdown. The diminished urine formation is usually associated with decreased glomerular filtration due to renal disease (e.g., glomerulonephritis), hypotension as in shock, dehydration, decreased renal blood supply or an obstruction within the tubules.

Polyuria, a volume of urine in excess of the normal (over 2000 ml. in 24 hours), may also indicate renal disturbance in which the ability of the tubules to reabsorb water and concentrate the solid wastes is limited. It is most often seen in chronic kidney disease. Nocturia (voiding during the night) usually accompanies polyuria. Inability of the kidneys to reabsorb the normal amount of water and to concentrate the wastes may be referred to as hyposthenuria. As well as the excessive volume, a low specific gravity of approximately 1.010 of the urine persists because the impaired tubules cannot concentrate or vary the amount of solids.

Abnormal Constituents in the Urine. Abnormal constituents revealed in urinalysis vary with the underlying renal disease. They include albumin, blood, casts, pus and organisms.

The large molecular structure of serum albumin inhibits its filtration through normal glomeruli. Its presence in urine almost always indicates damage to the glomeruli. Hematuria denotes blood in the urine and may be macroscopic or recognized only by microscopic examination. It indicates some pathological process within the kidney.

Urinary casts are microscopic cylindrical structures formed in the distal and collecting tubules by the agglutination of cells and cellular debris in a protein matrix. They are molded or cast in the shape of the tubule. Depending on their composition, casts are usually classified as red blood cell, epithelial, hyaline, granular or fatty. They point to the presence of some inflammatory or degenerative process within the tubules. Obviously, pus and bacteria in the urine indicate infection.

Azotemia. Metabolic wastes accumulate in the blood. Urea, creatinine and uric acid levels are elevated as well as the total concentration of protein metabolic waste, which is expressed as the blood urea nitrogen (BUN). In acute failure and anuria, the levels rise rapidly. In chronic kidney disease, even though there is polyuria, the blood urea progressively rises.

Fluid and Electrolyte Imbalances. Generalized edema may be one of the early symptoms of renal insufficiency and usually becomes apparent first around the eyes. It may be due to decreased glomerular filtration and the retention of water and sodium or to an abnormal permeability of the glomeruli to plasma proteins, especially serum albumin. The latter defect is associated with a condition known as nephrosis that occurs more often in children. The loss of plasma protein causes a decrease in the colloidal osmotic pressure of the blood, and an excess of water remains in the interstitial spaces. The urine is high in albumin, and the plasma protein is abnormally low.

In chronic renal failure due to impaired tubular function, the excessive volume of urine excreted (polyuria) may lead to dehydration unless there is a corresponding increase in the water intake.

Deficiencies or excesses of electrolytes may occur, depending on the nature of the renal disturbance and the degree of tissue damage. Failure of impaired tubules to secrete potassium ions is a serious development in renal insufficiency. Abnormal concentrations of sodium and calcium as well as hyperkalemia may also develop and may seriously affect cardiac function and threaten the patient's life.

Failure in the kidneys' capacity to excrete hydrogen ions by the formation and excretion of acid sodium phosphate and ammonia results in their accumulation in the blood and acidosis (see p. 63).

Vital Signs. An elevation of blood pressure occurs in most patients with renal insufficiency associated with parenchymal disease of the kidneys. It is attributed to an increase in the blood volume as a result of retention of sodium and water or a decrease in the renal blood flow and consequent secretion of renin by the juxtaglomerular cells. The renin combines with a blood protein to form angiotensin, which causes generalized vasoconstriction.

The pulse may become weak because of heart failure which may result from hypertension, excessive fluid load or disturbed electrolyte concentrations. Of all electrolyte disturbances, hyperkalemia (elevated serum potassium) is the most serious (see p. 58) for electrolyte imbalances).

The patient may experience dyspnea due to pulmonary edema. Kussmaul's breathing (deep rapid respirations), characteristic of acidosis, may be manifested. In advanced renal failure, the breath has an ammoniacal or "uremic" odor.

Fever is associated with infection in the kidneys or secondary infection, such as pneumonia, that may develop readily if pulmonary edema is present.

Gastrointestinal Disturbances. The patient experiences anorexia and, in the later stages of renal dysfunction, nausea and vomiting. Diarrhea may also be troublesome in the acute stage. Hiccups may develop in advanced failure, and the oral mucosa become sore and ulcerated.

Headache and Pain. Headache is an early complaint as a result of the hypertension and cerebral edema. Pain and tenderness in the back between the lower ribs and iliac crest occur in acute kidney disease because of the stretching of the renal capsule.

Visual Disturbances. The patient may complain of "spots before his eyes" or blurred vision which are attributed to edema of the optic papilla (papilledema). Loss of vision may actually occur as a result of a retinal hemorrhage.

Neurological Manifestations. Signs of both irritation and depression of the nervous system appear in renal failure. The patient becomes irritable, lethargic and drowsy. He may become disoriented and progress to a comatose state. Muscular twitching may be noticeable and, in advanced kidney disease, may be an indication of ensuing convulsions.

Skin Changes. In progressive renal insufficiency, the skin may take on a yellowish-brown discoloration. Dryness and scaliness are common with chronic disease and polyuria. The patient may complain of pruritus, and excoriated lesions may appear from scratching. In advanced failure, urea frost may be manifested, formed by deposits of small white crystals of urea excreted by the sweat glands. The frost is usually first seen around the mouth.

Anemia. Most patients with prolonged renal disease show a reduction in the production of red blood cells and a resultant anemia. It has been suggested that normal kidneys, as well as the liver, contribute erythropoietin which stimulates erythropoiesis. In the diseased kidney, this activity may be decreased. An increase in the rate of red blood cell destruction in renal insufficiency has also been demonstrated.[1]

Diagnostic Procedures

The investigation of renal dysfunction may include examination of urine specimens which may be voided or obtained by bladder or urethral catheterization, blood

chemistry determinations, renal function tests and roentgenographic studies.

Urine Examinations. The specimen of urine submitted for analysis is voided unless the physician requests that it be a midstream sample or collected by catheter. The voided specimen should be of the first voiding in the morning, since it provides some information about the kidneys' ability to concentrate wastes. Midstream and catheter samples are collected in sterile containers. All specimens are labeled clearly with the patient's name, time collected, method of collection and the examination required.

The color and clarity of the urine are noted, the reaction and specific gravity are determined, and tests are made for the presence of protein, sugar and ketone bodies (acetone, acetoacetic acid and hydroxybutyric acid). Microscopic examination of the urinary sediment, which is obtained by centrifuging the urine, may reveal abnormal constituents such as blood cells, casts, pus and bacteria.

If the urine is to be cultured, a midstream or a catheter specimen is collected. Catheterization is avoided if possible because of the danger of introducing infection into the urethra or bladder. To obtain a midstream sample from a female, the perineum and meatus are cleansed the same as for catheterization to prevent possible contamination from the perineum and vaginal secretion. In the case of the male, the external meatus is cleansed before voiding. Following the cleansing, the patient is instructed to void, and the first 50 ml. of urine are discarded to eliminate possible contamination by organisms that may be in the urethra.

A 24-hour collection of urine may be requested to be examined for quantitative determination of the total solid content or of specific substances such as protein, glucose, certain electrolytes and hormones. When the collection is started, the patient voids and that urine is discarded. At the end of the 24 hours he voids and the urine is included in the specimen. The urine is refrigerated or kept in a cool place. If the patient is ambulatory, it is made clear to him that all his urine is to be saved during the designated period.

Blood Chemistry Determinations. Impaired glomerular filtration and loss of tubular ability to discriminately reabsorb

---

[1] J. P. Merrill: *The Treatment of Renal Failure,* 2nd ed. New York, Grune and Stratton, 1965, p. 103.

and excrete lead to alterations in plasma composition. Blood specimens may be requested to determine the concentration of the following substances:

Protein Metabolic Nitrogenous Wastes
Urea nitrogen (BUN)—Normal: 10 to 20 mg. per cent
Creatinine—Normal: 0.5 to 1.5 mg. per cent
Uric acid—Normal: 2.5 to 6.0 mg. per cent

Electrolytes
Serum sodium—Normal: 135 to 145 mEq./L.
Serum potassium—Normal: 3.5 to 5.0 mEq./L.
Serum calcium—Normal: 4.5 to 6.0 mEq./L.
Serum phosphorous (inorganic)—Normal: 1.0 to 1.5 mEq./L. or 2.4 to 4.5 mg. per cent

Plasma Proteins—Normal: 6 to 8 Gm. per cent
Albumin—Normal: 3.5 to 5.5 Gm. per cent
Globulin—Normal: 1.5 to 3.0 Gm. per cent

Renal Function Tests

CONCENTRATION AND DILUTION TESTS. In the interest of maintaining homeostasis, normal kidney function is capable of varying the concentration of solid wastes and volume of urine according to the volume of body fluids. When there is an excessive loss of body fluid or a restricted intake, more water is reabsorbed by the renal tubules; the solid wastes are excreted in a smaller volume of urine and the specific gravity is high. Conversely, with a large fluid intake, less water is reabsorbed by the tubules, the volume of urine is greater and the specific gravity is lower than usual. This ability to appropriately vary the volume and concentration of the urine is impaired in tubular damage and may be tested by a concentration or dilution test.

The concentration test is designed to determine the kidney's ability to concentrate urine when the fluid intake is restricted. Fluids are restricted over a specified period. Then 2 or 3 urine specimens are collected, and the specific gravity of each is determined. If the kidneys are normal, the specific gravity is not less than 1.024. The procedure as to the period of fluid restriction and the number of specimens collected varies in different institutions. One procedure which is commonly used involves a dry evening meal and then no food or fluid until the test is completed the next morning. Three hourly urine specimens are collected in the morning (e.g., at 6, 7 and 8 A.M.). The time of voiding of each specimen is indicated on the labels. All the urine voided each time must be submitted to the laboratory. Previous to the commencement of the test, the patient receives an explanation so he will understand the fluid restriction and the collection of specimens.

The dilution test evaluates the ability of the kidneys to dilute the urine following a relatively large fluid intake. The procedure is as follows:

The patient remains in bed. On awakening in the morning, he voids and that urine is discarded. The test is explained to the patient, and he is then given 1 liter of fluid over a period of one-half hour. The fluid may be water, lemonade or clear weak tea. The patient voids in 1, 2, 3 and 4 hours, and all the urine voided each time is submitted to the laboratory. The time of voiding is indicated on each specimen. With normal kidney functioning, the specific gravity of the first specimen should be about 1.002 with a gradual increase occurring in the others.

CLEARANCE TESTS. In renal function, the removal or clearance of substances from the blood is achieved by glomerular filtration and tubular cell excretion. If a substance passes freely through the glomeruli and is neither reabsorbed or excreted by the tubules, the quantity appearing in the urine is the same as that filtered by the glomeruli. By measuring the amount that is excreted in the urine in a specified unit of time, information is obtained about the efficiency of glomerular filtration. The substances used for this evaluation may be creatinine or urea, which are naturally occurring metabolites, or rarely inulin (a polysaccharide), which is given intravenously.

Similarly, if a substance is cleared from the blood by tubular cell excretion, the amount in the urine and its rate of appearance indicates the excretory ability of the tubules. An intravenous injection of phenolsulfonphthalein (PSP) is used to test tubular clearance ability.

The urea clearance test involves the following procedure: Breakfast is usually withheld until the test is completed. The patient is given a minimum of 450 to 500 ml. of water to drink to promote urine formation. He is asked to void and this urine is discarded. The time is noted. A venous blood specimen is obtained for determination of the blood urea nitrogen. One hour after the discarded urine was voided the patient is asked to void again. All of this urine is sent to the laboratory. The specimen label will indicate the exact time the urine was collected. From the BUN and the concentration of urea in the urine formed in 1 hour, the laboratory calculates the volume of blood cleared of urea per minute. Normally 55 to 75 ml. of plasma are cleared of urea per minute.

In the creatinine clearance test, the patient is kept at rest during the test since endogenous creatinine is produced in muscular activity. Meat should be eliminated from the diet for a period of 48 hours before the test. A 24-hour specimen of urine and a venous blood specimen are collected for creatinine concentration determinations. The rate of urinary excretion per minute is calculated. The normal amount of creatinine excreted in 24 hours varies with age; in an adult the normal is about 1.2 to 1.7 Gm., and in a child it is approximately 0.36 Gm. Calculations are made to determine the volume of plasma cleared of creatinine per minute. "The product of urine concentration of creatinine (mg. %), multiplied by urine flow rate (ml. per minute), divided by the plasma concentration of creatinine (mg. %) gives the creatinine clearance rate. . . ."[2] The normal range is 90 to 140 ml. per minute. It is usually less for females (males have a greater muscle mass) and decreases with age.

The phenolsulfonphthalein (PSP) test indicates the excretory ability of the renal tubules. PSP is a red dye that is given intravenously and is completely excreted in a short time by normal kidneys. Less than total excretion of that given may indicate tubular damage and inefficiency or an obstruction of urinary flow through the renal pelves or lower urinary tract.

The procedure entails giving the patient

approximately 400 to 500 ml. of water and having him empty his bladder. This urine is discarded. The physician gives the prescribed amount (usually 1 ml.) of PSP intravenously and the exact time is noted. Urine specimens are then collected in 15, 30, 60 and 120 minutes after the dye was administered. All the urine voided each time is included in the specimens, and the time each was voided is clearly indicated on the labels. The intervals for the collection of urine specimens may vary in different situations; the nurse should receive a specific directive. Normally, 40 to 50 per cent of the dye is excreted over 1 hour and 75 per cent over 2 hours.

Radioactive Isotope Clearance Test. Renal function may also be studied by administering radioactive iodohippurate (Hippuran—I^{131}) intravenously and observing its elimination. As the Hippuran—I^{131} passes through the kidneys, scintillation probes or counters are placed over the kidneys to record the renal concentration of the radioactive substance in the form of a tracing called a renogram. A tracing is obtained for each kidney. From the renograms, the physician is able to assess the renal blood flow and kidney function.

Voided urine specimens may also be collected following the injection and are tested for the content of radioactive iodohippurate. Normally, about 75 per cent is excreted within 30 to 40 minutes.

Intravenous Pyelogram. A radiopaque substance that is eliminated by the kidneys is given intravenously, and a series of x-ray films are made at intervals to note the concentration of the contrast medium in the renal pelves, ureters and bladder.

Preparation for an intravenous pyelogram includes an explanation of the procedure to the patient and questioning as to whether he has any allergies or has ever had asthma or eczema. The physician is advised if any sensitivity or allergy is indicated by the patient. No fluids are given for 12 hours preceding the examination to provide a better concentration of the radiopaque substance. Castor oil or another laxative may be ordered the day before and an enema 2 to 3 hours before the test to cleanse the intestines of gas and feces, which produce shadows on the film. The vigorous catharsis may be quite exhausting to the

---

[2]C. C. Winter: Practical Urology. St. Louis, The C. V. Mosby Co., 1969, p. 55.

patient; he should be allowed to rest undisturbed as much as possible. If the patient is weak or elderly, he is advised to signal for the nurse so that assistance can be given when he goes to the bathroom. The laxative is contraindicated if the patient has a gastrointestinal condition such as peptic ulcer or colitis.

The contrast medium used is an iodide preparation, such as sodium diatrizoate (Hypaque) or sodium iodomethamate (Neo-Iopax), to which the patient may be sensitive. The physician gives a small intracutaneous dose of the dye first and observes the area for a reaction. If none is apparent, the radiopaque preparation is then given intravenously. The patient is advised that he is likely to experience a salty taste and a sudden flush of warmth for a brief period. He is observed closely for signs of respiratory distress, cold clammy perspiration and urticaria. These and any complaint of unusual sensations are promptly reported to the physician. An emergency tray or cart with epinephrine (Adrenalin), oxygen, antihistamine preparations such as tripelennamine hydrochloride (Pyribenzamine) and diphenhydramine hydrochloride (Benadryl), and cortisone preparations must be readily available for quick administration in the event of allergic manifestations.

Following the x-ray series, the patient is encouraged to take additional fluids to correct the dehydration incurred by the restriction of fluids and catharsis.

Cystoscopy and Retrograde Pyelogram. Cystoscopy involves the passage of a cystoscope through the urethra into the bladder. The instrument is equipped with a light which permits direct visualization of the internal surface of the bladder. A long fine catheter may also be introduced into each ureter through the cystoscope (ureteral catheterization) and a urine specimen collected from each kidney. The specimens must be labeled as to right or left ureter.

A radiopaque iodide preparation may then be introduced into the catheters, and x-rays are taken which will outline the renal pelves and ureters. This procedure is referred to as a retrograde pyelogram.

Preparation of the patient for a cytoscopy includes an explanation of the procedure. The well-prepared patient who knows what to expect is more relaxed, which lessens the spasms of the urethral sphincters and the discomfort. When the lithotomy position is described, he is assured that he will be draped so there will be minimal exposure. If there is an existing problem that interferes with comfortable flexion of the lower limbs, it is brought to the attention of the cystoscopy room staff so the positioning may be modified accordingly. The patient's signature indicating his consent for the examination is usually required. The patient is given extra fluids for several hours preceding the examination.

He may also receive a sedative such as sodium pentobarbital (Nembutal), sodium secobarbital (Seconal), or meperidine hydrochloride (Demerol) one-half hour before the cystoscopy to promote relaxation. Children usually receive a general anesthetic, so food and fluid are restricted for 6 to 8 hours preceding and intravenous fluid is administered to ensure urinary flow.

During the cystoscopy and ureteral catheterization, phenosulfonphthalein (PSP) may be given intravenously, and its appearance in the urine from each kidney noted and timed. Normally it appears in 4 to 6 minutes following the administration.

On completion of the examination, the patient rests in bed for a few hours. Discomfort in the back or bladder region may be relieved by local heat application (hot water bottle or electric heating pad) or a warm tub bath if the patient's condition permits. Additional fluids are encouraged. Any severe pain or persisting bright blood in the urine is reported to the doctor.

Renal Angiography. Renal blood vessels may be outlined on an x-ray film following the administration of a radiopaque substance such as sodium diatrizoate (Hypaque) into the aorta close to the source of the renal arteries. The contrast medium may be injected directly into the aorta by a long needle inserted through the lumbar region. An alternative method is the injection of the radiopaque liquid into the aorta via a small catheter introduced into a femoral artery and passed retrogradely into the aorta. Since the patient may be sensitive to the radiopaque iodide preparation, the same precautions as cited for intravenous pyelography are necessary.

Uremia

Uremia is not a disease entity but rather is a state or complex of symptoms reflecting failure of the kidneys to excrete the metabolic wastes and excess substances normally found in urine.[3] The uremic state may develop rapidly with acute renal failure or gradually over a period of months or years in chronic renal insufficiency.

The onset of uremia is usually marked by an increase in the patient's hypertension, nausea and vomiting, persisting severe headache, visual disturbances and weakness. Muscular twitching, disorientation, convulsions and coma are ominous signs. The volume of urinary output may be reduced; generalized edema, cardiac failure and pulmonary edema are likely to ensue as a result of the sodium, potassium and fluid retention.

Uremia may be corrected by treatment of the cause of impaired renal function. During this period, the blood level of wastes may be reduced by dialysis. In the case of chronic renal failure due to permanent kidney damage, the patient may be maintained on regular hemodialysis once or twice weekly and controlled dietary and fluid intake. The protein, sodium and potassium content of the diet is closely regulated according to the blood chemistry. The patient may be considered a candidate for a kidney transplant.

See nursing care in acute renal failure (p. 428) and chronic renal failure (p. 431). Dialysis procedures are discussed on pages 440 and 443.

Hydronephrosis

Hydronephrosis implies distention of the renal tubules, calyces and pelvis by the accumulation of fluid secondary to defective urinary drainage. The cause of the obstruction may be an intrinsic or extrinsic tumor, stricture of the ureter due to inflammation or fibrous scar tissue, or a calculus. In infants, it may develop as the result of a congenital developmental error in the form of a stricture or aberrant structure.

Hydronephrosis produces a palpable

---

[3]C. C. Winters: Practical Urology. St. Louis, The C. V. Mosby Co., 1969, p. 6.

mass, pain, and renal tissue damage by compression. The cause is sought and treated surgically.

If infection is the initiating factor or is superimposed, the accumulated fluid may be purulent. The condition may then be referred to as pyonephrosis.

Acute Renal Failure

Acute renal failure or insufficiency implies a sudden, severe interruption of kidney function and is frequently referred to as a renal shutdown.

Causes. The causes of acute renal insufficiency are numerous and may be extrarenal or primarily renal.

The more common extrarenal causes are a fall in arterial blood pressure (shock) or a reduction in the renal blood supply. These may be the result of hemorrhage; the loss of plasma as occurs in burns and massive crushing injuries; dehydration, which may be due to a deficient intake or excessive loss; septicemia or toxemia; or cardiac insufficiency. The fall in blood pressure reduces glomerular filtration, and if prolonged, the renal ischemia leads to renal tissue damage, especially tubular necrosis. Another extrarenal cause of acute renal failure is obstruction of the lower urinary tract. Interruption of the urinary flow may be the result of ureteral obstruction by calculi, intrinsic or extrinsic tumors and newgrowths, or severe infection (pyelonephritis).

Acute kidney failure caused by renal parenchymal damage may be due to acute glomerulonephritis (see p. 433), severe acute pyelonephritis (see p. 435) or tubular necrosis. As mentioned previously, prolonged renal ischemia may lead to the destruction of kidney tissue. The tubules are especially vulnerable since they are dependent upon the volume of blood that enters the efferent arterioles after glomerular filtration. Other causes of tubular necrosis include incompatible blood transfusions, crushing injuries and nephrotoxic chemicals. The exact mechanism that leads to tubular necrosis following a blood transfusion reaction is not understood. The incompatible blood causes the breakdown of a large number of red blood cells and the release of hemoglobin.

The molecules of hemoglobin pass through the glomeruli and become concentrated in the tubules, obstructing the flow of filtrate. Guyton states that with the hemolysis of erythrocytes, a vasoconstrictor agent is released into the blood stream, resulting in constriction of the renal arterioles and tubular ischemia.[4]

The tubular necrosis that follows a crushing injury is attributed to the concomitant shock and to the release of large amounts of myoglobin from the injured and necrotic muscle cells. The myoglobin enters the blood stream, passes through the glomeruli into the tubules where it becomes concentrated and accumulates, blocking the tubules. The person who has been "pinned down under a weight" for a period of time or who has been subjected to limb ischemia may appear in satisfactory condition when released but should be put to bed under close observation. He is likely to develop severe shock, acute renal failure and gross edema of the injured part hours later.

Certain chemicals and drugs may have a toxic effect on the renal tubules. Epithelial cells are destroyed, and the tubular lumen may be obliterated by swelling and edema of the tissues as well as by casts formed by the sloughed cells. Nephrotoxic chemicals, which may be taken accidentally or with suicidal intent, include carbon tetrachloride, ethylene glycol (a constituent of antifreeze), bichloride of mercury, chloroform and copper sulfate. Drugs which may prove toxic and damaging to the tubules include sulfonamides, salicylates, phenacetin and quinine. Generally these have been administered in excessive dosage, or the patient may have a hypersensitivity.

Signs and Symptoms. The first sign of acute renal failure is oliguria which may progress rapidly to anuria. In conditions in which renal insufficiency frequently occurs the physician may request an indwelling catheter so the hourly production of urine may be determined. An output of less than 30 ml. is an indication for concern and is reported immediately. If oliguria or anuria persists for a few days, manifestations of sodium, water and potassium retention, uremia and metabolic acidosis are likely to

develop. Sodium and water retention cause edema and unless the fluid intake is controlled, overhydration may lead to cardiac failure and pulmonary edema. The pulse becomes weak, and the respirations are labored and audibly moist. Elevation of the blood potassium may cause extreme weakness in the patient and a weak, irregular pulse. Cardiac arrest may occur suddenly.

The rate of the accumulation of nitrogenous wastes in the blood varies with the cause of the renal insufficiency. If there is rapid catabolism as in infection, fever, and pathological destruction of tissue, the blood concentration of nitrogenous wastes may rise more quickly. The onset of the uremic state is usually marked by mental changes, nausea and vomiting.

Metabolic acidosis develops because the hydrogen ions produced in metabolism are not being eliminated by the renal tubules. Respirations are increased in rate and depth, and an acidotic odor of the breath becomes noticeable.

If the renal failure persists, the patient may develop an increased bleeding tendency. Ulcerated areas in the mouth are common and may bleed. Vomitus may contain blood.

The patient becomes drowsy and may progress to a comatose state. Muscle twitching and convulsions may develop.

Nursing Care. The outcome in acute renal failure depends on the seriousness of the underlying cause, early recognition and prompt treatment. The nurse may play an important role in early recognition by being familiar with the possible causes of renal shutdown and by being alert to any significant decrease in a patient's urinary output.

Treatment is directed toward correcting the initiating cause of the renal insufficiency. If the renal shutdown is the result of hypotension, loss of blood, or dehydration, treatment will include the intravenous administration of blood, plasma, dextran, or electrolyte and glucose solutions. When renal failure is associated with severe infection, large doses of antibiotics are usually given intravenously. Antidotes may be appropriate in the case of poisoning, but the removal of some nephrotoxins from the blood may require hemodialysis. Surgical procedures are undertaken if obstructive uropathy is the etiologic factor in renal failure.

---

[4]A. C. Guyton: Textbook of Medical Physiology, 4th ed. Philadelphia, W. B. Saunders Co., 1971, p. 133.

The following discussion focuses on care related to the renal failure. Efforts are directed toward the maintenance of electrolyte concentrations within a range compatible with life, the prevention of overhydration and minimal production of nitrogenous wastes.

OBSERVATIONS. The patient with acute renal failure is seriously ill and requires constant nursing care and close observation for changes which may occur suddenly. An accurate record of the fluid intake and output is essential. An indwelling catheter may be used so that the hourly production of urine may be determined. As cited previously, an output of less than 30 ml. hourly or 500 ml. daily is ominous. Any evident perspiration is recorded, as this will be taken into consideration when estimating the volume of fluid the patient should have.

The pulse, respirations and blood pressure are checked frequently. Cardiac function may be impaired by the retention of potassium and fluid or by hypertension which may accompany renal parenchymal disease. Frequent electrocardiograms may be done to detect changes in the waves indicative of an elevated serum potassium level (hyperkalemia).

Any edema is noted, and the patient's weight may have to be recorded daily. A loss each day of approximately 0.2 to 0.3 kg. may be expected as a result of catabolism and the restricted intake. No loss or a gain usually indicates fluid retention. The respirations are observed for signs of developing pulmonary edema, which may result from overhydration and cardiac failure. A noticeable increase in the volume and depth of respirations may point to acidosis.

The blood pressure is taken at regular intervals to provide information on the patient's progress. A progressive rise in excess of normal levels is reported to the physician; it may point to increasing uremia. The temperature is taken every 4 hours even if normal, since a sudden elevation may occur and indicate complicating infection.

Muscular twitching, increasing drowsiness and disorientation are reported, since they may be manifestations of uremia, cerebral edema and approaching convulsions and coma.

FLUIDS AND NUTRITION. The daily fluid intake is limited to 500 ml. plus an amount equal to the urinary output of the preceding 24 hours. The 500 ml. replaces the obligatory loss through the skin and lungs. The fluids that may be given will depend on the serum electrolyte concentrations. Potassium and protein are restricted, and sodium may also be limited. If there is vomiting or diarrhea, the patient may require sodium chloride replacement. An explanation of the fluid restriction is made to the patient so he will understand why he may have only limited amounts distributed over 24 hours.

A minimum of 100 to 200 Gm. of carbohydrate is given daily to reduce the amount of tissue protein and fat broken down for energy. If the patient is not vomiting, it may be taken orally. A part of the carbohydrate may be administered as glucose dissolved in part of the allotted volume of water. A few drops of lemon juice may be added to make the solution less insipid. The physician may prefer to administer the carbohydrate by intravenous infusion of glucose in water, reserving only a small volume of water to be given orally.

REST. The patient's activity is restricted to minimize the production of metabolic wastes. The nurse explains the need for rest to the patient, bathes him and provides assistance in order to conserve his energy during necessary movement.

MOUTH AND SKIN CARE. In renal failure, the mouth requires special care. The tongue becomes coated, salivary secretion is reduced, and the mucosa and lips are dry and frequently encrusted. Ulcerative lesions may develop, and the patient may be distressed by the disagreeable taste frequently associated with uremia. Sordes predisposes him to respiratory infection and parotitis. Frequent cleansing of the mouth with hydrogen peroxide and rinsing with an antiseptic mouthwash are necessary, followed by a light application of mineral oil to which a few drops of lemon juice may be added. Petroleum jelly (vaseline) or cold cream is applied to the lips. Tart fruit candies such as "lemon drops" are helpful to stimulate secretions, reduce thirst and at the same time supply some sugar.

The patient is bathed daily to remove the increased wastes that may be excreted in perspiration and to provide comfort. His position is changed frequently, and pressure areas are gently massaged and are protected by squares of sheepskin to prevent pressure sores.

PREVENTION OF INFECTION. Infection is extremely hazardous in renal failure; the patient is more susceptible and handles it poorly. When it is possible, he is placed in a single room, and no one with an infection is permitted to care for or visit him. Frequent change of position, deep breathing and coughing are instituted to prevent pulmonary stasis and complications. The nurse who is also caring for other patients may be required to wear a mask and gown when giving care to the person with renal failure.

COMPLICATIONS. Complications which commonly develop in renal failure include hyperkalemia, cardiac insufficiency, convulsions and coma.

Since potassium is liberated from the cells in tissue breakdown and cannot be eliminated in renal failure, the extracellular concentration may reach toxic levels. Cardiac function becomes impaired, and failure or sudden cardiac arrest may occur. The nurse should be alert to possible clinical symptoms of potassium intoxication which include generalized muscular weakness, shallow respirations, complaints of tingling sensation or numbness in the limbs and around the mouth, a slow irregular pulse, and a fall in blood pressure.

As well as ensuring that no potassium is ingested in fluid or food, preventive measures may include the oral or rectal administration of a cation exchange resin, such as polystyrene sodium sulfonate (Kayexalate). The resin preparation combines with the potassium in the gastrointestinal secretions, preventing its absorption.

If hyperkalemia develops, an intravenous infusion of glucose with a dose of regular insulin may be given. This is to promote the deposition of the glucose as glycogen, a process which utilizes potassium. A solution of sodium bicarbonate or sodium lactate and probably calcium may be administered to counteract the effect of the excess potassium on the heart.

Cardiac insufficiency may occur as the result of the retention of sodium and water. The pulse may become weak and pulmonary edema be manifested in dyspnea and moist respirations. If hypertension is associated with the renal failure, it may also be a factor in heart failure. Digitalis may be prescribed to strengthen the heart, and aminophylline is given to relieve the respiratory distress. A phlebotomy may be done and 300 to 500 ml. of blood withdrawn to reduce the intravascular volume and venous return.

Convulsions may occur and are usually preceded by muscular twitching, persisting severe headache, severe hypertension, increasing edema and rising nonprotein nitrogen level. Padded crib sides are placed on the bed and a padded tongue depressor kept at the bedside. If a seizure develops, the tongue depressor is quickly placed between the patient's teeth to prevent biting of the tongue. If the teeth are clenched before the padded depressor can be introduced, no attempt should be made to force its entry as it may only incur injury to soft tissues or break a tooth. Only sufficient restraint is used to protect the patient from injury. Magnesium sulfate or sodium amytal may be ordered intramuscularly or intravenously and an antihypertensive drug such as reserpine (Serpasil) or hydralazine hydrochloride (Apresoline) may be given.

Increasing drowsiness may indicate increasing uremia and may progress to disorientation and coma. The delerious patient requires constant attendance, and a sedative such as paraldehyde or sodium amytal may be prescribed. If the patient becomes comatose, the care appropriate for any unconscious patient is applicable (see p. 103).

DIALYSIS. When the fluid and electrolyte imbalances and metabolic waste concentration threaten life, either peritoneal dialysis or hemodialysis may be instituted (see p. 440).

DIURETIC PHASE. Improvement in renal function is manifested by a steady increase in the volume of urine. The latter may rise rapidly to as much as 3000 to 3500 ml. in 24 hours. The diuresis is accompanied by marked losses of potassium, sodium and water because the tubules have not regained the ability to regulate the volume and composition of urine. Frequent serum electrolyte determinations continue, and necessary replacements are made either orally or intravenously. The fluid intake is increased to cover the volume lost. The nitrogenous waste concentration (BUN) decreases more slowly.

The patient receives a soft diet and then

a light diet with limited protein content, which is increased gradually as the blood urea level falls. The nurse continues to record the intake and output, and renal concentration tests may be done to determine if there is some residual insufficiency due to tubular necrosis.

Before being discharged from the hospital, the patient and his family are advised that activity should be resumed gradually and that extra rest will be necessary for several weeks. Dietary instructions are given, the importance of avoiding infection is stressed and suggestions are made as to the protective measures to use. The patient is advised of the date he is to see his physician or go to the clinic for a checkup and is told that he will be expected to take with him a specimen of the urine voided on rising that morning. The prolonged convalescence frequently causes socioeconomic problems for the patient and his family. The nurse may be able to assist by a referral to the social service or a welfare organization.

Chronic Renal Failure

Chronic renal insufficiency is due to progressive disease of both kidneys. Irreversible damage to nephrons occurs that eventually leads to uremia. The causes include chronic pyelonephritis, chronic glomerulonephritis, degenerative renal vascular changes (nephrosclerosis), polycystic disease and hydronephrosis.

The patient may pass through the early stage of chronic kidney impairment without the renal disease being recognized because the functioning nephrons compensate for those destroyed. The length of the period of compensation is dependent upon the rate of destruction of parenchymal tissue. Some live a normal active life for many years with compensated renal failure; others whose disease progresses rapidly may enter the advanced uremic phase in a matter of a few months.

Manifestations. Gradually, with increasing nephron destruction, the patient enters the phase in which renal compensation can no longer maintain homeostasis, and symptoms become apparent. Filtration is impaired, and there is a loss of tubular ability to vary the composition and volume of urine according to the need to conserve or eliminate urinary solutes and water.

The signs and symptoms vary considerably in patients in the early stage of uncompensated insufficiency but tend to become similar in the more advanced stage. An elevation in blood pressure, lassitude, headache and loss of weight may be the earliest manifestations. Urinalysis may reveal albumin due to increased permeability of glomeruli. The loss of plasma protein may be severe enough to produce the nephrotic syndrome (see p. 436). As more and more nephrons are destroyed, decreased filtration results in the retention of metabolic wastes. The blood urea and creatinine levels rise.

Tubular destruction causes electrolyte imbalances. There is usually an excessive loss of sodium which may produce hyponatremia unless there is adequate replacement. Potassium retention is not usually a problem until the terminal oliguric phase. In the advanced stage of failure, metabolic acidosis develops, and hypocalcemia may also be a problem, causing muscular twitching and general weakness.

The 24-hour urinary volume is increased and the patient experiences nocturia as a result of tubular inability to concentrate the glomerular filtrate. The concentration of solutes in the urine is invariable, producing a fixed specific gravity. If the fluid intake does not cover the increased fluid loss, the patient develops a negative fluid balance and the retention of solid wastes is increased.

Anemia is a common feature of chronic renal failure, contributing to the patient's fatigue, pallor and loss of efficiency.

Eventually, the urinary output is reduced, hypertension becomes severe, and the nitrogenous waste and potassium blood concentrations rise sharply. Late symptoms are persistent headache of increasing severity, nausea and vomiting, uremic frost, muscular twitching, convulsions, ulceration of the mouth, fetid breath, rapid deep respirations indicating acidosis, drowsiness, disorientation and coma. As a result of the severe hypertension and water retention, a cerebrovascular accident or cardiac failure and pulmonary edema may supervene.

Treatment and Nursing Care. The physician advises the patient and his family of the diagnosis, but it is frequently the nurse who must answer many of their questions, provide emotional support, and help them to understand and accept the prescribed regimen. The patient is usually in the hospital when the diagnosis of chronic renal disease is made, having probably had a series of kidney function tests. At first, he may be resentful and is unable to accept the fact that he has a progressive chronic disease. Instruction is likely to fall on deaf ears until he works through his immediate reactions. The nurse provides opportunities for him to verbalize his feelings and is alert for signs of his acceptance of his condition and readiness to learn how he may help himself.

DIET AND FLUIDS. The goal in dietary and fluid intake is to balance the intake with the output. A diet of 2000 calories is desirable to provide sufficient energy that will permit activity without the breakdown of tissue protein and fat. In the early stage of the disease, protein is limited to 30 to 50 Gm. daily to minimize the production of nitrogenous waste. The prescribed amount is adjusted periodically according to the BUN. Carbohydrate and fat provide the remaining calories. In the case of the patient who develops the nephrotic syndrome, protein is not restricted but instead is probably increased above the average dietary intake (see p. 436). Since the impaired tubular reabsorption usually results in an excessive loss of sodium, salt is not restricted in the diet unless there is edema or severe hypertension.

The fluid intake should cover the fluid loss. Tubular reabsorption of water is decreased in chronic renal failure, so the intake should be increased accordingly. Generally, a minimum of 2000 ml. is required to prevent dehydration from the increased urinary output. A record is made of the 24-hour intake and output. The patient is advised that he should not take more than 500 ml. in excess of his urinary output; as well as incurring edema, excessive water in the presence of the abnormal sodium loss may precipitate hyponatremia. Any significant decrease in the urinary output, indicating a negative fluid balance, is reported to the doctor, as it may signal more advanced failure. When oliguria supervenes, the fluid intake is adjusted according to the urinary output.

ACTIVITY. Although the patient's renal reserve is diminished, in the early stage of his disease his kidney function may be adequate as long as the prescribed diet and fluid intake are followed and metabolic extremes are avoided. The patient is encouraged to remain active within the limits of his strength but is advised to avoid undue fatigue. He requires more rest than the normal person. While still active, it is suggested that he should have 10 hours of sleep at night and should rest 1 hour during the morning and afternoon. The person at work may plan for 1 hour at noon and for 1 hour at the completion of his work day before his evening meal. Whether he is able to resume his former occupation or not depends on its demands. Certainly the ability to continue to be a useful, independent member of society provides self-esteem and emotional well-being. Suitable recreation and diversion in which the patient is interested should receive consideration. It lessens the focus on his disease and provides a more normal, balanced life.

HYPERTENSION AND ANEMIA. These are common concomitant problems of chronic renal insufficiency. The patient will probably be required to take an antihypertensive drug such as methyldopa (Aldomet), hydralazine (Apresoline) or guanethidine (Ismelin). The anemia is not responsive to the usual hematinic drugs; periodic blood transfusions may be necessary.

SKIN CARE. As the patient's blood urea accumulates, pruritus may become troublesome and uremic frost may appear. Bathing with a weak solution of vinegar in water (1 to 2 tablespoonfuls to a quart of water) will dissolve and remove the urea crystals deposited on the skin. An application of calamine lotion or caladryl may be used to provide relief of the itching.

INSTRUCTION AND SUPERVISION. Since the patient and his family must assume the responsibility for following the prescribed regimen, the nurse plans a program of instruction. A simple explanation of the role of the kidneys in eliminating body wastes is helpful before attempting to explain the importance of avoiding extra demands on the kidneys and how this is achieved. Diet outlines are reviewed, indicating food selection and preparation to meet the protein restriction and the daily calorie requirement. The measurement and distribution of the required fluid intake over the 24 hours are discussed. The patient is instructed to record his weight daily and to do this at the same time each day with the same amount of clothing. Any increase in his weight, puffiness around the eyes, swelling of the feet or hands, frequent headaches and increasing fatigue should be brought to the physician's attention. Measurement of his urinary output is recommended, and the patient is advised that an output of less than two-thirds of his intake should also be reported.

Infection increases the production of metabolic wastes, especially if accompanied by fever and a reduced fluid intake. The importance of avoiding chilling and exposure to persons with an infection is stressed. Practical suggestions are made as to how the possibility of exposure may be minimized. If the patient does develop a respiratory infection or any other disturbance, it is advisable to get in touch with the physician.

Frequent visits to the doctor or a clinic are necessary, and the patient is advised to take a urine specimen with him each time. His blood pressure and weight are checked, and the patient is questioned about his appetite and urinary volume. Blood specimens are taken to determine the hematocrit, hemoglobin level, and electrolyte and nonprotein nitrogen or urea concentrations.

In some instances, the patient and his family may be able to follow the therapeutic program, make necessary observations and recognize significant changes. Other patients may require a referral to a visiting nurse organization. The visiting nurse may assist with diet planning, check the patient's blood pressure and weight, counsel him as to activity and note any signs of deterioration. If the patient is returning to work, the occupational nurse at his place of employment is advised of the situation so she may provide the necessary assistance and follow the patient's progress.

It is very helpful if the patient and his family have the opportunity to discuss their problems and express their concerns with someone who shows an interest in them and will take the time to listen. Frequently problems are revealed to the nurse that she may be able to help solve, or significant information may be received that requires immediate referral to the physician.

ADVANCED RENAL FAILURE. In the oliguric and uremic phase of chronic renal disease, the care is similar to that cited for the patient with acute renal failure. Rest, more stringent dietary and fluid restrictions, special skin and mouth care and close observation for disorientation, convulsions, coma, cardiac failure and pulmonary edema are necessary.

When conservative treatment will no longer adequately control the blood concentration of wastes and the fluid and electrolyte balance within limits compatible with life, regular dialysis may be employed to maintain the patient. If both kidneys are severely damaged by infection, polycystic disease or newgrowths or if there is severe hypertension that cannot be controlled by conservative treatment, bilateral nephrectomy may be done, and the patient maintained entirely on hemodialysis 2 or 3 times weekly. Such a patient is a likely candidate for a kidney transplant. See the following section for a discussion of dialysis.

Acute Glomerulonephritis

At the onset, this disease is characterized by a diffuse, noninfectious inflammation of the glomeruli of both kidneys. Since the blood supply that supports the tubules normally passes through glomerular capillaries before reaching them, fibrous scarring and obliteration of some glomeruli lead to secondary degenerative changes in the associated tubules.

The inflammation is attributed to an antigen-antibody reaction following a beta type hemolytic streptococcal infection. It is suggested that the glomeruli release an altered protein in response to streptococcal toxin, which acts as an antigen. The antibodies that are then formed attack the glomeruli. The patient's history usually reveals that the renal disturbance follows a sore throat or respiratory infection of some form by a latent period of 2 to 4 weeks. In some instances, the infection may have been so mild that little or no attention was given to it at the time. Acute glomerulonephritis may develop in both sexes at any age but occurs more commonly in children and young adults; males are more often affected than females.

Signs and Symptoms. The onset is generally abrupt. The affected glomeruli are partially or completely obstructed, resulting in reduced filtration. Some rupture occurs, permitting the escape of blood into the tubules. The permeability of the glomeruli that remain patent is increased. The scant output of urine is cloudy and contains albumin, blood cells and casts. Edema develops and is usually seen first in the periorbital areas and ankles. The patient complains of pain and tenderness in the back, headache, weakness and perhaps visual disturbances. The blood pressure is elevated, and the decreased filtration results in a gradual accumulation of nitrogenous wastes in the blood (the BUN level is elevated).

Nasal and throat cultures may be done to determine if streptococci are still present. Examination of the blood may reveal an elevation in antistreptolysin O titer (ASO titer).

Neurological signs and symptoms corresponding to the degree of hypertension and cerebral edema may be present (see p. 430). Unless the renal insufficiency is reversed, uremia, pulmonary edema and cardiac failure may ensue.

Management. The treatment of patients with acute glomerulonephritis consists mainly of rest, fluid and diet regulation, and chemotherapy to eliminate possible residual streptococcal infection. The patient is confined to bed with restricted activity to minimize the production of metabolic wastes. The daily fluid intake is restricted to 400 to 500 ml. in excess of the urinary output of the previous 24 hours. The blood chemistry is followed closely and the sodium, potassium, and chloride intake regulated according to the findings. The patient is sustained chiefly on carbohydrate; a minimum of 100 Gm. is given daily to reduce the breakdown of tissue protein. Protein in the diet is regulated according to the BUN level and the amount of urea excreted in the urine. Similarly, salt restriction in the diet is regulated according to the degree of edema and hypertension.

If the low output of urine is prolonged and the blood potassium and nitrogenous waste levels are progressively increasing, either peritoneal dialysis or hemodialysis may be instituted (see p. 440).

Precautions are necessary to protect the patient from chilling and exposure to infection. A superimposed infection could aggravate the disease or produce pneumonia that could prove fatal.

The frequent association of glomerulonephritis with respiratory infections emphasizes their potential danger and the importance of prevention and prompt, adequate treatment of such infections. Too often they are ignored, considered as unavoidably seasonal and treated very lightly. Women who have a history of acute glomerulonephritis are advised to consult a doctor before planning a pregnancy, since they are more likely to develop toxemia and eclampsia.

According to the literature, the majority of patients with acute glomerulonephritis recover with no residual kidney damage. These patients generally show an increase in the volume of urine and a decrease in the blood pressure and BUN within 1 week. The albuminuria and microscopic hematuria may persist for much longer. A few patients progress through a subacute phase to chronic glomerulonephritis. Others may be asymptomatic for a period of months or years and then experience an insidious development of the chronic disease.

Chronic Glomerulonephritis

The persisting disease process of chronic glomerulonephritis and the repeated acute exacerbations which the patient may experience result in increasing numbers of glomeruli and tubules being destroyed. Renal function is progressively impaired, and the patient eventually reaches an end stage in which there is marked retention of metabolic wastes, chemical imbalance and severe hypertension. The course of the disease is rather unpredictable; the manifestations and rate of progression vary. A steady decrease in renal function may occur and prove fatal over a period of months. In other instances, progression of the disease may be insidious over years. Patients with chronic glomerulonephritis may have had an acute episode and entered the chronic phase or may have developed their disease without a history of any acute episodes.

Manifestations. In the early stage, the patient manifests some elevation of blood pressure, and the urinalysis reveals albumin, blood cells and casts. He is usually troubled by nocturia. Loss of tubular efficiency leads to inability to vary the water and electrolyte excretion. With reduced filtration the BUN progressively increases to levels above the normal. These early symptoms may remain mild over a varying length of time and then progressively become more dominant as renal damage increases. The urea blood level is markedly elevated, hypertension is severe, and anemia develops. The patient experiences easy fatigue, weakness, headache, anorexia and loss of weight. He may notice his vision is less acute and that his general tolerance and functional ability are reduced.

Reduced tubular ability to secrete hydrogen ions, form ammonia and conserve sodium and bicarbonate ions is likely to result in acidosis. Normal amounts of potassium are not excreted by the impaired tubules, producing serious cardiac arrhythmias and weakness. The pulse is likely to become slow and irregular with a prolonged diastole as a result of the elevated blood potassium concentration. The increasing retention of wastes leads to uremia, which is marked by persisting severe headache, edema and cerebral disturbances that are manifested by twitching, disorientation and convulsive seizures. The patient may soon progress to a state of coma, pulmonary edema and cardiac failure.

Management. In the early stages, the patient is treated by fluid and diet regulation based on frequent blood and urine reports. Rest and activity are adjusted to the degree of hypertension and renal insufficiency. As with the patient with acute glomerulonephritis, the prevention of respiratory infection is very important. When the kidneys can no longer keep the concentration of nonprotein nitrogenous wastes and the chemical composition of the blood within safe levels, regular dialysis may be instituted. At this time, the patient may become a candidate for a kidney transplant.

Pyelonephritis

This is an inflammation of the pelvis and parenchymal tissue of the kidney due to infection. The predominant causative organism is the Escherichia bacillus (*E. coli*), an inhabitant of the colon, which has invaded the lower urinary tract and ascended to the kidney via the ureter. In rare instances, the pathogen may be another organism, such as the staphylococcus or streptococcus, and may be blood-borne.

Significant predisposing factors are defective urinary drainage and reflux of urine from the bladder into the ureters. Obstructions to the flow of urine from the kidney may be the result of a renal calculus, newgrowth, stricture of a ureter due to pressure, scarring or congenital anomaly. Stasis of urine in the lower urinary tract due to bladder or urethral dysfunction may increase the intravesical pressure sufficiently to produce a reflux into the ureters.

Pyelonephritis is more common in females than males. The incidence is relatively high in female infants and children, due perhaps to fecal soiling and *E. coli* contamination of the urethral meatus. Its frequent occurrence in pregnant women is attributed to stasis of urine incurred by pressure from the enlarging uterus and atonia of the ureters due to the effect of progesterone. Pyelonephritis in males in the later years of life is generally associated with defective urinary drainage as a result of an enlarged prostate.

Manifestations. The onset is usually sudden. In children it may be accompanied by a convulsion. Manifestations include chills, fever, headache, nausea and vomiting, pain and tenderness in the loins, leukocytosis, frequent and painful micturition (dysuria). The urine is cloudy and contains bacteria, pus and blood, and epithelial cells.

Treatment. The patient is confined to bed and is encouraged to take liberal amounts of fluid unless there is complete obstruction of urinary drainage. An accurate record of the fluid intake and output is necessary. An antibiotic or sulfonamide preparation is prescribed. A urinary antiseptic such as methenamine mandelate (Mandelamine) or nitrofurantoin (Furadantin) may also be ordered. If nitrofurantoin or a sulfonamide preparation such as Gantrisin is used, the patient is observed for possible reactions which usually appear in the form of nausea and vomiting and a skin rash.

Unless there is complete eradication of the infection, pyelonephritis may become chronic with insidious destruction of nephrons, leading to uremia. Following the initial episode of acute pyelonephritis, the patient generally undergoes a thorough investigation for a predisposing obstructive lesion. Antimicrobial therapy and a high fluid intake are prolonged beyond the disappearance of acute signs and symptoms. Specimens of urine are examined and cultured at regular intervals after the antimicrobial drug is discontinued.

Tuberculosis of the Kidney

Tubercular infection in the kidney is usually secondary to tuberculosis elsewhere in the body. The tubercle bacilli are carried by the blood to the kidneys. Scattered characteristic granulomatous lesions (tubercles) develop, eroding renal tissue and leaving cavitations. The infection may involve pyramids and calyces, interfering with tubular drainage and leading to hydronephrosis. The infection may spread to involve the bladder.

The systemic symptoms characteristic of any tubercular infection are usually present—namely, low-grade fever, night sweats, loss of weight, fatigue and a positive tuberculin skin test. The urine contains pus and blood; smears and a culture reveal the presence of tubercle bacilli. The patient complains of back pain, which may become quite severe in advanced disease. An intravenous pyelogram is done to determine whether the disease is unilateral or bilateral.

The patient receives streptomycin, para-aminosalicylic acid (PAS) and isonicotinic acid hydrazide (Isoniazid). He is observed for possible reactions to the drugs which may take the form of dermatitis, fever, dizziness and impaired hearing. The patient may not be required to remain in bed but is placed on a regimen that will provide extra rest and prevent excessive exertion. A nutritious full diet is encouraged without restrictions if there is adequate renal function to prevent the accumulation of wastes in the blood. Frequent urine smears and cultures are made to determine the progress of the patient's disease. Treatment is continued for a lengthy period even if the cultures become negative for tubercle bacilli.

The Nephrotic Syndrome

The characteristic symptoms comprising the nephrotic syndrome are proteinuria, hypoproteinemia, generalized edema and usually hyperlipemia. It may develop in a patient with primary renal disease, or it may be associated with other conditions in which kidney involvement is secondary (e.g., disseminated lupus erythematosus). In many instances, the syndrome occurs without any known preceding primary or secondary renal impairment and is then referred to as idiopathic nephrosis or idiopathic nephrotic syndrome.

The idiopathic form has a much higher incidence in children, and males are more often affected than females. Several authors suggest that it may be the result of an immunologic process (antigen-antibody reaction).[5, 6, 7]

The proteinuria, which is chiefly albumin, is the result of some change in the glomeruli that causes an increase in their permeability to the plasma proteins. Obviously, the loss of the proteins reduces the colloidal osmotic pressure of the blood, contributing to increased movement of fluid into the interstitial spaces as well as to its decreased reabsorption into the capillaries (see p. 49). The resulting decrease in intravascular volume leads to retention of sodium and water by the kidneys. The excessive concentration of serum fatty components, which is determined by estimation of the cholesterol level, is not understood.

The urine is reduced in volume and usually contains casts as well as large amounts of albumin. In contrast with other forms of impaired renal function, the blood pressure and serum nitrogenous waste level (BUN) of patients with idiopathic nephrosis usually remain within a normal range in the absence of advanced damage to glomeruli.

The severity of the nephrotic syndrome is variable. In some, the edema may cause only slight puffiness in the periorbital areas and ankles, yet in others it may be so extreme that ascites (accumulation of fluid in the peritoneal cavity) and pleural effusion

[5] P. B. Beeson, and W. McDermott (Eds.): Cecil-Loeb Textbook of Medicine, 11th ed. Philadelphia, W. B. Saunders Co., 1963, p. 832.

[6] Sir Stanley Davidson (Ed.): The Principles and Practice of Medicine, 7th ed. Edinburgh, E. & S. Livingstone Ltd., 1965, p. 780.

[7] A. F. Michael, et al.: "Immunologic Basis of Renal Disease." Pediat. Clin. North Amer., Vol. 11, No. 3 (Aug. 1964), pp. 685–711.

develop. The edematous areas are generally soft and readily pit on pressure. The patient is usually pale, complains of fatigue and may experience anorexia, which further complicates the problem of hypoproteinemia. The onset may be insidious or abrupt.

When the nephrotic syndrome is secondary to renal disease, the treatment is directed toward the initial cause. The treatment of the idiopathic nephrotic syndrome includes the administration of an adrenal corticoid preparation such as prednisone or cortisone and a low-sodium, high-protein full diet. The recommended daily protein intake is usually 1 Gm. per kg. of body weight plus an amount equivalent to the daily loss in urine. This implies that 24-hour collections of urine are made for estimation of the amount of protein excreted. Because of the anorexia, it may be necessary to use low-sodium milk powder and protein concentrate in order to have the patient receive an adequate amount of protein. Intravenous infusions of plasma or albumin may be given. The patient is particularly susceptible to infection because of the lowered resistance of edematous tissues and reduced plasma gamma globulin which is essential in the formation of antibodies. Precautions are necessary to avoid exposure to infection. Prophylactic doses of an antimicrobial drug (antibiotic or sulfonamide) may be prescribed. A diuretic may be used in some instances if there is not a satisfactory response to the corticoid preparation and a reduction of the edema. Spironolactone (Aldactone), which counteracts the effect of aldosterone on the renal tubules, may be the drug of choice, or a thiazide preparation such as chlorothiazide (e.g., Diuril) may be indicated. The patient is not usually hospitalized after a satisfactory therapeutic regimen is established, nor is he confined to bed. Activity within his tolerance is encouraged. Treatment is generally required over a long period, and frequent medical checkups are necessary. A referral to a visiting nurse agency may be made to ensure regular supervision and guidance in dietary preparation, the taking of the prescribed drugs and the prevention of infection.

Nephrolithiasis (Renal Calculi)

Stones or small concretions may develop in the collecting tubules, calyces or the pelvis of a kidney. They are formed by the precipitation of urinary solids which adhere to a nucleus formed of sloughed tissue cells, pus, bacteria, blood or a combination of these. The precipitate may be calcium oxalate or phosphate, uric acid, or cystine, but most often stones are of mixed composition. They vary in size from tiny particles to large smooth or irregular masses. The irregular stone that forms in the pelvis and has projections into the calyces is referred to as a staghorn calculus.

Factors that predispose to renal calculus formation include infection, stasis of urine, hypercalcemia and hypercalciuria, and excessive excretion of uric acid (as in gout) and cystine. The latter may be the result of a disturbance in the metabolism of methionine (an amino acid) or faulty tubular reabsorption. Prolonged bed rest and immobility promote hypercalcemia and stasis of urine in the lower calyces. This emphasizes the importance of frequent change of position, range-of-motion exercises and a high fluid intake for patients who must be in bed. The immobile patient may be placed on a CircOlectric bed to facilitate renal drainage as well as promote circulation.

Renal calculi may obstruct renal drainage by impaction of the tubules, by completely filling calyces and the pelvis, or by lodging in a ureter. The urine accumulates in the pelvis and tubules, dilating them and creating a back pressure. This condition is known as hydronephrosis. Compression of the blood vessels and nephrons by the mass of fluid leads to their destruction and obliteration and to renal insufficiency.

Symptoms. The manifestations of renal calculus depend on the size of the stone and whether it remains stationary. It may remain silent over a long period, producing no symptoms. Small, gravel-like stones may be passed without any disturbance.

The majority cause some pain, hematuria, infection, and if large, kidney damage and renal insufficiency.

The patient may complain of pain in the back which may be caused by irritation of tissues by movement of the stone or the back pressure and accumulation of fluid if the stone is obstructing renal or ureteral outflow. A small stone may enter the ureter and initiate ureteral colic. The patient complains of excruciating pain radiating from the back to the front along the groin into the genitalia. He becomes pale, perspires, is extremely restless and may vomit. Frequently he thrashes about, assuming unusual positions in an attempt to obtain some relief.

Hematuria results from injury to the lining membrane of the pelvis or ureter. Infection is frequently associated with a calculus, and if present, chills, fever, leukocytosis and pyuria are likely to be manifested.

Complete obstruction of the kidney outflow is eventually reflected in renal insufficiency and a palpable mass in the renal area as a result of the hydronephrosis. The total volume of urine is less than normal, and blood investigations indicate reduced elimination of waste products.

Investigation of the patient for nephrolithiasis includes a simple roentgenogram of the kidneys, ureters and bladder. Preparation for this x-ray usually involves a cathartic the night before the x-ray followed by a cleansing enema in the morning. This is to prevent shadows on the film caused by feces and gas in the intestine. Calculi will show up as dense areas. More detailed information is then obtained from intravenous pyelography (see p. 425).

Treatment. If the pyelogram indicates that the calculus is small and may be passed by the patient, he is allowed up and encouraged to be active. Liberal amounts of fluids are given. All urine is strained through several layers of gauze and observation made for concretions.

During an attack of ureteral colic, the patient usually receives an analgesic such as meperidine hydrochloride (Demerol) to relieve the pain and an antispasmodic drug such as propantheline bromide (Pro-Banthine) to promote relaxation of the ureter. When the pain subsides, he is allowed to rest in bed and is given fluids.

If the stone is not passed and is lodged in the ureter, the physician may pass a ureteral catheter through a cystoscope past the calculus. It is usually left in place for 24 hours. This promotes drainage of urine from the renal pelvis and dilates the ureter. Instructions are usually left by the doctor about irrigating the catheter in the event that it becomes blocked by pus and blood in the urine. The patient remains in bed and pre-

cautions are taken to avoid dislodging the catheter. If patency of the catheter cannot be re-established by irrigation or the patient experiences pain, the physician is notified at once. When the catheter is removed, the calculus may pass spontaneously. If the calculus is in the lower third of the ureter, a special ureteral catheter with a looped or corkscrew tip may be passed, and an attempt is made to withdraw the stone.

When a stone in the kidney or ureter is too large to be passed, open surgery may be undertaken. Removal of a stone through the renal parenchyma is called a nephrolithotomy. Removal of a stone directly from the renal pelvis is known as a pyelolithotomy. The operation for extracting a stone from the ureter is a ureterolithotomy. If the calculus is in the lower part of the ureter, it is approached through an abdominal incision. When it is lodged in the upper part of the ureter, the approach is through an incision in the flank. For the nursing care of a patient undergoing renal surgery, see page 445.

Calculi are prone to recur in patients with a history of previous episodes. In an effort to prevent the formation of new stones or the enlargement of existing stones, the patient is advised that a high fluid intake of at least 3000 ml. daily is essential to maintain a dilute urine. A portion of this should be taken at bedtime and during the night to prevent the concentration of urine that normally occurs at night. If the climate or patient's occupation are such that there is an excessive loss of fluid in perspiration, the intake should be increased by 1000 ml.

In some instances, dietary restrictions may be prescribed as a prophylactic measure. If the principal component of the previous stone was calcium, foods high in calcium may be limited. If the ingredients of the stone precipitate readily in acid urine, an alkaline-ash diet* may be ordered. Conversely, if the elements of the calculus are precipitated readily in an alkaline urine, an acid-ash diet* may be recommended. In addition, drugs may be prescribed to maintain alkalinity or acidity of the urine according to whether the chemical of the calculus is more soluble in acid or alkaline urine.

---

*The reader is referred to a diet therapy text for details of these special diets.

The problem is that most stones are of mixed composition.

If the patient should become ill, prolonged immobility should be avoided. The patient is seen at frequent intervals by his physician, and roentgenograms at regular periods may be considered advisable.

Neoplasms in the Kidneys

Newgrowths in the adult kidney are of lower incidence than those in many other areas of the body. When they occur, they are usually malignant and are seen more often in males than in females. The most common form in adults is adenocarcinoma, which usually originates in the tubules. It readily invades the blood vessels, causing early metastasis to bones, lungs or liver, which may be the lesion that brings the person to the physician. Wilm's tumor is a highly malignant adenosarcoma which occurs in young children and may grow very large before being discovered.

In the adult, the first symptom is usually hematuria. As the neoplasm enlarges, the kidney becomes a palpable mass and the patient experiences pain, abdominal discomfort from pressure, anorexia and loss of weight. Ureteral colic may occur as a result of a blood clot entering the ureter. Polycythemia develops in some patients due to an overproduction of erythropoietin by the affected kidney. Others may have marked anemia. In children, the newgrowth is frequently first noted as an abdominal mass or swelling by the mother.

A cystoscopy with ureteral catheterization is done to determine if the source of the bleeding is unilateral or bilateral. Roentgenographic studies are made, using an intravenous or retrograde pyelogram to determine filling defects and the location of the neoplasm. A renal angiogram may also be done to assess the extent of blood vessel involvement.

If the disease is localized to one kidney, a nephrectomy is performed, followed by radiation or chemotherapy or both. If the renal pelvis is involved, the ureter is removed along with the kidney (nephro-ureterectomy). For nursing care required following renal surgery, see page 445. When both kidneys are affected or the patient's condition is considered inoperable, radia-tion and chemotherapy may be used. For the care of the patient receiving radiation and anticancer drug therapy, see Chapter 8.

Polycystic Disease of the Kidneys

This disorder is characterized by the widespread distribution of cysts of varying size throughout both kidneys. The disease is congenital and familial with equal affection of both sexes. It is predominant in infants and adults over 40 years of age. In infants and young children, other abnormalities may be present. The disease is often found in more than one member of a family and in successive generations. Because of the distinct difference in the age of the groups in which the disease has its greatest incidence, it is suggested that there are two different genetic types. When it occurs in infants and young children, it is considered to be autosomal recessive, but the polycystic disease which becomes manifest in adults is autosomal dominant.[8, 9]

The adult form is more common and progresses slowly; the patient remains asymptomatic during the first 3 to 4 decades of life. As the cysts enlarge, functional tissue and blood vessels are compressed, and eventually, serious renal insufficiency develops. Pressure on abdominal viscera may interfere with normal functioning and cause discomfort. The symptoms are intermittent gross hematuria from the rupture of blood vessels, pain in the back and abdomen and a palpable mass. The patient may experience episodes of ureteral colic due to blood clots entering the ureters. The degree of compression and damage of parenchymal tissue by the cysts determines the length of survival of the patient. With progression of the disease, he gradually manifests signs of increasing renal failure. The blood pressure and blood nitrogenous waste levels rise, electrolyte and fluid imbalances and anemia develop, and the patient eventually enters the terminal uremic phase.

Conservative treatment of the patient is

---

[8]W. L. Furlow, and L. F. Greene: "Congenital Polycystic Disease." Med. Clin. North Amer., Vol. 50, No. 4 (July 1966), p. 1102.

[9]W. A. Sodeman, and W. A. Sodeman, Jr.: Pathologic Physiology, 4th ed. Philadelphia, W. B. Saunders Co., 1967, p. 48.

similar to that for chronic glomerulonephritis. The patient may be maintained and kept active by regular hemodialysis. Various surgical procedures have been used and include incision and drainage of the cysts, application of sclerosing agents to the walls of the cysts, and decapsulation of the kidneys.

Since polycystic disease of the kidneys is a familial disorder, when a patient is discovered to be affected, other members of his family are examined and followed by routine checkups.

Trauma of the Kidneys

Accidental blows and injury to a kidney are not uncommon and may cause contusion, laceration or rupture of the capsule. In laceration and rupture, hemorrhage and the escape of urine into the surrounding tissues are serious problems. Gross or microscopic hematuria occurs and there is pain and tenderness in the kidney region. If the injury is severe and massive hemorrhage occurs, shock develops rapidly. Blood transfusions are given, and surgical intervention is used to bring the bleeding under control. The kidney may be repaired, or a partial or complete nephrectomy may be necessary, depending on the damage revealed. Contusion of the kidney will usually heal spontaneously. The patient is kept at rest, the fluid intake and output are recorded, and a frequent check is made of the urine for blood. If the damage is extensive, nephrons may be replaced by fibrous scar tissue, resulting in residual impaired function.

Hemodialysis

Hemodialysis is a procedure used in acute and chronic renal failure to lower the blood level of metabolic waste products (urea, creatinine and uric acid) and to correct abnormal electrolyte concentrations. Two methods currently in use are extracorporeal dialysis, which uses a machine referred to as the artificial kidney, and peritoneal dialysis. The term extracorporeal means that the dialysis takes place outside the body.

Both methods operate on the same principle. Dialysis implies the separation of 2 solutions by a semipermeable membrane. Molecules and ions of solutes pass through the membrane along a concentration gradient from higher to lower until an equilibrium is established on either side. The movement of a solute in dialysis depends on the size of its molecules as well as on its concentration on each side of the membrane. In hemodialysis, a porous membrane separates the circulating blood from a specially prepared dialyzing solution (dialysate) which usually contains specified amounts of sodium chloride, sodium bicarbonate, calcium chloride, magnesium chloride and glucose, all of which are normal plasma constituents.* By increasing or decreasing the amount of a solute in the dialysate in relation to its blood concentration, it will move into or out of the blood. For example, if the patient has been losing an excess of sodium in chronic renal failure, the sodium concentration of the dialysate is increased to a level above that of the blood to promote the diffusion of sodium ions into the blood. If hyperkalemia is a problem, the blood concentration is reduced by decreasing the amount of potassium added to the dialysate. Waste products (such as urea and creatinine) which are not being eliminated by the kidneys are not included in the dialysate, causing them to move out of the blood.

The porosity of the membrane used in hemodialysis only permits the transfer of small molecular solutes. Larger molecular substances, such as the plasma proteins, are held back.

Extracorporeal Hemodialysis. Various types of machines or dialyzers have been designed for extracorporeal hemodialysis, but all work on the same principle. In one widely used model, the blood is conducted out of a vessel into a long, porous, cellophane tube and is returned to a vein. The tube is encased in a supporting mesh and coiled on a drum which is suspended in a tank containing the dialyzing solution. The latter is kept in motion by a pump, is kept at body temperature, and is changed every 1 or 2 hours.

Before commencing dialysis, the cellophane tube is rinsed with sterile normal

---

*The inclusion of the calcium and magnesium salts may be influenced by the composition of the local water supply.

saline. It is then primed with 2 pints of blood which are compatible with each other as well as with the patient's blood. A further supply of compatible blood is kept readily available in case the patient's hematocrit indicates anemia that requires transfusion treatment or in the event of bleeding. Heparin is added to the priming blood and to the patient's inflow blood at intervals during the dialysis to prevent clotting within the extracorporeal circuit. The clotting time is checked frequently during the treatment. A bubble and clot trap is attached to the venous end of the line. Upon completion of the procedure, protamine sulfate may be injected into the venous end of the system to neutralize the circulating heparin. In some extracorporeal dialyses, regional heparinization may be used. This involves a steady infusion of heparin into the blood just after it leaves the patient and continuous neutralization of the heparin by the addition of protamine sulfate to the blood just before it re-enters the patient.

The rate at which the blood is pumped through the dialyzer is regulated according to the patient's body size and blood pressure, varying from 200 to 500 ml. per minute. A more rapid rate is usually used with a large person. It is limited at the commencement of dialysis and is gradually increased as the blood pressure stabilizes. A sharp fall in the blood pressure occurs if the blood flows out of the patient more rapidly than it is being returned or if there is an excessive loss of water into the dialysate, reducing the patient's total intravascular volume.

The pressure of the blood in the coil is monitored and can be raised by the application of a special clamp on the venous end of the tube. The latter procedure is used to establish a pressure gradient between the blood and dialysate for the purpose of increasing the filtration of water and salts from the blood. This process is referred to as ultrafiltration. In some instances, the dialysate may be made hypertonic to create an osmotic pressure that will remove excess water from the blood.

The length of time the patient is kept on the dialyzer varies with the patient's condition and type of machine used. The average range is 4 to 8 hours for patients on a regular dialysis program but may be longer for a patient with an acute renal shutdown. The frequency also varies with patients. In acute renal failure, daily dialysis may be necessary until renal function is re-established. Patients with chronic renal insufficiency are dialyzed 2 or 3 times weekly and probably lead a relatively normal productive life the remainder of the week. The chronic dialysis program may be long-term, extending over years, or may be a temporary measure for the patient who is awaiting a kidney transplant.

The patient and his family receive a simple explanation of the purpose of dialysis and what it involves. Prior to the initial treatment, if the patient's condition permits, he may visit the dialysis unit, meet the dialysis staff, and perhaps chat with a patient who is on a regular dialysis program; such preparation is helpful in reducing the patient's fears. A consent for the dialysis is signed by the patient or next of kin.

Preceding the first treatment, cutdowns are done to expose an artery and an adjacent vein. Either arm or leg vessels may be used. A cannula is introduced into each vessel, secured and attached to tubing which is brought out through the skin. An arteriovenous (A-V) shunt is established by connecting the tubes leading from the cannulae. The cannulae and tubing which are used are of inert synthetic materials (teflon and silastic) so that the shunt may remain permanently without causing reaction and deterioration. The incisions are sutured around the tubes, and sterile dressings and a bandage applied. Two clamps are attached to the bandage at all times so that they are readily available should the tubes become disconnected and bleeding occur. The distal loop of the **U**-shaped tube is left exposed so the patency of the shunt can be checked. If the patient is restless, it may be necessary to splint the limb. To start dialysis, the connecting tube on the A-V shunt is removed; the tube leading from the cannula in the artery is connected to the inflow tube of the dialyzer, and the tube leading from the cannula in the vein is fitted to the outflow tube of the machine.

Since available sites for establishing an A-V shunt are limited, certain precautions and care are necessary to prevent complications and maintain the patency of the bypass. The loop of the tube is checked at least every 2 hours for blood flow. Clotting in the shunt system and obstruction of the flow may occur with kinking or malalignment of the tubes or pressure being exerted on them. The blood becomes dark blue, and the bruit that is normally heard with a stethoscope over the venous side is absent. The tube must not be pinched to check cannula patency. If clotting is suspected, no attempt is made to clear the tube by "milking." The problem is reported immediately to the doctor or dialysis unit. Efforts will be made to remove the clots by aspiration and the use of heparinized saline.

The site is also checked for bleeding. If the tubes become disconnected, free bleeding is quickly recognized and the clamps previously mentioned are quickly applied to the tubes and the doctor notified. If the clamps do not control the bleeding, a tourniquet may be applied to the limb, releasing it every 5 minutes for 5 seconds. Subcutaneous bleeding may result from the displacement of a cannula or erosion of the artery or vein. This is reported promptly; pressure is applied over the site and a tourniquet used.

The limb in which there is an A-V shunt must not be used to determine blood pressure or administer intravenous infusions. Following the establishment of an A-V bypass in a leg, the patient is usually confined to bed, and all weight-bearing is avoided for about a week.

Specific directions are received from the doctor as to the care of the cannula site. Some suggest daily cleansing of the skin around the exit areas of the tubes with hexachlorophene solution or hydrogen peroxide. Others prefer that the site be cleansed and redressed only at dialysis unless there is infection or oozing of blood. If infection occurs, the skin of the area and the bypass tubing are cleansed daily with the prescribed antiseptic solution. Aseptic dressing technique is used, and a mask is worn by the person carrying out the procedure.

The patient is weighed just before and on completion of each dialysis. A weight loss indicates the fluid loss during the procedure. Blood specimens are taken prior to each dialysis for determining electrolyte concentrations, clotting time and the hematocrit. Adjustments may be necessary in the dialysate in accordance with the electrolyte values. Blood work may be repeated at intervals during the dialysis and on completion. As mentioned previously, the clotting time is usually checked hourly.

The patient is positioned comfortably on his back in bed, with the limb with the A-V shunt exposed and supported. Periodically during dialysis, the head of the bed may be raised or lowered if the blood pressure is satisfactory, the pillows are turned, gentle massage may be given to pressure areas and slight adjustments made to reduce the discomfort incurred by the hours of immobilization. A sedative may be prescribed if the patient is restless or extremely apprehensive.

The sphygmomanometer remains on the patient's arm throughout dialysis as frequent recordings of the blood pressure are necessary since the flow rate through the dialyzer is regulated accordingly. The pulse is checked at least every 15 minutes at first, gradually lengthening the interval to one-half hour if it is satisfactory. Continuous cardiac monitoring by oscillograph tracing may be required in some patients so there will be prompt recognition of a cardiac arrhythmia should it develop. The rate of respirations is noted and any difficulty in breathing, coughing or moist sounds are reported promptly.

Repeated checks are made for any indication of bleeding. The mouth, cannula sites, and all excreta are examined for any sign of blood. The dialyzing fluid is inspected frequently for any discoloration that would occur with the leaking of blood from the circuit.

Headache, vomiting and twitching may develop and should be brought to the physician's attention. Rarely, a patient becomes disoriented or has a convulsion. These disturbances are attributed to cerebral edema. Urea is cleared more rapidly from the blood than it crosses the brain-blood barrier. As a result, the higher concentration of urea in cerebral tissue fluid produces an osmotic pressure, resulting in the movement of water into the cerebral tissue.

Fluids are given, if tolerated, within the daily allowance. The patient is fed his regular meal, and in some instances, the dietary restriction on protein may be relaxed to some extent for that one meal. He is usually asked if there is something he would especially like to have.

If the bedpan is needed during dialysis, sufficient assistance is provided to prevent possible disturbance of the cannulae and tubes. The fluid intake and output are measured and recorded.

On completion of the dialysis, the shunt is re-established by attaching the connecting tube to the cannulae. Sterile dressings and a crepe or elasticized bandage are applied; again the nurse or assistant makes sure that the curved portion of the tube remains exposed and the emergency clamps are attached to the bandage. If the dialysis is not to be repeated, the cannulae are removed, the open areas sutured and pressure dressings and a snug bandage are applied. The site is checked frequently for possible hemorrhage.

An important role of the nurse working with a patient on a dialysis program is to provide psychological support and assistance with socioeconomic problems for him and his family. They very much need someone who indicates an appreciation of their problems, who is sincerely interested in the patient's progress and willing to help them, and in whom they have confidence. Dependence on a machine for survival is very threatening and difficult to accept. The patient and a family member receive detailed instruction about the dietary and fluid restrictions. These restrictions vary from patient to patient. Protein is limited to 40 to 60 Gm.; sodium and potassium may be restricted in some cases. Food values and meal planning are outlined. The relationship of the diet to the blood urea and potassium and of sodium to edema and blood pressure are discussed. (The fluid intake is based on the volume of urinary output.) The patient and his family need help in interpreting the patient's limitations and activities. His occupation and usual activities are determined, and suggestions are made as to advisable adjustments. In such discussions, it is important that suggestions include what the patient might do as well as what he should not do.

Care and maintenance of the A-V shunt are taught, and the patient takes over the necessary observations and care before his discharge from hospital. As well as the care procedure, the importance of observing the shunt every 1 to 2 hours, the recognition of complications (bleeding, clotting and in-fection) and the appropriate action should complications occur are discussed. Advice is given as to how the patient may protect the A-V bypass and also have maximum freedom.

The patient is given written instructions which outline the prescribed diet, fluid intake, activities and required rest, necessary observations, and the maintenance and care of the A-V shunt. In some instances, it is necessary to teach the patient and a family member how to take temperature and blood pressure.

After discharge from hospital, the dialysis unit may request the patient to record exactly the food and fluid taken between dialyses. This helps to determine if the restrictions are understood and being respected. The success of a dialysis program is largely dependent upon the ability of the patient to protect and maintain his shunt and upon his adherence to the dietary, fluid and activity regulations. This is tactfully conveyed to the patient and his family throughout the teaching and discussions.

A regular dialysis regimen has prolonged the life of many patients with chronic renal failure. It has permitted many of them to continue in their jobs and be independent, useful members of society. Although the hospital dialysis units have increased in number in recent years, particularly in larger medical centers, the number of patients that can be treated is still limited. The hospital-based unit usually necessitates the patient being away from his work at least 2 days a week. Because of this, the units' limitations, and the distance of many patients from a center, dialysis at home has been made possible for some patients. At present, the number is small but is steadily increasing. The references cited below feature hemodialysis in the home.[10, 11, 12, 13]

Peritoneal Dialysis. In this method of hemodialysis, the peritoneum and its capillaries are used as the dialyzing membrane

[10]A. Rae, et al.: "Hemodialysis in the Home," J.A.M.A., Vol. 206, No. 1 (Sept. 30, 1968), pp. 92–96.

[11]L. Schlotter: "Learning to be a Home Dialysis Patient," Nurs. Clin. North Amer., Vol. 4, No. 3 (Sept. 1969), pp. 419–428.

[12]B. M. Stewart: "Hemodialysis in the Home." Nurs. Clin. North Amer., Vol. 4, No. 3 (Sept. 1969), pp. 431–442.

[13]S. Wood: "Hemodialysis in the Home." Canad. Nurse, Vol. 65, No. 4 (Apr. 1969), pp. 42–44.

and the dialyzing solution is introduced into the peritoneal cavity. Just as in extracorporeal dialysis, small molecular solutes diffuse along a concentration gradient between the blood and the solution. If the patient is retaining an excess of fluid, the dialysate is made hypertonic and water is removed from the blood by osmosis.

An explanation of the purpose and the procedure is made to the patient and his family, and consent for the dialysis is obtained in writing. The patient is weighed before and on completion of the treatment, and blood levels of electrolytes, urea and creatinine are determined. The vital signs, including the blood pressure, are noted beforehand and serve as a comparative basis during and following the dialysis. The urinary bladder is emptied usually by catheter to prevent possible injury to the bladder by the trocar, and the patient is placed in the dorsal-recumbent position.

Following local anesthesia of the sub-umbilical site to be used, the physician makes a small skin incision and passes a trocar and cannula through the abdominal wall into the peritoneal cavity. The cannula is then replaced by a catheter, which has several openings and is secured to the abdominal wall by tape or a suture. A sterile dressing is fitted snugly around the tube to protect the incision. Two liters* of sterile dialysate (similar in composition to that used in extracorporeal hemodialysis) are warmed to body temperature and the flasks suspended on an infusion pole. Their tubes are connected by a Y tube which in turn connects to a tube leading to the catheter. The solution is allowed to flow rapidly into the peritoneal cavity and this generally takes 10 to 15 minutes. When the bottles are almost empty, the tubing is clamped; this leaves fluid in the system to initiate siphonage drainage later. The dialysate remains in the abdomen for a prescribed 30 to 90 minutes. The bottles are then lowered to the floor and the clamp released. It takes approximately 15 to 20 minutes for the solution to return. Fluid in excess of the volume initially introduced must be collected in another closed, sterile container and measured. The alternating infusion of fresh sterile dialysate and

*If the patient is a child, this amount is reduced to 1000 to 1500 ml.

drainage is repeated for the period of time specified by the physician which may vary from 10 to 36 hours. Should the drainage become very slow or stop before a minimum of 1800 ml. is returned, the openings into the catheter are likely to be blocked by omentum or viscera. *Gentle* pressure with the flat of the hand on the lower abdomen, or changing the patient's position may free the catheter and re-establish drainage. If these moves are not successful, the doctor is notified. The first return may be expected to be slightly tinged with blood from the parietal tissues. If this persists in subsequent exchanges, the doctor is consulted.

The blood pressure and pulse are recorded every 15 minutes during the first exchange, then every 30 to 60 minutes if they are stable. Any untoward signs or symptoms such as abdominal pain, vomiting, sharp rise or fall in blood pressure, rapid weak pulse, pallor, severe headache or reduced level of consciousness are reported promptly. If the dialysate is hypertonic, the blood pressure and pulse are recorded every 15 minutes throughout the entire procedure so that too great a loss of intravascular fluid will be quickly recognized before severe hypotension and shock develop. If the return fluid should reach 500 ml. in excess of the volume of dialysate used, the physician is consulted before any further exchange is undertaken. This indicates the necessity for an accurate record of the volume of dialysate infused and the amount returned with each exchange. Blood chemistry studies (BUN, electrolytes) are made at intervals during the dialysis and on completion.

Since the patient remains on his back during dialysis, frequent turning of his pillows, massage of pressure areas and limbs, the placing of sheepskin under the patient, and a brief change of position between exchanges are used to relieve the discomfort of the long periods of immobilization.

On completion of the treatment, the catheter is removed, and sterile gauze and dressing pads are applied. The site is observed at frequent intervals for drainage, and moist dressings are changed for sterile dry ones. The temperature and pulse are recorded every 3 or 4 hours. Fever, rapid pulse, complaints of abdominal pain and any abdominal rigidity are reported to the doctor since they may indicate complicating peritonitis.

Nursing in Renal Surgery

The more common surgical procedures used in the treatment of kidney disease include the following: nephrectomy (the removal of a kidney — may be partial or complete), nephrolithotomy (the removal of a calculus from the parenchymal portion of the kidney), pyelolithotomy (the removal of a calculus through an incision into the renal pelvis), nephrostomy (an incision into the kidney and the insertion of a tube for drainage) and nephro-ureterectomy (the removal of a kidney and its ureter).

Preoperative Preparation. Surgery on a kidney is preceded by a period of investigation of kidney function and the patient's general condition. If a nephrectomy is anticipated, the ability of the opposite kidney to compensate and assume the full responsibility for renal function must be determined. The patient and his family are generally very apprehensive of this major surgery. Aware of this, the nurse observes their behavior to determine their level of anxiety, concerns, and the reassurance needed. By showing an interest in them, providing opportunities for them to express their feelings, answering their questions and explaining what may be expected, the nurse helps to reduce the patient's and his family's anxiety and promotes their confidence in those responsible for his care. They may have been advised by the doctor that the removal of a kidney is necessary and need reassurance that normal function can be maintained by one kidney.

The physical preparation is similar to that cited in Chapter 10. Unless contraindicated by a condition such as hydronephrosis, the fluid intake is increased to promote the maximum excretion of metabolic wastes before surgery as well as optimal hydration. Since the incision is usually made in the flank of the affected side, the area of skin to be shaved and cleansed extends from the anterior midline to beyond the spine and from the nipple line to the symphysis pubis (see Fig. 10–1). The surgeon may request that an indwelling catheter and a nasogastric tube be passed the morning of operation. The latter is used because renal surgical patients are prone to develop a reduction or cessation of peristalsis and severe abdominal distention. The catheter is introduced so that a frequent check may be made of the urinary output.

Postoperative Care. The general nursing care presented in Chapter 10 is applicable to the patient who has had renal surgery. The nurse must be familiar with what was done at operation in order to understand the purposes and care of drainage tubes and make pertinent observations. The operative site is checked at frequent intervals for bleeding. If the kidney was removed, the wound may be sealed with only a tissue drain inserted. If the kidney remains, a tube may have been inserted, necessitating frequent observation for patency and characteristics of the drainage. The tube may become obstructed by a clot, which will cause back pressure unless promptly cleared. Irrigation with a small amount (approximately 10 ml.) of sterile normal saline may be ordered to remove clots. If the tube is connected to a drainage receptacle, the amount is measured and recorded every 6 to 8 hours. The volume of the urinary drainage from the indwelling catheter is noted, and less than 25 to 30 ml. per hour is reported. The urine is also checked for any sign of bleeding. An accurate record of the daily intake and output is kept and the balance estimated. A regular schedule of deep breathing, coughing and turning is established. A directive is received from the surgeon as to positioning. Some patients are not permitted to lie on the operative side for 36 to 48 hours; in other instances, the patient may be encouraged to lie on that side to promote drainage. With each change of position, caution must be used to avoid displacing the tube or leaving it compressed, kinked or with traction on it. Because of the location of the incision, deep breathing is likely to be painful, predisposing to shallow respirations and pulmonary complications. The nurse assists the patient and supports the operative area while prompting the patient to take 8 to 10 deep respirations and cough every 1 to 2 hours.

If the dressings become moist, they are reinforced and the surgeon consulted. He may not want them disturbed for the first day or two. If there is urine drainage, the dressings are changed frequently to prevent maceration of the skin and an offensive odor.

The patient is sustained on intravenous infusions for 36 to 48 hours. Clear fluids may then be given orally in small amounts and increased gradually as tolerated. Solid food is introduced as soon as intestinal peristalsis is re-established which is evident by the passage of flatus and absence of abdominal distention. If distention develops, the naso-gastric tube is left in place, and a rectal tube is inserted. A heat application (e.g., electric heating pad) to the abdomen may be ordered. An intramuscular injection of neostigmine (Prostigmin) may be prescribed to stimulate peristalsis, and a carminative enema is given.

Considerable pain is usually experienced in the first 2 to 3 days. Some aches and discomfort may be the result of the hyperextended lateral position used during operation. Support, change of position and analgesics are necessary. A small pillow placed between the lower costal margin and the iliac crest when the patient is on his side may reduce the discomfort by relieving strain on the incision.

Hospitalization for a minimum period of 12 to 14 days is usually considered necessary following renal surgery, since secondary hemorrhage may develop due to delayed healing and the sloughing of renal tissue. Necessary limitations of activity, any dietary restrictions, and the optimal fluid intake are discussed in detail with the patient and a family member before hospital discharge. If the wound still requires a dressing, they are taught how to care for it, or a referral is made to the visiting nurse agency. The expense of the necessary dressing supplies may pose a problem for the patient. An application may be made to an appropriate source of assistance, such as a service club or the community welfare organization.

Kidney Transplantation

The development of donor selection by tissue typing and the steady progress that has been made in managing the rejection process have resulted in an increase in kidney transplants. The candidates are carefully selected by a team of physicians, surgeons and a psychiatrist. Prospective recipients are persons whose life expectancy is limited to a few months at the most as a result of severe renal insufficiency or who have had a bilateral nephrectomy because of serious hypertension attributed to the release of excessive rennin by the kidneys. The patient must be free of chronic infection in other systems, and the lower urinary tract must be structurally normal and free of disease.

Rejection Process. The greatest hazard associated with any organ or tissue transplant from another person is the incompatibility of the recipient's tissue with that of the donor and the ensuing rejection process. Secondary to this are the consequences of the immunosuppressive drugs used to depress the rejection process, the most formidable one being the recipient's susceptibility to infection.

The rejection process is an antigen-antibody reaction or immune response. The present concept of the process suggests that cellular proteins, which are specific for each individual, act as antigens. They are released from the donor organ and transmitted to the lymphoid tissues (lymph nodes, spleen). The response is an increased production of lymphocytes and plasma cells which form antibodies to the foreign protein. These cells and antibodies are released into the circulation, invading and attacking the donor tissue. The kidney becomes swollen, edematous and congested. Thrombosis occurs in the blood vessels, and tissue necrosis due to ischemia follows. Rejection is manifested by fever, tenderness and swelling in the kidney region, general malaise, headache, anorexia, an elevation in the leukocyte count, decreased urinary output, edema, hypertension and elevated blood levels of urea, creatinine, sodium and potassium.

Because the cellular proteins are specific for each individual, donor tissue is rejected by the recipient's body unless it is taken from an identical twin. In this case, the transplant is compatible because the cellular proteins of both the host and donor are identical, having been determined by the same genetic blueprint of a single fertilized ovum. Such a graft (with identical cellular proteins or antigens) is referred to as an isograft. A graft between two genetically dissimilar persons is known as an allograft.

The intensity of the rejection process and the rapidity with which it develops correspond to the degree of difference in the structure of the cellular proteins of the recipient and donor; the greater the difference (or numbers of antigens), the more severe and rapid is the rejection. A method of tissue typing has been developed which has contributed greatly to the selection of more compatible donors. Tissue compatibility is tested on the basis of antigens carried by the lymphocytes. Not all the lymphocytic antigens have been identified, but to date, 12 types have been recognized. Currently, tissue matching is indicated as A, B, C or D. A represents the match characteristic of identical twins. B tissue indicates the presence of fewer antigens than a C match, and similarly, C has fewer than D.

Unless the organ is taken from an identical twin, some degree of rejection will occur. Fortunately, the process can be modified by therapeutic agents which depress the tissues responsible for the production of lymphocytes, plasma cells and antibodies. The immunosuppressive preparations used include azathioprine (Imuran), cortisone (prednisone), actinomycin C and antilymphocytic globulin (ALG). ALG is produced by the injection of washed lymphocytes into a horse, which reacts by forming antibodies against the antigens. Blood is then withdrawn from the horse and the globulin fraction extracted from the serum. Suppression of the patient's immune reaction makes him extremely vulnerable to any infection.

Donor. In early transplants, the kidney was obtained from a live, blood relative. Now cadavers serve as the principal donor source. The cadaver is frequently an accident victim or someone who has had a sudden death and who is known to have been in good health.

If a living donor is used, he is usually related to the patient. The donation is more likely to be successful if the relationship is close (e.g., sibling, parent) rather than a genetically nonrelated person (e.g., cousin, uncle by marriage). Obviously, the living donor must be in good health. He undergoes a thorough investigation which includes an intravenous urogram and an aortogram to ensure normal kidneys with a normal vascular supply. He must have volunteered willingly and made the decision without pressure from others. He is informed of the surgery he will undergo, the inherent risk in being left with one kidney, and the possibility of rejection of the allograft by the recipient.

When a cadaver is sought as a donor, the next of kin is approached when it is known that the patient cannot recover. Consent is obtained previous to actual decease, so that the organ can be removed promptly when death occurs to avoid damage from ischemia. Rarely have relatives been known to refuse.

Permission from the coroner is also necessary in the case of accidental and sudden death. Several persons are usually awaiting a kidney transplant. When a donor becomes imminent, a selection of 2 recipients is made on the basis of tissue matching, since both kidneys of the cadaver are usually used.

When death occurs, the kidneys are removed with their arteries, veins and ureters and are perfused with cold saline or lactated Ringer's solution containing heparin and procaine. The procaine promotes dilatation of the vessels. The donor kidney is placed in the recipient's iliac fossa on the side opposite to that from which it was taken. Its renal artery is anastomosed to the host's hypogastric artery and the renal vein of the graft is anastomosed to the common iliac vein. The ureter is implanted in the recipient's bladder, and his kidneys are removed because they are a potential source of infection. In some instances, the patient may have had a previous bilateral nephrectomy and was maintained entirely on hemodialysis.

Preoperative Preparation of the Recipient. When a person is selected as a candidate for a renal transplant, the physician discusses in detail with him and his family all that is involved. They are advised that his disease is irreversible and is likely to prove fatal before long. They are informed of what is entailed in the surgery; that the kidney graft may be rejected, necessitating the resumption of a chronic hemodialysis program; that continuous drug therapy and close supervision will be needed; and that precautions against infections will be necessary. A special consent is signed, indicating that the extent of his disease, the prognosis and what a transplant involves have been fully explained. If the patient has not been having hemodialysis, twice weekly treatments are instituted in an effort to bring him into an optimal condition for the transplant. Cultures are taken from the skin and all body orifices to check for infection. If any is found to be present, he receives appropriate antibiotic therapy. All personnel in contact with the patient should be free of colds and other infection, and strict medical asepsis is observed between patients. If the patient's anemia is severe, he may receive whole blood or packed cells, but generally transfusions are avoided because of the increased risk of sensitization and provoking an immunologic reaction. This predisposes the patient to more severe and rapid rejection of the donor kidney. The blood pressure, which is likely to be elevated, is followed closely. If an antihypertensive drug is being administered, the nurse is alert for side effects and sharp swings up or down. An accurate record is made of the fluid intake and output; the intake is regulated daily according to the output of the previous day to avoid overloading. Efforts are made to improve the patient's nutritional status and to meet his calorie requirements. His diet is catered to within the protein and sodium restrictions prescribed.

When the death of a suitable donor becomes imminent, the patient is started on immunosuppressive drugs. If the period is likely to be short, Imuran and Sulu-Cortef may be given intravenously. If the drugs are given orally over several days, the dosage may be adjusted according to the daily leukocyte count. The patient's hair is washed, and a hexachlorophene (pHisoHex) bath may be ordered to minimize the bacterial flora on the skin. The preoperative skin cleansing and shaving extend from the axillae to mid-thighs and include the perineum. A nasogastric tube may to passed to control postoperative vomiting and distention.

Postoperative Care. A unit and its content are thoroughly cleaned and disinfected in preparation to receive the transplant patient from the operating room. The care of the patient is assigned to one nurse (each shift), who does not participate in the care of other patients for several days to avoid possible cross infection. As well as the usual equipment necessary following any major surgery, the equipment assembled includes that required for protective isolation (sterile gowns, masks and gloves), collecting and measuring the urinary drainage (sterile connecting tubing and receptacle, sterile graduates, sterile specimen bottles including one for 24-hour collection, sterile water for rinsing), collecting and measuring gastric drainage (an intermittent gastric suction machine may be used), and special recording sheets (vital signs, hourly fluid intake and output, medication, doctor's orders, clinical nursing notes).

FLUID INTAKE AND OUTPUT. The patient returns from the operating room with an intravenous infusion running and an indwelling catheter in the bladder. The catheter is immediately connected to a sterile tubing and drainage receptacle. The nasogastric tube is attached to the suction machine or an appropriate receptacle. The urine is measured and recorded hourly, and frequent analysis is made for the specific gravity and protein, blood, sugar and acetone content. The gastric drainage is usually measured every 4 hours. The prescribed amount and composition of the fluid administered intravenously are based on the patient's fluid output (urinary and gastric drainage) and the urinalyses.

The transplanted kidney usually begins to excrete urine soon after the surgery. The volume may increase rapidly, resulting in profuse diuresis. Unless there is adequate replacement during this diuretic phase, dehydration, shock and electrolyte imbalance may develop. If the transplant fails to excrete sufficient urine for several days, hemodialysis may be used until the kidney function improves. A 24-hour collection of urine is continued for at least 10 to 14 days. Once the kidney function appears to be stabilized and the hourly measurement can be discontinued, the catheter is removed. The patient is encouraged to void frequently, and an aliquot of each voiding is analyzed. The nasogastric tube is usually removed within the 48 hours after surgery, and the patient receives clear fluids by mouth.

OBSERVATIONS. As well as the close check made of the patient's fluid intake and output, frequent monitoring of the vital signs is necessary. A daily leukocyte count is done, and frequent determinations are made of the blood levels of creatinine, urea and electrolytes. The patient is weighed each day at the same time, and any significant increase or decrease is reported. The nurse must be constantly alert for early signs and symptoms of the rejection process, infection, and side effects of the immunosuppressive drugs.

PROTECTION FROM INFECTION. Protective isolation technique is carried out for 1 to 2 weeks. Only personnel free of infection are allowed to enter the unit and give care to the patient. They are required to wear a sterile gown, gloves and mask. Close relatives permitted to visit the patient are screened for infection, are required to wear sterile gowns, caps and masks during the visit, and are not permitted direct contact with him. Originally, efforts were made to maintain an almost aseptic environment for transplant patients during their hospitalization. Some details have been relaxed since it was found that most complicating infections were endogenous.

The nurse must be constantly aware of the patient's lowered body resistance to infection due to depression of his most important defense mechanisms (lymphocytes and antibodies). The recognition of early signs of infection is necessary so that prompt antibiotic therapy may be instituted. Any oral or skin lesion, cough, nasal discharge, gastrointestinal disturbance, elevation of temperature or complaint of general malaise, pain or discomfort is promptly brought to the physician's attention. Following surgery, deep breathing and coughing every 1 to 2 hours are carried out until the patient is ambulatory to prevent the accumulation of mucus in the respiratory tract. Frequent cleansing and rinsing of the mouth with an oral antiseptic are important. A soft toothbrush is recommended to avoid trauma to the gums and oral mucosa.

MEDICATION. Following the surgery, the patient receives azathioprine (Imuran), corticoid preparation (prednisone) and antilymphocytic globulin at regular intervals. The frequency of the intramuscular injections of ALG is gradually decreased after 2 weeks and eventually discontinued. Imuran and prednisone are continued and their dosage is adjusted according to the leukocyte count and the patient's reactions to the drugs. It is necessary for the nurse to be familiar with the side effects of these drugs. Imuran may depress the bone marrow production of leukocytes and produce leukopenia. Reactions to prolonged administration of prednisone may include the retention of sodium and water, an elevation of the blood pressure, diabetes mellitus, hirsutism, the development of a round puffy face ("moon face"), euphoria, gastrointestinal ulceration, impaired liver and pancreatic function, and arrested growth in a child. Since ALG is a serum, one must be alert for an anaphylactic reaction; an intracutaneous sensitivity test is done before the initial dose.

The patient is observed closely for early manifestations of the rejection process (see p. 446), which may occur as early as the second or third day. Rejection is treated by increased dosage of the immunosuppressive drugs and the addition of actinomycin C. Local irradiation of the allograft area may also be used.

DIET. The diet progresses through fluids to soft foods and then to a light diet as tolerated. Roughage and highly seasoned foods are avoided because of the predisposition to gastrointestinal ulceration created by the prednisone. During a rejection crisis, renal function is impaired. The fluid intake and diet are adjusted to the reduced urinary output and changes in blood chemistry which occur. That is, the fluid intake will be approximately 400 ml. in excess of the volume of urine for the preceding day, and protein and sodium are restricted in the diet.

PREPARATION FOR DISCHARGE FROM HOSPITAL. The patient may become apprehensive about leaving the hospital and becoming independent. He is likely to become fearful as he learns he must follow a prescribed pattern of living indefinitely and be ever alert for early signs of rejection and complications. He and a member of his family receive a planned series of instruction which provides them with the opportunity to become informed about all aspects of his care.

A social service worker is usually available in a center where organ transplants are done and can be of considerable assistance to the patient and his family in planning for the future. The patient may not be able to resume his former occupation even if it is still available to him, since strenuous physical activity is not advisable. The social worker may provide assistance in finding suitable employment or, if work is not possible, may help in obtaining welfare assistance to provide for the patient and his family. For instance, the provision of his medications will be costly and may cause financial embarrassment for them.

The drugs which he must continue to take are fully discussed. It is helpful if a sample of each is attached to a card on which the name of the drug, its strength, and directions for taking are clearly printed. The nurse stresses the important role these drugs play and that if, because of illness, they cannot be taken or retained, the patient must promptly contact the physician or clinic. The cards are taken to the clinic or the doctor when visits are made so that if the dosage is changed, directions on the cards may be changed.

The patient is instructed to keep a daily record of his fluid output and to calculate his fluid intake on this basis. Verbal and written explanations are made of the content and preparation of his bland diet. Foods that are restricted are listed. Since the prednisone may increase his appetite, the patient is advised to guard against exceeding his normal weight.

Suggestions are made as to how he may protect himself as much as possible from infection. Close contact with persons with a cold or other types of infections should be avoided. Good hygiene practices in food handling and the frequent washing of the hands are stressed. A daily bath is recommended to minimize skin bacteria, and good oral hygiene is reviewed.

The early signs of rejection are reviewed with the patient and family. By this time, the patient is usually quite familiar with them through experience and realizes that prompt action is necessary. They are also cautioned to immediately report a cold, sore throat, fever, dysuria, frequency or other disturbances which may indicate infection.

The patient is usually in hospital for about 6 weeks. Following his discharge, he is followed closely by weekly visits to the clinic. If his progress is satisfactory, and he indicates understanding and efficient management of his care, the intervals between visits are gradually lengthened. A referral may be made to the visiting nurse association. Prior to visiting the patient at home, the visiting nurse is informed of his history and the details of his care regimen.

Fellowship develops between transplant patients while they are in hospital. They share common problems which include restrictions, fears and an uncertainty of life. Continued communication between these persons is encouraged; they can offer great support to one another.

DISORDERS OF THE BLADDER

Manifestations of Bladder Dysfunction

Retention of Urine. The inability of a patient to void is a relatively common problem. It may be due to obstructive disease of the bladder or urethra but occurs frequently after surgery, in acute illness and neurogenic disease, and as a postpartum complication. The resulting distention of the bladder and stasis of urine predispose to the development of ureteral back pressure, reflux of urine into the ureters, and infection of the bladder and kidneys. The reaction of the bladder to progressive obstruction of the outflow is hypertrophy of the detrusor muscle. Diverticula may develop; these are saccular protrusions of the mucosa between the muscle fibers. The sacs fill with urine which becomes stagnant and is readily infected. Calculi may also form within the diverticula.

The retention of urine is suspected if the patient has had a normal fluid intake and has not voided within a period of 8 to 10 hours. A distended bladder may also be manifested by frequent voiding of small amounts (30 to 50 ml.), which is termed retention with overflow. The patient may experience a constant desire to void but efforts to do so are ineffective.

Nursing measures used to induce voiding include increasing the fluid intake, providing adequate privacy, the pouring of warm water over the perineum, the application of heat (such as a hot water bottle or electric pad) over the bladder region (if permitted), having the patient hear running water and, unless contraindicated, assisting the patient to assume the normal position for voiding. The female patient may be supported in the sitting position in bed or may be allowed to use a commode at the bedside. The male patient may be allowed to stand beside the bed. A warm tub bath may prove effective with some patients.

When urethral catheterization is necessary, extreme precautions are used to avoid the introduction of organisms and trauma of the mucosa; sterile gloves are worn, and strict aseptic technique is observed throughout the procedure as well as gentle handling of the catheter to minimize trauma. If the retention has been acute and severe, then at first not more than 800 to 1000 ml. of urine is removed. The sudden, complete emptying of an overdistended bladder favors atony of the bladder wall and capillary bleeding. The sudden release of pressure on the blood vessels in the bladder region causes a sudden inflow of blood; the patient may experience faintness and some of the suddenly dilated capillaries in the mucosa may rupture, causing hematuria. The catheter is clamped and is opened hourly to drain off 100 ml. until the bladder is empty, or the catheter may be attached to decompression drainage. The latter method requires a **Y** tube positioned at a prescribed height (e.g., 5 to 6 inches) above bladder level; the catheter is attached to one arm of the **Y** tube. The tubing to the drainage receptacle is attached to the lower arm, while the third is left open to the air. Sufficient urine must collect in the bladder to raise the urine in the tube to the height of the **Y** tube before there is drainage. The access of air prevents a suction-siphonage action and complete emptying.

Frequency, Urgency and Dysuria. Irritation of the bladder or urethral mucosa may give rise to an abnormally frequent desire to void, urgency and painful micturition. The irritation is most frequently associated with infection in the lower urinary tract and less often with bladder calculi or chemicals excreted in the urine. The frequency of voiding may be increased by nervous apprehension or the taking of a diuretic or increased fluids but is not considered abnormal. Frequency due to a urological disturbance is generally accompanied by an urgency which implies that there is an intense desire to void immediately. The normal voluntary control to retain the urine cannot be maintained, and some urine may escape before the patient can reach the toilet or be placed on a bedpan.

When voiding is accompanied by pain or a burning, smarting sensation, the exact location and the time at which the discomfort occurs in relation to the flow of urine should be determined; that is, the patient must determine whether it is before, during or after the passage of urine that the pain occurs. This information may be helpful to the physician in locating the problem. Strangury is a term used occasionally when the dysuria is unusually severe and there is increasing frequency of decreasing amounts of urine.

Residual Urine. Micturition may not completely empty the bladder, leaving a residue of urine. It is recognized and the amount determined by catheterizing the patient immediately after he has voided. Residual urine is usually the result of an obstruction to the bladder outlet and causes a stagnation that predisposes to bladder infection and calculus formation.

Alterations in the Urinary Stream. The patient may have difficulty in initiating the urinary flow. This symptom of hesitancy is usually due to some obstruction in the bladder-urethral orifice or the urethra. Pressure within the bladder must be increased beyond the normal to force the urine past the obstructing lesion. This is most often seen in males as a result of prostatic hyperplasia but may also occur with newgrowths or constrictions resulting from scarring and fibrosis. The inability to maintain a continuous stream and dribbling may develop as the lesion encroaches further upon the outflow passage.

Intermittent abrupt cessation of the urinary stream during voiding may occur if the bladder-urethral orifice is suddenly occluded by a calculus or a portion of a papillary tumor near the orifice. This may also occur as a result of fatigue of the detrusor muscle. Because of resistance to the urinary outflow, the muscle tires before the bladder is empty; after a few moments, it contracts again and voiding is resumed.

Incontinence. As a symptom of dysfunction of the lower urinary system, the involuntary passage of urine is most often due to infection or irritation of the bladder or urethra. It may also be the result of some congenital anomaly (e.g., hypospadias) or incompetency of the bladder and urethral sphincters due to degenerative tissue changes (as seen in the elderly) or relaxation of the pelvic floor muscles. Incontinence is frequently associated with neurological disease or injury which results in loss of bladder sensation and voluntary control of micturition (e.g., spinal cord injury or cerebral damage). Reflex incontinence develops in which filling of the bladder initiates reflex emptying as occurs in infancy. Incontinence may also develop in any acute illness because of a loss of cerebral awareness.

Abnormal Constituents in Urine. Blood, pus, bacteria and mucus may be present in the urine as a result of infection, inflammation or tissue necrosis in the lower urinary tract. The urine may be cloudy and have an unpleasant or ammoniacal odor.

Cystitis

This is an acute or chronic inflammation of the urinary bladder characterized by frequency, urgency, dysuria and abnormal urinary constituents. It is most often due to infection caused by the ascent of organisms by way of the urethra, but it may also be associated with the administration of certain drugs (e.g., cyclophosphamide) and radiation therapy of the lower abdomen. Predisposing factors in infective cystitis are trauma of the tissues, stagnation of the urine, and distortion or compression of the bladder by an enlarged neighboring organ. The latter condition is a factor in the cystitis that not infrequently develops in the pregnant woman, especially in the last trimester; the enlarging uterus compresses the bladder. Cystitis has a higher incidence in females; this is attributed to the shorter urethra of a relatively wide caliber. Organisms from rectal and vaginal discharge can enter readily. In the male, it is usually secondary to prostatic hyperplasia or infection or to congenital malformation (e.g., hypospadias).

The inflammation is generally confined to the mucosa and submucosa which are hyperemic and edematous. Scattered hemorrhagic areas are present, and small ulcerative lesions may develop as a result of sloughing of the lining tissue. The urine contains blood cells, pus, bacteria and mucus. If cystitis becomes chronic, the inflammation may extend into the detrusor muscle. Fibrosing of the tissues occurs with the persisting inflammation, which reduces the bladder capacity and increases the problem of frequency.

Treatment. In some instances, cystitis is of brief duration, being resolved spontaneously. There is always the danger that the infection may ascend via the ureters and cause pyelonephritis. The infection is treated by the administration of a urinary antiseptic such as sulfonamide (Gantrisin), nitrofurantoin (Furadantin) and pyridium. A urine specimen obtained before any antimicrobial drug is given may be cultured to determine the infective organism and its sensitivity. A specific antibiotic may then be ordered. Sodium bicarbonate or sodium citrate may also be prescribed for the purpose of alkalinizing the urine to decrease the bladder irritation and dysuria. Warm sitz baths may reduce bladder spasm and provide considerable relief. The patient is encouraged to drink copious amounts of fluids which should include citrus fruit juices. He usually remains ambulatory unless there is fever.

If the condition persists, the cystitis is suspected of being secondary. The patient is then investigated for a primary condition which might be pyelonephritis, a bladder calculus, urethral stricture or, in the case of the male, an enlarged prostate.

Since cystitis is frequently the result of an ascending infection and occurs readily in females, good personal hygiene and efficient cleansing of the perineum, especially after defecation, are extremely important and require emphasis in health teaching. Adequate cleansing is often very difficult for the ill person who is weak or handicapped and confined to bed. It becomes the nurse's responsibility to see that the patient is kept thoroughly cleansed.

Bladder Calculi

Stones in the urinary bladder nearly always form as a result of urinary stasis as occurs in prostatic hypertrophy, neurological disease or injury that has resulted in the loss of voluntary bladder control or interruption of the sacral reflex arc, bladder diverticula, urethral stricture or prolonged immobility. The patient may complain of sudden cessation of the urinary flow before the bladder is emptied which is due to occlusion of the bladder-urethral orifice by the calculus. He may find that he is able to void only in certain positions, which are those that keep the stone away from the outlet. Irritation of the mucosa by the stone may result in hematuria, and infection is usually present. Small concretions may pass into the urethra and become lodged there, causing urinary obstruction and severe pain. A bladder calculus may be recognized on an x-ray film of the bladder or visualized by cystoscopy (see p. 426). The stone(s) may be removed through a suprapubic cystotomy (incision into the bladder) or by litholapaxy, depending on the size of the stone(s). For nursing care following a cystotomy, see page 456. Litholapaxy involves the passage of special crushing forceps (lithotrite) through a cystoscope into the bladder. The stone is grasped by the forceps and crushed. The bladder is then irrigated to wash out the concretions; the returned fluid is strained through gauze and the residue checked for amount and composition of the stone particles. The patient is given large amounts of fluids to help wash out the bladder.

Prior to the litholapaxy, the bladder is irrigated frequently with an acid solution (Suby's or G. solution)* which may soften the stones (depending on their composition), making them easier to crush. If the patient complains of irritation when the solution is instilled, it is reported to the physician and the composition of the solution may be adjusted to reduce the acidity.

The condition causing the stasis of urine which promotes calculi formation receives attention to avoid recurrence. If the patient has an obstructing prostate, it may be removed at the same time that the stone is removed. Patients who are immobilized must be turned and moved about frequently; a bed that can be tilted at different angles may be used. The patient who spends most of his day immobile in a wheelchair is equally as susceptible as the bed patient and should receive attention.

Bladder Injury

Accidental injury of the urinary bladder, causing perforation and extravasation of urine (escape of urine from the bladder), is not uncommon. It may occur when the pelvis is fractured or as a result of direct blows to the lower abdomen. If the bladder is full and distended at the time of the accident, it is more vulnerable.

If the laceration occurs in the upper portion, the rupture is intraperitoneal. Urine escapes into the peritoneal cavity and produces peritonitis. The patient exhibits shock (see p. 239) and experiences abdominal pain and tenderness. The abdomen becomes rigid and distended, and a paralytic ileus is likely to develop (see p. 371).

Rupture of the lower part of the bladder is usually extraperitoneal; urine escapes into the surrounding tissues, and infection, cellulitis and necrosis of tissue may ensue. Occasionally an abdominal or perineal fistula develops.

When there is a history of an injury or

blow to the lower abdomen followed by pain and tenderness, injury to the bladder is suspected. A urine specimen is obtained promptly, either by having the patient void or passing a catheter, to determine if there is hematuria. If blood is present in the urine, a cystogram may be done to confirm the diagnosis and locate the laceration. A cystogram is an x-ray of the bladder following the instillation of a radiopaque dye through a urethral catheter.

Treatment. The injury is a serious threat to life and requires prompt treatment. The shock and hemorrhage are treated with a blood transfusion and intravenous infusions. An indwelling catheter is placed in the bladder, and the patient is prepared for abdominal surgery. The site of injury is repaired and a temporary cystostomy (incision of the bladder and the introduction of a drainage tube) done to establish urinary drainage and prevent the possibility of pressure on the repair suture line. If the rupture was intraperitoneal, the extravasated fluid is aspirated before closure.

Following the surgery, the patient is observed closely for signs of infection. The patient may be placed on an antibiotic immediately. An accurate record of the fluid intake and all drainage is very important. (See section on nursing care of the patient having had a cystostomy, p. 456. For the care of the patient with peritonitis and paralytic ileus, see p. 374.)

Exstrophy of the Bladder

This is a developmental defect in which the anterior wall of the bladder has failed to fuse. The degree of failure of fusion varies. The opening may be small, forming a fistula that opens and drains urine onto the external surface of the abdomen; or the entire anterior bladder wall may be absent, accompanied by a wide defect in the abdominal wall, resulting in full exposure of the bladder interior. Urine spurts onto the abdominal wall from the ureters. The more extensive defects are nearly always associated with other anomalies in the genitourinary system. The pelvic bones may fail to meet to form the symphysis pubis. Epispadias (absence of the anterior wall of the male urethra) is a frequent counterpart. In the female, the urethra may be lacking. Exstro-

---

*Suby's or G. solution has a pH of 4 and contains citric acid (monohydrated), magnesium oxide (anhydrous) and sodium carbonate (anhydrous).

phy of the bladder is more common in males than females.

Infection of the bladder usually supervenes and may extend to the kidneys, seriously impairing their function. The corrective procedure used depends on the extent of the malformation and concomitant defects. If the exstrophy is not extensive, the bladder opening and the abdominal fistula are closed. If the defect is extensive, permanent urinary diversion may be undertaken (see p. 455). The defective bladder is removed and the abdominal wall repaired. The surgery is usually undertaken early in the child's life in order to prevent kidney infection and chronic renal failure.

Bladder Neoplasms

Newgrowths in the bladder may develop at any age but occur more frequently after the age of 50 and have a high incidence in males. The majority arise from the epithelial lining as papillomas and may be benign or malignant. Those that are benign and recur tend to eventually become malignant. Others appear as ulcers which are usually malignant and are more invasive of deeper tissue layers. Prolonged exposure to aniline dyes is recognized as a predisposing factor. It is recommended that the period of working with these chemicals should be limited to 3 years and that during this period such persons should have routine Papanicolaou smears made of their urine. They are also advised of the importance of prompt reporting of any blood in the urine or slight bladder irritation. Smoking has also been cited as a predisposing cause of bladder cancer.

The first symptom is usually intermittent, painless hematuria, or cystitis may be the initial factor that brings the patient to a physician. The lesion may encroach on the urethral orifice, giving rise to hesitancy and a decreased force and caliber of the urinary stream. Suprapubic pain and a palpable mass generally indicate that the condition is in an advanced stage. The patient may experience pain in the flank region if the growth obstructs a ureteral orifice, leading to hydronephrosis. The lesion ulcerates, which accounts for the hematuria, and readily becomes infected. If the infection is severe and anemia has developed, the patient manifests weakness and loss of weight.

Diagnostic procedures include a cystoscopy and biopsy. In some instances, the patient may be given several doses of tetracycline before a cystoscopic examination. The tetracycline produces fluorescence of the neoplastic tissue under the ultraviolet ray used in a special cystoscope. Cytological studies may also be made of a urine specimen.

Treatment. The treatment used depends upon whether the neoplasm is benign or malignant and, in the case of malignancy, upon the stage and the depth of the tissue involved. Surgery, radiation, chemotherapy, or a combination of these may be used. Small papillomatous newgrowths may be treated by transurethral resection followed by fulguration (electrocoagulation) of the base tissue. An indwelling catheter is placed in the bladder on completion of the operation, and the urinary drainage is observed frequently for possible bleeding. Bladder spasm and irritability may cause considerable discomfort which may be reduced by the application of a hot water bottle or heating pad to the lower abdomen or by a warm sitz bath. The patient is encouraged to take a minimum of 2000 ml. of fluids daily.

Since papillomas, benign as well as malignant, tend to recur, these patients are followed closely for 5 to 6 years. They are advised to report any bleeding or bladder irritability promptly. A cystoscopic examination is usually done every 3 months during the first year following the resection, every 6 months during the second year, and then annually for 3 or 4 years.

If the neoplasm is malignant, a partial (segmental) or total cystectomy (removal of the bladder) may be done. A partial cystectomy is only used if the cancer is in the upper part of the bladder well above the urethral orifices. At operation, a tube or catheter is placed in the bladder and brought out through the incision, and an indwelling catheter is also introduced through the urethra. Removal of a part of the bladder obviously reduces its capacity. Adequate drainage in the postoperative period is necessary to prevent distention and possible disruption of the suture line. The tube in the incision may be connected to gentle intermittent suction. The length of time it remains in the bladder will depend on the rate of healing.

The urethral catheter usually remains in place for approximately 2 to 4 weeks. On its removal, frequency becomes a problem for the patient because of the reduced bladder capacity. He is likely to become discouraged and depressed at this time, and understanding support from the nurse is essential. He may attempt to reduce the frequency by cutting down his fluid intake, which must be guarded against. The importance of a minimum of 2000 ml. and the spacing of the fluids so the intervals between voiding may be increased during certain periods (e.g., at night) are discussed with him. The traumatized bladder gradually becomes less irritable and increases its capacity.

A total cystectomy with ureteral transplantation for urinary diversion is used when the cancer is situated in the lower part of the bladder or is quite extensive. Permanent urinary diversion may be achieved by cutaneous ureterostomy, uretero-intestinal anastomosis, or the formation of an ileal conduit.

In cutaneous ureterostomy, the detached ends of the ureters are brought through the abdominal wall and secured at skin level. This is rarely the procedure of choice. Maintaining the patency of the ureters is difficult because of strictures that tend to develop. If catheters are placed in the ureters to maintain drainage, they readily block and are difficult to keep in place. Chronic kidney infection is a frequent complication with subsequent renal failure.

Uretero-intestinal anastomosis (ureterosigmoidostomy) provides a completely internal diversion. The ureters are implanted into the sigmoid colon and the urine and feces leave the body via a common channel — the rectum and anus. The urine draining from the ureters is retained in the lower bowel until approximately 200 ml. accumulate. The "defecation" impulse is initiated and the urine is expelled by voluntary relaxation of the anal sphincters. This is a more acceptable procedure to the patient; it eliminates an abdominal orifice, skin problems and the constant use of special drainage appliances. Unfortunately, the direct connection with the bowel predisposes the patient to ascending infection of the kidneys and subsequent renal insufficiency and to disturbances in blood chemistry. These disturbances are attributed to the absorption of substances from the accumulating urine in the intestine. Acidosis is a frequent problem, resulting from the reabsorption of chlorides.

In still another procedure that involves the lower bowel, the ureters are transplanted into the rectum which is severed from the sigmoid, forming what is sometimes referred to as an anal bladder. The free end of the colon is brought out to the skin surface, forming a colostomy. The urine and feces are kept separate by this method.

The ileal conduit (uretero-ileostomy) currently appears to be the procedure most favored. A segment of the ileum with its mesentery and blood supply is removed. The open ends of the ileum left by the resection are anastomosed to re-establish intestinal continuity. One end of the resected ileal section is closed. The open end is brought through the abdominal wall to the skin surface and secured. The detached ends of the ureters are implanted in the ileal segment near its closed end.

For the nursing care of a patient with urinary diversion, see page 459.

Internal or external radiation may be used in treating cancer of the bladder. It may be used alone, as an adjunct to surgery or with chemotherapy. Intracavitary radiation may be achieved by the enclosure of a radioisotope (e.g., Co^{60}, Au^{198}) in a catheter balloon which is placed within the bladder. The catheter is connected to a drainage receptacle, and all urine is saved and sent to the radioisotope department. In some instances, radon seeds or radiotantalum (Ta^{182}) needles may be implanted around the lesion. Certain precautions are necessary in the handling of these radioactive materials and are cited on page 92. Internal radiation causes cystitis, and the patient usually experiences considerable bladder spasms and discomfort. Fluids are given freely and analgesics may be necessary. The application of heat over the bladder region may provide some relief.

External radiation therapy is usually reserved for those patients whose cancer is deeply invasive and highly malignant. When it is used, the patient is likely to experience some gastrointestinal disturbances (nausea, vomiting and diarrhea) as well as cystitis, since the intestine proximal to the bladder will be exposed to the rays. For care of the patient receiving external radiation therapy, the reader is referred to page 90.

In advanced carcinoma of the bladder and when metastases are suspected, chemotherapy may be used as well as surgery and irradiation. The drugs used include 5-fluorouracil (5-FU), cyclophosphamide (Cytoxan) and amethopterin (Methotrexate).

Nursing the Patient Undergoing Bladder Surgery

Operative procedures used in the treatment of bladder disease may be transurethral or open surgery. Open surgery involves an incision through the abdominal wall. Transurethral operative procedures may be performed to obtain a biopsy, remove a neoplasm or calculus, or resect the prostate. The resectoscope, which is used to resect tissue, is similar to a cystoscope but has insulated walls and is equipped with a wire loop which is activated by a high frequency current to cut tissue and control hemorrhage by electrocoagulation. The procedure is referred to as a transurethral resection (TUR). For resection of the prostate, see page 511. A lithotrite, which is a special crushing instrument, is used to remove a stone, and the procedure is called litholapaxy.

Open surgery on the bladder may be undertaken for the repair of a perforation or laceration; the removal of a neoplasm, calculus, or the prostate gland; or a segmental resection or removal of the bladder. The open operative procedures include cystotomy (an incision into the bladder and closure without a drainage tube), cystostomy (an incision into the bladder and the insertion of a drainage tube which is brought out on to the abdominal surface), segmental cystectomy (the removal of a section of the bladder) and total cystectomy (the removal of the bladder, involving ureteral transplantation and urinary diversion). A suprapubic approach is most commonly used in open bladder surgery, with the bladder being opened below the peritoneum.

Nursing Care of the Patient Having a Cystotomy, Cystostomy or Segmental Cystectomy

Preoperative Preparation. Unless the bladder is injured or there is acute retention that cannot be relieved by urethral catheterization, the patient who is to have bladder surgery usually undergoes several days of investigation and preparation. Kidney function is assessed and certain blood chemistry levels are determined (e.g., urea, creatinine, potassium, sodium, chloride, calcium). The urine is examined microscopically, and if infection is present, a urinary antiseptic such as a sulfonamide preparation (e.g., Gantrisin) is prescribed. The patient is encouraged to take 2500 to 3000 ml. of fluid daily unless a large amount of fluid is contraindicated by cardiac or renal insufficiency. The fluid intake and output are recorded and the balance noted. The patient's nutritional status frequently requires attention. Many of these patients are elderly and the existing condition may have contributed to their lack of interest in food, resulting in deficiencies. In encouraging the patient to take nourishment, its importance in his recovery is explained. Dietary adjustments and supplements may be necessary to meet his nutritional needs.

During the preparatory period, an indwelling catheter may be used to provide adequate drainage and to reduce the residual urine. The patient is usually allowed to remain ambulatory. If there is an indwelling catheter, he is given a plastic drainage receptacle that may be attached to his thigh or gown while he is up. He should understand that it must be kept low enough to accommodate gravity drainage of the urine.

When the patient has been advised of the necessity for surgery, the nurse is alert to his need for psychological support. Opportunities are provided for him to express his feelings and concerns and to ask questions. He and his family are advised as to what may be expected following the operation. If the patient is to have a partial cystectomy, this explanation will include a discussion of the frequency of voiding that will be experienced when the tubes are removed because of the reduced capacity of the bladder. Reassurance is given that this gradually becomes less troublesome. If the period of waiting for the surgery is prolonged, some form of diversion in which the patient is interested may be provided, and his family is encouraged to visit regularly. If the patient's anxiety is interfering with his rest and he is unable to sleep, the physician is consulted, and a sedative may be ordered.

The immediate preparation for open bladder surgery is similar to that for any patient having abdominal surgery (see p. 107). The skin cleansing and shaving extend from the lower costal margin to mid-thighs and include the perineal area. If the operation is scheduled for late in the morning or for the afternoon, an intravenous infusion may be given earlier in the day to prevent preoperative dehydration.

Postoperative Nursing Care. Preparation to receive the patient after operation includes the assembling of sterile tubing and drainage receptacles ready for prompt connection to an indwelling urethral catheter and a cystostomy tube. A suction machine and bottles for setting up a closed drainage system may be necessary for the cystostomy. A tray of sterile equipment and solution (sterile water or normal saline) for irrigating the catheters in the event of obstruction by clots should be readily available.

DRAINAGE. The patient is returned from the operating room with an indwelling urethral catheter which is secured to the upper thigh to prevent traction. It is connected to sterile tubing leading to a sterile drainage receptacle which must have an air outlet to promote drainage by gravity. There is less danger of infection and better drainage if the end of the tube carrying the urine into the receptacle is kept above the level of the urine. The length of the tube should allow for turning and moving the patient without tension being exerted on the catheter. The excess tubing lies free on the bed and is secured so there is no loop between the bed and drainage receptacle; that is, the tube must hang straight from the edge of the bed for gravity drainage.

If there is a cystostomy as well, a tube is anchored in the bladder by a suture at the time of operation. This tube may be a special right-angled tube with a mushroom, winged or straight tip, or it may be a straight tube which requires a right-angled glass connecting tube. The cystostomy tube is attached to a sterile tube and receptacle, and the same precautions are necessary as those cited in the previous paragraph. Rarely, the cystostomy tube is connected to a suction machine which can be regulated to provide a *very low* constant or intermittent negative pressure. The amount of suction (negative pressure) is specified by the surgeon and does not usually exceed 5 cm. It must be carefully controlled to avoid trauma by suction of the bladder mucosa against the tube.

Both drainage systems are checked frequently (at least hourly for the first 36 to 48 hours) for patency. The characteristics (color, consistency, and content or sediment) of the drainage are noted at the same time. The urine will be blood-colored for the first 2 to 3 hours, gradually becoming lighter. The drainage is best examined at the glass connecting tubes before it becomes mixed with what is already in the receptacles.

The cystostomy tube, urethral catheter or the tubing may become obstructed by a blood clot. A sterile towel or pad is placed under the connecting tube and the catheter or cystostomy tube is disconnected and held over a sterile basin to see if it is draining. If blockage of the tubing is indicated, it may be "milked" or flushed with sterile water. The water is either collected in a separate container, or the exact amount used is noted if it is allowed to flow into the regular drainage receptacle. If the obstruction is within the catheter tube in the bladder, an order may be given to irrigate with sterile normal saline or sterile water. Fifty to 75 ml. of the fluid are introduced; if the initial fluid does not return, no more fluid is instilled and the doctor is consulted. Adequate postoperative drainage is very important to prevent bladder distention and pressure on the suture line.

The drainage from each system is measured and recorded every 6 to 8 hours. A fresh sterile receptacle replaces the one being emptied. Care of the tubing varies in different institutions; it may be replaced daily with a fresh sterile set or is changed every second day or twice weekly. The tubing that is removed is washed with a detergent and warm water and is usually flushed with 5 per cent acetic acid or full strength vinegar to remove deposits of urate crystals. It is then rinsed with water and sterilized.

The cystostomy tube usually remains in place from 4 to 7 days, depending on the patient's healing and progress. The urethral catheter is generally left for a few days longer or until the incisional opening in the bladder heals. When the cystostomy tube is removed, some urine will escape onto the dressing for a few days until the fistula heals over.

Following the removal of the urethral

catheter, a close check is made of the patient's frequency of voiding and the volume of the output for several days. If the patient is ambulatory, he is asked to record the necessary information. When a urethral catheter that has been in place for several days is removed, dribbling is not an unusual problem because the bladder-urethral sphincters have been continuously dilated for a period of time. Frequent perineal exercises, which consist of contracting the abdominal, gluteal and perineal muscles while continuing to breathe normally, may help the sphincters recover their tone and control. Occasionally, a patient may not be able to void and the catheter may have to be replaced if he has not voided within 8 hours.

A permanent cystostomy is sometimes done as a palliative measure with a patient who has an inoperable obstruction of the urethra (e.g., advanced carcinoma of the urethra, bladder neck or prostate). A urethral catheter is not inserted in this patient; bladder drainage is entirely dependent upon the cystostomy tube.

OBSERVATIONS. As well as frequent checking of the drainage system(s), the patient's blood pressure, pulse, color and level of consciousness are noted and recorded at frequent intervals, which are gradually lengthened if the vital signs are satisfactory. Hemorrhage and shock are not uncommon complications following either transurethral resection or open bladder surgery. Bleeding may be evident in the drainage, but the dressing, surrounding skin areas and groins are also examined.

The daily fluid intake and output are recorded for a longer period than with most surgical patients. The ratio of the intake to the output is examined by the nurse so that she is alert to possible renal insufficiency or retention of urine. The characteristics of the urine are noted for a period of 10 to 14 days. The appearance of sediment, blood, shreds of mucus-like material, cloudiness or unusual odor is reported. Sloughing and ensuing bleeding often occur 8 to 10 days following the removal of a lesion.

EXERCISE AND POSITIONING. The patient is urged to take 5 to 10 deep breaths and cough every 1 to 2 hours to prevent pulmonary complications until he becomes ambulatory and active. If approved by the surgeon, active flexion and extension of the feet and lower limbs are encouraged 3 or 4 times daily to prevent venous stasis. If these cannot be carried out actively, passive movement of the limbs through the normal range of motion is done by the nurse.

A regimen of turning every 1 to 2 hours is established; some patients may be able to assume responsibility for this soon after operation, but others, particularly elderly persons, may require assistance. Following each change of position the full length of each tube is checked to make sure it is not kinked, that it is not under the patient and being compressed, and that there is no loop between the bed and drainage receptacle. The patient is taught to make these checks when he changes his position.

The patient is allowed out of bed as soon as his condition permits, and ambulation is encouraged to promote normal physiological processes and prevent complications. When the patient is up, the drainage tubes may be connected to smaller plastic receptacles which may be attached to the patient's thigh or gown. When the patient becomes more independent in his activity, he must be advised that when he returns to bed, the drainage receptacle is transferred to the side of the bed in order to maintain gravity drainage.

DRESSINGS AND SKIN CARE. Compared with other abdominal surgery, the dressing is changed earlier and more frequently for patients who have had open bladder surgery. There is almost certain to be some leakage of urine through the incision and around the tube. The skin is cleansed of the urine frequently and is kept as dry as possible to prevent excoriation and infection. Following each cleansing, an application of a protective preparation such as petroleum jelly, zinc oxide ointment or karaya gum powder is made to the skin. The lower back, buttocks, groin, inner thighs and perineum are examined each time the dressing is changed. If any areas are moist with urine drainage, they are washed and thoroughly dried to prevent excoriation. The bedding is changed as often as is necessary to ensure dryness and comfort.

PAIN. Bladder trauma and irritation cause bladder spasms which are very painful, and the patient may also experience the desire to void frequently, even though the bladder is emptied by tube drainage. In the case of the sensation of frequency, it may be necessary to explain to the patient that the bladder is empty and that trying to void only increases bladder spasms and pain. An analgesic such as morphine or meperidine hydrochloride (Demerol) is usually necessary at intervals during the first 48 hours. If the pain and discomfort persist, the surgeon is consulted. Either the catheter or cystostomy tube may require adjusting to relieve the contact and pressure of its tip on the bladder wall.

FLUIDS AND NUTRITION. A daily fluid intake of at least 2500 to 3000 ml. (unless contraindicated by other coexisting disease) is necessary to ensure adequate irrigation of the bladder as well as to maintain satisfactory hydration. Most of it usually has to be administered by intravenous infusion the first day or two. A soft diet is given and is progressively increased to a regular diet as tolerated.

BOWEL ELIMINATION. The patient may be given a mild laxative after 2 days, or a cleansing enema may be given. Constipation and straining at stool are prevented, since they tend to increase the patient's pain.

PREPARATION FOR DISCHARGE FROM HOSPITAL. Most patients who have had a cystotomy or cystostomy remain in the hospital until the wound is healed and normal micturition is re-established. The nurse discusses the resumption of their previous activities with them and explains any restrictions indicated by the physician. They are advised to continue taking a minimum of 2000 to 2500 ml. of fluid daily. Some may require reassurance that no special care of the wound is necessary and that they may resume tub baths.

If the cystostomy is permanent or a urethral catheter is to remain in place, the patient and a member of his family are given detailed instruction about the necessary care. This instruction is given over several days and should be completed soon enough for the patient to carry out the care himself before going home. This gives him confidence and provides the opportunity to clarify certain points. Verbal and written instructions will include an explanation of the necessary equipment, its use and maintenance, how it may be acquired, and any precautions to be observed in its use. An inconspicuous, oval-shaped, plastic or rubber urinal (drainage receptacle) that may be strapped to the thigh is available. The inlet tube which is attached to the upper end of the bag is connected to the catheter or cystostomy tube by means of a glass connecting tube. The other end of the urinal has a screw stopper which permits emptying of the bag into a toilet at necessary intervals. The importance of thorough washing of the hands with soap and running water before connecting or disconnecting the equipment is stressed to reduce the possibility of ascending infection. The patient and a family member are also taught how to anchor the tube that is in the patient to the abdomen or thigh to prevent traction on it.

The bag and tubing are cleansed daily with a detergent and warm water, flushed with vinegar, thoroughly rinsed with water, and aired. They are advised to have 2 sets if possible so that one set may be well aired after the cleansing. This helps to prevent odor which could cause considerable embarassment and discouragement for the patient. The patient is reminded of the need to continue taking at least 2000 to 2500 ml. of fluid daily to provide adequate bladder irrigation. Odor is likely to be less of a problem with less concentrated urine, and there is less danger of infection with constant washing out of the bladder.

A referral may be made to a visiting nurse agency for assistance and supervision when the patient goes home. This is likely to be needed when the patient is elderly and finds it difficult to cope with the necessary care. The patient and family are advised as to how often the tube or catheter is to be changed at the clinic or by the doctor and of the need to promptly contact the doctor or clinic if the tube slips out of the bladder.

Nursing the Patient Who Has Had a Cystectomy and Ureteral Transplantation

Complete removal of the bladder necessitates establishing a new urinary outlet; this may be achieved by cutaneous ureterostomy, uretero-intestinal anastomosis (ureterosigmoidostomy) or ileal conduit (ureteroileostomy). For a description of these procedures, see page 455.

Following operation, the patient who undergoes a cystectomy and ureteral transplant is seriously ill. The amount of surgery usually involved predisposes the patient to severe shock. Frequently, considerable surrounding tissue is resected with the bladder (e.g., lymphatics, prostate gland), and if the ileal conduit procedure is used, an intestinal resection and anastomosis are done. The patient will have a large vertical or transverse incision through which the bladder is removed, the ureters are freed for transplant, and the intestine is resected. The stoma through which the urine will drain is made separately in the right abdominal wall. Care of the patient requires consideration of the needs incurred by the cystectomy, the intestinal surgery, the ureteral transplantation and urinary diversion as well as the individual patient's psychological and physiological responses to such radical surgery.

Preoperative Preparation. The operative procedure and the permanent change in urinary drainage that will ensue are explained to the patient and his family by the doctor. This is likely to produce considerable anxiety and despair and will prompt many questions. The nurse observes the patient closely for his reactions and conveys her acceptance and appreciation of his concerns. Opportunities are provided for him and his family to express their feelings and ask questions, and when they are ready, the necessary adjustments and care associated with urinary diversion are outlined in simple terms. They are told that a relatively normal, active life is possible. This may be reinforced by having a person who has had a permanent urinary diversion and has made a successful adjustment talk with them. If such a person is not available, someone with an ileostomy may prove helpful. The nurse who is willing to take time to talk freely with the patient, help him to make plans for his future, and is patient in repeating answers and reinforcing what has probably already been said can provide immeasurable support. A rapport is developed that contributes to acceptance of the situation and the development of positive attitudes on the part of the patient and his family.

There will be several days of investigation and preparation. Kidney function is evaluated and the blood levels of nonprotein nitrogenous wastes, potassium, sodium and chloride are determined. The patient usually receives a blood transfusion during and probably following the surgery, so typing and cross matching are necessary. At least 2500 ml. of fluid daily are given unless contraindicated by cardiac insufficiency or urinary obstruction.

If the intestine is to be entered, the patient receives a low-residue diet for 3 or 4 days, then clear fluids only on the day before operation to reduce the fecal content. The reasons for these restrictions are explained in order to gain the patient's cooperation and acceptance. Laxatives and enemas are also used for cleansing purposes, and a course of an antimicrobial drug that is poorly absorbed from the gastrointestinal tract is given orally to destroy intestinal organisms (e.g., Sulfasuxidine, Neomycin). The skin preparation includes the abdomen, upper thighs and perineum. The remainder of the preparation is similar to that for any major abdominal surgery (see p. 107).

The operation is a lengthy procedure; if the members of the family decide to go home, they are assured that they will be called as soon as the operation is over and advised of the patient's condition. If they choose to remain in the hospital, they are directed to a room where they may wait. A brief visit with them at intervals by the nurse and suggestions made as to where they may have a cup of coffee or lunch are appreciated and indicate a sympathetic understanding of their anxiety and concern.

The Patient with a Uretero-ileal Conduit. Preparation to receive the patient after operation includes the assembling of a sterile urinary drainage receptacle with tubing, gastrointestinal suction machine, intravenous infusion standard, sterile irrigation tray and sterile normal saline.

A large part of the required care is essentially the same as that for any patient having an intestinal resection, which is cited on page 374.

DRAINAGE. On completion of the operation, a catheter may be inserted into the ileal segment and anchored by a skin suture. The catheter is connected directly to sterile tubing leading to a drainage receptacle. The tubing should be long enough to permit turning the patient without traction being exerted on the catheter. Since the drainage is by gravity, the tube is positioned to hang straight from the bed to the drainage receptacle. The system is checked at least hourly, and the volume of urine is recorded; less than 15 ml. per hour is reported. The catheter may become obstructed by mucus secreted by the isolated ileal segment and may require periodic irrigation. If the nurse is responsible for the irrigations, a specified directive is received as to the quantity of sterile normal saline to be introduced at one time. The return is carefully measured. Distention of the ileal segment must be avoided; it causes pressure on the suture lines, urinary reflux and back pressure in the ureters. If the solution introduced is not returned, no more is added and the physician is consulted. The catheter is usually left in place 4 to 7 days, and then a disposable ileostomy bag is applied.

If a catheter is not inserted into the ileal conduit at operation, a disposable plastic ileostomy bag is secured to the skin around the stoma by means of an adhesive disk. The lower end of the bag is then connected to the tubing and drainage receptacle. With this arrangement, the ileostomy bag is examined when checking the drainage. The bag may require moving to empty any accumulation of urine into the lower bag. A cessation of drainage may indicate occlusion of the stoma by mucus or by swelling and edema of the tissues, and the physician is notified immediately. The stoma is usually dilated manually, and the bag is changed daily by the surgeon for a few days, after which the procedure may be repeated every 2 or 3 days by the nurse. A sterile rubber glove or finger cot is worn, and the finger used is lubricated with a water-soluble jelly and introduced gently. The interval is gradually lengthened and once weekly is usually sufficient as the tissues around the stoma heal and shrink. Eventually, this becomes a part of the care procedure taught to the patient and a family member. The stoma must be kept well dilated to promote free drainage and prevent an accumulation of urine in the ileal conduit. The doctor may insert a sterile catheter periodically to determine if there is residual urine. The temporary ileostomy bag is changed when dilatation of the stoma is done, and when this becomes less frequent, it is changed every 3 to 5 days. When the bag is removed, the stoma is covered with sterile wipes while the skin is gently washed and thoroughly dried. The skin is

likely to show some irritation, particularly during the first few weeks. A protective coating of tincture of benzoin, karaya gum powder (Protex powder, Derma-Guard) or neo-karaya (a combination of aluminum hydroxide gel and karaya) may be applied after each cleansing and before a new bag is applied. If excoriation of the skin persists or is severe, the doctor may decide to insert a catheter to prevent the escape of urine onto the skin, giving it a chance to heal.

When the stoma has shrunk to a permanent size and drainage is satisfactory, the patient is fitted for a permanent ileostomy bag (see p. 378).

Any abdominal pain, distention or rigidity, nausea, vomiting or fever is reported promptly. Any of these symptoms may indicate peritonitis, resulting from the escape of intestinal content from the site of the intestinal anastomosis or from a leakage of urine from the ileal conduit or ureters into the peritoneal cavity. The nurse is also constantly alert for a positive fluid balance, fever and any complaint of back pain, which might indicate renal infection or insufficiency.

POSITIONING AND AMBULATION. The patient is turned every 1 or 2 hours. Since the ileal conduit opens onto the right side of the abdomen, more complete drainage occurs when he is on his right side or back and the trunk is elevated. The doctor may suggest that the patient be turned on the left side for only very brief periods and that as soon as the blood pressure and pulse have stabilized, the head of the bed should be gradually elevated. With each change of position, the bag and tubing are checked for any kinks or compression.

Early ambulation is encouraged to foster adequate drainage as well as to promote normal physiological processes and prevent complications. If his condition is satisfactory, the patient will probably be allowed up 36 to 48 hours after operation. The plastic drainage receptacle may be carried by the nurse or may be attached to the patient's gown. If an ileostomy bag is applied to the stoma, the drainage tube may be detached while the patient is out of bed.

Gastrointestinal decompression suction is used to prevent vomiting and distention so that there is a minimum of pressure on the intestinal anastomosis site. The nasogastric tube remains in place for 3 to 4 days and the patient is given intravenous fluids. The suction is discontinued, and the patient is observed for any signs of distention. Small amounts of water are given and the tube is clamped. The physician usually listens for bowel sounds that indicate the re-establishment of peristalsis, and the nurse checks with the patient for the passing of flatus. If the water is tolerated and there is no distention, the nasogastric tube is removed. The intake of clear fluids is gradually increased and the diet progresses through soft foods to a light solid diet.

The patient and a family member are taught the care of the stoma, skin and appliance following the same plan as that outlined under instruction of the ileostomy patient on page 378. The patient should have his permanent appliance and the opportunity to develop complete familiarity with the necessary care, including dilation of the stoma, before being discharged from the hospital. During this period, he is advised of the importance of continuing a daily intake of 2500 to 3000 ml. to keep the ureters and ileal conduit well irrigated. The patient and family are cautioned that the physician is to be consulted immediately if there is a decrease in urinary drainage, abnormal constituents such as blood in the urine, fever, pain in the back or abdomen, severe skin excoriation or general malaise. The patient is followed closely after hospital discharge. A referral may be made to a visiting nurse association, and the patient is seen at regular intervals at the clinic or by his physician. These visits may be frequent at first, and the intervals are gradually increased to 3 to 6 months if the patient's progress is satisfactory.

The Patient with a Ureterosigmoidostomy. The patient who has the ureters transplanted into the sigmoid has the advantage of not having continuous external urinary drainage. No special appliance is necessary, and the problem of skin irritation is eliminated. The colon retains the urine drainage from the ureters, and the anal sphincters control the expelling of urine just as they do feces. Approximately 200 ml. of urine collect between anal voidings. The patient's stool becomes softer or liquid as the feces become mixed with urine.

A rectal tube with several openings is inserted when the operation is completed and remains in place for several days. It may be anchored by a suture or by securing the ends of a tape which circles the tube to the thighs. The tube is connected to a sterile tube leading to a drainage receptacle. Irrigations of sterile normal saline or water may be ordered to keep the tube clear of mucus and feces. Not more than 30 ml. are introduced at one time. Distention of the intestine is avoided to prevent pressure on the suture lines at the sites of the ureteral implants as well as reflux from the bowel into the ureters. The drainage is checked hourly the first 2 or 3 days and is measured and recorded. If at any time there is no drainage for 1 hour, the doctor is notified.

When the tube is removed, the patient is instructed to establish a voiding schedule. The urine should be expelled at least every 4 hours to minimize the reabsorption of urinary waste products (e.g., chlorides and urea). The amount is measured and recorded each time. The patient may be wakened at regular intervals at night, or the doctor may order a rectal tube inserted each night at bedtime to prevent an over-accumulation of urine in the colon. The tube is connected to a receptacle at the bedside. The patient is taught to insert and care for the tube, since the procedure is usually continued when he goes home.

After the operation, the patient receives only clear fluids for 2 to 3 days, then a low-residue diet for 4 to 6 days to minimize the fecal content of the large intestine. The antimicrobial drug given preoperatively may be continued postoperatively for several days. A daily intake of 2500 to 3000 ml. fluid is necessary, and the patient is told of the importance of continuing this after his discharge from the hospital. The fluid intake and output are measured and the balance noted.

A family member and the patient are also instructed to report promptly any pain, fever, nausea, vomiting or generalized weakness. These symptoms may indicate kidney infection or electrolyte imbalance. The latter may occur as a result of reabsorption of urinary constituents from the bowel. Laxatives should not be taken without a doctor's order; if one is necessary, a small dose of milk of magnesia may be prescribed. An adequate balanced diet and the suggested fluid intake generally are sufficient to promote normal bowel elimination.

If a surgical procedure which establishes an "anal bladder" and a permanent colostomy is used, the care relating to the urinary excretion is similar to that cited following a ureterosigmoidostomy. The patient will also require the nursing considerations as outlined on page 378 because of the colostomy.

The Patient with Cutaneous Ureterostomy. This method of urinary diversion is used less often than the others because it is difficult to maintain adequate drainage. Stenosis of the ureters is prone to develop. The detached end of each ureter is brought out to the skin surface and everted to form a slightly protruding ureteral bud. The patient comes from the operating room with a catheter secured in each ureter. These are labeled right and left, corresponding to the ureters, and are connected to separate drainage receptacles which are also labeled, respectively, right and left. The drainage is checked frequently, and if either catheter stops draining, the doctor is notified and sterile equipment is prepared for irrigation. The catheters are left in place 7 to 12 days to minimize the urinary flow over the stomata while healing of the ureters to the abdominal wall takes place. The surgeon may order the application of normal saline compresses to the stomata around the catheters to prevent drying of the mucous membrane of the ureteral buds.

When the catheters are removed, an ileostomy bag may be applied over the stomata. The free end of the bag has an opening by which the urine drains into a connecting tubing and larger drainage receptacle. When the patient is ambulatory, the tubing may be connected to a plastic urinal strapped to the patient's thigh. There is also a special ureterostomy cup available, which is placed over the ureteral buds and may be held in place by a strap around the patient or by adhesive disks similar to those used with ileostomy bags. The cup is connected to a rubber or plastic urinary bag that can be attached to the patient's thigh. The urinal bag is replaced at night by a drainage receptacle at the side of the bed. The bag or cup is changed every 2 or 3 days, and the connecting tubing and bag are changed daily. If an adhesive disk is used to hold the appliance in place, it is removed with a special commercial solvent available from the companies supplying the equipment. The skin around the ureteral buds requires frequent examination and attention. It is washed and thoroughly dried with each change of the appliance, and requires the application of a protective preparation such as tincture of benzoin, karaya gum powder or zinc oxide ointment. If the skin becomes excoriated, the physician is consulted. Exposures of 15 to 20 minutes to a radiant heat lamp may be ordered. Precautions must be taken to cover the stomata with sterile gauze during the treatment, and to prevent burning, the lamp should not be closer than 24 inches to the site.

The patient and a member of his family are given detailed instruction in the care of the stomata, skin and appliance. Two sets of equipment are desirable to allow efficient cleansing and airing. Opportunities are provided for the patient to become competent in the necessary care before he is discharged from the hospital. As with other methods of urinary diversion, the importance of a daily fluid intake of 2500 to 3000 ml. is stressed. There is always the danger that a patient may restrict his fluids so he will have less drainage to cope with, not realizing the need for continuous internal irrigation of the ureters. The patient and his family are cautioned to get in touch with the doctor at once if drainage from either stoma stops, fever develops, or pain in the back or abdomen is experienced. Continuous drainage of urine from both ureters is necessary to prevent back pressure and ensuing hydronephrosis as well as ascending infection of the kidneys. The patient is followed closely; the stomata may require periodic dilatation. A referral to a visiting nurse agency for frequent supervision is recommended, and the patient is seen regularly in the clinic, or by his doctor.

Summary Concerning Urinary Diversion. Factors to be considered in caring for a patient who undergoes permanent urinary diversion, regardless of the method used, include the following:

The patient's psychological reaction to a change in body image and normal pattern of function requires thoughtful understanding on the part of the nurse with sincere efforts to reduce the patient's despair and promote acceptance and motivation.

Preoperative cleansing and sterilization

of the bowel are necessary if the operative procedure involves resection of or entry into the intestine.

Maintenance of continuous, adequate urinary drainage from the ureters postoperatively is essential to prevent renal complications.

Drainage of urine through an opening onto the skin requires special skin care to prevent excoriation and maceration.

Drainage of urine into the sigmoid or rectum and its accumulation there necessitates scheduled anal voiding at least every 4 hours to minimize the reabsorption of urinary waste products which may incur electrolyte imbalance, acidosis and an elevation of blood urea.

A daily fluid intake of 2500 to 3000 ml. of fluid is important to provide good internal irrigation of the renal pelves and ureters.

A planned program of instruction in the care of stomata, skin and appliance is given to the patient and a family member. It should be given over a period of time that will allow them to acquire a satisfactory understanding and competence by the time the patient leaves the hospital. The instruction includes an explanation of the need for ample fluids and prompt reporting of decreased urinary drainage and significant symptoms.

Information about the patient's previous employment is obtained, and consideration is given as to whether it is suitable for him to resume his position or whether a referral to a social service worker would be of assistance in finding another occupation.

The patient requires a close follow-up. Frequent home visits by a visiting nurse, especially during the first few weeks after leaving the hospital, can provide assistance and considerable support to the patient and his family. Regular visits to a clinic or the doctor are necessary.

DISORDERS OF THE URETHRA

Urethritis

Inflammation of the urethra is most often due to infection but may also follow trauma.

The patient complains of dysuria and frequency. The causative organism may be identified by cultures and smears of the urine or discharge from the urinary meatus. A urinary antiseptic or an antibiotic (depending on the causative organism) is prescribed, and the patient is encouraged to force fluids.

Urethral Stricture

Stricture of the urethra may be congenital or acquired. A congenital stricture may go unrecognized for a period of time and is probably only discovered when it causes retention and stasis of urine that lead to urethritis or cystitis. An acquired stricture is usually the result of infection or trauma which has caused inflammation and ensuing fibrous scarring. The patient with a stricture may experience hesitancy in initiating voiding and a small, slow urinary stream.

Treatment consists of gradual dilatation by the introduction of bougies or catheters weekly or every 2 weeks over several months. In some instances, a catheter may be left in place to maintain dilatation or to provide adequate urinary drainage. Rarely, a temporary cystostomy is necessary because of severe retention.

Urethral Caruncle

A caruncle is a small, vascular, benign tumor that develops on the urethral wall near the urinary meatus. It occurs in females, usually appearing after the menopause. It bleeds easily and may be very sensitive. The patient may compain of pain on voiding and while sitting.

The caruncle is removed by cautery or excision. An indwelling catheter may be inserted and left in place for 24 to 48 hours because edema of the urethral tissues may interfere with voiding. The patient may find the pressure of the catheter on the site very uncomfortable. For this reason, some doctors avoid the use of a catheter unless acute retention develops. A dressing of petroleum jelly is applied to the site to avoid irritation and friction until the area heals.

References

BOOKS

Beeson, P. B., and McDermott, W. (Eds.): Cecil-Loeb Textbook of Medicine, 13th ed. Philadelphia, W. B. Saunders Co., 1971, pp. 1139–1232.

Bergerson, B. S., Anderson, E. H., et al. (Eds.): Current Concepts in Clinical Nursing. St. Louis, The C. V. Mosby Co., 1967. Chapter 2 (Patients with Kidney Transplants).

de Wardener, H. E.: The Kidney, 3rd ed. London, J. & A. Churchill Ltd., 1967.

Douglas, A. P., and Kerr, D. N. S.: A Short Textbook of Kidney Disease. London, Pitman Medical Publishing Co., Ltd., 1968.

Ham, F. C., and Weinberg, S. R.: Urology in Medical Practice, 2nd ed. Montreal, J. B. Lippincott Co., 1962.

Harrison, T. R., et al. (Eds.): Principles of Internal Medicine, 4th ed. New York, The Blakiston Division, McGraw-Hill Book Co., Inc., 1962, pp. 1473–1507.

Hirschhorn, R. C.: Handbook of Practical Urology. Philadelphia, Lea and Febiger, 1965.

Merrill, J. P.: The Treatment of Renal Failure, 2nd ed. New York, Grune and Stratton, 1965.

Smith, D. R.: General Urology. Los Altos, California, Lange Medical Publications, 1966.

Sodeman, W. A., and Sodeman, W. A., Jr.: Pathologic Physiology, 4th ed. Philadelphia, W. B. Saunders Co., 1967. Chapter 29.

Sutton, A. L.: Bedside Nursing Techniques in Medicine and Surgery, 2nd ed. Philadelphia, W. B. Saunders Co., 1969. Chapter 15.

Winter, C. C., and Roehm, M. M.: Care of Patients with Urologic Diseases, 2nd ed. St. Louis, The C. V. Mosby Co., 1968.

Winter, C. C.: Practical Urology. St. Louis, The C. V. Mosby Co., 1969.

PERIODICALS

Baltzan, R. B.: "Glomerulonephritis." Canad. Nurse, Vol. 62, No. 8 (Aug. 1966), pp. 45–47.

Berman, H. I.: "Urinary Diversion in the Treatment of Carcinoma of Bladder." Surg. Clin. North Amer., Vol. 45, No. 6 (Dec. 1965), pp. 1495–1506.

Bois, M. S., et al.: "Nursing Care of Patients Having Kidney Transplants." Amer. J. Nurs., Vol. 68, No. 6 (June 1968), pp. 1238–1247.

Calcagno, P. L. (Ed.): "Symposium on Renal Disorders." Pediat. Clin. North Amer., Vol. 11, No. 3 (Aug. 1964).

Clark, J. E., and Soricelli, R. R.: "Indications for Dialysis." Med. Clin. North Amer., Vol. 49, No. 5 (Sept. 1965), pp. 1213–1234.

Dosseter, J. B.: "Present Status of Renal Transplantation." Canad. Nurse, Vol. 63, No. 10 (Oct. 1967), pp. 32–34.

Downing, S. R.: "Nursing Support in Early Renal Failure." Amer. J. Nurs., Vol. 69, No. 6 (June 1969), pp. 1212–1216.

Fellows, B. J.: "The Role of the Nurse in a Chronic Dialysis Unit." Nurs. Clin. North Amer., Vol. 1, No. 4 (Dec. 1966), pp. 577–586.

Frenay, A. C.: "A Dynamic Approach to the Ileal Conduit Patient." Amer. J. Nurs., Vol. 64, No. 1 (Jan. 1964), pp. 80–84.

Furlow, W. L., and Greene, L. F.: "Congenital Polycystic Renal Disease." Med. Clin. North Amer., Vol. 50, No. 4 (July 1966), pp. 1101–1116.

Holden, H. M., et al.: "Peritoneal Dialysis." Canad. Nurse, Vol. 62, No. 3 (Mar. 1966), pp. 40–43.

Martin, A. J.: "Renal Transplantation." Amer. J. Nurs., Vol. 68, No. 6 (June 1968), pp. 1240–1241.

McDonald, J.: "Nursing Care in Renal Transplantation." Canad. Nurse, Vol. 63, No. 10 (Oct. 1967), pp. 35–39.

Melick, W. F., and Naryka, J. J.: "Carcinoma in Situ of the Bladder in Workers with Xenylamine: Diagnosis by Ultraviolet Light Cystoscopy." J. Urol., Vol. 99, No. 2 (Feb. 1968), pp. 178–182.

Nesbitt, L.: "Nursing the Patient on a Long-Term Hemodialysis." Canad. Nurse, Vol. 63, No. 10 (Oct. 1967), pp. 40–41.

Schlotter, L.: "Learning to be a Home Dialysis Patient." Nurs. Clin. North Amer., Vol. 4, No. 3 (Sept. 1969), pp. 419–428.

Stewart, B. M.: "Hemodialysis in the Home." Nurs. Clin. North Amer., Vol. 4, No. 3 (Sept. 1969), pp. 431–442.

Tests of Renal Function. Nurs. Clin. North Amer., Vol. 2, No. 4 (Dec. 1967), pp. 800–803.

Trusk, C. W.: "Hemodialysis for Acute Renal Failure." Amer. J. Nurs., Vol. 65, No. 2 (Feb. 1965), pp. 80–85.

Watson, I.: "Nursing Care of Patient with Glomerulonephritis." Canad. Nurse, Vol. 62, No. 8 (Aug. 1966), pp. 48–49.

Wood, S.: "Hemodialysis in the Home." Canad. Nurse, Vol. 65, No. 4 (Apr. 1969), pp. 42–44.

19
Nursing in Disorders
of the Reproductive System

by Donna Shields, B.Sc.N., C.N.M., M.S.N.

EMBRYOLOGY

The reproductive system is unique in mammals in that it differs markedly between sexes. Sex is determined at the time of fertilization by the inclusion of the XX chromosomal pair of the female or the XY genotype of the male. In this early period of human development, sex differentiation can be determined microscopically by the presence or absence of Barr bodies in a cell nucleus which has been taken from the embryo. These Barr bodies, which are always one less than the number of X chromosomes, indicate the genotype of the embryo.

As the embryo grows, a genital ridge develops but remains undifferentiated in either sex until the seventh week of intrauterine life. At this time sex differentiation can be made morphologically for the genital ridges of the embryo, accompanied by the primordial germ cells, have grown and differentiated into a rudimentary testis or ovary, depending on the sex of the cell.

An elaborate bilateral duct system also develops. In the male much of this duct system degenerates, and the remaining portion forms the epididymis and ductus

deferens which then join the male urethra. In the female the duct systems develop bilaterally, and as growth continues, the two ducts meet and fuse in the midline. The portion which fuses becomes the uterus, cervix and vagina. This process of fusion takes some weeks to complete and, indeed, may never occur, giving rise to paired uteri and vaginas. Fusion may be incomplete, causing some abnormalities of the uterus (Fig. 19–1).

While internal development proceeds the external genitalia are also becoming differentiated. In the "neuter" phase of development three small protuberances appear caudally on the external surface of the embryo. These protuberances consist of the "genital tubercle" and, on either side of this tubercle, the genital swellings. In the male the tubercle becomes elongated and develops into the male phallus while the genital swellings become the scrotal tissue. These two swellings must develop, descend and fuse, closing the urethra in the male penis and forming the pendulant scrotum. Should fusion not be complete on the dorsal surface, a condition known as hypospadias occurs (Fig. 19–2). Epispadias, a rarer

466

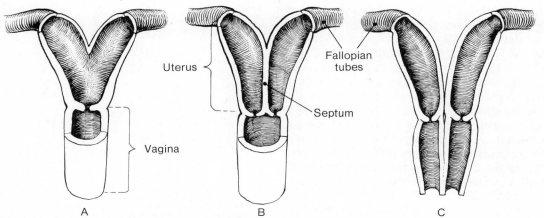

Figure 19–1 Some abnormalities of the uterus resulting from incomplete fusion of the ducts. *A*, Bicornate uterus. *B*, Uterus septus and a double cervix. *C*, Double uterus, cervix and vagina.

malformation, may also occur. Here the failure of the urethra to fuse completely occurs on the ventral side of the penis. From these swellings, the prepuce, or fore-skin, of the penis also arises. The foreskin is attached to the penile shaft at the base of the glans. The foreskin then drops down like a hood over the glans and remains partially fixed until sometime between birth and 3 years of age. During this time the congenital adhesions break down and the prepuce is then easily retractable over the glans penis.

The female genitalia arise from the same three ridges. The tubercle becomes the clitoris, and the genital swellings develop into the labia majora and minora. As the labia meet anteriorly, they form a loose-fitting, hood-like fold over the clitoris. This fold is similar to the prepuce of the male penis. Posteriorly, the labial folds fuse just before the anus. Thus, male and female reproductive systems have homologous counterparts.

By the sixteenth week of embryological life the sex of the infant can be determined externally. At this time the testes of the male, which normally reside in the scrotum, are not there. In early development the testis and ovary are abdominal organs. As further growth takes place, they descend over the pelvic brim in the case of the ovaries or into the scrotum in the case of the testes. The

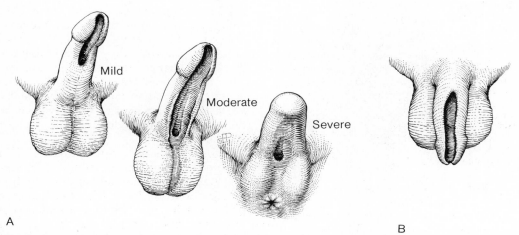

Figure 19–2 *A*, Hypospadias—mild, moderate and severe. In severe hypospadias note the similarity to the female. *B*, Epispadias.

descent of the testes appears to be in response to hormonal and mechanical control. As the fetal testes begin to produce testosterone, in about the seventh month of fetal life, descent occurs, and they pass through the inguinal canal and the external inguinal ring to enter the scrotum by the ninth month. During descent the testis is surrounded by a tube of peritoneum known as the processus vaginalis. After descent has occurred, this tissue generally becomes obliterated, leaving the testis covered by the tunica vaginalis. Following descent, the testis shows a decline in its production of testosterone until puberty. As in all processes, descent may not occur or may occur imperfectly. This may result in maldescent of the testes.

PHYSIOLOGY OF THE MALE REPRODUCTIVE SYSTEM

The system consists of the paired testes, epididymis, vas deferens, common ejaculatory ducts, urethra, penis and the scrotum. The accessory organs are the seminal vesicles, prostate gland and the bulbo-urethral glands (Fig. 19–3). A cross section of the testis (Fig. 19–4) demonstrates the relationships between the seminiferous tubule, rete testis, efferent ductules, epididymis and vas deferens.

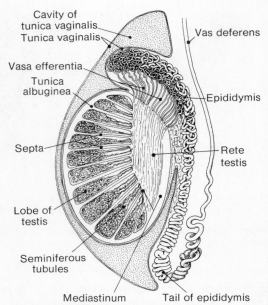

Figure 19–4 Section of the testis.

The Testes

Each lobe of the testis contains a seminiferous tubule surrounded by tissue. In this tissue are interstitial, or Leydig, cells, which are endocrine in action, producing the male hormones of which testosterone is the most prominent. These cells become activated to produce some androgens in the fetal period but remain nearly dormant until puberty. At puberty, under the complex control of the hypothalamus and pituitary glands, the testes are stimulated to produce male hormones. Under the influence of these androgens, the boy begins the process of puberty. The external organs of reproduction grow and develop. The distribution of body hair changes to that of the adult male. The larynx and musculoskeletal systems develop and change. Concurrently, the testes begin to produce sperm. Puberty ends with the sexual and reproductive maturity of the individual.

Spermatogenesis. Spermatogenesis begins in the seminiferous tubule (Fig. 19–5). Here a basilar membrane around the lumen of the tubule is lined with two major cell types which project into the lumen of the tube. The first of these, the germ cells, are called spermatogonia. These cells undergo growth and multiplication to become primary

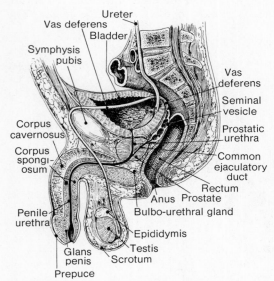

Figure 19–3 Sagittal view of the male reproductive system and pelvis.

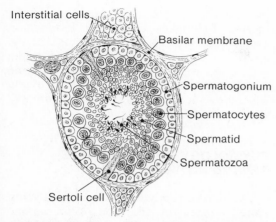

Interstitial cells

Basilar membrane

Spermatogonium

Spermatocytes

Spermatid

Spermatozoa

Sertoli cell

Figure 19–5 Transverse section of a seminiferous tubule in the interstitial tissue of the testis.

and secondary spermatocytes and then spermatids. Until this phase is complete the cell appears to have sufficient nutrients in itself. Now, however, the second type of cell, the Sertoli or sustentacular cell, is apparently necessary to provide nutrition for the spermatid. The spermatid is engulfed by the sustentacular cell and begins a metamorphosis which produces viable spermatozoa. When growth is complete the sperm is released into the lumen of the seminiferous tubule and is rapidly transported to the epididymis and thence through the duct system. Although sperm may appear to be mature at the time of release into the tubule, they do undergo further maturation, increasing in fertility and vigor as they progress through the ducts. Sperm removed from the tail of the epididymis rather than the head are more fertile. If sperm are not ejaculated, they rapidly degenerate and are absorbed. Spermatogenesis is continuous and new sperm are constantly being produced. The exact time of spermatogenesis is unknown but the whole process probably takes some days. This is in contrast to the female who does not produce ova throughout her lifetime but merely matures ova present from her own primordial germ cells.

Spermatogenesis is also sensitive to heat and occurs at a temperature a few degrees lower than body temperature. It is for this apparent reason that the testes are suspended in the scrotum, allowing the temperature of the testes to be regulated by the body. The dartos muscle within the scrotum contracts or relaxes in response to varying temperatures. Coldness causes it to contract bringing the testes closer to the body for extra warmth. The reverse is true in heat. It is also known that men with uncorrected cryptorchism remain sterile possibly because the body temperature intra-abdominally is incompatible with successful spermatogenesis.

Duct System and Accessory Glands

The viable sperm must be transported from the testis to the penis and thence to the female reproductive tract so that fertilization may take place. Here the duct system and the accessory glands play a major role. As the vas deferens ascends into the pelvic cavity, it widens into a broad ampulla. The duct of each seminal vesicle and the ampulla of the adjacent vas deferens meet to form the common ejaculatory duct. As a secretory organ, the seminal vesicle does not store sperm but rather produces a fluid which is rich in nutrients. These nutrients provide for the sperm until fertilization. At ejaculation, the seminal vesicles contract and seminal fluid is forced into the common ejaculatory ducts and into the prostatic urethra where the prostate gland also discharges its fluid.

The prostate gland which is fused to the neck of the bladder is divided into three lobes which surround the urethra. The prostate develops in puberty and is easily palpable on rectal examination. During the years of sexual maturity the prostate secretes a thin, milky-looking solution. This solution is alkaline and is believed to reduce the acidity of seminal fluid and vaginal secretions. This is an important reproductive function, as the motility and viability of sperm are greatly reduced in an acid solution. Sperm are more motile in a neutral or slightly alkaline solution. At ejaculation the muscle layers of the prostate gland contract rhythmically, forcing prostatic fluid into that portion of the urethra near the prostate. Simultaneously with these contractions of prostatic muscle, the fibers at the neck of the bladder continuous with muscle fibers in the prostate gland also contract, closing the internal urethral orifice.

Further fluid is added to the semen by the bulbo-urethral glands. These paired glands lie posterior to the urethra and discharge their fluid into it when they contract at ejaculation. This fluid seems to function merely as a lubricant and fluid medium for the sperm.

When all fluids are pooled in the prostatic portion of the urethra the first phase of ejaculation has been completed. The next phase is accomplished by powerful rhythmic contractions. The result is that the semen is forced along the length of the urethra in the erect penis and expelled from the urinary meatus under pressure.

Deposition of the semen in the vagina of the female is one function of the penis. The penis also serves as an excretory organ. In order to obtain intromission, the penis must move from its normally flaccid state to one of erection. Such a change is due to engorgement with blood of the corpora cavernosa and the corpus spongiosum.

Semen is a milky, viscous fluid varying at one ejaculation from 2 to 7 ml. in quantity and containing about 60,000,000 to 100,000,000 sperm per ml. The alkaline fluid is rich in nutrients and minerals to support the sperm. It coagulates a few minutes after ejaculation and then reliquefies later. The sperm, which are actively motile by lashing their tails, move slowly up through the uterus into the outer one-third of the uterine (Fallopian) tube where fertilization usually takes place. It is believed that the acrosome or projection on the head of the sperm releases hyaluronidase, an enzyme which dissolves the outer wall of the ovum. This allows a sperm to enter the ovum and fertilization to take place.

PHYSIOLOGY OF THE FEMALE REPRODUCTIVE SYSTEM

The female reproductive tract consists of paired ovaries, uterine tubes, a uterus and vagina (Fig. 19–6). Externally, the labia, clitoris, and Skene's and Bartholin's glands are part of the reproductive system (Fig. 19–7). The external area may be collectively referred to as the vulva, perineum or pudenda. Generally, perineum refers to the area stretching from the symphysis pubis laterally to the thighs and posteriorly to the tip of the coccyx. This is arbitrarily divided into the anterior and posterior perineum by an imaginary line drawn between the ischial tuberosities. Anteriorly, this contains the urogenital triangle and posterially the rectal triangle, including the perineal body. The

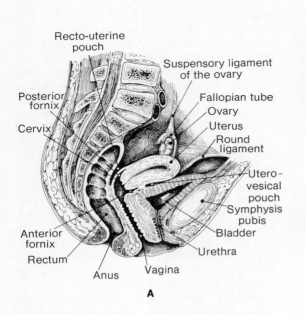

A

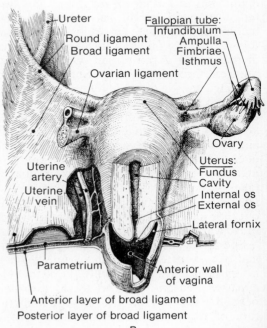

B

Figure 19–6 *A,* Median sagittal section of the female pelvis. *B,* Uterus and adnexa, posterior view (uterus, cervix and vagina wedge sectioned).

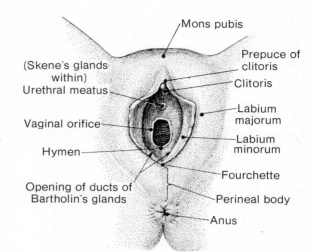

Figure 19–7 Female external genitalia.

area between the labia majora is referred to as the pudendal cleft. That area which lies between the labia minora and extends from the clitoris to the fourchet is referred to as the vestibule. Bartholin's glands, whose ducts open into the vestibule, may be referred to as the greater vestibular glands, Skene's being the lesser.

The female reproductive system functions to produce the female hormones (estrogen and progesterone), to ripen ova for fertilization, and for intercourse which permits fertilization of ova and the release of sexual tension. In addition, the organs of reproduction incubate the human conceptus, providing it with safety and nourishment until the fetus is expelled from the uterus to continue its growth and development externally.

The Ovary

The ovary is a small, almond-shaped organ lying posterior to the broad ligament of the uterus and attached to it by the mesovarium. Cross sections of the ovary show a cortex and a medulla. The cortex, or outer layer, is composed of connective tissue and cells among which are scattered the ova and developing follicles. Over this outer layer of the cortex is a thin layer of germinal epithelium. The medulla is composed of connective tissue containing blood vessels and smooth muscle fibers.

The fetal ovary is recognizable very early. By the fourth month of intrauterine life some cells in the ovary have differentiated enough to be recognizable as primary oocytes. Current belief holds that such oocytes, numbering only 300 to 400 in each woman, are determined at fertilization. Throughout childhood certain of these oocytes develop but never reach maturity and ovulate. Then, under the influence of the maturing hypothalamus, which stimulates the anterior lobe of the pituitary to produce hormones, puberty begins.

The secondary sex characteristics begin to develop. First there is growth and development of the breast tissue. Pubic hair appears and the internal and external organs of reproduction become fully developed and functional. The vagina under the influence of estrogens thickens and develops several layers of squamous epithelium. This makes it more resistant to infection. Previously, the vaginal pH had been neutral or alkaline; now it becomes acidic. This is largely due to Döderlein's bacillus which oxidizes the glycogen which has been deposited in the vagina to form lactic acid. Concurrently, the ovaries are developing and menarche, or the beginning of menstruation, occurs.

The Ovarian Cycle

Under the influence of the follicle-stimulating hormone (FSH) produced by the pituitary gland, the primary follicle begins to mature. The primary follicle is composed of an oocyte and follicular cells. Growth is eccentric and the oocyte or ovum gradually comes to lie at one side of the group of follicular cells. Fluid collects between these cells and the ovum. A clear membrane, the zona pellucida, develops and surrounds the ovum. As the follicle grows, the cells surrounding it begin to form and are termed thecal cells. Now the interstitial cell stimulating hormone (ICSH, luteinizing hormone) works with the FSH to allow the thecal cells to function. These cells, which are similar to the Leydig cells of the male, produce estrogens which are released into the blood. As this estrogen circulates, it signals to the anterior pituitary gland to reduce the production of FSH. ICSH continues to be produced. Many follicles may start to ripen, but usually only one continues on to ovulation. The others undergo degeneration in the ovary. The thecal cells surrounding these degenerated (atretic) follicles also produce estrogens. The mature follicle may now be termed a Graafian follicle after de Graaf who first described it in 1672 (Fig. 19–8).

As the Graafian follicle approaches ovulation, it comes to lie close to the surface of the ovary. The tissue over it becomes thin and taut. Soon the follicle wall ruptures and the ovum, surrounded by the zona pellucida and some attached granulosa cells, is expelled into the abdominal cavity. The time of rupture is designated as ovulation. Although it is felt that a buildup of pressure within the follicle is not the principal cause of rupture, the precise mechanism is still not perfectly understood. Some authors believe that necrosis of tissue over the taut area is a more likely reason for the freeing of the ovum into the abdominal cavity.

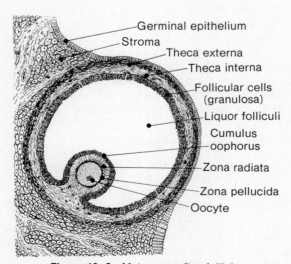

Figure 19–8 Mature graafian follicle.

Germinal epithelium
Stroma
Theca externa
Theca interna
Follicular cells (granulosa)
Liquor folliculi
Cumulus oophorus
Zona radiata
Zona pellucida
Oocyte

However it is accomplished, ovulation marks the end of the preovulatory, or follicular, phase.

The ovary now embarks on the luteal phase of its cycle. Immediately following ovulation, the wall of the follicle collapses inward and some hemorrhage may occur into this cavity. In a few hours the remaining granulosa cells hypertrophy and begin to show the characteristic yellow of the corpus luteum. These yellowed granulosa cells are now called luteal cells. The luteal cells are stimulated by ICSH to become the corpus luteum and to begin producing progesterone. Estrogen continues to be produced as well. The corpus luteum reaches full maturity by about the ninth day following ovulation. At this time it is easily recognizable on the surface of the ovary as a raised yellowed area and may constitute nearly one-half of the volume of the ovary. Near this time, by unknown methods, the corpus luteum apparently receives a message that the ovum has been fertilized. If it does so, the corpus luteum is maintained and becomes known as the corpus luteum of pregnancy. If fertilization does not occur, the luteal site begins to degenerate, and progesterone production drops. As the site degenerates, so do the thecal cells. Estrogen production from this source declines. The luteal site shrinks to form a small mass of whitish scar tissue on the surface of the ovary which is known as the corpus albicans.

In response to the falling estrogen and progesterone levels, the hypothalamus signals the pituitary gland to release FSH and ICSH and the cycle repeats itself. This cycle recurs roughly every 28 to 32 days in the vast majority of adult women from menarche to menopause unless it is interrupted by periods of pregnancy. However, in response to this cycle, the endometrium of the uterus also undergoes cyclic phenomena. These phenomena are known as the uterine cycle. The two cycles, uterine and ovarian, are intimately related and occur simultaneously.

The Uterus

The uterus is a thick-walled, muscular, pear-shaped organ about 3 inches in length in the adult virgin. It is held in position by its ligaments and by the pelvic floor. The uterus is composed of three layers: an inner mucous layer, or endometrium; a middle muscular layer, or myometrium; and an outer serous layer which covers the entire body of the uterus except where it is reflected up and over the bladder. The uterus is divided into two distinct parts: the body and the cervix.

The cervix projects into the vagina. It appears to be mainly connective tissue, and only 10 per cent is muscle. The endometrial lining of the body of the uterus extends downward, undergoing certain modifications in the cervical canal and terminating just above the external os of the cervix where it meets the stratified squamous epithelium of the vaginal wall.

The Uterine Cycle

In the uterine cycle the endometrium plays a major role. The endometrium is a thin, pink membrane which is attached directly to the underlying muscle layer. It is composed of surface epithelium, uterine glands and connective tissue and is richly supplied with blood vessels and tissue spaces. The thickness of the endometrium varies with the cycle. At the beginning of a new cycle it is probably about 0.5 mm. thick. In response to the estrogens of the preovulatory phase of the ovary it begins to proliferate and continues to do so throughout the cycle until it reaches a peak of proliferation and secretion several days following ovulation. In addition to the effect of estrogen, the progesterone released in the luteal phase of the ovary further promotes the secretory activity of the endometrium. In this secretory stage the endometrium is edematous, the glands are large and sacculated, the arteries have developed their typical coiled, tortuous pattern and some connective tissue has undergone hypertrophic stages. The rich, succulent endometrium now contains much glycogen. At this time the endometrium may be 5 to 6 mm. in depth. In short, all is ready for the implantation of the fertilized ovum should it appear. In perfect timing the endometrium reaches its peak development approximately 7 to 8 days following ovulation, or just when the fertilized ovum should appear in the uterine cavity ready for implantation.

If the ovum has been fertilized and the corpus luteum is continuing to secrete progesterone, the endometrium is maintained and implantation may occur successfully. However, should the corpus luteum not receive this message, it begins to degenerate. Estrogen and progesterone production decline. This decline in progesterone causes the endometrium to retract and degenerate. Vasoconstriction of blood vessels occurs and the uterus becomes ischemic. Shortly thereafter the endometrium begins to slough away and menstruation begins. The process of sloughing takes from 3 to 7 days with each woman usually establishing her own pattern. Menstrual flow is composed of endometrial tissue, mucus and some blood. As the tiny arterioles constrict and relax, bleeding occurs. Usually not more than 50 to 60 cc. of blood per menstrual period is lost. At the completion of menstruation the endometrium has returned to its unproliferative state. It is now ready to respond again to the rising estrogen levels.

The Menstrual Cycle

The uterine and ovarian cycles are often referred to as the menstrual cycle. This cycle begins on day one, which is the day menstruation begins, and continues until the day before menstruation begins again. Ovulation occurs on or around the fourteenth day of the cycle. However, this is subject to many factors and the timing of ovulation in any one woman is often a matter of considerable variation.

Anovulation

Not all cycles are ovulatory and it is known that women can have an anovulatory cycle and still menstruate. The precise mechanisms for these phenomena are not clearly understood. Some believe that in such cases a follicle develops, becomes cystic and degenerates. Certainly, some such mechanism appears possible, particularly in adolescent girls, in whom the first menstrual periods may be anovulatory, and at the menopause.

Cervical, Vaginal and Tubal Cycles

Changes also occur in the cervix, vagina, and uterine tubes in response to these stimuli from the ovary. Estrogen prompts the endocervical glands to respond by increasing their secretions and developing in length and tortuosity. This is accompanied by increased vascularity and tumescence of the cervix. From about the seventh day of the menstrual cycle to about the twenty-first the cervical mucus gradually increases in amount. The mucus contains an increasing concentration of sodium chloride which causes it to show a typical ferning pattern when allowed to dry on a slide. During the other periods of the cycle and during pregnancy the dried cervical mucus shows a beaded pattern. The mucus reaches its peak of production at ovulation. The consistency changes at ovulation and becomes thinner and can be drawn out into long, thin threads. This is called Spinnbarkeit. These changes demonstrate the timing of the body as the mucus will permit easy entry of the sperm at ovulation, the most logical time. Indeed it appears that the cervical mucus permits passage of sperm through the cervix only at this particular time.

Changes in the vagina and uterine tube are minimal compared to the changes in the ovary, uterus and cervix. The vaginal epithelium proliferates and reaches a peak at ovulation time. The uterine tube becomes swollen. Its secretory cells enlarge and project beyond the ciliated cells. Maximum development is timed to occur simultaneously with ovulation and the passage of the ovum through the tube. The ovum is also assisted in its passage by the wave-like contractions of the uterine tube and the beating of the tubal cilia toward the uterus. These contractions appear to be under the influence of estrogens. The uterine tube secretes fluids which provide nutrients first for the ovum and then for the conceptus until implantation occurs.

The Vagina

The vagina, a fibromuscular tube from 3 to 4 inches long, is the female organ of intercourse. Here sperm are deposited. It also serves as a passage for the fetus from intrauterine to extrauterine life. The vagina is protected by the labia, which usually remain in close approximation over the introitus. During sexual excitement the labia become engorged and swollen and gape, thus exposing the vestibule.

Under neural stimulus, Bartholin's glands secrete a fluid which serves to lubricate the vaginal introitus. However, the mucus these vulvovaginal glands secrete is minimal and not of sufficient quantity to lubricate the entire vagina. Hence most vaginal lubrication arises from the vaginal walls themselves. Very quickly following sexual stimulation the vaginal walls exhibit a "sweating" like appearance as beads of mucoid material appear throughout the rugal folds. Soon the droplets run together and form a complete coat of lubrication over the inner surface of the vagina. Since there are no glandular elements in the vaginal wall, it is hypothesized that the exudation is a result of marked dilatation of the venous system which surrounds the vagina. The cervix, once thought to be the source of much of the lubrication of the vagina, also appears to play a relatively minor role. This appears to be confirmed by the fact that little or no secretory activity of the cervix has been observed during sexual activity. Also, women who have undergone total hysterectomy and bilateral salpingo-oophorectomy produce reasonable vaginal lubrication in response to sexual stimulation. Indeed the same response will develop in artificially constructed vaginas, and the source of the lubricating material is presumed to be the same.

The vagina also responds to sexual stimuli by enlarging. The inner two-thirds of the vagina expands and lengthens, forming a basin for the seminal pool which will form in the posterior fornix of the vagina just below the cervical os. The outer third of the vagina becomes engorged and constricted, serving to assist the vagina to form a reservoir for the semen. Engorgement of pelvic organs also results in a slight elevation of the uterus and cervix.

An orgasm may occur as a generalized systemic feeling with sensation localized in the clitoris and rhythmic muscular contractions of the outer third of the vagina and the uterus. With orgasm, pelvic engorgement of blood vessels is rapidly resolved. This causes the uterus to return to its normal position, placing the cervix very near to or in the seminal pool, thus facilitating movement of sperm through the cervix.

The clitoris seems to be a unique organ in human anatomy. As the primary focus of sensual response, it appears to serve no other function. Made of fibrous tissue with two corpora cavernosa and richly innervated, it undergoes engorgement and enlargement when the female is sexually stimulated either physically or mentally. It also appears to be the translator of sexual stimuli to other organs of the reproductive tract. There is no apparent observable response in the clitoris at orgasm.

The Menopause

The reproductive functions of the male and female continue throughout adult life. Given health and opportunity, the male's sexual and reproductive capabilities may extend well into the eighth decade of life with the only major change being a slowing of sexual response and a gradual reduction in libido (sexual drive).

Women, however, present a different picture. Reproductive function, usually demonstrated by menses, continues until middle age. Then, at the average age of 47, women cease menstruating. The climacteric or cessation of menstruation is perhaps the most obvious sign of the menopause, or "change of life." Actually, the menopause in onset and duration resembles puberty, which was a gradual awakening of reproductive function over a period of 6 months to 2 years. The menopause also may take a few months to several years and is the result of decreasing estrogen production. Ovarian follicles cease to ripen. The endometrium does not respond as richly, and menstruation becomes scantier and shorter in duration. The woman may have several anovulatory cycles, just as she may have had in puberty. Eventually the menses may become irregular and finally cease. Dropping estrogen levels stimulate gonadotrophic hormones (FSH, ICSH) which show a proportionate rise, but the ovary does not respond fully. The vascular system, once functioning smoothly under hormonal control, begins to respond to these imbalances and the woman may experience "hot flashes," feelings of tingling and faintness. She may have periods of sweating, especially at night. Hypertension may develop, for estrogen appears to have inhibiting effects on the development of atherosclerosis. Osteoporosis has also been linked to declining estrogen levels. She may feel depressed and experience swings in mood for no apparent reason. Much of this may be unsettling to the woman, especially when accompanied by cessation of reproductive function and fears of loss of usefulness, sexual function, love of her husband and advancing age. Most women accept the changes with some minor disturbances. It would seem that an understanding of the menopause and some reassurance of her usefulness and worth will help most women. Only about 25 per cent of women require hormone replacement treatment. This is always in the form of short-term therapy with oral estrogens. The dosage is individualized to relieve the symptoms and is continued for 2 to 3 months, at which time a reassessment is made to decide whether to continue or stop treatment. It should be understood that all estrogen production does not cease at menopause. The ovaries do not appear to be inert postmenopausally, and it is thought that they continue to excrete small amounts of hormones. This is in addition to estrogens from the adrenal gland. Over the years estrogen production declines further and the development of other organ changes occurs. The vulva become atrophic and thin from a resorption of fatty tissue. The uterus decreases in size; the endometrium becomes thin and atrophic. The vaginal epithelium thins out and is more susceptible to injury and infection. Lubrication of the vagina may require supplementation so that dyspareunia (painful sexual intercourse) need not occur. Sexual function can continue with little change in the vast majority of postmenopausal women. The most important factors in the continuance of sexual function appear to be the opportunity for and the frequency of intercourse so that the changes of the menopause themselves do not mean this phase of a woman's life must cease. Indeed, relief from fear of pregnancy may make the experience a more enjoyable one.

GENERAL NURSING CONSIDERATIONS

The patient with a disorder of the reproductive tract presents some special concerns for the nurse. In many ways a human being is defined by his sex. Knowing he or she is a man or a woman gives the person a set of behaviors, culturally and physiologically determined, which help to guide his or her actions. The normal functioning of the reproductive tract gives constant reassurance of a person's essential maleness or femaleness. The distortion or interruption of these processes may prove very disturbing to the individual and his family.

The person may fear loss of reproductive function. The ability to reproduce is seen by many as a criterion of usefulness and sexuality. The loss of function may be followed by feelings of uselessness or of being only half a person. These feelings can be particularly distressing to the woman who has defined herself in terms of her reproducing and sexual function. To her the removal of her uterus or ovaries may be tantamount to removing her femaleness. Because she may feel less a woman, she fears her husband will see her as less a woman. Indeed, in some unfortunate situations, he may. Thus, to the fear of loss of reproductive function may be added the fear of loss of a loved one. For some the fear of loss of libido as well as sexual function may be very frightening and can cause the patient much anguish.

Also, most patients have been culturally conditioned to the idea that these areas of the body should not be discussed, much less exposed, in examination or discussion. Thus, it should not be difficult for a nurse to understand why a patient may be nervous, anxious, embarrassed and perhaps uncooperative, demanding or irritable.

The nursing approach to all patients requires a double focus. With one inner eye the nurse must see the disease and understand the nature of its cause, transmission, course and resolution. Accompanying this must be a knowledge of the nursing care as well as some understanding of the medical treatment and prevention for the disease. With the other inner eye the nurse must focus on the patient. It is the ability to apply this double focus which seems to allow the nurse to remain sensitive to the patient as an individual; to see, always, a person with a disease, a person sick, a person in the hospital.

As each human being is a unique individual, so shall each person's response to a life situation be a unique one. Illness is another life experience to which a person responds. This response is governed by many factors.

The person's age, past experiences, cultural group and social class are but a few. Some reactions are personality characteristics either inborn or learned. Others are responses to transient stresses and pressures on the patient which appear prominent at that time and place. These stresses may be so important to the patient that they appear to dominate his thoughts, preventing him from concentrating on other situations. The patient's response to his illness and hospitalization, and the resulting effect of this response on the course of the disease and the effectiveness of medical treatment, has long been hotly debated and ill defined. Research does indicate that very anxious preoperative patients do not tolerate surgical procedures and anesthesia as well as calm, confident patients. One nursing study (Dumas et al.) indicates that the incidence of postoperative vomiting could be reduced by a nursing approach which deliberately set out to explore the patient's worries preoperatively. Unfortunately, too little study has been done to show the relationship between the response to illness or medical therapeutics and the course of the patient's illness.

The nurse is frequently left with a frightened, lonely patient who, too often, is confounded by the strange processes, which, unasked for, have gripped his or her body, and by the hospital and its therapeutics which hope to restore the patient to health. A nurse who approaches the patient warmly and with a general air of confidence usually communicates these feelings to the patient. With the patient who talks freely and verbalizes well, she usually has an easier time and can offer her explanations and interpretations of the illness and treatments in response to the patient's particular need and at a time which appears appropriate. With other patients who are more reserved, verbalize less easily or who are more timid, she may have to work harder. Here a nonverbal approach such as touching the hand, providing physical care and answering the call bell readily and willingly will communicate much to the patient. As a result, the patient becomes more relaxed and secure in the environment. Anticipating the need for explanations and interpretations may have to be done, for the patient may not realize that an explanation would help to ease his tensions and feelings of insecurity or helplessness. Generally, relatives need as much consideration and nursing as the patient. Since the lives of family members are so intimately interwoven, a crisis for one is a crisis for all. By reassuring the relatives, you may be reassuring the patient, as often the anxiety and tension of one family member is easily communicated to the others. Allowing the family to work together to cope with a situation with some assistance from the medical team may also be a wise adjunct to therapy. Many families have faced other crises together and have developed methods of handling crises which were compatible with their way of life.

As in all things, knowledge will help the patient. Such knowledge should ideally begin at an early age. The nurse has a role to play in the teaching of the normal anatomy and physiology of reproduction to all age groups in whatever professional capacity she occupies at the time, i.e., public health nurse, occupational health nurse, etc. In addition, she must deliberately provide opportunities for patients in the hospital to ask her questions and to help provide solutions and interpretations. This will require skill in interviewing in order to determine what the patient really wants to know and skill in phrasing answers, since the nurse must communicate with the patient. The nurse must also cope with her own feelings and culturally determined responses. Her sense of modesty may be offended. She may have difficulty accepting attitudes which differ radically from her own. This conflict may be particularly acute when she is nursing patients who have obtained abortions, contracted venereal disease or pelvic inflammatory disease. A non-judgmental acceptance of the patient is required of the nurse. However, the nurse may find this difficult until she has reconciled her own feelings with the requirements of a professional in the situation.

CONGENITAL ANOMALIES OF THE MALE

Maldescent of Testes

Approximately 4 per cent of newborn males will exhibit some form of maldescent of the testes. Unilateral maldescent of testis is about 4 times as prevalent as bilateral maldescent. The cause of this condition is not known but may be related to defects in the surrounding structures of the fetal testes, defects in the testes themselves or hormonal deficiencies. The majority of testes descend during the first 3 months of extrauterine life. Many more descend at puberty under the influence of rising testosterone levels. Probably less than 1 per cent of men remain with undescended testes following puberty. The principal sign is an inability to palpate one or both testes in the scrotal sac.

It is important to distinguish between three possible types of maldescent. Retractile testes are those which, under the influence of a strong muscular reflex, are drawn up to the external inguinal ring. This gives a false impression on palpation that the testes are not in the scrotum. No treatment is required. Ectopic testes are those which have descended to an abnormal site. Commonly this is the superficial inguinal pouch but may be almost anywhere near the normal path of descent. Cryptorchism is a condition in which the descent of the testis is interrupted anywhere along the normal path of descent.

Treatment of ectopic or cryptorchid testes may consist of first administering chorionic gonadotropins or methyltestosterone for short periods of time. This is usually more successful in bilateral undescended testes, indicating that these testes would probably have descended spontaneously at puberty. Because histological changes can be observed in undescended testes as early as 6 years of age, treatment is usually initiated earlier than puberty to ensure maximum functioning of the testes. Should hormone therapy be unsuccessful, orchiopexy (surgical placement and fixation of the testis in the scrotal sac) is indicated. Hernioplasty may also be done to repair the inguinal hernia which is often present in these cases. The patient will be on bed rest or bed rest with restricted activity for several days. Thereafter excessive physical activity should be avoided for about 6 weeks.

Should the condition not be diagnosed until after puberty, most authorities agree that orchiopexy is indicated even though the man may be sterile. First, the Leydig cells of the testes continue to produce male hormones which will sustain the secondary sex characteristics. Secondly, such testes have a higher incidence of malignancy than do normally positioned testes and can be more easily examined yearly for malignancy in the scrotum than in the abdomen. In unilateral conditions, the extrascrotal testis will be removed to further reduce the possibility of malignancy. This leaves the man with one functioning testis as a source of sperm and male hormones.

Absence or Duplication of Organs

Congenital absence of the penis, scrotum and vas deferens are very rare. However, in certain genetically determined syndromes the testicular tissue may be absent or nonfunctioning. One such example is Klinefelter's syndrome. The person with this syndrome has an XXY genotype. This produces atrophic testes and sterility. The person may also have eunuchoid development, and mental retardation may or may not be present. Androgens are administered to prevent feminization. Other examples are hermaphrodites, or persons who have some characteristics of both sexes. This could be genetically determined as a true hermaphrodite or could be due to a feminizing lesion, producing a pseudohermaphrodite.

Hypospadias

Hypospadias arises from a failure of the folds to fuse (Fig. 19–2). Chordee, a curvature of the penis, usually accompanies hypospadias and epispadias. Since the sex of the child may be doubtful, chromosome studies will be carried out and treatment based on the results of these findings. In mild cases of hypospadias, no treatment is necessary, as function is usually not impaired. In more severe cases, surgical repair will be necessary. This repair will straighten the penile shaft so that normal intercourse is possible. In addition a urethra will be formed which extends as near as possible to the tip of the glans so that semen is deposited deep in the vagina. Surgery is usually not immediately indicated and may be done in a series of operations beginning at about the age of 2 in a child in whom the condition has been detected early. In a few unfortunate cases the child is assumed to be female from birth and these extreme cases

may not be discovered until puberty and the development of secondary sex characteristics. For this reason, it is important that the nurse carefully examine the external genitalia of the newborn and report to its physician any baby which she feels does not appear normal.

Epispadias

Epispadias is much rarer than hypospadias and is often associated with exstrophy of the bladder (Fig. 19–2). Because of the possible bladder involvement, the patient may be incontinent as a result of imperfect or absent urethral sphincters. Surgical repair provides the child with a functioning penis and urethra.

Preoperatively, a cystostomy may be done (p. 456). The patient may also return from the operating room with a splinting catheter in the urethra until healing takes place. If the patient is discharged home with a cystostomy, the parents will need instruction in the care of the child.

CONGENITAL ANOMALIES IN THE FEMALE

Absence or Duplication of Organs

The uterus, cervix and vagina can undergo duplication or incomplete fusion (Fig. 19–1). The exact incidence of such anomalies is unknown, since they are largely asymptomatic. Some may cause sterility in women or an increased risk of abortion. Rarely an organ is completely absent. Also, as in the male, some absence (agenesis) or maldevelopment of tissue (dysgenesis) is genetically determined. Ovarian agenesis may be the result of an XO genotype (Turner's syndrome). The patient with this genotype may present a characteristic appearance from birth with a webbed neck, multiple anomalies, small birth weight or irregularities of the hairline. However, in others the patient may present in adolescence because of the failure of the menarche to appear. Treatment is usually estrogen replacement therapy, with 1 mg. being given every day for 3 weeks followed by withdrawal. Withdrawal of estrogen permits the endometrium to slough away, thus simulating a menstrual period. Because the ovaries do not exist, the patient remains sterile.

Imperforate Hymen

Normally the hymen is patent. Rarely, it may not be. Usually the condition is not discovered until adolescence when the girl may present herself because of absence of menstrual flow. Menstruation occurs but the menstrual blood is retained behind the closed hymen. The patient may complain of crampy, lower abdominal pain occurring monthly. She may also notice dysuria, frequency, and urinary retention as the growing mass of retained menstrual blood accumulates in the vagina, putting increasing pressure on the bladder and urethra. Treatment consists of a cross-shaped incision of the hymen which allows drainage of the debris. This debris is often a thick, chocolate-like material. Because of this old blood, the risk of postoperative infection is greatly increased. Antibiotics are usually ordered. The nurse must pay careful attention to good aseptic technique postoperatively to further reduce the risk of infection. She must see that adequate drainage is maintained; that frequent cleansing of the perineum occurs; and that perineal dressings are changed frequently.

The hymen may also be rigid. This is usually discovered when the patient presents with a complaint of dyspareunia. In mild cases the patient will be instructed to dilate the hymen digitally usually while sitting in a tub of warm water. In difficult cases, hymenotomy is performed. This is one rationale for a premarital examination. The discovery of a rigid hymen and its treatment premaritally may be of great importance to a newly married couple.

FERTILITY AND INFERTILITY

CONTROL OF FERTILITY

Perhaps one of the greatest problems facing the world today is the control of fertility. Constantly, one is bombarded with news of the population explosion and its disastrous implications for the future of the world. These implications have usually been stated in terms of the developing nations, but more recently they have taken on a global context. In addition, there is a growing feeling that contraception be considered a matter of personal decision—that it can exercise an important liberalizing potential for the family or the single person. In the light of these discussions it would seem that the health professional has a responsibility to extend the knowledge and availability of contraception to anyone who requests it. With more family practice units and conception control clinics in the outpatient department or the public health department the nurse has an expanding role in the control of fertility.

Nursing Responsibilities

Generally, the nursing responsibilities include referral of the patient to the appropriate clinic or doctor, education and interpretation. Depending on the nurse's situation and knowledge, these may be taken care of in an initial interview (or group discussion) with a patient (or a group of patients) seeking birth control advice. The nurse can assist the patient or couple in making a decision by presenting concise, factual information about the methods available. The couple should choose a method which will be most compatible with their personal circumstances. Most certainly this should be the one they will use and feel comfortable in using. No method of birth control is effective unless it is used constantly. This final decision is usually made with medical counsel. As the doctor reviews the patient's history, he may make other recommendations which will affect the person's or couple's choice. The patient or couple will need counsel in the proper use of the method they have chosen and what to expect in the period of initial adjustment. The nurse should validate the patient's real understanding of the method chosen and provide explanations and interpretations if necessary. In a simple fashion the knowledge of an alternate emergency method should be provided as well, for it is this which may prevent a pregnancy. Emergencies do occur. The patient forgets to take her pills to the cottage, or she discovers the intrauterine device is missing at 1:30 A.M. and is too embarrassed to call the doctor at that hour. Be sure the patient leaves the clinic or office with the knowledge of this alternate method. Usually, the use of spermicidal foam or the use of a condom by the husband will overcome these situations. The nurse is responsible for gaining sufficient knowledge of the complex subject of contraception to be able to present factual knowledge to couples and to discuss the pros and cons of each method. In addition, the nurse will need to understand much of the emotional, social and religious aspects of contraception. A detailed presentation of family planning is beyond the scope of this work, but a brief outline of methods follows.

Methods of Contraception

Coitus Interruptus. This method consists of the male withdrawing his penis from the vagina before ejaculation occurs and ejaculating outside the vagina. Coitus interruptus, or withdrawal, is better than no attempt at birth control but is still very unreliable. Care must be taken not to ejaculate on or near the vulva, as the sperm may make their way into the vagina and pregnancy can result. The method requires the man to have advance awareness of ejaculation. This control and knowledge may be difficult to establish and may require more sexual experience than the man or couple possesses. Also, some sperm may escape before ejaculation occurs. The method has also come under considerable criticism for its psychological effects. These have been associated principally with frustration as a result of unresolved sexual tensions on the part of one or both partners. However, if the method is accepted by the couple and orgasm and ejaculation do occur, the resulting psychological stresses are probably minimal.

Condom. The condom is a thin rubber sheath which is placed over the penis before intromission. It prevents pregnancy by acting as a mechanical barrier to the sperm. Proper use includes application before intromission to avoid the possibility of a pre-ejaculatory emission of semen into the vagina and careful withdrawal of the penis and condom following intercourse to be sure that some semen is not lost into the vagina or over the vulva. Some doctors advise the use of a spermicidal jelly as a lubricating agent over the condom. This is a method of additional safety, particularly if the condom should be defective. However, newer methods of manufacture have greatly reduced this hazard. The condom is reasonably priced and is available without prescription. This greatly increases its availability and hence makes it one of the most widely used methods in the world.

Some couples find it objectionable as a method of birth control because it may interrupt sexual foreplay; it can lessen sensation; and its effective use relies heavily on the motivation of the male. These objections can be overcome if it is used by a highly motivated man who is taking mature responsibility for his behavior. Fortunately, many such men exist and the condom is classified as a highly effective form of birth control.

Diaphragm. The diaphragm is a thin rubber cap which is inserted into the vagina by the woman and placed over the cervical os. The cap provides a mechanical barrier to the sperm. In addition a spermicidal jelly is placed in the dome of the cap. When the diaphragm is in place the spermicidal jelly will be in touch with the cervix.

The diaphragm is not dispensed without a prescription and requires individual fittings by a doctor initially, after a few months of use and following pregnancy or miscarriage. The woman also requires careful teaching in the proper insertion and care of the diaphragm. The diaphragm is inserted manually or with an inserter which is provided. The position of the diaphragm should be checked following each insertion. The woman stands with one foot elevated or squats. The diaphragm is squeezed between two fingers thus narrowing it, and the drop of jelly is kept facing up as the woman slips the diaphragm into her vagina. In its proper position, the diaphragm cups the cervix with its anterior side behind the pubic bone and its posterior side in the posterior fornix of the vagina. Following insertion the woman must be taught to check the position of the diaphragm to see that it is properly situated. Properly positioned, it is not felt by either partner. It can be left in place for 24 hours but should then be removed and cleansed with soap and water. Removal should not take place until at least 6 hours post coitus to ensure death of all sperm present in the vagina.

Used by intelligent, well instructed, highly motivated women it is a highly effective method of birth control. However, some women find it distasteful to insert the diaphragm and to check its position. For these women it is probably a very poor method of birth control.

Spermicidal Preparations. In more recent years chemicals with a spermicidal action have been placed in gels, creams, aerosol foams, suppositories and foam tablets. These are inserted into the vagina about one-half hour before intercourse. The foam or jelly coats the cervix and inner vaginal walls. It should remain in the vagina for at least 6 hours to be sure that all sperm are dead. Used consistently, the method is very effective. Objections to the method center around the messiness which can result after coitus and a distaste in some people for the idea of killing a living sperm. Some men may complain of a slight urethral irritation when some foaming types of preparations are used.

Douche. The vaginal douche or irrigation may be used for cleanliness following coitus or may be considered to be a method of birth control by those who are under the impression that it "washes the sperm away." In fact, it may force the sperm into the uterine cavity and merely speed them on their way. It is not a reliable method of contraception.

Breast-feeding. Under the stimulus of breast-feeding many women remain anovulatory for several months. Others quickly regain their fertility. Hence, breast-feeding should not be considered a method of birth control.

The Rhythm Method. This method requires temporary abstinence from coitus during the possible ovulation time of the woman. It is the only method of birth control officially sanctioned by all religions. The rationale for the method is based on several assumptions. First, a woman is only fertile at the time of ovulation, which occurs once monthly at a predictable time, and the ovum lives for approximately 24 hours. Secondly, sperm will survive in the genital tract for only 3 days. Placing these facts together and allowing 3 days before and after ovulation for the life span of the sperm we arrive at 6 days. Since we know that the time of ovulation varies in any one woman we must allow 1 or 2 days for extra safety on either side. This now gives us a fertile period of approximately 8 days' duration, falling near the middle of the menstrual cycle. The crux

of the problem is the timing of ovulation. Since no anticipatory method of timing ovulation has been discovered, we must rely on a retrospective view of the time of ovulation in any one woman. Under the influence of the rising progesterone levels following ovulation, the basal body temperature in women shows a rise. This rise should be noticeable within the first 24 hours following ovulation. The temperature remains slightly elevated for the remainder of the cycle (Fig. 19–9). Most physicians will attempt to predict the time of ovulation for any one woman after she has carefully recorded the dates of her menstrual periods and her temperatures taken daily at a uniform time. Depending on the woman, the doctor or the clinic, this may be done for 3 to 6 months. An average is then calculated from these dates and her individual period of likely fertility is plotted. In the graph (Fig. 19–9) the fertile period can be seen for a regular 28-day cycle. The calculated fertile period should be reviewed at specified intervals by the woman and her doctor. At periods of her life when ovulation is being established or re-established, i.e., during postpartum and lactation or menopause, the method is highly unreliable. In women of very regular periods and with high motivation the method has had considerable success. However, until a foolproof method of anticipating ovulation is achieved, this method will have to be regarded merely as reliable even in highly motivated couples. One major objection by some couples is that the period of abstinence is long and occurs at a time when the libido in the woman may be very high.

The Intrauterine Device. An intrauterine device is an object placed inside the uterus which remains in the uterus and prevents pregnancy. The action is not completely understood. Some doctors feel that the pregnancy is prevented by the intrauterine device (IUD) causing rapid contractions of the uterine tube such that the ovum is moved along the tube too rapidly, making it unsuitable for fertilization. Others feel that it is implantation which is prevented.

Most intrauterine devices used today are usually made of a flexible plastic and are in several shapes. The device must be inserted by a doctor. It is a sterile procedure.

First, the doctor will sound the uterus, confirming its depth. Then, having threaded

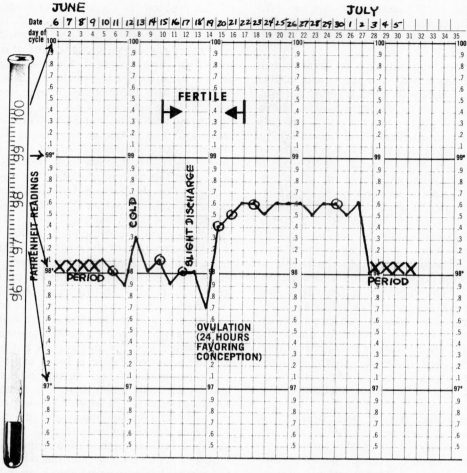

Figure 19–9 Basal body temperature chart showing fertile period. (Modified from Bleier, I.: Maternity Nursing, 3rd ed. Philadelphia, W. B. Saunders Co., 1971, p. 188.)

the IUD into the inserter he will insert this through the cervix, push down the plunger and retract the inserter. The use of the uterine sound and the skill of the inserter greatly reduce the risk of perforating the uterus. However, uterine perforation remains a rare complication of the IUD. Removal of the device is by a small hook. Many devices are equipped with strings which hang into the vagina just below the cervix. The device can usually be removed by gentle traction on the strings. The woman is also taught to check for the presence of these strings weekly; during her menstrual period she checks them daily. If she checks her pad or tampon, she usually satisfies this safety precaution. IUD's can be expelled from the uterus, and this is most likely to occur during the menstrual period. Women who have never been pregnant have an increased tendency to expel the device as do women who have previously expelled it. Also, because of the tightness of the cervical os in the nullipara, insertion and removal of the IUD may be more difficult. For these reasons some doctors will not recommend an IUD for nulliparous women. If the woman notices that the IUD appears to have been expelled, she should report this to the doctor so that he may confirm this. In some women the IUD causes cramping and spotting. Also, the first menstrual periods following insertion may be considerably heavier. The patient should report these to her doctor. In earlier years infection associated with IUD's discouraged their use. This has not proven to be a problem in recent years.

Pregnancies do occur in about 2 to 3 per cent of women using an intrauterine device. The device is left in place and is removed following the birth of the placenta. No damage to the fetus has been reported.

However, the IUD does rank as a very effective method of birth control in about 80 per cent of the women who try it. The 20 per cent failure rate arises from pregnancies, expulsions and removals because of cramping or bleeding.

Oral Contraceptives. Birth control pills are synthetic chemical hormones which resemble the female hormones of the ovary. In suppressing ovulation they mimic the action of pregnancy. The high hormone levels inhibit the production of pituitary gonadotropins which stimulate ovulation. Thus the woman is anovulatory. Protection is established as soon as the woman begins taking the pills.

The pills are divided into two types: the combined form and sequential form. The combined pill contains synthetic estrogen and progesterone hormones in each pill. This pill is more effective in preventing pregnancy apparently because it induces changes in the cervix, making the mucus thicker and more impenetrable by sperm. Also, changes occur in the endometrium which would discourage implantation should fertilization occur.

The sequential pills are given in sequence. The first 14 pills contain estrogen only, and the last 7 pills contain a combination of estrogen and progesterone. The sequential pills appear to be slightly less effective than the combined ones. Pregnancies have occurred with women following the sequential regimen. However, the risk of pregnancy in both types is minimal if used as prescribed. If taken correctly, the pills are the most effective method of contraception today.

Both types of pills are dispensed in the same way. The oldest method is a pill a day for 21 days (sometimes 20) and no pill for the next 7 days regardless of the woman's period. Confusion frequently arises over when to start the pill. Initially, the first pill is taken on the last day of the woman's menstrual period unless she has an unusually long one. Then the fifth day of the menstrual

cycle is used as a beginning day for the pill. Now the pills will regulate her menstrual cycle and she takes them as prescribed. It is wise for her to cross them off on a calendar or devise a method of knowing when to start again because each succeeding 21-day series of pills is started on the basis of when she took the last pill, not on her subsequent menstrual period. She begins again regardless of the state of her menstrual period.

To make this regime easier a more recent regimen is the "pill a day" packet. This contains 28 pills. The final 7 pills are placebos and simply correspond to the 7 pill-free days of the other method. This does make it much easier for women to follow, for no timing, counting or remembering other than to take the pill is required. Also, to maintain consistently high hormonal levels in the body, the pill should be taken at approximately the same time each day.

Withdrawal bleeding is regulated by the pill and occurs regularly at some time during the 7 pill-free days. This withdrawal bleeding simulates true menstruation. With the withdrawal of the high hormone levels, the endometrium sloughs away. However, menstruation is usually scantier and shorter, since the endometrium is thinner and scantier. A woman may miss one period, but should she miss two, this should be reported to the doctor immediately.

Much discussion has occurred over the possible side effects or complications attendant on the use of oral contraceptives. For many women adjustment to oral contraceptives may take some months. During that time she may experience nausea, fullness and tingling in her breasts, headache, some spotting between menstrual periods, weight gain, chloasma or masking of pregnancy, acne, loss of libido or changes in vaginal discharge. On the other hand she may feel better, have relief from menstrual cramps and have an increased libido. Sometimes changes in dosages or in the timing of taking the pill helps. If she takes the pill with supper or lunch, she may feel less nauseated later.

The major complications of the pill are very rare. In certain situations the risk of the pill may be considerably less than the hazard of a pregnancy. Major concern has centered around the increased incidence of thromboembolic disease in women using the pill. Because of this, patients who may be susceptible to thromboembolic disease may be advised to use another method of birth control. Oral contraceptives would also be contraindicated in patients with already existing lesions which might be aggravated by high levels of estrogen.

The missed pill is cause for concern in many women. The woman should take the pill when she remembers it and take the next pill as she is accustomed to do. This may mean taking two pills in one day. On the sequentials, the omission is more serious. The couple should plan to use an additional method of birth control for the remainder of that cycle. Should more than one pill be missed in either the combined or sequential pills, then the couple should use an alternate form of birth control for the remainder of that cycle. If several pills are missed, the doctor should be consulted as the cycles may be sufficiently interrupted as to require some further regulating under medical supervision.

Sterilization. Sterilization means the termination of reproductive capacity and is the most extreme case of fertility control. However, it may be chosen as a method of birth control. In other cases when the hazards of pregnancy are life threatening, it may be strongly indicated. In others, it is a sad sequel to necessary treatment to save or prolong the life of the patient.

Removal of any or all of the major organs of reproduction in either male or female results in sterility. Generally that is considered too extreme. A simple method of mechanically barring sperm and egg from meeting is required which will neither reduce natural hormone levels nor affect sexual capacity.

VASECTOMY. In men vasectomy will accomplish this purpose. This simple operation can be done in the doctor's office. On the surface of the scrotum the ascending spermatic cord is palpated and identified. Under local anesthetic a small incision is made slightly to one side of each cord. The vas deferens is dissected and ligated in two places. It may or may not be severed after ligation. Thus, sperm are barred from reaching the vagina. Some cases are recorded of reconstructing the vas deferens. However, the rate of successful reconstruction is low. Thus, the patient should regard a vasectomy as irreversible. A vasectomy may also be done abdominally.

TUBAL LIGATION. Tubal ligation is the comparable operation in women. It can be done vaginally but is usually done abdominally. Under a general anesthetic two small incisions are made in the abdomen. The uterine tube is dissected, a loop of tube is lifted up, ligated, and above the ligation is either crushed with a clamp or severed. In some operations the uterine end of the tube may be turned back and embedded in the posterior wall of the uterus. Various names for these techniques include Madlener, Pomeroy and Irving respectively. As in the male the tubes can be reconstructed, but the incidence is not high. Thus, the patient should see the operation as irreversible. The operation is not entirely harmless. Rare major complications postoperatively can be pulmonary embolism and later tubal pregnancy. These make the operation a more hazardous procedure than a vasectomy.

Nursing responsibilities in both operations include regular pre- and postoperative care (see p. 107). However, in addition to the consent for operation, there is a separate consent for sterilization which must be signed by both husband and wife before the operation.

INFERTILITY

Infertility is defined as the failure to conceive after 12 months of adequate exposure without the use of contraceptives. Primary infertility refers to a couple who has never conceived. Secondary infertility refers to a couple who has had a previous pregnancy but now cannot conceive. Approximately 12 per cent of couples prove infertile. Of this 12 per cent about 40 per cent of the problem rests with the man, 40 per cent with the woman and from 5 to 10 per cent with the couple as a unit.

Causes of Infertility

The possible causes of infertility are too numerous to list. However, the major causes can be grouped under several headings. Any impairment of ovarian function which interrupts ovulation creates infertility. This may be caused by hormonal imbalances or may be due to some intrinsic defect in the ovaries themselves. The same is true of the testes.

The conducting system may not be patent. Infections leading to adhesions are a major cause in both men and women. Malformations or displacements of the organs of the reproductive tract may contribute to infertility. The problem may arise because of unique factors particular to the union. Vaginal secretions may not be compatible with the seminal fluid, causing the sperm to die.

Nursing Responsibilities

The patient will usually go through a series of investigative tests. During these tests the nurse's supportive presence is of great value. The nurse should understand the technique and procedure well enough to prepare the patient for the test or to teach the patient how to perform some tests. Some women may feel more at ease discussing such problems with the nurse. Use should be made of this opportunity to listen and reassure the patient. This may happen when the nurse is told several facts which the patient "forgot" to tell the doctor. Also, the nurse may be asked questions which the patient hesitated to ask the doctor. Any pertinent information should be relayed to the appropriate medical advisor as well as those questions the nurse did not feel capable of answering.

The Investigation

The investigation usually begins when the woman presents herself to the gynecologist with a complaint of failure to conceive. By this time the problem may have become a nagging fear for both her and her husband. Often reassurance and ventilation of the anxiety seem to help the patient, for many patients are reported as returning shortly thereafter as pregnant. A persistent infertility case will require thorough investigation. Many gynecologists prefer to see the couple together so that both partners may receive an outline and discussion of the approach which will be used. The doctor's assessment of the possible cause of the infertility will guide the direction of the investigation. Some techniques which are used in investigating infertility are described.

Medical History and Physical Examination. A detailed medical history and physical examination is done for both partners. Par-

ticular attention will be paid to the development of the secondary sex characteristics and any evidence of virilizing or feminizing effects. Any history of infections and injuries involving the generative tract will be carefully noted. In addition the doctor will take a marital history to gain an adequate picture of the couple's sexual pattern. The woman will be asked to give a detailed menstrual history. At this point some education in human reproduction may help the couple.

Before other tests are begun, infections, particularly cervicitis and prostatitis, are likely to be treated as they may contribute to infertility. Anemia, poor health, exhaustion, overwork, stress and other psychosocial situations all may be causative factors, and the doctor often tries to relieve these first if they seem of sufficient magnitude to be affecting the sexual adjustment of the couple.

Ovulation. Whether or not ovulation occurs monthly may have to be established. The patient is asked to keep a basal body temperature chart. This also helps the doctor to estimate hormone levels. The woman is asked to come to the office or clinic near ovulation time. Cervical smears will be taken and tested for spinnbarkeit and ferning. Respectively these tests help to time ovulation and indicate how receptive the cervical mucus is to sperm. If ferning appears to be unsatisfactory, the patient may be given small oral doses of stilbestrol daily for several cycles. The patient may be requested to return for serial vaginal smears, which give indications of ovulation.

Urinalysis. Urine tests may be done to determine whether adequate levels of pituitary gonadotropins are present, and if the doctor feels it is warranted, the presence and amount of 17-ketosteroids are established. This may be done for both partners.

Endometrial Biopsy. This may be done at approximately the twenty-first day of the menstrual cycle and indicates whether or not a healthy endometrium is present. If it is not, then the problem may be one of failure of the fertilized ovum to achieve successful implantation.

Patency of the Tubes. The Rubin test is performed by insufflating the uterine tubes with carbon dioxide under pressure. It may or may not be done under anesthesia and is frequently done on an outpatient basis.

It is a sterile procedure. As the carbon dioxide is injected, the results are traced on a graph and show normal wave-like patterns or abnormal patterns. The test is considered positive by observing the graph patterns, auscultating sounds of gas bubbling through the tubes, complaints of referred shoulder pain by the patient or x-ray evidence of air beneath the diaphragm. The shoulder pain is the result of the gas escaping from the ends of the patent tube and exerting pressure on the phrenic nerve which is felt as referred pain to the shoulder. The test may be done more than once and dilation of the cervix may be done on succeeding attempts. Carbon dioxide is used to avoid the possibility of an air embolism.

Hysterosalpingogram. A hysterosalpingogram is the injection of a radiopaque dye into the genital tract. It serves to outline the uterine cavity and the uterine tubes. The patient may not be anesthetized. The test is done in the x-ray department under sterile technique. The patient is usually asked to move from side to side after the injection in order to promote spilling of the dye into the abdominal cavity. This test is considered a more informative one because the exact location of any lesion is noted.

POSSIBLE COMPLICATIONS OF TUBAL PATENCY TESTS. Pain, collapse and vomiting may be experienced shortly after the test is done, especially in women who were not anesthetized. The patient should be observed for these signs for approximately 3 hours following the test. Helping the patient to assume a knee-chest position for a few minutes before standing up may prevent further discomfort. Cramps and vomiting may be more prevalent following cervical dilatation.

Other complications may include exacerbation of pelvic infections, air embolism or sensitivity reactions to the dye and inadvertent abortion.

On the other hand, either of the tests may be therapeutic because they may have opened the tract. This is supported by many patients who conceive with no further treatment.

Sims-Huhner Postcoital Test. Postcoitally, a specimen of seminal fluid from the posterior fornix of the vagina and the cervical canal is aspirated. The specimen is examined for motility of the sperm and their ability to survive in the cervix or vagina. This test is best performed at the time of ovulation. The patient will be instructed not to douche or to use lubricants for 2 days before the test. Following intercourse she will remain supine, hips elevated on a pillow for 30 minutes. Within the next 2 to 4 hours she will come to the doctor's office or the fertility clinic at which time the specimen will be taken. A reading will assess how many live, motile sperm are in the specimen. Should the sperm not be present, the investigation may be directed toward the male. Does he have sperm? If he does, why is he not capable of depositing them near the cervix? If they are dead or nonmotile, the vaginal environment may be hostile to them. One such reaction is due to the stimulus a foreign protein (sperm) evokes in the woman's body. Consequently, antibodies develop. The antibodies in the female inactivate the sperm before fertilization takes place. Following a 3- to 6-month period of abstinence or the use of a condom by the male, circulating antibodies may be sufficiently reduced to permit sperm to live in order to fertilize.

Semen Analysis. A specimen of seminal fluid will be examined for volume and the number, morphology and mobility of sperm. Ideally, 2 to 5 cc. of fluid should be present. The fluid should gel and then reliquefy after 15 to 20 minutes. The sperm should number above 60 million per cc. of ejaculate, and 60 per cent should still show vigorous activity when examined at room temperature 2 hours after ejaculation. Not more than 20 per cent of the sperm should show abnormal forms.

The specimen is collected after a 3-day period of abstinence from coitus. It is collected in a dry, sterile jar by masturbation or coitus interruptus and is brought to the clinic for examination within 2 hours of collection.

If no sperm are present in the ejaculate, the patency of the duct system may be assessed. Testicular biopsy may be indicated. If the biopsy shows living sperm, then the failure of the sperm to arrive in the seminal fluid may be due to a blockage in the tube.

Treatment

Surgery. In both male and female, surgery is aimed at restoring function. Adhesions may be released; the ducts are reconstructed. In certain cases polyethylene tubes are inserted into the uterine tubes to help maintain patency. Cysts and tumors are removed as indicated. The nursing care would be the same as that for any pelvic operative procedure.

Alpha Amylase. Should the seminal fluid not reliquefy, a suspension of alpha amylase introduced into the vagina postcoitally has attained some success. The woman must be instructed to insert 1 cc. of the suspension into her vagina and to remain supine with hips elevated for 30 minutes following insertion. The solution should be kept refrigerated.

Hormone Therapy

CLOMIPHENE. Hormones may be administered to induce ovulation. Clomid or clomiphene is an estrogen-like synthetic which stimulates the hypothalamus to stimulate the pituitary to increase the output of gonadotropins. The dose prescribed is highly individualized and is given on a short-term basis. As a preparation to its use, the couple must know about ovulation time so that coitus could be planned for that time of the month.

The drug does stimulate the growth of benign ovarian cysts which usually disappear after its use. The incidence of multiple births is increased in couples using this medication. There do not appear to be any long-term effects.

GONADOTROPINS. Should attempts to stimulate the pituitary to produce gonadotropins fail, then the gonadotropins may be supplied artificially. Human pituitary gonadotropins made from freeze-dried human pituitaries may be administered. These are in effect the FSH and ICSH hormones. Both are needed to ripen the oocytes, as they promote release of the ripened egg or stimulate ovulation. Human menopausal gonadotropins taken from the urine of menopausal women will also work on the ripened oocyte. Perganol is an example. However, there must be an oocyte, for it will not stimulate the development of one. Ovarian cysts also follow its use as do multiple pregnancies. The doses are highly individualized, but 50 per cent pregnancy rates have been recorded following the use of these drugs.

Hormone therapy may also be instituted in the man. Gonadotropins may be prescribed in individualized doses. Sometimes vitamin B will be prescribed to ensure the normal inactivation of estrogens by the liver. Varying doses of testosterone may be tried with varying rates of success.

DISORDERS OF THE MENSTRUAL CYCLE AND MENSTRUATION

Mittelschmerz

Mittelschmerz is a feeling of lower abdominal pain on one side on or near ovulation day. It is thought to be caused by fluid or blood escaping from the ruptured follicle site and causing peritoneal irritation. It occurs in about 25 per cent of women. Occasionally, when the right side is involved, fear of appendicitis may bring the woman to the doctor.

Premenstrual Tension

This syndrome is probably experienced by most women in mild forms. However, extreme cases are seen. The symptomatology includes a feeling of fullness or heaviness in the lower abdomen, backache, painful breasts, irritability, headache, weight gain premenstrually, nervousness, depression and insomnia.

The favored etiology relates the symptoms to an imbalance in the estrogen-progesterone ratio. The high levels of estrogen result in sodium retention, which is characterized by increased intercellular fluid and edema. This edema gives the bloated feeling, headaches, irritability and breast tenderness. Secondary to these hormonal imbalances, the patient may become hypoglycemic. This accounts for feelings of faintness and weakness. Other theories on the possible etiology are concerned with overproduction of the antidiuretic hormones and adrenocortical hyperactivity.

Treatment consists in taking a sympathetic and understanding approach, as the patient may be very upset by the changes of mood and behavior which she experiences. The patient will be instructed to restrict sodium intake in the latter half of the cycle. She may also be given oral diuretics for some days immediately before menstruation. In most cases the nurse is responsible for giving the patient whatever guidance in food selection and preparation that the patient requires to assist her to follow this regimen. While she is on diuretics, it is also wise to instruct the patient to take her pill with orange juice. This guards against possible excessive loss of potassium from the use of diuretics. In conjunction with this treatment, the doctor may prescribe a mild tranquilizer to ease her nervousness.

Dysmenorrhea

Dysmenorrhea is defined as pain with menstruation. Two types, primary and secondary dysmenorrhea, are commonly distinguished.

Primary Dysmenorrhea. Primary dysmenorrhea is a spasmodic type of pain, occurring at the onset of the menstrual period and lasting from 1 to 24 hours. It is most common among young girls, rarely beginning with the menarche and fading away spontaneously around 24 years of age or following the delivery of a full-term infant. No pathology in pelvic structures is associated with this type of dysmenorrhea. In addition to the cramps, there may be shivering, a feeling of tension, nausea, vomiting and pallor. Some girls faint easily at this time.

The etiology remains unclear. It appears to be connected to ovulation, as anovulatory cycles are rarely accompanied by dysmenorrhea. This probably explains why the first few cycles are pain-free and dysmenorrhea in some girls is synchronous with ovulation. Also, the daughters of women who suffer or have suffered from dysmenorrhea are more frequently dysmenorrheic. Whether this is learned or inherited is still disputed. In any case the psyche can play a role in aggravating the symptoms but is very rarely the sole explanation. A woman's personal tolerance for discomfort undoubtedly affects her response to any pain, dysmenorrhea being no exception.

The prevalent physiological explanation involves ischemia of the uterine muscle. The uterus does undergo contractions which can be demonstrated by placing a bag of fluid in the uterine cavity and measuring the pressure in milligrams of mercury. The myometrium exhibits hypercontractibility, and the strong contractions squeeze the

blood vessels dry, causing intermittent muscle ischemia. In addition, we know that some vasoconstriction occurs which may contribute to the ischemia. The hypercontractibility is probably caused by transitory hormonal imbalances. The syndrome may be aggravated by pelvic congestion due to a mild degree of premenstrual tension. This may cause a dull ache as well as cramps. Most authorities do not accept that dysmenorrhea is due to faulty innervation of the uterus, cervical stenosis or excessive progesterone. Also, the small cochleate (extremely anteflexed) uterus is usually not considered to be responsible for dysmenorrhea.

Treatment consists of a kind and sympathetic approach by all members of the health team. Vasodilators, antispasmodics and mild analgesics may be prescribed. If the patient has some fluid retention premenstrually, a diuretic may be prescribed as well. Often, the doctor may prescribe a 3-to 6-month course of oral contraceptives. This induces anovulatory periods and may be followed by very good results. It may also be diagnostic. Should dysmenorrhea continue, the physician may look for other causes. In more extreme cases, surgery may be chosen. The cervix is dilated with varying success. A presacral sympathectomy or, in desperation, a hysterectomy may be done.

NURSING RESPONSIBILITIES. The school and occupational health nurses commonly deal with the girl or young woman suffering from dysmenorrhea. She may present herself in their office, or the nurse may be asked to interview the girl or woman who frequently misses school or work because of dysmenorrhea. Frequent, severe dysmenorrhea should always be investigated by the physician, and it is the nurse's responsibility to suggest this to the patient and assist her in obtaining this care.

In regard to general care, the patient may need instruction in the normal anatomy and physiology of menstruation. This serves to eradicate misconceptions and lessen the fear and anxiety which may be associated with her periods. She may need some instruction in menstrual hygiene so that her period does not seem distasteful and restricting. This may simply mean a switch from sanitary pads to tampons, frequent bathing or the use of a deodorizer. The patient may need to be encouraged to get more exercise and be sure that she is not constipated before her period.

Immediate care involves providing a sympathetic, understanding approach; a place to lie down; a warm blanket, if necessary; and usually a mild analgesic. When the symptoms are relieved, the girl often continues with her work. However, before returning to work or home, she might appreciate a cup of tea. If the patient has been given a prescription for medication, she should be instructed to take the tablet before dysmenorrhea becomes acute. This will prevent the symptoms and has the double advantage of breaking a cycle. The girl can feel some control over the events which are happening to her rather than being totally subject to them.

Secondary Dysmenorrhea. Secondary dysmenorrhea is a congestive, constant type of pain which often starts 2 to 3 days before the period and persists well past the first day. It may continue for a day or two following the period. Pain may radiate through the abdomen into the back and down the legs. It occurs after several years of normal painless menses and is frequently associated with pelvic pathology. The most frequent causes are tumors, inflammatory diseases, emdometriosis and fixed malpositions of the uterus. It is essentially a symptom of disease. Should the nurse be consulted by a woman describing these symptoms, the woman should be referred to a doctor immediately.

Abnormal Uterine Bleeding

Abnormal uterine bleeding is always symptomatic of another cause. Many of the disorders of the reproductive tract or of pregnancy can give rise to some type of abnormal bleeding per vaginam.

Amenorrhea

Amenorrhea, or absence of menstruation, may be primary or secondary. Secondary amenorrhea is that which occurs after several months or years of normal menses.

Menorrhagia

Menorrhagia is excessive bleeding at the time of normal menses.

Polymenorrhea

Polymenorrhea refers to cyclic bleeding which is normal in amount but occurs too frequently.

Epimenorrhagia

Epimenorrhagia is cyclic bleeding which is both excessive and too frequent.

Metrorrhagia

Metrorrhagia refers to any bleeding which occurs between menstrual periods. Any bleeding per vaginam at any time other than a normal menses is included, even if it amounts only to slight staining.

Dysfunctional Uterine Bleeding

True dysfunctional uterine bleeding refers to that which occurs in the presence of endocrine dysfunction rather than organic disease. It can present a very real challenge to the physician, as the cause of the bleeding is often difficult to discern. It may be seen as chronic epimenorrhagia or as an episode of acute bleeding. In certain cases Premarin may be given. This is a conjugated estrogenic substance which promotes hemostasis. It is particularly good in controlling cases of capillary bleeding.

Endometriosis

Endometriosis is the location of endometrial-like tissue outside the uterine cavity. Although the location may be varied, the most frequent locations are in or near the ovaries, the uterosacral ligaments and the uterovesical peritoneum. Extrapelvic sites may be as varied as the umbilicus, an old laparotomy scar, vulva or even lungs. The tissue responds to the hormones of the ovarian cycle and undergoes a small menstruation just like the uterine endometrium. Statistics vary, but perhaps 5 per cent of all patients seen by the gynecologist suffer from endometriosis.

Etiology may be varied. Two major theories are prevalent. One concludes that small bits of endometrial tissue are forced or regurgitated back up the uterine tube and escape into the abdomen during menstruation. The other theory points out that the peritoneum and reproductive tract derive from the same early embryological tissues. Some of the tissue may be misplanted from that early time. Under sufficient stimulation, such as prolonged estrogen stimulation unrelieved by the amenorrhea of pregnancy, these cells respond and differentiate into a functioning endometrial tag. Rare cases seem to be caused by small pieces of endometrium being transported to other parts of the body through the lymphatics or by the blood. This seems to be true of endometrial tissue in the limbs or in lung tissue. As the ectopic endometrium menstruates, the blood collects in little cyst-like nodules which have a characteristic bluish-black look. Usually they are pea-sized but may be much larger. Those in the ovary and uterosacral area often attain a size of 3 to 6 cm. These ovarian cysts are sometimes termed "chocolate cysts" because of the thick, chocolate-colored material which they contain. The cysts become surrounded by fibrous tissue which makes them easy to palpate, as they feel firm and well defined. Frequently the cyst perforates and spills its sticky contents into the abdomen. The resulting irritation promotes the formation of adhesions which readily fix the ovary or the affected area to the broad ligament or other pelvic structures.

The disease is seen most frequently in the white, nulliparous woman, aged 30 to 40. It occurs more commonly in the upper economic and social groups, presumably because of less frequent and later childbearing.

The patient may have no symptomatology, and the disease may only be discovered incidental to abdominal surgery. More commonly, the patient complains of pain. Secondary dysmenorrhea may appear with pain becoming severe 1 to 2 days before menstruation. The pain gradually becomes worse and may be described as "boring." This is due to the distention and pain of the swollen, shedding areas contained within the fibrous capsule of the cysts. The patient may also complain of backache, dyspareunia of a deep nature localized in the posterior fornix of the vagina or persistent lower abdominal pain occurring throughout the cycle. Pain may be of an acute nature, localized in the abdomen when a cyst ruptures. The physician may suspect endometriosis when a patient is infertile, since this is a common symptom of this group. Sometimes the adhesions become severe enough to cause a bowel obstruction or painful micturition.

Diagnosis is frequently confirmed on bimanual examination when firm nodular lumps are felt in the adnexa. Visualizing the typical bluish nodules may be done by culdoscopy, laparoscopy or during a laparotomy. Treatment is based on the age of the patient, her desire for more children and the severity of the disease. Pregnancy relieves the symptoms and may be advised if the couple wants more children. Pseudopregnancy may be achieved by the administration of progesterone for varying periods of time.

Treatment may be surgical and is directed at preserving reproductive function. Affected areas are removed, and fixed organs released. Infertility often ceases following surgery. In severe cases a hysterectomy may be done. Depending on the extent of the cystic involvement, oophorectomy may also be performed. The symptoms usually disappear at the menopause as ovarian atrophy begins and hormonal stimulation declines.

Adenomyosis Uteri

This condition is similar to endometriosis in that it is characterized by ectopic endometrium within the muscular wall of the uterus or the uterine tube. While it is often classified as "intrauterine endometriosis," Novak suggests that the disease processes are quite different. Adenomyoma is also a poor way of referring to the process, for it is not a true tumor. The cause is unknown. In any case, the uterine endometrium appears to grow downward between the muscle bundles of the myometrium. This produces a uniform, moderate enlargement of the uterus. The patient may complain of menorrhagia and secondary dysmenorrhea. Often pelvic endometriosis is also present. Then the uterus may be fixed (frozen) in the pelvis, and pelvic nodules may be palpated. The patient may complain of pain in the sacral or coccygeal area as well.

INTERRUPTIONS OF PREGNANCY

Abortion

An abortion is the termination of a pregnancy before the fetus is viable. Some confusion exists over when a fetus becomes viable. Arbitrarily, viability has been set as above 20 weeks of gestation, 500 Gm. of weight or a crown-rump length of 18 cm. The definition is not universal and varies from country to country. "Miscarriage" also refers to abortion but is the lay term for designating lack of criminal involvement.

The incidence of abortion is difficult to state accurately. Estimates place it at between 10 to 20 per cent of all conceptions.

Causes. Most known causes can be separated into three major groups: fetal, maternal and faulty environment. Fetal causes are often associated with chromosomal or other abnormalities which are incompatible with life. This has been considered to be as high as 40 per cent of all causes of abortion. Maternal and faulty environment causes are more varied. Endotoxins, as a result of severe infections in the mother, may invade the fetus, usually causing its death and later expulsion. Drugs ingested by the mother may damage the fetus directly or may damage the placenta and hence the nutrition of the fetus. Hormonal imbalances may be the cause of some abortions, especially in cases in which the thyroid gland is involved. Lack of progesterone may result in a poorly developed endometrium. As a result, nidation does not occur or does so ineffectively. Anatomic uterine defects or uterine pathology causes some abortions. Nutritional factors are linked to abortion and premature labor, for adequate nutrition of the woman bears an important part in her reproductive capacity. The emotional state of the woman is also considered a possible contributing factor. This often centers around fear, grief or emotional trauma in susceptible women. Physical trauma can also induce an abortion. This may be true of surgery performed during pregnancy.

A threatened abortion is one in which the threat to the pregnancy is slight. With care, the woman may carry the pregnancy to term. Since any bleeding, however minor, per vaginam is abnormal in the pregnant woman, any evidence of such bleeding is taken as a sign of threatened abortion until proven otherwise. In addition, some backache or mild intermittent lower abdominal pain may be present. If the abortion is not to be immediate, cramping and bleeding may stop. Should the cramping and bleeding increase in spite of treatment, the abortion may now be called imminent. It becomes inevitable when bleeding continues, cramps become stronger and regular, the cervix dilates and the membranes rupture. The inevitable abortion becomes the complete abortion when all products of conception are expelled. This usually occurs before the twelfth week of gestation. The abortion is incomplete when some of the products of conception are retained. This is usually the placenta and membranes and is more fre-

TABLE 19–1 CLASSIFICATION OF ABORTIONS

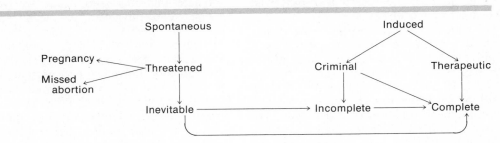

quent following the twelfth week when the placenta is more firmly embedded. The umbilical cord breaks, leaving the placenta and membranes in utero. A missed abortion is one in which the fetus dies; symptoms of abortion cease and the products of conception are retained in the uterus for 2 or more months. Following this, the uterus is not observed to increase in size. Indeed, it begins to regress slightly as the amniotic fluid is absorbed. No fetal heart is heard. The patient remains amenorrheic, and the breasts regress. The abortus is usually expelled spontaneously but may be retained for many months or years. In such cases it becomes a shriveled sac with areas of dense calcification.

A woman is considered to be an habitual aborter when she aborts 3 or more consecutive pregnancies. The causes can be any of the causes of a single abortion but persist through several pregnancies. In addition, an incompetent cervix is frequently sited as a cause of habitual abortion. Possibly because of inherent problems in the cervix or trauma to the cervix during surgery, the cervix dilates easily and will not retain the pregnancy. Loss of the pregnancy usually occurs later at about 16 to 20 weeks. Dilation of the cervix is rapid, with little pain and bleeding. Rupture of the membranes occurs, followed by the expulsion of the fetus.

Treatment and Nursing Care

THREATENED ABORTION. The treatment of threatened abortion is aimed at preserving the pregnancy. Every pregnant patient should be told the danger signs of pregnancy. Often this instruction is the responsibility of the nurse in either the clinic or the office. Thus, the woman should recognize bleeding as abnormal and be aware that she should notify her doctor immediately. She should then go to bed and rest unless otherwise instructed by her physician.

On admission to the hospital, the patient is placed on bedrest. Temperature, pulse and blood pressure are noted as frequently as the patient's condition warrants. All the pads, linens and clothing stained with blood are kept for inspection by the doctor. This helps in the estimation of blood loss. The possibility of losing the pregnancy may be very distressing to most women. The patient should be given sympathy, reassur-

ance and support. This assists in keeping the patient quiet and calm and allows her to get the physical and mental rest which is considered advisable. Sedatives may be ordered. In addition, the patient is observed for any increased bleeding or cramping which would indicate a change in status. A diet low in roughage is usually ordered with supplementary iron and vitamin C. Purgatives and enemas are avoided in order to avoid stimulation of the uterus. Rectal and vaginal examinations are contraindicated. Bleeding usually ceases within 24 to 48 hours if the pregnancy is going to continue. At this time the doctor will probably perform a careful speculum and bimanual examination, since other possible causes of bleeding must be ruled out. These causes could be carcinoma or other complications of pregnancy.

Opinion is divided on the success or failure of hormonal methods used in attempting to prevent loss of the pregnancy. Sometimes progesterone preparations like Delalutin may be prescribed in the hopes of retaining the pregnancy. Others feel this is of little value.

On discharge home the patient is instructed to get extra rest and to avoid strenuous exercise, heavy lifting, excitement or fatigue. Coitus may be restricted for a period of 2 weeks or longer. Should bleeding recur, the patient is advised to notify her doctor and remain in bed.

MISSED ABORTION. The patient will be followed by her doctor to see that the pregnancy progresses normally. If it does not, and a persistent brownish discharge recurs, missed abortion may be suspected. The diagnosis may be difficult for the physician to make until it is quite clear that the uterus has ceased to enlarge and that the fetus is dead. A positive pregnancy test may only indicate that placental tissue still remains living. The physician is faced with the choice of interfering to evacuate the uterus or waiting until it is done spontaneously. Physically, there is usually no pressing need. Emotionally, however, it is very distressing to the woman and her family to know that she is carrying a dead fetus. The danger from afibrinogenemia as a complicating factor to intervention by the physician increases as the dead fetus is retained. Presumably this occurs as some of the degenerating products of the fetus enter the maternal blood stream. This danger appears to be most serious about 4 to 6 weeks after fetal death. Therefore fribrinogen studies may be done before intervention is attempted.

For these reasons the physician usually intervenes approximately 2 weeks after death of the fetus. The dead fetus may be aborted by means of an intravenous oxytocic administered in high concentrations. The patient may be started on 20 I.U. of Pitocin in 1000 ml. of 5 per cent dextrose in water. Each hour the dose may be increased until effective contractions occur. The therapy will continue until abortion ensues or for 8 to 10 hours. Then the drip may be discontinued and resumed at the original beginning levels of Pitocin the next day. The procedure is emotionally and physically exhausting for the patient. She requires much supportive nursing care. Also, the contractions are painful, and some analgesic should be administered. Since no danger can result to the fetus, the mother need not suffer unduly. Close observation of the patient's condition for overhydration is necessary because of the danger of overhydrating her with large amounts of fluid containing Pitocin which has an antidiuretic action. An intake and output record should be kept.

INEVITABLE ABORTION. The treatment of an inevitable abortion is similar to that of a threatened abortion. The patient is placed on bed rest. Blood will be taken for hemoglobin, typing and cross matching. The amount and character of the bleeding is observed carefully. Blood pressure and pulse may need to be taken every 10 minutes if bleeding is profuse, and the patient must be observed for other signs of shock. Any tissue or suspicious clots are saved to be examined for traces of fetus and placenta. Good perineal care is maintained by frequent cleansing of the vulva to reduce the risk of infection and to promote the patient's comfort. Procedures for perineal care will vary. Generally, soap and water are sufficient. The perineum is swabbed from the pubes to the perineal body (front to back) and from the vulva out to the thigh. The rectal area is washed last. This is to prevent the spread of bacteria from the rectum upward into the vagina and thence to the endometrium. A perineal shave prep may be ordered. Support and encouragement are provided by the nursing and medical staff, as the patient may be very distraught at the impending loss of her infant. If the abortion seems to be approaching a conclusion, it is not assisted. However, with the membranes ruptured, the cervix dilated and contractions tapering off, the process may be hastened by the administration of intravenous Pitocin.

If the abortion has been complete and the physician is satisfied of this, the woman is treated similarly to a postpartum patient. A slight lochial discharge is expected and the woman must be taught perineal care. She will be discharged home in 3 to 4 days, depending on the state of her health. Coitus may be contraindicated for 4 to 6 weeks to reduce the chance of an infection.

When the products of conception are retained, the uterus must be emptied. Two of the major causes of bleeding associated with pregnancy result from the partially separated placenta and retained fragments of conception. The uterus cannot contract effectively; the torn blood vessels remain open and bleed. Also, the risk of infection is much increased by the debris lying in the uterus. If the bleeding is acute, the patient is usually taken to the operating room and an emergency dilatation and curettage (D and C) is done. Under a general anesthesia, the cervix is gently dilated until the passage of a curette is possible. Dilatation is accomplished by using the dilators or by the use of a special vibrating dilator. The curette is used to scrape the tissue from the walls of the uterus.

Following this operation the patient receives perineal care and is observed for signs of hemorrhage and infection. She may receive an intravenous oxytocic solution to help involution of the uterus. Because of the danger of accidental perforation of the uterus with the instruments, the patient is observed postoperatively for signs of peritoneal irritation or abdominal (concealed) hemorrhage. Packing may or may not have been inserted in the vagina to help control or prevent hemorrhage. This should be carefully noted on the chart. If packing was inserted, the nurse must watch the patient even more carefully for signs of shock, since any bleeding may be concealed by the packing. If there is packing, it will have to be removed within several hours to allow free drainage of lochia and thus help prevent infection. The nurse should anticipate some postoperative vomiting, since these women appear to have an increased incidence of vomiting postoperatively. Good preoperative care may do a great deal to present us with a more relaxed, confident patient. This may lessen vomiting to some extent. However, often the patient goes to the operating room on an emergency basis, either to control hemorrhage or to prevent its occurrence. To prepare this patient for the operating room adequately requires a smooth blending of supportive nursing care and the accomplishment of all the necessary tasks as quickly as possible. The easiest and least skilled method is to do the technical tasks efficiently. The most accomplished method, and therefore the most difficult, is to do the necessary preparation efficiently and at the same time to reassure the patient and explain the procedure to her while going about these tasks in a calm, quiet manner. This invites the respect and confidence of the patient and her family.

INCOMPETENT CERVICAL OS. The patient who has had several abortions will probably receive a thorough assessment between pregnancies in an attempt to ascertain her problem. Should the cause be considered an incompetent cervical os, the physician may attempt to tighten the cervix with a suture. This is usually done during the twelfth to sixteenth week of pregnancy. The Shirodkar technique consists of running a nondissolving suture around the cervix like a drawstring or purse string. The Lash operation involves removing a small piece of tissue from the cervix and closing the gap with sutures. The Lash operation particularly may be done between pregnancies.

On return from the operating room, the pregnant patient is observed for signs of labor and imminent abortion. Should the abortion appear inevitable, the suture must be removed or serious tearing of the cervix might occur. At term, the suture is removed and vaginal delivery follows, or the suture is retained and delivery is by cesarean section.

The patient who has aborted will often be distraught at losing another pregnancy. She may experience the loss of the desired child acutely, and in the immediate period following the abortion she may derive little con-

solation from being told that she can have other children or that she has children at home. It is the loss of this child which she feels. Sympathy, understanding and someone to talk to are greatly appreciated by these women. The nurse who deals with these patients should further acquaint herself with the patterns of normal grieving so that she may understand these patients more fully.

Baptism of Fetus. If the patient who aborts is Roman Catholic, the fetus must be baptized. In addition, some Protestants may feel strongly that the fetus should be baptized. The nurse may ascertain this by tactfully inquiring what the patient's wishes are. Baptism may be performed by any person, regardless of his religious beliefs. If a clergyman is immediately available, he should be asked to perform this rite. In his absence, the nurse may have to baptize the fetus. Clear water must be poured over the head of the fetus while the nurse pronounces the words, "I baptize you in the name of the Father and of the Son and of the Holy Spirit." The water must come into direct contact with the fetus. Therefore, if the fetus is still in the amniotic sac, the sac must be broken before baptism is performed. The procedure is similar for all religions. If the fetus is very small, it may have to be immersed in water to ensure that water reaches the head. Sometimes a conditional baptism is given with the words, "If thou art living, I baptize thee. . . ." This is done in cases in which the fetus may have died before delivery, but the exact state is unknown.

Therapeutic Abortion. Occasionally, an abortion is induced by the physician as a means of treatment for the patient. Because an abortion concerns the life and death of at least two people, it is governed by religious and legal codes. Very complex issues surround the topic of induced abortions, and a discussion of all are beyond the scope of this work. Only a brief discussion of the law and the medical and nursing management of such a situation is presented here. To understand the religious, social, humanistic, philosophical, legal, psychological and medical considerations the nurse must delve into the related literature in these disciplines.

The laws governing abortions vary from country to country and, at the present time, are undergoing much revision in all nations.

In the United States, laws will vary from state to state. American and Canadian laws are similar, but Canadian law is described because this author is most familiar with it. Canadian law states that therapeutic abortions may be performed legally, subject to certain stated conditions, in cases in which the continuation of the pregnancy would endanger the life and health of the mother. Certain stated conditions include that the abortion must be performed in an accredited or approved hospital by a qualified medical practitioner after a certificate in writing stating that the pregnancy is injurious to the woman has been obtained from the therapeutic abortion committee of that hospital. The committee must exist and be composed of a minimum of three physicians qualified in the field. A majority vote is required to obtain permission. All other abortions are illegal and, if performed, constitute a grave breach of the law. Assisting a patient to procure an abortion outside the limits of the legal condition is also a serious offense punishable by law.

In practice, most therapeutic abortion committees liberally interpret the law. A recent survey in Toronto shows that abortions have been obtained legally for such things as rape, extreme youth of the mother, incest, substantial congenital defects of the fetus, rubella in the mother before 13 weeks of pregnancy, mental retardation and some humanistic reasons such as multiple sclerosis. These are obviously in addition to such basic medical reasons as cardiac disease, renal disease, diabetes or mental illness, all of which may be aggravated by the added burden of a pregnancy.

The majority of therapeutic abortions are performed before 12 weeks of pregnancy. Usually a careful dilatation and curettage is done, and the pregnancy is discontinued in this manner. A suction D and C may be done. A suction tip, looking much like a Hegar dilator, is slipped through the cervix. It is attached to a special electric vacuum pump which sucks out the uterine contents. The pressure of the pump is carefully regulated.

When the pregnancy is above 12 to 14 weeks this procedure becomes more difficult. Other methods may be selected by the physician. He may decide to induce labor by the use of an intra-amniotic injection. The technique and preparation are similar to a paracentesis, but an amniocentesis is done. With strict sterile technique the patient's abdomen is prepared and draped. A skin wheal is made with a local anesthetic agent. Then a needle is inserted through the abdomen, and into the amniotic cavity. Some amniotic fluid is withdrawn and replaced with either a 50 per cent dextrose solution or 20 per cent saline solution. The fetus dies, and the uterus is apparently irritated and begins to contract within 36 to 48 hours. The contractions may need to be assisted with an oxytocic medication given intravenously. Complications may include infection following dextrose or absorption of the hypertonic saline into the circulatory system.

Later pregnancies of 16 to 20 weeks' gestation may be terminated by the performance of a hysterotomy. This means that an incision is made into the uterus and the contents removed. It is a miniature cesarean section. The pre- and postoperative care is similar to abdominal surgery. However, perineal and abdominal shave preparations may be ordered. Postoperatively, the fundus must be checked for firmness and position. Lochia is observed for color, amount and odor, since hemorrhage or infection may occur postoperatively. Perineal care is as described on page 493.

The therapeutic abortion is not a totally benign procedure. Physical and mental complications may arise. The patient may feel guilty at the destruction of a human life. Thus, the decision to do an abortion is a weighty one for the doctor as it is for the patient. She and her family will need support and acceptance.

Criminal Abortion. The criminal abortion is a dangerous procedure. Often women attempt to abort themselves by the use of strong douches or instruments which they insert into the uterus. Frequently, the instrument used punctures the posterior fornix of the vagina, the cervix or perforates the uterus. The bowel may be involved should the instrument be inserted far enough. Conditions are furtive; untrained people frequently officiate; and sterility is not maintained. These patients frequently contract an infection and may present a grave situation. The situation is known as a septic abortion. Infection is essentially an endometritis, which may spread to peritonitis or to septicemia.

Ectopic Pregnancy

Implantation of the fertilized ovum anywhere outside the uterine cavity is considered an ectopic pregnancy. Most frequently this occurs in the ampullary portion of the uterine tube, but it may be ovarian, abdominal or cervical. Ectopic pregnancies are estimated as occurring once in every 250 pregnancies. Women with a history of 1 ectopic pregnancy have an increased risk of having a second one.

An ectopic pregnancy results when the passage of the zygote to the uterine cavity is impeded or slowed. Any blocking of the tube or reduction in tubal peristalsis will achieve this. Former salpingitis, tumors and hormonal imbalances may all play a part.

As implantation occurs, the chorionic villi burrow into the thin tubal wall. Eventually, they burrow into a blood vessel, and bleeding occurs. If the bleeding is sufficient, the fetus dies. This is the fate of most. The abortus may be retained in the tube as a tubal mole or may be extruded through the end of the uterine tube as a tubal abortion. Occasionally, the trophoblast burrows through the wall of the tube and out into the peritoneal cavity. This is known as a ruptured tubal pregnancy and often occurs as the result of a pregnancy in the narrow isthmus of the tube. A secondary abdominal pregnancy may follow if the chorionic villi settle elsewhere in the abdominal cavity and begin to grow. This is rare.

Signs and Symptoms. The accurate diagnosis of an existing ectopic pregnancy or a recently aborted ectopic pregnancy may require much skill, since the picture may be confusing. Fortunately, many are diagnosed by bimanual examination of the early pregnant woman. Others abort before the patient sees a physician. These women may first be seen in the emergency department or in the clinic with a variety of symptoms.

The woman has a history of the early signs of pregnancy, including amenorrhea usually of 6 to 10 weeks' duration. Soon after her first missed period she may have complaints of a localized pain on one side due probably to the distension of the tube. Following this she may have sharper intermittent pain in the same area. This may be due to strong peristaltic waves of the tube attempting to pass the embryo or abortus along the tube. At some point the patient may experience a sharp, severe pain. This is probably synchronous with separation of the embryo and some hemorrhage. The sharp pain may be followed by generalized abdominal discomfort as blood spills into the abdomen. Referred shoulder pain may occur. Four or five days following this episode there is bleeding per vaginam due to falling hormone levels, which occur following the death of the fetus and cause the endometrium to regress and menstruation to occur.

Acute Ruptured Tubal Pregnancy. Sometimes the patient reports no early symptoms but experiences one episode of acute abdominal pain shortly after her missed period. This acute pain is often accompanied by vomiting and fainting. Some vaginal bleeding may be present but appears too minimal to warrant the reaction of the patient. The patient may rapidly go into shock with a drop in blood pressure, rapid weak pulse, pallor, sweating, low temperature and cold extremities. The abdomen is distended with blood and may be tight and tender to the touch. A pelvic examination of the patient may be difficult because of the exquisite tenderness. The patient presents as an emergency situation.

NURSING RESPONSIBILITIES. Nursing care includes notifying the physician immediately and treating the patient for shock by elevating the foot of the bed, using warm blankets and checking vital signs every 10 minutes. The nurse will be responsible for having equipment on hand for the doctor to start an intravenous infusion and to take blood for hemoglobin, typing and cross matching. Catheterization is usually ordered. The nurse should be ready to prepare this patient for surgery, which is frequently a laparotomy.

Examination Under Anesthesia (E.U.A.). In other situations, the patient presents with many atypical signs. The symptoms may be common to many conditions such as pelvic inflammations, appendicitis, tumors or abortions. A thorough investigation is necessary to establish the true diagnosis. Since these women often experience extreme tenderness on bimanual examination, the physician may feel an examination under anesthesia is required. The patient is prepared for surgery. A combined perineal and abdominal shave preparation is usually ordered.

COLPOTOMY. Under anesthesia careful speculum and bimanual examinations are performed. To assist in performing these examinations a colpotomy may be necessary. A small horizontal incision is made in the posterior fornix of the vagina. The surgeon slips a finger through this incision into the cul-de-sac and palpates the adnexa. He may obtain dark, clotted blood from the pelvic hematocele which may have formed in the cul-de-sac following tubal abortion. Through the colpotomy incision a culdoscope is inserted, and direct visualization of the contents of the pelvis is then possible. The incision is closed with 2 or 3 sutures. If drainage is desired, a Penrose drain may be inserted. Antibiotics may be given for prophylaxis.

CULDOCENTESIS. A needle is injected into the cul-de-sac and any contents are aspirated. Blood is indicative of a hemorrhage. Culdocentesis may be done on an outpatient basis. The patient first empties her bladder and then assumes a lithotomy position with assistance from the nurse. Sterile technique is employed. The posterior vaginal wall is exposed; a local anesthesia administered; the needle is inserted, and the contents of the cul-de-sac are aspirated.

All of the above techniques are frequently employed to investigate other pelvic conditions. Usually they are not performed in the presence of an acute vaginal infection. When the diagnosis of a tubal pregnancy is confirmed, a salpingectomy (removal of uterine tube) with the removal of the fetus is performed. This is usually done within 24 to 48 hours of diagnosis unless the situation is acute, in which case it will be done immediately.

Ectopic pregnancies in other locations will be investigated in a similar fashion. Treatment is usually surgical removal of the fetus. However, abdominal pregnancies have carried to term and been delivered by laparotomies.

Hydatidiform Mole

Hydatidiform mole is an abnormal development of the chorionic villi of the conceptus. It begins to form about the fifth week of embryological life. The mole appears to occur when the fetal cardiovascular structure fails to develop, but an intact trophoblast and a functioning maternal structure remain. As the fluid accumulates, the chorionic villi distend into small clear vesicles, clinging to thin shreads of connective tissue in a grape-like pattern. Few blood vessels are present in the mass. Characteristically, there is no fetus. Rarely, some mole-like degeneration may be present on one part of an otherwise normal placenta.

The condition is rare in North America, occurring about once in every 2500 pregnancies. However, it is more prevalent in the Far East. The reason for this is not known.

Signs and Symptoms. The patient exhibits the signs and symptoms of early pregnancy. Vomiting may be more frequent. The uterus is often much larger than expected for the weeks of gestation. About the twelfth week, some vaginal bleeding may occur, and this is often the first sign of some abnormality. No fetal movements are reported by the mother, and no fetal parts can be palpated. On palpation the uterus may have an elastic consistency. There is an increased incidence of pre-eclampsia. Urine tests for the quantity of chorionic gonadotropins excreted show very high titers which persist and do not fall as is usual in a normal pregnancy. These high levels also stimulate the formation of theca lutein cysts in the ovary. The cysts regress following the abortion of the mole.

Treatment and Nursing Responsibilities. The patient is usually admitted to the hospital and nursed as a threatened abortion (p. 492) until proven otherwise. All perineal pads are carefully inspected for pieces of the mole, as this would be diagnostic.

An ultrasonic scan of the abdomen will most likely be done. The scan plots a "snowflake" pattern, which is typical of a mole and is considered diagnostic. Thyroid function tests may also be ordered with an expectation of some hyperthyroidism.

Often the mole is partially aborted spontaneously. Hemorrhage may be acute. Oxytocics will be given to control the bleeding, and a careful and complete evacuation of the uterus will be done. Because of the danger of perforating the uterus in areas weakened by the erosion of the mole, a curette is usually not used. Instead, sponge forceps may be used to gently wipe away the tissue. Postoperatively the patient must be observed for signs of hemorrhage.

Because approximately 50 per cent of all cases of chorionepithelioma are preceded by a mole, the patient will receive close follow-up care during the year following the mole. Often, the first sign of the recurrence of the mole or the development of a malignancy is a rising chorionic gonadotropin level. Therefore, levels will be taken every 2 weeks for 3 months and monthly thereafter for a further 6 to 9 months. The patient will be advised against pregnancy during this follow-up period as early pregnancy also produces high chorionic gonadotropin levels which could mask the signs.

Chorionepithelioma Malignum

Chorionepithelioma is a malignant tumor of the embryonic chorion and is marked by invasion of the uterine musculature by malignant trophoblastic cells which have lost their original villous pattern. Destruction of uterine tissues with accompanying necrosis and hemorrhage is the result. The growth quickly metastasizes, and the most frequent site is the lung. The condition is extremely rare but because of its rapid advancement is considered to be one of the most malignant of all pelvic neoplasms. Death usually occurs within 12 months unless the patient receives early treatment. Endometrial biopsy taken at a diagnostic dilatation and curettage may confirm the diagnosis.

The chemotherapeutic agent methotrexate is the treatment of choice but may be combined with surgery. The drug is a folic acid antagonist and may be administered orally or parenterally in individualized doses up to 25 mg. per day. This dose is administered for 5 consecutive days and then withdrawn for a week. The course may need to be repeated several times if chorionic gonadotropin titers do not regress. Actinomycin-D may also be used alone or in combination with methotrexate. These measures are used in the younger woman. In the woman over 40 the treatment would probably be a combination of chemotherapy and surgery.

INFECTIONS OF THE MALE REPRODUCTIVE TRACT

Balanitis

Balanitis* is an infection of the glans penis. Many different organisms may be causative. It is generally associated with poor personal hygiene in the uncircumcised male, but it may be due to venereal diseases. Symptoms include redness, swelling, pain and a purulent discharge. The disease may be chronic and may cause the formation of adhesions and scarring.

Treatment. The infection is treated with the appropriate antibiotic following culture and sensitivity tests. Once the inflammatory process is controlled, circumcision, the excision of the prepuce, is advised.

On return from the operating room, the patient has a small petrolatum gauze dressing which is changed following each voiding. The patient may be taught to do this and how to care for the dressing at home.

Should bleeding occur, a pressure dressing is applied. The dressing may make voiding impossible or difficult. Usually the dressing can be removed within a short period of time.

PHIMOSIS. Phimosis is a condition in which the preputial orifice is too small to permit retraction over the glans. It may be congenital but is most frequently a sequel to infection or trauma. Circumcision is advised.

PARAPHIMOSIS. Paraphimosis occurs when a narrowed prepuce is either forced back over the glans or is gradually retracted over it. It then forms a tight, constricting band around the glans; venous return is impaired, and swelling and pain follow. Usually pain is too severe to permit manipulation, so a general anesthetic is given, and the foreskin is pulled forward. Occasionally the foreskin may have to be incised, and a slit is made up the dorsal surface. This is usually followed by circumcision after the treatment of any infection which may have been present.

Balanos is the Greek work meaning acorn; in reference to the glans, it is a combining form indicating relationship to the glans penis.

Prostatitis

Prostatitis is usually an ascending infection of the genitourinary tract, but it may also be the result of the hematogenous spread of the organism. It is often secondary to urethritis or instrumentation of the urethra, as occurs in the use of an indwelling catheter.

In the acute stage, fever and chills are accompanied by hematuria, frequency and dysuria. A urethral discharge may be noted. Rectal examination usually reveals an enlarged, tender "hot" prostate. Since infection of the seminal vesicles almost invariably accompanies prostatitis, the seminal vesicles can be palpated as well. Prostatic massage and instrumentation of the urethra are avoided to prevent possible spread of the infection to the epididymis, bladder and kidney. Exceptions are made only to relieve acute urinary retention, which may be a sequel to the enlarged prostate. A small urethral catheter will be used. In severe cases, drainage may be by suprapubic cystostomy rather than by catheterization. Prostatic abscesses may develop and usually drain through the urethra. Occasionally, excision and drainage are required.

The patient is placed on bed rest. Appropriate antibiotic therapy is ordered, and the tetracyclines are frequently chosen first. The patient is in considerable pain. The nurse often sees a tense, anxious and frightened patient who needs reassurance and support. Explanations to clarify that the infection is not venereal may be necessary. Analgesics, warm sitz baths and rectal irrigations help to relieve the pain and bladder spasms. The irritable bladder may require special attention, and antispasmodics and bladder sedatives are frequently ordered. Fruit juices and bicarbonate of soda help to alkalininize the urine.

In cases in which treatment is early, excellent results usually follow. However, the acute picture may become chronic. The symptoms are mild and include a low-grade fever and some bacteria and pus in the urine. Fertility and potency are usually not affected unless complications ensue. The chronic infection does not respond well to treatment. Antibiotics and chemotherapy are given. Prostatic massage 4 to 5 times every 7 to 14 days is done by the physician and helps by draining the bacteria away. Sexual intercourse accomplishes the same purpose. Daily sitz baths also help resolve the infection, and the patient will need instruction in taking a sitz bath at home.

Epididymitis

Epididymitis may be caused by any pyogenic organism. It frequently follows prostatitis and may be a complication of prostatectomy. Fever, malaise and chills accompany swelling and pain in the scrotum. The patient may be so uncomfortable that he may walk in a waddling fashion. Symptoms of cystitis may be present, and a hydrocele often develops. The swelling and irritation cause congestion of the testes which impedes the circulation of blood. Sterility follows from necrosis of the tubular epithelium and fibrosis which occludes the ducts.

The patient is placed on bed rest. The scrotum is elevated on towel rolls or with a Bellevue bridge during the acute stage. Local applications of heat or cold may be ordered. Sitz baths often relieve symptoms of congestion and pain. After the patient is ambulant, a roomy scrotal support is worn.

Antibiotics are given but are not usually curative. If the disease is diagnosed early, a local anesthetic agent is injected into the spermatic cord above the testes. Symptoms are usually absent in a day or two following this treatment. Chronic epididymitis may follow an acute episode. If the involvement is bilateral, sterility follows.

Orchitis

Inflammation of the testes may follow any infectious disease or may be acquired as an ascending infection from the genital tract. Most commonly it follows mumps parotitis. The mumps virus is excreted in the urine; therefore, the spread to the testes in this case appears to be by descent. The onset is sudden, manifested by pain and swelling of the scrotum followed by fever and prostration. Urinary symptoms are usually not present. A hydrocele may develop, and the involvement may be unilateral or bilateral. Sterility probably follows death of the spermatogenic cells from ischemia. Bed rest, scrotal support and local applications of heat are necessary. A padded athletic support may be worn continuously.

Antibiotics are used in some situations but are not of value against the mumps virus. Local infiltration of the spermatic cord with a local anesthetic may relieve the symptoms. The prevention of mumps in the postpubertal male has some value. If a man who has not previously had mumps has been in contact with the virus, gamma globulin is usually administered.

INFLAMMATORY PROCESSES OF THE FEMALE REPRODUCTIVE TRACT

Kraurosis Vulvae

Kraurosis vulvae describes the shrinkage which occurs in vulvar structures as a result of atrophy. The lesions remain localized in the vestibule and on examination appear smooth and "angry" red. As the condition progresses, increasing atrophy causes shrinking of the introitus. Dyspareunia, itching and soreness are frequent complaints. Treatment begins with good perineal hygiene. Lubricants are advised to relieve the dyspareunia. Local applications of estrogen preparations achieve good results. The condition does not appear to have any connection with future malignancies of the vulva.

Leukoplakia Vulvae

Leukoplakia shows typical areas of thickened gray patches of epithelium scattered over the vulva and perineum. These initial patches crack easily, and fissures and excoriated areas develop. Pruritus is common, and secondary infection of the scratched lesions occurs. Ulcerations may develop. The disease is remarkable in that three-quarters of vulvar carcinoma shows evidence of previous leukoplakia. The exact connection is unknown, but the patient must be carefully followed to detect any malignancy.

Treatment begins with careful perineal care. Following every voiding, vulval cleansing is performed using cotton balls and a mild soap. Hot sitz baths may be prescribed, and cornstarch may be used to keep the vulva dry. Antibiotics and hydrocortisone cream assist in the healing. If the pruritus is severe, topical anesthetics may be applied in conjunction with the administration of mild sedatives. Screening tests for cancer are done. If the condition resists treatment, a simple vulvectomy is performed.

Bartholinitis

Bartholinitis is an infection of the greater vestibular gland and may or may not be gonorrheal in origin. The infection is an ascending one, progressing up the ducts to the gland. Symptoms are usually those of an acute infection — pain, swelling, inflammation and a purulent discharge. Cellulitis of the surrounding tissues aggravates the situation, but the infection may localize and become an abscess. This is usually excised and drained. Sometimes the infection subsides, leaving the duct scarred and occluded. This may be followed by a cyst filled with the secretions of the gland which now cannot escape. The cyst is usually a painless swelling in the lower third of the labium minus. Treatment is to excise the cyst and gland. Alternatively, a marsupialization of the cystic duct may be done. This leaves the functioning gland in place.

Hot sitz baths or saline soaks may be ordered following surgery. The patient may need instruction on how to take a sitz bath at home. Following the daily bath, a fresh tub of hot water is run. The patient sits in this for 10 to 15 minutes. The water is not above the level of the iliac crest.

Vaginitis

Physiologic Leukorrhea. Physiologic leukorrhea is a normal whitish discharge which helps to keep the vagina moist. It is composed of endocervical secretions, leukocytes, desquamated epithelial cells and other normal flora of the vaginal tract. The pH is normally 4 to 5 but varies during the life cycle of the woman. At birth, it may be as low as 5 under the hormonal stimulus of the mother. As a child it is 6 to 7. At menarche the pH becomes acidic again, and assumes the adult pH of 4 to 5. Postmenopausally, estrogen is withdrawn, and the pH rises to 6 to 7 again. The quantity of the discharge also varies among women, during stages of the menstrual cycle and during pregnancy. An increase is usually noticed at ovulation, during sexual stimulation and during pregnancy. The most characteristic symptom of a vaginitis is a change in the normal vaginal discharge.

Trichomoniasis. The most common cause of vaginitis is a flagellated protozoon, known as a trichomona, which grows and thrives in a vaginal pH of 5 to 6. Trichomonas may be found in the large bowel and occasionally in the bladder and vestibular glands. They can be transmitted to a man at intercourse and from him can be communicated to other women or serve as a source of reinfection. In men, trichomonas may be harbored in the urethra, bladder or prostate.

The woman presents with symptoms of a heavy, yellow, frothy discharge which has a slight odor. This heavy discharge may be irritating to the vulva, causing pruritus and excoriation. The vaginal mucosa is reddened and is slightly edematous. The patient may complain of dyspareunia and, if the bladder is involved, of dysuria and frequency. As the condition becomes chronic, the woman has fewer symptoms. Diagnosis is confirmed when trichomonas are seen microscopically in a vaginal smear.

Men frequently have few symptoms. There may be some urethral itching and a slight discharge. Invasion of the bladder may produce frequency and burning on micturition. Wet smears are made of the urethral discharge, and the protozoa seen microscopically confirm the diagnosis.

Treatment is usually the oral administration of metronidazole (Flagyl) 250 mg. three times a day for 10 days. Repeat smears will then be done, and a repeat course of therapy may be necessary. During the treatment, a condom should be worn until both partners are considered cured. Women may be given vaginal suppositories instead of oral therapy. A suppository is inserted morning and night, daily for 4 to 8 weeks. This is continued through the menstrual period, for the menstrual flow is alkaline and provides an excellent medium for the protozoa. Insertion is like that of a vaginal tampon. The patient is instructed to remain flat for about 10 minutes following insertion.

Monilial Vaginitis. Monilial vaginitis occurs when the vagina is invaded by the fungus *Candida albicans*. The vaginal pH is usually 5 to 7. Pregnant women and diabetics are predisposed because of glycosuria and the increased glycogen present

in the vagina during pregnancy. Contamination may be from the rectum. A thick, white, curdy vaginal discharge is present which frequently causes pruritus and irritation of the vulva. The vaginal walls are reddened and covered with typical white patches. When the patches are swabbed off, bleeding may occur. Diagnosis is confirmed microscopically from a vaginal smear.

The patient is instructed in careful perineal care and hand washing to avoid reinfection and spread of the fungus to others, especially children. The vagina and labia are cleaned, and the white patches are removed. Following this, the soap is removed with normal saline. The area is painted with 1 per cent gentian violet and is allowed to dry for 5 minutes. Since the dye may stain the patient's clothing, she is given a pad to wear and is advised to wear old underwear until the treatment is completed. At home the nonpregnant woman may be asked to take daily, weak vinegar douches followed by the insertion of gentian violet jelly for 14 days. Mycostatin orally or in suppository form achieves good results. It may be given to pregnant women.

Atrophic Vaginitis (Senile). Because of hormonal changes following the menopause, the pH rises and the glycogen stores are reduced in the vagina. The vagina loses its rugae and becomes smooth and shiny. It is now more susceptible to invasion by organisms. A sticky, mucoid discharge may appear. The patient complains of a burning in the vagina, dyspareunia and pruritus of the vulva. Occasionally, the discharge is blood-flecked, as areas of the vagina ulcerate and adhesions develop and tear. Infection is controlled by the use of systemic antibiotics or sulpha drugs. Estrogens are administered orally or vaginally. When the vaginitis is relieved, medication is stopped, and the patient may be advised to have cleansing vinegar douches periodically.

Cervicitis

The cervix is the main barrier against ascending infections of the genital tract. As such it is exposed to many insults. The majority of these are small lacerations which occur during childbirth or injuries associated with surgery, instrumentation or venereal disease. Bacteria invade these slits in the cervix. When the cervical epithelium is damaged, the infection easily spreads to the endocervix. Congestion and edema follow. An increase in cervical mucus results in an elevation in vaginal pH. The cells of the endocervix begin growing out around the external os. This outgrowth of cells produces a red, granular raised lesion. As the cervix is exposed to further trauma, the eroded areas become infected again and again. Chronic cervicitis results.

The symptoms vary. Usually a heavy vaginal discharge exists. The patient may notice deep dyspareunia or some blood-stained discharge following intercourse or douching.

The diagnosis depends on the characteristic appearance of the lesion. Cytological studies are usually done to distinguish cervicitis from early carcinoma. When carcinoma is ruled out, the condition is generally treated by cautery of the endocervix. After cautery the old tissue sloughs away followed by the regeneration of the new from the outside edges of the lesion. The patient should expect a brownish discharge for 1 to 2 weeks as the old tissue sloughs away.

Often patients with cervicitis need to be taught proper perineal care. The use of strong, irritating douches should be discouraged, and perineal hygiene is stressed.

Pelvic Inflammatory Disease (P.I.D.)

Pelvic inflammatory disease has come to mean all ascending pelvic infections once they are beyond the cervix. Many organisms may be responsible for the symptoms. However, among the most frequent are the gonococcus and *Staphylococcus aureus*. On occasion, tuberculosis and anaerobic bacteria can be causative. Symptoms may follow labor and delivery, a criminally induced abortion, surgical procedures, a contact with gonorrhea or cervicitis. Other, rarer causes exist as well. The condition may be acute or chronic.

Signs and Symptoms. The typical picture is one of a systemic infection with fever, chills, malaise, anorexia, nausea and vomiting. This is usually accompanied by lower abdominal pain which is either unilateral or bilateral. In more chronic cases, this pain is increased before and during menstruation.

Pain is experienced on movement of the cervix. Leukorrhea is present. With gonorrheal or staphylococcal infections the discharge is usually heavy and purulent; streptococcal infections cause a thinner, more mucoid discharge.

Spread of the infection occurs by two typical routes, which are demonstrated in Figure 19–10. Symptoms depend on which route the infection follows. In Route I the bacteria spread along the surface of the endometrium to the tubes and into the peritoneum. The consequences of this route may be adhesions or cysts of the tube with consequent infertility. In more advanced cases abscesses develop about the ovary or in the cul-de-sac. Infection following Route II is spread mainly through the lymphatics and produces a pelvic cellulitis in contrast to the more localized endometritis or salpingitis (infection of the uterine tube) of Route I. Thrombophlebitis may follow this cellulitis. Advanced and virulent infections admitted by either route may become systemic and may show all the signs of septicemia.

Treatment and Nursing Care. The patient with an acute episode is usually admitted to the hospital. She may or may not be isolated, depending on the cause of her infection. The patient is placed on bed rest in semi-Fowler's position to promote drain-

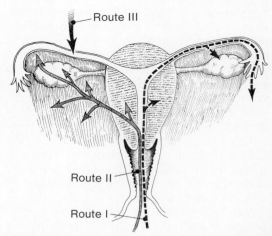

Figure 19–10 Common routes of the spread of pelvic inflammatory disease. Route I: commonly gonococcus and staphylococcus. Route II: frequently streptococcus. Route III: tuberculosis, usually a descending infection from another source.

age of pus into the vagina and the cul-de-sac. Perineal care should be done as needed to keep the patient clean and comfortable. Douching is usually avoided, since it may only advance the infection further. Heat to the lower back and abdomen may be soothing. Analgesics and sedation may be ordered. The patient will receive antibiotics following culture and sensitivity studies. In some cases blood cultures may be obtained. Surgical treatment is deferred, if possible, until the infection is controlled. A culdocentesis or colpotomy may be done to drain a pelvic abscess. Tubo-ovarian abscesses may require an abdominal approach. In cases of prolonged, debilitating infections which are resistant to conservative treatment, salpingectomy or hysterectomy may be done.

VENEREAL DISEASE

The most common venereal diseases are gonorrhea and syphilis. A brief review of these follows.

Gonorrhea

The specific organism causing gonorrhea is *Neisseria gonorrhoeae,* and it is transmitted almost exclusively by sexual intercourse. The organism dies quickly when not harbored in the human body.

Signs and Symptoms. Symptoms appear 4 to 10 days after the initial contact. In the male, urethritis occurs, heralded by a purulent urethral discharge. Some itching and burning about the meatus are also present. The urethral meatus is red and edematous. The infection may remain localized. However, an ascending infection involving the prostate, seminal vesicles, bladder and epididymus may result. If adhesions develop, they may damage the urethra and duct system with consequent urethral stricture and infertility.

Diagnosis is confirmed when the gonococcus is seen microscopically in smears on cultures taken from the urethra. If discharge is slight, the first urethral washings may be used. These are obtained by collecting the first portion of a voided urine specimen. The penis is not swabbed off before collecting the specimen.

In the adult female the vagina with its layers of squamous epithelium is resistant to the gonococcus. Therefore, the vulnerable areas are the vestibular glands, the urethra and the endocervix. The glands become red, swollen and sore. A purulent discharge may drain from the urethra and the ducts of the glands. Leukorrhea is present in cases in which cervicitis accompanies the picture. Dysuria and frequency often occur. Sometimes the symptoms may be mild and vague in the female. The infection may ascend above the cervix and may form the characteristic picture described in pelvic inflammatory disease.

Diagnosis is made on the basis of organisms seen in smears or cultures. To obtain these specimens the patient is instructed not to void or douche for approximately 2 hours before the cultures are taken. The vulva are not cleansed first. With the patient in a lithotomy position, smears are taken from the urethra, cervix and the ducts of the vestibular glands.

Treatment. Treatment with antibiotics, notably penicillin, is highly successful and has succeeded in reducing the incidence of complications. However, there is evidence of strains of gonococcus showing an increasing resistance to penicillin. Other antibiotics can be employed if penicillin does not eradicate the infection. Treatment is successful in cases in which repeated cultures are judged to be negative.

Syphilis

Syphilis is a more serious disease and, fortunately, is less common than gonorrhea. The causative organism is the spirochete *Treponema pallidum.*

Signs and Symptoms. Incubation varies between 2 to 4 weeks. In most cases the disease is spread by sexual intercourse. As with the gonococcus, the spirochete does not survive outside the host. In the untreated condition, three stages are distinguished. The primary lesion is a small, painless chancre or ulcer. It is deep and has indurated edges. Usually this chancre heals spontaneously, giving the false impression that the disease is cured. This primary lesion appears most commonly on the penis of the male. In the female, it may appear on the labia, vagina or cervix. The secondary stage is usually characterized by a rash appearing over the body. This rash may be accompanied by condylomata lata on the female vulva. This is a cauliflower-appearing collection of flat, gray vulvar warts. As are all lesions of syphilis, these are teeming with spirochetes and are highly infectious. The rash is usually accompanied by malaise and fever. In a short period, this rash regresses and the patient enters the tertiary stage. The bones, heart and central nervous system, including the brain, are affected. Personality disorders arise and the typical ataxic gait of the tertiary syphilitic appears. A large, ulcerating necrotic lesion known as a gumma now occurs. Rarely is it seen in the genital tract, but it may occur on the vulva or in the testes. At this stage the disease may be arrested but not reversed.

Diagnosis is made by a careful history, clinical findings, and cultures or biopsies from the lesions. Blood serology is also assessed. Since blood serology is not positive for about 4 weeks after the onset of the disease, the early diagnosis is made from scrapings of the lesions. They can be seen on dark-field examination. These scrapings are made before antibiotic therapy is initiated so that the diagnosis can be confirmed. Blood serology tests such as the Kahn, Wassermann and VDRL are all reliable.

Treatment and Nursing Care. Treatment is by antibiotic, and penicillin is the drug of choice. Usually a series of injections is necessary.

Most cases of venereal disease are treated on an outpatient basis, and the patient must be taught how to protect himself and others. First the nature and transmission of the disease should be understood. No immunity develops and reinfection can occur easily. Strict personal and perineal hygiene should be observed. Hand washing following any handling of the genitalia is imperative, as the gonococcus can be readily carried to the eye, which quickly becomes infected. Blindness may ensue if treatment is not received. Women who are handling small children need to be especially careful. Also, the vagina of a prepubertal girl is extremely sensitive to the gonococcus because it lacks the protective layers of squamous epithelium. A particularly distressing form of vulvovaginitis may occur as a result of contamination from a family member. Sexual contacts are to be avoided until the physician notifies the patient he or she is cured. The nurse must practice all she teaches by following strict medical asepsis while caring for patients who are in the infectious stages of the disease. All equipment must be sterilized following use, and dressings or swabs are disposed of in a safe way. The disease may be transmitted by direct contamination with living spirochetes of a laceration. For this reason, the nurse who has a break in her skin must be very careful when dealing with the lesions of syphilis. Gloves may be indicated. Once therapy has been initiated, the patient is usually noninfectious within 48 hours.

The disease may be very distressing to the patient. The patient may experience guilt feelings, and marital difficulties may arise when one partner infects the other. The disease carries a social stigma. For these reasons, confidentiality must be maintained by the nurse at all times. Indeed, the issue is protected by law. However, the disease is reportable. Contacts must be identified and discreetly followed by the public health nurse. The nurse, by explaining the nature of the disease, usually obtains the patient's cooperation in identifying contacts. In addition, the nurse should include venereal disease in any lectures she prepares on general health education in the schools so that the population may become more aware of the signs and symptoms as well as the modes of transmission of these diseases.

DISPLACEMENTS AND RELAXATIONS OF THE FEMALE GENITAL ORGANS

Retroversion and Retroflexion of the Uterus

The normal position of the uterus is one of some anteversion and anteflexion (Fig. 19-11). It is not a fixed organ. The filling of the bladder or bowel may cause a change in uterine position. On occasion, the uterus assumes a retroverted or retroflexed position. When retroverted, the fundus points toward the sacrum and the cervix toward the anterior vaginal wall. Retroflexion refers to the position of the fundus of the uterus in relation to the cervix. In retroflexion the fundus bends back over the cervix (Fig.

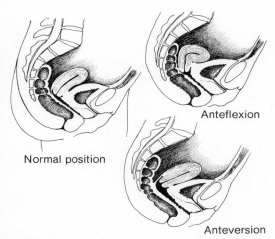

Figure 19–11 Normal position of the uterus, anteflexion, and anteversion.

19-12). Degrees of retroversion and retroflexion are possible so that the case may be mild or extreme.

The etiology appears to lie in a weakness of the supporting structures which may be either congenital or acquired. The acquired weakness is frequently due to injuries during the maternity cycle. Adhesions and tumors may pull or push the uterus into this position.

The patient may complain of backache, infertility, dyspareunia or secondary dysmenorrhea, but she is frequently symptomless unless the situation is extreme. Backache and dysmenorrhea are probably associated with pelvic congestion. Infer-

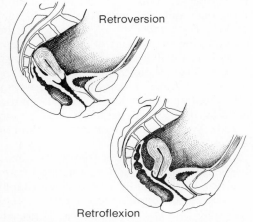

Figure 19–12 Retroversion and retroflexion of the uterus.

tility may arise because the cervix does not reach the seminal pool. Frequently, the ovaries prolapse into the cul-de-sac and become congested and enlarged. Because of this, intercourse may be painful.

Treatment and Nursing Responsibilities. Usually the uterus is manually replaced, and a vaginal pessary is inserted to hold the uterus in place. The most common pessaries used are the Smith-Hodge type. The pessary functions by holding the cervix in a posterior position. This in turn rotates the uterus forward. When the pessary is properly in position, the patient is unaware of its presence and no difficulty is experienced on voiding or during intercourse. The patient will return in about 4 to 6 weeks to have the pessary checked and removed for cleaning. The physician may then give the patient a 6-week trial period without the pessary to see if she remains free of symptoms. If not, a further trial with the pessary may be given.

The nurse frequently has to instruct the patient in proper personal hygiene after the insertion of the pessary. All pessaries are irritating, especially those which are rubber and have some degree of movement. An offensive smelling leukorrhea usually develops, and chronic ulceration may occur. The patient will need to return for checkups as advised. Also, she will be instructed to douche every 2 to 3 days. This is best done when lying flat in the bathtub. The douche can is held about 2 feet above the vagina and the inflow is by gravity. Occasionally, if warm water seems inadequate, a weak (0.5 per cent) solution of lactic acid may be used.

In other cases the uterus may be surgically suspended by shortening the round ligaments. This is not usually the first choice of treatment.

Prolapse, Cystocele and Rectocele

Uterine prolapse refers to the downward displacement of the entire organ. Prolapse (Fig. 19–13) may occur in varying degrees. First-degree prolapse describes the condition existing when the uterus descends within the vagina. Second-degree prolapse occurs when the cervix protrudes through the introitus. Procidentia, or third degree prolapse, refers to the entire uterus protruding through the introitus with total inversion of the vagina.

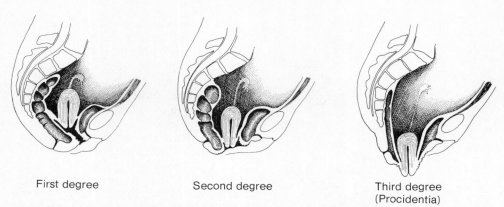

First degree

Second degree

Third degree
(Procidentia)

Figure 19–13 Uterine prolapse, showing first-, second- and third-degree (procidentia) prolapse.

Cystocele, urethrocele, rectocele and enterocele refer to herniations or relaxations of the bladder, urethra, rectum and small bowel into the vagina (Fig. 19–14). They may occur singly or in combinations with some degree of uterine prolapse.

The single most important etiologic factor in the development of these conditions is thought to be injury at childbirth. The pelvic floor and supporting structures may be stretched and torn during the process of delivery and are thereby weakened. Further relaxation results after the menopause as the tissues atrophy following estrogen withdrawal. Large intra-abdominal tumors may also place an added strain on already weakened tissue. In some rare cases, the structures seem to be congenitally weak.

The patient with a prolapse often complains of a feeling of "something coming down." She may have a dragging or heavy

feeling in the pelvis, accompanied by backache. She may have bladder symptoms of either retaining or losing urine. She may have recurrent cystitis. When the cervix protrudes through the introitus, it may become ulcerated from constant friction. This may produce pain and bleeding. The patient with a cystocele frequently has symptoms of stress incontinence.

Diagnosis is usually confirmed by bimanual and rectal examinations. The patient will be asked to bear down, cough or strain while the doctor estimates the degree of prolapse or herniation.

Treatment and Nursing Responsibilities. The best treatment is prevention. Better care during the maternity cycle has helped to reduce the incidence of these complications. Exercises should be taught by the nurse to all patients in the postpartum period and the same exercises may be taught to help relieve mild prolapse. These consist of alternately tightening and relaxing the gluteal and perineal floor muscles. Practicing starting and stopping the stream of urine also helps the patient regain good perineal muscle tone. She should continue to practice these exercises several times a day for several weeks.

In situations in which surgery is contraindicated, the use of pessaries may be employed. A variety are available for different degrees of prolapse.

Surgical intervention is frequently necessary to correct the situation. An anterior and posterior colporrhaphy and perineorrhaphy repair a cystocele and rectocele respectively.

If some prolapse of the uterus is present and future childbearing is not an issue, a Manchester repair may be done. This com-

Cystocele

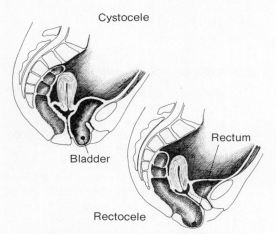

Bladder

Rectum

Rectocele

Figure 19–14 Cystocele and rectocele.

bines the amputation of an elongated cervix and shortening of the cardinal ligaments with an anterior and posterior repair. Although childbearing is not precluded by an anterior and posterior repair, delivery by cesarian section is usually recommended in order to retain this repair. Vaginal hysterectomy with an anterior and posterior repair is usually performed for more severe uterine prolapse. The uterine tubes and the uterus with all or part of the cervix will be removed. The ligaments and blood vessels are ligated, and a cuff is made in the upper portion of the vagina.

The nursing care of these patients is similar to that given to any patient undergoing surgery. However, the patient will receive a perineal shave preparation. Catheterization is usually performed preoperatively. Orders may be given outlining special perineal or vaginal preparations. The nurse should assist the patient in understanding the limitations, if any, surgery will impose on sexual and reproductive capacity, since many misunderstandings frequently occur.

During surgery the patient may receive intravenous vasoconstrictors to reduce the danger of hemorrhage. Blood loss during vaginal surgery tends to be heavy and is heavier still in premenopausal women.

The patient's legs are carefully lifted together to be placed into and removed from the stirrups. No one should lean or apply pressure on the anesthetized leg. These measures will reduce postoperative discomfort, avoid strain on the repaired perineal muscles and help reduce the incidence of postoperative emboli. These same measures should be used whenever a patient's legs are placed in stirrups.

Following vaginal surgery, the nurse observes the patient for signs and symptoms of hemorrhage, urinary tract infection, thromboemboli and infections at the surgical site. Hemorrhage may be frank, oozing or in the form of a large hematoma. The oozing of blood may not be readily noticed by the patient or the staff; therefore, the nurse must be careful to observe the estimated blood loss over a period of time, not just each time she checks the patient. A hematoma is a form of concealed hemorrhage; the blood vessels bleed into the tissue of the vagina or perineum. The patient complains of discomfort or pain over the site. The tissue

bulges and may be so taut as to glisten. The nurse should notify the doctor immediately and be prepared to assist with treatment and the possible return of the patient to the operating room. Blood transfusions may be required. The clot may be evacuated, the bleeding vessels ligated or the site firmly packed. Antibiotics may be ordered to lessen the chance of infection.

The patient may return with a urinary catheter attached to drainage. This usually remains in place for 7 to 9 days until the edema is resolved. The patient without a catheter must be observed for signs of adequate bladder function. Voiding in sufficient quantities should occur at least every 6 hours. To induce the patient who is unable to void to do so requires all the nurse's skill in an attempt to avoid catheterization. Patients are usually ambulated early and getting up to void helps. If sitz baths or perineal irrigations are allowed, having the patient take one immediately before attempting to void usually helps. When catheterization is necessary, the strictest aseptic technique should be followed.

Perineal care is important to the prevention of infection. Depending on the extent of the surgery, sterile technique may be required. It should be as frequent as necessary to keep the perineal area clean and dry. General principles of working from front to back are followed. In addition, sterile pads are applied. Sitz baths may be ordered. The patient sits in a tub of water up to the level of the iliac crest. An irrigation may be ordered with sterile or plain water or some solutions. The nurse or patient runs the solution from a bag and tubing over the perineum into a basin. If the patient is well enough, she is frequently taught how to do these procedures.

Straining at stool is avoided by a low residue diet and the avoidance of constipation.

On discharge the patient may receive further instructions; some physicians definitely restrict heavy lifting and prolonged standing, walking and sitting. Intercourse is contraindicated for approximately 6 weeks.

Stress Incontinence

Stress incontinence is the involuntary loss of small amounts of urine when a woman

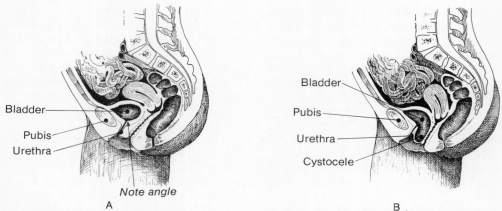

Figure 19–15 *A*, The bladder at ease—no stress incontinence. *B*, Cystocele without stress incontinence.

coughs, sneezes or otherwise suddenly increases the intra-abdominal pressure and, therefore, the intravesical pressure. It should be distinguished from urge incontinence and frequency.

Continence is thought to be maintained at the junction of the urethra and the bladder. Assistance is also received from the muscles surrounding the urethra as well as a tight supporting perineal floor. In the continent woman the angle between the urethra and posterior wall of the bladder is approximately 90° (Fig. 19–15). Normally, this angle is only obliterated at micturition (Fig. 19–16). However, in stress incontinence the slight effort of straining, coughing or sneezing is sufficient to reduce this angle, and an involuntary loss of urine occurs. This explanation is thought to describe about 90 per cent of stress incontinence. A woman may have a cystocele (Fig. 19–15) and still be continent if the angle is maintained.

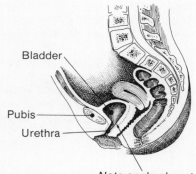

Note angle absent

Figure 19–16 The bladder during micturition.

However, many women with a cystocele also have accompanying stress incontinence.

Occasionally, stress incontinence follows a cystocele repair. This is probably due to elevation of the bladder to a position which obliterates the angle. For this reason many surgeons check the angle following repair to be sure it will be adequate.

The symptoms may become distressing to the woman. Frequently small dribbles of urine cause wetness, irritation and an offensive odor. The woman may have to wear a perineal pad or plastic pants continuously. Gradually she may become shy of social contacts and may confine herself to home.

Diagnosis is made on examination by the doctor. Cystourethrograms may also be indicated. In this procedure a dye outlines the urethra and bladder, demonstrating the state of the angle at rest, during straining and, if possible, on micturition. A small chain may also be inserted to further outline the urethra on x-ray.

Treatment and Nursing Responsibilities. Treatment consists of prevention of injury by good maternity care and the practice of postpartum exercises in the immediate postpartum period. In some mild cases exercises may be prescribed and will help if practiced. In the older woman, the symptoms seem to be aggravated by a weakening of structures secondary to reduced estrogen stimulation; in these cases, estrogen suppositories may be given. Oral synthetic estrogens, such as diethylstilbestrol, may be given as well.

Surgery may be necessary in order to

elevate the urethra and restore the proper urethrovesical relationship. Two types of operations are commonly used to restore the angle.

In the Aldridge sling operation the surgeon makes a sling of fascia. This sling is then attached to the anterior abdominal wall. This serves to elevate the urethra and restore the angle. The approach may be abdominal, vaginal or both. Occasionally, the sling is too tight and the patient has difficulty micturating and emptying the bladder properly. Cystitis and other complications may occur. Teaching the patient to bend her body forward when attempting to void postoperatively helps. This relaxes the muscles of the abdomen, thereby loosening the sling and obliterating the angle.

The Marshall-Marchetti-Krantz operation elevates the urethra by suturing the anterior vaginal wall on each side to the periosteum of the pubic bone and the anterior wall of the bladder to the pubic bone. A catheter with a large (30 cc.) bag is inserted preoperatively to serve as a landmark during surgery. Postoperatively, the nurse will be responsible for catheter care. On some occasions the patient returns home with the catheter in place. The nurse must teach the patient how to care for her catheter at home.

Fistulae

Fistulae may occur between the vagina or uterus and the bladder, urethra or rectum (Fig. 19–17). They can occur as a sequel to injury during labor and delivery, surgery, disease processes such as carcinoma and radiation therapy.

When urinary fistulae develop, some urine leaks into the vagina or uterus. Rectal fistulae cause the escape of flatus and feces into the vagina. In both instances, irritation to the tissues occurs. An offensive odor develops and causes much embarrassment for the patient. Since many fistulae spontaneously heal within a matter of several weeks, treatment may be postponed. During that period nursing care is very important to the patient. Frequent perineal care is required to keep the patient clean. Cleansing and deodorizing douches may be ordered. High enemas may be given to reduce the constant flow of feces. Care should be taken to go above the fistula with the rectal tube. If the

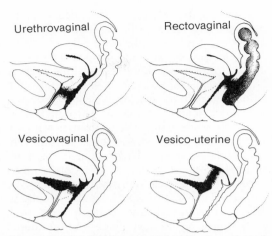

Figure 19–17 Fistulae: urethrovaginal; rectovaginal; vesicovaginal; and vesicouterine.

fistula does not heal spontaneously, surgery may be indicated. Following surgery involving the bladder, the patient may return from the operating room with a urethral as well as a suprapubic catheter. Drainage must be maintained so that pressure on the repaired area is kept at a minimum. Repair may also include implantation of the ureters elsewhere. Rectal fistulae may be repaired and a temporary colostomy established in order to provide time to heal. Ambulation may be postponed for a few days. The woman may be discharged home on restricted activity until the doctor advises that the repair is complete.

BENIGN AND MALIGNANT DISORDERS OF THE MALE REPRODUCTIVE TRACT

Spermatocele

A spermatocele is a cyst of the spermatic cord which contains sperm in a thin white fluid. It lies above the testis and is separate from it. The mass will transilluminate. Usually a spermatocele requires no treatment. Sometimes it may become large enough to be confused with hydrocele and to be aggravating to the patient. Then it may be excised. The etiology is unclear.

Varicocele

Varicocele is the dilatation of the venous plexus about the testis. It occurs most frequently on the left side. Its appearance on the right side may indicate that a tumor is occluding the vein above the level of the scrotum. Some testicular atrophy may occur if the circulation is impeded for long periods of time. This may result in sub-fertility. On palpation behind and above the testis the physician feels a mass of tortuous veins which empties when the patient lies down.

Treatment may consist of a scrotal support which relieves the dragging sensation. If fertility is an issue or the condition is severe, the internal spermatic vein may be ligated. The results are usually excellent. A scrotal support may be worn for 4 to 5 days following surgery since scrotal edema may be present.

Hydrocele

A hydrocele is a collection of fluid in the tunica vaginalis. It may occur following local injury, infection or a neoplasm and may be unilateral or bilateral. More often it is chronic, and the cause is unknown. In newborn babies, the cause is usually a late closure of the processus vaginalis. This frequently closes spontaneously. In some young men a chronic type exists because the processus vaginalis never closes completely, and a connection remains between the peritoneal cavity and the tunica vaginalis.

Treatment is not required unless circulation to the testis is impaired or the hydrocele becomes large, unsightly and uncomfortable. Then the hydrocele is aspirated, and a sclerosing drug may be injected. In chronic cases the tunica vaginalis is excised (hydrocelectomy). Postoperatively the scrotum is elevated on a pillow or bridge dressing, and a pressure dressing is applied. Depending on the operation, there may or may not be a drain present in the incision. The patient must be observed for hemorrhage which may be concealed in the hydrocele sac. When ambulatory the patient usually requires a fresh scrotal support daily. Immediately after the operation he may need a larger support than usual.

Torsion of the Testes

Torsion of the testis occurs when the testis rotates within the tunica vaginalis. Often this is due to spasm of the cremaster muscle which rotates the testis in what is often an abnormally large vaginalis. The young man experiences a sudden severe pain in the area of the testis which is unrelieved by rest or support. Because the torsion reduces the blood supply to the testis, testicular atrophy follows rapidly. Sometimes under local anesthesia the doctor will attempt to reduce torsion. If this is unsuccessful, surgical reduction follows.

Benign Hyperplasia of the Prostate

The reason benign enlargement of the prostate gland occurs is unknown. However, it is estimated that over 50 per cent of men over 60 show some signs of prostatic enlargement. Of these, about one-quarter will require treatment.

In the young adult male the prostate gland is encased in a thin capsular membrane which is closely adherent to the underlying tissue. Gradually the tissue begins to enlarge by new growth (hyperplasia) and the capsule of the prostate becomes thick and is loosely attached to the underlying tissue. This inner tissue can now be easily stripped away, leaving the thickened capsule intact. The enlarging prostate encroaches on the urethra and the base of the bladder, producing certain symptoms.

Signs and Symptoms. Gradually, the man may experience hesitancy in beginning the flow of urine. The stream of urine is reduced in force and size. Incomplete emptying of the bladder produces residual urine which reduces bladder capacity so that urgency and frequency result. Nocturia occurring 3 or more times in one night is a good indication of frequency. Often, cystitis occurs as well. In severe cases, the bladder becomes overdistended, and hypertrophy and small diverticula follow as weakened areas of bladder mucosa bulge out between the bands of muscle fibers. The backup of urine causes hydroureter or even hydronephrosis. Over long periods of time renal function may be impaired.

Frequently, the patient does not seek medical attention until acute retention of urine occurs. Overdistension of the bladder is usually the precipitating factor. The patient is catheterized and decompressed. Decompression allows for the slow release of urine from the bladder. This prevents a sudden release of pressure in the abdomen which could cause shock and hemorrhage. Shock follows the rush of blood from vital centers to fill the newly released blood vessels. This sudden filling may cause small blood vessels in the bladder mucosa to rupture. The catheter remains in place for 2 to 3 days after which normal voiding patterns usually return.

Backache and sciatica may also bring the patient to the doctor, since the enlarged prostate exerts pressure on nerves.

Diagnosis and Treatment. Treatment is indicated to relieve the symptoms and to prevent infections of the urinary tract and renal damage. If the amount of residual urine in the bladder is above 75 to 100 cc., the physician may feel treatment is necessary even though the symptoms are not severe. Residual urine is estimated in several ways. Immediately after voiding, a catheter may be passed and any remaining urine is drawn off and measured. A radiopaque dye can be injected into the bladder. The man is then asked to void and postvoiding films are made. Direct visualization of the bladder may be done by cystoscope, and any bladder changes will be noted. Intravenous pyelograms will indicate the extent of ureter and kidney involvement. Renal function tests may be ordered as well.

Treatment is usually surgical removal of the enlarged structures. A period of preoperative preparation may be necessary. Residual urine and hydroureter are treated by catheterization for a period of 1 to 2 weeks. The patient is prepared for surgery by explaining what may follow the operation so that the postoperative period is not so traumatic. Because of the incidence of post-prostatectomy epididymitis, the vas deferens may be ligated to prevent this complication. The operation may be done concurrently or preoperatively. A signed consent is required.

Several operations are commonly used to treat this condition. The choice of operation seems to depend on the size of the prostate, the condition of the patient and the preference of the surgeon. A prostate in excess of 50 Gm. is considered by most surgeons to be too difficult to remove transurethrally. Therefore, an open route is chosen.

TRANSURETHRAL PROSTATECTOMY. This procedure is the most frequently performed operation and is the closed method. Postoperative recovery is usually rapid; potency is maintained, and urinary results are good. The operation is performed with a resectoscope, an instrument similar to a cystoscope but equipped with cutting and cauterizing attachments. This slender instrument is inserted up the urethra to the prostatic urethra, and the enlarged prostate is chipped away. The capsule remains intact. During the operation, the bladder and urethra are continuously irrigated with a sterile, isotonic, nonconductive clear fluid. In this manner, debris and blood are washed away. Following removal of the intracapsular tissue, a Foley catheter with a 30 cc. bag is passed. The catheter bag is pulled down into the prostatic fossa where it exerts pressure on blood vessels and helps to prevent hemorrhage. The catheter is usually attached to straight drainage, but it may be attached to medium or high decompression drainage.

The decompression drainage aids hemostasis by keeping constant pressure on the prostatic fossa. Also, the partially full bladder may help reduce bladder spasm. However, care should be taken to check that the catheter is draining and that the bladder is not full. A full bladder may cause hemorrhage by "milking" the blood vessels in the fossa.

Immediately after the operation the catheter drainage is bloody. The nurse must be alert for signs of hemorrhage by paying close attention to the blood pressure and pulse of the patient and the amount of drainage. Frequent irrigations of the catheter are usually ordered. If the catheter becomes plugged, the doctor is notified.

The fluid used to irrigate the bladder during the operation may be absorbed, causing hemodilution. The signs and symptoms of this may be those of sodium deficiency or excessive blood volume. Complaints of headache, nausea, vomiting or muscle weakness should not be ignored by the nurse but must be reported. Hypertension, restlessness, apprehension, shortness of breath or blurred vision likewise should be reported. If the physician expects that the operation may be more than 2 hours long, fluid intake may be restricted for 12 hours before the operation. Following the operation, 200 to 300 ml. of normal saline may be given intravenously over 2 hours. The nurse must observe the patient for signs of pulmonary edema.

Frequently, the irritation of the catheter gives the patient the urge to void. With a properly draining catheter this usually passes. However, if the patient attempts to void around the catheter, the bladder muscles contract and make the patient more uncomfortable. Careful preoperative preparation of the patient so that he understands the phenomenon and therefore does not try to void postoperatively usually is the greatest help to the patient. In severe cases, the patient will need sedation or an analgesic to obtain relief. If the catheter causes the patient great discomfort postoperatively, the nurse should check for other causes. Frequently, this increased discomfort is due to an overdistended bladder produced from a catheter which is not draining properly or from hemorrhage into the bladder. Occasionally, the bladder has been perforated during the operation and the hemorrhage is perfusing into the abdominal cavity. All of these require immediate attention—complaints of pain by the patient should never be ignored or go uninvestigated by the nurse.

Because hemorrhage remains a threat, even in the later postoperative period, care is taken to prevent its occurrence. The patient is cautioned against straining to pass stool, and a light diet is usually ordered. Enemas, rectal tubes and rectal thermometers are frequently contraindicated during the first postoperative week.

Because of the danger of a urinary tract infection, prophylactic antibiotics are frequently given for approximately 2 weeks postoperatively. The catheter is removed 3 to 7 days postoperatively, and for a short period following this, the patient is usually instructed to record and measure each voiding. If difficulty in voiding is still present, the catheter may be reinserted. The nurse should watch for signs of incontinence which may follow or signs of urinary retention which may indicate a urethral stricture. Before being discharged the patient should be told that an episode of bleeding may occur about the second to fourth week postoperatively. In that event, he should contact his physician and come to the emergency department of the hospital. Also he is warned to avoid any straining, heavy lifting or vigorous exercise for about 1 month postoperatively.

SUPRAPUBIC PROSTATECTOMY. This operation may be chosen when the prostate is large and when some bladder surgery is indicated as well. This is probably the second most frequent operation after the transurethral method. Potency is maintained following the operation.

A small abdominal incision is made above the pubis and directly over the bladder. The bladder is opened, and through another incision into the urethral mucosa, the prostate is excised. The prostatic capsule remains intact. Various methods of draining the bladder and applying pressure to the operative site may be used postoperatively. A Foley catheter with a large bag and a cystostomy tube may be used. Sometimes a cystostomy tube with packing or a hemostatic bag in the prostatic fossa is used. Traction to maintain pressure on the hemostatic bag is achieved by attaching it to a bird cage apparatus which is placed between the patient's thighs. The packing and the hemostatic bag may have to be removed in the operating room at a later date. Sometimes only a Penrose drain in the abdominal incision is all that is judged necessary. It is usually removed after 36 hours. Special urethrostomy cups may have to be used in these cases to keep the patient dry and to collect urine for measurement. If a cystostomy tube is present, it is removed 3 to 4 days postoperatively. The indwelling catheter usually stays until the abdominal incision is nearly healed. The suprapubic incision may take time to heal. The nurse will need to have skill in keeping the patient dry and odorless. Bladder spasm is a frequent difficulty to these patients. Usually the muscles become fatigued in 24 to 48 hours and the bladder spasms become fewer. Recovery may be prolonged, since ambulation is slower.

RETROPUBIC PROSTATECTOMY. This method is preferred by some surgeons. Urinary results are excellent and potency is maintained. An abdominal incision is made above the bladder. The bladder is not incised, but the surgeon dissects down between the pubis and the bladder to reach the prostate. The capsule is opened and the tissue is removed. A large Foley catheter is inserted postoperatively. Since the bladder has not been opened, discharge on the abdominal dressing should not contain urine. If it does, the surgeon should be notified. The postoperative care is the same as for any prostatectomy patient. These patients seem to have fewer bladder spasms and less difficulty voiding.

PERINEAL PROSTATECTOMY. In a perineal prostatectomy the surgeon excises the prostate through a semicircular incision in the perineal body. The prostatic capsule is opened and the gland is removed. The pre- and postoperative care resembles that of other prostatectomies. A perineal shave preparation will be necessary. Because of the risk of rectourethral fistula, the large bowel may be surgically prepared preoperatively (p. 374). Unfortunately, after this operation is performed the patient may be impotent, and some difficulty may be experienced in establishing urinary continence following surgery.

Carcinoma of the Prostate

Carcinoma of the prostate gland is one of the most common tumors seen in men. Perhaps 20 per cent of all malignancies in the adult male are due to prostatic lesions. It is frequently seen in association with benign hyperplasia but does not result from it. Because of its frequency and the fact that early diagnosis can be made in many cases by a rectal examination, all men should be advised to have an annual checkup after the age of 40. Nurses are advised to include this advice whenever it is related in their health teaching to the community.

Signs and Symptoms. The symptoms are essentially those of benign enlargement of the prostate. On rectal examination, the surgeon palpates a hard nodule. Since the nodule may resemble other conditions, a biopsy is often done. Two types are commonly used. A *needle biopsy* is safely done on an outpatient basis. The perineum is cleansed and draped. The surgeon palpates the nodule with one finger in the rectum, and simultaneously guides a needle, passed through the perineum, to the site. Several samples are usually collected. On discharge, the patient is instructed to watch the injection site for signs of redness, pain and swelling and to report their occurrence to his physi-

cian. This technique is not judged to be as complete as *direct biopsy*. Under anesthesia, the perineum is cleansed, and a small incision is made. Direct biopsy of the prostate is made and sent to the laboratory. If immediate results are positive, a prostatectomy may be done before the patient leaves the operating room. If negative, the incision is closed, and the surgeon awaits the more extensive laboratory report. Because of the possibility of an immediate prostatectomy, the patient is prepared for the operating room as if he were undergoing major surgery.

Classification, Treatment and Nursing Care. Carcinoma of the prostate is classified into four stages. These stages are based on the results of rectal examinations, serum acid phosphatase levels, x-rays of the skeleton and metastases. Stage I or carcinoma in situ is often called latent, or focal. Usually there are no symptoms. In Stage II the nodule may be palpated on rectal examination. When Stage III is reached, the growth has spread to the seminal vesicles, the base of the bladder and outside the prostatic capsule, but no distant metastases are present and acid phosphatase levels are probably not elevated significantly. Serum acid phosphatase is normally very high in prostatic secretions, however it does not circulate in the blood. With Stage IV carcinoma excessive levels of serum acid phosphatase are produced which are circulated in the blood stream. Previously the thick prostatic capsule has kept the lesion localized and prevented spread into the abdominal cavity. Now the blood and lymphatics carry the disease to distant sites. The bones of the pelvis are most frequently affected. Also, because of bone and liver involvement, severe anemia may occur, accompanied by the other symptoms of a terminal disease.

Stages I and II are treatable. Stages III and IV usually receive palliative therapy. Treatment is by radical prostatectomy by the retropubic or perineal routes. The entire gland and seminal vesicles are removed. The bladder neck is sutured to the urethral stump. A large Foley catheter is inserted which serves as a splint for the urethra as well as a drain for the bladder. Drains may be placed in the incision lines as well. Pre- and postoperative care are similar to that of any prostatectomy.

Incontinence may follow temporarily or

on a longer basis. Immediately after the operation the man may be incontinent of feces as well. The patient is usually greatly relieved to be assured that this is usually temporary and that control can be regained by practicing perineal floor tightening and relaxing a few times periodically throughout the day. This also aids in the re-establishment of urinary continence. Some surgeons ban the use of incontinence clamps or bags, feeling that the patient comes to rely on them and will never regain function. In particularly resistant cases, a prosthesis with an inflatable bulb may be inserted below the urethra in an attempt to restore normal anatomy. Hopefully, this will restore continence.

If the perineal route was used, care must be taken to avoid infection. The incision must be kept clean by frequent cleansing following bowel movements. A heat lamp may be ordered for several days postoperatively. The scrotum may be elevated on an adhesive bridge in order to acquire adequate exposure of the incision. In the presence of hemorrhoids, a heat lamp is usually contraindicated.

In Stages III and IV palliative therapy usually includes the administration of estrogens and an orchiectomy because carcinoma of the prostate is aggravated by androgens. The effect of estrogens may distress the man as he may have swelling of breast tissue and some nausea and vomiting. This combination of estrogens and orchiectomy (removal of testes) may produce good results for about 18 months. Then the adrenals seem to recover from the estrogen induced hormonal imbalance and begin producing androgens again. Cortisone may be given now in an attempt to depress this source of androgens. In extreme situations an adrenalectomy may be performed. Deep x-ray therapy reduces discomfort from bone metastases. Radioactive phosphate given orally or intravenously also lodges in the bone, bringing relief from pain. In the case of a bladder obstruction, a transurethral prostatectomy is done. Since the operation is merely palliative, no attempt is made to remove all of the growth.

The patient will require nursing care related to the special needs of the terminally ill and to the aforementioned prostatectomy therapies.

Carcinoma of the Testes and Penis

Most tumors of the testes are malignant. However, only about 0.5 per cent of all malignancies occur in this area. Frequently, the man is in the prime of his reproductive years. Treatment is bilateral orchiectomy.

Malignancies of the penis are essentially malignancies of the skin. The glans and prepuce are nearly always affected. The development of carcinoma of the penis seems to be directly related to chronic infections of the area. The disease is also less frequent among circumcised men. Treatment is by excision of the affected areas or by partial or total amputation of the penis, depending on the progression of the condition.

BENIGN AND MALIGNANT DISORDERS OF THE FEMALE REPRODUCTIVE TRACT

Polyps

Polyps are common benign growths occurring mainly in the endometrium and cervix. The polyp has a characteristic smooth, shiny surface and is pink to deep red in color. They are small in size, seldom exceeding more than 3 cm. in length. The cause is unknown. No symptoms are usually present, but occasionally postcoital bleeding occurs. Treatment is by surgical excision of cervical polyps and may be followed by dilatation and curettage to remove endometrial polyps. The patient receives nursing care as for minor vaginal surgery.

Myomas of the Uterus

A myoma (fibromyoma, liomyoma) is a benign tumor of the uterus composed of myometrium and fibrous tissue. Colloquially, myomas are known as "fibroids." At least one-quarter of women over 35 years of age show some evidence of myomas. The cause is unknown.

Myomas occur mainly in the uterine body. According to their position they are classified as subserous, submucous and intramural (Fig. 19–18) and may become pedunculated. A pedunculated fibroid in the uterine cavity may be referred to as a fibroid polyp. This may be extruded through the cervix and may

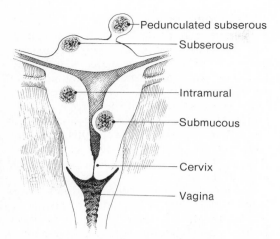

Figure 19–18 Uterine fibroids.

come to lie in the vagina. Myomas in the broad ligament or cervix are recorded, but these locations are rare. Several fibroids of varying sizes may be present in any one uterus. As the fibroids become larger, their blood supply may be reduced, causing some degeneration. The most common is a hyaline degeneration in the middle of the myoma. This causes a loss of cellular structure and, in extreme cases, a collection of gelatinous fluid lies at the center. Sometimes the tumor shows signs of fatty changes and may even become calcified (womb-stone). A so-called red degeneration may occur usually in association with pregnancy. The tumor looks like raw beef on the inside. The patient shows signs of malaise with fever, rapid pulse and pain over the fibroid. Following the menopause all myomas atrophy and show slight shrinkage.

Signs and Symptoms. Symptoms vary with the size and location of the tumor. Frequently with small tumors, there are no symptoms. Occasionally hypermenorrhea occurs. Pain is rarely a symptom but most frequently is associated with torsion of a pedunculated myoma. Sometimes the myoma passing through the cervix causes cramps. Secondary dysmenorrhea may occur as a result of mechanical interference. Large myomas can cause frequency or retention of urine. Pressure on veins, lymphatics, and nerves of the pelvis may cause varicosities, unilateral or bilateral edema of the lower extremities, or a radiating pain through the thighs. Occasionally, these tu-

mors may be the cause of abortions or infertility. Some tumors become infected.

Treatment. Treatment depends on the age of the woman, her desire for more children and the size of the myoma. In the young woman who wishes children, a myomectomy is usually done. This is the enucleation of the myoma, but the uterus is retained. Blood loss during the operation may be extensive as the surgeon excises multiple myomas from a large uterus which may not contract efficiently. Persistent oozing of blood may occur postoperatively for the same reasons. The nurse should be alert to this possibility. In cases of very large myomas the treatment is hysterectomy.

In the young woman, myomas are not a contraindication to pregnancy and usually cause no difficulty. Rarely, they may obstruct labor or cause a postpartum hemorrhage.

Tumors of the Ovary

Tumors of the ovary are many and varied. The etiology of most is unknown. For purposes of clarity they are roughly divided into non-neoplasms and neoplasms. Only a few are described in each group.

Non-neoplasms. Non-neoplasms are usually simple cysts or collections of fluid surrounded by a thin capsule. They do not grow but expand only as more fluid accumulates. These physiologic cysts are seen mainly during the reproductive years. The follicular cyst is the most common of this group. Corpus luteum cysts may occur as well. Theca lutein cysts develop under the stimulation of high levels of chorionic gonadotrophins.

Occasionally, the Stein-Leventhal syndrome or polycystic disease of the ovary is distinguished. The syndrome appears in the late teens and early twenties with variable symptoms. These may include a history of sterility, secondary amenorrhea, hirsutism and bilateral cysts in the ovary. The ovary shows some enlargement and presents a glistening white appearance. Microscopically, many atretic follicular cysts are present. The syndrome is thought to follow an endocrine imbalance probably arising in the ovary but affecting the hypothalamus. Treatment is usually surgical, and a wedge resection of the ovary is performed. Ovulation, menstruation and pregnancy may follow a wedge resection in a sizable proportion of cases. The nursing of the patient is the same as that for any patient undergoing abdominal surgery.

Neoplasms. Pseudomucinous cystadenomas are the single most common neoplasms, occurring in about 40 per cent of patients with a neoplastic ovarian growth. Also, they may attain the largest size of any ovarian tumor. The tumor is characterized by multiple pockets filled with a thick fluid called pseudomucin. They may be bilateral and may become malignant.

Serous cystadenoma is the second most common of this group and appears to arise from germinal epithelium. The cyst contains a serous fluid. These cysts are frequently bilateral and frequently become malignant.

The dermoid cyst or teratoma may be cystic or solid. When it is soft, the cyst is filled with sebaceous material, hair and ordinary skin. The solid cyst frequently contains cartilage, bone, teeth, thyroid, and similar material. Rarely is the cyst malignant. It occurs most frequently in young women and may be bilateral.

Neoplasms of the ovary may also be divided into those which have some hormonal effect and those which do not. One tumor with no hormonal effect is a *dysgerminoma*. It arises from the primitive germ cells and is usually malignant. A *fibroma* is a benign solid neoplasm occurring most frequently in the postmenopausal patient. The fibroma arises from connective tissue in the ovary and may be associated with Meig's syndrome, which is characterized by ascites and pleural effusion.

Those tumors which have hormonal effects may be further subdivided into feminizing and virilizing lesions. The most common of the rare feminizing tumors is the *granulosa cell tumor.* The tumor produces estrogen and may induce precocious puberty or cause hypermenorrhea or post-menopausal bleeding. It may be malignant or may be associated with carcinoma of the endometrium. The most common of the even rarer masculinizing tumors is *arrhenoblastoma.* By the production of androgens, presumably from the primitive male cell elements in the ovary, the woman is masculinized. In about 15 to 25 per cent of cases it proves to be malignant.

Carcinoma of the Ovary

Primary carcinoma of the ovary is usually the common adenocarcinoma. However, a review of ovarian growths is indicated, as almost any one of them has the potential to become malignant. The most common malignancy arises from the serous cystadenoma. Only one ovary may be affected, but the other quickly follows, apparently because of the close lymphatic connections. About 5 per cent of all cancers in the female arise in the ovary.

Secondary tumors represent metastases from almost any other cancer. However, the Krukenberg tumor deserves mention. In this case bilateral, equal involvement is usually secondary to tumors in the stomach or gallbladder. Backup of the lymphatic drainage appears responsible for this particular tumor, especially since other metastases usually occur later.

Signs and Symptoms. The ovarian tumor in its early stages is often symptomless. The symptoms commonly result from the size of the tumor or its position. An increase in girth may be noticed but ignored. Pressure on the bladder causes frequency or a feeling of fullness. Constipation, edema of the legs, anorexia and a full feeling in the abdomen may be present. Pain may be associated with stretching of the tissues as the tumor enlarges. Ascites may be present, accompanied by difficulty in breathing. At regular yearly checkups, palpation of the adnexa will reveal a mass. Often this may be the first discovery of the tumor.

Treatment. Because of the danger of malignant growth, any ovarian mass is observed suspiciously. A rule of thumb says that any soft mass below 5 cm. may be watched closely for 2 to 3 months. If no further growth occurs, then conservative treatment may be considered. Other tumors demand biopsy, and a laparotomy is indicated. Following diagnosis, the surgeon strives to preserve as much ovarian function as is possible. In premenopausal women benign growths, if size permits, will be enucleated and ovarian function retained. Malignant growths are treated with total hysterectomy and bilateral salpingo-oophorectomy (removal of the tubes and ovaries). Surgery is followed by irradiation. Unfortunately, many malignancies have metastasized before discovery of the tumor. Prognosis is poor and surgery may only be palliative. Further treatment is directed toward relieving the symptoms of the terminally ill patient. Recurrent ascites may be a problem, and frequent paracentesis may be indicated. Occasionally intraperitoneal colloidal gold or chemotherapy will be used.

Complications of Ovarian Tumors. Torsion or twisting of the growth on its stalk frequently occurs. Circulation is impeded, and necrosis may follow. The patient usually feels a sudden severe pain in the lower abdomen. Treatment is by excision of the tumor at an immediate laparotomy.

The cyst may rupture. Often the "chocolate cyst" of endometriosis ruptures and drains fluid into the abdomen. Again the patient may present with an "acute abdomen."

Hemorrhage and infection occur in tumors as well. Usually, they are more common in the malignant tumor.

Postsurgical menopause is the result of a bilateral oophorectomy. The symptoms are similar to those of the regular menopause, but may be more severe because of the sudden withdrawal of hormones. Replacement therapy with estrogens may begin before the patient leaves the hospital if it is not contraindicated by malignancies which are aggravated by estrogens.

Carcinoma of the Cervix

Carcinoma of the cervix is the second most frequent malignancy in women. The woman who has borne children, married young, or had an early active sex life with several partners and some degree of chronic cervicitis is more apt to develop the disease. Poor hygiene in the uncircumcised male also seems to raise the incidence of the disease in women. The woman is more likely to be above the age of 35.

Because 5-year survival rates are excellent in those cases which are discovered early, all women over the age of 25 should have yearly medical examinations and Pap smears (p. 88). The nurse has a responsibility to disseminate this knowledge. The nurse should dwell on the hopeful aspects of cure following cases of early recognition. This may encourage more women to seek medical attention by reducing their anxiety, since knowledge does not always ensure that the patient will seek medical attention. Fear of what she may discover often seems to prevent the patient from consulting her physician. The nurse should do her utmost to persuade the woman confiding irregular bleeding to her to seek medical attention immediately.

Signs and Symptoms. The malignant change usually occurs at the squamocolumnar junction of the cervix (Fig. 19–19). A small lesion develops which, in the early stages, can be confused with other cervical conditions. The early stages may be asymptomatic, but eventually some bleeding from the vagina occurs. An unusual vaginal discharge may be present. This may become foul smelling, suggesting an infection. Pain is a late symptom and is followed by weight loss, anorexia and cachexia.

Carcinoma of the cervix is divided into stages. Stage 0 is carcinoma in situ, or focal carcinoma. The only symptoms are histologic. Stage I is carcinoma confined to the cervix. A small lesion similar to an erosion is present. In Stage II the carcinoma has spread to close adjacent structures, and the upper third of the vagina may be involved. By Stage III invasion has reached the pelvic walls and lower vagina. Stage IV is marked by extensive pelvic involvement, including the bladder or bowel, and distant metastases may be present.

Treatment and Nursing Care. Treatment is usually guided by the stage assigned to the situation by the physician. Since the main method of diagnosing Stage 0 car-

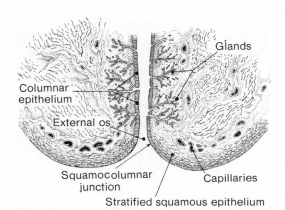

Figure 19–19 Squamocolumnar junction of the cervix.

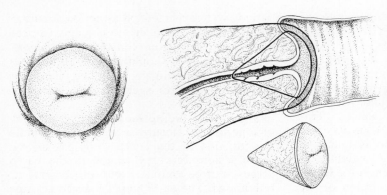

Figure 19–20 Cone biopsy of the cervix.

cinoma is the Pap smear, the results of this test help to guide treatment. In Classes I and II the cells are nonmalignant, and no treatment is usually necessary. Classes III and IV are usually followed by a biopsy.

A *punch biopsy* may be done with special punch biopsy forceps. Because of the paucity of nerve endings in the cervix, the biopsy may be done with relative comfort for the patient. She may feel something like a pinch when the biopsy is taken. A Schiller test can be done. Normally the cervix contains glycogen. This is depleted in areas of abnormal cell change. When Lugol's solution (iodine in potassium iodide) is swabbed on the cervix, the normal epithelium stains a dark brown. Glycogen-deficient areas are a pale color by contrast, and these are the areas biopsied.

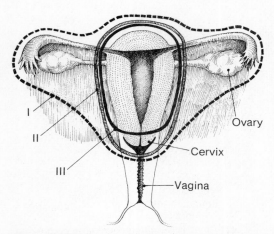

Figure 19–21 Types of hysterectomy. I: total hysterectomy with bilateral salpingo-oophorectomy (pan-hysterectomy). II: total hysterectomy. III: subtotal hysterectomy.

Further treatment may be a *cone biopsy*. It is an operative procedure in which a cone-shaped segment of the central cervix is removed. The internal os remains intact (Fig. 19–20). On examination the section may contain all of the malignant area. In these cases the biopsy may be considered sufficient treatment. Pre- and postoperative care for the biopsy is similar to any minor vaginal surgery. The major difference is that these patients face the threat of a malignant disease and may be extremely anxious. Considerable skill in providing supportive nursing will be demanded of the nurse.

In older patients a total hysterectomy and bilateral salpingo-oophorectomy (panhysterectomy) is often performed following a positive Pap smear or biopsy (Fig. 19–21). A total hysterectomy includes removal of the cervix and the upper third of the vagina. A subtotal hysterectomy includes removal of only the uterine corpus and the upper portion of the cervix, leaving a generous vaginal cuff. Some surgeons prefer to remove the cervix at every hysterectomy because of the possibility of carcinoma arising in the cervical stump at a later date.

The patient is prepared as for abdominal surgery. A perineal shave preparation may be ordered as well, and the mons pubis, vulva, perineal body, and the upper third of the thighs are shaved. Postoperatively, any vaginal discharge must be observed. Some staining may occur from the vaginal cuff. A Foley catheter may be inserted and may remain in place for 1 or 2 days postoperatively. The nurse should be alert to possible signs of hormonal imbalance following removal of the ovaries as well as signs of a urinary tract infection and thromboemboli.

Later stages of carcinoma will be treated with radical surgery, such as the Wertheim's operation. In this operation a total hysterectomy, bilateral salpingo-oophorectomy, partial vaginectomy and pelvic lymph node dissection are performed. Extensive dissection is required. Often the ureters and bladder have been handled and may be atonic following surgery. Care must be taken to see that the catheter is draining properly and that bladder distention does not occur. Early ambulation is encouraged. Special attention should be directed toward observing for signs of thromboemboli postoperatively. Femoral areas as well as the calves should be observed. Otherwise, the postoperative care is the same as that for other surgical patients.

In even more extreme cases, a pelvic exenteration may be done. This operation includes all of the Wertheim's operation plus a total vaginectomy and removal of bladder and bowel. The patient may return postoperatively with an ileostomy, a colostomy or an ileal conduit. Nursing care for such conditions is elaborated elsewhere (p. 377). In these operations preoperative bowel preparations are done. Postoperatively, drains may be left in areas of node dissection to prevent the pooling of blood and serum which may easily lead to infection. The drains may be draining freely or may be attached to suction. Usually they are advanced daily and removed by the fifth postoperative day.

The postoperative adjustment to life may be difficult. Preoperative discussions with the physician and nurse should help to prepare the patient. Sexual function is lost. The menopause may occur as estrogen therapy is frequently contraindicated. The care of the colostomy or ileostomy must be learned and accepted. The patient will require much understanding and support from the nursing staff while the nurses gently encourage her to retain as much independence as is compatible with her situation.

Frequently external and internal radiation therapy is used in conjunction with, or instead of, surgery for these patients. Radium in special containers is inserted into the cervical canal and into the lateral fornices of the vagina. The insertion of the radium is an operative procedure. The patient receives a cleansing enema the day before and a perineal shave preparation. During the procedure a urinary catheter with a small bag is passed. This prevents a distended bladder from coming into contact with the radium which would greatly increase the chance of a vesicovaginal fistula. After the radium is inserted, packing is placed in the vagina and may be sutured in place to maintain the position of the radium. Postoperatively the patient remains on bed rest with head and shoulders nearly flat. A slipper bedpan is used, and straining at stool is discouraged. The catheter is checked to ensure that it is draining. These measures help to ensure that the radium remains where it has been placed. Complaints of pain and any bloody discharge should be reported to the physician. The time for removal should be carefully observed. Removal may be uncomfortable for the patient because of the tight packing, and the patient may need an analgesic for this. Care must be taken to dispose of the radium in a safe manner. The nurse must also protect herself while taking care of the patient and must teach visitors to protect themselves as well. The patient and her family will need explanations of the procedures and understanding from the nurse. In later observations the nurse watches for signs of radiation sickness (p. 92). Also, any leaking of urine may indicate a fistula is forming and should be reported to the physician.

Carcinoma of the Endometrium

This is also a frequently occurring malignancy. Symptoms may be delayed until the disease has made considerable progress. A painless, bloody vaginal discharge may be the first sign of any abnormality. Treatment is surgical removal of the involved structures. Where radium is inserted, several containers attached to strings may be placed in the body of the uterus to irradiate the endometrium.

Carcinoma of the Vagina and Uterine Tubes

Both of these conditions are rare. Treatment is by surgical excision.

Carcinoma of the Vulva

Carcinoma of the vulva is a less frequent malignancy, occurring mainly among women in their fifth and sixth decades of life. It is frequently preceded by such conditions as leukoplakia or chronic ulceration of the vulva. Because of the possibility of these lesions becoming cancerous, the physician may elect to treat them by a simple vulvectomy which removes only the vulva. Carcinoma, however, is treated by radical vulvectomy. Here the dissection is extensive for the clitoris, labia and all the perineal subcutaneous tissue; all the perineal glands and the femoral and inguinal lymphatics are removed.

Preoperative preparation includes all the measures common for perineal and abdominal surgery. The patient and nursing staff may react with repugnance at the thought of this surgery. It is frequently seen as mutilating. However, the results of the operation are quite favorable. Sexual function is retained, as the vagina is not removed. Young women have conceived following simple vulvectomy and have been delivered by cesarean section.

Postoperatively, the patient returns to the ward with an indwelling catheter. Much edema is present, and great care must be taken not to dislodge the catheter. It may be very difficult to replace. The operation may be done in two stages or all at once. In the former, the patient returns with an open area, requiring future skin grafting. Barrier isolation may be required for this patient both before and after skin grafting. A bed cradle over the pubic area will keep bed linen away. When the procedure is completed in one operation the patient may return with a bulky pressure dressing held in place by a **T** binding. In other cases there are bilateral stab wounds near the iliac fossa containing drains which are attached to a suction machine; this arrangement may replace the pressure bandage. Thus, the fluid is drained away and the skin flap is kept in close approximation to the underlying tissue so that it becomes firmly attached to the tissue. Some necrosis along the incision lines may be expected, and occasionally skin grafting may be necessary to replace a necrotic area. The stitches are usually not removed for 2 to 3 weeks. Close observation must be maintained for thromboemboli. Once ambulation is begun, the patient may need elastic stockings to avoid swelling of her legs. Standing for long periods of time should be avoided.

References

BOOKS

Behrman, S. J., and Gosling, J. R.: Fundamentals of Gynecology, 2nd ed. New York, Oxford University Press, 1966.

——————————: Birth Control Handbook. Montreal, Students' Society of McGill University, September, 1969.

Ellis, H., and Calne, R. Y.: Lecture Notes on General Surgery. Oxford, Blackwell Scientific Publications, 1966.

Eastman, N. J., and Hellman, L. M.: Williams Obstetrics, 13th ed. New York, Appleton-Century-Crofts, 1966.

Everett, H. S., and Ridley, J. H.: Female Urology. New York, Harper and Row, 1968.

Fitzpatrick, G. M.: Gynecologic Nursing. New York, The Macmillan Co., 1965.

Garland, G., and Quixley, J.: Obstetrics and Gynaecology for Nurses. London, English Universities Press Ltd., 1956.

Guyton, A. C.: Textbook of Medical Physiology, 4th ed. Philadelphia, W. B. Saunders Co., 1971.

Hamilton, W. J., Boyd, J. D., and Mossman, H. W.: Human Embryology. Baltimore, The Williams and Wilkins Co., 1962.

Jacob, S. W., and Francone, C. A.: Structure and Function in Man, 2nd ed. Philadelphia, W. B. Saunders Co., 1970.

Jeffcoate, T. N. A.: Principles of Gynaecology. London, Butterworth and Co., Ltd., 1957.

Lockhart, R. D., Hamilton, G. F., and Fyfe, F. W.: Anatomy of the Human Body. London, Faber and Faber Ltd., 1959.

Loraine, J. A., and Bell, E. T.: Fertility and Contraception in the Human Female. Edinburgh, E. and S. Livingstone Ltd., 1968.

Masters, Wm. H., and Johnson, V. E.: Human Sexual Response. Boston, Little, Brown and Co., 1966.

Myles, M.: Textbook for Midwives, 6th ed. Edinburgh, E. and S. Livingstone Ltd., 1968.

Novak, R., and Woodruff, J. D.: Novak's Gynecologic and Obstetric Pathology, 6th ed. Philadelphia, W. B. Saunders Co., 1967.

Sawyer, J. R.: Nursing Care of Patients with Urologic Diseases. St. Louis, The C. V. Mosby Co., 1963.

Smith, D. R.: General Urology. Los Altos, Lange Medical Publications, 1966.

Te Linde, R. W.: Operative Gynecology, 2nd ed. Philadelphia, J. B. Lippincott Co., 1953.

Thomas, J. B.: Introduction to Human Embryology. Philadelphia, Lea and Febiger, 1968.

PERIODICALS

Alford, D. M.: "Nursing Care of the Patient with Endometriosis." Nurs. Clin. North Amer. Vol. 3, No. 2 (June 1968), pp. 217–27.

Barglow, P., et al.: "Hysterectomy and Tubal Ligation: A Psychiatric Comparison." Obstet. & Gynecol., Vol. 25, No. 4 (April 1965), pp. 520–27.

Bennett, E. A.: "Abortion." Nurs. Clin. North Amer., Vol. 3, No. 2 (June 1968), pp. 243–51.

Berry, J. L.: "Postprostatectomy Urinary Incontinence and Some Experiences with the Berry Procedure." Surg. Clin. North Amer., Vol. 45, No. 6 (Dec. 1965), pp. 1481.

Blanchet, J.: "Estrogen and the Menopause." Canad. Nurse, Vol. 63, No. 2 (Feb. 1967), pp. 38–39.

Cavanagh, D.: "The Vaginal Examination." Hosp. Med., Vol. 5, No. 1 (Jan. 1969), pp. 35–51.

Clark, M. M., and Storrs, J. A.: "The Prevention of Postoperative Vomiting After Abortion: Metoclopramide." Brit. J. Anaesth., Vol. 41 (Oct. 1969), pp. 890–93.

Doe, R., and Seal, U.: "Acid Phosphatase in Urology." Surg. Clin. North Amer., Vol. 45, No. 6 (Dec. 1965), pp. 1455.

Dumas, R. C., et al.: "The Importance of the Expressive Function in Preoperative Preparation." *In* Skipper, J. K., and Leonard, R. C. (Eds.): Social Interaction and Patient Care. Philadelphia, J. B. Lippincott Co., 1965.

Durbin, Sister M. S.: "Geriatric Gynecology." Nurs. Clin. North Amer., Vol. 3, No. 2 (June 1968), pp. 253–61.

Frank, I.: "The Cytodiagnosis of Prostatic Carcinoma." J.A.M.A., Vol. 209, No. 11 (Sept. 15, 1969), pp. 1698.

Franklin, R. R., and McIlhaney, J. S.: "Anomalies of the Female Genital Tract." Nurs. Clin. North Amer., Vol. 3, No. 2 (June 1968), pp. 205–15.

Goldfarb, A. F., and Crawford, R.: "Polycystic Ovarian Disease, Clomiphene, and Multiple Pregnancies." Obstet. & Gynecol., Vol. 34, No. 3 (Sept. 1969), pp. 307–9.

Gonder, M.: "Prostatitis." Surg. Clin. North Amer., Vol. 45, No. 6 (Dec. 1965), pp. 1449.

Gray, L.: "Views and Reviews, Indications, Techniques and Complications in Vaginal Hysterectomy." Obstet. & Gynecol., Vol. 28, No. 5 (Nov. 1966), pp. 714–22.

Green, T.: "Radical Vulvectomy." Clin. Obstet. & Gynec., Vol. 8, No. 3 (Sept. 1965), pp. 642.

Greenblatt, R. M.: "Infertility." Seminar Report, Vol. 5, No. 5 (Winter 1960), p. 9 (Edited by Merck, Sharp and Dohme Research Laboratories).

Gunn, A. D. G.: "The Legal Termination of Pregnancy." Nurs. Times, Vol. 65, No. 36 (Sept. 4, 1969), pp. 1130–32.

Haltiwanger, E.: "Management of Benign Prostatic Hypertrophy." Surg. Clin. North Amer., Vol. 45, No. 6 (Dec. 1965), pp. 1441.

Hofmeister, F. J., and Reik, R. P.: "Vulvectomy." Amer J. Nurs., Vol. 60, No. 5 (May 1960), pp. 666–68.

Jordan, W. P.: "Hydroceles and Varicoceles." Surg. Clin. North Amer., Vol. 45, No. 6 (Dec. 1965), pp. 1535–46.

Lane, M. E.: "Emotional Aspects of Contraception." Bull. Amer. Coll. Nurse-Midwives, Vol. 15 No. 1 (Feb. 1970), pp. 16–25.

MacLean, M. A.: "Carcinoma of the Cervix." Canad. Nurse, Vol. 61, No. 12 (Dec. 1965), pp. 968–71.

McEwan, D. C.: "Estrogen Replacement Therapy at Menopause." Canad. Nurse, Vol. 63, No. 2 (Feb. 1967), pp. 32–6.

Maudsley, R. F., and Robertson, M. B.: "Common Complications of Hysterectomy." Canad. Med. Ass. J., Vol. 92 (April 24, 1965), pp. 908–11.

Mayo, P., and Wilkey, N.: "Prevention of Carcinoma of the Breast and Cervix." Nurs. Clin. North Amer., Vol. 3, No. 2 (June 1968), pp. 229–41.

Mellinger, G. T.: "Carcinoma of the Prostate." Surg. Clin. North Amer., Vol. 45, No. 6 (Dec. 1965), pp. 1413.

Montagu, G. B.: "Psychiatric Illness After Hysterectomy." Brit. Med. J., Vol. 2 (April 1968), pp. 91–5.

Prout, G. R.: "Chemical Tests in the Diagnosis of Prostatic Cancer." J.A.M.A., Vol. 209, No. 11 (Sept. 15, 1969), pp. 1699.

Shipkowitz, I., and Mengert, Wm.: "Urinary Bladder Care After Vaginal Operation." Amer. J. Obstet. & Gynec., Vol. 97 (Mar. 15, 1967), pp. 828.

Spivak, M. M.: "Therapeutic Abortion. A Twelve-Year Review at Toronto General Hospital, 1954–65." Amer. J. Obstet. & Gynec., Vol. 97 (Feb. 1, 1967), pp. 316.

Sturgis, S. H.: "Treatment of Ovarian Insufficiency." Amer. J. Nurs., Vol. 64, No. 1 (Jan. 1964), pp. 113–16.

Tan, P., Ratnam, S. S., and Quek, S. P.: "Vacuum Aspiration in the Treatment of Incomplete Abortion." J. Obstet. & Gynaec. Brit. Comm., Vol. 76 (Sept. 1969), pp. 834–36.

Valk, Wm. L., and Melsust, W. K.: "The Management of the Prostatic Nodule." J.A.M.A., Vol. 209, No. 11 (Sept. 15, 1969), pp. 1697.

Walker, A. H. C.: "Why Perform a Hysterectomy?" Nurs. Times, Vol. 63 (Jan. 6, 1967), pp. 12–14.

Williams, T. J.: "Preoperative and Postoperative Care in Radical Pelvic Surgery." Clin. Obstet. & Gynec., Vol. 8, No. 3 (Sept. 1965), pp. 629.

20
Nursing in Disorders of the Breast

THE NORMAL BREAST

The breasts, or mammary glands, lie on the anterior chest wall. The base of each rests on the fascia of the pectoralis major muscle, and supporting ligaments extend from the skin through the breast to the fascia. They are undeveloped in both sexes until puberty. At this time, the female breasts enlarge and develop secreting cells and ducts in response to increased concentrations of ovarian and certain adenohypophyseal (anterior pituitary) hormones. Estrogen is responsible for the growth of the duct system, and the luteotrophic hormone and progesterone are considered the chief stimulants for the development of the secreting cells. The cylindrical projection on the skin surface forms the nipple, which is perforated by duct orifices. The pinkish area of skin around it is referred to as the areola; it becomes markedly pigmented during pregnancy and retains the darker color following delivery. The male breasts remain rudimentary throughout life.

Following growth and maturation, the female breast is composed of 15 to 20 lobes, each with a duct that opens on to the surface of the nipple. Each lobe consists of clusters of secreting cells which form lobules. The main ducts (lactiferous ducts) are formed by the union of smaller ducts which drain the lobules. They are dilated just before entering the base of the nipple to form reservoirs, or ampullae, for the milk during active secretion. The lobes and ducts are separated and supported by areolar, fibrous and fatty tissues. The size of the breasts is mainly determined by the amount of fatty tissue rather than by glandular tissue.

The blood supply to the breasts is abundant and is derived from the internal mam-

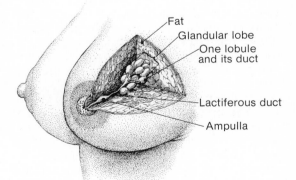

Figure 20–1 Section of a breast showing lobular cluster of cells and lactiferous duct.

mary arteries and branches of the thoracic and intercostal arteries. A large proportion of the lymph in the breasts is channeled through the axillary lymph nodes; the remainder drains through mediastinal nodes.

The breasts are subject to menstrual, cyclic changes associated with alterations in the concentrations of various hormones. Varying degrees of enlargement, tenderness and discomfort develop during the few days preceding menstruation and disappear in a day or two.

During pregnancy, the lobes and ducts enlarge in preparation for the secretion of milk. Lactation is the function of the breasts and occurs only after the birth of a child, continuing as long as the milk is withdrawn. After the menopause, the lobes and ducts undergo some atrophy and replacement with fibrous tissue.

DISORDERS OF THE BREASTS

The most common disorders of the breasts are fibrocystic disease, fibroadenoma, carcinoma and infection. The symptoms which most commonly lead to investigation include a lump or mass in the breast, nipple bleeding or discharge, nipple retraction, a lump (enlarged lymph node) in the axilla or supraclavicular region, change in breast contour due to dimpling or retraction of an area, pain and tenderness, an inflamed area and an ulcerated area.

Diagnostic Procedures

Investigation of the patient for breast disease includes inspection first with the arms at the side and then with them raised above the head. The size and contour of the two breasts and nipples are noted and compared. The physician looks for any discoloration, discharge, retracted areas, dilated subcutaneous veins and localized swelling. The breasts are palpated first while the patient is in the sitting position and then while she is in the supine position with a small pillow or folded towel under the shoulder on the side being examined to balance the breast upon the chest wall. The axillary and supraclavicular areas are then checked for enlarged lymph nodes. The

physician may ask the patient to stand and bend forward with her arms extended so that he may detect dimpling or retraction of an area of skin. Special diagnostic procedures used are mammography, transillumination and biopsy. A mammogram is a series of roentgenograms of the breast which are examined for any areas of increased density and, if present, their characteristics (e.g., location, size, shape, regularity of borders). Transillumination of the breast is performed in a darkened room by directing a strong, cool light upward from beneath the breasts. The examiner looks for dense areas, and the examination may be used as an aid to differentiating between a cyst and a solid mass.

Biopsy provides a specimen of tissue for cytological examination and may be obtained by aspiration, resection or excision. In the case of breast tumors, most physicians prefer an excision biopsy, since it permits an examination of the complete tumor.

Self-Examination of the Breast

Early recognition and prompt treatment of cancer offer the patient the most promise for control of the disease. Women are urged to examine their breasts monthly and to see a physician promptly if any changes are observed. They are also advised of the necessity of an annual examination by the doctor.

Every nurse has the responsibility as well as frequent opportunity to teach patients and friends the importance and the procedure of regular self-examination of the breasts. A pamphlet outlining the process is published by the National Cancer Society and is available for distribution, free of charge, from the local branches. A film demonstrating the procedure is also available from the same source.

The examination should be made regularly each month a few days after menstruation and should be continued after the menopause. With arms at the sides, the woman inspects her breasts before a mirror for symmetry in size and contour, dimpling of the skin and changes in the nipples. The process is then repeated with the arms raised above the head. She then assumes the supine position with a small pillow or folded towel under the shoulder on the same side as the breast to be examined. The arm is raised over the head and the inner half of the breast is gently palpated with the flat of the fingers for any mass. The arm is lowered to the side and the outer half of the breast is palpated. The process is then repeated with the other breast.

FIBROCYSTIC DISEASE (MAMMARY DYSPLASIA)

This is a relatively common disorder of the female breast and is characterized predominantly by fibroplasia, epithelial hyperplasia and the formation of cysts. It is attributed to a hormonal imbalance, is usually bilateral and occurs most often in women 30 to 50 years of age with a higher incidence in those approaching menopause. A painless mass is usually the first and only manifestation; occasionally there may be some tenderness. The patient may experience more severe soreness and pain of the breasts than is usual in the premenstrual period.

The cysts may be aspirated under local anesthesia. If a solid mass is encountered or the aspirated fluid contains blood, an incisional biopsy may be done to rule out carcinoma. Following the initial aspiration, the patient is re-examined periodically and aspiration of recurrent or newly formed cysts may be necessary. The disease regresses with the onset of menopause.

FIBROADENOMA

Fibroadenoma is a benign tumor which develops most frequently in young women. It generally occurs singly, but rarely there may be more than one. Although it is not usually encapsulated, it remains localized and is freely movable. Medical authors indicate no increased tendency to subsequent carcinoma in patients who have had a fibroadenoma.

The treatment consists of local excision of the tumor, which is submitted for cytological examination for confirmation of the diagnosis of nonmalignancy.

CARCINOMA

The breast is the most common site of cancer in the female. The incidence is high;

approximately 4 per cent of adult women develop the disease,[1] and it accounts for a large number of deaths annually. It rarely occurs under the age of 25 years, and the incidence progressively increases with age.

Most breast cancers originate in the epithelial tissue of the ducts; the remainder arise from the secreting cells of the lobules. The cause is unknown. As with cancer of other areas, heredity may have some influence as there is significant evidence of familial incidence; that is, a person is more likely to develop cancer of the breast if there is a family history of the disease.[2] Many malignant tumors of the breast appear to be influenced by ovarian hormones, especially estrogen. It has been demonstrated that some patients with cancer of the breast have a remission of their disease when the estrogen concentration is reduced by oophorectomy, adrenalectomy, hypophysectomy or by the administration of androgens (male hormones).

Manifestations

The earliest symptom is generally a single, painless, nontender mass which is poorly circumscribed and may have a nodular surface. It is usually discovered by the patient when bathing or during a routine examination. Other symptoms which may develop include a change in the size or contour of the affected breast, retraction of the nipple or an area of the skin over the breast, bleeding or discharge from the nipple, a scaly rash around the nipple, enlargement of axillary or supraclavicular lymph nodes or a bleeding, ulcerated area on the breast surface.

As the cancer grows, it spreads to adjacent tissues, such as the skin and underlying fascia and muscle. Retraction is due to involvement of the supporting fibrous tissue; there is a proliferation of fibroblasts and ensuing scar tissue within the breast and fascia of the chest muscles. The breast becomes firmer and cannot be moved as freely. Ulceration is associated with advanced disease which has spread to involve the skin.

---

[1] C. D. Haagensen: Carcinoma of the Breast (Monograph). New York, American Cancer Society, Inc., 1958, p. 12.

[2] R. T. Shackleford: Diagnosis of Surgical Disease. Philadelphia, W. B. Saunders Co., 1968, Vol. 1, p. 495.

Metastases

Cancer of the breast may spread directly into adjacent structures or may metastasize to distant structures by emboli of tumor cells being transported through the lymphatics or the blood vessels. The axillary, supra-clavicular or mediastinal lymph nodes are usually the first site of secondary involvement. Other structures which frequently become the site of metastases are the lungs, liver, spine, pelvic bones and femura.

Types of Breast Cancer

Cancers of the breast may be classified according to certain tissue changes. The most common type is scirrhous carcinoma, which is characterized by marked fibrosing and hardness. The medullary breast cancer grows rapidly, forming a larger mass, which is softer in consistency than the scirrhous type. There is less fixation of the breast. A third type which occurs rarely is known as mucoid or colloid because its cells secrete mucin. Papillary carcinoma is characterized by small papillary growths within the duct system and usually causes bleeding from the nipple. Paget's disease is an intraductal cancer that extends to involve the nipple and areola. A scaly rash and erosion of the nipple accompany this type.

Treatment

The forms of treatment used in carcinoma of the breast are surgical removal (mastectomy), radiation, alteration of hormonal concentrations either by the administration of certain hormones or by the removal of certain hormone-producing structures, and chemotherapy. The choice is influenced by the extent of the disease (that is, whether it appears to be localized or has metastasized to regional lymph nodes or distant structures), the age and general condition of the patient, and the physician's personal philosophy as to the best therapy. In relation to the latter, radical mastectomy may be advocated, or a modified radical or simple mastectomy may be the selected procedure.[3]

---

[3]D. C. Sabiston, and W. W. Shingleton: "The Surgical Management of Breast Cancer." Surg. Clin. North Amer., Vol. 46, No. 5 (Oct. 1966), pp. 1270–1276.

Surgical Treatment. Radical mastectomy is the operation adopted by most surgeons and involves removal of the complete breast, the underlying pectoralis muscles and the axillary lymphatics and lymph nodes. A large area of the overlying skin is removed, and if the remaining skin flaps cannot be approximated without a good deal of tension, a skin graft is done. The anterior surface of the thigh is usually used as the donor site.

A more conservative form of radical mastectomy in which the underlying muscles are not removed may be used (modified radical mastectomy), or a simple mastectomy which consists of removal of the breast without axillary and muscle dissection may be performed.

Radiation Therapy. External radiation therapy may be used as an adjunct to surgery or alone in cases in which the disease is advanced and inoperable or in which there is a local recurrence after surgery. For the care of the patient receiving radiation therapy, the reader is referred to page 90.

Hormonal Therapy. As cited earlier, some patients with carcinoma of the breast experience a remission of their disease when the concentration of certain hormones is altered (mainly estrogen). Their cancer is said to be hormone-dependent. Hormonal therapy is not curative but, hopefully, palliative. A change in the hormonal concentration may be achieved surgically or by the administration of certain hormones.

The patient may have an oophorectomy (removal of the ovaries), especially if she is premenopausal. This reduces the production of both estrogen and progesterone. An adrenalectomy or hypophysectomy may also be done to decrease the production of estrogen if the patient has shown a favorable response to an oophorectomy. The patient who has an adrenalectomy will require cortisone replacement therapy (see p. 559 for care following adrenalectomy). If a complete hypophysectomy is done, the administration of cortisone and thyroid extract will be necessary, because of the removal of the respective trophic hormones (ACTH and TSH), as well as a pitressin preparation to replace the antidiuretic hormone (ADH).

The administration of an androgen (male hormone) such as testosterone may be prescribed alone or in conjunction with one of the above surgical procedures. Androgen therapy is likely to cause masculinization; there is a deepening of the voice, growth of hair on the face and the development of other secondary male characteristics. Cortisone may be ordered even though no adrenalectomy is done; it suppresses adrenocortical activity, thus reducing the secretion of sex hormones. Occasionally, estrogen may be given to women in the older age group.

Chemotherapy. The patient with widespread metastases may be treated by the use of an anticancer drug. The drug is circulated in the blood and is toxic to normal as well as cancerous cells. See page 94 for information regarding chemotherapy in cancer.

Breast Cancer in the Male

Carcinoma of the breast is relatively rare in the male, usually occurring in the fifth or sixth decade. The course of the disease is similar to that in the female; it readily metastasizes to regional lymph nodes and other structures. It is often unrecognized and neglected in the early stage because of the low incidence in men; as a result, metastases have frequently developed when the patient is first seen. Treatment involves radical mastectomy and radiation therapy. A bilateral orchidectomy (removal of the testes) and hormonal therapy may also be used.

Nursing Care in Breast Surgery

Preoperative Preparation. If there has not been a previous biopsy to determine if the mass is benign or malignant, the patient is prepared as for a radical mastectomy. The tumor is excised and the surgical team waits while a quick frozen section is examined by the pathologist (see p. 87). If the mass indicates malignancy, a radical mastectomy is then performed. Before operation, the surgeon explains to the patient and the family the procedure that will be followed, and the operative consent indicates "biopsy and possible radical mastectomy."

PSYCHOLOGICAL PREPARATION. The general public has become more aware of cancer, but unfortunately, many persons do not realize that a goodly number of cancer patients who receive early treatment are cured. To many, the word cancer only implies suffering, mutilation and death. Not infrequently, fear of learning the truth leads to delay in seeking medical advice.

The impact of being advised of the need for a biopsy and possible radical mastectomy (if the mass is cancerous) understandably evokes fears and emotional reactions in the patient. Her anxiety may be focussed upon suffering, disfigurement, loss of femininity, or death. How she will react is unpredictable; responses and behavior are individualized, depending on background and previous experiences. One patient may appear quite unconcerned but actually is in turmoil underneath her composure. Some may be withdrawn and unresponsive; others are resentful that this should happen to them; and a few may be actually disorganized. The patient may have feelings of helplessness, loneliness and abandonment. Each patient requires the support of a nurse who understands and appreciates what the implications of the situation may be for her and her family.

The nurse needs to know what the doctor has told the patient and should observe her closely for her reactions. The patient is encouraged and is given opportunities to talk about the situation and ask questions. In this way, the nurse learns of the patient's particular concerns and can discuss them, appropriately clarifying misconceptions and informing the patient that she will be able to resume former activities, that excellent prostheses are available, and that hopefully her tumor is one in which good results can be expected. Being able to express her fears openly and being aware of the nurse's understanding and available support generally help to reduce the patient's level of anxiety.

PHYSICAL PREPARATION. Usually, there is a minimal period of preparation; the surgery is considered urgent in order to prevent spread of the disease, if possible. A chest x-ray and possibly liver function tests may be done to detect metastases in the lungs and liver. The patient's blood is typed and crossmatched, and blood is made available for transfusion. Her general condition is assessed, and erythrocyte and hemoglobin estimations are made. If anemia is present, a transfusion may be ordered preoperatively. The fluid intake is increased to ensure optimum hydration.

An explanation is made to the patient of

what she may expect following operation. This will include the deep breathing, coughing and exercises that she will be required to do.

The local skin preparation (shaving and cleansing) extends from above the clavicle to the umbilical level and from the nipple line on the unaffected side to the back on the affected side and includes the axilla and the arm to the elbow. If the surgeon anticipates the need for skin grafting, preparation of an indicated donor site will be necessary. A sedative is generally given the night before operation to ensure adequate rest. The remainder of the preparation conforms to general preoperative preparation (see Chapter 10).

Postoperative Care. If the patient's surgery involves only resection of a tumor and not mastectomy, no special care is required. A nurse remains with the patient until she recovers from the anesthetic; she is then made comfortable and is left to rest. The doctor visits to advise her of the pathological findings. She may be permitted to be up later that day or the next morning, and if no further surgery is required, she is usually discharged from the hospital on the second or third postoperative day. The sutures are removed in 5 to 7 days in the doctor's office or surgical clinic.

If a mastectomy was done, care includes the following considerations:

OBSERVATIONS. The breast has an abundant blood supply, which increases the blood loss during surgery and the risk of postoperative hemorrhage. Close observation of the patient is maintained during the first 36 to 48 hours to detect early signs of shock or hemorrhage. The dressings are inspected for blood, and the bedding under the affected side is also checked, since blood may not be visible on the dressing because of its flow over the patient's side or from the axillary area. The space between the chest wall and the skin may be drained by a tube brought out through a stab wound. The surgeon may request that it be attached to a closed drainage system or to a suction machine. The amount and color of the drainage are noted at frequent intervals, and any indication of bleeding is reported at once.

The patient's blood pressure, pulse, color and responses are recorded at frequent intervals. Her reaction to the mastectomy is also noted, since emotional disturbance may contribute to shock. Throughout the patient's hospitalization, the affected arm is checked frequently for edema.

POSITIONING. When the patient is fully responding, the head of the bed is gradually elevated to promote wound drainage. The patient is turned on the unaffected side every 2 or 3 hours. The affected arm is immobilized for 36 to 48 hours to prevent hemorrhage and wound strain. The immobilization is usually achieved by enclosing the arm within the strapping or binder that is used to hold the dressings in place. If it is not incorporated with the dressing, the arm is supported and elevated on a pillow above the level of the right atrium to promote lymphatic and venous drainage. The hand is raised so that it is higher than the elbow. When moving or turning the patient, the arm is gently lifted, and any abduction and extension that might increase wound tension are avoided. After 2 or 3 days, the doctor usually permits some movement. The patient tends to hold the arm close to the trunk, predisposing to contracture and limited range of shoulder movement. To prevent this a firm pillow is placed between the trunk and the arm to maintain abduction.

RELIEF OF PAIN. An analgesic such as morphine or meperidine (Demerol) is prescribed for the relief of pain during the first 48 hours. A milder analgesic such as codeine or an aspirin and codeine compound is then used if necessary. Turning the patient, slight change of position and flexion of the fingers and hand and forearm of the affected arm or adjustment of supporting pillows may also contribute to the relief of discomfort.

DEEP BREATHING AND COUGHING. The respirations are likely to be shallow because of the chest wound. To prevent pulmonary complications, the patient is encouraged to take several deep breaths and cough at frequent intervals during the period she is confined to bed. Gentle support to the affected side while deep breathing and coughing may lessen the discomfort and be reassuring to the patient.

FLUIDS AND NUTRITION. There is a considerable loss of blood and fluid during a radical mastectomy. A blood transfusion is frequently given during the surgery or immediately after. Fluids are given intravenously the day of operation to replace the loss and may be continued until sufficient quantities are taken orally. The patient is given fluids by mouth as soon as she can tolerate them and is progressed to a regular diet accordingly.

DRESSING. The dressing is quite bulky and, unless there is bleeding, is usually left undisturbed for several days. The drainage tube may be removed the second or third day, depending on the amount of drainage. Sutures are removed in 7 to 9 days; the surgeon may remove every other one, leaving the remainder for a few days longer, depending on the healing that has taken place and the degree of tension on the incision. If a skin graft has been done, the donor site dressing may be removed in 3 or 4 days, leaving the area exposed. It may be quite sensitive and require protection from the bedding. The patient is encouraged to view the wound while it is being dressed so that she gradually becomes accustomed to the permanent change in her appearance prior to discharge from hospital.

AMBULATION AND EXERCISES. The patient is usually assisted out of bed the day after the operation. If the arm is not incorporated in the dressing, it is supported in a sling the first few times she is up. A nurse remains with her to determine her reaction and provides support when she is walking or going to the toilet because her balance and accustomed pattern of movement are interfered with by the immobilization of the arm. Exercise of the affected arm is necessary soon after the operation to prevent contracture and limited range of movement and to restore normal function. The surgeon indicates when exercises may commence. This may vary from a few days to a week or two, depending on the condition of the wound.

During the first week, the patient is encouraged to alternately extend and flex the fingers, hand and forearm several times, 3 or 4 times a day. Then gradual abduction of the arm and raising it over the head are introduced when indicated. The purpose of the exercises is explained, and she is advised that to regain the full use of her arm, she must begin to use it now. The initial exercises are begun slowly; the frequency and vigor may be increased from day to day according to the patient's tolerance. Using the affected arm in the performance of self-

care activities such as washing the face, bathing, cleaning the teeth and brushing and combing the hair is encouraged by the nurse.

A more formalized program of exercises is planned and started with the consent of the surgeon. These generally include pulley motion, rope turning, pendulum swinging, climbing the wall with the hands, and rod-raising. Additional exercises may be included later.

Pulley motion is achieved by throwing a rope over a shower curtain rod or overhead bed bar. The patient takes an end of the rope in each hand, stands straight with arms abducted and extended and pulls the rope up and down in see-saw fashion. When one arm is pulling the rope down, the other arm is raised.

The rope turning exercise involves circumduction of the arm. A 7- or 8-foot rope is tied to a door knob or a firm, stationary object. The loose end of the rope is held in the hand of the affected arm, which is kept straight. The rope is then swung around in circles as one turns a skipping rope. The range may be limited at first, but the patient is encouraged to progressively make larger circles.

In pendulum swinging, the patient bends forward from the waist, allowing her arms to fall forward in front of her. They are then swung from side to side in a pendulum motion.

Climbing the walls with the hands requires the patient to stand close to and face a wall and place the palms of her hands against it at shoulder level. Using the fingers in a crawling motion, the hands are moved up the wall as far as she can reach and then down again to shoulder level. The objective is to reach full extension of the arm.

In the rod-raising exercise, a rod (similar to a broom handle) approximately 4 feet long is grasped with the hands as far apart as possible. It is raised over the head, lowered behind the head, raised again and returned to the original position. An exercise which may be substituted for this one entails raising the arms out from the sides to shoulder level, placing the hands behind the neck, extending the arms again, and then lowering them to place the hands behind the lumbar region of the back.

All exercises are done only twice the first day, then gradually they are increased from day to day until each is repeated 10 times 2 or 3 times daily. When the patient is discharged a written outline of the exercises which she is expected to continue is prepared for her and reviewed by the nurse. The local branches of the National Cancer Society have a booklet entitled "Help Yourself to Recovery." This illustrates and gives directions for postmastectomy exercises and activities as well as useful information on prostheses. A supply of these booklets should be kept available on the surgical ward for use by the nurse in teaching the patient exercises. A copy is also given to the patient if her physician approves.

EDEMA OF THE ARM. The removal of axillary lymphatics in radical mastectomy occasionally causes edema and swelling of the arm after operation. If it develops, an elastic or crepe bandage is applied, extending from the wrist to the shoulder. The arm is elevated on pillows during the night. During the day, it is recommended that the patient rest the arm on the back of a sofa or a table or something comparable for a brief period several times. If edema becomes severe, a diuretic such as chlorothiazide (Diuril) may be ordered.

PROSTHESIS AND CARE OF THE WOUND AREA. Before the patient is discharged from the hospital, she is advised as to how to care for the wound area. The area may be bathed as usual but should be gently patted dry. Vigorous rubbing is discouraged in case of wound separation. Gentle massage of the area with vaseline or cocoa butter may be suggested to increase the elasticity of the skin, which is generally drawn very tightly over the chest wall. The patient is cautioned that if any irritation, redness, open sore or swelling occurs she should see her physician. She is also advised that if swelling (edema) of the arm occurs, it should be reported.

The patient is encouraged to be fitted for a brassiere with a prosthesis. The improvement it makes to her general appearance will raise her morale. The various types of prostheses (e.g., sponge rubber, semiliquid, padded) may be described and a list of reliable supply firms with experienced fitters is given to the patient. The nurse shows the patient how to pad the brassieres she has with absorbent cotton covered with soft cotton so they can be used until a properly fitted prosthesis can be worn. The surgeon will indicate when the wound is sufficiently healed that she may wear a prosthesis. The nurse avails herself of the opportunity to describe the wound to the patient's husband or a close relative and emphasizes that the patient may be sensitive about this alteration in her appearance.

If the wound is not completely healed and requires cleansing and dressing, the patient or a member of her family is taught the necessary procedure, or a referral may be made to the visiting nurse agency. A visiting nurse may also be helpful in supervising the patient's exercise program and care during radiation therapy if it is given.

If a series of radiation treatments is to be given, the surgeon discusses this with the patient and advises her when the first treatment will be given. It is not usually instituted until the wound is firmly healed and is generally given on an outpatient basis (see p. 90). The doctor also informs the patient as to when she may resume her household activities or return to her former occupation. The resumption of former activities is encouraged just as soon as the patient is well enough. It relieves her depression and leaves her less time to concentrate on her disease.

A close follow-up is done on the patient; she is required to make frequent visits to her doctor or the cancer clinic during the first year or two. Then, if there has been no evidence of recurrence of her disease. the interval between examinations is lengthened.

INFECTION OF THE BREAST

Infection of the breast causes acute mastitis and most commonly occurs during lactation. The causative organism enters through a fissure or abrasion of the nipple which might have been prevented by careful cleansing and protection. The patient's temperature is elevated, and the breast becomes firm, red, painful and very tender. The patient is given an antibiotic and kept at rest. The baby is taken off the breast temporarily, and hot or cold applications may be ordered. Unless the infection is checked in the early stage, suppuration may develop, necessitating surgical drainage.

References

BOOKS

Cole, W. H. and Zollinger, R. M.: Textbook of Surgery, 8th ed. New York, Appleton-Century-Crofts, 1963. Chapter 35.

Davis, L. (Ed.): Christopher's Textbook of Surgery, 9th ed. Philadelphia, W. B. Saunders Co., 1968. Chapter 18.

Haagensen, C. D.: Carcinoma of the Breast (a monograph). New York, The American Cancer Society, Inc., 1958.

New York City Cancer Committee: Essentials of Cancer Nursing, New York, The American Cancer Society, Inc., 1963.

Shackleford, R. T.: Diagnosis of Surgical Disease, Vol. 1, Philadelphia, W. B. Saunders Co., 1968. Chapter 9.

Southwick, H. W., Slaughter, D. P., and Humphrey, L. J.: Surgery of the Breast. Chicago, Year Book Medical Publishers, Inc., 1968.

PERIODICALS AND PAMPHLETS

*American Cancer Society: "The Nurse and Breast Self-Examination." New York, The American Cancer Society, Inc.

*_____ "Help Yourself to Recovery." New York, The American Cancer Society, 1957.

Lippincott, R. C.: "The Physician's Approach to the Patient with Cancer." Surg. Clin. North Amer., Vol. 47, No. 3 (June 1967), pp. 559–564.

Sedgwick, C. E.: "Management of Carcinoma of the Breast." Surg. Clin. North Amer., Vol. 47, No. 3 (June 1967), pp. 707–722.

---

*Available from the local branches of the National Cancer Society.

21
Nursing in Disorders of the Endocrine System

THE ENDOCRINE SYSTEM

A gland is an organ which extracts substances from the blood and produces one or more new chemical substances, referred to as secretions. Glands may be classified as exocrine or endocrine. The secretion of an exocrine gland is carried along a duct into a body cavity or to the external surface of the body. Examples of such glands are the salivary, gastric, mammary and sweat glands. Endocrine glands do not have ducts; their secretions, which are called hormones, pass directly into the blood and act on remote tissues.

The glands usually cited as comprising the endocrine system are the hypophysis (pituitary gland), thyroid gland, 4 parathyroid glands, 2 adrenal (suprarenal) glands, islets of Langerhans and 2 gonads (ovaries and testes). Unlike other body systems in which the component organs are located close together and are connected, the glands are situated in various parts of the body. There are other organs which are known to demonstrate endocrine action through their liberation of chemical agents into the blood. They are not considered to be part of the endocrine system since they are a more integral part of other major systems. These include the gastrointestinal glands, which secrete gastrin, secretin and pancreozymin (see p. 322), and the kidneys, which secrete rennin into the blood (see p. 417). The placenta, formed in pregnancy, also serves as an endocrine gland because of its production of progesterone, estrogen and chorionic gonadotrophin.

Coordination and integration of the development and functions of the body are dependent upon the nervous system and the endocrine system. The endocrine system is concerned mainly with growth, maturation, metabolic processes and reproduction. The action of each hormone is specific. One hormone may modify the activity of all body cells (e.g., thyroxine); others affect the activity of only one particular organ (e.g., adrenocorticotrophin). The site of action of any hormone is referred to as the target organ or tissue. Some hormones are necessary for survival (e.g., adrenal corticoid); others are not essential to life (e.g., gonadal secretions).

The production of endocrine secretions is generally controlled according to the need for their action; that is, production and release into the blood stream are stimulated

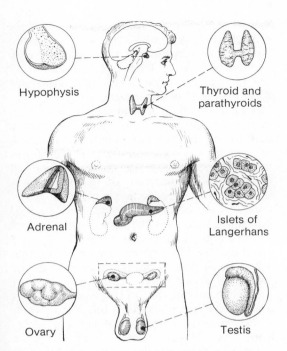

Figure 21–1 Locations of glands in the body.

when their action is needed and are inhibited when the effect is achieved. The control mechanism may be mediated by the blood concentration of the target organ or by physicochemical processes. For example, regulation of secretion by the thyroid, adrenal cortices and the gonads is maintained by hormones which are produced by the adenohypophysis (anterior pituitary gland) and are liberated in response to the blood concentration of the hormones of those glands. To illustrate, the adenohypophysis secretes a thyroid-stimulating hormone (thyrotrophin), and in turn, the output of thyrotrophin is controlled by the level of thyroid hormones in the blood. This reciprocal arrangement is referred to as a feedback mechanism. A hormone which stimulates the secretion of another hormone is referred to as a trophic hormone. An example of control by a physicochemical process is the influence of the osmotic pressure of the blood on the output of the antidiuretic hormone (see p. 52).

Disorders of an endocrine gland may incur an excess or deficiency of its hormone(s). Signs and symptoms of the disorder are predominantly manifestations of dysfunction in the target organ or tissues.

HYPOPHYSIS (PITUITARY GLAND)

The hypophysis is a very small gland located at the base of the brain in the sella turcica, a depression in the sphenoid bone. It is attached to the brain by a stalk, the infundibulum, which contains nerve fibers and blood vessels. The gland has two distinct parts: the anterior lobe, or adenohypophysis, and the posterior or neural lobe, or neurohypophysis. The adenohypophysis is an embryological outgrowth of the roof of the mouth and is completely separated from its origin. The neurohypophysis develops from the base of the brain, remaining connected to the hypothalamus by the infundibulum.

The cells of the adenohypophysis are truly glandular, in that they extract substances from the blood and secrete new chemicals (hormones). The neurohypophysis consists mainly of many terminal nerve fibers which originate with nerve cells (neurons) in the hypothalamus. The fibers are supported by nonsecreting cells called pituicytes. The hormones released by the neurohypophysis are secreted by the neurons.

Adenohypophysis (Anterior Pituitary Lobe)

The anterior lobe of the pituitary gland consists of 3 major types of cells, classified according to their stainability by certain dyes: acidophils or alpha cells, basophils or beta cells, and chromophobes.* The cells are arranged in columns or groups surrounding blood sinuses. This portion of the gland is responsible for the secretion of 6 hormones: somatotrophin or growth hormone (STH or GH), thyrotrophin (TSH), corticotrophin or adrenocorticotrophic hormone (ACTH), and 3 gonadotrophins [follicle-stimulating hormone (FSH), luteotrophin (LTH) and luteinizing hormone (LH)]. The last 5 of these (TSH, ACTH, FSH, LTH and LH) stimulate other glands; STH acts directly on almost all tissues of the body.

A branch of the internal carotid artery supplies the adenohypophysis but the blood is circulated through the lower hypothala-

---

*Pituitary neoplasms are frequently indicated as being eosinophilic, basophilic or chromophobic.

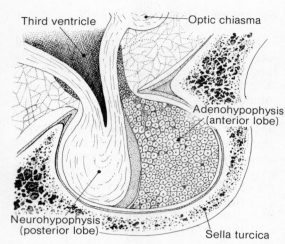

Figure 21-2 The hypophysis.

mic tissue before entering the gland. It is carried from the hypothalamus in hypothalamic-hypophyseal portal vessels in the infundibulum (pituitary stalk) to the sinusoids of the adenohypophysis. Control of the various adenohypophyseal secretions is mediated by neurosecretory substances or releasing factors which are liberated by special hypothalamic neurons into the hypothalamic-hypophyseal portal system. On reaching the sinusoids, these substances influence the secretory activity of the glandular cells.

Functions of the Adenohypophyseal Hormones. Somatotrophin is concerned with the growth of the body and plays an important role in determining the size of a person. It is most freely secreted from infancy until late adolescence. The most striking effect of the hormone is evidenced on the skeleton. Bones increase in length and thickness, the muscles enlarge and there is a corresponding growth of the viscera. Metabolism is accelerated by STH, and a positive nitrogen balance develops because of the increased use of proteins in tissue synthesis. Growth is also dependent upon the secretion of normal amounts of other hormones. The thyroid hormones are necessary to maintain an adequate metabolic rate, and insulin must be available to promote glucose metabolism for the provision of energy. Overproduction of the growth hormone can have a diabetogenic effect; an excess of the hormone results in decreased carbohydrate utilization, an elevated blood sugar level, glycosuria

and increased utilization of fat. If an excessive concentration of STH is prolonged, the islets of Langerhans of the pancreas may become exhausted from overstimulation by the high blood sugar level, and permanent diabetes mellitus may ensue.

Thyrotrophin (thyroid-stimulating hormone) promotes the growth and secretory activity of the thyroid gland, the function of which is the production of hormones which regulate the metabolic rate of all tissues. The production of thyrotrophin is regulated by a feedback mechanism. A decrease in the blood concentration of thyroid hormones increases the secretory output of thyrotrophin; conversely, when the thyroid hormones reach a normal or above normal level, there is a reciprocal decrease in the release of thyrotrophin.

Corticotrophin (ACTH) has as its target organ the adrenal cortices, influencing their secretory output of several cortical secretions. ACTH secretion is regulated by a corticotrophin-releasing factor produced in the hypothalamus in response to a decreased blood level of cortisone, or to nerve impulses initiated by biological stress (e.g., trauma, pain).

The follicle-stimulating hormone (FSH) causes the development of the ovarian follicle and the secretion of estrogen. The secretion of FSH is reciprocally related to the blood level of estrogen; FSH production is increased as the estrogen level declines. (See p. 473 for details of its role in the female menstrual cycle.) In the male, FSH promotes the production of spermatozoa in conjunction with the male hormone testosterone.

The luteinizing hormone (LH) promotes ovulation and is necessary for the formation of the corpus luteum in the ruptured follicle. When the corpus luteum develops and secretes progesterone, the production of LH is suppressed. In the male, this hormone may be called the interstitial cell-stimulating hormone (ICSH) because it stimulates the production of the male hormone testosterone by the interstitial cells of the testes.

Luteotrophin (LTH) stimulates the corpus luteum to secrete progesterone and initiates the secretion of the mammary glands which have undergone preparatory changes in response to the estrogen and progesterone blood levels. Because of this latter function, the hormone is sometimes called the lacto-genic hormone or prolactin. Its action in the male, if any, is undetermined.

A seventh adenohypophyseal hormone which is normally secreted in very small amounts in man is the melanocyte-stimu-lating hormone (MSH). In lower animals, especially Amphibia, the hormone regulates the production of pigment by cells in the skin. Its chemical structure is similar to that of ACTH, and pigmentation of the skin may occur in the human with a high blood con-centration of ACTH. Pigmented areas of the skin are frequently seen in persons with a deficiency of adrenal cortical secretion which results in an increased, compensatory output of ACTH.

Neurohypophysis (Posterior Pituitary Lobe)

Two hormones, the antidiuretic hormone (ADH) and oxytocin, are released by the neurohypophysis. The antidiuretic hormone, also called vasopressin, increases the permeability of the distal and collecting tubules of the kidneys, resulting in increased reabsorption of water. Release of ADH by the posterior pituitary lobe is regulated by osmoreceptors in the hypothalamus. When the osmotic pressure of the blood is elevated (for example, because of dehydration or in-creased salt concentration), the neurons sensitive to changes in the osmotic pressure of the blood transmit impulses to the neuro-hypophysis to release ADH into the circu-lating blood. Conversely, if the solute con-centration of the blood is below normal, nerve impulses are not produced and release of ADH is inhibited. The reduction in the blood concentration of ADH decreases the permeability of the renal tubules to water. This hormone plays an important role in maintaining normal fluid balance. When it is present in large amounts, ADH stimulates a relatively transient, generalized vasocon-striction, hence the term vasopressin. It is not considered to have any significant role in regulating blood pressure. ADH released into the general circulation is destroyed rapidly by enzymatic action, mainly in the liver and kidneys.

Oxytocin excites contractions of the pregnant uterus, especially during the latter part of gestation. It also stimulates other smooth muscle in the body to a lesser extent, which accounts for its use occasionally to stimulate peristalsis in abdominal distention. The mechanism that prompts the release of oxytocin to initiate labor contractions is not known. Sensitivity of the uterine muscle to the hormone is thought to gradually increase throughout pregnancy, reaching a maximum at term.[1] This hormone plays an important role in lactation; suckling initiates afferent nerve impulses which on reaching the hypo-thalamus bring about the liberation of oxytocin from the neurohypophysis. The hormone is carried by the blood to the mammary glands, stimulating the release and flow of milk.

Disorders of the Hypophysis (Pituitary Gland)

Manifestations of disorders of the hypo-physis vary greatly, depending on which lobe is involved, the nature of the disease (hyperplasia, neoplasm or destruction of tissue), and the particular type of cell of the adenohypophysis that is involved. Dysfunc-tion may be manifested in one or more of the gland's target organs, reflecting either an excessive or deficient output of one or more hypophyseal hormones. Secondary neuro-logical disturbances may also occur as a result of pressure on neighboring brain tis-sue by a pituitary neoplasm. For example, early symptoms may be persisting headache or visual disturbances. The visual disturb-ances frequently occur because of the prox-imity of the visual tract. Conversely, primary pathological lesions in the brain, especially in the hypothalamic region, may cause secondary involvement of the hypo-physis.

The more commonly recognized disease entities associated with the adenohypo-physis include: gigantism, the result of an excessive secretion of somatotrophin in childhood; acromegaly, due to an excessive secretion of somatotrophin commencing in adulthood; dwarfism, resulting from a defi-ciency of somatotrophin in childhood; Cush-ing's disease, the result of a hypersecretion

---

[1]J. H. V. Brown, and S. B. Barker: Basic Endocrinol-ogy, 2nd ed. Philadelphia, F. A. Davis Co., 1966, p. 52.

of adrenocorticotrophin; and Simmond's disease, which occurs with a deficiency of all the adenohypophyseal hormones. Hyperthyroidism (Graves' disease) may also be secondary to an excessive production of thyrotrophin or an abnormal form of the hormone and is discussed under Disorders of the Thyroid, page 544.

The most common disorder associated with the neurohypophysis is diabetes insipidus, which is a result of a deficiency of the antidiuretic hormone.

Gigantism and Acromegaly

An overproduction of somatotrophin before closure of the epiphyses causes a rapid overgrowth of the bones, producing the condition known as gigantism. It may commence in early childhood or not until adolescence. A person with this disturbance may attain a height of 7 to 8 feet. Most cases are attributed to an adenoma of the acidophilic cells (eosinophils). When the person passes adolescence, acromegaly is superimposed on the gigantism.

If the adenoma develops after the epiphyses have closed, longitudinal growth cannot occur, but marked thickening of the bones develops. Enlargement of the head, jaws, hands and feet becomes apparent. Increased growth of cartilage produces an increase in the size of the nose, ears, costal cartilages and larynx. Hypertrophy of the larynx may be accompanied by a deepening of the voice, and the change in the costal cartilages results in an increase in the thoracic circumference. The skin, subcutaneous tissues and lips thicken, the chin lengthens and the lower teeth separate because of the overgrowth of the mandible. Viscera enlarge and may become overactive, leading to disturbances. Allbright states: "The excessive secretion of growth hormone appears to affect all organs and tissues except the brain."[2]

As well as the evident skeletal changes and alteration in appearance, the patient experiences lethargy, weakness, increased metabolic rate and excessive sweating due to hypertrophy of the thyroid, joint pains and stiffness in the limbs, tingling or numbness in the hands, and impaired carbohydrate metabolism and hyperglycemia due to the diabetogenic effect of STH. Pressure from the expanding neoplasm may cause headache, insomnia and loss of visual acuity. Increased gonadal function may be associated with the early stage of acromegaly, but later, loss of libido and amenorrhea are common. Osteoporosis, rarefaction of bones due to loss of calcium, may develop, especially in the vertebrae, and kyphosis (forward curvature of the spine) may be seen in the advanced stage. Hypertension is a common complication. The course of the disease varies considerably from one patient to another; it may develop slowly over many years in some, but in others it may prove fatal in 3 or 4 years. Destruction of hypophyseal tissue by progressive growth and spread of the tumor may cause a general hypopituitarism.

Gigantism and acromegaly may be treated by external or internal irradiation of the hypophysis or by an hypophysectomy (see p. 538). Internal radiation may be achieved by the implantation of radioactive gold (Au^{198}) or yttrium (Y^{90}) seeds in the hypophysis. The gland is approached through the nasal cavity and sphenoid bone. The disease is likely to cause emotional reactions and depression in the patient and his family. Support and understanding from the nurse may help them to accept and adjust to the situation. A high-calorie well-balanced diet is necessary to meet the increased metabolic rate. With some it may have to be modified because of the decreased carbohydrate metabolism. Substitution hormonal preparations are prescribed if an hypophysectomy is done or if the patient manifests insulin, thyroid, adrenal or gonadal insufficiency in the advanced stage of the disease.

Cushing's Disease

A basophilic tumor or disturbance in the hypothalamus may give rise to an excessive production of ACTH and, in turn, hyperactivity of the adrenal cortices. The adrenal cortices respond by hyperplasia and an excessive secretion of glucocorticoids, producing the characteristic features of Cushing's disease. The syndrome is more often a consequence of a primary disorder of the adrenal gland; the reader is referred to page 566.

[2]P. B. Beeson, and W. McDermott (Eds.): Cecil-Loeb Textbook of Medicine, 11th ed. Philadelphia, W. B. Saunders Co., 1963, p. 1359.

Pituitary Dwarfism

A deficiency of somatotrophin in childhood produces dwarfism. The deficiency most often becomes apparent when the child is 2 to 4 years of age. He may be normally formed, but his proportions are not characteristic of the age at which growth ceases and the head is relatively larger than the rest of the body. In some instances, the head and trunk develop normally, but growth of the legs and arms is stunted. Dwarfism due to a somatotrophic deficiency is differentiated from that due to a deficiency of the thyroid hormone (cretinism) in that the mental development is normal. The deficiency in some patients may be limited to somatotrophin or it may involve other hormones. Sexual development and maturity may or may not be normal.

A second type of dwarfism which is rarely seen is referred to as Fröhlich's syndrome, in which there is obesity and failure of sexual development; mental retardation may be present in some. An adult form of Fröhlich's syndrome occurs in which obesity, atrophy of the genitals and loss of reproductive ability occur. The obesity in Fröhlich's disease is attributed to hypothalamic involvement.

Simmond's Disease (Panhypopituitarism)

This disease denotes a deficiency of all the adenohypophyseal hormones. The condition may be the result of a primary lesion, such as a tumor or cyst, within the anterior lobe itself, or it may be secondary to a space-occupying lesion in neighboring structures or to interference with its blood supply. The latter may occur with thrombosis of the hypophyseal vessels rarely associated with postpartum shock (Sheehan's syndrome). Frequently the causative lesion is a craniopharyngioma which is derived from vestigial cells of Rathke's pouch.* This tumor occurs most often in children but may not give rise to symptoms until adulthood because it grows slowly. A second neoplasm that may

be responsible for panhypopituitarism is an adenoma of the chromophobe cells. The cells of both these tumors are nonsecreting, and as they enlarge, they compress and destroy the acidophilic cells (eosinophils) and basophils. Surgical excision or irradiation of the gland for the purpose of suppressing the secretion of certain hormones in the treatment of carcinoma of the breast (see p. 526) or acromegaly may incur hyposecretion of all the adenohypophyseal hormones.

The multiple hormone deficiency results in a lack of stimulation to the thyroid, adrenal cortices and gonads. Secondary atrophy and a hyposecretion of their hormones ensue. If the condition occurs in childhood, failure of the secretion of somatotrophin along with the others produces dwarfism. Growth and development are arrested, the skin becomes wrinkled and the child develops an appearance characteristic of a "wizened old person." In the adult, there is also a general wasting of all body tissues and the person exhibits emaciation and severe weight loss. The skin is dry and wrinkled and may assume a yellowish cast. The body hair becomes sparse. Decreased thyroid activity causes a reduction in the metabolic rate, leading to a subnormal temperature and extreme weakness. Arrested function of the gonads results in failure of ovulation, amenorrhea, an absence of spermatogenesis and impotence. Concomitant hypoglycemia and hypotension are seen and may lead to shock and coma. The low blood sugar is attributed to the decreased adrenal corticoid secretion. If the panhypopituitarism is due to an expanding neoplasm, the neurohypophysis and the infundibulum (neural stalk) may become involved, manifested by polyuria and extreme thirst, which is characteristic of a deficiency of the antidiuretic hormone. The hypothalamus may also be affected and varied neurological disturbances become evident; for example, the patient may experience severe anorexia.

Treatment and Nursing Care. Treatment includes the administration of substitution hormones of the target glands. The patient receives cortisone and dessicated thyroid in dosages adjusted to his individual needs. Gonadal hormones may be prescribed, depending on the patient's age. Grollman suggests that the administration of testo-

---

*Rathke's pouch is the embryological structure which arises from the roof of the mouth to form the adenohypophysis.

sterone (male hormone) to both sexes is of value for its anabolic effect.[3]

The nurse plays an important role in encouraging these patients to take a high-calorie, high-vitamin diet. Since anorexia is a frequent problem, resourcefulness is necessary to gain the patient's cooperation and to tempt him to take adequate nourishment. Various methods and approaches must be tried. It is usually helpful to provide small servings of high-calorie foods at frequent intervals rather than the usual 3 or 4 regular meals. Varying the foods, adding concentrates to fluids, determining the patient's preferences, having favorite "dishes" prepared at home and brought to him, eating with others and a change of environment are just a few suggestions that may prove beneficial. If the patient is emaciated and inactive or confined to bed, bony prominences and pressure areas require frequent and special care to prevent pressure sores. The lethargy and apathy generally associated with Simmond's disease predisposes to the patient's immobility. Prompting the patient to change his position and exercise within his tolerance is necessary to stimulate circulation and prevent complications.

Diabetes Insipidus

The etiological factor in this disorder may be a deficiency of the antidiuretic hormone (ADH or vasopressin) or failure of the renal tubules to respond to ADH. The latter is a rare hereditary condition present at birth. A deficiency of ADH is most commonly due to hypoactivity or destruction of a part of the hypothalamic-neurohypophyseal system resulting from primary or metastatic neoplasms. In some instances, no apparent cause can be identified.

Diabetes insipidus is characterized by a very large urinary output (polyuria) and extreme thirst (polydipsia). The daily output may range from 8 to 20 liters and the patient may experience anorexia, loss of weight and strength, and electrolyte imbalance. The urine has an abnormally low specific gravity and does not contain any abnormal constituents. If fluid is withheld or does not keep pace with the output, an excessive loss of urine continues, leading to severe dehydration. The persisting symptoms of polyuria and polydipsia day and night interfere with rest and normal activities.

The patient is treated by replacement therapy; a preparation of posterior pituitary extract or vasopressin is prescribed. The preparations used include dessicated posterior pituitary powder which is applied to the nasal mucosa every 6 to 8 hours, aqueous solution of vasopressin (Pitressin) which is given daily by subcutaneous or intramuscular injection, and vasopressin tannate in oil which is given intramuscularly every 2 or 3 days. The latter preparation is absorbed more slowly; less frequent administration is necessary, since one dose can be large enough to provide the relief of symptoms over a longer period. The use of the powdered extract in the nose is more convenient and economical, but irritation of the mucosa may contravene its continued application.

The patient is usually hospitalized during diagnostic investigation and regulation of the optimal dosage of the substitutional hormone. It is difficult for the patient to accept the fact that he will most likely be dependent on the drug for the remainder of his life. The nurse can help the patient to plan for necessary readjustments and should reassure him that he can resume a normal pattern of life. The patient and a family member are taught the details of how to administer the drug, including care of the equipment. They may require further explanation of the disorder to appreciate the importance of regular administration of the drug and should be advised that it is ineffective if taken orally because it is inactivitated by the digestive enzymes. Since the preparations are relatively costly and may pose an economic problem for the family, it may be necessary to arrange for assistance for them through a social service agency. A referral may also be made to a visiting nurse association so that supervision and direction are provided in administration of a parenteral preparation when the patient goes home.

Hypophysectomy

The hypophysis (pituitary gland) may be removed because of hyperfunction or a neoplasm of the gland. Hypophysectomy is also

---

[3]A. Grollman: Clinical Endocrinology and Its Physiologic Basis. Philadelphia, J. B. Lippincott Co., 1964, p. 69.

employed in the treatment of cancer of the breast and prostate. Malignant disease of these organs is supported by the sex hormones estrogens and androgens respectively. Removal of the source of gonadotrophic hormones reduces support of the primary neoplasm and its metastasis. Withdrawal of the hormones does not cure the disease, but usually produces a remission for a period of several months. The hypophysis is removed by a frontal intracranial operation. In some instances, the neural stalk which transmits the nerve fibers from the hypothalamus to the neurohypophysis may be preserved at operation, thus preventing diabetes insipidus. Hypophysectomy results in the withdrawal of the adrenocorticotrophic hormone (ACTH), the thyroid-stimulating hormone (TSH), and probably the antidiuretic hormone (ADH), as well as the gonadotrophins. The patient requires cortisol, thyroxine and possibly ADH replacement for the remainder of his life. Gonadal function ceases, and the patient becomes infertile. If the surgery was done because of disease of the hypophysis, the male patient may be given testosterone to prevent impotence.

Preoperative Preparation. Because of the location and the infrequency of this particular operation, the patient and his family are very apprehensive. The nurse, cognizant of their anxiety, encourages them to verbalize their fears and ask questions and provides necessary emotional support. The permanent results of the surgery will have been explained by the physician, but the nurse, knowing what the patient has been told, is prepared to answer their questions and explain the hormonal replacement.

Specific directions are received from the surgeon for the skin preparation. Usually, an area of approximately 2 inches from the hairline across the front of the head is shaved and cleansed. The patient is advised that there will be frequent recording of his blood pressure, temperature, pulse and respirations following the operation and that he may not receive anything by mouth for a day or two but that his fluid and nutritional needs will be met by continuous intravenous infusion. Cortisol is usually given the day before operation and again before going to the operating room. An indwelling catheter may be passed before the surgery so that a frequent, accurate check may be made of the urinary output to determine the need for ADH replacement. A venous cutdown with the insertion of a cannula and continuous intravenous infusion may be ordered to establish a route for the quick administration of drugs and fluids as needed.

Postoperative Care. The care following a hypophysectomy is similar to that of any patient who has had intracranial surgery (see p. 637). Close observation will be made for early signs of acute adrenal insufficiency (see p. 555) or fluid imbalance. Cortisol is given intravenously until the patient can tolerate it orally. The dose is gradually decreased until the maintenance dose is established. Pitressin is usually necessary to control the fluid loss; the dosage is adjusted to the urinary volume (see Diabetes Insipidus, p. 538). Thyroid extract is generally started orally on the second or third postoperative day.

The patient is allowed out of bed with assistance on the second or third postoperative day. The period of hospitalization is relatively short (approximately 10 days); instruction about the taking of the necessary hormones (cortisol, pitressin and thyroxine) is begun as soon as the patient is well enough.

THYROID GLAND

The thyroid is a **V**-shaped gland situated in the neck. It consists of 2 lateral lobes, one on each side of the trachea immediately below the larynx. These lobes are connected by a middle lobe or isthmus lying across the anterior surface of the trachea. The lobes contain numerous vesicles or follicles which are lined by secreting thyroid cells. The follicles contain a clear, colloidal protein-iodine compound called thyroglobulin. The gland has an abundant blood supply; paired superior and inferior thyroid arteries arise from the external carotid and subclavian arteries.

Two hormones are produced and released into the blood; these are triiodothyronine (T_3) and tetraiodothyronine (thyroxine, T_4). The latter (T_4) occurs in greater amounts than the former (T_3). The thyroid hormones are formed by the combination of the amino acid tyroxine and iodine. The tyrosin molecule first combines with 1 or 2 iodine atoms

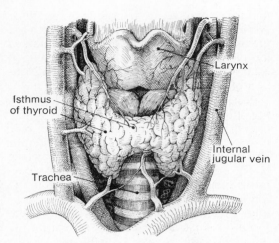

Figure 21-3 The thyroid gland.

to form monoiodotyrosine (MIT) or diiodo-tyrosine (DIT) respectively. Oxidative reactions, promoted by enzymes, combine these compounds to form triiodothyronine and thyroxine (MIT + DIT → T_3; DIT + DIT → T_4). T_3 and T_4 are stored in the thyroglobulin in the follicles. They are freed from the thyroglobulin and released into the blood as needed. In the blood most of the thyroid hormone combines loosely with a globulin fraction of the blood proteins from which it readily separates at cellular level.

The thyroid hormones (T_3 and T_4) increase the metabolic rate in most of the cells by stimulating oxidative processes. There is a notable increase in cellular activity, oxygen consumption and heat production. The hormones are essential for normal physical growth, maturation and mental development. The activity of the thyroid gland is controlled by thyrotrophin (TSH) secreted by the adenohypophysis. It may also be influenced indirectly by the nervous system through the hypothalamus, which is closely linked with the adenohypophysis. TSH promotes the uptake of available tyrosine and iodine as well as the release of the hormones from the thyroglobulin into the blood. A reciprocal or feedback relationship exists between thyrotrophin and the thyroid hormones. When the blood concentration of the thyroid hormones decreases, the hypothalamus produces a releasing factor which alerts the adenohypophysis to secrete thyrotrophin. Conversely, with an increase in the thyroidal hormone concentration of the

blood, a corresponding decrease of the thyrotrophin output occurs.

The thyroid gland has recently been considered to be the source of a third hormone called thyrocalcitonin. It is secreted in response to an elevation in the blood calcium, and by promoting the movement of calcium into the bones, it lowers the amount of calcium in the blood.[4, 5]

Disorders of the Thyroid

Disease of the thyroid may cause a hyposecretion or hypersecretion of the thyroid hormones and a change in the size and contour of the gland. A deficiency in the secretion is called hypothyroidism; an excessive secretion is referred to as hyperthyroidism. The normally functioning gland is designated as euthyroid.

Tests Used in Assessing Thyroid Function

Serum Protein-Bound Iodine (PBI) Test. Since most of the thyroid hormone in circulation is bound to plasma protein, a measurement of the iodine precipitated with plasma protein provides information about the amount being produced. False results are presented if the patient has received iodine in the form of a medication or radiopaque contrast dye within the preceding month or two. The PBI level is also higher in the second and third trimesters of pregnancy. Normal value: 4.0 to 8.0 micrograms per cent.

Basal Metabolic Rate. Measurement of the patient's oxygen consumption over a given period of time when he is at rest provides an indirect estimate of the amount of heat produced by cellular activity. Since heat production is influenced by the thyroid hormones, the amount produced reflects the amount of these hormones in circulation. The person's temperature must be normal, and an undisturbed rest period of at least 1 hour and a fasting period of 14 hours precede the test. A record is made of his height,

---

[4]A. C. Guyton: Textbook of Medical Physiology, 4th ed. Philadelphia, W. B. Saunders Co., 1971, p. 906.
[5]E. E. Chaffee, and E. M. Greisheimer: Basic Physiology and Anatomy, 2nd ed., Philadelphia, J. B. Lippincott Co., 1969, p. 556.

weight and age. An explanation of what the test involves is made to the patient to reduce apprehension which could influence the results obtained. The test is done in the morning in a comfortably warm room, and the patient remains lying down at complete rest. A clamp is placed on the nostrils and he is asked to breathe through his mouth from a tube supplying oxygen, usually for 6 minutes. A table of the mean oxygen consumption according to sex, weight and height has been compiled with which those of the patient are compared. The difference in his oxygen consumption (which represents his heat production and metabolic cellular activity) with the comparable mean is expressed as a percentage above or below the normal. Because of the influence of subjective factors, the test is not considered particularly reliable unless repeated several times. Usually, those subsequent to the first test provide lower results because the patient is less apprehensive of the procedure.

Normal value: 10 to 15 per cent above or below the normal for the patient's sex, height and weight.

Radioactive Iodine Thyroid Uptake (RAIU). This test determines the rate at which the thyroid is removing iodine from the blood and utilizing it. The patient receives a small (tracer) oral dose of radioiodine (I^{131}) in water. The amount concentrated in the thyroid in 6 hours and in 24 hours is estimated by placing a Geiger counter over the neck. A hyperactive thyroid will have a high uptake, and an underactive gland will show a lower concentration than normal. The distribution of radioactivity may also indicate a difference in the degree of activity in different areas of the gland. The uptake of the radioiodine may also be determined by measuring the amount excreted in the urine in 24 or 48 hours. The patient voids when the iodine is administered and that urine is discarded. All urine is then saved for the prescribed 24 or 48 hours and submitted to the isotope laboratory. The fraction of the dose of I^{131} not excreted is assumed to have been localized within the thyroid.

Normal value: 15 to 45 per cent of that administered is taken up within 24 hours.

Radioiodide Suppression Test. This test of thyroid function is based on the homeostatic balance between the production and release of thyroid hormones and their blood concentration which is regulated by the hypothalamic-adenohypophyseal system. When a preparation of thyroid hormone is administered, raising the blood concentration of the hormone, the activity of a euthyroid is suppressed; the output of hormones is decreased in order to establish the normal blood level. If the thyroid is hyperactive, the administration of thyroid hormone will not suppress its activity.

The suppression test involves a 24-hour radioiodide uptake test which is followed by the daily administration of thyroid hormone for 7 days. The RAIU test is then repeated. The uptake of the normal thyroid will be considerably less than in the second test. Failure of the increased blood concentration of the hormone to decrease thyroid activity and the iodine uptake indicates hyperthyroidism.

Red Blood Cell and T$_3$ Tagged with I^{131}. In this test, triiodothyronine tagged with radioiodine is added to a specimen of the patient's blood. The amount of binding of the hormone by the erythrocytes is noted. In hyperthyroidism, the binding is high; conversely, it is low in hypothyroidism.

Thyroid Scan. The uptake or lack of uptake of radioiodide by a limited area of the thyroid can be determined by a scan or scintigram. Following the administration of a tracer dose of I^{131} a scanner is passed over the thyroid and automatically makes a graphic record of the radiation emitted, showing the distribution of the isotope in the gland. Areas of greater concentration show greater density on the record. This procedure is helpful in determining the presence of a localized hyperactive lesion such as an adenoma.

Achilles Tendon Reflex. The extent of the response of the foot to a tap on the Achilles tendon and the time involved in the rise and fall of the foot are measured and recorded by a special machine. The patient with an overactive thyroid records a more rapid and greater response; a lesser response over a longer period is characteristic of hypothyroidism.

Thyroid Stimulation Test. This test is used to determine if the cause of hypothyroidism is within the thyroid or is secondary to a deficiency of thyrotrophin. The response of the thyroid to an injection of thyrotrophin (TSH) is measured by a radioiodine uptake or by a serum protein-bound iodine estimation. Obviously, if the uptake of I^{131} or the PBI remain abnormally low, the problem is primarily in the thyroid. If the radioiodide uptake and PBI are normal following the thyrotrophin injection, the problem may be attributed to a deficient secretion of thyrotrophin by the adenohypophysis.

Hypothyroidism

The effects and manifestations of a deficiency of thyroid hormone differ with the age at which it develops as well as with its degree and duration. If the dysfunction is congenital or develops in infancy or early childhood, it gives rise to cretinism. In the adult it produces myxedema.

Cretinism. A deficiency of thyroid hormone in infancy or childhood is characterized by the failure to achieve normal physical growth and mental development. The child may become a mentally deficient dwarf. The symptoms of cretinism are rarely present in the newborn but more often appear gradually in infancy or early childhood. Suggestive signs include: limpness and inactivity; feeding problems; pale, dry, cool skin; thick tongue, coarse features; coarse hair; and a puffy appearance. The circulation is sluggish, the temperature is usually subnormal and the pulse slow. Constipation is a common problem. The child's growth is stunted, and there is a distinct lag in the development of normal behavioral responses. If the deficiency is recognized in the early stages and a thyroid preparation administered, normal growth and development may occur. If the deficiency is allowed to persist, irreversible damage results, and both physical growth and mental development are retarded.

The fact that cretinism may be corrected if recognized and treated early emphasizes the nurse's role in promoting adequate infant and child supervision. Mothers should be taught the characteristics of normal growth and development. Simple, authentic information is available to parents in pamphlets and booklets published by provincial and state health departments. The mother is encouraged to take the child to well-baby or pediatric clinics for regular examinations.

Myxedema. Adult hypothyroidism is known as myxedema. The symptoms and the rate at which they develop correspond to the degree of thyroid inactivity. An abnormal decrease in thyroid hormone causes a general reduction in cellular metabolism, producing mental and physical sluggishness. The person gradually exhibits apathy and slowness in responses. An abnormal deposition of a mucopolysaccharide, which tends to hold water, occurs in the subcutaneous tissues, giving the person an edematous appearance. The skin becomes dry and thick, the face (particularly the eyelids) appears puffy and the lips and tongue enlarge. The person experiences weakness, fatigue and an increased sensitivity to cold. His appetite is poor although he may show a gain in weight. The temperature, pulse and blood pressure are abnormally low. Mental processes are retarded, and the patient sleeps a lot. Impaired function of the reproductive system is manifested by menstrual disorders, such as metrorrhagia and amenorrhea, and loss of sexual drive. Hoarseness and slow, monotonous speech may be noted. Because of his complacency and dull mental processes, the condition is of much less concern to the patient than to his family or friends witnessing the changes. Allowed to progress, the disorder may lead to arteriosclerotic changes, cardiac insufficiency or coma.

Causes of hypothyroidism include destruction of the gland by a disease such as thyroiditis and Hashimoto's disease (see p. 549), irradiation, prolonged iodine deficiency, a disorder of the hypothalamic-adenohypophyseal system which results in a deficiency of thyrotrophin, and complete thyroidectomy.

Treatment and Nursing Care. Hypothyroidism is treated favorably by the administration of thyroid extract or thyroxine. Preparations used are dessicated thyroid (thyroid), thyroglobulin (Proloid), sodium levothyroxine (Synthroid) and sodium liothyronine (Cytomel). Sodium liothyronine is a preparation of triiodothyronine (T_3) and acts very rapidly, but the effect is sustained for a shorter period than the others, which are not fully effective before 7 to 10 days. The dosage is usually small to start with and is gradually increased to guard against a too sudden and excessive demand on the heart by rapid acceleration of metabolism. The pulse is checked and recorded frequently until the maintenance dose is established. Reactions to overdosage include rapid pulse rate, palpitation, restlessness or hyperactivity, nervousness and insomnia. The maintenance dose is individualized on the basis of the responses observed and recorded.

It may be necessary for the nurse to explain the condition to the patient and his family and emphasize that replacement therapy must be continued indefinitely. The patient may neglect taking the medication when he feels better. During the myxedematous state, it is important that the family appreciate that the patient's lethargy and dullness are a part of his disease. They may be prone to criticize and drive the patient. The nurse and his family must be patient and tolerant of his slowness. He should be encouraged and given time to complete responses and activities. Early indications of improvement and response to the drug therapy may be pointed out to them for reassurance that the condition is reversible.

Much of the nursing care is symptomatic. For example, extra warmth is provided because of the patient's lower tolerance to cold. Without extra clothing and bedding, he may be uncomfortable in an environmental temperature that is comfortable to others. A minimum of soap is used on the patient's skin, and oily lotions or creams are applied to relieve the dryness. A low-calorie, high-protein diet is served with added roughage to combat the problem of constipation. Laxatives or enemas may be necessary to avoid impaction. The hypothyroid patient is seen at the clinic or by his physician at regular intervals; adjustment of the drug dosage may be necessary from time to time.

Goiter

The term goiter simply indicates enlargement of the thyroid gland. It may be a compensatory hypertrophy as occurs in iodine deficiency or in cases in which there is an increased demand for the thyroid hormone, as in pregnancy and puberty. Enlargement may be the result of a neoplasm, thyroiditis or hyperplasia associated with pathological hyperactivity, as in Graves' disease (exophthalmic goiter). Rarely, it is due to a congenital defect in which a specific enzyme which is necessary in the process of forming the hormones is missing or defective. A goiter may be classified as diffuse or nodular; endemic or sporadic, depending on the frequency with which it occurs in a given area; and toxic, nontoxic or simple, depending on whether the enlargement is accompanied by hyperthyroidism.

Goiter most commonly refers to an enlargement that is endemic and due to a deficiency in the natural supply of iodine in the water and soil. It is seen most often in mountainous areas and inland areas distant from the sea (e.g., Great Lakes districts, Rocky Mountains and Alps). Terms used to describe it include simple endemic goiter, iron-deficient goiter, and simple colloid or nontoxic goiter. In most areas where the natural source is inadequate, the simple, inexpensive prophylactic measure of adding iodine to salt used in food has been adopted. Residents of such districts should be informed of the significance of using iodized salt.

The enlargement of the thyroid in iodine deficiency occurs because of stimulation by an increased release of thyrotrophin by the adenohypophysis in response to the low hormone concentration of the blood. The follicles increase in number and size and the thyroid becomes more vascular. If the iron deficiency and excessive thyrotrophin stimulation are prolonged, the gland tends to develop nodules which contain greatly distended follicles that may eventually undergo degeneration.

The enlarged gland may cause disfigurement which creates embarrassment for the person. More serious symptoms are pressure on the larynx and trachea manifested by a chronic cough and respiratory difficulty, interference with swallowing, and compression of nerves in the area.

The simple nontoxic goiter is treated with an iodide preparation (e.g., potassium iodide), or if there is evidence of hypothyroidism, the patient receives a thyroid preparation. In the early stages, with an adequate supply of iodine, the goiter gradually becomes smaller. If the gland has been enlarged over a period of years and has become nodular, drug therapy is likely to be less effective. The gland remains large and surgical removal of a large portion may be indicated to relieve pressure on the trachea, larynx, esophagus or nerves and to improve the patient's appearance.

Hyperthyroidism

Hyperthyroidism implies an excessive secretion of the thyroid hormones and may be called thyrotoxicosis, toxic goiter, exophthalmic goiter, Graves' disease or Basedow's disease. The terms exophthalmic goiter, Graves' disease or Basedow's disease are reserved for hyperthyroidism that is accompanied by exophthalmos and extreme nervousness.

The exact cause of hyperactivity of the thyroid is not clear. It is suggested that it may be due to a primary disorder within the gland, an excessive secretion of thyrotrophin (TSH), or the production of an abnormal form of the trophic hormone.[6, 7] The disease affects females more often than males and is rare in childhood. Frequently the onset is closely related to an emotional crisis in the person's life.

Manifestations. Some enlargement of the gland is evident and may be due to a diffuse hyperplasia of the gland or the development of one or more adenomas. The increased blood level of thyroid hormones accelerates the metabolic rate. The patient's appetite increases, and unless the food intake keeps pace with the rapid metabolic rate, there is a marked loss of weight. Lowered heat tolerance and excessive sweating are manifested. The hyperthyroid patient is uncomfortably warm in an environmental temperature quite acceptable to others. Nervousness, apprehension, emotional instability and restlessness are evident, and the hands are warm and moist in contrast to the cold, moist extremities associated with anxiety. Although the patient is eating more, he complains of weakness and quick fatigue. The pulse is rapid and exhibits a sharp rise on exertion. Shortness of breath on exertion and palpitation are experienced. The diastolic blood pressure is usually lower than normal because of widespread vasodilation. A fine, rapid tremor develops in the hands and is accentuated when they are outstretched. Diarrhea, resulting from increased gastrointestinal activity, may be troublesome. Menstrual disorders, such as oligomenorrhea (scant flow) or amenorrhea, are common. The gland shows some enlargement and may be readily seen to move upward with the larynx in swallowing. Eye changes may appear in hyperthyroidism (Graves' disease or exophthalmic goiter), which is considered secondary to a disturbance in the hypothalamic-adenohypophyseal system that causes excessive stimulation of the thyroid. Exophthalmos, a protrusion of the eyeballs, occurs. The upper eyelids are retracted, showing the upper sclerae. The lids fail to follow the movement of the eyes when the person looks down (von Graefe's sign).

Treatment. Hyperthyroidism may be treated by antithyroid drugs, radioactive iodine (I^{131}) or surgery. The drugs used interfere with the formation of the thyroid hormones. They include methimazole (Tapazole) and the thiouracil derivatives—propylthiouracil, methylthiouracil (Methiacil, Thimecil) and iothiouracil (Itrumil). The antithyroid drugs may be used to prepare a patient for surgery or as definitive treatment. In the latter case, they are given over a prolonged period of 1 to 2 years. Side effects which may develop are agranulocytosis, dermatitis and hepatitis. The patient is advised to promptly report a sore throat, swollen tender "neck glands," fever, rash or jaundice. It is important that he understand the necessity for taking the drugs regularly and on the hours suggested in order to obtain the desired effect and prevent a remission. Some compensatory enlargement of the gland usually occurs, and the patient may be reassured that this is not serious.

Treatment by radioiodine (I^{131}) is very simple and has proved very effective, largely replacing surgery and prolonged antithyroid drug administration. It is given orally, and the radioiodine is trapped in the thyroid where its radiations destroy tissue, reducing the functioning mass. Improvement is usually evident in 3 weeks, and the metabolic rate is expected to reach a normal level in 2 to 3 months. Radioiodine is not generally given for therapeutic purposes to persons under 20 years of age, and it is never given during pregnancy. Some physicians question its use during the reproductive years because of the risk of genetic mutation.

The patient who receives a therapeutic dose of radioiodine is isolated in a single unit

[6]W. A. Sodeman, and W. A. Sodeman, Jr.: Pathologic Physiology, 4th ed. Philadelphia, W. B. Saunders Co., 1967, p. 181.

[7]T. R. Harrison, et al. (Eds.): Principles of Internal Medicine, 4th ed. New York, The Blakiston Div., McGraw-Hill Book Co., Inc., 1962, p. 589.

for 8 days (half-life of I¹³¹), and the necessary precautions are taken to protect personnel (see p. 92). Specific directives should be obtained from the radioisotope laboratory as to the collection and disposal of the patient's urine in which the iodine is eliminated. The patient is observed closely for signs of aggravation of his disease. Rarely, a thyroid storm (thyrotoxic crisis) may develop (see p. 549). Following discharge from the hospital, regular visits to the clinic or the physician are necessary. The patient is examined for remission of his disease and possible hypothyroidism. The protein-bound iodine blood level is determined and the basal metabolic rate may be checked. If hypothyroidism is indicated, a replacement preparation (e.g., desiccated thyroid) is prescribed.

A partial thyroidectomy may be done if antithyroid drug sensitivity precludes its prolonged administration, if radioactive iodine is contraindicated or if the gland is very large, causing disfigurement or pressure on the respiratory tract or on the esophagus. In hyperthyroidism, approximately three-quarters of the gland is removed; in the case of cancer of the thyroid, a complete thyroidectomy is done which necessitates continuous replacement therapy during the remainder of the patient's life.

Nursing the Patient with Hyperthyroidism. The care of a hyperthyroid patient, whether in the hospital or at home, requires the following considerations.

ENVIRONMENT. Because of the patient's nervousness and hyperexcitability, quietness and serenity in his environment are very important. An established routine, so that he knows what to expect and what is expected of him at given times may prevent unnecessary disturbance which only aggravates his condition. If the patient is being cared for at home, the family must be made fully aware of these needs. They are advised that his irritability, restlessness, and emotional lability are characteristic of his illness and that to argue with him or criticize him will worsen it. In the hospital, the patient is placed in a single room; if this is not possible, careful consideration is given to his placement on the ward. Exposure to very ill, talkative or otherwise disturbing patients is avoided. Since the patient is producing more than the normal amount of body heat, he is only comfortable in an environment of lower temperature than normal persons tolerate. Scant, lightweight bedding is used, and the room is kept well ventilated.

OBSERVATIONS. An accurate record of the patient's temperature, pulse and respirations is made at least every 4 hours, and the patient's responses and degree of restlessness and agitation are noted frequently. This is necessary so that any early indication of increasing thyrotoxicosis and cardiac insufficiency may be recognized and receive prompt attention. The patient is told that his vital signs will be checked at regular intervals so he will not be unduly apprehensive about his condition because of the frequent checking. The physician may request the recording of a sleeping pulse; in hyperthyroidism, the elevated rate persists during sleep. The patient is weighed daily or every second day to determine if his calorie intake is keeping pace with his metabolic rate. Reactions to visitors are noted; an elevation in pulse rate and increased agitation and excitement may indicate the need for additional limitations on visitors.

REST AND ACTIVITY. Activity is restricted because it increases the metabolic rate, but the patient's nervous excitability makes it difficult for him to rest. Efforts are made to provide some interest or occupational therapy that expends little energy. Depending on the severity of the patient's condition and his pulse rate, he may be allowed up, since enforced confinement to bed may cause greater irritation and restlessness. He is discouraged from wandering about the ward aimlessly. Regular doses of a sedative, such as phenobarbital (Luminal) or amobarbital sodium (Sodium Amytal), may be ordered at regular intervals. A stronger preparation may be necessary at bedtime to ensure adequate sleep; examples of drugs administered at bedtime include secobarbital sodium (Seconal) and pentobarbital sodium (Nembutal).

Keeping the patient as comfortable as possible by frequent turning of the pillows, changing of the bed linen and patient's gown when they become moist because of the excessive perspiration, and gentle soothing back rubs help to promote rest. Situations which tend to annoy or frustrate the patient are avoided. Needs should be anticipated, and things that prove awkward for him because of tremor are unobtrusively done for him. Whenever possible, the same nurse cares for the patient, since adjusting to strange personnel may be stressful.

DIET. The patient requires a high-protein, high-carbohydrate, high-calorie diet (4000 to 5000 calories) to prevent tissue breakdown by the high metabolic demand and to satisfy the patient's increased appetite. A snack between meals and at bedtime is provided. Tea and coffee are usually restricted to eliminate caffein stimulation. Decaffeinated coffee may be used as a substitute.

FLUIDS. The patient's excessive heat production and resulting perspiration increases his fluid loss, necessitating extra fluids. Also, there is an increased production of metabolic wastes, requiring dilution for elimination by the kidneys. A minimum intake of 3000 to 4000 ml. daily is recommended. An explanation of the importance of this amount of fluid is made to the patient to gain his cooperation, and a variety of fluids are provided.

SKIN CARE. A daily bath is necessary because of the profuse perspiration. If the patient is extremely restless and is confined to bed, special attention is given to the pressure areas. Soft linen is selected and talcum applied to the skin to prevent friction irritation.

VISITORS. Visitors are restricted to those persons who do not excite the patient and who use judgment in their conversation with him. Obviously, those who focus on the patient's condition, transmit disturbing information, or are themselves excitable could aggravate the patient's symptoms.

Nursing the Patient Who Has Thyroid Surgery. In caring for the patient who has had a thyroidectomy, pertinent factors to be kept in mind are the location of the gland in relation to the trachea and larynx, its proximity to the recurrent laryngeal nerve which controls the vocal cords, its abundant blood supply, and that the parathyroid glands, which influence neuromuscular irritability through their control of the blood calcium level, lie on the posterior surface of the thyroid. The nurse must be constantly alert for manifestations of disturbances due to these factors.

PREOPERATIVE PREPARATION. The hyperthyroid patient who is to have surgery is given an antithyroid drug for several weeks prior to operation to reduce the metabolic rate. During this period, whether at home or in the hospital, the care cited in the preceding section is applicable. The antithyroid drugs produce some compensatory enlargement of the gland and an increased blood supply. When the metabolic rate has been reduced to a satisfactory level, the drug is discontinued. Then in a few days, a course of Lugol's solution (a strong iodine preparation) is commenced and continued for approximately 10 days. This reduces the size and vascularity of the gland, facilitating surgery and lessening the problem of bleeding. Since Lugol's solution has a disagreeable taste and may also irritate the mucous membrane, it is well diluted in fruit juice (e.g., grape juice) or milk.

Preparation includes an electrocardiogram to obtain further information about the patient's cardiac status and blood typing and cross matching for transfusion. The female patient may have some concern for the cosmetic effect of the operation. She is assured that consideration is given to this and that the scar becomes barely perceptible in a few months. During the interval, it may be concealed by a scarf or necklace. Remembering that the hyperthyroid patient is hyperexcitable and apprehensive, judicious explanations are made of what may be expected after the operation. If the patient still responds by extreme nervous reactions and tachycardia to stressful situations, the surgeon may consider it inadvisable to inform the patient of the exact day of operation. An intravenous infusion of normal saline or glucose in normal saline may be ordered for 2 or 3 mornings and is given before the patient's breakfast. Then on the day of operation, instead of the usual solution, he receives an intravenous anesthetic, usually thiopental sodium (Sodium Pentothal), and is unconscious when taken to the operating room. Specific orders are received about the local skin preparation. For the female patient, the surgeon may require only thorough cleansing of the entire neck, upper shoulder aspect and upper chest. In the case of the male patient, shaving as well as cleansing is necessary.

The family are informed when the surgery is to be done, and their cooperation is sought when the patient is not to know the day of operation. The nurse sees that the operative consent is signed well ahead of time.

PREPARATION TO RECEIVE THE PATIENT AFTER OPERATION. Special equipment to be assembled and ready for use when preparing to receive a patient following a thyroidectomy includes: sandbags or small firm pillows to immobilize the head; suction machine and catheters for clearing mucus from the throat; steam inhalation to facilitate the patient's breathing and removal of mucus; intravenous infusion equipment; a sterile emergency tracheostomy tray in the event of respiratory obstruction; equipment for quickly obtaining a blood specimen for blood calcium determination; and ampules of calcium chloride or calcium gluconate with the necessary equipment for intravenous administration in the event of the complication tetany (hypocalcemia).

POSTOPERATIVE CARE. A nurse remains in close attendance on the thyroidectomy patient, especially during the first postoperative 48 hours. He is usually very apprehensive, and serious complications may develop rapidly.

Observations. The blood pressure, pulse and respirations are recorded every 15 minutes; the frequency is gradually reduced if they remain stable. The rectal temperature is recorded every 4 hours; after the second day the temperature may be taken orally. The degree of restlessness and apprehension is noted and, if not relieved by the prescribed sedation, is brought to the surgeon's attention. Particular attention is paid to the patient's respirations; any complaint or sign of respiratory distress and cyanosis are reported promptly, since they may indicate laryngeal paralysis or compression of the trachea by accumulating blood. Some hoarseness is common and is due to irritation of the larynx by the surgery and the endotracheal tube used in administering the anesthetic. The physician is advised if the hoarseness and weakness of the voice persist beyond 3 or 4 days. The fluid intake and output are measured, and the balance is noted.

Positioning and Activity. When the patient has recovered from the anesthetic, he is placed on his back and the head of the bed is moderately elevated. The head and neck are supported by a pillow and are positioned in good alignment, preventing flexion and hyperextension. A sandbag or firm pillow is placed on either side of the head for immobilization. The patient is advised not to move his head but to relax, since it is adequately supported. He tends to develop tension in an effort to keep it still. Gentle massage of the back of the neck may promote relaxation and reduce his discomfort. When the patient's position is changed, the nurse lifts and supports the head, preserving good alignment. After the first or second postoperative day, if his progress is satisfactory, the patient is taught to lift and support his head by placing his hands at the back of his head when he wishes to move.

While the patient is confined to bed, foot and leg exercises are encouraged, as with other surgical patients. If the vital signs are stabilized and normal, the patient is assisted out of bed on the second or third postoperative day.

Following removal of the sutures or skin clips and firm healing of the incision, head exercises which include flexion (forward and lateral), hyperextension and turning are gradually introduced with the surgeon's approval. To prevent contraction, the patient may be taught to gently massage the neck twice daily, using lanolin, cold cream or an oily lotion.

Respiratory Secretions. There is likely to be increased mucus secretion in the respiratory tract which proves troublesome and difficult to raise. The patient is helped by suctioning and by being assisted to a sitting position with support given to his head and neck while he coughs and clears away secretions.

The throat may be sore, and tracheal irritation may also be a source of discomfort. Analgesic throat lozenges and steam in the room may be ordered to provide some relief. The steam may also help to make the secretions less tenacious and easier to raise.

Fluids and Food. Some difficulty in swallowing is usually experienced for a day or two, but fluids by mouth are encouraged as soon as tolerated. Intravenous fluids are given until an adequate amount can be taken orally. The patient progresses through a soft diet to a full diet in 2 to 3 days.

Medication. Meperidine hydrochloride (Demerol) or morphine may be ordered to keep the patient comfortable and less apprehensive during the first 48 hours. Judicious use must be made of the narcotic; the drug is not repeated without consulting the physician if there is evident depression of the respirations to 12 or less per minute or if there is increased difficulty in raising mucus secretions. On the other hand, unnecessary withholding of sedation increases the patient's metabolism and restlessness and may precipitate tachycardia.

Complications. The nurse must be aware that hemorrhage, respiratory difficulty, loss of voice and tetany are serious complications which may occur following thyroid surgery. The first three may develop with startling rapidity and are usually seen within 48 hours of operation.

Hemorrhage may be manifested by a rapid thin pulse, fall in blood pressure and evident bleeding. The bleeding may only be discovered by frequent checking of the dressing and by sliding the hands under the shoulders and behind the neck. Blood may collect quickly within the tissues and cause pressure on the trachea. The patient may complain of a choking sensation and shortness of breath; cyanosis and dyspnea develop, and unless the pressure is relieved quickly, asphyxia may occur. The doctor is notified immediately at the earliest sign or change. The dressing is loosened to promote freer, outward drainage. Instruments for removing the sutures or skin clips are brought to the bedside, and the emergency tracheostomy tray is made ready, since the doctor may consider an immediate tracheostomy necessary. On reporting the situation, the nurse may be instructed to remove the skin clips to allow the escape of blood. A thick sterile dressing is then applied until the doctor arrives. The patient will probably be returned to the operating room where the bleeding is brought under control. Blood replacement may be necessary.

Occasionally, injury to one or both recurrent laryngeal nerves may occur during thyroid surgery. These nerves control laryngeal muscles, the opening of the glottis and voice production. Injury to one nerve produces hoarseness and weakness of the voice but no serious respiratory disturbance. Bilateral nerve injury causes paralysis of muscles on both sides of the larynx, resulting in closure of the glottis and respiratory obstruction. The patient is unable to speak, the respirations suddenly become stridulous (i.e., have a shrill, crowing sound), cyanosis develops and loss of consciousness ensues unless respirations are quickly re-established. Prompt endotracheal intubation or emergency tracheostomy is done, and oxygen is administered via either tube. The injury and paralysis are rarely permanent; function is usually gradually restored, and the tracheostomy tube is removed.

During surgery, interference with the blood supply to the parathyroid glands or injury or removal of parathyroid tissue may occur which depresses secretion by the glands. Decreased parathyroid hormone concentration leads to hypocalcemia, resulting in increased neuromuscular irritability and the condition known as tetany. Early signs of this complication include complaints of numbness and tingling in the hands or feet, muscle twitching and spasms, and gastrointestinal cramps. A change may be evident in the voice, which may become high-pitched and shrill because of spasm of the vocal cords. To confirm increased neuromuscular irritability due to hypocalcemia, the patient is examined for a positive Chvostek's or Trousseau's sign. Chvostek's sign is demonstrated by twitching of the upper lip and contraction of the facial muscles in response to tapping of the facial nerve in front of the ear. Trousseau's sign is elicited by the inflation of a blood pressure cuff around an arm; if the blood calcium level is low, spasmodic contraction of the forearm muscles occurs, producing a claw-like flexure of the hand and fingers. A blood specimen is obtained for serum calcium determination with the appearance of early symptoms. Calcium gluconate is then given orally until normal parathyroid function is resumed.

CARE AFTER DISCHARGE FROM HOSPITAL. The patient's hospitalization is usually brief if no complications develop. Information as to the amount of activity he may resume is obtained from the doctor and discussed with the patient. Extra rest will still be necessary, and the patient is advised to continue neck exercises until there is freedom of movement without any feeling of pulling. He is usually followed at the clinic or by the physician for about a year, being examined for any residual laryngeal damage and hypoparathyroidism, recurring hyperthyroidism, or developing hypothyroidism.

Thyroid Storm (Thyrotoxic Crisis)

This is a serious complication of hyperthyroidism that usually proves fatal, but fortunately, it is rarely seen since the advent of antithyroid drugs and radioiodine. The crisis may be precipitated in a hyperthyroid person by a severe infection, such as pneumonia, or by an emotional crisis. It must also be kept in mind as a possible, but rare, complication of a subtotal thyroidectomy or radioiodine treatment.

It is attributed to the sudden release of large amounts of the thyroid hormones into the circulation. The metabolic rate rises rapidly and the patient manifests hyperpyrexia, an extremely rapid pulse, inordinate restlessness, disorientation, diarrhea and vomiting, and eventually shock and coma due to heart failure and circulatory collapse.

The patient receives a continuous intravenous infusion of solutions of glucose and necessary electrolytes. Sedatives or tranquilizers, cortisone, digitalis or quinidine, and sodium iodide are administered, and the patient is placed in an oxygen tent. Hypothermia, ice packs or cold sponges are used in an effort to lower the temperature. Intensive nursing care and constant attendance at the bedside are necessary.

Thyroiditis

Inflammation of the thyroid occurs rarely and may be acute or chronic. Acute thyroiditis may be the result of viral or bacterial infection or may follow irradiation therapy of the gland. The thyroid area of the neck is tender, warm and reddened; the temperature is elevated and signs of hyperthyroidism may develop. The patient may be treated by bed rest, an antimicrobial preparation if the condition is of infectious origin, and local cold applications.

Chronic thyroiditis occurs in a form which may be referred to as Hashimoto's disease. This disease is an autoimmune reaction; that is, the patient develops antibodies in response to antigens originating in his own thyroid. It is suggested that substances which normally remain within the thyro-

globin escape into the general circulation. The production of lymphocytes and plasma cells with antibodies is stimulated, and these cells infiltrate and attack the thyroid, resulting in destruction of the functioning tissue. The gland becomes swollen and congested, and eventually hypothyroidism develops. The condition may be treated with cortisone, or because of the increased incidence of cancer in Hashimoto's disease, a complete thyroidectomy may be done. Replacement therapy is used for the associated hormone deficiency.

A second type of chronic thyroiditis, which is extremely rare, is known as Reidel's struma. The etiology is unknown. The condition is characterized by "the slowly progressive invasion of part or all of the thyroid and adjacent cervical tissues by dense fibrous or collagenous connective tissue."[8] The affected area becomes very hard and may cause pressure on the trachea and esophagus. Surgical resection may be undertaken.

Carcinoma of the Thyroid

The most common malignancy of the thyroid is adenocarcinoma. Signs and symptoms include rapid and progressive enlargement of the gland without an appreciable increase or decrease in thyroid hormone secretion, hardness and fixation of the gland, lymph node enlargement in the neck and supraclavicular areas, hoarseness due to involvement of the recurrent laryngeal nerve, and respiratory distress because of pressure on the trachea.

The condition may be treated with internal radiation by the administration of radioiodine (I^{131}), relatively large doses of desiccated thyroid to suppress the gland's activity, or total thyroidectomy followed by radiation therapy and hormonal replacement.

PARATHYROID GLANDS

The parathyroid glands are small oval bodies attached to the posterior surface of

[8]A. Grollman: Clinical Endocrinology and Its Physiologic Basis. Philadelphia, J. B. Lippincott Co., 1964, p. 173.

the lateral lobes of the thyroid. The number may vary but is usually four. They secrete the hormone parathormone (PTH), which controls the concentration of calcium and inorganic phosphorus in the blood through its action on the intestine, bone tissue and the kidneys. It promotes absorption of calcium in the intestine and demineralization of bone and the movement of the calcium and phosphorus into the extracellular fluid. In the kidneys, the hormone increases the excretion of phosphorus by decreasing its reabsorption from the glomerular filtrate; conversely, the reabsorption of calcium is increased, decreasing its excretion in urine.

Parathormone, through its regulation of blood calcium and phosphorus, plays an important role in normal physiology. A normal concentration of calcium is essential for the normal structure of bones and teeth, coagulation of blood, maintenance of normal cardiac rhythmicity, normal neuromuscular excitability and cellular membrane permeability. The greater part of the absorbed calcium is deposited in bones. The optimal blood calcium level for meeting these functions is 9 to 11 mg. per cent (5 mEq. per L.). Phosphorus functions in cellular metabolism, bone structure and the maintenance of a normal pH of body fluids. The normal blood concentration of inorganic phosphorus is 3 to 4 mg. per cent (2 mEq. per L.).

The rate of secretion of the parathyroid hormone is controlled by the concentration of calcium in the blood. When the calcium level rises above normal, the glands are inhibited and less hormone is produced. A fall in the blood calcium level stimulates the glands, resulting in an increased output of parathormone.

In summary, a feedback system exists between the parathyroid glands and circulating calcium level. Following a decrease in calcium concentration, the increased secretion of parathormone causes the release of calcium and phosphorus from the bones, increased calcium absorption from the intestine, and increased reabsorption of calcium and decreased reabsorption of phosphorus by the renal tubules. When the blood calcium is increased, there is decreased secretion of parathormone, and the above responses are reversed.

Parathyroid Disorders

Primary disease of the parathyroid glands is rare; the disturbances seen are most often secondary to thyroid disease.

Hypoparathyroidism

Parathyroid insufficiency may be the result of idiopathic atrophy of the glands or surgery on the thyroid. In the case of surgery, there may have been interference with the blood supply to the glands, injury which inhibits secretion or, rarely, inadvertent removal of them. The deficiency of parathormone causes hypocalcemia, and symptoms of increased neuromuscular excitability are usually the first manifestations (see p. 59). Less calcium is excreted in the urine because of the low blood calcium, and the bones tend to become more dense. If the deficiency is prolonged, calcium deposition may develop in the lens and conjunctiva of the eyes, the brain, lungs or gastric mucosa. The hair becomes thin and gray.

The hypocalcemia is corrected initially by the intravenous administration of calcium gluconate or calcium chloride. The patient is then given regular oral doses of a calcium salt such as gluconate or lactate along with a preparation of vitamin D or dihydrotachysterol (A.T. 10). Vitamin D and A.T. 10 promote the absorption of the calcium.

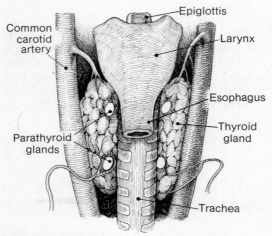

Figure 21–4 Posterior surface of the thyroid gland, showing the parathyroid glands.

Hyperparathyroidism

The cause of an excessive secretion of parathormone is usually an adenoma but may rarely be hyperplasia or carcinoma of the glands. The blood calcium level is high, and the blood level of inorganic phosphorus falls as renal excretion of it increases. Because of the hypercalcemia, the concentration of calcium in the glomerular filtrate is higher than normal, predisposing the formation of renal calculi. Neuromuscular excitability is depressed and loss of muscle tone is evident. Demineralization of the bones may be so marked that fibrous cystic areas develop, which frequently lead to deformities and pathological fractures. In some instances bone tumors consisting of an overgrowth of osteoclasts develop.

The patient may complain of muscular weakness, loss of appetite, nausea, vomiting and constipation. The urinary volume is usually increased because of the excessive calcium and phosphorus to be excreted. Renal function may become impaired; the tubular epithelium may be damaged by the excessive excretion of calcium or the formation of renal calculi. When bone changes occur, the disorder may be referred to as von Recklinghausen's disease or osteitis fibrosa cystica, and the patient may experience tenderness and pain in the bones, especially with weight-bearing. Frequently, the disease is only recognized when some deformity develops or a pathological fracture occurs.

The patient with hyperparathyroidism should receive 3000 to 4000 ml. of fluid daily. If anorexia, nausea and vomiting are problems, intravenous infusions are given to ensure an adequate intake. Foods containing calcium are restricted in the diet.

Hyperparathyroidism is treated by surgical excision of the gland with the adenoma or, in the case of hyperplasia, removal of all the glands but one. Following surgery, the patient is observed closely for the early signs of possible hypocalcemia (tetany) cited on page 59. A diet high in calcium and phosphorus is usually given to restore normal bone structure.

ADRENAL GLANDS

The two adrenal or suprarenal glands are situated immediately above the kidneys. Each one is enclosed within a capsule and consists of 2 distinct parts, the cortex and medulla, which are functionally unrelated and are of different embryological origin. The cortex develops from germinal mesodermal cells. The medulla is derived from the ectoderm in close association with the sympathetic division of the autonomic nervous system with which it is functionally related. The adrenal glands have an abundant blood supply through branches of the aorta and the inferior phrenic and renal arteries.

The Adrenal Cortex

The cortex forms the outer part as well as the greater portion of the gland and produces hormones essential to life. These are steroids and collectively are called the adrenocorticoids, corticosteroids or corticoids. Cells of the cortex have a high cholesterol and vitamin C content. These substances are used in the formation of the hormones. The corticoids are divided into 3 groups—namely, the mineralocorticoids, glucocorticoids and sex hormones.

Mineralocorticoids. The most significant mineralocorticoid is aldosterone, which influences electrolyte concentrations and fluid volume. It stimulates the renal tubules to reabsorb sodium and excrete potassium, and it decreases the sodium concentration while increasing the potassium content of saliva and sweat. An increase in the level of circulating aldosterone causes an increase in the sodium concentration of extracellular fluids. The consequent elevation in their osmotic pressure causes an increased release of the antidiuretic hormone and a resultant retention of water. Conversely, a decreased output of aldosterone reverses these reactions.

The secretion of aldosterone is regulated in the interest of maintaining "normal sodium concentration in the extracellular fluids and normal extracellular fluid volume."[9] Factors which influence the amount of aldosterone released are the blood sodium and potassium levels and the blood volume. A decrease in the sodium concentration stimulates an increased output of aldosterone, and conversely, a rise in sodium to above the normal

[9]A. C. Guyton: Textbook of Medical Physiology, 4th ed. Philadelphia, W. B. Saunders Co., 1971, p. 889.

level decreases the output of the hormone. The effect of potassium is the reverse of that of sodium; that is, the adrenal cortices respond to an elevated potassium concentration by an increased secretion of aldosterone, and vice versa. A decreased blood volume or fall in arterial blood pressure to below normal brings about increased aldosterone secretion.

Glucocorticoids. Several glucocorticoids have been recognized, but cortisol (hydrocortisone) is considered to be the most important, since it is produced in much greater amounts than the others. Cortisol influences the metabolism of glucose, protein and fat and is concerned with the body's responses to physical and mental stress. Its actions are complex and not clearly understood; for example, it enables a person to deal more effectively with stress, but how this is achieved is not known. Cortisol elevates the blood sugar level, and the liver glycogen stores are increased. Tissue protein is broken down and the amino acids are converted to glycogen or glucose in the liver (gluconeogenesis). Fat is also mobilized, some of which is also converted to glucose.

Glucocorticoids are secreted in response to circulating adrenocorticotrophic hormone (ACTH). In turn, the production and release of ACTH by the adenohypophysis depends upon the concentration of glucocorticoids in the blood, establishing a feedback mechanism. When the glucocorticoid blood level falls, the hypothalamus produces a corticotrophin-releasing factor, which is transmitted via the hypothalamic-hypophyseal portal system to the adenohypophysis, initiating a release of ACTH. With an elevation of blood glucocorticoids, the output of ACTH is depressed.

Of clinical significance, a concentration of cortisol in excess of the normal secretion suppresses local inflammatory responses to irritating substances (anti-inflammatory effect), delays healing through depressed fibroplasia and reduces tissue sensitivity reactions to antigens (anti-allergic reaction). Other effects also associated with an excess of this steroid are atrophy of the lymphoid tissues, a decreased production of lymphocytes and eosinophils, an increased secretion of gastric hydrochloric acid and pepsinogen which predisposes to the development of ulcers, and increased cerebral excitability manifested by restlessness and euphoria. The glucocorticoids, as well as the mineralocorticoids, may also cause some sodium retention, resulting in a positive fluid balance.

Adrenal Sex Hormones. The adrenal cortices of both sexes secrete both male and female hormones—namely, androgens, estrogen and progesterone. Estrogen and progesterone are produced in lesser amounts than the androgens, but normally, the quantity of any of these hormones is considered to be physiologically insignificant compared with the amounts produced by the gonads. Occasionally, tumors of the adrenal cortex may result in an excessive production of the sex hormones, leading to precocious sexual development in childhood, masculinizing changes in the female adult or feminization in the case of an adult male.

Adrenal Medulla

The medulla forms the central portion of each adrenal gland and is comprised of specialized neurons (nerve cells) which secrete two hormones, epinephrine (adrenaline) and norepinephrine (noradrenaline). Because of their chemical composition, they are frequently referred to as catecholamines. During any stress or threat to the organism, the hormones are released and serve with the autonomic nervous system to produce defensive reactions throughout the body. Their production is controlled by nerve impulses transmitted to the medullae by sympathetic nerve fibers, and their effects are similar to those produced by sympathetic innervation. Approximately 80 per cent of the secretion is epinephrine, and the remainder is norepinephrine.

Epinephrine causes constriction of the peripheral and renal blood vessels and dilatation of the coronary and skeletal muscle vessels. The rate and force of contraction of the heart and skeletal muscle capacity are increased. The smooth muscle of the bronchioles, gastrointestinal tract and urinary bladder relaxes. The dilator muscle fibers of the irises contract, resulting in dilatation of the pupils. The blood sugar is elevated by increased glycogenolysis (conversion of glycogen to glucose) in both the liver and skeletal muscles. The metabolic rate is accelerated, and there is an increased alertness and awareness due to stimulation of the brain. Epinephrine also promotes the release of adrenocorticotrophin which in turn increases the secretion of glucocorticoids.

Norepinephrine causes a more generalized vasoconstriction and does not cause dilatation of any vessels. Because of this action, it is more effective in raising the blood pressure. It does not affect carbohydrate metabolism or contribute to elevation of the blood sugar level.

Disorders of the Adrenal Cortices

As with other endocrine glands, dysfunction of the adrenal cortices may involve hyposecretion or hypersecretion of their hormones. Adrenocortical hypofunction produces Addison's disease. Hyperfunction may cause Cushing's disease or primary aldosteronism.

Assessment of Adrenocortical Function

Investigation of adrenocortical activity includes the following tests:

Urinary Excretion of 17-Ketosteroids. An estimation of the concentration of 17-ketosteroids in a 24-hour urine collection provides some indication of the secretory activity of the adrenal cortices. These ketosteroids are metabolic products of androgens and glucocorticoids. If the concentration is less than normal, an intravenous infusion of ACTH in normal saline is given slowly over 8 hours, and the urine is collected for a second 24-hour specimen. If the low level of 17-ketosteroids still persists, it suggests dysfunction of the adrenal cortices. An elevation in the urinary steroids following the administration of the ACTH indicates a deficiency in the secretion of ACTH by the adenohypophysis.

Normal 24-hour urinary steroids: adult male, 8 to 20 mg. per 24 hours; adult female, 6 to 15 mg. per 24 hours.

Eosinophil Count. Normally, an elevated concentration of glucocorticoids reduces the number of circulating eosinophils. Using this as a means of testing adrenocortical function, the eosinophil count is taken in the morning before breakfast. Then the patient receives an intramuscular injection of ACTH. The response of normal adrenal cortices is an increased output of glucocorticoids and a corresponding fall in eosinophils. If there is no appreciable decrease in the circulating eosinophils, it suggests adrenocortical hypofunction.

Normal eosinophil count: 200 per cu. mm. or 1 to 3 per cent of leukocytes.

Normal following ACTH injection: approximately 20 to 30 per cent decrease of the initial count.

Water Excretion Test. Adrenocorticoid insufficiency reduces the renal ability to excrete water rapidly. The patient is given 1500 ml. of water in the fasting state. Normally, the urinary output will be 1000 ml. or more within 5 hours. A decrease to 50 per cent or less of the volume of water given is common in adrenocortical hypofunction.

Blood Chemistry. Blood electrolyte concentrations are determined, and the ratio of sodium to potassium is noted. In adrenocortical insufficiency, the sodium level is below normal and that of potassium is elevated, decreasing the ratio of sodium to potassium.

Normal sodium: 132 to 142 mEq./L.
Normal potassium: 3.5 to 5.0 mEq./L.
Normal ratio Na:K — Approximately 1:30.

The fasting blood sugar is determined and is found to be below normal with decreased adrenocorticoid secretion and above normal with hypersecretion.

Normal blood sugar: 70 to 100 mg. per cent.

Addison's Disease

Primary failure of the adrenal cortices to produce corticoids is most often the result of atrophy of the glands but may also be caused by tubercular infection or a neoplasm. Atrophy of the glands is thought to develop from an auto-immune reaction; antigens escape from the adrenals, resulting in infiltration and ultimate destruction of the glands by lymphocytes, plasma cells and antibodies. Secondary hypofunction of the adrenal cortices occurs with hypopituitarism and the concomitant deficiency of adrenocorticotrophin.

The resultant deficiency of glucocorticoids interferes with the maintenance of a normal sugar level; the body cannot compensate by gluconeogenesis, and hypoglycemia develops, especially between meals. There is a general depression of metabolic activity and energy production. The ability to cope with even mild stress is greatly diminished, and minor infections, slight injuries, exposure to extremes of temperature, or emotional problems that are relatively insignificant to the normal person may prove very serious to these persons.

The aldosterone deficiency incurs decreased reabsorption of sodium by the renal tubules with a consequent excessive loss of water as well as sodium in the urine. Severe dehydration may develop, leading to a depletion of the intravascular volume and ensuing reduced cardiac output, hypotension and shock. There is not the normal exchange of hydrogen ions for reabsorbed sodium ions in the kidneys, and acidosis may develop. Increased reabsorption of potassium by the tubules produces an elevated blood level, and hyperkalemia may develop (see p. 58).

The adrenocortical insufficiency causes an outpouring of the adrenocorticotrophic hormone (ACTH). As noted earlier in this chapter, ACTH is similar in chemical structure to the melanocyte-stimulating hormone (MSH) and in high concentration may produce similar effects. As a result, pigmented areas of the skin are common to the patient with Addison's disease.

The disease has an insidious onset; according to Grollman, it is not usually manifested before nine-tenths of the cortical tissue is destroyed.[10] The patient complains of weakness and constant fatigue which become progressively more severe and incapacitating unless treatment in instituted. Listlessness, irritability and impaired mental ability may be manifested. Anorexia, nausea and constipation alternating with diarrhea are common complaints. The skin takes on a dusky, bronze hue, and brown pigmented areas appear, especially in sites normally exposed to light pressure or friction such as the backs of the hands (particularly over the knuckles), face, neck, axillae and "belt" areas. Patchy areas of pigmentation may also be observed in the oral mucosa and conjunctivae.

Treatment and Nursing Care. Addison's disease is treated by maintenance doses of

corticoid preparations. The glucocorticoids are replaced by the oral administration of hydrocortisone (cortisol) 2 or 3 times daily. To avoid gastric irritation, the drug is taken with meals. The deficiency of mineralocorticoid (aldosterone) is met by the giving of desoxycorticosterone intramuscularly or fludrocortisone (synthetic aldosterone) orally once daily. If desoxycorticosterone is used, after the maintenance dose is determined, a preparation in which the drug is carried in an oil solution (desoxycorticosterone trimethylacetate) may be given intramuscularly at intervals of 3 or 4 weeks instead of the daily dose.

The nurse caring for a patient receiving corticoid preparations must be familiar with the potential adverse effects of these drugs. If the patient receives corticoids in doses even slightly in excess of the amounts normally secreted, certain changes are likely to occur, especially with prolonged administration. Constant observation is necessary for early signs of side effects. Restlessness, insomnia, euphoria and swings in mood may be manifested. The patient's susceptibility to infection may be markedly increased by the drug's suppression of lymphocyte and antibody production and local inflammatory responses. Muscle wasting and weakness may occur as a result of an excessive protein breakdown and increased loss of potassium in the urine. Sodium and water retention may be evidenced by edema. Increased fat deposition on the trunk and face may develop, changing the patient's general appearance. Increased fullness and rounding of the face produces the characteristic change referred to as the "moon facies." Females may develop secondary male characteristics accompanied by growth of hair on the face, and growth of the breasts in males is occasionally seen. Prolonged administration of corticoids in excess of normal secretion may also produce hyperglycemia and glycosuria. The patient also becomes predisposed to the development of gastrointestinal lesions, such as peptic ulcers.

The patient with Addison's disease is encouraged to take a high-carbohydrate, high-protein diet. The danger of hypoglycemia which may occur with glucocorticoid deficiency may be offset by the patient taking nourishment between meals and at bedtime. A directive as to the amount of salt

---

[10] A. Grollman: Clinical Endocrinology and Its Physiologic Basis. Philadelphia, J. B. Lippincott Co., 1964, p. 290.

to be included in the diet should be received from the physician. Some patients may require additional salt; for others, the average amount served with meals is sufficient.

Acute corticoid insufficiency, which is also referred to as Addisonian crisis, may develop when corticoid replacement is inadequate or omitted, or it may be what brings the patient for medical attention before the disease is diagnosed. Frequently a crisis is precipitated by some physical or psychological stress such as infection, exposure to extremes of temperature, gastrointestinal upset (e.g., vomiting and diarrhea), fever, profuse perspiration, strenuous activity, anxiety or grief. Acute insufficiency is serious, and unless treated promptly, it can rapidly lead to death. Early symptoms are nausea, vomiting, diarrhea, abdominal pain, fever and extreme weakness. Severe hypoglycemia and dehydration develop rapidly; the blood pressure falls, and shock and coma may follow.

Addisonian crisis is treated by continuous intravenous infusion of dextrose in normal saline to which hydrocortisone (cortisol) is added for at least the first 24 hours. Hydrocortisone is also given orally or intramuscularly. The large doses of hydrocortisone which the patient receives usually exert sufficient sodium-retaining effect, eliminating the need for supplementary administration of a mineralocorticoid preparation. A vasopressor such as levarterenol (Levophed) or metarminol (Aramine) may be ordered intravenously to raise the blood pressure. This will be given in a separate intravenous solution, since the rate of flow must be carefully controlled according to the blood pressure. Frequent recordings of the blood pressure, temperature, pulse, respirations and level of response are made. The patient is kept at absolute rest to avoid expenditure of energy and is turned, bathed and fed by the nurse. He is kept flat, and any change of position is made slowly because of the hypotension. Frequent, high-carbohydrate feedings are given as soon as they can be tolerated. When the patient's blood pressure and other vital signs have returned to normal and are sustained, and the condition which precipitated the crisis has been controlled, the corticoid dosage is gradually reduced to maintenance level.

An important nursing function in caring for the patient with Addison's disease is teaching him and his family about his disease and the necessary care. A simple explanation is given of the nature of the condition, and he is told that, although hormone replacement will be necessary during the remainder of his life, if the prescribed therapeutic regimen is followed, he can live a relatively normal life. The importance of regular and adequate hours of rest, stopping activities short of fatigue and the avoidance of exposure to cold are stressed, indicating the effect of exposure and overexertion on cellular activity and the blood sugar level. No medications, including laxatives, except those ordered by the physician should be taken. Explicit instructions are given regarding the taking of the prescribed corticoid preparations; directions are written clearly, and the importance of taking the exact amounts at the prescribed times is emphasized. If the patient is to have desoxycorticosterone acetate in oil intramuscularly every 3 or 4 weeks instead of fludrocortisone by mouth, a referral is made to a clinic or to a visiting nurse agency for the administration. The high-carbohydrate, high-protein diet with the amount of sodium recommended by the physician is discussed in detail, explaining the need for nourishment between meals and at bedtime to maintain a normal blood sugar level. The patient and family are advised of the need for avoiding contact with those with an infection as much as possible, and suggestions are made as to how this may be achieved. They should understand that a stressful situation or illness demands more corticoids. To prevent a serious crisis or acute corticoid insufficiency, prompt medical attention is necessary with any disorder such as a respiratory infection, vomiting, diarrhea, fainting or sudden weakness. The role of worry and emotional situations in precipitating a crisis is emphasized.

The patient with Addison's disease should always carry an identification card or wear a Medic-Alert bracelet or pendant which clearly indicates that he has a corticoid insufficiency and what should be done in the event of injury or sudden collapse. The nurse does not attempt to provide all the necessary information at one time. The instruction is planned to cover several periods; salient points are clarified and reinforced by repetition, and opportunities are provided for the patient and family members to ask questions.

Cushing's Disease

This is a rare disorder which is more common to females and results from an excessive secretion of adrenal corticoids. It may be due to primary hyperfunction of one or both of the adrenal cortices or may be secondary to a pathological hypersecretion of adrenocorticotrophin (ACTH) by the adenohypophysis. Primary hyperactivity of the adrenal cortex is usually caused by a neoplasm, most frequently an adenoma, but may also occur as a result of unexplained hyperplasia.

The manifestations will vary in individual patients according to age and the amount of corticoid being produced in excess of the normal. The increased output of cortisol causes excessive protein catabolism, gluconeogenesis, an abnormal distribution of fat and atrophy of lymphoid tissue. The patient manifests a decreased glucose tolerance, hyperglycemia, and muscle wasting and weakness. His appearance changes because of the increased deposition of fat on the trunk, thin wasted limbs, and a round, bloated looking face ("moon" face). Purple striae may appear, notably on the abdomen, buttocks and thighs, and are due to increased fragility of the blood vessels and atrophy of the skin. The production of lymphocytes is suppressed, increasing the patient's susceptibility to infection. Osteoporosis may occur, usually in the vertebrae, because of calcium mobilization; the patient frequently complains of backache.

The excessive secretion of mineralocorticoids results in electrolyte, fluid and acid-base imbalances. Hypernatremia, water retention and hypokalemia develop. The increased reabsorption by the renal tubules of sodium ions in exchange for hydrogen ions (see p. 64) depletes the acid ions, producing alkalosis. The low blood level of potassium causes extreme weakness and cardiac dysfunction. Hypertension is common due to the sodium and water retention.

As a consequence of the increased production of androgens, the female patient develops secondary male characteristics. There is a marked growth of hair on the face, the voice deepens, breasts atrophy, amenorrhea occurs and the clitoris may enlarge. If the disease occurs in childhood, precocious sexual development is evident in the male. The female child manifests masculinization with marked enlargement of the clitoris.

If the disease is secondary to a hypersecretion of ACTH, the disturbances are associated with an excessive production of the glucocorticoids only.

Treatment and Nursing Care. The treatment of Cushing's disease depends upon whether the hypersecretion of corticoids is due to primary dysfunction of the adrenal cortices or is the result of a hypersecretion of ACTH. In the case of an adrenocortical neoplasm, the affected gland is removed. If the cause is hyperplasia, a bilateral adrenalectomy is usually done. The patient then receives hormonal replacement therapy as outlined under Addison's disease on page 554. If the condition is secondary to a pituitary tumor, the tumor is usually treated by irradiation or surgical removal.

Nursing care of the patient with Cushing's disease is mainly symptomatic. If he is ambulatory, precautions are necessary to prevent accidental falls which may occur because of his weakness. The fluid intake and output are recorded to determine the amount of water retention, and the sodium intake is restricted. The blood pressure and pulse are taken at regular intervals so that early changes may be detected. Changes in mood and behavior are common and should be reported. Exposure to persons with infection is avoided because of the patient's lowered resistance.

Primary Aldosteronism

Rarely, an excessive production of aldosterone occurs and is usually caused by an adenoma or hyperplasia of the particular adrenocortical cells which secrete the hormone. The most striking features of the disease are the excessive renal loss of potassium and hypertension. The patient experiences severe generalized muscular weakness. Depletion of the body potassium reduces the kidneys' ability to concentrate the urine, and polyuria occurs. Alkalosis develops and may incur tetany and paresthesias. Despite an increased retention of salt, there is not a corresponding retention of water or edema. This is attributed to an increased glomerular filtration rate and the polyuria. As a result of the hypernatremia and polyuria, the patient usually experiences severe thirst. An elevation of arterial blood pressure is common. Treatment consists of surgical removal of the adenoma or affected gland preceded by administration of potassium salts.

Dysfunction of the Adrenal Medullae

Pheochromocytoma

Disease of the adrenal medullae is very rare and occurs in the form of a neoplasm known as a pheochromocytoma, which produces an excessive amount of epinephrine and norepinephrine. The tumor is usually unilateral, benign and causes hypertension, hyperglycemia and hypermetabolism. The increased liberation of large amounts of the hormones is usually paroxysmal at first, lasting from a few minutes to hours, but is likely to eventually become persistent. The patient frequently complains of a pounding headache, nausea, vomiting, palpitation, air hunger, nervousness, tremor and weakness. Sweating, pallor, dilatation of the pupils, tachycardia and a sharp rise in the blood pressure are also manifested. The increased glucogenolysis and subsequent elevated blood sugar may result in glucosuria.

Tests used to establish the diagnosis of pheochromocytoma include the phentolamine (Regitine) test and estimation of the blood and urinary content of the hormones or their major metabolite. Phentolamine is given intravenously and neutralizes circulating epinephrine. If the hypertension is due to a pheochromocytoma, there is a rapid, brief decline in the blood pressure. The pressure usually returns to its previous level in 10 to 15 minutes. The patient lies flat in bed during the test, and vasopressor drugs (e.g., Levophed) should be available for prompt administration in the event of a vasomotor collapse and hypotension.

Determination of the catecholamines in the urine is usually done on a 24-hour specimen. The normal varies from 8 to 165 micrograms per 24 hours; this may range from 300 to 4000 micrograms in the case of pheochromocytoma. The normal blood content is 0.2 to 7.0 micrograms per liter. The principal metabolite of the hormones is vanillyl mandelic acid (VMA) and is excreted in the urine. An estimation of the amount of VMA in a 24-hour specimen may be done. Normally 2 to 9 mg. are excreted in 24 hours; this is markedly increased in patients with pheochromocytoma. The patient with pheochromocytoma is treated by surgical removal of the tumor or the affected gland.

Nursing in Adrenal Surgery

Surgery of the adrenal glands may be done on patients with hypersecretion of hormones due to hyperplasia or tumors of one or both glands. The procedure may involve the removal of both adrenal glands (bilateral or total adrenalectomy), the removal of one gland (unilateral adrenalectomy) or resection of a part of a gland (subtotal adrenalectomy). Bilateral adrenalectomy is frequently undertaken with patients with cancer of the breast and occasionally on those with cancer of the prostate. Malignant disease of these organs is dependent to some extent on sex hormones, and since the adrenal cortices produce both estrogens and androgens, their removal eliminates a source of the supporting hormones. In the case of cancer of the breast, adrenalectomy is preceded by oophorectomy (removal of the ovaries). The patient with cancer of the prostate undergoes orchidectomy (removal of the testicles) before adrenalectomy is considered.

Preoperative Preparation. Preparation of the patient for adrenal surgery includes the general preparation cited in Chapter 10. Blood studies are done to determine electrolyte concentrations, and corrections are made as indicated. Because of an excessive potassium excretion, a solution of potassium chloride may be ordered to restore the normal level of potassium in the blood. The blood sugar level and glucose tolerance are investigated. The patient is given a high-protein diet because of the protein depletion due to excessive glucocorticoid secretion. The fluid intake and output are measured, and the balance is noted. The blood pressure is recorded at least once daily to serve as a postoperative comparative base-line. The patient with hyperfunction of the adrenal cortices frequently has experienced hypertension for some time. Too rapid a fall postoperatively to an actual normal level could be indicative of vasomotor collapse and hypotension in such a person.

If both adrenal glands are to be removed, the patient and his family must understand that constant hormone replacement will be necessary for the remainder of the patient's life. They may indicate some concern about meeting the expense of the drugs; the nurse may suggest sources of assistance or refer the problem to the social service department.

After operation, the patient's respirations tend to be shallow because the incision is close to the diaphragm. In discussions with the patient as to what he may expect postoperatively, emphasis is placed on the need for frequent deep breathing and coughing to prevent complications. He is taught how to cough and is assured of support.

The surgeon's approach to the adrenal gland is usually through a high flank incision or occasionally through the abdomen. When a bilateral adrenalectomy is done, two incisions are made unless the transabdominal approach is used. The entire trunk from the nipple line down to and including the pubis is shaved and cleansed. A nasogastric tube is passed before the sedative is given on the morning of operation. This prevents postoperative vomiting and abdominal distention.

Cortisol may be administered before and during as well as following the operation to prevent adrenal insufficiency in the immediate postoperative period. A venous cutdown with the introduction of a cannula into the vein may be ordered, and an intravenous solution run slowly and continuously. This is in preparation for prompt administration of corticoids or a vasopressor as indicated.

Postoperative Care. During the first few postoperative days, and until the maintenance dosages of cortisol and desoxycorticosterone or fludrocortisone are established in the case of adrenalectomy, special attention is paid to the patient's blood pressure, fluid balance and blood chemistry. Constant nursing care is necessary until the vital signs and the corticoid concentrations are stabilized. The blood pressure, respirations and pulse are recorded every 15 minutes for several hours and the interval gradually lengthened if they remain satisfactory. Any rapid or significant fall in the blood pressure, dyspnea or tachycardia is reported promptly.

The fluid intake and output are accurately measured, and any imbalance is brought to the physician's attention. Frequent checks may be made of the blood sodium, potassium and glucose levels, which influence the amount of corticoids given. Vomiting after the nasogastric tube is removed, increased weakness, hypotension and an elevated temperature may indicate acute corticoid insufficiency.

As indicated previously, deep breathing and coughing are very important while the patient is confined to bed and are encouraged at least every 2 hours. The patient's position is also changed every 1 to 2 hours. A portable chest x-ray may be ordered. Any dyspnea or complaint of chest pain is reported at once.

Intravenous corticoids are given continuously for a day or two with the dosage and rate of flow adjusted to the patient's clinical manifestations and the electrolyte and fluid balances. Oral doses of cortisol are started as soon as tolerated by the patient; a daily intramuscular injection of desoxycorticosterone is also given and is usually replaced by oral fludrocortisone in a few days. The dosage of both corticoid preparations is gradually tapered until maintenance amounts are established. When the intravenous corticoids are withdrawn, an intravenous infusion of glucose in water or normal saline is continued slowly even though the patient may be tolerating fluids by mouth. The purpose of this is to keep the route available for quick administration of corticoids or a vasopressor (e.g., Levophed, Aramine) if needed. The patient's condition tends to be labile and may change quickly. The nurse must be constantly alert for signs of corticoid insufficiency or indications of excessive corticoid administration. When the nasogastric tube is removed, the patient is started on fluids containing glucose and progresses to a regular diet as tolerated.

When surgery is performed to remove a pheochromocytoma, a marked rise in the blood pressure may occur during or immediately following surgery because of an excessive liberation of epinephrine and norepinephrine from the tumor during the removal. An adrenergic blocking agent such as phentolamine (Regitine) is kept available for quick intravenous administration to neutralize the medullary hormones.

More often the problem following the surgery is severe hypotension. The blood pressure is maintained by the giving of a vasopressor such as levarterenol (Levophed) or metaraminol (Aramine, Presonex) in an intravenous solution. The rate of flow must be carefully controlled and adjusted according to frequent blood pressure recordings and the doctor's directives. The patient is kept flat, and any change in position achieved slowly.

When unilateral adrenalectomy or a subtotal resection of one or both glands is done, the patient may receive some cortisol following operation. Less will be required than in total adrenalectomy and is gradually withdrawn.

Following adrenal surgery, the patient usually remains in bed for 2 or 3 days or until the blood pressure remains at a satisfactory level. Before commencing ambulation, the head of the bed is elevated and the blood pressure checked. When the patient is permitted to get out of bed, a nurse remains with him, and the blood pressure is checked every 15 minutes the first time he is up. If a significant decrease in blood pressure occurs, the patient is returned to bed and kept flat. The application of elastic or crepe bandages to the lower extremities may be made before getting the patient up in order to maintain a greater blood volume in vital areas.

In preparation for discharge, the patient who has had a bilateral adrenalectomy receives the same instruction as the patient with Addison's disease (see p. 555). If he has had one gland removed or a subtotal resection done, he is cautioned to avoid overfatigue, exposure to extremes of temperature (especially cold), infections, and emotional disturbances as much as possible. It is possible that stress may precipitate an acute adrenal insufficiency or crisis because the remaining adrenal tissue cannot meet the increased hormonal demand. He is advised to contact his doctor immediately if he experiences weakness, fainting, fever, or nausea and vomiting as he may require a corticoid supplement. Following any adrenal surgery, the patient should resume activity very gradually and is followed closely at the clinic or by his physician. Usually several months are required to satisfactorily adjust the hormonal replacement. The patient who has had hypertension due to pheochromocytoma usually does not regain a normal blood pressure level for 3 to 4 months.

ISLETS OF LANGERHANS

The pancreas is both an exocrine and endocrine gland. Its exocrine secretions are carried by a system of ducts to the duodenum and contain enzymes which play an important role in digestion (see p. 322). The islets of Langerhans form the endocrine component of the pancreas and consist of irregularly scattered groups of cells which are totally independent of the pancreatic system of ducts (see Fig. 21–5). The islets are highly vascularized and consist mainly of two types of cells — alpha cells, which secrete the hormone glucagon, and beta cells, which produce insulin. Both of these hormones are protein and are rendered inactive in the gastrointestinal tract by the proteolytic enzymes; therefore, they must be administered parenterally.

Insulin. This hormone plays a dominant role in carbohydrate metabolism. It promotes the transfer of glucose across the cell membrane. Those especially affected are muscle cells, where glucose is converted to glycogen, and adipose tissue cells, where the glucose is changed to fat and stored as such. Liver cells are freely permeable to glucose, and with insulin present, it is suggested that the activity of the hepatic enzyme glucokinase

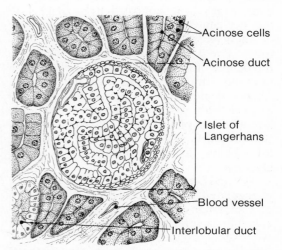

Figure 21–5 Location of cells of islets of Langerhans between lobules of pancreas.

is increased, stimulating the conversion of glucose to glycogen, which is then stored within the hepatic cells. The action of a second hepatic enzyme, glucose-6-phosphate, which promotes the conversion of glycogen to glucose and its release into the blood, is decreased by insulin. These effects result in a lowering of the amount of glucose in the blood.

Insulin also stimulates the uptake of amino acids, especially by muscle cells, where they are used to form tissue proteins. Because insulin favors the entrance of glucose and its conversion to fat in adipose tissue cells, fat mobilization is inhibited, and consequently, the fat content in the blood is kept at a lower level.

The secretion of insulin is regulated by the concentration of the blood glucose. An elevation increases the production of insulin, and conversely, a decrease below the normal blood level of glucose suppresses its secretion. Thus, a feedback mechanism is established to control the output of insulin in order to maintain the blood sugar level within a normal range.

Glucagon. This hormone may also be referred to as the hyperglycemic factor, since its primary effect is stimulation of glycogenolysis (the conversion of glycogen to glucose and its release into the blood) by the liver to increase the blood glucose concentration. Its secretion by the alpha cells is stimulated by a low blood sugar level.

Blood Sugar Level. The normal blood sugar (glucose) level 3 to 4 hours after a meal varies from approximately 70 to 110 mg. per cent. Fluctuations occur as a result of energy expenditure and the ingestion of foods. The types of food taken also influence the degree of change; obviously, a meal high in carbohydrate produces a greater concentration of glucose for a period of time than a meal with a low carbohydrate content. An elevation of the blood sugar level above the normal is known as hyperglycemia. A level below normal is referred to as hypoglycemia.

As cited previously, the blood sugar level is regulated by the hormones of the islets of Langerhans. It may, however, be influenced by several other endocrine secretions. An excess of the somatotrophic hormone (growth hormone) produces a tendency toward hyperglycemia by decreasing the utilization of glucose and stimulating the production of glucagon. The release of glucocorticoids (cortisol) by the adrenal cortices promotes gluconeogenesis (formation of glucose from amino acids and the glycerol portion of fat), resulting in an elevation of the blood sugar. Epinephrine and norepinephrine stimulate liver glycogenolysis and this metabolism of muscle glycogen to lactic acid, which is then converted to glucose by the liver. The thyroid hormones also increase the blood sugar level by an acceleration of gluconeogenesis.

Disorders of Islets of Langerhans

Diabetes Mellitus

Diabetes mellitus is a chronic disorder of carbohydrate, fat and protein metabolism due to an insufficient secretion of insulin or a diminished effectiveness of that secreted. As a result of the absolute or relative deficiency of insulin, there is an inadequate transfer of glucose into the cells; the utilization of glucose for energy and cellular products and its conversion to glycogen or fat and storage as such are depressed. Glucose accumulates in the blood, causing hyperglycemia.

Fat may be mobilized from adipose tissue and broken down to provide a source of energy. The mobilized fat is withdrawn from the blood by the liver and broken down to glycerol and fatty acids. The fatty acids are oxidized by the hepatic cells to ketone bodies (aceto-acetic acid, oxybutyric acid and acetone), which are then circulated and may be metabolized by cells to produce energy, carbon dioxide and water. According to Keele and Neil, only a limited amount of ketone acids can be utilized by the cells.[11] If ketogenesis proceeds rapidly, exceeding the rate at which they can be metabolized, the ketone acids accumulate in the blood, causing ketosis or ketone acidosis.

Tissue protein may also be broken down to amino acids which are deaminized by the liver to form glucose, contributing to

---

[11]C. A. Keele, and E. Neil: Samson Wright's Applied Physiology, 10th ed. Toronto, Oxford University Press, 1961, p. 418

TABLE 21–1 ENDOCRINE GLANDS, THEIR HORMONES AND ASSOCIATED DISORDERS

GLAND	HORMONES	FUNCTIONS	DISORDERS
Hypophysis A. Adenohypophysis (anterior lobe)			Simmond's disease—decrease of all adenohypophyseal hormones
	Somatotrophin (growth hormone, STH, GH)	Growth, aids in determining size; accelerates metabolism; diabetogenic action	Giantism—increase of STH in childhood Acromegaly—increase of STH in adulthood Dwarfism—decrease of STH in adulthood
	Thyrotrophin (TSH)	Promotes growth and secretory activity of the thyroid	Hyperthyroidism (Graves' disease)—secondary to increase of TSH
	Corticotrophin (adrenocorticotrophic hormone, ACTH)	Influences adrenal cortices	Cushing's disease—increase of ACTH
	Gonadotrophins 1. Follicle-stimulating hormone (FSH)	Causes development of ovarian follicle, secretion of estrogen	
	2. Leutrotrophin (LTH)	Promotes ovulation; required for formation of corpus luteum	
	3. Leuteinizing hormone (LH) (lactogenic hormone, prolactin)	Stimulates secretion of progesterone; initiates secretion of mammary glands	
	4. Melanocyte-stimulating hormone (MSH)	Regulates production of pigment by cells in skin	
B. Neurohypophysis (posterior lobe)	Antidiuretic hormone (vasopressin, ADH)	Increases permeability of distal and collecting tubules of kidneys; therefore, increases reabsorption of water	Diabetes insipidus—decrease of ADH
	Oxytocin	Excites contraction of pregnant uterus; some effect on smooth muscle; stimulates release and flow of milk	
Thyroid	Triiodothyronine (T_3) Tetraiodothyronine (T_4)	Increases metabolic rate by stimulating oxidative processes; promotes normal physical growth, maturation, mental development	Hypothyroidism Cretinism in child Myxedema in adult Goiter Hyperthyroidism Thyroid storm Thyroiditis Carcinoma
Parathyroid	Parathormone (PTH)	Controls concentration of calcium and inorganic phosphorus in blood.	Hypoparathyroidism Hyperparathyroidism
Adrenal glands A. Adrenal cortex	Adrenocorticoids (corticosteroids, corticoids)		Addison's disease (hypofunction of cortices) Cushing's disease (hyperfunction of cortices)
	1. Mineralocorticoids, aldosterone	Influences electrolyte concentration and fluid volume	Primary aldosteronism (increase of aldosterone)
	2. Glucocorticoids, cortisol (hydrocortisone)	Influences metabolism of glucose, protein and fat; concerned with body's responses to physical and mental stress	
	3. Sex hormones (androgens, estrogen and progesterone)		
B. Adrenal medulla	Epinephrine (adrenalin)	Constricts peripheral and renal blood vessels; dilates coronary and skeletal muscle vessels; relaxes smooth muscle of bronchioles, gastrointestinal tract, urinary bladder; dilates pupils; elevates blood sugar; promotes release of adrenocorticotrophin; accelerates metabolic rate	Pheochromocytoma (increase of production of both hormones)
	Norepinephrin (noradrenalin)	Generalized vasoconstriction	
Islets of Langerhans	Insulin	Role in carbohydrate metabolism	Diabetes mellitus

the hyperglycemia. Both the uptake of amino acids by the cells and body protein synthesis are decreased.

Incidence. Diabetes mellitus is more common in middle-aged and older persons but cannot be considered rare in children and young adults. The incidence is higher in women than men, in persons who are obese or have a history of obesity, and among relatives of diabetics. The figures are also higher in urban populations and among those in sedentary occupations.

The disorder is very prevalent, affecting 1 in 35 persons.[12] Many thousands are known diabetics, and it is believed that those diagnosed represent only a relatively small fraction of those undetected. The WHO Expert Committee on Diabetes Mellitus reported that there is an increasing incidence of diabetes in most parts of the world and that the increase corresponds with "increased food consumption, reduced physical exercise and obesity."[13] The increased number of diabetics may also be attributed to (1) increased longevity—more persons survive to the high-incidence age; (2) the lower mortality rate among young diabetics because of improved treatment and control of their disease; (3) extended education of the public about the disease; and (4) the increased number of detection facilities.

Etiological Factors

INSULIN DEFICIENCY. A common factor in all diabetes mellitus is a lack of sufficient metabolically effective insulin to promote normal carbohydrate metabolism and maintain a normal blood sugar level. The deficiency may be absolute or relative. An absolute deficiency implies that the beta cells of the islets of Langerhans are not actually producing sufficient insulin to meet the demand. This may occur as the result of degeneration of beta cells. A relative deficiency occurs as a result of insulin antagonists which are substances that modify or combine with insulin, making it ineffective, or block its use at the site of action. Little is known of these substances as yet, but much research is presently concentrated on this area of diabetes. Some authors include those hormones such as the glucocorticoids, epinephrine, glucagon and somatotrophin as insulin antagonists because of their hyperglycemic effect through their promotion of gluconeogenesis or glycogenolysis. More often the term insulin antagonist is reserved for a substance which interferes with the action of insulin. Substances, such as the hormones cited, which effect a persisting hyperglycemia are more likely to produce an absolute deficiency of insulin through creating an excessive demand for insulin which eventually "burns out" or exhausts the beta cells. The resulting diabetes is secondary to the condition, causing the hypersecretion of the hyperglycemic hormone.

HEREDITY. It is now generally accepted that persons who develop primary diabetes mellitus have an inherited predisposition to the disease. It is transmitted as a recessive genetic trait, which implies that those likely to develop diabetes must have received a defective gene from each parent. The penetrance of the defective genes appears to vary; some homozygotes (persons who have inherited a gene for the predisposition from each parent) do not develop the disease even in their advanced years. The expected incidence according to the Mendelian law of heredity is as follows: if both parents are diabetic, all of their children will most likely become diabetic if they live long enough. When a diabetic marries a carrier,* there is a 50 per cent chance that each child will develop diabetes. If he does not receive a defective gene from each parent, he will receive one from the diabetic parent and be a carrier. If both parents are carriers, the child has a 25 per cent chance of being a diabetic, a 50 per cent chance of being a carrier and a 25 per cent chance of receiving normal genes. In the case of a marriage of a diabetic to a noncarrier, none of their children will become diabetic, but they will all be carriers (see Table 21–2).

OBESITY. The majority of diabetics who develop their disease after the age of 40 are obese or have a history of obesity. The relationship is not understood. It is thought that probably persons with a predisposition to the disease who take an excess of food

---

[12]The Canadian Diabetic Association, 1969.

[13]World Health Organization Expert Committee on Diabetes Mellitus: Diabetes Mellitus. WHO Technical Report Series, No. 310. Geneva, WHO, 1965, p. 5.

---

*A carrier is a person who is free of the disease but has one gene bearing the predisposition to diabetes.

TABLE 21–2 GENETIC COMPOSITION OF OFFSPRING WHEN PARENTS ARE (*A*) A DIABETIC AND A CARRIER, (*B*) TWO CARRIERS, (*C*) A PROBABLE DIABETIC AND A NONCARRIER

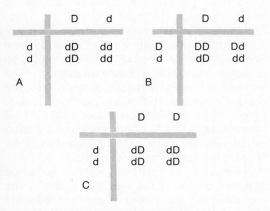

KEY D = dominant normal gene; d = recessive gene for predisposition to diabetes
DD = Noncarrier
Dd = Carrier
dd = Person likely to develop diabetes

create increased demands for insulin which results in eventual exhaustion of the beta cells of the islets. The association of diabetes with obesity is very significant in considering prevention.

Manifestations. Diabetes mellitus in young persons usually has a sudden onset in a severe, acute form. In older persons, the onset is most frequently insidious, going undetected and untreated for a considerable period of time. Their diabetes may be recognized in a routine examination in which glucosuria is discovered, or eventually a distressing symptom presents which prompts them to consult a doctor.

Although the most striking symptoms are the result of abnormal carbohydrate metabolism and the resultant hyperglycemia, the disorder is also marked by disturbances in protein and fat metabolism and degenerative changes, especially in the vascular system. The patient excretes an excessive volume of urine (polyuria) as a result of the increased concentration of glucose in the glomerular filtrate. The glucose increases the osmotic pressure of the filtrate, preventing the reabsorption of water. As a result of the excessive water loss, the patient ex-

periences a persisting thirst (polydipsia), and dehydration and electrolyte imbalance may develop. The blood sugar concentration exceeds the capacity of the renal tubules to reabsorb it from the glomerular filtrate, and sugar is excreted in the urine (glucosuria). The maximum capacity of the renal tubules to reabsorb glucose represents what is referred to as the glucose renal threshold. The normal is 165 to 180 mg. per cent.

Weakness and fatigue are common complaints because the glucose cannot be utilized to produce energy. There is a loss of weight which is attributed to the mobilization of fat from adipose tissue and the breakdown of protein. Some patients also experience an increased appetite (polyphagia).

Older female patients may develop pruritus of the vulva; this is usually due to infection by fungi which thrive on the glucose deposit from the urine. The vulva becomes swollen and inflamed. In some instances, it is this distressing condition that brings the patient to the doctor and leads to the diagnosis of her diabetes. Rarely, male patients develop pruritus and inflammation of the prepuce and glans penis.

Other manifestations associated with long-term disease are impaired vision due to retinal changes and opacity of the lens (cataract) and pain, numbness and tingling in the extremities due to peripheral neuritis.

Diagnostic Procedures. The diagnostic procedures used in the investigation for diabetes mellitus are simple in comparison with those used for many other conditions. They involve the following urine and blood tests.

URINALYSIS. A urine specimen is examined for the presence of glucose and ketone bodies (acetone, aceto-acetic and β-oxybutyric acid). Normally, glucose is almost completely reabsorbed from the glomerular filtrate by the renal tubules and what remains in the urine is insignificant and not detected by the usual tests. If sugar is present (glucosuria), the amount is noted on the basis of the intensity of the reaction and is indicated as a trace, one plus, two plus, and so on. Simple, quick methods of testing the urine for sugar have been devised in the form of a tablet, powder or a strip of paper impregnated with the necessary reagent. Directions for their use and a color comparison chart accompany each product. The color chart indicates the characteristic color change associated with certain glucose concentrations. The presence of glucose in the urine may only be suggestive of diabetes mellitus; for instance, the person may have a low glucose renal threshold. If glucose is found, blood sugar determinations are then made for more conclusive evidence.

A 24-hour urine specimen may be ordered to determine the amount of sugar the patient excretes in that period. The collection usually begins in the morning. The patient voids and that urine is discarded. The time is noted and all urine that is voided until that time the next morning is saved. The patient is asked to empty his bladder at the time the test is completed, and that urine is included in the specimen.

Ketone bodies may be present in the urine of a diabetic because of the mobilization and breakdown of fat. Ketonuria occurring with glucosuria generally indicates the presence of diabetes mellitus. Materials similar to those cited in testing for sugar are available for simple quick testing for ketonuria.

BLOOD SUGAR. A blood sugar determination is made from a specimen of venous blood following a period of 4 to 8 hours of fasting. The normal range is 70 to 110 mg. per cent. In mass surveys for diabetes mellitus and in detection clinics, the blood specimen does not provide a fasting blood sugar level, but the patient is questioned as to when he last ate; a note is made of this and the information is taken into consideration when assessing the report. Persons with abnormally high or borderline levels are followed for further investigation.

GLUCOSE TOLERANCE TEST. This test determines the patient's ability to clear the blood of excess glucose following the ingestion of sugar and to return the blood sugar to a normal level. Preferably, the patient should receive approximately 250 Gm. of carbohydrate in his diet for 2 or 3 days preceding the test. Food is then withheld overnight, and in the morning a urine specimen and venous blood sample are collected for glucose determinations. The patient then receives by mouth 100 Gm. of glucose dissolved in 300 to 500 ml. of water, which may be flavored with lemon juice. Urine and blood specimens are collected in 1/2, 1, 2 and 3 hours after the ingestion of the glucose. These are examined for the glucose concentration. Normally, the blood sugar level rises to approximately 140 to 160 mg. per cent but returns to normal within 2 hours. In the diabetic, the elevation in the blood sugar will be much higher and several hours (3 to 5) may be required for the original level to be resumed.

Rarely, glucose may be given intravenously rather than orally, and urine and blood specimens are collected 30, 60, 90 and 150 minutes following the administration. The amount of glucose used is based on the patient's weight (0.5 Gm. per kg.) and is given in sterile distilled water (20 Gm. of glucose to 100 ml. of water) over a period of 30 minutes. The blood sugar should resume a normal level in 90 minutes.

Normally, with either method, no sugar appears in the urine. In the diabetic, the elevation in the blood sugar exceeds the glucose renal threshold and glucosuria occurs.

TOLBUTAMIDE TEST. This test determines the patient's response to an intravenous injection of sodium tolbutamide which normally results in an increased secretion of insulin. After an overnight fast, blood is taken for blood sugar determination, and the patient is then given 1 Gm. of sodium tolbutamide dissolved in 10 or 11 ml. of sterile distilled water over a period of 2 minutes. The blood sugar level is obtained in 20, 30, 40 and 60 minutes following the tolbutamide administration. The blood sugar falls rapidly in normal persons. In diabetes, even in those with a very mild form of the disease, the decrease in blood sugar is less and the decline takes longer.

Stages of Diabetes.[14] Potential diabetic or prediabetic stage are terms applied to persons who are known to have an inherited predisposition to developing diabetes. In this stage, which may be of short duration or persist until the later years of life, they are asymptomatic and have a normal glucose tolerance test. Potential diabetics include the identical twin of a diabetic, a person of diabetic parents, a person with one diabetic parent and one nondiabetic parent who has a close relative who is a diabetic (e.g., parent, sibling, niece or nephew), and a woman who

---

[14]WHO Expert Committee on Diabetes Mellitus, op. cit., pp. 7–8.

J. Malins: Clinical Diabetes. London, Eyre and Spottiswoode, 1968, p. 2.

has given birth to a live or stillborn child weighing 4.5 kg. (10 lb.) or more at birth.

Latent diabetes is the stage in which a potential diabetic has (1) a normal glucose tolerance test but a history of having had a diabetic response to the test when obese or during a stress situation such as infection or pregnancy or (2) an abnormal blood sugar response, similar to that found in diabetes mellitus, to a provocative test such as the intravenous sodium tolbutamide test.

Subclinical or asymptomatic diabetes is the stage in which the person's fasting blood sugar may or may not be elevated above the normal level, but a glucose tolerance test shows a diabetic response. Degenerative vascular changes may occur in this stage as well as in more advanced diabetes.

The clinical stage of diabetes is that phase of the disease in which the characteristic symptoms are manifested. Glucosuria occurs, the fasting blood sugar is above normal and the glucose tolerance test is abnormal.

Diabetes mellitus may also be classified as primary (essential) or secondary. Primary or essential diabetes is that which develops as a result of an inherited predisposition. Secondary diabetes may develop as a result of a persisting hyperglycemia incurred by an endocrine disorder (e.g., hypersecretion of the adrenal cortices, hyperpituitarism) or excision or destruction of the islets of Langerhans.

Prevention and Case-Finding. With the present state of knowledge, preventive measures in diabetes mellitus are limited chiefly to the prevention and correction of obesity. This is especially important for those with a family history of diabetes or a suggestive obstetrical history. As indicated previously, the majority of diabetics are either obese at the time their disease is manifested or have a history of obesity. The incidence of diabetes among women who have previously given birth to an infant of 4.5 kg. or more is sufficiently significant to recommend that they maintain their ideal weight and be checked annually for diabetes mellitus. The hospital and visiting nurse have a responsibility to advise persons who are overweight of the many adverse effects of obesity and that they are possible candidates for diabetes mellitus. Occasionally, the nurse is questioned by a diabetic about whether he should marry and whether his children will be diabetic. The hereditary predisposition and the possible chances of transmission may be explained; with that information, the persons concerned must decide for themselves. They are also urged to discuss the problem with a physician or may be referred to a genetic counseling clinic.

Programs for case-finding and education of the general public about diabetes mellitus are organized by the national diabetic associations and their local branches. The nurse should be familiar with these associations so that patients and their families may be advised to avail themselves of the services. Detection clinics may be set up, or industrial or community surveys made by mobile laboratory units. A blood sugar is done on each registrant, and those with a definite or borderline elevation are followed. Obese persons, those in the most susceptible age group (over 40 years of age), those with a family history of diabetes, and women with a history of having had a large baby are urged to visit the clinic or participate in the survey.

Informing the public as to the characteristics of diabetes mellitus, susceptibility factors (obesity and family history), possible consequences of undetected and uncontrolled diabetes and available sources of screening is being promoted by the distribution of brochures by the diabetic associations and life insurance companies and through the use of mass media.

Treatment and Nursing Care. When the diagnosis of diabetes mellitus is made, the patient must be reassured that, although his disease cannot be cured, it can be controlled so that he can live a reasonably normal life. Treatment is directed toward correcting the hyperglycemia and glucosuria, maintaining the patient's normal weight and strength (and in the case of a child, normal growth and development), encouraging appropriate activity and the prevention of complications commonly associated with diabetes. The treatment of all patients includes a carefully regulated diet, moderate exercise and education about the disease and necessary care; for some it may include the administration of insulin or an oral hypoglycemic drug. The plan of treatment is determined on an individual basis; the therapeutic requirements for control in the case of one diabetic may be quite different to those of another.

DIET. Diabetes does not preclude the need for all the essential food principles, but it does necessitate careful selection and control of the amounts of the major food elements to provide a balance between the caloric intake and energy expenditure. The caloric intake should equal the energy output to avoid a positive balance with a resultant hyperglycemia and weight increase or a negative balance that may lead to an excessive fat breakdown with the risk of ketoacidosis. The diet can be quite similar to that of the normal person and provide sufficient variety to make it appetizing and palatable.

The dietary prescription indicates the number of calories required each day and the proportions of these calories to be allocated to carbohydrates, protein and fat. The number of calories is determined by the patient's ideal weight,* age and activity. Principles and methods used in the calculation of the diabetic diet vary among physicians. Joslin and White suggest the following as a basis for calculating the adult diabetic's caloric requirements: 30 calories per kg. (14 calories per lb.) of the ideal weight for the sedentary individual; 40 calories per kg. for the more active person; 20 calories per kg. if the patient is on bed rest; and 15 calories per kg. if the person is overweight.[15] In the case of a heavy laborer, 45 to 60 calories per kg. of his body weight may be needed to meet his increased expenditure of energy. The diabetic child's caloric intake must provide for growth and considerable activity and may be based on the rule of 1000 calories for the child at the age of 1 year plus 100 calories for each additional year; that is, the 2-year-old would receive 1100 calories, the 3-year-old 1200 calories and so on. The child's caloric requirement may also be calculated on weight; 100 calories per kg. of weight at the age of 1 year, 75 calories per kg. at 5 years, 50 calories per kg. at 10 years, and 40 calories per kg. at 15 years.[16, 17]

*The ideal weight is obtained from a standard table of weights according to sex, height and build.

[15]A. P. Joslin, and P. White: The Dietary Management of Diabetes. Med. Clin. North Amer., Vol. 49, No. 4 (July 1965), p. 905.

[16]Ibid.

[17]P. White: The Child with Diabetes. Med. Clin. North Amer., Vol. 49, No. 4 (July 1965), p. 1073.

Apportionment of the calories into carbohydrate, protein and fat differs from the normal diet in that the carbohydrate is usually lower. The protein allowance is usually the same as that recommended for the normal diet: 1.0 to 1.5 Gm. per kg. of body weight for adults and 2.0 to 3.0 Gm. per kg. for children. Generally, 40 per cent of the adult diabetic's caloric intake is provided as carbohydrate; this is about 10 per cent less than in the normal diet. The remaining calories are then made up in fat. This works out to approximately 15 per cent of the total calories in protein, 40 per cent in carbohydrate, and 45 per cent in fat. For children, the amount of carbohydrate prescribed is usually within normal limits (i.e., 50 per cent of the caloric requirement) because of their activity and growth.

In providing the necessary carbohydrates, concentrated forms such as sugar, candy, jams, honey, ice cream, sherbets, pastries, cake, and sweetened beverages are avoided. The carbohydrates most commonly used are bread, cereals, milk, fruits and vegetables. In the selection of fat, the substitution of unsaturated for saturated fats is usually recommended because of the diabetic's predisposition to the development of atherosclerosis and vascular lesions.

As a guide for selecting the kinds and amounts of food in the diabetic diet in keeping with the physician's dietary prescription, foods have been divided into 6 basic classes—namely, milk, vegetables, fruits, breads, meats and fats. The vegetables are subdivided into classes A and B according to their nutrient value. Foods have been listed in each class, indicating the amount in household measurements of each which comprise one serving and the value of one serving in terms of Gm. of carbohydrate, protein and fat. These lists are referred to as exchange lists, and one serving is called an exchange. All exchanges in a list are equal in value; thus one may be substituted for another in the amount indicated. The exchange system permits the diet to be varied and planned according to the availability of foods as well as to the patient's preferences. To illustrate, if the patient's meal allows one fruit exchange, he may select 1/2 cup of unsweetened applesauce, one small orange, 1 cup of raspberries, or 1/2 of a small banana from the multiple exchange list of fruits; each has the same value of 10 Gm. of carbohydrate and provides 40 calories.

The patient's daily food allowance is outlined as to the amount of food or number of exchanges he may have from each exchange list. This must then be allocated to his meals and snacks. The division of the day's allowance depends upon the associated treatment. If diet is used without insulin or a hypoglycemic drug, it is simply divided into 3 equal parts and intermediate snacks. When insulin is used, the division of the carbohydrate and the number of feedings are specified by the physician. The exchange lists and sample menus for various daily caloric requirements (1000 to 3000 calories) are available from the Diet Counseling Service of national and local diabetic associations,[18] hospital dietary departments and diabetic clinics, diet therapy textbooks,[19] and reference books written primarily for diatics.[20, 21, 22]

It must be impressed upon the patient that all of his daily food allowance should be eaten and that nothing else of caloric value is taken. When the patient is unable to take a portion of his diet, the caloric requirement is made up in some way (e.g., orange juice, milk), especially if he is receiving insulin. Meals should be taken regularly; the delay or missing of a meal may upset the blood sugar level and promote the breakdown of fat. The carbohydrate is distributed over the day to avoid abnormal fluctuation in the blood sugar concentration. Foods of no significant nutrient value which the patient may have as desired include clear broths and consommé, clear tea and coffee, jello made with sugarless jelly powder, tomato juice, and artificially sweetened carbonated beverage. Several commercial sweetening agents which are of no nutritional value are available; one is saccharin which can only be added to the food after it is cooked; another

commonly used sweetener is sodium or calcium cyclamate.* Some physicians discourage the patient from using a sweetener on the basis that if he becomes accustomed to unsweetened foods, he is less likely to be tempted to take those sweetened with sugar. Commercially prepared dietetic foods are available. An artificial sweetener is used in these, and they tend to be expensive. However, they may help to vary the patient's diet occasionally. If the patient becomes ill and cannot tolerate solid foods, he may be given fruit juices (unless diarrhea is a problem), ginger ale, gruel and milk.† If these are not tolerated, intravenous infusions of glucose may have to be administered.

The diabetic diet is very much an individual factor. Following the initial dietary prescription, the patient is followed closely to determine if it is satisfactory; the urine is checked daily for sugar, frequent blood sugar determinations are made, his weight is recorded daily, and his general reactions (physical and psychological) are noted. Adjustments of the total caloric intake and in the amount of carbohydrate and fat may be necessary. Consideration is given to adapting the prescribed diet to the patient's food habits which are influenced by his cultural and economic background, family, and individual preferences.

INSULIN. If the diabetic on a regulated diet does not have sufficient effective insulin in his body to use and store his carbohydrate requirement and prevent fat and protein catabolism, insulin may be prescribed. The majority of diabetics requiring insulin therapy tend to be children and adults who have developed their disease before the age of 40. The person whose diabetes is normally controlled by diet regulation may require insulin during periods of increased body demands and stress (e.g., infection, surgery, pregnancy).

Insulin is a protein which is still being

[18]American Diabetes Association, New York, N.Y., U.S.A. The Canadian Diabetic Association, Toronto, Ontario, Canada.

[19]S. R. Williams: Nutrition and Diet Therapy. St. Louis, The C. V. Mosby Co., 1969.

[20]E. P. Joslin: Diabetic Manual, 10th ed. Philadelphia, Lea and Febiger, 1960.

[21]H. Rosenthal and J. Rosenthal: Diabetic Care in Pictures, 4th ed. Philadelphia, J. B. Lippincott, 1968.

[22]G. F. Schmitt: Diabetes for Diabetics, 2nd ed. Miami, The Diabetic Press of America, 1968.

*This chemical has recently been considered to be a possible carcinogen and has been banned from some markets.

†One-half cup orange juice is equivalent to 10 Gm. of carbohydrate and provides 40 calories; 6 oz. ginger ale is equivalent to 1 slice of bread and has 15 Gm. of carbohydrate (60 calories); ½ cup gruel is equivalent to 15 Gm. of carbohydrate and 2 Gm. of protein (70 calories); 1 cup skim milk is equivalent to 12 Gm. of carbohydrate and 8 Gm. of protein (80 calories).

TABLE 21–3   ONSET, PEAK AND DURATION OF VARIOUS INSULINS

TYPE	ONSET OF ACTION AFTER INJECTION (HOURS)	PEAK OF ACTION (HOURS)	DURATION OF ACTION (HOURS)
Rapid-acting:			
Regular (unmodified crystalline)	$1/2$–1	2–4	6–8
Semi-lente	1–2	5–7	12–18
Intermediary-acting:			
Globin	2–4	10–14	10–22
NPH (isophane)	1–2	10–20	20–32
Lente	1–2	14–18	26–30
Slow-acting:			
Protamine zinc	4–8	16–24	24–36
Ultra-lente	4–8	16–24	24–36

prepared from a natural source, namely the pancreas of cattle, hogs and sheep. The preparation of a synthetic form has been reported, but the product, as yet, is not being marketed.[23] Being protein, insulin is destroyed in the gastrointestinal tract by proteinases; therefore, it must be given parenterally. Several types are available and may be classified as rapid-acting with shorter period of action, intermediate-acting with longer period of action, and slow-acting with prolonged period of action. The rapid-acting preparations include regular (unmodified, crystalline) and semi-lente insulins. The intermediate-acting insulins include globin, neutral protamine Hagedorn (NPH, isophane) and lente; those which are absorbed more slowly and have a prolonged effect on lowering blood sugar are protamine zinc insulin and ultra-lente insulin. See Table 21–3 for the onset and duration of action of each type of insulin.[24] These figures are approximate, since individual differences in responses do occur.

It is important that the nurse caring for or counseling diabetics be familiar with the action characteristics of the various types of insulin so that complaints and disturbances can be considered in relation to the onset, peak and duration of the type being received. A summary of these, kept readily accessible for reference on the hospital ward, in the clinic or in the visiting nurse's bag can prove very helpful.

Insulin is measured in units. One unit of insulin promotes the metabolism of approximately 1.5 Gm. of glucose.[25] Dosage is determined individually on the basis of the amount of glucose in the diet which the person is unable to metabolize as manifested by the blood sugar level and glucosuria. Insulin is supplied in 10-ml. (cc.) vials in 2 strengths: one has a concentration of 40 units per ml. (cc.), and the other contains 80 units per ml. (cc.). The latter is usually used when the patient requires more than 40 units in one dose; the more concentrated insulin reduces the volume of solution to be injected. Insulin syringes may be calibrated for the measuring of units of both strengths, necessitating careful checking to be certain

[23]Canadian Diabetic Association (Report of an address by C. Best), C.D.A. Newsletter, Vol. 16, No. 2. Second Quarter, 1969, p. 16.

[24]H. Rosenthal, and J. Rosenthal, op. cit., pp. 91–97. W. B. Hadley: Insulin Treatment of Diabetes Mellitus. Med. Clin. North Amer., Vol. 49, No. 4 (July 1965), p. 922.

[25]American Society of Pharmacists, Committee on Pharmacy and Pharmaceuticals: Hospital Formulary, Vol. 2. American Society of Hospital Pharmacists, 68:20, 1969.

that the scale used corresponds to the strength of the insulin being used and that ordered. The time and frequency of administration depend on the type of insulin and the patient's response. Quick-acting insulin is given 20 to 30 minutes before breakfast and may be repeated before lunch and supper if the urine still shows sugar. Following the administration of rapid-acting insulin, food must be given within 1 hour to prevent hypoglycemia. The slower-acting insulins are generally only given once daily, usually in the morning at breakfast time. If the patient is ill and cannot take his meal or for some reason the meal is delayed, the insulin is omitted. If it is given and the patient does not eat or he vomits, the incident is reported promptly and the patient is given glucose in some form to prevent hypoglycemia.

Insulin is given by hypodermic below the subcutaneous fat to prevent lipodystrophy. The arms, thighs and abdomen are the areas used, and the site is rotated. Too frequent use of one site causes fibrosing and scarring which delay absorption as well as make the injection more difficult.

All insulin other than the regular must be thoroughly mixed before use to ensure uniform suspension and concentration throughout. This is done by rotating the bottle and inverting it from end to end; vigorous shaking is avoided. Some patients require a combination of fast-acting and slower-acting insulins. The strengths of the two insulins (i.e., the units per ml.) should be the same. Before mixing two types for one administration, the nurse checks with the physician; some prefer to have them given separately. Generally, regular insulin may be mixed with protamine zinc, NPH or lente insulin. To avoid contamination of the regular insulin, it is drawn into the syringe first or separate needles may be used. When both are loaded, the syringe is then slowly tipped up and down until the two preparations are well mixed.

Each bottle of insulin bears an expiration date beyond which the content should not be used. Insulin should be kept in a cool place, preferably a refrigerator. Extremes of temperature and exposure to sunlight are likely to cause deterioration.

Various local and general reactions to insulin may occur. The local reactions are minor in nature and include local sensitivity, lipodystrophy and fibrosis. Frequently, when insulin therapy is first started, sensitivity may be manifested at the site of injection because the insulin is a foreign protein and antigenic. The area becomes red, swollen and itchy but the response is generally temporary and disappears as the patient becomes desensitized by the repeated doses of insulin.

The local action of insulin on the adipose tissue cells may incur a swelling of the fatty tissue followed by atrophy which leaves a hollow space in the area. These atrophic areas are not serious but present an undesirable cosmetic effect. They may be prevented by making sure that the insulin is introduced below the subcutaneous tissue. Frequent and repeated injections into one area of tissue may result in fibrosing of the tissue and induration of the site. Fibrous tissue has poor vascularization which decreases the rate of absorption of the insulin. This complication may be prevented by systematic rotation of the injection sites, avoiding the use of any one spot oftener than once every 2 to 3 weeks.

General insulin reactions include insulin resistance and hypoglycemia. Insulin resistance is said to be present when diabetes cannot be controlled with less than 200 units of insulin per day.[26, 27] It may occur secondary to some other diseases such as severe adrenal cortical hyperfunction, acromegaly and thyrotoxicosis. As a primary condition, it is attributed to an antigen-antibody reaction. Antibodies are developed in response to the foreign protein (insulin). It is more likely to occur with insulin extracted from cattle than with that prepared from the pancreas of hogs. Insulin resistance usually develops insidiously several months after insulin treatment has begun. Treatment includes the use of pork insulin and cortisone to reduce the patient's antibody production.

Hypoglycemia is discussed on page 577.

ORAL HYPOGLYCEMIC DRUGS. There are two groups of drugs which lower blood sugar — sulfonylurea compounds and bigua-

---

[26]T. R. Harrison, et al. (Eds.): Principles of Internal Medicine, 4th ed. New York, the Blakiston Division, McGraw-Hill Book Co., Inc., 1962, p. 647.

[27]J. S. Soeldner, and J. Steinke: Insulin Resistance. Med. Clin. North Amer., Vol. 49, No. 4 (July 1965), p. 939.

TABLE 21–4   ORAL HYPOGLYCEMIC DRUGS

GROUP	DURATION	ACTION
Sulfonylurea compounds		Stimulate the secretion of insulin
Tolbutamide (Orinase)	6–12 hours	
Chlorpropamide (Diabinese)	up to 60 hours	
Acetohexamide (Dymelor)	12–24 hours	
Biguanide preparations		Thought to enhance effectiveness
Phenformin (DBI)	4–6 hours	of insulin, increasing cellular
Long-acting phenformin (DBI-TD)	8–12 hours	uptake of glucose

nides. The fact that they may be taken orally provides a distinct advantage. Their use is limited mainly to diabetics whose disease is mild, stable and generally has developed after the age of 40.

The sulfonylurea compounds lower the blood sugar by stimulating the secretion of insulin. These preparations include tolbutamide (Orinase), chlorpropamide (Diabinese) and acetohexamide (Dymelor). The principal difference between these preparations is in the duration of their action: tolbutamide has some effect in lowering the blood sugar for 6 to 12 hours; chlorpropamide is effective up to 60 hours; and acetohexamide acts for 12 to 24 hours. The biguanide preparations are phenformin (DBI), which is effective for 4 to 6 hours, and long-acting phenformin (DBI-TD), which is effective in lowering the blood sugar over a period of 8 to 12 hours. The action of the biguanide preparation is not clearly understood, but it is thought to enhance the effectiveness of insulin, increasing the cellular uptake of glucose.

It must be remembered that it is still important for the patient receiving oral hypoglycemic agents to respect his prescribed diet, exercise and supervision. Although the risk of hypoglycemia is less than with insulin therapy, it may occur, and the patient must be made aware of the early manifestations. Occasionally, the oral hypoglycemic agents produce some side effects such as gastrointestinal disturbances (heartburn, nausea, vomiting, diarrhea), headache, skin rash and itching.

GENERAL HYGIENIC MEASURES.   During hospitalization, particular attention is paid to the patient's skin and feet, especially if he spends the greater part of the day in bed. The diabetic's skin is less resistant to pressure and irritation, and when broken, it readily becomes infected and is difficult to heal. It is kept clean and dry; a mild soap is used for bathing, and a light application of lanolin or oils may be made to prevent cracking if the skin is dry. Foot soaks and oiling may be necessary to remove thick dry skin, calluses and corns. The toenails are cut straight across to avoid ingrown toenails and possible infection. For the bed patient, a footboard is used to relieve the weight of bedding on the feet, and a routine of frequent, regular foot and leg exercises is established, especially with older persons. Vulnerable pressure areas are gently massaged every 3 or 4 hours and are protected by frequent turning and the placing of a square of synthetic sheepskin under the patient.

Exposure to infection is avoided since any infection tends to increase the demand for insulin and may interfere with the diabetic's normal food intake, predisposing him to ketosis. Any indication of a respiratory infection, gastrointestinal disturbance or skin lesion is promptly brought to the physician's attention, since such conditions require more prompt and careful attention than in the nondiabetic.

EXERCISE.   A moderate amount of exercise is an important part of diabetic treatment. It promotes the use of glucose and may diminish the amount of insulin or oral hypoglycemic needed to control the blood sugar level. It also stimulates and improves the circulation, helps to maintain muscle tone and prevents obesity. Some diabetics have sufficient exercise in their occupation, but those in sedentary jobs or who are retired should have a planned program which is introduced gradually. Since the prescription for diet and a hypoglycemic is based on the patient's physical activity, the regimen should be the same each day to minimize fluctuations in the blood sugar concentration. When variations in daily energy expenditure are necessary, adjustments in the diet may be needed. Extra carbohydrate in the form of fruit, milk or bread may be added if activity is increased. When the usual amount of activity is decreased for some reason, (other than illness or infection) some decrease in the caloric intake is usually indicated.

Active exercise at regular intervals is encouraged during hospitalization unless contraindicated for other physical reasons. With an anticipated increase of activity on discharge from the hospital, the insulin dosage may be decreased and the carbohydrate and fat intake may be increased. For the older diabetic a daily routine of walking and light home chores (house and garden) is recommended.

The aim is to maintain a balance between energy expenditure and the prescribed treatment (diet and insulin or oral hypoglycemic). More than the usual amount of exercise lowers the blood sugar; less than the usual amount will raise it.

The diabetic participating in strenuous activity, particularly if he is on insulin therapy, should advise a coworker or, in the case of sports, a friend or sports supervisor that he is a diabetic. He should also carry sugar cubes or candy which he can take at the first sign of weakness and hypoglycemic reaction. When making a change in occupation that involves either a decrease or increase in activity, the diabetic should have his plan of therapy reviewed by his physician or at the clinic.

EDUCATION. Diabetes mellitus is a disease with which the patient will have to live the rest of his life. To maintain successful control of his disease which will permit him to live an independent satisfying life, the diabetic must have an understanding of his disease, the treatment and care prescribed for him and the possible complications. Patient and family education is a responsibility of the nurse caring for the diabetic and plays as important a role in successful treatment as diet and insulin.

Before launching a program of instruction, it is necessary to assess the patient's attitude toward his disease and to determine his readiness to accept the teaching. The patient may become quite emotional when told he has diabetes and its implications. His behavior may manifest depression, fear, withdrawal or resentment that this has happened to him. The nurse, recognizing the patient's reaction, conveys to him a willingness to listen and to talk about his future when he is ready. Most patients work through their immediate reactions and reach a phase in which they verbalize their feelings and are prepared to listen and accept the reassurance that their disease can be controlled and that the necessary treatment and care will become a routine part of their life without seriously altering it.

In planning the instruction, it is necessary to know the patient's background so that care can be adapted as much as possible to his accustomed way of life. The physician and dietitian may participate in the program, but the nurse should be familiar with their advice so that she can answer the patient's and his family's questions and reinforce certain areas when necessary. The amount of information given at one time depends on the patient's ability and willingness to receive it. Generally, brief periods of discussion are more effective than the presentation of a large amount of information at one time. Group instruction may be used in the hospital or clinic for some topics, but it must be remembered that each diabetic's treatment is individualized. A large part of the discussion must be on an individual basis.

Teaching is begun as soon as possible to avoid giving too much at one time, leading to confusion and discouragement, and to allow time for the patient to practice self-care, read and ask questions.

Explanations are made in simple lay terms; and demonstrations are broken into steps, made slowly, repeated as often as necessary, and sufficient opportunity is provided for the patient to practice. Illustrations and written explanations and directions are used for clarification. Reading material (books, pamphlets) written for diabetics should be made available; examples of such publications are listed below.

The instruction program covers the following: an explanation of diabetes; diet; insulin therapy; urine testing; hypoglycemia; uncontrolled diabetes; identification card, special personal care; regular supervision; and sources of information and assistance.

A simple basic explanation is made of the nature of diabetes, relating it to the symptoms experienced by the patient. To illustrate, the patient may be told that the sugar and starches (such as bread and cereal) are converted by digestion to a simple form of sugar called glucose, which is the body's chief source of energy. In order for the cells to extract it from the blood and use it, the chemical insulin is necessary. In diabetes, there is not sufficient insulin being produced to use the amount of sugar and starches being taken, so glucose accumulates in the blood in excess of the normal. The kidneys remove some of the excess which is the reason why the diabetic voids a lot and the urine contains sugar. The loss of large amounts of urine results in thirst. Weakness, fatigue and hunger occur because the sugar is not being burned to produce energy. The body, in an effort to provide energy, may break down body tissue, causing a loss of weight. Some diabetics produce enough insulin to handle the amount of sugar they actually need to still maintain their normal weight. Others may require more glucose because of their activities but are not producing sufficient insulin to use that amount, so they require a drug which may be taken by mouth or insulin, which must be taken by an injection.

The prescribed diet must be clearly and carefully interpreted to the patient. The initial instruction is usually given by a dietitian, but considerable clarification and reinforcement by the nurse, who is with the patient more often, is usually necessary. The prescription, sample meal plan and exchange lists are explained. The foods allowed each day, their division into meals and snacks, and the selection from exchange lists are reviewed several times. It is helpful to have the patient plan meals for several days. The purchase and preparation of his food and how it may be worked in with the family meals are discussed. The following general principles which apply to the diabetic diet are cited: only standard measuring cups and spoons are used; amounts used should be accurate and correspond with that indicated on the exchange list; concentrated sweets such as sugar, candy, jams, honey, cake and pastries should be avoided; labels are carefully read when purchasing canned and prepared foods, and only those indicating that no sugar has been added are used; to satisfy hunger, foods of no caloric value may be taken which include clear tea and coffee, sugarless jelly powder, consommé, clear broth, bouillon or oxo and artificially sweetened beverages; the daily food allowance should all be eaten; and meals should be taken at regular hours. A frequent question raised by patients is whether liquor, beer and wine are allowed. The question is referred to the attending physician; if an alcoholic beverage is permitted, it should be counted in the total caloric intake, since it is fairly high in calories.* The patient is encouraged to read and obtain for his personal use books and pamphlets which contain considerable detail on diabetic diets. The national diabetic associations have a Diet Counseling department which is prepared to provide assistance in meal planning.

If the patient is on insulin therapy, he is advised of the necessary equipment and where it may be obtained. An explanation is made of what insulin is and of the several

American Diabetes Association, New York: Facts about Diabetes; ADA Forecast (bimonthly publication).

Ames Co. of Canada (Division of Miles Lab. Ltd.), Toronto: Guidebook for the New Diabetic Patient.

Canadian Diabetic Association, Toronto: Manual for Diabetics in Canada; Meal Planning Booklet; Diabetes—A Question and Answer Book; CDA Newsletter (quarterly publication); Cookbook for Diabetics.

Connaught Medical Research Laboratories: Insulin—A Handbook for Diabetic Patients, 10th ed. Toronto, Connaught Laboratories, 1967.

E. P. Joslin: Diabetic Manual, 10th ed. Philadelphia, Lea and Febiger, 1960.

H. Rosenthal, and J. Rosenthal: Diabetic Care in Pictures, 4th ed. Philadelphia, J. B. Lippincott Co., 1968.

G. F. Schmitt: Diabetes for Diabetics, 2nd ed. Miami, Florida, The Diabetic Press of America Inc., 1968.

*Caloric value of 240 ml. (8 oz.) of beer is 114; 45 ml. (1½ oz.) of whiskey is 120 calories; and 120 ml. (4 oz.) of wine is 114 calories.

types and strengths, indicating the name, nature and strength of that prescribed for him and how it is identified. Measurement by units is demonstrated, and the patient is encouraged to practice the handling of the syringe and needle and the measurement of his prescribed dose. Instruction and demonstrations are then given to familiarize him with the sterilization of the equipment, aseptic handling, rotating of the vial to equalize the suspension of insulin, withdrawal of the required amount of insulin, the necessary rotation and cleansing of sites for injection, the actual injection and the aftercare of the equipment. Storage and maintenance of an adequate supply of insulin are discussed. Free insulin is available to many patients but can usually only be obtained by a special requisition form signed by the patient's physician. Automatic injectors are available which may be of assistance to those patients who find the injection of the needle difficult. The injector has a mechanically controlled spring which, when released, pushes the needle quickly through the skin. If it is used, a metal-tipped syringe is usually necessary.

If an oral hypoglycemic is prescribed, the importance of taking the drug in the exact dosage at the times ordered is stressed. Written directions are given, and the patient is advised that if headache, nausea, vomiting or other disturbances are experienced, he should contact the doctor.

The diabetic may be required to test his urine regularly for sugar and ketone bodies using one of the commercial preparations (e.g., Clinitest, Clinistix or Tes-Tape), and the procedure and interpretation of the result are demonstrated. Occasionally, the patient may have to be taught to adjust his insulin dosage according to the results of the urine tests.

The diabetic who is receiving insulin or an oral hypoglycemic should know that under certain circumstances, the blood sugar may fall below normal levels, resulting in what is called an insulin or hypoglycemic reaction. The patient and family should be familiar with the symptoms (see p. 577) and know what to do. The causes of hypoglycemia are cited (see p. 577), and the patient is advised that on experiencing early symptoms, he should immediately take a concentrated form of sugar that is quickly available.

Two or 3 cubes of sugar, tea or coffee with 2 or 3 teaspoonsful of sugar, 2 or 3 small candies, orange juice or grape juice (4 oz.), or a teaspoonful of honey, corn syrup or jelly may be used. If the symptoms do not disappear in 10 minutes, the administration is repeated. The patient on insulin is advised to always carry lump sugar or hard candies with him. Following a reaction, he should rest for 2 or 3 hours to reduce the demand on his blood sugar and should take some form of protein (cheese, milk or peanut butter). It will slowly provide some glucose and contribute to the maintenance of a more constant blood sugar level. The family should know that if the diabetic cannot swallow or retain sugar, a physician is called at once, or he is taken as quickly as possible to a hospital emergency department. Friends and associates as well as the family should know that the diabetic receives insulin and may experience a reaction. The patient is advised that insulin reactions should be reported to the doctor; his insulin dosage or diet may require adjustment.

The patient should also be able to recognize early symptoms of uncontrolled diabetes, which causes hyperglycemia. If it is not corrected in the early stage it may lead to the serious complications of diabetic acidosis and coma. Hyperglycemia and ketosis develop more slowly than hypoglycemia—usually over several days. The disturbance is usually manifested by loss of appetite, nausea, vomiting, thirst, weakness, drowsiness and general malaise. Sugar will be present in the urine. It is frequently associated with infection or stress or may be due to dietary indiscretion or omission of insulin or oral hypoglycemic. The patient is advised that his physician is contacted as soon as symptoms are experienced. Until medical attention is obtained he should remain in bed, keep warm, drink hot clear fluids without sugar freely and repeat them even if he vomits; if possible, someone should remain with him.

Every diabetic should carry a diabetic identification card at all times so that his condition will be made known quickly in the event of a reaction, illness or accident. Cards which carry appropriate information are available from physicians, the diabetic clinic and the National Diabetic Association or its local branches; a written one may be carried temporarily. The diabetic may also acquire a membership in the Medic-Alert Foundation, which provides a Medic-Alert emblem in the form of a bracelet or medallion to be worn at all times. The emblem indicates the medical problem and the number of the diabetic's file from which information can be obtained at any time.

The patient is advised that, because of his diabetes, he may be more susceptible to infections and will tend to heal more slowly when breaks occur in the skin. Any infection predisposes to uncontrolled diabetes, and persons whose disease is uncontrolled appear to develop infection more readily. The diabetic avoids contact with persons who have an infection as much as possible. The skin should be kept clean, warm and free of irritation and pressure as much as possible, and precautions are taken to prevent cracks and breaks in the skin. Scratches, cuts, abrasions and hangnails are cleansed with alcohol or a solution of hexachlorophene and are protected by a dressing. The use of strong antiseptics (such as iodine) and adhesive is avoided. Prolonged exposure to sunlight and the use of local heat applications (electric heating pad, hot water bottle) are discouraged. If heat applications are necessary, extra precautions are necessary; a lower degree of heat and extra covers are used.

The adult diabetic's feet require constant special attention because of the increased susceptibility to circulatory disorders as well as infections. The patient is directed to bathe his feet daily with warm (not hot) water using a mild soap and to dry them thoroughly, especially the areas between the toes, using gentle pressure rather than vigorous rubbing. Talcum powder may be used sparingly or alcohol is applied if his feet tend to be moist and perspire; if they are dry and scaly, a light application of lanolin is rubbed into the skin. The toenails are cut straight across with scissors. If calluses and corns cannot be controlled by rubbing them with a pumice stone, they should be treated by a chiropodist who is advised of the person's diabetes. Stockings or socks should fit well to avoid any constriction or wrinkles that might cause irritation or pressure and are changed daily. To prevent possible interference with the circulation, round garters are not worn.

Shoes should be well-fitting so there is no irritation or pressure on any part of the foot, and new shoes are worn only for brief periods until broken in. The foot and leg exercises introduced during hospitalization should be continued, particularly if the patient is likely to be inactive. Walking barefoot, the use of commercial corn remedies and the application of heating appliances are discouraged. Numbness, persisting coldness, discoloration, a burning feeling, pain or any unusual condition of the lower limbs is reported to the physician.

It is advisable for the diabetic to have an annual eye examination because of the predisposition to visual change which can only be detected by an ophthalmologist.

The newly diagnosed diabetic will be required to make more frequent visits to his physician or the clinic. These will become fewer as his disease and treatment are stabilized. The patient is instructed to take a urine specimen with him on each visit. The nurse in either situation checks with him as to how he is managing and gives him the opportunity to ask questions. Some phase of his care may require repetition and reinforcement. Before leaving the hospital, the importance of keeping the scheduled appointment is stressed. In the case of older persons, assistance may be necessary in making some arrangements for transportation to the clinic.

The patient and his family are made aware of the available sources of help and information. These include the national and local diabetic associations, the visiting nurse agency and public health nursing department. The services provided by the various organizations and recommended publications are cited. Patients are encouraged to obtain a membership in a diabetic association, which may be obtained through a local chapter or directly from the national association. This entitles them to the regular periodical and additional literature published by the association.

The care of the child or adolescent diabetic requires the understanding and cooperation of the entire family. Because of their growth and the vigorous activity characteristic of these young persons, closer medical supervision is necessary. They tend to be less stable and more frequent adjustments in their insulin dosage and diet are necessary. The child is taught self-care and self-administration of his insulin as soon as possible. He must be able to recognize early symptoms of hypoglycemia and know when to take the sugar cubes or concentrate form of glucose that he always carries with him. It must be emphasized in discussions with the parents that the child be encouraged to assume responsibility for his own care and that he be permitted to live as much like a normal child as possible so that he and his associates will not think of him as being "different."

Throughout all patient and family education, emphasis is placed on the positive — that is, control can be maintained, permitting the diabetic to carry on an active satisfying life. Certainly they must be made familiar with signs of certain complications and know what action to take to avoid serious consequences, but one must guard against creating unnecessary anxiety and discouragement.

Complications of Diabetes Mellitus. The most common complications of diabetes are diabetic acidosis, degenerative changes and hypoglycemia. Hypoglycemia occurs in those receiving insulin or oral hypoglycemic therapy.

DIABETIC ACIDOSIS (KETOSIS). Diabetic acidosis is a serious complication which develops in uncontrolled diabetes. The glucose in the blood cannot be utilized by the cells, and fat becomes the major source of energy. Fat is mobilized and broken down rapidly, producing ketone bodies (aceto-acetic acid, β-oxybutyric acid and acetone) in excess of the tissue cells' ability to utilize them. The acids and acetone accumulate in the blood. At first the normal pH is maintained by the buffer systems,* but eventually the alkali reserve becomes depleted and the pH of the body fluids falls, resulting in acidosis. At the same time, the increased concentration of glucose causes an increased output of urine (osmotic diuresis), and de-

---

*Example of the type of reaction that takes place:

$NaHCO_3$ (sodium bicarbonate) + aceto-acetic acid $\rightarrow$
Na aceto-acetate + H_2CO_3 (carbonic acid)

The sodium aceto-acetate is excreted in the urine, causing a loss of the base sodium. The weaker carbonic acid dissociates to H_2O and CO_2 and the CO_2 is eliminated through ventilation.

hydration develops. The increased osmotic pressures of the extracellular fluid result in the movement of fluid out of the cells accompanied by electrolytes. Serious sodium, potassium and phosphate deficiencies develop.

Ketosis has an insidious onset over several days, being preceded by symptoms characteristic of uncontrolled diabetes (polyuria, thirst, glucosuria, weakness). The symptoms related to the accumulation of ketones and reduced alkalinity of body fluids include anorexia, nausea, vomiting, deep and rapid respirations (Kussmaul's breathing), drowsiness, weakness which progresses to prostration, and abdominal pain or muscular cramps. The skin and mouth are dry, and the eyeballs are soft because of dehydration. The patient may appear flushed in the early stages but later becomes pale due to hypotension. The pulse is rapid and may be weak because of severe dehydration and the reduced intravascular volume. Unless the condition is recognized and treated promptly, the blood pressure falls, the patient becomes comatose, and his condition is critical.

The patient's urine shows a high concentration of sugar and ketones. The blood sugar is elevated and the sodium and chloride blood levels are lower. The potassium level may be elevated at first due to hemoconcentration and loss of the electrolyte from the cells but later falls below normal. The blood urea level is usually higher, and the leukocyte count is generally elevated. The carbon dioxide concentration and combining power are lowered as well as the pH.

The most common causes of diabetic acidosis are acute infection and gastrointestinal disorders. These conditions not only incur metabolic changes and demands but may lead to neglect of diet and insulin therapy. Other causes include dietary indiscretion, omission of insulin doses and undiagnosed diabetes mellitus.

The patient with diabetic acidosis requires immediate treatment which is directed toward stimulating the utilization of glucose by the cells, decreasing the production of ketone bodies by the administration of insulin, and correction of dehydration and the electrolyte imbalance. Any causative disorder is also treated.

The nurse who is notified that a patient

with ketosis is awaiting the doctor may assemble the following equipment to prevent delay in treatment: regular insulin; vasopressor drugs; intravenous infusion equipment; sterile syringes and needles for subcutaneous and intravenous injections; necessary equipment for taking blood samples; catheterization tray with an indwelling catheter and urine drainage receptacle; sphygmomanometer and stethoscope; and mouth care tray.

Immediate blood determinations are made of the glucose, carbon dioxide, specific electrolytes and urea concentrations. The hematocrit is also checked to determine hemoconcentration. An indwelling catheter is passed, and the urine is examined for glucose and ketones. The patient receives repeated doses of regular (quick-acting) insulin intravenously and a continuous intravenous infusion. The solution for the infusion and the dosage of insulin are based on the laboratory blood and urine findings. An electrocardiogram is done to detect changes in heart action characteristic of a low potassium blood level. The initial solution used is usually normal saline; sodium lactate or sodium bicarbonate and potassium chloride or potassium phosphate may be added later. Repeated blood sugar determinations and urinalyses are done. When the blood sugar level approaches normal, the frequency of administration and the dosage of insulin are decreased, and an intravenous glucose solution (5 per cent in water or saline) is usually ordered. If the patient's blood pressure is low and shock is present, a blood transfusion may be given, or a vasopressor such as levarterenol (Levophed) or metaraminol (Aramine) may be administered intravenously. This administration will necessitate frequent checking of the blood pressure, since the rate of flow of the solution containing the vasopressor is regulated according to the blood pressure response.

If the patient is comatose, the positioning, precautions to maintain respiration and prevent aspiration, safety measures (crib sides), frequent change of position and constant nursing attention which are appropriate for any unconscious patient must be applied (see p. 103). The blood pressure, pulse and respirations are recorded every 30 to 60 minutes; the temperature is recorded every 2 to 3 hours; an hourly check is made of the urinary output; and the patient's level of consciousness is noted. A gastric lavage may be done by the physician to reduce the risk of aspiration if the patient is vomiting frequently.

The patient should be kept warm with extra blankets. Frequent mouth cleansing and the application of an oil or cream to the lips are necessary. As soon as the patient regains consciousness and oral fluids can be tolerated, water, salty broth, orange juice, ginger ale, sweetened tea, milk and gruel are given freely. The fluid intake and output are recorded, and the balance is noted. As soon as possible, the patient receives a prescribed soft diet, and if tolerated, it is increased to a prescribed light diet. When the patient is taking sufficient nourishment by mouth and a satisfactory blood sugar level is maintained, intravenous infusions are discontinued and regular subcutaneous doses of insulin re-established.

Unless the cause of the ketosis was evident at the onset, efforts are made to determine why it occurred. Further patient and family education may be indicated.

DEGENERATIVE CHANGES. The blood vessels of practically all diabetics undergo degenerative changes to some extent. Atherosclerosis (deposits of the fatty substance cholesterol) develops in the arteries, narrowing their lumen, and the endothelial walls of the capillaries thicken. These changes may eventually interfere with the normal cellular nutrition and oxygen supply, contributing to tissue change and impaired function. The structures which most frequently manifest lesions and reduced efficiency are the eyes, coronary arteries, kidneys, lower limbs and nerves.

The higher incidence of these vascular changes in diabetics is not understood, nor is there agreement as to whether the severity and rate of progression may be correlated with the control of the diabetes.[28, 29, 30]

[28]Sir Stanley Davidson (Ed.): The Principles and Practice of Medicine, 7th ed. Edinburgh, E. & S. Livingstone Ltd., 1965, p. 747.

[29]A. Marble: Relation of Control of Diabetes to Vascular Sequelae. Med. Clin. North Amer. Vol. 49, No. 4 (July 1965), pp. 1137–1144.

[30]T. R. Harrison, et al. (Eds.): Principles of Internal Medicine, 4th ed. New York, The Blakiston Division, McGraw-Hill Book Co., Inc., 1962, p. 655.

Diabetic retinopathy occurs in the form of minute aneurysms in the retinal vessels. These dilatations are prone to rupture and cause a hemorrhage into the eye. The condition is only revealed by ophthalmoscopic examination. Depending on the location of the lesions, the diabetic's vision may or may not be affected.

Atherosclerosis of the coronary arteries of the diabetic frequently leads to angina pectoris and myocardial infarction, especially in older persons.

Renal function may be slowly impaired by changes in the glomerular capillaries (intercapillary glomerulosclerosis or Kimmelstiel-Wilson syndrome) and by sclerotic changes in the larger renal vessels. The patient may manifest albuminuria and some degree of hypertension.

Defective circulation, due to vascular changes in the lower limbs, frequently leads to gangrene. A small superficial injury may be a precipitating factor. The gangrene may necessitate the amputation of a toe, foot or leg. Restricted circulation may be manifested by abnormal coldness of the extremities, numbness, discoloration, muscular cramps, weakness, burning pain or a small ulcer that does not heal. When impaired circulation is manifested, Buerger's exercises may be recommended; while the patient lies on his back, he raises one or both legs, allowing them to rest on a support until they blanch (approximately 1 to 3 minutes). A straight-backed chair, which is padded, may be used as a support; the top of the back and the front of the seat rest on the bed. A regular Buerger board may be available and can be adjusted to different heights (45° to 60° angle). Following the elevation and blanching of the limbs, the patient sits up, allowing the legs to hang over the side of the bed until they become red (5 to 10 minutes). The doctor may suggest that repeated flexion, extension, and inward and outward rotation of the feet be carried out while in this position. When color is restored to the legs and feet, the patient lies in the horizontal position for a few minutes (5 to 7 minutes) before repeating the exercise. The doctor indicates the number of times the exercise is to be done and may state a specific number of minutes for each stage.

Peripheral neuritis is a painful complication of diabetes. The patient may experience muscular cramps, tingling, numbness or burning pain in the extremities; this is usually most troublesome at night. The condition frequently responds to vitamin supplements, especially the vitamin B complex, increased protein in the diet, and better control of the diabetes.

HYPOGLYCEMIA. Hypoglycemia implies an abnormally low blood sugar concentration. Signs and symptoms usually begin to appear when the blood sugar falls below 60 mg. per cent. The onset of symptoms, however, varies with individuals — some may develop symptoms at a higher level of blood sugar; others may not manifest the disturbance until a lower level is reached. Adults tend to have symptoms earlier than child diabetics.

The causes of hypoglycemia in the diabetic may be the delay or omission of a meal after having taken insulin or an oral hypoglycemic agent; an undue amount of energy expenditure; an overdosage of insulin; a gastrointestinal disorder which produces anorexia, vomiting or diarrhea; or improvement in the diabetic's ability to utilize glucose.

A hypoglycemic reaction in a patient receiving regular insulin usually occurs approximately 2 to 6 hours after the injection. In the patient receiving an intermediate-acting insulin given in the morning it happens more commonly in the afternoon or evening. Hypoglycemic reaction to a slow-acting insulin generally occurs during the night or early in the morning of the following day.

It should be kept in mind that it is possible for the patient receiving an oral hypoglycemic to develop hypoglycemia. It develops insidiously and may occasionally go unrecognized.

The signs and symptoms manifested by an abnormally low blood sugar are a reflection of its effect on the central nervous system. The brain is very dependent on a constant, adequate supply of glucose. Any deprivation, even for a relatively brief period may seriously impair cerebral activity and result in permanent damage. Similarly, repeated occurrences of hypoglycemia, even of short duration, especially in children, may incur some permanent cerebral impairment. The manifestations of hypoglycemia vary from one patient to another but tend to be the same with each reaction for the same person which makes it more easily recognizable by him. The earlier signs and symptoms include sweating, tremor, apprehension, hunger, weakness, tachycardia and palpitation. More advanced symptoms are faintness or dizziness, blurring of vision or diplopia, headache, slow reactions, uncoordinated movement which occasionally leads to mistaking the patient's condition for alcohol intoxication, muscular twitching that may progress to convulsions especially in children, disorientation and confusion, stupor and eventual loss of consciousness. The urine will be negative for sugar. All diabetics, their immediate family and close associates should be familiar with the early signs and symptoms of hypoglycemia and should know what to do.

If the patient can still swallow, he is immediately given some form of rapidly absorbable concentrated sugar. Ten to 15 Gm. of carbohydrate are usually sufficient to restore the blood sugar level. Orange juice (120 ml.) or other sweetened fruit juice or 2 teaspoonfuls of corn syrup, honey or sugar with a glass of water may be used. If there is no improvement in 5 to 10 minutes, the administration is repeated. If the patient is unconscious or uncooperative, 30 to 50 ml. of 50 per cent glucose are given intravenously. Glucagon (1 to 2 mg.) or epinephrine 1:1000 (0.5 ml.) subcutaneously may be ordered to promote glycogenolysis and subsequent increase in blood glucose. A venous blood specimen is collected as soon as possible and is repeated at frequent intervals until the patient is stabilized.

Following a reaction, the patient is encouraged to rest for several hours in order to decrease the utilization of his blood glucose. Some form of protein (cheese or milk) should be given the patient to provide additional glucose which is produced slowly over a period from protein metabolism. The nurse always checks with the physician before giving the next scheduled dose of insulin. Adjustments are usually made in the carbohydrate content of the diet and in the insulin dosage. The patient may learn from the experience if encouraged to examine the reaction in retrospect. A discussion of the possible cause and the early symptoms may be helpful in preventing further reactions and in having the patient recognize hypoglycemia at the onset.

Diabetes Mellitus and Pregnancy. In recent years, the diabetic woman whose disease is well controlled and relatively stable is not usually advised against pregnancy. Occasionally, the nurse may be asked about this, and she should advise the woman to consult her physician. Pregnancy does affect diabetes and does carry certain risks, but with close medical supervision throughout the gestation period and strict adherence by the patient to the prescribed regimen, a successful pregnancy may be anticipated with most diabetic women.

The diabetic should report to her physician as soon as she suspects she is pregnant. She is then usually referred to an obstetrician who works closely with the internist during the entire pregnancy. The patient is required to make frequent visits, usually weekly or every 2 weeks, to the physicians. Her blood sugar and urea levels, blood pressure and weight are followed, and the urine is examined for sugar, acetone and albumin. The increase in the size of the uterus and the presence or absence of fetal heart sounds are noted on each visit.

The carbohydrate and protein portions of the diet are increased at the onset, and rarely, the insulin dosage is increased also. Further adjustments are made at intervals based on the findings at each visit. Additional insulin is usually necessary in the second and third trimesters. Sodium is usually restricted to 1.5 to 2.0 Gm. daily. A diuretic may be prescribed if the patient shows an excessive weight gain due to fluid retention. The clinic nurse or a visiting nurse should review the required self-care with the patient and help her establish a satisfactory daily regimen. Control of her diabetes is essential; hypoglycemia or diabetic acidosis may threaten the patient's life as well as that of the fetus. She is advised of ominous signs and symptoms (e.g., ketonuria, rapid gain in weight, pain) and the importance of promptly reporting them to the doctor. The patient is hospitalized 1 to 2 weeks prior to the predetermined delivery date. The pregnancy is usually terminated at the completion of the 36th or 37th week either by cesarean section or induction of labor. The fetus tends to be overweight, and the mortality rate in babies of diabetic mothers is higher than in those of nondiabetics. The insulin dosage is reduced previous to induction of labor or the cesarean section because the requirement falls to prepregnancy levels quickly with delivery. Intravenous glucose 5 per cent in water is given during labor or preoperatively and is repeated during the immediate postpartum or postoperative period. Frequent urinalyses are done for sugar and acetone; the findings along with the blood sugar level serve as the bases for the insulin dosage and the amount of glucose to be given. The newborn infant requires special attention because of its prematurity and increased susceptibility to neonatal complications.

Surgery and Diabetes Mellitus. The emotional stress, physical trauma and physiological responses associated with surgery present a greater problem for the diabetic than for the normal person. A decrease in the utilization of glucose and an increased demand for insulin are likely to occur, predisposing the diabetic to acidosis. The diabetic who is to have elective surgery is hospitalized several days before the operation. During this period, his diabetes is thoroughly checked and brought under optimum control. The blood sugar is brought within normal range, and the urine must be free of sugar and ketones. The patient undergoes a thorough investigation for complications of his disease (degenerative changes), and his fluid and electrolyte balances and nutritional status are assessed. The total caloric intake and the carbohydrate and protein portions of the diet may be increased; this may necessitate additional insulin to ensure metabolism. The increase in carbohydrate is to provide an adequate reserve of liver and muscle glycogen.

The morning of operation, intravenous glucose 5 per cent in normal saline and a dose of regular insulin may be ordered. If a long operative period is anticipated, an indwelling catheter may be passed so that a urine specimen may be analyzed during surgery and additional intravenous solutions and insulin given if indicated.

Postoperatively, constant nursing attention is necessary; responses and reactions vary greatly with individuals. The insulin requirement may increase sharply with some patients and not with others. The pulse, respirations and blood pressure are usually recorded frequently for a longer period than usual, and a frequent check is made of the patient's level of consciousness. If the patient does not recover consciousness following the operation in a reasonable period of time, it is brought to the physician's attention. An indwelling catheter is passed if drainage was not established before operation. Blood and urine specimens are obtained immediately after operation and are repeated every 2 to 4 hours. Intravenous solutions and regular insulin are usually given; the type of solution and insulin dosage are based on the urine and blood findings. The nurse must be constantly alert for signs of hypoglycemia and acidosis.

Oral feedings are started just as soon as they can be tolerated, and specific orders are given as to what liquids may be given and how much the patient is to receive. The sooner he is returned to his usual diet the better. Frequent foot and leg exercises are especially important because of the diabetic's predisposition to vascular changes and circulatory problems. Precautions are taken to provide the maximum protection against infection; any slight indication of possible infection such as an elevation of temperature, cough or sore throat is reported immediately. Early ambulation is encouraged to promote greater utilization of glucose as well as to stimulate the patient's circulation.

Hyperinsulinism

An excessive secretion of insulin by the islets of Langerhans occurs rarely. It may be due to a functioning-cell neoplasm in the pancreas, involving the islet cells, or to an unexplained hyperactivity of the islets. The overproduction of insulin produces periodic hypoglycemic episodes which are usually precipitated by fasting or exercise. The patient manifests the signs and symptoms cited on page 577. Because of the repeated attacks, changes in personality and reduced intellectual ability may be evident as a result of permanent brain damage. The patient is treated by surgical excision of the newgrowth or a subtotal pancreatectomy.

References

BOOKS

Beeson, P. B., and McDermott, W. (Eds.): Cecil-Loeb Textbook of Medicine, 13th ed. Philadelphia, W. B. Saunders Co., 1971, pp. 1718–1855 and 1639–1664 (Diabetes Mellitus).

Brown, J. H. V., and Barker, S. B.: Basic Endocrinology. Philadelphia, F. A. Davis Co., 1962.

Davidson, Sir S.: The Principles and Practice of Medicine, 7th ed. Edinburgh, E. & S. Livingstone Ltd., 1965, pp. 655–757.

*Dolger, H., and Seeman, B.: How to Live with Diabetes. New York, Pyramid Books, 1966.

Green, J. H.: An Introduction to Human Physiology, 2nd ed. Toronto, Oxford University Press, 1968. Chapter 15.

Grollman, A.: Clinical Endocrinology and Its Physiologic Basis. Philadelphia, J. B. Lippincott Co., 1964.

Guyton, A. C.: Textbook of Medical Physiology, 4th ed. Philadelphia, W. B. Saunders Co., 1971. Chapters 75, 76, 77, 78 and 79.

Harrison, T. R., et al., (Eds.): Principles of Internal Medicine, 4th ed. New York, The Blakiston Division, McGraw-Hill Book Co., Inc., 1962, pp. 561–663.

*Joslin, E. P.: Diabetic Manual, 10th ed. Philadelphia, Lea and Febiger, 1960.

Langley, L. L.: Outline of Physiology, 2nd ed. New York, The Blakiston Division, McGraw-Hill Book Co., 1965. Chapters 27, 28, 29, 30 and 33.

*Malins, J.: Clinical Diabetes Mellitus. London, Eyre and Spottiswoode, 1968.

Netter, F. H.: Endocrine System and Selected Metabolic Conditions. The Ciba Collection of Medical Illustrations, Vol. 4: Ciba Pharmaceutical Co., 1965.

Proudfit, F. T., and Robinson, C. H.: Normal and Therapeutic Nutrition, 12th ed. New York, The Macmillan Co., 1964. Chapter 33.

Ralli, E. P.: The Management of the Diabetic Patient. New York, G. P. Putnam's Sons, 1965.

*Rosenthal, H., and Rosenthal, J.: Diabetic Care in Pictures, 4th ed. Philadelphia, J. B. Lippincott Co., 1968.

*Schmitt, G. G.: Diabetes for Diabetics, 2nd ed. Miami, The Diabetic Press of America Inc., 1968.

Sodeman, W. A., and Sodeman, W. A., Jr.: Pathologic Physiology, 4th ed. Philadelphia, W. B. Saunders Co., 1967. Chapter 8.

*The Canadian Diabetic Association: Manual for Diabetics in Canada, 2nd ed. Toronto, The Canadian Diabetic Association, 1965.

PERIODICALS

Abbott, M. M., et al.: "Diabetes Mellitus and Its Complications in an Elderly Population." Canad. Med. Ass. J., Mar. 21, 1964, p. 726.

Bell, G. O.: "Hashimoto's Thyroiditis." Surg. Clin. North Amer., Vol. 42, No. 3 (June 1962), pp. 647–652.

Belmonte, M. M.: "Diabetes in Childhood." Canad. Nurse, Vol. 59, No. 2 (Feb. 1963), pp. 143–145.

Daughaday, W. H., and Frawley, T. F. (Eds.): "Symposium on Endocrine Disorders." Med. Clin. North Amer., Vol. 52, No. 2 (Mar. 1968).

Fager, C. A.: "Surgical Ablation of the Pituitary Gland." Surg. Clin. North Amer., Vol. 45, No. 3 (June 1965), pp. 697–703.

Lubic, R. W.: "Nursing Care after Adrenalectomy or Hypophysectomy." Amer. J. Nurs., Vol. 62, No. 4 (Apr. 1962), pp. 80–84.

Martin, M. M.: "Insulin Reactions." Amer. J. Nurs., Vol. 67, No. 2 (Feb. 1967), pp. 328–331.

––––––––––– "New Trends in Diabetes Detection." Amer. J. Nurs., Vol. 63, No. 8 (Aug. 1963), pp. 101–103.

––––––––––– "Diabetes Mellitus: Current Concepts." Amer. J. Nurs., Vol. 66, No. 3 (Mar. 1966), pp. 510–514.

Moore, M. L.: "Diabetes in Children." Amer. J. Nurs., Vol. 67, No. 1 (Jan. 1967), pp. 104–107.

Nordyke, R. A.: "The Overactive and the Underactive Thyroid." Amer. J. Nurs., Vol. 63, No. 5 (May 1963), pp. 66–71.

Pearson, O. H.: "Adrenalectomy and Hypophysectomy." Amer. J. Nurs., Vol. 62, No. 4 (Apr. 1962), pp. 80–84.

Shea, K. M., et al.: "Teaching a Patient to Live with Adrenal Insufficiency." Amer. J. Nurs., Vol. 65, No. 12 (Dec. 1965), pp. 80–85.

White, P. (Ed.): "Symposium on Diabetes." Med. Clin. North Amer., Vol. 49, No. 4 (July 1965).

––––––––––––––––––––––

*Useful books for diabetics.

22
Nursing in Disorders of
The Nervous System

INTRODUCTION

The nervous system is the dominant system of the body. It provides an elaborate communication system and directs and integrates (along with the endocrine system) body activities.

The manifestations of dysfunction within the nervous system depend on the location of the lesion. This necessitates some understanding of the areas of the nervous system involved in various activities. Space does not permit an extensive review of the anatomy and physiology of this system, but some basic information of selected areas, especially pertinent to nursing, is presented.

All body movement, including much of the visceral activity, is brought about by contraction of muscle tissue which, in practically all instances* is initiated and coordinated by the nervous system. Relatively few primary disorders of muscle activity occur, but loss of movement (paralysis) and abnormal movement (e.g., spasticity) resulting from nervous dysfunction are common. For this reason, this section includes a brief consideration of muscle tissue.

---

*Exceptions: Inherent capacity of cardiac and intestinal muscle.

THE NERVOUS SYSTEM

The component structural parts of the nervous system are the brain, spinal cord, nerves, ganglia, receptors and effectors. The brain and spinal cord comprise the central nervous system; the other parts form the peripheral nervous system. There are two main functional divisions: the cerebrospinal or somatic nervous system, which is concerned mainly with activities at conscious level (perception and willed responses), and the autonomic or involuntary nervous system, which innervates visceral muscle and glands. These divisions are useful for descriptive purposes; the activities of the total system are interrelated.

Neuron

The microscopic structural unit of the nervous system is the neuron (nerve cell), which consists of a cell body and cytoplasmic processes. Each neuron has a single process called an axon, which conducts impulses away from the cell body, and one or more processes known as dendrites that carry impulses toward the cell body. Dendrites have many branches, increasing the

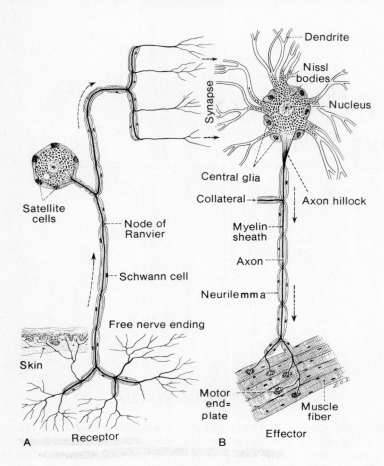

Figure 22–1 Diagram of a neuron. (From King, B. G., and Showers, M. J.: Human Anatomy and Physiology, 6th ed. Philadelphia, W. B. Saunders Co., 1969, p. 59.)

surface area over which impulses may be picked up. Axons frequently extend over great distances and give off branches nearer to their terminations. The processes (axons and dendrites) may be referred to as nerve fibers.

Unlike most body cells, neurons are incapable of reproduction by mitosis; when they are destroyed they are not replaced. A process may be replaced under favorable conditions (see p. 590).

Nerve cells may be classified as motor (efferent), sensory (afferent) or connecting (internuncial). The axon of a motor neuron transmits impulses which leave the central nervous system to stimulate muscle or glandular tissue. The sensory neuron's axon transmits impulses to all areas of the brain or spinal cord. One or more of its dendrites end in a receptor of some type in the periphery. Connecting neurons occur only in the gray matter of the brain and spinal cord. Nerve impulses must pass from the sensory neuron through one or more connecting neurons before being dispatched to a muscle or gland by a motor neuron. These play an important role, especially within the cerebral cortex, since they comprise the association areas which are discussed with the cerebral cortex. They "decide" the responses to the incoming (sensory) impulses and prompt the initiation of the particular motor neuron response.

Nerve Impulse

The functions of the nerve cells are to receive, initiate and conduct "messages" known as nerve impulses. An impulse is a physicochemical process. It occurs as the result of a mechanical, chemical or electrical change at some point in the immediate environment of the neuron. This change temporarily alters the permeability of the cell membrane at that point and is referred to as the stimulus. The series of events that result from the change in the membrane permeability produce an electrical current.

When a normal neuron is in a resting state, the outer surface of its membrane is electropositive, but the inner surface is electronegative. As a result, it is said to be polarized. This electrical polarity is attributed to the selective action of the cell membrane by which a higher concentration of sodium ions is maintained outside the cell. The positive sodium ions, which are normally attracted to the negative ions within the cell, are not allowed to cross the membrane; if they do so, they are ejected by the cell membrane. The electronegativity within the cell is mainly due to the nondiffusable protein anions and retained chlorine anions. When the stimulus occurs, the membrane becomes permeable to sodium. The influx of cations depolarizes the membrane; a reversal of the electrical potential develops as the outer surface of the membrane becomes electronegative and the inner surface becomes electropositive. This change alters the electrical relationship of the excited area to the adjacent portions; the shift of ions acts as a stimulus, and a wave of depolarization passes along the length of the neuronal process. In a fraction of a second, following depolarization, the membrane recovers its normal permeability and the resting electrical polarity is restored. The electrical currents that are generated as impulses sweep over the fibers and may be recorded and used in assessing function (e.g., electroencephalogram).

During the conduction of impulses, the neurons consume oxygen and glucose and produce heat and carbon dioxide. Impulse velocity is determined by the size of the neuronal process (nerve fiber) and whether or not it has a myelin sheath. The smaller unmyelinated fibers conduct more slowly than the larger, myelinated ones.

Synapse. Neurons occur in a chain-like arrangement to provide a pathway for impulses. The axon of one neuron passes the impulse to a dendrite or the cell body of the successive neuron in the pathway. The point of transmission is referred to as a synapse. A slight gap exists between the end of the axon and receptive neuron. The transmission is brought about by the release of a chemical from the terminal portion of the axon which acts as a stimulus to initiate the impulse in the succeeding neuron. The chemical transmitter is then rapidly destroyed or removed.

Reflex Arc, Receptor, Effector. The functional unit of the nervous system is called a reflex arc; structurally, it consists of the pathway over which impulses are conducted from a receptor to an effector. At the ending of afferent (sensory) fibers in the peripheral nervous system are receptors. A receptor, in a few instances, consists of bare nerve fibers; in others the afferent fibers end in specialized structures which are sensitive to specific stimuli. When the receptor is stimulated by a change in its environment (pressure, temperature, chemical, stretching) it evokes an impulse in the nerve fibers. The impulse is carried through the cell body of the sensory neuron and via its axon into the central nervous system. Here, it may pass through one, several or many connecting neurons before it excites a motor neuron

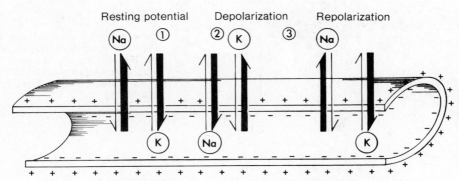

Figure 22–2 Resting state, depolarization and repolarization.

whose axon (efferent or motor fiber) carries the impulse out of the central nervous system to muscular or glandular tissue. The terminal portion of the efferent fiber releases a chemical at its junction with the effector, initiating its response. This response is contraction in the case of muscle and is secretion if it is a gland that is innervated.

Neuroglia

Lying among the neurons of the central nervous system are supporting cells referred to collectively as neuroglia. There are 3 types of glial cells, which vary in size, shape and function, but all have many processes which interlace with the neuronal processes. The astrocytes are star-shaped, and some of their processes attach to adjacent small blood vessels. Oligodendroglia have fewer and shorter processes, and the third type, which are smaller, are called microglia. Knowledge of the function of the glial cells is limited. The astrocytes increase during infection and probably play a role in transporting fluid and nutrients from the blood into the neurons. The microglia are capable of enlarging and becoming phagocytic to remove exudate and degenerative tissue following injury. It has been suggested that the oligodendrocytes play a role in the formation and maintenance of the myelin around the neuron processes. It is also thought that the glial cells contribute to the blood-brain barrier by which certain substances in the blood are prevented from entering the brain neurons. In contradistinction to the neurons, glial cells can divide and multiply; the majority of brain tumors arise from the uncontrolled growth of neuroglia.

THE CENTRAL NERVOUS SYSTEM

Brain

The brain is protected by the skull and for purposes of description may be divided into the cerebrum, basal ganglia, thalami, hypothalamus, midbrain, pons varoli, medulla oblongata and cerebellum.

Cerebrum. The cerebrum is divided by a longitudinal fissure into 2 hemispheres which are joined at their bases by bands of nerve fibers, collectively forming the corpus callosum. Each hemisphere is subdivided into 4 main lobes: frontal, parietal, temporal and occipital, corresponding approximately in location with the overlying skull bones. The lobes are separated by fissures: the central fissure (fissure of Rolando) lies between the frontal and parietal lobes; the lateral fissure (fissure of Sylvius) separates the temporal from the parietal and frontal lobes; and the parieto-occipital fissure separates the occipital from the parietal and temporal lobes.

The brain contains areas of gray and white matter. The gray matter is an aggregation of neuronal bodies and unmyelinated pro-

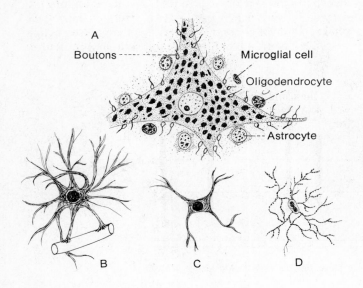

A
Boutons
Microglial cell
Oligodendrocyte
Astrocyte

B   C   D

Figure 22-3 *A,* Neuroglial cells. *B,* Astrocyte. *C,* Oligodendrocyte. *D,* Microglial cell. (From King, B. G., and Showers, M. J.: Human Anatomy and Physiology, 6th ed. Philadelphia, W. B. Saunders Co., 1969, p. 58.)

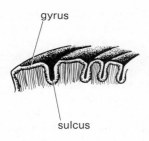

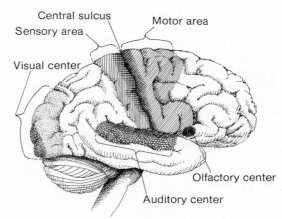

Figure 22–5 Portions of the brain.

cesses; the white matter consists primarily of myelinated fibers. The surface of the cerebrum (cerebral cortex) consists of gray matter which is arranged in a series of coil-like elevations called gyri. The shallow crevices between the gyri are sulci.

The cerebral cortex is a highly specialized area involved in all conscious processes. It is responsible for the intellectual processes such as learning, thought, memory, reasoning, verbalization and willed (voluntary) body movement, all of which are dependent on the information received through the afferent pathways.

Some parts of the cortex are receptive areas for incoming impulses and are called sensory areas or centers; others are concerned with dispatching outgoing impulses to prompt action responses in peripheral structures and are referred to as motor areas or centers. Around the sensory and motor areas lie the association areas, which occupy the greater portion of the cortex. A maze of connections exists between the association areas themselves as well as between them and sensory and motor centers. The asso-

ciation areas "analyze" the data received by the sensory areas, giving them meaning and making decisions as to appropriate responses which are then initiated. In some instances, the response may be to store the perception in memory; in others, it may involve stimulation of motor centers to bring about body movement or speech.

Certain areas of the cerebral cortex have been recognized as being primarily responsible for particular functions. The motor area that initiates all voluntary movements of the body occupies the strip of the frontal lobe immediately in front of the central fissure. The area in one hemisphere controls the movements on the opposite side of the body. The muscles are represented from the lower lateral surface of the lobe medially in the following order: head, throat, hand, arm, trunk, thigh, leg and foot.

The medial end of the motor strip terminates on the surface of the lobe in the longitudinal fissure. The size of the cortical area representing the muscular control in the various parts of the body is quite irregular and is proportional to their functional importance. The muscles of the fingers and hands have a large representation because of the frequent activity and precision movements. Similarly, the areas innervating the muscles involved in the highly developed function of speech (larynx, tongue, lips) are large. The area in front of the primary motor area is known as the premotor or secondary motor area. It is thought to be involved in patterns of movement requiring the coordinated contraction of groups of muscles.

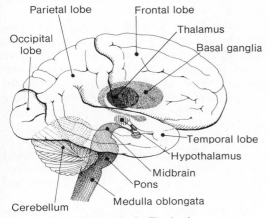

Figure 22–4 The brain.

It has connecting pathways with the primary motor area and lower levels of the brain.

The sensory impulses that enter the cortex are conducted to various areas, depending on their origin. The impulses concerned with touch, pressure, temperature, pain and the sense of position of the body and its parts (collectively referred to as the somesthetic senses) are received in the area of the parietal lobe just behind the central fissure. As with the motor areas, sensations from the lower part of the body are received at the medial portion lying within the longitudinal fissure. Those from the head are received at the lower lateral part of the strip. Sensations from the right side of the body are transmitted to the left hemisphere and vice versa.

Impulses originating in the retinae of the eyes are transmitted to the posterior part of the occipital lobe, resulting in vision. The visual center in the right occipital lobe receives impulses from the right half of the retina of each eye, and conversely, the left cerebral visual center receives those from the left half of each eye.

The centers for hearing lie in the superior parts of the temporal lobes. Impulses from both ears are received in both the right and left auditory centers. The sense of smell (olfactory sense) is also represented in the temporal lobe. The frontal lobes anterior to the motor areas are concerned with the personality, emotional reactions, initiative and sense of responsibility for socially acceptable standards. Persons who undergo prefrontal lobotomy, in which the severing of fibers interrupts many association pathways, frequently exhibit a complete change of personality, loss of judgment and inhibitions, and reduced efficiency.

The abstract mental activities such as thought, learning, reasoning, memory and emotions involve widespread cortical activity rather than a definitive local area. Associative memory is constantly used; it provides the knowledge that a person has. For example, vision stored as memory, auditory sensation stored as memory and other sensory experiences in memory may all be recalled and associated to give incoming impulses meaning and provide an appropriate response. To illustrate, if one has been introduced to a person and gains information about him at some time, he recognizes that person when he meets him again and recalls what he knows about him. One hemisphere tends to be dominant; in right-handed persons, the left hemisphere is dominant and vice versa.

The interior of the cerebrum consists mainly of white matter. Myelinated neuronal processes (nerve fibers) are arranged in functionally related bundles called tracts. These are classified as commissural, association and projection tracts. The commissural tracts transmit impulses between the two hemispheres. The association tracts carry impulses from one area of the cerebral cortex to another in the same hemisphere. Projection tracts are ascending and descending pathways from one level of the central nervous system to another. One of the most important of these is the internal capsule.

Basal Ganglia (Nuclei). Embedded within the cerebral white matter of each hemisphere are 4 irregular masses of gray matter, collectively referred to as the basal ganglia, or nuclei. Singly, they are the lentiform nucleus, caudate nucleus, amygdaloid body and the claustrum. The lentiform nucleus is subdivided into the putamen and globus pallidus. The lentiform and caudate nuclei and the segment of the internal capsule which separates them constitute what may be called the corpus striatum. The functions of the basal nuclei are not clearly understood. The corpus striatum is concerned with skeletal muscle tone and inhibitions essential to orderly, smooth patterns of movement. Injury and degenerative changes within the striatum cause increased muscular tone, rigidity and disturbed movements. The amygdaloid and claustrum are thought to be concerned with emotion and autonomic nervous system function.

Thalami. A large oval mass of gray matter lies at the base of each hemisphere and forms the lateral walls of the third ventricle. Each is referred to as a thalamus and serves as an important relay center for all afferent impulses. The impulses are "sorted" and forwarded to appropriate cerebral cortical areas. Each thalamus is capable of producing a crude uncritical awareness of pain, temperature and pressure; refinement of the sensation as to precise location, quality and intensity is made at cerebral cortical level.

Hypothalamus. Lying below the thalami

and forming the floor of the third ventricle is an important gray mass called the hypothalamus. It has extensive connections with higher and lower levels of the central nervous system and with the posterior lobe of the pituitary gland (neurohypophysis). The hypothalamus integrates and coordinates the responses of the autonomic nervous system, regulating visceral activities; for example, it exerts a control on vasomotor tone, gastrointestinal motility and heart rate. It contains groups of neurons responsible for temperature regulation. Through connections with the thalami and cerebral cortex, the hypothalamus' regulation of visceral activities may be influenced by emotional impulses.

Neurons in the hypothalamus also serve as osmoreceptors (cells sensitive to changes in the osmotic pressure of body fluid) and regulate the production and release of the antidiuretic hormone, which plays an important role in maintaining fluid balance. The production and release of oxytocin (see p. 535) is also influenced by the hypothalamus. This area of the brain also has control centers concerned with appetite and sleeping and waking mechanisms.

Midbrain. This portion of the brain is a short segment below the thalami and is comprised of a number of ascending and descending pathways. A narrow canal, the cerebral aqueduct, passes through the center, connecting the third and fourth ventricles. Groups of neurons form the corpora quadrigemina, which is comprised of 2 superior colliculi and 2 inferior colliculi. The superior colliculi correlate eye movements with movements of the head and trunk and initiate protective reflexes (blinking, closure of eyelids). The inferior colliculi are groups of neurons concerned with auditory reflexes such as the startle reflex on hearing a sudden sound and the turning of the head to improve the hearing of a sound. Centers (groups of neurons) for postural and righting reflexes also occur in the midbrain.

Brain Stem. The midbrain continues downward into the pons varoli, which consists almost entirely of tracts linking the various parts of the brain and serving as a conduction pathway. The pons also contains groups of neurons (nuclei) which give rise to some cranial nerves (V, VI, VII and VIII).

Below the pons lies the medulla oblongata, which continues down to connect with the spinal cord. It is comprised of ascending and descending conduction pathways and several important regulating centers. Groups of neurons form the vital cardiac, respiratory and vasomotor regulation centers. It also contains reflex centers for salivation, sneezing, vomiting, coughing and swallowing as well as the nuclei for a number of cranial nerves (IX, X, XI and XII).

Cerebellum. This portion of the brain lies under the posterior portion of the cerebrum posterior to the pons and medulla. It is separated from the cerebrum by a fold of meningeal membrane (dura mater) called the tentorium cerebelli. A fissure divides the cerebellum into hemispheres which are connected at their base. The outer surface consists of smooth layers of gray matter, and the interior consists mainly of white matter. The cerebellum has wide connections with other parts of the brain and with the spinal cord through tracts running through the pons. It is linked with the motor centers of the cerebral cortex, and it functions in the coordination of muscular activity. Afferent impulses are received from the proprioceptors in the skeletal muscles which result in impulses being delivered to the cerebral motor centers to provide synergic control in movements in which several muscles are involved. For example, antagonist muscles are inhibited and relax to allow contraction of the prime movers; the cerebellum is largely responsible for this type of integration to provide smooth, effective patterns of movement. Afferent impulses are also delivered to the cerebellum from the labyrinth of each internal ear. These impulses prompt appropriate reflex muscle responses to maintain balance of position or postural equilibrium.

Reticular Formation. A core of gray matter extending from the spinal cord through the medulla, pons, midbrain and into the hypothalamus comprises the reticular formation. It has widespread afferent connections, receiving sensory impulses from all over the body. It initiates impulses which are transmitted via subcortical relay areas to most of the cortex, alerting it to deal with ensuing impulses. In this way, it is said to produce an awareness or state of wakefulness. The neurons of this area

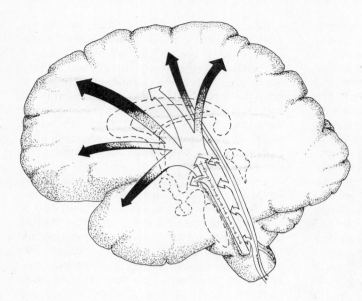

Figure 22–6. The reticular activating system.

learn to be selective, making judgment as to whether the cortex should be alerted or not. For example, a mother may not be awakened by heavy, noisy traffic, but she is aroused by the slightest whimper from her infant. Injury to this area produces loss of consciousness. The reticular formation also contributes to smooth, orderly motor performance, both reflex and voluntary.

Blood Supply to the Brain. The blood supply to the brain is derived from the 2 internal carotid arteries and the 2 vertebral arteries which arise from the subclavian arteries. At the base of the brain, the carotids give off anterior and middle cerebral arteries. The vertebrals, on reaching the brain, unite to form the basilar artery which gives rise to posterior cerebral arteries. The cerebral arteries are connected by communicating arteries, forming an arterial circle at the base of the brain called the circle of Willis. Branches of the cerebral arteries extend throughout the brain. Blood from the capillaries enters veins which empty into sinuses in the dura mater (outer meningeal membrane). The sinuses are drained by the internal jugular veins.

Ventricles and Cerebrospinal Fluid. Within the brain are a series of cavities called ventricles which originate with the embryonic, neural tube. There are 2 lateral ventricles, one in each cerebral hemisphere. Each lateral ventricle communicates with the third ventricle by means of an inter-

ventricular foramen (foramen of Munro). The third ventricle is a small and slit-like space between the thalami, and the larger fourth ventricle lies between the pons and the cerebellum. The third and fourth ventricles are united by a narrow channel called the cerebral aqueduct (aqueduct of

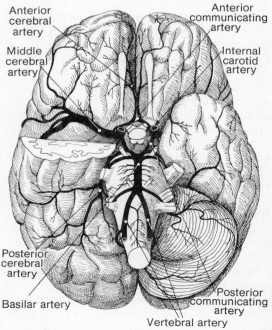

Anterior cerebral artery
Middle cerebral artery
Anterior communicating artery
Internal carotid artery
Posterior cerebral artery
Basilar artery
Posterior communicating artery
Vertebral artery

Figure 22–7 The blood supply to the brain.

Sylvius). The fourth ventricle has openings into the subarachnoid space (see meninges) and is continuous with the narrow central canal of the medulla and the spinal cord.

Within the ventricles, complex networks of capillaries (choroid plexuses) occur from which fluid escapes into the cavities, forming what is referred to as the cerebrospinal fluid. The fluid flows through the communicating channels and eventually escapes from the fourth ventricle into the subarachnoid space to surround the brain and spinal cord. This distribution of the fluid provides a protective cushion for the brain and cord.

The cerebrospinal fluid is steadily and slowly absorbed from the subarachnoid space into the venous sinuses. Any interruption within the cerebrospinal fluid circuit, such as occurs with a congenital absence of openings between the fourth ventricle and subarachnoid space, results in an excessive accumulation of fluid within the ventricles. The condition is referred to as hydrocephalus. The brain tissue becomes compressed between the skull and the expanding volume of fluid.

Meninges. The brain and spinal cord are enclosed in 3 layers of membranous tissue known as the meninges. The tough outermost layer is the dura mater. The cranial portion of the dura mater occurs in 2 layers; the external layer is adherent to the skull bones and does not continue into the spinal region. The 2 cranial layers are closely connected except where they form sinuses to receive the venous blood from cerebral vessels.

The middle membrane is called the arachnoid; it is much thinner and lies free. The potential space between the dura mater and arachnoid is known as the subdural space.

The innermost membrane is the pia mater and is thin, reticular and elastic; it is closely applied to the surface of the brain and cord, dipping into the fissures and sulci. The space between the arachnoid and pia mater is referred to as the subarachnoid space and contains the cerebrospinal fluid.

Spinal Cord

The cord, continuous with the medulla oblongata, originates at the foramen magnum of the skull and extends downward in the vertebral canal to approximately the

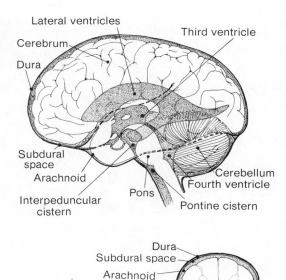

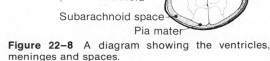

Figure 22-8 A diagram showing the ventricles, meninges and spaces.

second lumbar vertebra. It tapers off into a fine cord called the filum terminale. A ventral and a dorsal fissure incompletely divide the cord into lateral halves.

The cord consists of gray and white matter, but in contrast with the cerebrum, the gray matter is concentrated in the interior, roughly in the form of an **H**. White matter comprised of tracts is on the outside. Afferent impulses are received by neurons in the posterior columns or horns of gray matter. Efferent impulses are discharged by neurons in the anterior columns or horns of the gray matter. The gray matter also contains neurons which may transmit impulses from one lateral half of the cord to the other, from dorsal to ventral and to other levels of the central nervous system. The cord consists of 31 segments, each of which gives rise to a pair of spinal nerves. Two notable enlargements occur—one is in the cervical region corresponding to the origin of the upper limb nerves, and the other is in the lumbar region and gives origin to the nerves supplying the lower extremities.

The spinal cord provides conduction pathways to and from the brain and func-

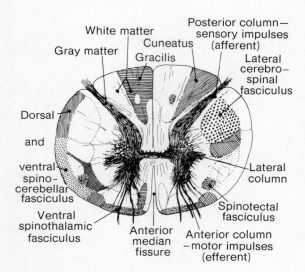

White matter
Gray matter
Cuneatus
Gracilis
Posterior column—
sensory impulses
(afferent)
Lateral
cerebro-
spinal
fasciculus
Dorsal
and
ventral
spino-
cerebellar
fasiculus
Ventral
spinothalamic
fasciculus
Anterior
median
fissure
Anterior column
—motor impulses
(efferent)
Spinotectal
fasciculus
Lateral
column

Figure 22–9 Cross section of the spinal cord.

tions as a center for reflex actions which are involuntary responses following the reception of certain afferent impulses.

Nerves and Tracts

The term nerve refers to a bundle of nerve fibers which extends beyond the central nervous system. Nerves consisting only of afferent fibers which transmit impulses from the periphery to the central nervous system are called sensory nerves. Motor nerves are comprised entirely of efferent fibers, which transmit impulses from the central nervous system out into the periphery. Many of the nerves—for example, all the spinal nerves—contain both efferent and afferent fibers and are known as mixed nerves.

Structurally, 3 types of nerve fibers occur; one is enclosed in a sheath of fatty substance, myelin, and an outer membranous sheath called the neurilemma (sheath of Schwann) and is known as a myelinated or medullated fiber. The other type has no myelin sheath but does have a neurilemma and is referred to as a nonmyelinated or nonmedullated fiber. Most unmyelinated fibers belong to the autonomic nervous system, which is concerned with visceral action. A third type of nerve fiber lacks a neurilemma. All fibers within the central nervous system and those of the optic and auditory nerves have no neurilemma. An injured nerve fiber cannot be regenerated in the absence of the neurilemmal sheath.

Nerve tracts are bundles of nerve fibers within the brain or spinal cord that transmit impulses that are usually similar in origin, termination and function. The origin and destination may be determined from the name of the tract. For example, the corticospinal tract carries impulses originating in the cerebral cortex to the spinal cord; the spinothalamic tract transmits sensory impulses from the spinal cord to the thalamus.

Nerve Regeneration. Unlike most cells in the body, the adult nerve cells cannot reproduce by mitosis to replace any that are destroyed. Nerve fibers are outgrowths of the cell body of the neuron. If a fiber's connection with the cell body is interrupted, the distal fragment ceases to function and degenerates. The fiber may regenerate and restore function, providing it has a neurilemma. Since nerve fibers within the central nervous system have no neurilemma, they cannot regenerate to re-establish function.

When a fiber with a neurilemma is damaged, the distal fragment disintegrates and the debris is removed by phagocytic cells. The Schwann cells of the neurilemma proliferate, forming strands and a pathway along the course of the degenerated portion of the fiber. The distal tip of the viable portion of the fiber begins to extend buds or branches; one of these finds and extends into

TABLE 22–1   ORIGIN AND FUNCTIONS OF CRANIAL NERVES (12 PAIRS)

NUMBER	NAME	ORIGIN OF MAIN NERVE FIBERS	FUNCTION
I	Olfactory	Sensory fibers: neurons in nasal mucosa	Olfactory sense (sense of smell)
II	Optic	Sensory fibers: neurons of retina	Vision
III	Oculomotor	Motor fibers*: nucleus in midbrain	Movements of the eyeball and upper eyelid; size of the pupil of iris (i.e., constriction and dilation of pupil to regulate amount of light admitted); control of ciliary muscle to regulate degree of refraction by the lens
IV	Trochlear	Motor fibers: nucleus in midbrain	Movement of eyeball by superior oblique muscles
V	Trigeminal	Motor fibers: nucleus in pons	Motor function: mastication
	Largest cranial nerve; has 3 sensory divisions— ophthalmic, maxillary and mandibular	Sensory fibers: gasserian or semilunar ganglion in temporal bone	Sensory function: sensations (pain, touch, temperature) of the face, nose, teeth and mouth
VI	Abducens	Motor fibers: nucleus in pons	Movement of the eyeball by lateral rectus muscle
VII	Facial	Motor fibers: nucleus in pons	Motor function: contraction of facial and scalp muscles (facial expression); secretion of saliva by submaxillary and sublingual glands
		Sensory fibers: geniculate ganglion in temporal bone	Sensory function: taste (from anterior two-thirds of tongue)
VIII	Auditory (acoustic) Has 2 divisions: vestibular cochlear	Sensory fibers: vestibular branch: vestibular ganglion in internal ear cochlear branch: spiral ganglion in internal ear	Sensory function: vestibular branch: equilibrium (position balance) cochlear division: sense of hearing
IX	Glossopharyngeal	Motor fibers: nucleus in medulla	Motor function: swallowing; reflex control of blood pressure through connection with carotid pressoreceptors; salivary secretion by parotid glands
		Sensory fibers: jugular and petrous ganglia	Sensory functions: taste and oral and pharyngeal sensations
X	Vagus Has very wide distribution	Motor fibers: nuclei in medulla	Motor function: muscles of pharynx, larynx, thoracic and abdominal viscera (e.g., regulates gastrointestinal motility or peristalsis; influences cardiac rate); secretion by gastric, intestinal and pancreatic glands
		Sensory fibers: jugular and nodosa ganglia	Sensory function: sensations in pharynx, larynx, and thoracic and abdominal viscera
XI	Accessory	Motor fibers: nucleus in medulla and the spinal cord	Movement of shoulder and head by trapezius and sternocleidomastoid muscles
XII	Hypoglossal	Motor fibers: nucleus in medulla	Movements of the tongue

*Most motor nerves are considered to also contain some sensory fibers by which information as to the existing conditions in the muscles concerned (proprioceptive data) is transmitted into the central nervous system. The proprioceptive impulses result in appropriate motor responses to facilitate the required pattern of movement.

the tube-like pathway formed by the strands of Schwann cells and continues to grow until it reaches the peripheral destination. This is a slow process; Gardner suggests that when the fiber starts to grow it "regenerates at the rate of a few millimeters a day," but then slows up.[1] Nonmyelinated fibers regenerate more rapidly than those that must form a myelin sheath. When a peripheral nerve is severed, this means that a great many fibers are separated from their cell bodies. If the 2 cut ends of the nerve are approximated and sutured, less scar tissue forms, favoring the regenerative process. Occasionally, because of fibrous scar tissue, a branch or bud of the viable fiber stump may not find its way into the "tube" of Schwann cells which is essential to the growing fiber. In such an instance, multiple growing tips may be produced by the fiber stump and may form a small mass referred to as a neuroma.

THE PERIPHERAL NERVOUS SYSTEM

The peripheral nervous system consists of nerves and ganglia. The nerves may be divided into 2 main groups—namely, the cranial and spinal nerves—according to whether they emerge from the central nervous system at the cranial or spinal level.

Cranial Nerves

Twelve pairs emerge from the undersurface of the brain and are numbered according to the order in which they arise from the front to back. They are also named according to their function or distribution. Some of the cranial nerves consist mainly of efferent (motor) fibers, three are comprised of afferent (sensory) fibers only (I, II and VIII), and others are made up of both motor and sensory fibers (mixed nerves). Cell bodies of the motor fibers form nuclei within the pons or medulla. Sensory fibers originate in ganglia (groups of neurons outside the central nervous system) (see Table 22–1).

[1]E. Gardner: Fundamentals of Neurology, 5th ed. Philadelphia, W. B. Saunders Co., 1968, p. 89.

Spinal Nerves

Thirty-one pairs of nerves arise from the spinal cord and are numbered and named according to the order in which they arise and the vertebral level at which they emerge. There are 8 cervical, 12 thoracic, 5 lumbar and 5 sacral pairs and 1 coccygeal pair. The cervical and thoracic nerves emerge from the vertebral column at the level they arise from the cord. The lumbar, sacral and coccygeal descend from the lower end of the cord (which terminates at first or second lumbar vertebra) and emerge from the vertebral canal at their respective vertebral level.

All spinal nerves are mixed, and each one has 2 origins which are referred to as the ventral and dorsal roots. The ventral root of a spinal nerve is comprised of neurons in the ventral column or horn of gray matter. The axons of the neurons emerge from the cord carrying efferent impulses and join with afferent fibers to form a spinal nerve just before emerging from the vertebral column. The dorsal root of a spinal nerve is formed by a ganglion (dorsal root or spinal ganglion) lying just outside the spinal cord. The dendrites of the neurons of the ganglion form the afferent (sensory) fibers of the nerve. The axons of the neurons carry the impulses into the dorsal column of gray matter of the cord (see Fig. 22–10).

After emerging from the vertebral canal each spinal nerve divides into 2 major branches, the anterior and posterior rami. The posterior rami divide into smaller branches which go directly to the muscles and skin of the posterior portions of the head, neck and trunk.

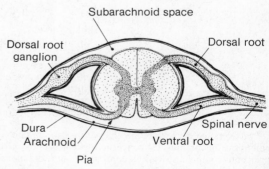

Figure 22–10 A spinal nerve, its dorsal root ganglion, dorsal root and ventral root.

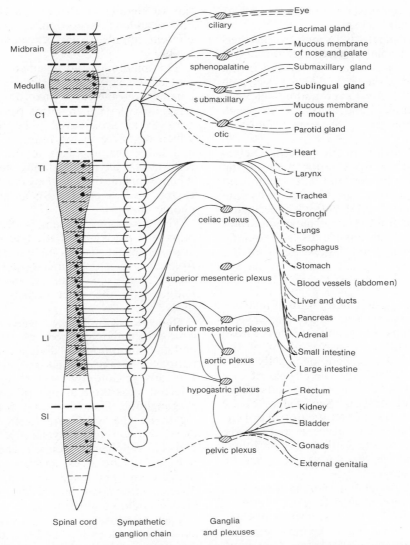

Midbrain

Medulla

C1

TI

LI

SI

Spinal cord   Sympathetic   Ganglia
               ganglion chain   and plexuses

Eye
ciliary
Lacrimal gland
Mucous membrane
of nose and palate
sphenopalatine
Submaxillary gland
Sublingual gland
submaxillary
Mucous membrane
of mouth
otic
Parotid gland
Heart
Larynx
Trachea
Bronchi
celiac plexus
Lungs
Esophagus
Stomach
superior mesenteric plexus
Blood vessels (abdomen)
Liver and ducts
Pancreas
inferior mesenteric plexus
Adrenal
Small intestine
aortic plexus
Large intestine
hypogastric plexus
Rectum
Kidney
Bladder
Gonads
pelvic plexus
External genitalia

Figure 22–11   Ganglia associated with the sympathetic division of the autonomic nervous system.

The anterior rami supply all the structures of the extremities and lateral and anterior portions of the trunk. These branches tend to form plexuses before going to the structures they innervate. A plexus is an intermixing of several nerves, forming a network. Several nerves emerge from the plexus; each nerve and its branches are named according to the regions they supply (e.g., femoral, ulnar, radial). Four main plexuses are formed by the anterior rami of spinal nerves—the cervical, brachial, lumbar and sacral plexuses. The cervical plexus is formed by the anterior rami of the first 4 cervical spinal nerves. The most important branch arising from this plexus is the phrenic nerve, which supplies the diaphragm. It contains fibers from the third, fourth and fifth cervical nerves. Injury to the spinal cord above these levels may result in respiratory paralysis.

The brachial plexus, which is located in the shoulder region, is formed by the anterior rami of the fifth, sixth, seventh and eighth cervical nerves and the first thoracic. The nerves derived from the plexus supply the upper extremity (musculocutaneous, median, ulnar and radial nerves).

The lumbar plexus is formed by the intermingling of the anterior rami of the first 4 lumbar spinal nerves and is located in the lumbar region of the back. The nerves which emerge supply the lower abdominal wall, external genitalia, and parts of the thigh and leg (femoral, saphenous, obturator nerves).

The sacral plexus in the posterior pelvic cavity is formed by anterior rami of the fourth and fifth lumbar and first, second and third sacral spinal nerves. The nerves leaving the plexus supply the buttocks, perineum and lower extremities. The most important nerve derived from this plexus is the sciatic nerve, the longest and largest nerve of the body.

Ganglia

A ganglion consists of a group of neurons outside the central nervous system. Several different groups of ganglia occur. Those associated with the sensory fibers of the cranial nerves are named specifically (e.g., gasserian ganglion, the dendrites of the neurons form the 3 sensory divisions of the trigeminal (V) nerve). (See Table 22–1.)

The ganglia which form the dorsal or sensory root of the spinal nerves lie just outside the spinal cord and within the vertebral column. These are known as the spinal or dorsal root ganglia.

The ganglia associated with the autonomic (visceral) nervous system (Fig. 22–11) may be divided into 3 groups according to their location. The vertebral, sympathetic or lateral ganglia occur in 2 chains; 1 chain of 22 ganglia lies on each side of the vertebral column (3 cervical, 11 thoracic, 4 lumbar and 4 sacral). A second group of autonomic ganglia are called the collateral or prevertebral ganglia. They lie in front of the vertebral column and close to large arteries for which they are named (e.g., iliac, mesenteric, splanchnic ganglia). A third group are referred to as the terminal ganglia and lie close to or within the viscera which the nerve fibers supply.

The Autonomic Nervous System

The autonomic or visceral division of the nervous system is responsible for the regulation of smooth and cardiac muscle activity and glandular secretion. It carries only efferent impulses, and the actions are unwilled.

The anatomical arrangement differs from that of the voluntary system. Impulses are carried from the central nervous system to a ganglion from which axons pass to the viscera to be innervated. The nerve fibers which originate in the brain or spinal cord and carry the impulses to the ganglia are referred to as preganglionic fibers. Those which transmit the impulses from the ganglia to the viscera are known as the postganglionic fibers.

The autonomic system is divided into 2 parts: the parasympathetic and sympathetic systems. Most viscera have a nerve supply from each division; impulses delivered from one system excite activity, and those originating with the other division inhibit activity.

The Parasympathetic Nervous System. The preganglionic fibers of the parasympathetic autonomic division enter the periphery at the cranial and sacral levels. For this reason, the system may also be referred to as the craniosacral division. The preganglionic fibers are quite long, extending to ganglia which are located within or close to the viscera they supply. The cranial division supplies the ciliary and sphincter muscles of the eyes, salivary glands and thoracic and abdominal viscera. The sacral division innervates the muscle tissue of the bladder, colon and rectum.

The responses to parasympathetic innervation are localized and specific for various parts of the body. One part alone may receive impulses. Generally, the activities promote a normal state; they are concerned with the restoration and conservation of body energy and elimination of body wastes. For example, parasympathetic impulses slow the heart rate and conserve cardiac energy when necessary.

The Sympathetic Nervous System. The preganglionic fibers of this autonomic division are short and are derived from the thoracic and lumbar regions of the spinal cord. Because of these origins, the system is also referred to as the thoracolumbar nervous system. The associated ganglia lie in 2 chains of approximately 22 ganglia each, extending along either side of the vertebral column from the base of the skull to the coccygeal region (3 cervical, 11 thoracic, 4 lumbar and 4 sacral). These ganglia are known as the sympathetic or vertebral ganglia. Those in each chain are connected by nerve fibers (preganglionic fibers) passing up or down to higher or lower ganglia. Most of the axons of the ganglionic neurons are distributed in the spinal nerves; a few are distributed separately and directly to the viscera concerned.

The sympathetic nervous system produces generalized physiological responses rather than specific localized ones. It responds to stress, strong emotions (e.g., fear, anger), severe pain, cold, or any threat. The purpose of the responses induced is to mobilize the body's resources for defensive action ("fight or flight"). It produces vasoconstriction of superficial and abdominal viscera, increasing the volume to the heart, skeletal muscles and brain. Glycogenolysis is promoted, sweat gland and adrenal medullary secretions are increased, and the bronchioles and pupils of the eyes dilate. The heart rate, cardiac output and arterial blood pressure are increased.

The responses to sympathetic nervous impulses are augmented by the release of epinephrine and norepinephrine by the adrenal medullae. Stimulation of the sympathetic nervous system results in stimulation of the adrenal medullae. Their secretions are released into the blood stream, producing generalized "defensive" responses similar to those produced by sympathetic innervation.

CHEMICAL MEDIATORS. Transmission of impulses from the preganglionic fibers to the ganglia in both the sympathetic and parasympathetic nervous systems is dependent upon the release of acetylcholine by the terminal portion of the preganglionic axons. The postganglionic fibers of the parasympathetic system also release acetylcholine at their junction with the effector organs to facilitate the transmission of their impulses. The fibers which release the chemical mediator, acetylcholine, are said to be cholinergic. Most of the postganglionic fibers of the sympathetic system are adrenergic; they release sympathin (norepinephrine) at their junction with the effector organs or tissues.

REGULATION OF AUTONOMIC INNERVATION. Regulation and integration of autonomic activity is attributed mainly to the hypothalamus. Although the responses are unwilled, they may be influenced by cerebral cortical activity. Tracts from the cortex to the hypothalamus deliver impulses which frequently arise from emotional stress that may result in overstimulation of either the parasympathetic or sympathetic nervous system. For instance, chronic emotional stress resulting in excessive parasympathetic stimulation of gastric glands is thought to play an important causative role in peptic ulcer.

MUSCLE TISSUE AND ACTIVITY

Most of man's activities, and indeed his survival, depend on functioning muscle tissue. This tissue performs vital activities such as circulation of the blood, respiration and peristaltic movement of food through the gastrointestinal tract; it also maintains posture against gravity and is responsible for movements of a part of the body as well as the mobility of the body as a whole. The capacity of the body to carry out these activities is directly dependent upon the specialized physiological properties peculiar to muscle tissue. These are: *contractility,* which is a shortening and thickening of muscle cells as a result of their ability to convert chemical energy to mechanical energy; *extensibility,* which indicates the capacity of stretching; *elasticity,* the ability to resume their original length after a stretching force is removed; *excitability or sensitivity,* which is the capability to respond by contraction to a change in the environment which may be initiated by a nerve impulse, pressure, stretching, chemical changes (e.g., calcium concentration) or temperature changes (e.g., cold stimulates contraction); and *tonus,* which is a continuous partial contraction maintained by groups of muscle cells contracting in relays.

During muscle contraction, the chemical reactions which occur liberate both mechanical and heat energy. The heat energy contributes to the maintenance of normal body temperature. At rest, most of the body heat is produced by metabolic activities within visceral cells such as occur in the liver.

Muscle cells, because of their elongated shape, may be referred to as muscle fibers.

The cell membrane is called the sarcolemma. Since varying degrees of muscular performance are needed throughout the body for its diversified activities, different types of muscle tissue with different types of control occur. These are cardiac, smooth (visceral) and striated (skeletal or voluntary) muscle tissues. Cardiac muscle tissue has been discussed in Chapter 13. Smooth muscle tissue is found in viscera (e.g., blood vessels, gastrointestinal tract, bladder) and is under autonomic nervous control. The muscle cells are smaller and are arranged in sheets or layers, and their sarcolemmae are not as well defined as in skeletal muscle.

Skeletal muscle tissue forms what is generally referred to as the muscle system. It comprises the muscles which are attached to the bones and are responsible for external body movements and the maintenance of position against gravity. Each muscle fiber presents the microscopic appearance of being striated. Its cytoplasm, which may be called sarcoplasm, contains many myofibrils and its sarcolemma is well defined. In contradistinction to most body cells, each striated muscle fiber has several nuclei. A skeletal muscle consists of several bundles of muscle fibers or fasciculi. Each bundle or fasciculus is enclosed in a sheath of connective tissue (perimysium) and the several bundles which comprise the muscle are also enclosed in strong connective tissue (epimysium) and may also have a tough fibrous coating, called the fascia. Prolongations of the connective tissue extending beyond the actual muscle fibers form the tendinous attachments to bones. Each skeletal muscle has an origin, which is the fixed point of attachment, and an insertion, which is the attachment to the movable part. When the muscle contracts, the insertion is pulled toward the origin. The thick part of the muscle consisting of the bundles of fibers may be referred to as the body of the muscle.

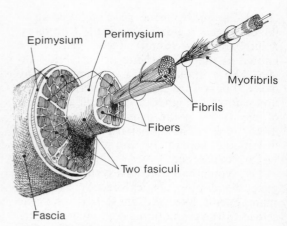

Figure 22–12 Cross section of a skeletal muscle.

Contractions are usually voluntarily produced, since the motor centers lie within the cerebral cortex. Involuntary (unwilled) contractions do occur in the form of reflex responses (see p. 599).

Each motor nerve fiber divides into many branches when it reaches the muscle, and an unmyelinated branch is distributed to each muscle fiber. The point of contact between the nerve fibril and muscle fiber is known as the myoneural or neuromuscular junction or motor end-plate. When a nerve impulse reaches a myoneural junction, acetylcholine is released by the terminal portion of the nerve fiber. The sarcolemma is electrically polarized; the inside is negative to the outside. The acetylcholine initiates a wave of depolarization which sweeps over the fiber. Depolarization is followed by a series of chemical reactions within the cell which result in the release of mechanical and heat energy and the shortening and increased tension of the fiber characteristic of contraction. The acetylcholine is quickly destroyed by the enzyme cholinesterase, the cell membrane becomes repolarized and the fiber relaxes.

Motor Innervation of Skeletal Muscles

Contraction of skeletal muscles normally only results from nerve impulses which are discharged by motor neurons within the central nervous system and are transmitted along peripheral nerve fibers to the muscle.

Sensory Innervation of Skeletal Muscles

Afferent nerve fibers carry sensory impulses from the skeletal muscles to the central nervous system, informing it of stretching of the muscle fibers, tension of tendons, and of pain. The end organs (receptors) which are sensitive to these changes and initiate the impulses are classified as proprioceptors. Muscle spindles, which are excited by stretching, lie between the muscle fibers and are associated with the stretch reflex (see p. 600). Golgi bodies are the proprioceptors located in the tendons which are sensitive to tension; when the tension becomes excessive, impulses are initiated that result in inhibition of muscle contraction. Free nerve endings are also distributed within the muscle that give rise to pain impulses.

Chemical Composition and Contraction

About 20 per cent of a muscle fiber is represented by the proteins myoglobin, actin and myosin. Actin, myosin and adenosinetriphosphate (ATP) are the main contractile elements of muscle fiber. Water accounts for about 75 per cent of the tissue, and the remaining 5 per cent includes carbohydrate (glycogen), phosphocreatine, creatine and inorganic salts (potassium, sodium, calcium, magnesium chloride).

The source of the energy for muscle contraction is a series of chemical reactions within the muscle fibers. Briefly, these include the following: the motor nerve impulse causes depolarization of the sarcolemma, leading to the sudden breakdown of adenosinetriphosphate (ATP) to adenosinediphosphate (ADP) and the release of phosphate and energy; the energy promotes the interaction of actin and myosin filaments which produces the actual shortening and thickening of the muscle (contraction); phosphocreatine is hydrolyzed and gives up phosphate, which combines with ADP to quickly restore the ATP so that a constant source of energy for contraction is maintained; glycogen is then broken down, releasing phosphate and lactic acid; the phosphate molecules combine with creatine to replenish the phosphocreatine; about one-fifth of the lactic acid is oxidized to energy, carbon dioxide and water; and the remainder of the lactic acid is reconverted to glycogen. The initial reactions which provide instantaneous energy for contraction do not utilize oxygen (anaerobic). The oxidation of lactic acid requires oxygen and the energy released is utilized in the resynthesis of the basic compounds used during contraction. In strenuous exercise, the oxygen supply is generally inadequate to oxidize lactic acid and provide the required energy for resynthesis. Lactic acid accumulates and the exercise is said to have incurred an oxygen debt; that is, the oxygen provided was not sufficient to keep pace with the production of lactic acid.

The strength of the contraction of a muscle depends on the number of fibers excited; a maximal or intense stimulus involves all fibers. When stimulated, each fiber responds on the all-or-none principle; it contracts to its fullest capacity. The force of contraction of a fiber increases proportionately with its length up to a certain point, after which it decreases. The size of the muscle also influences the force of the contraction. The larger the mass, the greater amount of energy produced. A muscle responds to repeated increased demands by hypertrophy of the individual fibers. If demands are decreased, the cells store less substance for energy and become smaller, producing muscular atrophy.

A single stimulus to a muscle produces a quick jerky contraction referred to as a twitch. A tetanic contraction is a sustained contraction with no apparent relaxation; it results from a rapid succession of stimuli being delivered to the muscle. When a muscle shortens and produces movement but the tension remains much the same, the contraction is said to be isotonic. An iso-

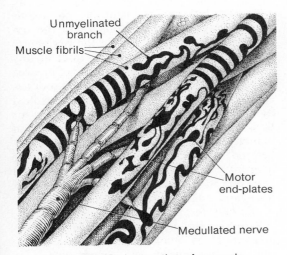

Unmyelinated branch

Muscle fibrils

Motor end-plates

Medullated nerve

Figure 22–13 Innervation of a muscle.

metric contraction is one in which the length of the muscle does not change, but its tension is noticeably increased.

Muscles are arranged to function in pairs; the contraction of one of the pair is accompanied by relaxation of the other (reciprocal inhibition). For example, if the biceps is to contract to flex the forearm, the triceps must relax. The muscle which contracts is called the prime mover, and the one which relaxes at the same time is known as the antagonist. Other muscles may be necessary in certain patterns of movement and may be classified as synergists or stabilizers. They facilitate the work of the prime mover.

Voluntary Movement

Normal voluntary movements (as well as many involuntary movements) are the result of controlled contraction and relaxation of groups of muscles. All willed movements, from the simplest (which involves only a prime mover and its antagonist) to the most complex refined activity involving various groups of muscles, depend upon excitation of neurons within the cerebral cortex (upper motor neurons) and at a lower level (lower motor neurons). The neurons at a lower level may be cranial nerve nuclei in the brain stem or may be in the spinal cord. Two motor pathways are involved within the central nervous system—the pyramidal and extrapyramidal tracts or systems.

Pyramidal Tract (Corticospinal Tract). Willed movement begins with the stimulation of a specific area of neurons in the motor area of the cerebral cortex (see p. 585). If the movement applies to only muscles on one side of the body, only the motor area of the cerebral hemisphere on the opposite side will be involved. The axons of the motor neurons of each hemisphere converge in the interior of the cerebrum, coming together in a compact mass referred to as the internal capsule. The fibers continue down through the midbrain and brain stem. In the lower part of the medulla most of them (75 to 80 per cent) cross to the opposite side before descending into the spinal cord. At various levels in the cord, the fibers synapse with neurons in the anterior column or horn of gray matter. The axons of these neurons form the motor fibers of the

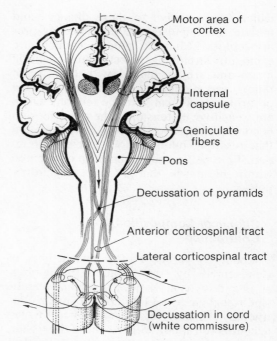

Figure 22–14 The pyramidal tract (corticospinal tract).

peripheral nerves by which the impulses are delivered to the muscle fibers. Some fibers in the tract may synapse in the brain stem with nuclei of cranial nerves. The impulses are then carried out to a muscle by motor fibers of a peripheral cranial nerve.

The neurons in the cerebral cortical motor areas are referred to as the upper motor neurons. Those with which the axons of the upper motor neurons synapse are called the lower motor neurons. The axons of the lower motor neurons carry the impulses to skeletal muscles in the periphery. Interruption of the pyramidal tract at any level produces paralysis. Damage of an area above the lower motor neurons produces spastic paralysis. The muscles controlled by the affected upper motor neurons or their axons resist passive movement and exhibit increased muscle tone and exaggerated reflexes. Injury of lower motor neurons or their axons results in flaccid paralysis in the respective muscles, loss of tone and reflexes, and wasting (atrophy) of the muscles.

Extrapyramidal System. Willed movement involves much more than just activation of the pyramidal system which is mainly concerned with initiating the contraction of prime movers. Excitation of upper and lower motor neurons alone cannot achieve even the simplest movement. When a specific activity is performed, a pattern of movement occurs which requires a varying number of muscular responses. As well as reciprocal relaxation of the antagonist muscle(s), the pattern of movement may include the contraction of a group of muscles simultaneously or in coordinated, timed sequence, the stabilization of a neighboring joint, and adjustments in posture. Some movements require rapid relaxation of the antagonists; others need slow, gradual relaxation in order to provide smooth precise movement. These essential components — inhibition, facilitation and coordination — are controlled by the extrapyramidal system, which is more complex than the pyramidal system. Extrapyramidal impulses are initiated in several different areas of the brain below conscious level. They may originate in the basal ganglia (caudate nucleus, putamen, globus pallidus), cerebellum and reticular formation and may be influenced by impulses from the premotor areas of the frontal lobe. All of the impulses synapse in the reticular formation and are transmitted by reticulospinal tracts to lower motor neurons. The lower motor neurons provide the final common pathway for all afferent impulses (both pyramidal and extrapyramidal) to skeletal muscles.

Disturbance within the extrapyramidal system or interruption of a tract does not cause paralysis but may produce abnormal movements. There may be slowness of response, tremors, lack of coordination or excessive muscle tone.

The following activity illustrates the role of the pyramidal and extrapyramidal tracts in voluntary movement. If a person who is standing reaches out to pick up a pen from a table, he consciously concentrates on the action of his fingers and thumb necessary to grasp the object. Several muscle responses are involved as well as the flexion of fingers and thumb. The forearm is extended to reach the pen (the biceps relaxes and the triceps contracts); muscles contract to stabilize the shoulder and wrist; leaning forward to reach the pen may be necessary, so the trunk flexes and shifts the center of gravity, necessitating muscle action in the trunk and lower extremities to insure the maintenance of the upright position.

The pyramidal tract transmits the impulses which were consciously initiated to produce the actual picking up of the pen by the fingers and thumb. The other essential components of the total movement (reciprocal relaxation, correlation, stabilization and adjustments in posture) are automatically contributed by the extrapyramidal system.

Reflexes

A reflex is an involuntary response which tends to be specific, or of fixed pattern for a given stimulus. Nerve impulses initiated in the periphery enter the central nervous system and automatically activate a certain response in a peripheral structure. The response may involve the contraction of muscle tissue or the secretion of a gland. The nervous pathway over which the impulses pass is called a reflex arc. The arc is comprised of receptors (e.g., proprioceptors in a muscle, cutaneous pain receptors), an afferent pathway (sensory nerve fibers), central nervous system connections (e.g.,

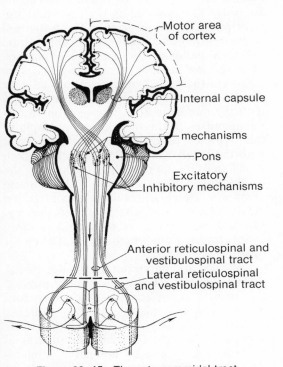

Motor area of cortex

Internal capsule

mechanisms

Pons

Excitatory
Inhibitory mechanisms

Anterior reticulospinal and vestibulospinal tract
Lateral reticulospinal and vestibulospinal tract

Figure 22–15 The extrapyramidal tract.

connecting or internuncial neurons of the spinal cord), motor neurons (e.g., lower motor neurons in anterior columns of spinal cord), efferent pathway (motor nerve fibers) and effector organ (muscle fibers or glandular cells).

Reflexes occur without conscious or willed initiation, but the person usually becomes conscious of the reflex activity because the impulses reach the cerebral cortex and are interpreted as sensation. For example, when a person touches a hot stove, his hand is withdrawn before he is fully aware of the burn sensation.

Reflex responses are either protective or postural. Protective reflexes are produced in response to irritating or painful stimuli. Examples are the closing of the eyelids when the cornea is lightly touched, excessive lacrimal secretion when the eye is irritated by a foreign particle, muscle spasm around an injured area (e.g., rigidity of abdominal wall), contraction of underlying muscles when the abdomen is stroked with a sharp object (withdrawal reflex) and rapid withdrawal of the hand from a hot stove.

Postural reflexes maintain an appropriate degree of muscle tone which is essential in supporting the body against gravity and maintaining an upright position. The body is subjected to the pull of gravity at all times. The only way the body can stay upright is by muscles exerting a continual pull on bones in the opposite direction from gravity. Two reflex mechanisms operate in regulating the muscle contraction necessary to provide the antigravity force. They are the stretch (myotatic) reflex and impulses which originate in the internal ear. When a person bends over or changes his position, movement of the fluid in the semicircular canals in the ear gives rise to sensory impulses which are transmitted by the vestibular fibers of the eighth cranial (auditory) nerve to nuclei in the brain stem. Impulses are then transmitted via vestibulospinal tracts from the nuclei to motor neurons which discharge impulses to certain muscles, resulting in an increase in their tone in support of the body's upright position.

If muscle fibers are stretched, they usually oppose the stretching force by quickly contracting. When the muscle is stretched, proprioceptors (spindles) are stimulated and initiate impulses which are transmitted to the spinal cord. In the cord, the afferent fibers synapse with connecting neurons which in turn synapse with motor neurons whose axons conduct the impulses out to the muscle. If the reflex arc for the stretch reflex is interrupted, the muscle becomes atonic and flaccid. An extremely strong contraction exerts an excessive tension in the muscle's tendon, causing tendon proprioceptors (Golgi bodies) to initiate afferent impulses. These impulses bring about inhibition of the motor neurons concerned, reducing the strength of the contraction.

Even the simplest reflex muscle response or movement involves more than the primary contracting muscle. For instance, the antagonist must reciprocate with relaxation; this necessitates inhibition of its tone. This inhibition takes place in the central nervous system and is imposed on the lower motor neurons which innervate the muscle whose fibers are to relax. The exact inhibitory mechanism is not clear. A reflex may be complex, involving responses in several muscles, some of which may be contralateral. To illustrate, if a person steps on something sharp, the limb is quickly drawn up. The person avoids putting it down and placing his weight on the injured area again. In order to maintain his balance and upright position, the muscles in the trunk and opposite limb must adjust and compensate.

Reflex pathways or arcs are comprised of a varying number of neurons. The simplest consists of 2 neurons; the afferent fibers which enter the cord synapse directly with the motor neurons whose axons transmit impulses to the muscle. An example of this type of reflex arc is that associated with the patellar reflex ("knee jerk") which is elicited by tapping the tendon of the quadriceps femoris muscle. The muscle fibers are stretched, resulting in contraction of the muscle and extension of the leg. More often, a reflex arc includes 1 or more connecting neurons which activate the motor neurons.

Reflexes are important clinically; deviations from normal responses may provide information about the location and nature of neurological disorders. The reflexes observed clinically may be classified as superficial, deep or pathological. Superficial reflexes are evoked by cutaneous stimulation. Deep reflexes are produced by tapping a tendon. Pathological reflexes are responses not normally present. These reflexes are discussed on page 604.

NEUROLOGICAL DISORDERS

The cause of organic disease of the nervous system, as with other systems, may be congenital, vascular, degenerative, infectious, traumatic or neoplastic. Since it is the main control system of the body, the problems associated with a neurological disorder can be varied, multiple and complex, involving several different parts and systems. The resulting disturbances depend primarily on the area(s) of the nervous system affected, the extent of the lesion and to a lesser degree, on the nature of the pathological process. The lesion may diminish or abolish normal responses or cause defective or excessive activity.

Neurological disorders are many and complex. This section presents a discussion of only those which are most commonly encountered and their implications for nursing.

Manifestations of Neurological Disorders

The diagnosis of neurological disease frequently includes a prolonged period of observation of the patient's responses and behavior. The nurse may make an important contribution by making close, accurate observations and detailed, meaningful records. This necessitates a knowledge of what is relevant and significant and the ability in many instances to elicit responses in order to observe and assess the patient. Knowledge of the rate at which functional changes and defects develop is important. Certain conditions are known to have a sudden onset with signs and symptoms reaching maximum intensity very rapidly (e.g., traumatic and severe cerebral vascular lesions). Others have an insidious, prolonged onset with the changes in actions and behavior occurring so gradually that they may be unnoticed and are recognized only in retrospect by the patient, his family and associates.

Motor Dysfunction. Significant factors to be noted in relation to a patient's motor ability include the size, tone and strength of his muscles, his performance (pattern, accuracy and success) of common purposive movements, the ease and smoothness of passive and active movements, his posture and gait, the presence and character of involuntary, purposeless movements, and any asymmetry between the two sides of the body.

Paralysis and abnormal movements are common symptoms of neurological disease.

PARALYSIS. Paralysis implies the loss of power of muscular contraction. It may be partial (exhibited by weakness) or complete and may be classified according to its location. Monoplegia indicates paralysis of one limb. Hemiplegia signifies the loss of muscular power in the limbs on one side of the body. It may also involve the muscles on one side of the face; if it affects the side of the face opposite to that of the paralyzed limbs, the term alternate hemiplegia may be used. Paraplegia denotes paralysis of both lower extremities, and quadriplegia means paralysis of all 4 limbs. Isolated paralysis indicates the loss of the contractile ability of one muscle of a group; this symptom is usually associated with peripheral nerve injury rather than with a lesion of the central nervous system and is usually accompanied by loss of sensation in the area supplied by the affected nerve.

Paralysis may also be classified as that due to an upper or lower motor neuron lesion. Damage to the motor areas of the cerebral cortex or their projection pathways (corticospinal or pyramidal tracts) produces paralysis due to an upper motor neuron lesion or what may also be termed spastic paralysis. Since the lower motor neurons and reflex arc are intact, the affected muscles are still capable of reflex movements and exhibit hypertonicity (spasticity) as well as exaggerated reflexes. There is increased activity of postural (stretch) and protective reflexes (see Table 22–2). Paralysis resulting from injury of the motor neurons in the nuclei of cranial nerves or in the anterior horns or columns of gray matter in the spinal cord or damage to their axons in the periphery may be referred to as that due to a lower motor neuron lesion or as flaccid paralysis. Flaccidity occurs because the reflex arc is interrupted; there is a lack of reflex innervation and responses (see Table 22–2).

ABNORMAL MOVEMENTS. Excessive

TABLE 22–2 COMPARISON OF PARALYSIS OF UPPER AND LOWER MOTOR NEURON ORIGIN

	UPPER MOTOR NEURON LESION	LOWER MOTOR NEURON LESION
Involvement	Muscle groups affected	Individual muscles may be involved
Tonus	Increased; muscles spastic; resist passive movement	Absent; muscles flaccid; no resistance offered
Reflexes:		
Normal	Normal tendon reflexes exaggerated (hyperactive); abdominal reflex absent or diminished on affected side	Tendon reflexes absent; abdominal reflexes diminished if lesion is at thoracic level
Pathological	Babinski's sign present; i.e., dorsiflexion of toes, especially the great toe, in response to scratching sole of the foot	Babinski's sign absent; normal response (plantar flexion of toes) present
	Hoffmann's sign present in hand (flexion of thumb and index finger following sudden release of terminal phalanx of middle finger after it has been flexed)	Hoffmann's sign absent
Muscle atrophy	Only slight atrophy	Marked muscle wasting
Fasciculations (involuntary contractions of small groups of muscle fibers in a muscle)	Absent	May be present

muscle tone, loss of integration and coordination, and involuntary purposeless movements are also expressions of disordered nervous function.

Hypertonicity may cause spasticity or rigidity in muscles. In spasticity, there is quick contraction of the antagonist muscle in response to sudden passive movement (resistance is offered to passive movement). After a few seconds or minutes the opposing muscle relaxes and the desired movement is achieved. Rigidity results from a steady, excessive contraction of flexor and extensor muscles; as a result, movement is inhibited.

Failure of coordination and the normal sequence of activities of a group of muscles seriously impairs movements. The disturbance may be manifested in the gait, inability to achieve the desired range in a movement (dysmetria), jerky irregular movements and a lack of steadiness and control of speed.

Spontaneous involuntary movements associated with impaired nervous function include a variety of tremors, athetoid and choreiform movements, spasms, tics and convulsions. Tremors are rhythmic movements due to alternate contractions and relaxations of prime movers and antagonists. They are seen most often in the distal portions of the extremities, but the head, jaws, lips and rarely the trunk may also be affected. The tremor is observed as to amplitude, frequency, distribution and its relationship to rest and voluntary movement. A fine rapid tremor, especially of the hands, is commonly associated with anxiety, fatigue and toxic conditions such as thyrotoxicosis, uremia and alcoholism. Intention or cerebellar tremor begins after a willed movement is initiated and is intensified as the action continues, especially where increasing precision is required. It may be seen when the person is reaching for a specific object or attempting to arrive at a definite goal. This tremor may be noted in the patient with multiple sclerosis. Static tremor is coarse and occurs with the part at rest. It is suppressed by willed movement but disappears also when the patient is asleep. The "shaking" is commonly seen first in the hands or the head. This tremor is usually due to degenerative changes in the region of the basal ganglia and is characteristic of Parkinson's disease. An action tremor is one which develops only when the limbs assume and maintain a certain position. It has a familial tendency and may appear in early adulthood.

Athetoid movements are stereotyped, slow and writhing, following a definite pattern in the individual patient. They are continuously repeated, ceasing only during sleep, and are commonly seen in persons with cerebral palsy. Athetosis may be unilateral or bilateral.

Choreiform movements are rapid, arrhythmic and forceful. They begin abruptly, are variable in pattern and distribution, and may occur when the patient is asleep. The limbs, face and tongue are most frequently involved. The forcefulness of the movements may lead to injury unless adequate protection is provided.

Spasms or cramps are produced by the involuntary contraction of a large muscle or group of muscles. Sites which are frequently affected are the leg, foot, arm and neck. The cause may be a lesion within the central nervous system (e.g., degenerative change in the extrapyramidal system), a deficient blood supply to the muscle(s), overstretching and injury of the muscle fibers, or a blood calcium or sodium deficiency.

Dystonic movements involve spasms in the proximal portions of the limbs as well as the trunk. The result is usually slow, grotesque, twisting movements and abnormal posture.

A tic or habit spasm is a stereotyped, repetitious, purposeless pattern of movement which is functional in origin. The form is variable from one person to another. The tic usually develops in childhood or adolescence and is thought to be often a symptom of underlying tension or excitement.

Apraxia is a term used to describe motor dysfunction when the person is unable to carry out, on request, a skilled or complex movement. Isolated movements which are a part of the more complex pattern may be achieved but the total cannot be put together. In some patients, this is attributed to an inability to grasp or retain the idea of the desired act. In others it is attributed to the memory loss of the established pattern of movement which is learned in early childhood and normally retained.

Central nervous system disturbances may be manifested by convulsions or seizures, which are uncoordinated, purposeless contractions of muscles. Convulsive movements may involve the entire body or only a part, and may be clonic or tonic. The term tonic is used to describe a rigid spasm resulting from prime movers and antagonists contracting simultaneously. A clonic seizure is characterized by alternate contraction and relaxation of the muscles. Generalized convulsions are accompanied by loss of consciousness.

ABNORMAL GAITS. Locomotion depends upon a normal degree of tone and close integration and coordination of the action of the involved muscles of the lower limbs and trunk. These factors are primarily dependent upon normal innervation. In neurological diseases, various abnormal gaits may be manifested.

The ataxic gait is associated with a loss of the proprioceptive sense in the extremities and a lack of coordination of muscle action. The person is not sure of the position of his lower limbs and is unable to judge or control placement or length of steps. As a result, he tends to watch his feet when walking. The gait is clumsy, the base too wide (the feet are placed abnormally far apart), and the feet are lifted abnormally high and slapped down hard. The steps are unsure and unevenly spaced and may deviate to one side. The ataxia is more pronounced in the dark.

The steppage gait (foot drop gait) is characterized by foot drop due to paralysis of the anterior tibial muscles and by the person lifting the legs abnormally high to avoid dragging and stumbling.

A cerebellar gait is marked by staggering, erratic steps and reeling or deviation to one side. The legs are vigorously moved forward and the feet forcefully slapped to the floor.

The gait characteristic of patients with Parkinson's disease may be referred to as a propulsion or festination gait. The trunk is flexed forward, the steps are short and shuffling, and the speed of walking progressively accelerates.

The scissors gait occurs as a result of spasticity in the lower limbs. The thighs and legs are adducted and movement is difficult, slow and irregular. When the person walks, one leg is placed directly in front of the other, and the knees rub with each step. The steps are short and jerky and may be accompanied by compensatory, forward movements of the trunk and hip.

Abnormal Reflexes. Exaggerated or diminished responses of normal reflexes and the presence of pathological reflexes are frequently among the earliest indications of a neurological disturbance. Those which are most commonly checked during the examination of a patient include the following deep (tendon) and superficial reflexes. The maxillary reflex is elicited by tapping the middle of the chin when the upper and lower teeth are separated and the jaw relaxed; the normal response is quick closure of the jaw. The biceps reflex is tested by striking the biceps tendon when the forearm is extended; the normal response is flexion of the arm at the elbow. Similarly, the triceps jerk is examined by the tapping of the triceps tendon, with the forearm flexed; extension at the elbow may be expected. Extension or flexion of the wrist normally occurs when the corresponding tendon is tapped.

Stroking of the abdomen normally elicits tensing of the abdominal muscles on the side being stroked. The response may be diminished or absent in lesions of the corticospinal tracts above the lumbar level of the cord.

The patellar reflex (knee jerk) is tested by striking the patellar tendon; the normal response is quick contraction of the quadriceps femoris muscle, resulting in extension of the leg. Tapping of the Achilles tendon normally produces contraction of the calf muscles (gastrocnemius and soleus) and plantar flexion of the foot (ankle jerk).

Other reflexes commonly tested are the corneal and pupillary reflexes. Normally the eyelids close when the conjunctiva is irritated by gentle touch. The pupil of the eye normally constricts when light is flashed on the eye.

The more common pathological reflexes tested in examining the patient include Hoffmann's sign, Babinski's sign, ankle clonus and Brudzinski's sign. Hoffmann's sign is present when the thumb and fingers flex in response to flicking of the distal phalanx of the middle finger or to its flexion and sudden release by the examiner. Babinski's sign is the extension of the great toe and probably fanning of the other toes in response to stroking of the sole of the foot. Normally, flexion of the toes occurs. Ankle clonus is characterized by repetitive, rapid flexion and extension of the foot in response to forceful, quick dorsiflexion of the foot while the leg is relaxed and extended. Brudzinski's sign is elicited by the forward flexion of the patient's head by the examiner; the abnormal response is flexion of the ankle, knee or thigh.

Disturbance of Sensation. A neurological lesion may cause abnormalities of sensation characterized by a dulling, loss or intensification of one or more senses. In checking the patient's senses the physician explores the face, trunk and limbs. A sensory disturbance may be localized to one particular area of the body because of the different sensory pathways being associated with different parts. Hypo- or hypersensitivity of a particular area may provide information about the location of a lesion.

The patient's superficial (exteroceptive) sensations of pain, temperature and touch are noted. Impairment of the sense of position may be demonstrated by the patient's inability to recognize the position of a limb which has been moved by the examiner. A disturbance in his sense of movement may be noted by his lack of perception of passive movement of a digit or limb. A disturbance in the patient's sensory system may also be manifested by his inability to recognize a familiar object by the feel of its shape, size and texture, or by his inability to detect that a stimulus is being applied at 2 points simultaneously. The capacity to recognize the shape, size and texture of objects and identify them by touch is referred to as stereognosis.

During tests which are made to evaluate the patient's sensations, his eyes must be closed.

Normally, a person is aware of vibrations when a tuning fork with a frequency of 512 cycles per second is applied to a body prominence such as the clavicle and iliac crest. Loss of sensory acuity may be detected by the physician testing the patient's appreciation of vibration following the application of the tuning fork to several bony prominences.

Visual Disturbances. Neurological lesions, especially within the brain, frequently cause disturbances in vision, in the movements of the eye and eyelids, and in the pupillary and corneal reflexes. Edema of the optic disks may also occur. The patient may experience reduced visual acuity, diplopia (double vision), blurring of vision, or loss of vision in part or all of the visual field in one or both eyes. On examination, the pupils may be uneven in size, and one or both may remain fixed, not reacting to light. The corneal reflex may be abolished, exposing the eye to injury. Normal movements of the eyeball may not be possible because of interference with motor innervation to the extrinsic muscles. Ptosis (lid drop) due to paralysis of the muscle responsible (levator palpebrae) may be evident. Involuntary movement of the eyeballs may occur and is referred to as nystagmus. It may take the form of side-to-side, up-and-down or rotating movements. Some neurological patients manifest the inability to follow the examiner's moving finger.

Ophthalmoscopic examination of the fundus may reveal swelling, pallor and edema of the papilla or optic disk which may be associated with increased intracranial pressure.

Auditory Disturbance. Loss of hearing may be a symptom of a disorder in the middle ear, damage to the cochlear portion of an auditory nerve, or a lesion affecting the auditory pathway within the brain. Deafness due to external or middle ear disease is classified as conduction deafness; that due to nerve damage or a brain lesion is known as perception deafness.

Any complaint of a constant or recurring abnormal sound, which the patient may describe as roaring, ringing, buzzing or swishing is recorded and brought to the physician's attention.

Vestibular Disturbance. The most common symptoms produced by a disturbance in the semicircular canals of the internal ear or of the vestibular nerve (part of auditory nerve) or pathway within the brain are dizziness and loss of position balance (equilibrium). Nystagmus, nausea and vomiting may also be present.

Speech Dysfunction. Intracranial lesions frequently cause aphasia, which is the loss of the ability to understand words or use them to communicate. It occurs frequently in persons who have suffered a cerebral hemorrhage or thrombosis or who have a brain tumor. Aphasia may be classified as motor (expressive) or sensory (receptive). Motor aphasia implies the inability to speak or write; the sensory type is the inability to understand the written or spoken word. Mixed forms of disturbances occur, depending upon the location, size and nature of the lesions. A patient may experience both motor and sensory aphasia. Another may understand what is said and written but is unable to express his thoughts in words or writing. Another may be able to interpret the written and spoken word and communicate by writing but cannot speak. Still another patient may be able to speak but his responses are inappropriate and meaningless, or he may use one or two words repeatedly though attempting to express different ideas.

Impaired Intellectual Ability. The patient may manifest impaired reasoning or judgment, unjustified fears, distorted ideas and loss of memory. His attention span may be abnormally short, and he may be unable to do very simple calculations or identify normally familiar objects or sounds.

Emotional Lability. Disordered emotional reactions may be evident in the patient's fluctuating attitudes. There may be inappropriate laughing, crying, irritability, hostility or anger. Sharp swings in mood may occur; the patient who is withdrawn and depressed or anxious may suddenly become excited or euphoric.

Impaired Awareness. Confusion and disorientation as to time, place and persons may occur in cerebral lesions. The patient may be stuporous (can be roused) or unconscious. He may be semicomatose, a state in which there are responses to painful stimuli, or in deep coma in which there are no responses at reflex level.

Change in Appearance. Frequently, the family of a patient with a neurological disorder comments on the change in his appearance which has probably taken place over a period of time. His face may have become inexpressive (as in Parkinson's disease); his posture may have altered; or he may have become careless about his personal care and grooming.

Change in Food Habits. Anorexia may be a problem, or the reverse (excessive appetite) may develop if the disorder is in the region of the hypothalamus. The patient may experience a loss of taste because of involvement of one or both of the seventh (facial) cranial nerves or their nuclei. Dysphagia (difficulty in swallowing) may occur because of interference with motor innervation to the muscle tissue of the soft palate and pharynx (glossopharyngeal nerves). Nausea and vomiting may be symptoms of increased intracranial pressure, cerebral irritation or disorders of the vestibular system. Vomiting of cerebral origin is frequently projectile and may not be preceded by nausea.

Abnormal Vital Signs. A combination of an abnormally slow pulse and increased arterial blood pressure is usually associated with increased intracranial pressure. A high temperature may indicate infection or loss of control by the body temperature center in the hypothalamus.

Impaired Autonomic Function. Local or general flushing, a difference in the skin temperature in one area to that of others, and the absence of or excessive skin moisture (sweating) may be symptoms of disturbed autonomic nervous system function.

Incontinence. Bladder and bowel incontinence are common in disease of the brain or spinal cord.

Changes Associated with Pituitary Dysfunction. Manifestations of pituitary hormonal imbalance may be symptoms of a brain lesion in the hypothalamic and pituitary region. The pituitary disturbance is secondary to a primary neurological disorder. (See Chapter 21 for discussion of pituitary dysfunction.)

Failure of Growth and Development. In an infant or child, a neurological disorder may be manifested by failure of the child to grow and develop or by the development of a deformity (e.g., abnormally large head).

Disturbances in Cranial Nerve Innervation. Disturbances in innervation by one or more of the cranial nerves may be a symptom of neurological disease and assists in localizing the lesion. In examining the patient, the physician evaluates the cranial nerves consecutively. Beginning with the olfactory nerves (I), the patient's sense of smell in each nostril is tested, using odorous substances such as coffee, peppermint and oil of cloves. Then optic nerve (II) function is assessed by examining the eyes and determining the patient's visual acuity and fields. Functions of the oculomotor (III), trochlear (IV) and abduceus (VI) cranial nerves are tested together by examining eye movements and pupillary reaction. Sensory function of the trigeminal (V) nerves is evaluated by testing both sides of the face and mouth for touch, temperature and pain senses and the cornea for the normal reflex response of closing the eye. Their motor function is tested by requesting maxillary movements. Sensory function of the facial nerves (VII) is studied by testing the taste by using bitter, salty, sweet and sour stimuli in turn. Motor function is assessed by requesting him to perform certain facial activities (e.g., smile, frown, pucker the lips, close the eyelids). Both hearing and equilibrium functions associated with the auditory nerves (VIII) are tested. Caloric and rotation tests (see p. 610) may be done to assess the vestibular system. The glossopharyngeal (IX) and the vagus (X) nerves are tested together by observing the gag reflex, the ability to swallow, and the strength and quality of the patient's voice. His ability to turn his head and shrug his shoulders provides information of the innervation of the sternocleidomastoid and trapezius muscles by the spinal accessory (XI) nerves. Hypoglossal (XII) nerve function is assessed by requesting and observing various movements of the tongue.

Diagnostic Procedures

Certain special investigative procedures may be used by the physician to aid in determining the location and nature of neurological lesions.

Lumbar Puncture. This procedure involves the introduction of a needle into the lumbar subarachnoid space below the termination of the spinal cord. It is passed through the intervertebral space between the third and fourth or fourth and fifth lumbar vertebrae. The purposes of the puncture in diagnosis are to determine the pressure of the cerebrospinal fluid and to obtain specimens of the fluid.

A signed consent for the lumbar puncture

is obtained; the procedure and the importance of his relaxation and remaining still during it are explained to the patient. He is placed in a lateral, horizontal position with his back at the edge of the bed. The lower limbs are flexed, the knees drawn up toward his chin, and the head and trunk are flexed forward. The purpose of the flexions is to separate the spinous processes, making it easier to insert the needle. Strict asepsis is necessary to prevent possible introduction of infection into the spinal canal. The pressure of the fluid is measured by a manometer which attaches to the needle when the stilette is removed. One or two specimens are then collected in sterile containers and are carefully sealed and labeled.

Normally, the pressure of the cerebrospinal fluid, in the recumbent position, ranges between 60 to 180 mm. of fluid. An abnormal elevation in the pressure may be due to an intracranial, space-occupying lesion such as a tumor, edema of the brain, intracranial hemorrhage or an infection such as meningitis. An abnormally low pressure may be the result of a block in the subarachnoid space above the site of the puncture.

The pressure of the fluid normally fluctuates slightly with respirations and rises quickly with coughing and abdominal compression. Measurement of the pressure may include the Queckenstedt test, which determines whether or not there is free passage of fluid from the cranial cavity to the site of the puncture. The nurse applies pressure to the jugular veins in the neck for 6 to 10 seconds. This raises the intracranial venous pressure which is quickly reflected in the pressure of the cerebrospinal fluid. Normally the fluid in the manometer rises quickly by approximately 100 mm. and falls readily upon the release of the jugular compression.

The cerebrospinal fluid specimens may be examined for color (normally clear and colorless), leukocyte count (normal: 0 to 5 lymphocytes), glucose concentration (normal: 50 to 80 mg. per cent), protein concentration (normal: 15 to 40 mg. per cent, mainly albumin), chloride concentration (normal: 725 to 750 mg. per cent) and the presence of pathological organisms. The colloidal-gold reaction test for syphilis may also be done on the cerebrospinal fluid specimen.

Following a lumbar puncture, the patient is kept flat and at rest for several hours. He may develop a severe headache, which is attributed to a reduction in the volume of the cerebrospinal fluid either by removal at the time of the puncture or later leakage into the tissue. The patient remains flat in bed, an ice bag is applied to the head and an analgesic (e.g., acetylsalicylic acid) is administered.

Cisternal Puncture. This procedure is similar to the lumbar puncture, but a shorter needle is introduced below the occipital bone into the cistern magna (subarachnoid space between the undersurface of the cerebellum and posterior surface of the medulla). Preparation of the patient includes shaving the nape of the neck up to the occipital protuberance. The patient is placed on his side with his head flexed. The patient is observed very closely; any dyspnea or respiratory irregularity is reported promptly. It may indicate injury to the medulla by the needle.

Roentgenograms. X-rays of the skull and spine are used to detect such abnormalities as fractures, congenital deformities, unusual intracranial calcified areas and osteoporosis (demineralization of vertebrae).

Cerebral Angiogram (Arteriogram). A radiopaque, iodide preparation (e.g., Hypaque, Diodrast) is injected into a carotid artery or, less frequently, into a vertebral artery for the purpose of visualizing the cerebral vascular system. X-ray films are made of the head and neck during and on completion of the injection of the contrast material. The presence of an aneurysm, occlusion of a vessel, or displacement of blood vessels by an intracranial mass may be demonstrated.

An explanation of the procedure is made to the patient and his family, and a written consent is obtained. Since some patients are sensitive and react to the iodide contrast preparation, any history of allergy, asthma, eczema or known sensitivity is brought to the physician's attention and clearly recorded in a conspicuous place on the patient's chart. A small test dose of the dye may be given routinely before the arteriogram is done, and the patient is observed for signs of sensitivity. If the patient is to receive a general anesthetic (which depends on his ability to cooperate), food and fluid are withheld for 6 hours previous to the procedure. If the patient is a male adult, the neck must be shaved before the examination. In the case of a female, all hair pins and bobby pins are removed, and the hair is secured within a cap. A sedative (e.g., Demerol) and atropine may be given 30 or 60 minutes before the scheduled time for the arteriogram. Artificial dentures are removed. The vital signs, including the blood pressure, and facial symmetry are noted to serve as a comparative base-line during and after the procedure.

Preparation to receive the patient after the procedure includes the making of an anesthetic bed, placing crib sides on the bed and the assembling of emergency equipment in the event of complications. Emergency equipment includes a tracheotomy tray; drugs used in sudden, allergic reaction and anaphylactic shock such as epinephrine hydrochloride (Adrenalin) 1:1000, aminophylline, levarterenol (Levophed) and antihistamines (e.g., Benadryl); and the syringes, needles and other equipment that would be necessary for parenteral administration of drugs.

Following the arteriogram, if the patient received a general anesthetic, he is placed in a semiprone or lateral position. When consciousness is regained, he is usually positioned with his head and shoulders slightly elevated. The application of an ice bag to the site of the injection into the artery may be ordered to prevent edema and bleeding. The patient is observed very closely for several hours for early signs of possible complications. Vasospasm within the cerebral vascular system may occur, manifested by weakness or paralysis of limbs, facial paralysis, speech or swallowing difficulty, disorientation or changes in level of consciousness. There may be hemorrhage from the arterial puncture site; the blood collects in the tissue, forming a hematoma, which may compress the trachea, necessitating an emergency tracheotomy. A delayed sensitivity reaction may develop which may be manifested by repeated sneezing, pruritus, urticaria (hives), pallor or cyanosis, complaints of tightness and irritation in the chest, faintness, or respiratory difficulty. The blood pressure, pulse and respirations are recorded at frequent intervals, and the injection site in the neck examined for swelling and discoloration. Movements and strength of the limbs are tested regularly, and the face is observed for any sign of paralysis. If there are no complications, the patient resumes his previous routine in 12 to 24 hours.

Pneumoencephalogram. In this investigative procedure, air or oxygen is introduced into the subarachnoid space through a lumbar or cisternal puncture. Twenty to 30 ml. of cerebrospinal fluid are withdrawn and replaced by an equal volume of gas, which serves as a contrast medium so that the ventricles, their aqueducts and the cranial subarachnoid space can be visualized by x-rays. The patient is placed in a sitting position, and the gas rises when injected into the subarachnoid space. Abnormal shape, size or displacement of the ventricles or their failure to fill may indicate a congenital anomaly, atrophic or scarred areas of the brain, or a space-occupying lesion. Similarly, distortion of the spinal subarachnoid space or failure to fill may demonstrate a lesion.

An explanation of the procedure is made to the patient and a close relative, and written permission for the examination is obtained. The patient is advised that he will be required to remain quiet for 2 or 3 days and is likely to experience a headache for a day or two. The vital signs are noted for comparison later. Food and fluid are withheld for 6 hours before the encephalogram, and dentures are removed. A sedative is usually given 30 or 60 minutes before the examination.

After a pneumoencephalogram, the vital signs are recorded at frequent intervals (every 15 minutes for 2 hours, then every hour for 6 to 8 hours or until stabilized) so that early signs of increased intracranial pressure may be detected. Headache, nausea and vomiting are common; the patient is kept flat* in bed for at least 24 to 48 hours and is kept as quiet and undisturbed as possible. Crib sides may be necessary for safety if the patient is very distraught because of the headache or shows any signs of disorientation or confusion. An ice bag and analgesics are used to relieve the headache. He is given fluids as tolerated

---

*Some difference exists as to whether the patient should be kept flat or have his head slightly elevated. It is advisable to obtain a directive from the patient's physician.

and is provided with the necessary assistance in taking them to avoid raising his head. If prolonged nausea and vomiting result in an inadequate fluid intake, it is brought to the doctor's attention so that parenteral fluids may be given to prevent dehydration.

Ventriculogram. A roentgenogram of the skull is made following the direct replacement of cerebrospinal fluid in the lateral ventricles with air or another contrast medium. It involves the making of 2 burr holes (trephine openings) in the skull. A needle is then passed into each lateral ventricle, and the contrast medium is introduced following the removal of the fluid. The purpose is to visualize the ventricular system; the size, shape and filling of the ventricles are noted.

The preparation of the patient is similar to that cited above for pneumoencephalogram. The posterior third of the head is shaved, and the whole head is thoroughly cleansed before operation.

Following the ventriculogram, the vital signs are taken every 15 minutes for the first hour and then every half hour for 2 hours. If they remain satisfactory, the interval is then gradually increased. The patient may experience headache, nausea and vomiting, but these discomforts are usually less severe and of shorter duration with a ventriculogram than following a pneumoencephalogram. The scalp wounds are examined daily, and the sutures are usually removed in 4 to 5 days.

Myelogram. This procedure is a roentgenographic study of the spinal subarachnoid space and is used to detect and localize lesions which are compressing the spinal cord or nerves. A radiopaque liquid is injected into the subarachnoid space in the lumbar region. The flow of the contrast medium up and down the canal on tilting the table is observed by fluoroscope. A series of x-ray films is also taken. If the canal is blocked above the lumbar region, the radiopaque liquid is injected by cisternal puncture. On completion of the x-rays, the radiopaque substance is aspirated to prevent meningeal irritation.

As with other diagnostic procedures, an explanation is made to the patient so that he will know what to expect. Consent to the examination is signed. Food and fluid are withheld for 4 to 6 hours preceding the test in case of nausea and vomiting.

Following the myelogram, the patient remains flat in bed for several hours. He is observed for 2 or 3 days for signs of meningeal irritation. Persisting headache and pain and stiffness of the neck, especially on flexion of the head, are reported. If the contrast material is not removed, the patient's head and shoulders are elevated to prevent the fluid from rising to the cranial subarachnoid space.

Electroencephalogram (EEG). This is a graphic record of the electrical activity of the brain. Several electrodes are placed in standard positions on the head; they are distributed over the frontal, parietal, occipital and temporal areas, and one is attached to each ear lobe. The action potentials carried by the leads from the electrodes are amplified 10,000,000 times and then recorded. Some electrical activity is recorded at all times by the brain except during very deep anesthesia and during a severe depletion of blood to the brain.

The waves in the tracings are observed for their frequency per second, amplitude, wave forms (spike, flat, serrated), rhythm and distribution of the activity. An EEG is of value in diagnosing epilepsy, tumors and hematoma. For example, it is of assistance in localizing an area of electrically inactive tissue, such as a tumor.

The procedure is explained to the patient beforehand so that he will not be fearful of "receiving a shock." He should be relaxed; apprehension and fear will influence brain activity. If the patient has been receiving an anticonvulsant, the physician may order it to be omitted during the 24 or 36 hours preceding the EEG. The recording is made in a special insulated room. The patient is recumbent or seated comfortably with his eyes closed. Periodically various forms of stimulation may be used to evoke or intensify abnormal responses. The stimuli may include opening of the eyes, side-to-side and up-and-down eye movements, hyperventilation, clenching of the jaw and light flashes. No special care is necessary following an EEG.

Echoencephalogram. This diagnostic procedure involves the direction of a beam of ultrasonic waves (high frequency sound waves not perceptible to the normal human ear) horizontally through the skull and an oscilloscope recording of the echoes. The waves normally are reflected by midline structures. The time taken for the reflected waves to return can be projected, and on this basis, a shift of the midline structures can be demonstrated and may confirm the presence of a space-occupying lesion.

Brain Scan (Radioisotope Uptake). The presence of a brain tumor, hematoma or area of inactive or degenerative tissue may be demonstrated by an increased focal uptake. Normal brain cells form a blood-brain barrier and prevent the isotopes that are used from entering the cells. The radioactive substances commonly used are mercury (Hg^{197} or Hg^{203}) and radioiodinated serum albumin. The mercury is administered intravenously in the form of Hg^{203}- or Hg^{197}-labeled chlormerodrin (Neohydrin), and scans are made in 15 to 30 minutes. When radioiodinated serum albumin is used, the patient usually receives a relatively large dose of Lugol's solution the day previous to the scan to prevent thyroid uptake of the iodinated serum albumin.

Caloric Test. Neurological investigation may include a caloric test to assess the function of the vestibular portion of the acoustic (VIII) cranial nerve and the vestibular system. The test consists of thermal stimulation of the auditory canals and observance of the patient's reactions. Hot or cold water introduced into the external ear produces changes in the temperature of the endolymph (fluid within the semicircular canals) and sets it in motion, giving rise to certain impulses.

Before the test the patient is advised as to what will be done and that he should indicate any discomfort such as dizziness, nausea and vomiting that he experiences during it. He is tested for past pointing and Romberg's sign for comparison with the responses to the caloric test. Romberg's sign is the falling or swaying to one side when the patient stands with his feet together and his eyes closed. The past pointing test involves having the patient direct a finger to a particular mark with his eyes closed. Past pointing is manifested by deviation of the finger from the mark. Food and fluids are withheld for 4 to 6 hours before the test because of the likely responses of nausea and vomiting.

The patient may be placed in a sitting position with the head tilted backward at an angle of 60 degrees. If the recumbent position is used, the head is flexed forward at an angle of 30 degrees. The two ears are tested independently with cold water, 20° to 21° C. (68° to 70° F.), and then with hot water, 40° to 45° C. (104° to 113° F.). The solution is introduced slowly and is discontinued with the initial response. Observations are made for nystagmus; its duration is timed, and the direction of the quick phase is noted. Complaints of dizziness, nausea and vomiting are recorded. Normally, stimulation with cold water produces nystagmus with the rapid phase of the movement directed toward the side opposite to that being stimulated, past pointing deviation and postural deviation (Romberg's sign) to the side stimulated, vertigo, and probably nausea and vomiting. The characteristics of the normal responses to stimulation with hot water are nystagmus with the rapid component directed to the side of stimulation, past pointing and postural deviation to the side opposite to that stimulated, vertigo, and probably nausea and vomiting. Pathological lesions interfering with the function of the vestibular system produce an absence of or diminishment in the responses to thermal stimulation.

Following the caloric test, the patient remains in bed with a minimum of disturbance until free of dizziness, nausea and vomiting.

Electromyogram (EMG). This is a record of the electrical activity of a muscle. Surface electrodes are rarely used; needle electrodes are more commonly placed in the muscle. Normal voluntary muscle is electrically inactive when at rest but demonstrates a characteristic pattern when contracting. The procedure is of value in the investigation of peripheral nerve injuries and of primary disease of the muscle (e.g., dystrophy).

CEREBROVASCULAR DISEASE

The most common cerebrovascular disorders include cerebral atherosclerosis, cerebral aneurysm, cerebral infarction and cerebral hemorrhage. Infarction and hemorrhage cause what is commonly referred to as a cerebrovascular accident, or stroke, and are most frequently sequelae to cerebral atherosclerosis or aneurysm.

Cerebral Atherosclerosis (Arteriosclerosis)

Atherosclerosis of the cerebral vessels is a chronic degenerative process characterized by the gradual development of atheroma (fatty plaques) in the intima and subsequent roughening and destruction of the endothelium, narrowing of the lumen and weakening of the vascular wall. These degenerative changes predispose to cerebral ischemia, thrombosis with regional infarction and hemorrhage. The atheromatous plaques tend to predominately form in the carotid, vertebral and larger cerebral arteries but may be diffuse, involving both large and small cerebral vessels. The disease tends to develop more rapidly in persons with hypertension, diabetes mellitus, obesity and heart disease, and who are heavy smokers.

Generalized atherosclerosis develops insidiously and increases progressively after the age of 45 to 50. Resultant physical and mental changes may be quite marked in some persons. If cerebral atheroma are predominate, changes in brain function become evident. Reduced intellectual ability, loss of memory for recent events, resistance to change, exaggerated emotional responses, confusion and personality changes may be manifested. Recurrent transient ischemia from which the person recovers may occur; he may complain of sudden brief weakness and numbness of a limb, lightheadedness, vertigo or blurring of vision; he may stumble and even fall or have difficulty with his speech. Gradually more permanent changes may develop, or the person suffers a cardiovascular accident (stroke).

The person who experiences any of the above symptoms is encouraged to seek medical advice. Although there is no specific treatment, progress of the degenerative vascular changes may be delayed and serious sequelae avoided (e.g., stroke). If the patient is overweight, a reduced calorie intake is advisable. A diet which is low in cholesterol and saturated fats (animal fat) may also be instituted. If he is found to have hypertension, a hypotensive drug may be prescribed. Confusing situations, excessive physical exertion and emotional stress are avoided,

but activity within the patient's capacity is encouraged. His family is helped to understand the disorder and to develop tolerance and patience. Increasing guidance and assistance with personal care may be necessary on their part.

The patient, especially if young, may be considered a candidate for surgery in which an endarterectomy is done. This surgical procedure involves opening of the artery, removal of the atheromatous intima and reconstruction of the vessel. The site of the incision may be reinforced by a patch of Teflon or a graft taken from a vein.

Cerebral Aneurysm

An aneurysm is a localized outpouching of the wall of an artery. It is most commonly due to a congenital weakness in the vascular structure but may also develop as a result of degenerative changes (atherosclerosis) in the vessel or arteritis. Generally, the aneurysm is single, but occasionally there may be more than one. The congenital form is frequently referred to as a berry aneurysm. The defect may be asymptomatic, only giving rise to disturbances when the blood pressure becomes elevated or degenerative vascular changes develop in later life.

An aneurysm remaining intact may gradually enlarge, causing pressure on adjacent tissue and producing symptoms which depend on its location. Frequently, these premonitory symptoms are headache, drowsiness, facial pain and disturbed vision, ptosis and dilatation of the pupil in one or both eyes. In some instances, the aneurysm ruptures suddenly without having produced previous symptoms. The patient may experience sudden severe pain in the head, vomiting and rapid loss of consciousness, presenting the clinical picture of a stroke (see p. 613). If it is a small hemorrhage, the patient may manifest only a dulling of consciousness or may remain fully conscious. Restlessness, disorientation and other mental disturbances may be exhibited. As with all focal brain lesions, the signs and symptoms will vary with the location of the aneurysm. A lumbar puncture is usually done to determine if there is bleeding into the subarachnoid space (subarachnoid hemorrhage), which is most commonly due to a ruptured aneurysm. This may be followed by an arteriogram to determine the site of the defect.

Care of the patient with an aneurysm that is causing pressure or has ruptured involves complete bed rest for a period of 3 to 4 weeks. If the patient is unconscious, the care will include that which is applicable to any unconscious patient (see p. 103).

The patient is kept flat and exposed to a minimum of stimuli. Even if he is conscious, everything must be done for him to avoid exertion that might precipitate bleeding. His vital signs are recorded at frequent intervals and any significant change, such as an increasing elevation or sudden fall in the blood pressure, is reported promptly. The patient is turned gently every 2 hours and is given skin care to prevent pressure sores. Generally, only fluids are permitted for several days, and they are given through a straw by the nurse to avoid having the patient raise his head. The intake is measured, and if inadequate, or if the patient is comatose, intravenous fluids may be given. These are administered very slowly and in limited amounts to prevent a rapid increase in the intravascular volume and an elevation of the blood pressure. Vomiting is controlled to avoid increased intracranial pressure; if the patient is nauseated, oral fluids are withheld and an antiemetic such as dimenhydrinate (Dramamine) may be prescribed.

An indwelling catheter may be used with the female patient to prevent the exertion of using a bedpan. Constipation and straining at stool must be avoided because of the danger of increasing intracranial pressure. Glycerine or medicated suppositories such as bisacodyl (Dulcolax) or a mild bulk laxative is used. A mild sedative such as phenobarbital may be ordered to reduce restlessness. The patient is likely to experience headache, and a mild analgesic may be prescribed. The physician is usually reluctant to have the patient receive some analgesic preparations because they tend to mask significant neurological changes. An ice bag is used to provide some relief for the patient's headache.

The importance and purpose of strict bed rest, avoidance of coughing, straining and physical exertion, and the restriction of visitors are explained to the patient and his family at the onset to ensure cooperation.

Surgical treatment of the aneurysm may be undertaken, depending on its size and location and the condition of the patient. If the aneurysm is accessible, various procedures are used to obliterate the sac. These include the placing of a ligature or clip on the stalk, the application of 2 clips or ligatures to the parent artery on either side of the sac, wrapping the aneurysm in fascia or muscle tissue, or spraying the aneurysm with a plastic material. A less direct procedure involves the clamping or ligation of the carotid artery; ligation of the artery is permitted by the establishment of a collateral circulation from the opposite carotid artery through the circle of Willis. The clamp that is placed on the carotid artery is so designed that it is adjusted daily to produce gradual occlusion over a period of days while the collateral circulation is taking over. During this period, the patient is observed closely for signs of cerebral ischemia, which may be manifested by motor or sensory deficits, disturbances in mental responses or level of consciousness, or significant changes in vital signs. For nursing care of the patient undergoing surgery, see page 637.

Cerebrovascular Accident (Stroke)

A cerebrovascular accident, or stroke, may be defined as a sudden interruption of the blood supply to a part of the brain. It may be due to a thrombosis, hemorrhage or, rarely, an embolism. The site of the lesion may be an internal carotid or vertebral artery, the basilar artery, circle of Willis or a cerebral artery. The disorder may also be referred to as apoplexy.

Cerebral thrombosis is most often associated with atherosclerosis; the lumen of the vessel is narrowed, impeding the flow of blood. The circulatory stasis leads to thrombus formation, occlusion of the vessel and ischemia of an area of brain tissue. Narrowing of the vessel and ensuing thrombosis may occasionally be the result of vasculitis or outside pressure by a space-occupying lesion. An inadequate delivery of blood to the brain, secondary to cardiac insufficiency, shock or reduced intravascular volume, may also cause stasis and subsequent thrombosis. The onset of a stroke due to thrombosis may be relatively gradual and usually occurs when the person is at rest. If the occlusion of the vessel persists, necrosis of the tissue follows; the infarct eventually liquefies and is absorbed. Glial and fibrous scar tissue replaces the brain tissue which was destroyed.

When a cerebral hemorrhage occurs, the artery which ruptures has usually been vulnerable because of degenerative changes (atherosclerosis) in its walls or because of the presence of an aneurysm (a weak, saccular, vascular area). The hemorrhage may have been precipitated by an elevation of blood pressure. The escaping blood forms a hematoma which presses on the surrounding tissue. The pressure, along with the deficit in the blood supply, leads to destruction of adjacent brain tissue. The onset of a stroke caused by a cerebral hemorrhage is sudden and is usually associated with physical activity or emotional stress.

Cerebral embolism is the occlusion of a cerebral vessel by a blood clot, a clump of fat or tumor cells, or bacteria which has been carried by the circulation from another area of the body. Blood clots which form emboli may originate in the heart as a result of cardiac disease or in the saphenous or femoral veins due to circulatory stasis. A fat embolism most often follows a fracture; an embolism formed of tumor cells may arise from a malignant neoplasm. An infected embolus may be associated with bacterial endocarditis. The stroke due to an embolism occurs suddenly.

Incidence. Cerebrovascular accidents account for a large proportion of neurological disease and are responsible for many deaths, and mental and physical disability. It is thought the majority of strokes result from cerebral thrombosis. They have their highest incidence in those over 60 years of age. The principal predisposing factors are atherosclerosis, hypertension, congenital aneurysm and conditions which provide a possible source of emboli.

Effects and Manifestations. Obviously, the effects of a cerebrovascular accident depend upon the site of the lesion and the amount of brain tissue affected. The damage may be so severe that death ensues within a few hours or days, or the injury may be so slight that the symptoms are transient and may even go unrecognized. Between these extremes are many variants. Certain patterns of defects have been recognized as being associated with a cerebrovascular accident involving specific vessels and areas.

The following clinical features are common to the majority of patients who suffer a cerebrovascular accident.

PREMONITORY SYMPTOMS. Premonitory manifestations may be experienced which might include persistent headache, dizziness or "lightheadedness," fleeting loss of consciousness or "blackout," brief confusion, blurring of vision in one or both eyes, stumbling of speech or "thickness" of the tongue, or transient local sensory and motor deficits. Any of these symptoms are especially important and should serve as a warning, especially if the patient is known to have hypertension, arteriosclerosis or a condition which may give rise to an embolus.

LOSS OF CONSCIOUSNESS. A period of unconsciousness is common to stroke patients and may vary from hours to days. Coma lasting longer than 24 to 36 hours presents a grave prognosis. A few patients experience only a clouding of consciousness and confusion.

CONVULSIVE MOVEMENTS. The immediate onset may be accompanied by convulsive movements which may be local or general.

HEADACHE AND VOMITING. If the patient remains conscious, he may complain of severe headache as a result of increased intracranial pressure. Vomiting frequently occurs with the initial onset and may be recurring in the conscious patient.

VITAL SIGNS. The respirations are usually slow and stertorous or may be Cheyne-Stokes. The pulse is generally slow, full and bounding. The temperature may be normal during the first few hours, then becomes elevated. Progressive hyperpyrexia is considered an unfavorable sign.

MOTOR AND SENSORY DEFICITS. Hemiplegia is one of the most common effects of a stroke. For a few days, there is a marked loss of tone in the affected structures and an absence of normal reflexes. Babinski's sign is present in the paralyzed limb. Even with the patient in coma, one may recognize a greater loss of tone in the muscles of the paralyzed limbs; when the limbs are flexed, the affected one falls more quickly in a limp, lifeless manner. Later this flaccidity in the affected limbs is replaced by spasticity and hyperactive reflexes characteristic of upper motor neuron lesions. One side of the face may be paralyzed, resulting in that side blowing out and in with each respiration. The mouth may also be drawn to one side. When conscious, the patient may experience difficulty in swallowing (dysphagia), indicating some paralysis of the swallowing muscles. There may also be loss of sensation in some parts. Motor and sensory deficits in the limbs occur on the side of the body opposite to the lesion.

SPEECH DEFECT. There may be complete or partial loss of speech. The defect may take various forms (see p. 605); he may not only be unable to communicate verbally but may manifest some impairment in comprehension of either verbal or written communication.

EYE CHANGES. The eyes as well as the head tend to turn to the side of the lesion in the early stage; later, the deviation may be reversed and the head and eyes are probably turned to the side of the paralysis. The pupils may be uneven or constricted to "pin point" size, the corneal and pupillary reflexes are most likely absent, and the physician's examination of the fundus may reveal papilledema resulting from increased intracranial pressure. The conscious patient may indicate impaired vision, and there may be a defective movement of one or both eyes.

OTHER SYMPTOMS. The face may be flushed, and stiffness of the neck (nuchal rigidity) may be present. Incontinence is common. After the acute stage, it may become evident that the patient has suffered some mental impairment.

Treatment and Nursing Care. At the onset, the outcome as to residual disability is unpredictable. The degree of recovery will depend on the size of the infarction or hemorrhage. When the patient regains consciousness, some functional recovery may be expected as the pressure and edema in the area of the brain lesion subside. The permanent disability is generally not confirmed for several days. If function is regained, it tends to follow a general pattern in which the facial and swallowing muscles recover first and then those of the lower limbs. Speech and arm function are regained more slowly and less completely.

During the acute phase of the illness following a cerebrovascular accident the care is principally supportive and is directed toward preventing complications and damage that may interfere later with maximum rehabilitation (e.g., subluxation and contractures). When the patient is comatose, the care will include that which is applicable to any unconscious patient as cited in Chapter 9. Following the acute phase, care emphasizes rehabilitation of the patient to a reasonably active, independent life compatible with his residual disabilities.

POSITIONING. While unconscious, the patient is placed in a semiprone or lateral position to facilitate breathing and prevent the aspiration of mucus and vomitus. A pharyngeal airway may be introduced to permit unobstructed breathing. Suction equipment is kept at the bedside to remove mucus and any vomitus when necessary. Good alignment of the head is maintained to avoid compression of the neck vessels; flexion may interfere with cerebral venous drainage, favoring cerebral congestion and increased intracranial pressure. The physician may want the patient kept turned on the side of his lesion and minimal moving of the patient for several hours to prevent the possibility of increased intracranial bleeding.

Crib sides are placed on the bed in the event of recovery of consciousness accompanied by disorientation and restlessness. These remain on the bed until the patient is sufficiently rehabilitated that he can turn and sit up in bed without danger of losing his balance.

OBSERVATIONS. In the initial acute phase, the vital signs are recorded at frequent intervals. An abnormal elevation of the blood pressure, a decrease in the pulse and slow or Cheyne-Stokes respirations may indicate increasing intracranial pressure. An abnormal fall in the blood pressure and weakening of the pulse may point to circulatory collapse. A progressively rising temperature to levels of hyperpyrexia is an unfavorable sign, generally pointing to interference with the body temperature regulating center and loss of the controlling reflexes.

The size of both pupils is observed and checked at intervals for changes, the level of consciousness is noted by being alert to any movements made by the patient and to responses such as resistance or withdrawal offered to passive movement or other forms of care.

FLUIDS AND NUTRITION. During the

first 24 to 48 hours fluids may be administered intravenously. The rate of flow and volume are carefully controlled to avoid too rapid an increase in the intravascular volume and blood pressure. If coma is prolonged, or the patient has considerable dysphagia, nasogastric feedings may be introduced to provide sufficient nutrients (see p. 339). An accurate record of the patient's fluid intake and output in the acute phase is necessary.

When consciousness is regained, the swallowing reflex is tested before giving any fluids orally. If the patient can swallow, a soft diet is given and is progressively increased to a full, balanced diet as soon as tolerated. The patient will probably have to be fed at first, particularly if the area he is accustomed to using is paralyzed, but with the necessary assistance, he is encouraged to feed himself as soon as possible to establish independence. If one side of the face is paralyzed, food is placed in the opposite side of the mouth to make swallowing easier. Mouth care is then given following the meal to remove retained food particles from the weak side.

REACTION AND BEHAVIOR. Emotionally a stroke is devastating to a patient, and usually, the more intellectually intact he is, the greater is the psychological impact. On regaining consciousness, he may be confused at first, but as his thoughts clear, he is shocked to find himself in a totally strange environment, unable to communicate or to move one side of his body. The depression and resentment or hostility that the patient is likely to manifest are normal responses. His immediate thought is likely to be that life is no longer worth living. The patient gradually works his way through his depression and becomes interested and cooperative as his rehabilitative program is introduced.

He requires an explanation of what happened to him and what is going to be done for him. At this time, he is greatly in need of understanding and psychological support. A visit from a member of his family may now provide considerable reassurance. Continuing care by the same personnel as much as possible is helpful. If he is in a single room, he will probably be less apprehensive if transferred to a room where there is at least one other patient. Isolation tends to contribute to greater despair, but conver-

sation with others provides verbal stimulation which plays a role in speech therapy if necessary. Taking time to converse with the patient as a normal person may convey some assurance to him that he is still worthwhile and that people are interested in him. Such courtesy and respect are likely to promote a more positive attitude in the patient toward his recovery and usefulness.

A lack of concern for his disability may reflect brain damage. Similarly, responses such as uncontrolled crying and inappropriate laughter may be manifested and are likely to be very distressing to the family. It is impressed on the family that the patient's behavior does not necessarily represent his true feelings and that such responses may disappear or become less marked. The patient may exhibit impaired intellectual ability which may affect certain areas of mental activity such as judgment, reasoning and comprehension. This intellectual loss combined with impaired physical and possible language abilities may prevent the patient from resuming previous activities and responsibilities—for example, his return to gainful employment. The family is alerted to these facts so that they may avoid ensuing problems as much as possible.

Some stroke patients develop fixed ideas and rigid behavior which also relate to changes in the brain, and these persons are not apt to respond to verbal entreaties. Relatives are helped to understand and accept these as sequelae of the disease process.

ORAL AND SKIN CARE. During the acute stage, the mouth requires frequent cleansing (every 2 to 3 hours) with a mild, antiseptic mouthwash to prevent the accumulation of secretions. Good oral hygiene plays an important role in preventing parotitis to which older patients seem to have a greater predisposition. Mineral oil or petroleum jelly is applied to the lips. Later, because of the hemiplegia, the patient may find cleaning his teeth difficult and require some assistance until he becomes more adept with the functioning arm and hand.

Because of their inability to turn and move in bed, especially in the early phases of their illness, stroke patients are particularly prone to develop presure sores. The majority of these patients are in the older age group which increases the predisposition because their skin is less resistant and develops local anemia more readily when subjected to pressure. While confined to bed, the patient is turned every 2 hours. The vulnerable bony prominences (sacral and lateral hip areas, heels, malleoli and shoulder and scapular areas) are kept clean and dry and are massaged gently to stimulate circulation. A protective emollient or lotion may be applied if the skin is dry. An air mattress or squares of sheepskin may be used to protect pressure areas. When the patient is allowed out of bed, precautions are still necessary to prevent prolonged sitting; he must be taught to stand or shift his weight from one hip to another at intervals to relieve compression of vessels in the area.

ELIMINATION. During the acute phase, an indwelling catheter is used to prevent skin irritation by involuntary voiding. It is used for as brief a period as possible because of the chance of urethral and bladder irritation and developing infection. When the catheter is removed, the patient is placed on the bedpan or toilet at frequent, regular intervals, gradually decreasing the frequency as control is re-established. During rehabilitation, stress incontinence is likely to occur at times when the patient becomes emotional and frustrated, further increasing the patient's discouragement. Reassurance and psychological support from the nurse are needed in these situations.

The enforced inactivity associated with hemiplegia frequently gives rise to constipation. The nurse must be alert to the possibility of impaction. An enema, laxative, or glycerine or bisacodyl (Dulcolax) suppository may be necessary at first but increased dietary roughage and fluid intake should be used to resolve the problem as soon as possible.

MEDICATIONS. On regaining consciousness, the patient may complain of severe headache. Acetylsalicylic acid or acetylsalicylic acid compounds may be prescribed, but strong analgesics are generally withheld because they tend to mask neurological symptoms. If hypertension persists following a cerebrovascular accident, a hypotensive drug such as reserpine (Serpasil) may be prescribed.

APHASIA. The aphasia associated with a cerebrovascular accident is usually expressive in type (see p. 605). It occurs most frequently in those whose lesion is in the left cerebral hemisphere. Right hemispheric lesions tend to produce dysarthria in which the muscles involved in articulation (e.g., larynx, tongue) are affected.

The sudden loss of the ability to communicate creates fear and frustration in the patient, especially in the initial phase. He feels isolated, lonely and threatened. The nurse endeavors to allay some of the patient's anxiety by anticipating his needs as much as possible, acknowledging his difficulty and concern, and indicating support in working through his problem. He is likely to benefit psychologically from knowing that someone understands and is interested in helping. Most aphasic patients can recover their ability to communicate to some degree. It is not possible to predict the extent of this at the onset; speech is usually recovered very gradually and slowly and requires the assistance of those around the patient. The nurse avoids conveying what may be false optimism at first but reassures the patient and his family that special assistance will be given to help in the recovery of speech. In the early stage of recovery from the stroke, patient's gestures to indicate needs and wishes may be encouraged but should not be accepted indefinitely, since established use of them may inhibit his efforts to verbalize.

If the services of a speech therapist are available, an assessment of the patient's language capacity is made and a retraining program planned. In many situations, the nurse will be mainly responsible for helping him recover the ability to communicate. It is necessary, as soon as possible, to determine whether the patient can express his ideas verbally or by written word and whether he understands what is said to him and, if so, whether his comprehension is limited to short simple phrases or single words. Rarely, intellectual impairment occurs which precludes speech rehabilitation.

It is important to talk normally and with ease to the patient. Auditory stimulation and socialization play important roles and are considered as valuable as structured remedial drills. For this reason, following recovery from the acute stage of the illness, he is better off in a room with others. It must be remembered that the fact that he cannot speak is no indication that his intelligence, comprehension and hearing are impaired. The patient should not be discussed within his hearing as though he does not hear or understand. This was a very disturbing factor cited by Buck in writing of his experiences.[2] The aphasic patient should receive the courtesy and respect due every patient and be included in the conversation taking place in his presence. The nurse is cautioned against treating him as a child, since he does not necessarily think as a child. In chatting, use short simple sentences; if there is evidence of difficulty in comprehension, they should relate to the present and his immediate environment as much as possible.

When helping the patient to recover his speech, the vocabulary selected is kept to a simple, functional level. Emphasis is placed on nouns and simple responses such as "yes" and "no" first, then progression through verbs and adjectives to short sentences is used, much the same as the process used with the young child learning to communicate. The use of several sensory avenues is usually more effective than the use of just one at a time. Hearing words in direct association with the objects they represent and the printed words contributes to recovery. As care is given, names of articles being used are enunciated slowly and clearly. The vocabulary is gradually extended to other useful words by placing actual objects or pictures of the objects and the printed name before the patient and repeating the name several times. He is asked to say the word and is given plenty of time to respond. The patient should be rested and relaxed and in a quiet undistracting setting during the periods of instruction, which are kept brief as he tires easily and his attention span is likely to be short. He should never be pressured to the point of frustration which leads to discouragement and withdrawal. Emphasis on exact pronunciation is avoided. Some speech therapy departments use a special language machine which may be left with the patient to use on his own. It presents a picture of an object and its name in print at the same time that the word is presented audibly. When advised as to the use of it, the patient is of course instructed to "speak" the word. The repetitive association of the object with the written and spoken word does facilitate recovery, especially in those who are highly motivated and not easily discouraged.

After the first 2 or 3 weeks, at which time the patient is returned to his home, most of the assistance in the recovery of speech must come from the family. Early in the illness, family members are helped to understand the patient's communication problem and their role in the rehabilitation program. Frequently, the patient makes more rapid progress when he goes home to the familiar relaxed environment. The importance of conversing normally with the patient, expecting a response and giving him plenty of time to respond are discussed with the family. The methods and details related to periods of instruction are explained, and it is helpful if at least one member observes a teaching session carried out in the hospital or rehabilitation center. An excellent reference and guide which the family may be given is the booklet "Aphasia and the Family."[3] This may be reviewed with them by the nurse and clarification of details made whenever necessary. Emphasis is placed on the need for patience and effort on the part of all concerned and on the need of providing opportunities for the patient to practice and use what speech he has. The family is advised that progress is likely to be slow and may require many months. They are cautioned against placing excessive demands on the patient, which may have demoralizing effects. The patient will be slow in responding or expressing himself; but if he is cut off, he readily becomes discouraged and gives up. Progress should be acknowledged because it encourages him and prompts motivation for continued effort.

FAMILY. A stroke is usually as much of a shock and tragedy to the family as it is to the victim. Buck, a physician writing about his personal experience following a stroke, makes the following statement: "A stroke is actually a family illness and continuous counseling should be readily avail-

[2] M. Buck: "Adjustments During Recovery from Stroke." Amer. J. Nurs., Vol. 64, No. 10 (Oct. 1964), pp. 92–95.

[3] American Heart Association: Aphasia and the Family. New York, American Heart Association, 1965. Available in Canada from the Canadian Heart Foundation and its branches.

able for the entire household.''[4] The nurse has a responsibility to talk with them, answer their questions when possible and discuss how they may help the patient and each other. If it is the wage-earner who has been stricken, economic hardships may be imposed on the family. A discussion with a social service worker may be arranged or a referral to a social welfare agency made. As well as the disability, the patient may exhibit inappropriate or bizarre behavior which the family finds very distressing and hard to understand and accept. An effort is made to explain that this is due to actual tissue damage and is not controllable by the patient.

Members of the family who are informed and develop an acceptance of the situation with a positive attitude play an important role in motivating and assisting the patient to regain functions and independence. To fill this role, they require the guidance and support of the health team. This is particularly important when the patient leaves the hospital. Too often the family and the patient are left to carry on entirely on their own when the patient leaves the hospital. Some follow-up should be arranged with a visiting nurse agency.

REHABILITATION. Certain aspects of the care that the stroke patient receives in the early stage of his illness play an important role in his rehabilitation. As cited previously, the muscles of the affected limbs are flaccid for a few days, then become spastic. The paralyzed arm is adducted, and flexion occurs at the elbow, wrist, finger and thumb joints. The lower limb assumes a position of external rotation at the hip, flexion of the thigh and leg, and plantar flexion of the foot. With immobility, muscles atrophy and the collagen fibers of the connective tissue of tendons, ligaments and joint capsules tend to shorten and become dense and firm. The process may be hastened by circulatory stasis, edema and trauma. As a result, if the affected limbs are permitted to remain immobile in the positions they automatically assume, contractures and reduced range of motion may become permanent, making rehabilitation difficult and possibly creating deformities which actually increase the patient's disability. Maintenance of joint mo-

[4]M. Buck: op. cit., p. 93.

tion, support to prevent the pull of gravity on joints and subsequent subluxation, and positioning to prevent contractures and maintain good alignment are essential from the onset of the illness. In the supine position, the paralyzed arm is abducted to a 90° angle, and a pillow is placed along the chest into the axilla. Internal rotation of the shoulder is avoided. The arm and hand are supported on a pillow; a roll is placed in the hand to preserve the normal position. In some instances, marked spasticity may necessitate the use of a padded splint, especially at night, to prevent flexure contractures of the wrist and hand. If the hand is edematous, the hand and arm are elevated above the level of the heart to promote venous and lymphatic drainage and reduce stasis. A long sand bag or firm roll is placed along the outer side of the lower limb to counteract external rotation. To be effective, the sand bag must extend from above the greater trochanter to the external malleolus. The foot is kept at right angles to the leg by the use of a footboard.

When the patient lies on his unaffected side, his paralyzed limbs are supported in good alignment on pillows to prevent strain on the shoulder and hip joints. Two or 3 times a day, the patient is placed in the prone position for 30 minutes. The affected arm is adducted and extended, palm down and the roll is kept in place. A folded bath towel or small pillow is placed under each shoulder to avoid inward rotation. A small flat pillow is placed under the ankles, and the feet are extended beyond the mattress to prevent plantar flexion. The limbs are passively moved through a full range of motion 2 or 3 times daily. While the patient is helpless and confined to bed, his position is changed every 2 hours; he is encouraged to take 8 or 10 deep respirations and cough each time he changes position. Bedrest and immobility promote stasis and retention of pulmonary secretions which predispose to infection.

The stroke patient is usually assisted out of bed for progressively increasing periods as soon as his vital signs have returned to normal. This lessens muscle deterioration and the possibility of pulmonary complications, facilitates the recovery of postural reflexes, and promotes a more positive attitude on the part of the patient toward his future. When the patient is up, the affected arm is placed in a sling to prevent subluxation of the shoulder joint.

As soon as the patient is well enough, an assessment is made of his remaining abilities and disabilities to determine his rehabilitation potential. Each one must be evaluated and treated on an individual basis.

As cited previously, the location and extent of brain damage influence the nature of impaired function. Most hemiplegic patients fortunately experience extensor spasm of the affected knee and hip with weight-bearing which stabilizes the leg as the good leg is carried through a forward step. Instead of this extensor spasm, in response to the weight-bearing, some experience spasm of the flexor muscles. When the patient attempts to walk, the knee and hip flex and will not support him. This necessitates the application of a leg brace for stabilization. Others, because of interference with the blood supply to the cerebellum, suffer ataxia and marked loss of balance. This is likely to preclude ambulation, and the patient remains in a wheelchair.

Sensory function may also be impaired; as well as a reduced sensitivity to pain, pressure and temperature, there may be a loss of the ability to know the location of parts of his body in space, making movement difficult. The ability to recognize objects by touch (sterognosis) may also be impaired.

A stroke may cause intellectual damage; reasoning, judgment and normal responses may be impaired and will limit the level to which the patient may be rehabilitated.

Once this assessment of the patient's abilities and disabilities is completed, a plan is made and instituted for exercises and teaching to assist the patient to function within the framework of his disability. He should be given every opportunity to recover as great a degree of independence as possible to make life more tolerable for him and his family. The program, in which the nurse has an important role, is directed toward assisting the patient to achieve self-care and mobility and regain verbal communication if speech has been impaired. A physiotherapist, in cooperation with the physician, may plan and introduce the program, but frequently it is the nurse who must follow

it up and give the necessary guidance and support to the patient and his family.

As soon as possible, the retraining for self-care is begun while the patient is still in bed. He learns to feed himself and to care for his person (washing himself, combing his hair, dressing and undressing). He is taught how to change his position in bed and to pull himself to a sitting position through the help of an overhead bar attached to the bed or a rope secured to the foot of the bed. Crib sides on the bed also provide assistance in sitting up and ensure safety against falls until he can maintain his balance. A schedule of exercises is established to strengthen the trunk and unaffected muscles so they may compensate for those paralyzed. Passive movements of the affected limbs are carried out to prevent contractures and stimulate circulation as a part of the exercise schedule. The patient is taught to do the exercises on his own, and he also learns how to do the passive movements of the affected limbs with his good limbs. Progressively, he learns to sit on the side of the bed, to stand, to transfer to a chair or commode, and eventually to walk using a walker or a regular or wide quadruple base cane for support. When assisting the patient in walking, the nurse or family member supports him from his affected side. A leg brace may be necessary if the patient has the previously cited problem of flexor spasm in the paralyzed leg, and he will require instruction in applying it. If plantar flexion and toe-dragging interfere with walking and tend to trip the patient, a drop-foot splint may be used. The bed is lowered and made stationary when transfer techniques are being carried out.

Rehabilitation also includes retraining in simple useful functions (activities of daily living) on which every person is so dependent in normal living. These include such activities as opening doors, using the telephone, writing his name if the dominant hand has been paralyzed, handling various articles (e.g., wallet) and turning on the radio or television. The housewife is assisted in learning to use various pieces of household equipment and is advised of simpler ways of performing some housekeeping tasks; suggestions are made for reorganizing the kitchen and other facilities so that she may be less dependent.

In relation to the aphasia which the patient may experience, the suggestions cited under speech impairment are continued. Efforts to have them regain some speech must not be abandoned too soon because of lack of early improvement.

As a guide to the exercises used for hemiplegic patients and the retraining for the activities of daily living and for suggestions for adaptations and special devices to promote independence and usefulness, the references cited below should be familiar to the nurse.[5] These booklets are readily available and may be used by the patient and his family. Other useful references which are applicable to the rehabilitation of the stroke patient are also included at the end of this chapter.

The total rehabilitation program is fully discussed with a member of the family. This person should be familiar with the exercise and passive movement regimen and should understand the importance of encouraging and permitting the patient to do things for himself. The family members, as do many nurses, find it difficult to stand back, leaving the patient to persevere and struggle with activities. The brochure entitled "Strokes—A Guide for the Family," which is published by the American Heart Association, may be helpful to the family and should be made available.

When the rehabilitation plan is instituted, the stroke patient is usually discharged from the hospital. Both the patient and his family still require considerable support and assistance. Following discussions with the family, a referral may be made to a visiting nurse agency. It is helpful in many instances if a visit is made to the home before the patient is discharged so that the situation may be assessed and modifications of the environment suggested to facilitate the patient's care and independence. These may include the changing of rooms, hand rails beside the toilet and bath tub, the placement of articles for ready accessibility to the patient, making the bed stationary, arranging for a footboard, the removal of scatter rugs and wax from floors, and selection of a chair that will promote good posture and also allow the patient to rise from it with a minimum of difficulty. The visiting nurse becomes familiar with the patient's history, his potential and the rehabilitation program planned so she can provide the necessary supervision. Assistance may be given in solving the social and economic problems imposed on the family by this illness and disability. Financial supplements may be arranged, and the nurse may help the family to organize so that all share in the increased responsibility. Early signs of resentment may be recognized, and by listening to the family members' points of view and explaining the patient's condition and unusual behavior, complete rejection of him may be prevented.

The patient is encouraged to develop interests and worthwhile hobbies and to gradually assume responsibility for some household chores within his physical and intellectual capacity. The performance of some useful tasks, remunerative or otherwise, promotes the patient's morale and greater harmony within the family.

The goals of rehabilitation are not achieved in a few weeks; in most instances, attainment requires months of perseverence and patience. The patient and his family naturally experience periods of depression, frustration and pessimism. The established goals should not exceed the possibility of realization. Activities are taken in steps so achievement may be experienced. Demanding too much at one time fatigues and discourages the patient, defeating progress. Complete restoration to his previous functional ability is seldom possible, but much can be done to restore the patient to a degree of independence that makes life more tolerable for him and his family.

DEGENERATIVE DISEASES OF THE NERVOUS SYSTEM

Paralysis Agitans (Parkinson's Disease)

Paralysis agitans is a progressive degenerative disease within the brain that causes

---

[5] Chronic Disease Program, Public Health Service, U.S.: Strike Back at Stroke. Washington, U. S. Department of Health, Education and Welfare.

————————: Up and Around. Washington, U.S. Department of Health, Education and Welfare.

American Heart Association: Do it Yourself Again. New York, American Heart Association.

These booklets are distributed by the American Heart Association and the Canadian Heart Foundation.

dysfunction of the extrapyramidal system, resulting in muscular rigidity, difficulty in initiating voluntary movements, tremor and disturbed autonomic nervous function.

Etiology and Incidence. For a long period this disease was attributed chiefly to degenerative changes in the basal ganglia. Recently, failure of the substantia nigra to produce normal amounts of the chemical dopamine is considered to play an important etiological role. The substantia nigra (meaning black substance) is a nucleus in the midbrain and consists of neurons distinctly characterized by their high pigment (melanin) content. These cells produce dopamine and deliver it via their axons to the basal ganglia which function as part of the extrapyramidal system. The chemical appears to be essential for normal functioning of the basal ganglia. It is excreted from the body in the urine. Patients with Parkinson's disease show reduced urinary levels, and autopsies have revealed an abnormally low amount of melanin in the substantia nigra of these patients.[6, 7]

This disease, which is relatively common, usually has its onset between the ages of 50 and 60 and has a slightly higher incidence in males.

Symptoms. Tremor and muscular rigidity develop insidiously and at the onset are usually unilateral with involvement of the other side developing later. The fine tremor occurs when the part is at rest, is arrested with voluntary movement and when the person is asleep, and becomes more pronounced with emotional stress and fatigue. The tremor develops initially in the distal portions of the limbs and eventually involves the head, lips and tongue. In the upper limbs the involuntary movements are confined mainly to the wrist, fingers and thumb; in the legs, flexion and extension at the ankle occur. Tremor of the fingers and thumb produce the characteristic "pill-rolling" movement.

In the early stage of the muscular rigidity, the patient may complain of stiffness on moving, but gradually as tonic contraction of

skeletal muscle increases, voluntary movements become slow and difficult. There is marked resistance of the limbs to passive movement. The patient may have difficulty in starting to walk, and his gait is characterized by short, shuffling steps. The trunk and head are flexed forward, causing a progressive acceleration of his steps (festination gait), difficulty in stopping and a predisposition to falling. The arms are adducted and semiflexed, and their normal swing during walking is absent. He may have difficulty in assuming any change in position such as sitting down, rising from the sitting position and turning in bed. Finger movements are impaired as evidenced by the patient's small cramped writing and difficulty with tying his shoes or closing fasteners on his clothing.

Rigidity of the facial muscles produces a mask-like, inexpressive appearance. Speech becomes weak, slurred and monotonous (devoid of inflections) as the muscles concerned with articulation become involved. Late in the disease, the patient may experience difficulty in mastication and swallowing. The respiratory excursion and the ability to cough are diminished, predisposing the patient to chest complications. Pain and easy fatigue due to the continuous increased traction of muscles on their attachments are common. Dryness of the skin, coldness of the extremities and an excessive secretion of saliva may occur due to disturbances in the autonomic nervous system.

Treatment and Nursing Care. The patient with paralysis agitans is encouraged to remain active for as long as reasonably possible. Because the condition progresses slowly, generally over years, he is usually able to continue his gainful occupation. As the tremor and slower movements become more troublesome, he may have to change his occupation, depending on its nature, and may eventually be forced to give it up. It should be remembered that the patient's mask-like expression and motor impairment belie his mental capacity, which suffers no deterioration until the very late stage.

Currently, treatment falls into 3 categories—namely, drug therapy, physical therapy and surgery. These do not cure the disease but may be effective in reducing the distressing tremor and muscular rigidity.

DRUG THERAPY. The drugs used in treatment of Parkinson's disease include natural

[6]A. Fangman, and W. E. O'Malley: "L-Dopa and the Patient with Parkinson's Disease." Amer. J. Nurs., Vol. 69, No. 7 (July 1969), p. 1455.

[7]J. Gilroy, and J. S. Meyer: Medical Neurology. New York, The MacMillan Co., 1969, p. 171.

and synthetic anticholinergic preparations, antihistamines, and dihydroxyphenylalanine (L-dopa).

The anticholinergic preparations are thought to inhibit the transmission of the abnormal impulses responsible for the excessive muscular contraction and tremor. The natural antiparkinsonism drugs, such as tincture and extract of belladonna, atropine, scopolamine and stramonium, are employed less often now because the synthetic preparations generally produce fewer and less severe side effects. The synthetic preparations include trihexyphenidyl (Artane), benztropine mesylate (Cogentin), cycrimine hydrochloride (Pagitane) and procyclidine hydrochloride (Kemadrin). A patient receiving a natural or synthetic anticholinergic drug is observed for side effects which commonly are dryness of the mouth and skin, blurring of vision, headache, retention of urine, tachycardia and palpitation. The patient is generally started on a small dose of the prescribed preparation, which is gradually increased until side effects appear. The dosage is then slightly reduced and maintained at a level at which the patient is free of side effects. An antihistamine, such as diphenhydramine hydrochloride (Benadryl), may also be ordered; this assists in reducing the patient's tremor and anxiety. Side effects of this drug may be lightheadedness and drowsiness.

L-Dopa is a new experimental drug which is still under investigation. Its initial use was based on studies which indicated that patients with paralysis agitans have less than the normal amounts of dopamine in their substantia nigra and basal ganglia. Dopamine, as such, is not given, since it does not cross the blood-brain barrier; dihydroxyphenylalanine (L-dopa) is given and is absorbed by the substantia nigra which then produces dopamine.[8]

Reports on clinical investigations of the use of this new drug indicate promising effects.[8] Tremor and muscular rigidity are markedly reduced, facilitating normal movements and independence, and the face loses the inexpressiveness. At first the patient receives a small dose which is progressively increased over several days. He is hospitalized during this period, since some side effects of varying intensity may be experienced. These may be manifested in gastrointestinal or cardiovascular disturbances. He is observed for hypotension, pulse changes, anorexia, nausea, vomiting, marked weakness, restlessness, abnormal patterns of movement (e.g., athetosis), behavioral changes, confusion, and swings in mood. Frequent blood counts are made since some patients have shown a fall in granulocytes.

PHYSICAL THERAPY. Because of the difficulty in moving associated with the muscular rigidity, the patient is prone to remain immobile. As a result the normal range of joint movement may be lost and contractures develop. A program of physical therapy is instituted when the patient's disease has advanced to the stage when even slight difficulty in activity is manifested. A schedule of exercises is planned and initiated in a rehabilitation or physical therapy department. The types of exercises are prescribed according to the patient's disability and are designed to promote independence and self-care within the limits of his potential capacity. The family and visiting nurse must be familiar with the program, since the patient may reach a stage at which he is not sufficiently self-motivated to carry out the daily exercises and requires prompting and encouragement. Progression of the disease may necessitate periodic adjustments in the prescribed program.

SURGICAL TREATMENT. Certain patients may be treated by pallidotomy or thalamotomy, which may alleviate tremor and muscular rigidity; results vary. The pallidotomy procedure produces a lesion in the globus pallidus; in the case of the thalamotomy, the lesion is produced in the ventrolateral portion of the thalamus. The thalamic surgery appears to be the surgery of choice in recent years. Either procedure is performed under local anesthesia and involves the destruction of a well-defined area of tissue by the introduction of absolute alcohol, electro-

[8]Fangman and O'Malley, loc. cit., p. 1457.

Gilroy and Meyer, loc. cit., p. 176.

G. C. Cotzias, et al.: "Modification of Parkinsonism—Chronic Treatment with L-Dopa." New Eng. J. of Med., Vol. 280, No. 7 (Feb. 13, 1969), pp. 337–344.

Editors: "Changing the Outlook for Parkinson Patients." Med. World News, Nov. 29, 1968, pp. 32–35.

coagulation, freezing by means of liquid nitrogen (cryosurgery) or separation from adjacent tissue using a leukotome (fine blunt wire). The surgery is performed on the side opposite to the limbs with the greater rigidity and tremor. If this results in improvement, and there is bilateral involvement, the operation may be undertaken on the other side a few months later.

The patients for surgical therapy are carefully selected. Preferably the candidates are those who are 50 to 60 years of age who are not responding to drug therapy, are not fully incapacitated and whose disease is unilateral. In preparation for surgery, anti-parkinsonism drugs are usually discontinued several days preceding the scheduled date. General preoperative preparation is applicable, and a specific directive is given as to the necessary local skin preparation. The usual procedure is to shampoo the patient's hair the afternoon or evening before the scheduled operation using hexachlorophene. A small area of the scalp is then shaved in the operating room, preceding the making of a burr hole through which the surgeon works. The patient is advised that local anesthesia will be used and that he will be requested, during the procedure, to perform movements such as opening and clenching his hand or raising his arm on the side opposite to the surgery. These are made to assist in localizing the area of tissue to be treated. An explanation is also made of the frequent checking of his vital signs and responses that will be made after the operation.

Following the surgery, the head of the bed is elevated to promote venous drainage and prevent cerebral edema and increased intracranial pressure. The vital signs are recorded every half hour for several hours; the interval is gradually increased if they remain normal. Frequent observations are made of the patient's level of consciousness; pupillary reactions, size and equality; and orientation. Tests are made for any indication of loss of motor and sensory function. Crib sides are placed on the bed in the event of mental confusion or sudden seizure. A suction apparatus and padded tongue depressor should be readily available in the event of a convulsion. The patient is usually assisted out of bed in 36 to 48 hours and is helped to walk. The limbs are passively moved through a full range of motion 2 or 3 times daily, and an active exercise program is instituted as soon as the patient's condition permits.

GENERAL NURSING CONSIDERATIONS. The majority of persons suffering from paralysis agitans are cared for at home until the advanced stage of their disease leads to marked disability and helplessness. The clinic or visiting nurse assumes the major role in providing the necessary counseling and guidance for the patient and his family at the onset and through the successive months and years. It is important that the nurse understand the nature of the patient's disease and recognize the emotional, physical and socioeconomic problems incurred by it. The fact that his intellect is unimpaired must be kept in mind as well as his tendency to become very self-conscious, depressed and withdrawn because of his appearance and limitations. The reader will find it helpful to read Margaret Bourke-White's "My Mysterious Malady" to receive first hand the thoughts and reactions of a person with Parkinson's disease.[9]

The nurse helps the family and those around the patient to understand his problems and emphasizes his need to be treated normally, to socialize, and to do things for himself even though he may take much longer than usual. The environment should be quiet, cheerful and free of haste and confusion, since emotional stress and fatigue aggravate his tremor and rigidity. As the disease progresses, certain aspects of his care require increasing attention and modification.

The patient is encouraged to feed himself, and provision is made for the fact that he takes longer, spills food and probably has difficulty in chewing and swallowing. His nutritional status and weight are followed, since he may consume only a small part of his meals because of depression and fatigue. Inadequate food intake weakens the patient and influences his capacity to participate in an exercise program and other activities. A schedule of frequent smaller meals may be helpful and he may find it

---

[9]Margaret Bourke-White: My Mysterious Malady. Chicago, United Parkinson's Disease Foundation. (Taken from "Portrait of Myself" published by Simon Schuster Inc., 1963.)

easier to take strained or chopped foods or food prepared in a blender. The patient may be less self-conscious and take more if privacy is ensured while he is eating. His clothing is protected during the meal so that traces of his incapacity do not remain to increase his concern. Eventually, he may require assistance, especially with fluids.

Constipation is a frequent problem because of the reduced activity, tension, prescribed drugs and limited bulk in the diet. Impaction may develop. Additional fluids, fruits and vegetables may be included in the diet, and a bulk-producing laxative may be prescribed to establish regular bowel movements.

The patient sits for prolonged periods and may also be unable to change his position in bed because of the rigidity. Obviously, this predisposes to circulatory stasis and pressure sores. Assistance at regular intervals to prevent these prolonged periods of immobility is necessary. Assistive devices, such as a rope secured to the end of the bed or suspended from an overhead bar, may be helpful for the patient to raise himself to a sitting position from which he can shift his weight. When he is up, arms on his chair may permit him to raise himself to a standing position.

Excessive salivation and difficulty in swallowing may cause drooling, which is extremely uncomfortable and embarrassing for the patient, An adequate supply of available soft tissues, skin care with the application of a protective lotion or ointment, and frequent changes of the pillow cover are necessary.

The patient's forward flexion of the trunk, shuffling gait, and slowness of righting reflexes to maintain his balance predispose him to falls. Some simple modifications within his environment may prevent such accidents. Floors should not be waxed. Hazards such as scatter rugs, small stools and other articles which might trip him are removed. A straight chair that is not likely to tip or move as he lowers himself into it or rises from it is provided. A raised toilet seat and hand bars in appropriate places in the bathroom facilitate self-care and prevent falls. The patient's belongings and articles he is likely to need are kept in places which are easily accessible to him.

Clothing with zippers rather than buttons and pull-on shoes instead of those with laces are suggested so that the patient can maintain his independence in dressing and undressing as long as possible. By being able to achieve these tasks, he is likely to be more interested in his personal appearance and is less likely to drift into the habit of remaining in pajamas and a dressing gown throughout the day. The male patient usually becomes dependent on others to shave him before many other self-care activities are relinquished. A schedule is planned for a member of his family to assume this responsibility regularly so that the patient does not feel neglected or that he is a nuisance.

Participation in activities and socialization with the family and others in the home and outside are promoted. Otherwise, the Parkinson's disease patient becomes a very lonely, disillusioned person. Personality changes are fostered by isolation and frequently lead to difficult patient-family relationships. The results of group involvement in exercises and planned recreation in institutions have demonstrated the benefits derived from socialization and being one of the group.

Multiple Sclerosis (Disseminated Sclerosis)

Multiple sclerosis is a degenerative disease characterized by demyelination of nerve fibers within the spinal cord and brain. The lesions are irregular and scattered which accounts for the term disseminated. Destruction of an area of a myelin sheath occurs, followed by a proliferation of neuroglial cells, scar formation, and damage to the nerve fiber with ensuing loss of transmission of impulses.

Etiology and Incidence. The cause of multiple sclerosis is unknown despite prolonged and continuous research. At present, theories undergoing investigation are concerned with auto-immunity, viruses and neurobiochemistry as possible etiological factors.

The disease is more prevalent in colder climates, but once established, climate does not appear to influence its progress. It has a slightly higher incidence in females and most frequently has its onset in persons between 20 and 40 years of age.

Course and Manifestations. Multiple sclerosis is characterized by remissions and relapses, and the course is extremely variable and unpredictable. Spontaneous remissions of varying length are common, especially in the early years of the disease. The manifestations may vary from one relapse to another as a result of lesions developed in tracts other than those previously involved. Gradually, the cumulative, residual effects of nerve fiber damage from recurring exacerbations lead to a chronic incapacitated state in which the patient is helpless and is confined to a wheelchair.

Early symptoms usually include transient tingling sensations, numbness and muscular weakness in one or both arms and legs and visual disturbances which may take the form of nystagmus, diplopia or blurring of the vision. The patient may manifest emotional lability, evidenced by alternating periods of euphoria (false sense of well-being), depression and irritability. Later, with repeated relapses and increasing damage, the patient may develop paralysis, impaired speech, dysphagia, increasing loss of sensation, bladder and bowel incontinence, increasing visual difficulties, personality changes and intellectual impairment. Weakness of the respiratory muscles and cough reflex may also be present, predisposing him to pulmonary complications.

At present, there are no specific diagnostic tests for multiple sclerosis. The cerebrospinal fluid of many of these patients shows an elevated gamma globulin level and a positive colloidal gold precipitation test (Lange colloidal gold curve).

Treatment and Nursing Care. There is no specific treatment for multiple sclerosis, but good counseling and care may contribute to the prevention of relapses and complications as well as help to keep the patient active and independent as long as possible. Management comprises mainly general supportive measures and symptomatic care which increase in amount and complexity with the progression of the patient's disease. He is cared for at home through the early stages of his disease and as long as the family can provide adequate care. Hospitalization or care in a nursing home usually becomes necessary when complete dependence has been reached or when secondary conditions such as bladder or pulmonary infection or decubitus ulcers intervene. While being cared for at home, regular supervision and assistance by a visiting nurse should be provided. It may be necessary for the hospital or clinic nurse to inform the family of this available service and make the initial referral. If the illness poses socioeconomic problems for the patient and his family, a social worker may be brought in to counsel them, or they may be advised of welfare agencies from which assistance may be obtained. They are told of the Multiple Sclerosis Society[10] and of the services it provides and are urged to avail themselves of these. As well as promoting research of the disease, the association assists in securing a wheelchair and self-help devices, transports patients to clinics, contacts sources of welfare if needed, and has voluntary workers who make home visits and plan occupational therapy and recreational programs for multiple sclerosis patients.

A plan of care for the patient with multiple sclerosis includes the following considerations.

DURING REMISSIONS. In early remissions when the residual effects are likely to be minimal, the patient is encouraged to resume his usual pattern of life, modifying it as necessary to avoid overfatigue, emotional stress and infections, since these frequently precipitate an exacerbation. A well-balanced diet, adequate, regular rest and learning to accept what cannot be readily changed to avoid emotional upsets are stressed. In the case of a married woman, the physician usually advises her of the increased risk of a relapse incurred by pregnancy. A visit to the physician or clinic at regular intervals is recommended.

REST. During a relapse, the patient is confined to bed for a period of 2 to 3 weeks or until symptoms begin to disappear. The promotion of rest and alleviation of the patient's likely psychological concern for his condition are a challenge to the nurse. Warm baths, massage, pleasant quiet surroundings, encouraging reading and listening to the radio and taking time to visit and chat with the patient to avoid long periods of

---

[10]Multiple Sclerosis Society of Canada, 76 Avenue Road, Toronto, Canada

The National Multiple Sclerosis Society, 257 Park Ave. South, New York, U.S.A.

Both national associations have local chapters or branches throughout the provinces and states.

isolation may promote relaxation and rest. The limbs are passively moved through a full range of motion twice daily but active exercises are only permitted later when indicated by the doctor.

STEROID THERAPY. An adrenocorticoid preparation such as dexamethasone (Decadron) or adrenocorticotrophin (ACTH) may be used to treat acute exacerbation. The response to this therapy varies with patients; some manifest a remission of symptoms fairly quickly, but others may show little improvement. Generally, at first the patient receives fairly large doses, which are gradually decreased over a number of weeks. The drug may then be discontinued or a maintenance dose of dexamethasone prescribed. He is observed closely when receiving the drug for changes in his symptoms as well as for side effects.

PSYCHOLOGICAL FACTORS. Those associated with the patient should be aware of the possible personality and behavioral changes that are likely to develop. Frequently, relationships become strained and "scenes" and situations develop because of a lack of understanding that the patient's reactions and swings in mood are an actual part of his illness. If marked depression is evident, he is not left alone, and precautions are instituted to guard against suicide. Hobbies and interests are fostered to keep the patient occupied, remembering of course that fatigue is to be avoided. A quiet, cheerful environment, free of confusion, is important; the patient is likely to become emotional when exposed to an atmosphere of pressure or haste.

MOTOR DISABILITY. The patient is kept ambulatory as long as is reasonably possible. Spasticity and muscle spasms, especially in the lower limbs, are prone to develop in the advanced stages of the disease, and walking becomes increasingly difficult. In order to prevent falls, floors are not waxed and are kept clear of scatter rugs, stools, electric light cords, and other articles over which the patient might trip. It is helpful if hand rails are installed in appropriate places to facilitate continued mobility and independence. When stairs become difficult for the patient, consideration should be given to having the patient's room on the main floor. This may necessitate additional bathroom facilities, or moving to another house or an apartment. Articles he is likely to need for self-care or for the performance of small chores are kept within easy reach.

When walking becomes impossible, a wheelchair is provided, and the patient is taught to transfer himself from the bed to chair if he has sufficient strength in his arms and trunk. He is taught to maneuver the chair from room to room and outside if possible in order to widen his horizon and prevent isolation.

In the case of the homemaker, adjustments in the kitchen may be made to permit the patient to work from her wheelchair. Rehabilitation centers usually have personnel who will assess the situation and make work simplification suggestions.

The family members require instructions on how to transfer the patient from the bed to a chair and on guarding against injury to him in the process.

A carefully controlled program of physical therapy may be prescribed after an acute exacerbation and continued within the patient's tolerance. It is introduced very gradually, and the patient is observed for regressive symptoms. Walking between parallel bars or with the aid of a walker may be helpful in rehabilitating the patient. He and his family are instructed as to the continuance of the program at home.

When spasticity develops in the paralyzed limbs, massage, passive movements and careful positioning similar to that used with the hemiplegic patient (see p. 619) are used to prevent contractures, joint immobility and deformities.

LOSS OF SENSATION. The interruption of sensory pathways may result in the patient's loss of awareness of temperature, pressure, pain, and position of limbs. Precautions are necessary to protect the patient; local heat applications are not used, and the temperature of the bath water must be carefully controlled; prolonged pressure and malpositioning are avoided.

SKIN CARE AND MOUTH CARE. As the patient becomes increasingly inactive, the skin requires frequent care and protection from prolonged pressure to prevent decubitus ulcers. His position is changed every 2 hours, and the skin is kept clean and dry and is gently massaged to stimulate circulation. Pressure is relieved by the use of pieces of sheepskin or sponge rubber and an air mattress. A footboard or cradle is provided to keep the weight of the bedding off the feet.

Muscular weakness or paralysis of the arms may prevent the patient from cleaning his teeth himself. He may also have some difficulty in swallowing which results in the accumulation of mucus and food particles in the mouth, leading to sordes. His teeth and mouth should be cleansed after each meal or oftener if indicated.

ELIMINATION. In the early stages of multiple sclerosis, the patient may experience urgency and occasional incontinency, which he finds very distressing. Atropine or propantheline (Pro-Banthine) may be prescribed to relax the detrusor muscle and increase the bladder capacity. Rarely, a patient may develop retention of urine during an acute relapse of his disease, necessitating catheterization. In the advanced stage of the disease, sphincter control is usually lost. An indwelling catheter may be used for a period of time to protect the skin. As soon as possible it is replaced by an attachable rubber or plastic urinal, and efforts are made to establish an automatic bladder (see p. 15).

Constipation is a common problem as a result of inactivity and weakness of the abdominal muscles. The fluid intake and roughage in the diet are increased, and a stool softener or bulk-producing laxative may be ordered. If the patient has incontinence of feces, regular use of a glycerine or bisacodyl (Dulcolax) suppository each morning stimulates evacuation at a convenient and predictable time.

PREVENTION OF PULMONARY COMPLICATIONS. Weakness of respiratory muscles results in shallow breathing and difficulty in coughing up secretions, predisposing the patient to chest infection. He is instructed to breathe deeply and encouraged to cough several times every 2 to 3 hours. In late stages of the disease, suctioning may be helpful. The patient with multiple sclerosis is protected as much as possible from contact with persons with infection.

Myasthenia Gravis

This is a chronic disease in which there is muscular weakness due to failure of the transmission of the nerve impulse at the myoneural junction. The cause of the myoneural block is unknown. It is suggested there may be a deficiency of effective acetylcholine released by the nerve fiber ending (synaptic knob), excessive cholinesterase (the enzyme which inactivates acetylcholine), or a defect in the motor end plate which reduces its ability to respond. An autoimmune reaction is suspected of producing antibodies which interfere with motor end plate activity. Myasthenia gravis is in some way related to a disorder of the thymus.*

Incidence and Manifestations. Myasthenia gravis is relatively uncommon and is seen more often in women. The onset in females is usually between the ages of 20 to 30 and between 60 to 70 years of age in males. The course, severity, symptoms and extent of involvement vary. The primary manifestation of the disease is skeletal muscle weakness which may affect an isolated group of muscles or may be fairly general. Movements may be initiated, but exhaustion rapidly intervenes. Some patients experience remissions and exacerbations; in others there may be progressive involvement and severity. The weakness is less marked following a period of rest, becoming more intense toward the end of the day.

Most frequently, the external ocular, pharyngeal, jaw, shoulder and arm muscles are the first to be affected. The patient manifests ptosis, diplopia, difficulty in chewing and swallowing, progressive weakness of the voice, and difficulty in performing activities, such as combing his hair or shaving, which requires the raising of his arms. In more serious cases, the trunk and lower limb muscles become involved, causing respiratory insufficiency or complete failure and paraplegia.

Investigation of the patient for myasthenia gravis usually includes roentgenograms of the chest to determine if there is any enlargement of the thymus. A second diagnostic procedure that is frequently used is the edrophonium (Tensilon) test. Following an intravenous injection of this anticholinesterase drug, the response of the affected

---

*The thymus is a mass of lymphoid tissue located posterior to the sternum in the upper mediastinal region of the thorax. It progressively increases in size to the age of puberty, then gradually atrophies. Its function is not clearly understood. Currently, it is thought to be primarily concerned with the production of lymphocytes and antibodies.

muscles is observed. Edrophonium is quick-acting and has a very transient effect of approximately 15 to 30 minutes. Prompt improvement in the strength of the affected muscles occurs in myasthenia gravis.

Treatment and Nursing Care. Care of the patient is naturally defined by the severity and course of the disease. The principal treatment is the continuous use of an anti-cholinesterase drug, which does not cure the disease but controls the muscular weakness sufficiently to permit many patients to resume their gainful employment and live a normal life. The drug preparations most commonly employed include neostigmine (Prostigmin), ambenonium chloride (Myte-lase) and pyridostigmine bromide (Mesti-non). The dosage is adjusted to the needs of each patient, being based on the control of muscular weakness and on the appearance of side effects such as abdominal cramps, diarrhea, and increased sweating, salivation and bronchial secretions. Since the effect of these drugs lasts only 4 to 6 hours, that which is prescribed is taken orally 3 or 4 times daily unless the slow-release preparation of pyridostigmine is used which reduces the frequency of the dosage. Before leaving the hospital, the patient learns the details of adjusting the dosage according to evident needs. Such factors as increased physical activity, emotional stress, infection and menstruation can alter the daily requirements.

Treatment may include radiation of the thymus or thymectomy. Results vary; in relation to thymectomy, Gilroy and Meyer state that "the best results occur in patients under 40 years of age who have had their disease for less than 5 years."[11]

The implications for nursing include the following factors:

REST. Extra rest is very important to the patient with myasthenia gravis. At the onset of the disease, if the symptoms are mild and not seriously incapacitating, the nurse helps the patient to plan his day so that he will get extra rest and avoid fatigue. A regular rest period before or during the lunch period and again during the afternoon are advisable if possible, and a minimum of 8 hours of sleep each night is recommended. It may be necessary for him to change his occupation or accept part-time employment because of the restrictions imposed by his disease. During an exacerbation, the patient is kept in bed, and the nurse gives complete care to conserve his strength. Care is planned to ensure uninterrupted intervals of rest. With improvement, he gradually assumes self-care, and the reaction to the increased activity is observed.

OBSERVATIONS. The nurse is responsible for noting and recording accurately the patient's response to the drug therapy. Side effects of the drug, increasing intensity in his symptoms or the appearance of new manifestations are reported promptly. Particular attention is paid to the patient's respirations; weakness of the respiratory muscles may develop rapidly, or weakness in the ability to cough and remove secretions may lead to pulmonary insufficiency and respiratory infection.

DIET. Modifications in the diet are necessary if difficulty in chewing and swallowing are experienced. Soft, strained foods, blender prepared foods and concentrated nutritious fluids may be used. The prescribed anticholinesterase drug is usually administered 30 or 45 minutes before the meal so that fatigability is reduced and the patient is able to take a normal amount. It is also helpful if a rest period is planned to precede the meal hour. In acute episodes, he must be fed slowly. If the dysphagia is such that sufficient nourishment cannot be taken, a nasogastric tube is passed, and tube feedings are given at regular intervals (see p. 339). The fluid intake is checked as the patient may tend to neglect taking an adequate amount because of the effort involved.

PREVENTION OF INFECTION. In the hospital precautions are necessary to protect the patient from exposure to infection. Respiratory infection is particularly serious because of his inability to cough and raise secretions. The disease usually worsens with any type of infection. The patient and his family are advised of the importance of avoiding possible contacts and the appropriate preventive measures. If infection develops, the physician should be notified promptly so that early antimicrobial therapy may be instituted. The patient is cautioned against self-medication; no drugs other than those prescribed should be taken at any time.

---

[11] J. Gilroy, and J. S. Meyer: op. cit., p. 686.

MYASTHENIA GRAVIS FOUNDATION. The patient and his family are informed of the services of the Myasthenia Gravis Foundation[12] and are given a copy of the helpful brochures published by the organization.

MYASTHENIC CRISIS. An acute episode with respiratory insufficiency is an emergency demanding prompt intensive care. The crisis may occur spontaneously but more often is precipitated by an infection, physical or emotional stress, reduced effectiveness of the anticholinesterase drug, or excessive dosage of anticholinesterase drugs which causes what is referred to as a cholinergic crisis. The crisis is characterized by extreme generalized muscular weakness, which poses as great a threat to the patient's life as the acute relapse of his disease because of the interference with breathing. The patient in a cholinergic crisis also manifests constricted pupils, excessive sweating, salivation and bronchial secretions, abdominal cramps, diarrhea and difficulty in swallowing.

Serious respiratory involvement necessitates prompt intratracheal intubation or tracheostomy and the use of a mechanical respirator. Frequent, deep suctioning is necessary to clear the airway; manual or mouth-to-mouth artificial respirations may be necessary to sustain the patient until he reaches the hospital and the respirator is operating. If the patient is known to have been receiving an anticholinesterase drug, an edrophonium (Tensilon) test is done. If the cause of the crisis is associated with a deficiency of the anticholinesterase drug, a prompt improvement is likely to be manifested. The patient is then given neostigmine intramuscularly. If there is no improvement in the patient's symptoms in the Tensilon test, the crisis is attributed to overdosage of an anticholinesterase preparation. A dose of atropine sulphate may be ordered if there is excessive salivation and bronchial secretion. A nasogastric tube is passed, and a tube feeding is given every 2 to 3 hours to sustain the patient.

With improvement, the use of the respirator is discontinued for brief periods. If the patient's respirations are adequate, these periods are progressively lengthened until the patient can get along without the respirator.

Following a crisis, further instruction on the general management of the patient's life and drug therapy may be indicated.

NEOPLASMS OF THE NERVOUS SYSTEM

Intracranial Newgrowths

Primary intracranial newgrowths most commonly arise from the neuroglial tissue, meninges, cerebral blood vessels, hypophysis and nerve fibers. They are named according to their tissue origin and may be benign or malignant. See Table 22–3 for the names, origins and most frequent sites of intracranial tumors. The brain is not an infrequent location for metastatic tumors; the most frequent sites of the primary malignancy are the lungs, breast, skin, gastrointestinal tract and the kidneys. Primary malignant neoplasms of the brain differ from those elsewhere in the body in that they rarely metastasize to other parts.

Manifestations. The signs and symptoms of an intracranial neoplasm are extremely variable and are classified as general or focal. Focal symptoms are the result of the local effects of the neoplasm and reflect its location. The compression or tissue destruction that it causes interferes with the function(s) of that particular area of the brain and may be motor, sensory or psychological. Examples of focal manifestations include weakness or paralysis of a limb, ataxia, convulsions, aphasia, change in personality, disorientation, impaired intellect, impaired vision, loss of hearing, facial paralysis and loss of sensations. They usually develop gradually and may be single or multiple from the onset.

General symptoms occur as a result of increased intracranial pressure and ensuing compression of brain tissue. The increase in the pressure may be due directly to the space-occupying lesion within the rigid cranium or to the associated cerebral edema, venous congestion or an obstruction in the cerebrospinal fluid pathway.

---

[12] The Myasthenia Gravis Foundation, 53 Sunnycrest Rd., Willowdale, Ontario, Canada

The Myasthenia Gravis Foundation, Incorporated, 2 East 103rd St., New York, U.S.A.

TABLE 22–3   INTRACRANIAL TUMORS[12]

NAME OF NEOPLASM	ORIGIN	MOST FREQUENT SITES	COMMENTS
Gliomas	Neuroglial tissue		Commonest type of intracranial neoplasm; rate of growth varies with type of glioma
Astrocytoma	Astrocytes	Adults—cerebrum Children—Cerebellum	Most common glioma; grows very slowly; infiltrates surrounding tissue
Glioblastoma	Undifferentiated glial cells	Frontal, parietal and temporal lobes	Highly malignant
Medulloblastoma	Undifferentiated glial cells	Cerebellum	Rapid extension; highly malignant
Ependymoma	Ependymal cells of the lining of the ventricles and aqueducts.	Fourth ventricle	Rare; frequently papillomatous; may obstruct flow of CSF
Oligodendroglioma	Oligodendrocytes	Cerebral hemispheres	Rare; grows very slowly; tends to calcify
Meningioma	Meninges	Along the course of the intracranial venous sinuses	Are extracerebral, causing compression of brain tissue; usually encapsulated; grow slowly
Hemangiomas Angioma	Blood vessel wall	Middle cerebral artery	(Not a true neoplasm) Congenital mass of tortuous, enlarged vessels; benign, but may interfere with adjacent tissues
Angioblastoma	Blood vessel wall	Cerebellum	Tendency to form cysts
Pituitary adenomas Chromophobe adenoma	Adenohypophyseal glandular tissue	Anterior pituitary lobe (adenohypophysis)	Encapsulated; compresses pituitary gland tissue and optic nerves, leading to hypopituitarism and impaired vision
Chromophil adenoma (acidophilic adenoma)	Adenohypophyseal glandular tissue	Anterior pituitary lobe (adenohypophysis)	Seen less often than chromophobe adenoma; causes hyperpituitarism (giantism or acromegaly)
Craniopharyngioma	Embryological defect in craniopharyngeal duct	Anterior to the pituitary stalk	Produces pressure on surrounding structures, interfering with function
Acoustic Neuroma	Eighth cranial (acoustic) nerve		Encapsulated

[12]Information compiled from:
A. B. Baker (Ed.): Clinical Neurology. Vol. 1, New York, Hoeber-Harper, 1955. Chapter 5.
Lord Brain: Clinical Neurology, 2nd ed. New York, Oxford University Press, 1964. Chapter 9.
M. E. Leavens: "Brain Tumors." Amer. J. Nurs., Vol. 64, No. 3 (Mar. 1964), p. 80.

Manifestations of increasing intracranial pressure due to an intracranial tumor may include the following:

Headache, which may also be due to traction on pain-sensitive structures such as blood vessels and cranial nerves, is usually one of the early symptoms and is intensified by activities such as coughing, vomiting, straining at stool and lowering of the head.

Mental disturbances. These gradually appear and may be mild at the onset, probably taking the form of fatigue, listlessness, a short attention span, restlessness, irritability or emotional instability. They become more marked as the pressure increases and may progress through disorientation and stupor to an eventual loss of consciousness.

Vomiting due to pressure on the vomiting

center in the medulla. It may not be preceded by nausea and usually occurs during the night or early morning.

Papilledema and *visual disturbances.*

Changes in vital signs occur as a result of pressure on the brain stem and venous congestion. The blood pressure rises and is accompanied by a slowing of the pulse rate. The respirations tend to become slower, then irregular or Cheyne-Stokes.

Dilation and *failing reaction to light of one or both pupils* due to pressure on the third cranial (oculomotor) nerve.

Progressive loss of function of limbs.

The patient undergoes an extensive neurological examination for motor sensory and intellectual functions. Various diagnostic procedures are done which may include roentgenograms, an arteriogram, ventriculogram, brain scan using a radioisotope, electroencephalogram and biopsy (see p. 606).

Treatment and Nursing Care. The type of treatment used for the patient with an intracranial neoplasm depends on the location and type of tumor, and his general condition. Surgery or radiation may be used. Whenever possible, surgical excision of the neoplasm is the method of choice, but in many instances, the neoplasm may be inaccessible or may involve vital areas, making removal impossible. Radiation therapy may then be used. The tumors most successfully treated by surgery are meningiomas, acoustic neuromas, pituitary adenomas, and astrocytomas; these tumors, with the exception of the astrocytomas, are extracerebral. In the case of an inoperable neoplasm which is obstructing the cerebrospinal fluid pathway, a tube may be placed between the lateral ventricle and the cisterna magna (subarachnoid space in posterior area below the brain) to bypass the obstruction (Torkildsen operation). When the lesion is inaccessible or cannot be removed because of a vital area (such as the midbrain) being involved, a palliative decompression operation may be performed in which a portion of the skull is removed to reduce the intracranial pressure. This retards brain damage and relieves headache and papilledema.

The nurse carefully notes and records the patient's motor and sensory functions, speech ability, complaints such as headache, dizziness, tingling or numbness of a part, responses and behavior, orientation, ability to carry out usual daily activities, pupillary size and reaction to light, and vital signs. Observation is an ongoing process through successive contacts so that changes and newly developed symptoms may be promptly recognized. The nurse's recognition and accurate recording of deviant physical and behavioral factors may play an important role in the diagnosis and localization of the intracranial newgrowth. Knowing that a space-occupying growth is suspect, the nurse is especially alert for signs of increasing intracranial pressure. Measures such as crib sides on the bed are used to prevent possible accidents, and a wrapped tongue depressor is kept available at the bedside in the event of a seizure.

The nursing care is planned according to the patient's needs which are determined mainly by the disturbances, dysfunction and dependencies caused by the intracranial lesion. He is kept ambulatory if his condition permits. If confined to bed, the head of the bed is elevated to promote cerebral venous drainage, which helps to reduce the intracranial pressure and headache. The nurse changes his position at regular, frequent intervals if the patient is lethargic, listless or semiconscious and tends to remain immobile. Particular attention is paid to his nutritional status; an adequate intake is especially important if surgery is anticipated.

The patient may be very upset emotionally and in despair about his future. Acknowledging his fear as understandable, encouraging him to talk about the situation and his feelings, and adequate explanations in preparation for the various diagnostic procedures may reduce his insecurity. The family's anxiety is understandable. Recognition of their concerns, stopping to talk with them and keeping them informed about the patient and what is being done for him instills confidence and helps them to accept the situation. In some instances, it is necessary to suggest that they avoid conveying their emotions to the patient, explaining that he is in need of their support and positive attitude.

A mild analgesic such as acetylsalicylic acid may be used for the relief of headache. Diphenylhydantoin sodium (Dilantin) may be prescribed for oral or intravenous administration to control seizures. To reduce intracranial pressure, osmotic diuresis may be induced by the intravenous injection of mannitol (Osmitrol) or a hypertonic solution of urea and glucose (Urevert). These preparations are not reabsorbed by the renal tubules, and by their osmotic action, they reduce the amount of water reabsorbed from the glomerular filtrate and increase the urinary output. Dexamethasone (Decadron), which is an adrenocorticosteroid drug, is frequently prescribed for patients with an intracranial lesion to control intracranial pressure that may be aggravated by the inflammatory process. It may be administered orally or by intramuscular injections.

Spinal Neoplasms

Newgrowths which arise within or encroach upon the spinal cord may be benign or malignant, primary or secondary (metastatic), and may be classified according to their origin as extradural or intradural. The extradural neoplasms occur in the vertebrae or the space between the dura mater and vertebrae and are most commonly metastases. Intradural tumors are extramedullary (outside the spinal cord) or intramedullary (arise within the cord). The intradural-extramedullary type constitutes about 50 per cent of all spinal neoplasms. They may arise from the meninges (meningiomas), nerve roots (neuromas or neurofibromas) or blood vessels (hemangiomas). Gliomas comprise the majority of intramedullary newgrowths.

Manifestations. The compression of nerve roots or tracts and neurons within the cord by a neoplasm is manifested by sensory and motor dysfunction. The parts of the body affected depend upon the level of the lesion. In the case of nerve root involvement, the affected areas correspond to those innervated by those particular spinal nerve fibers. Involvement of cord tracts and neurons may interfere with functions in all parts on one or both sides of the body which derive their innervation from the cord below the level of the lesion.

Damage and eventual loss of impulse conduction in the anterior (motor) nerve roots by an extramedullary growth produce progressive muscle weakness, flaccid paralysis, loss of tendon reflexes and muscle wasting comparable to lower motor neuron paralysis (see p. 602). Irritation of the posterior (sensory) nerve roots causes pain and abnormal sensations (e.g., tingling, "pins and needles"). Eventually as the neoplasm extends, interruption of the impulses results in a loss of sensations.

Newgrowths within the cord or compression by an extramedullary tumor may involve sensory or motor tracts. Pain, pressure and temperature sensations may be dulled or lost, and the patient may be unable to appreciate the position of affected limbs due to interference with proprioception impulse pathways. Damage to the pyramidal tracts (corticospinal motor tracts) produces muscle weakness at first, then spastic paralysis, exaggerated tendon reflexes, and bladder and bowel dysfunction similar to that of an upper motor neuron lesion (see p. 602).

Disturbed motor or sensory function may involve parts of one or both sides of the body, depending on the extent of the compression.

Investigation procedures usually include a lumbar puncture and Queckenstedt's test to determine possible obstruction to the cerebrospinal flow, roentgenograms of the spine, and a myelogram (see p. 609).

Treatment and Nursing Care. Primary extramedullary neoplasms are removed by surgery as soon as diagnosed; unnecessary delay may result in permanent paralysis. Intramedullary growths are more difficult to remove without seriously damaging the spinal cord and interrupting motor and sensory tracts. When the spinal neoplasm is inoperable or metastatic, relief of compression by laminectomy and probably partial resection of the newgrowth may be done. Radiation therapy of the involved area may be used as an adjunct to surgery or alone if the lesion is inoperable. For preoperative preparation of the patient for spinal surgery and postoperative nursing care, see page 652.

The care required by the patient who is inoperable or during investigation depends on the discomfort and disability he experiences. Loss of voluntary muscle power may vary from slight loss of strength in one group of muscles to paraplegia or quadriplegia and complete dependence (see p. 647).

Close observation is made for exaggeration of the patient's symptoms and for the appearance of new ones, indicating compression and damage. Significant factors to be noted are his motor abilities (strength, coordination and motion); complaints of pain; abnormal sensations or loss of feeling; bladder dysfunction, which may be manifested by frequency, urgency incontinence or retention; bowel dysfunction (constipation or fecal incontinence); condition of the skin, especially over the vulnerable bony prominences; and the patient's reactions to his illness.

TRAUMA OF THE NERVOUS SYSTEM

Head Injuries

Head injuries have become a major problem because of the present-day mechanization and the increasing number of automobile accidents. An accident may result in laceration of the scalp, skull fracture or brain injury. If there is a wound in the scalp and a fracture of the skull permitting communication between the air outside and the cranial cavity, the injury is termed open. Conversely, a closed injury is one in which the skull remains intact.

Laceration of the Scalp. The scalp is quite vascular, and when lacerated or torn away from the skull, it bleeds readily. The wound is cleaned thoroughly and sutured. Repair is usually delayed if fracture of the skull and brain injury are suspected or if the patient is in shock. In such cases the wound is cleansed, and a sterile dressing is applied. Efforts are made to determine if the patient has had immunizing tetanus toxoid injections. If he has, a booster dose of the toxoid may be ordered; if there has been no previous immunization, a prophylactic dose of tetanus antitoxin will be prescribed. Before this is given, the patient or his family is questioned as to any history of allergic reactions, eczema and asthma, and a small test dose is administered intracutaneously (see p. 39).

Fracture of the Skull. When a patient is known to have received a blow on the head or is unconscious following an accident, roentgenograms are made of the skull and examined for possible fracture. A skull fracture may be classified as linear, comminuted, compound or depressed. A linear or simple fracture is one in which these are two fragments which remain in apposition or are not displaced. In a comminuted fracture, multiple linear fractures occur, but the fragments are not displaced. No specific treatment is used for a simple linear or comminuted skull fracture, but the patient is kept at rest and the head of his bed is elevated. He is under close observation because a fracture rarely occurs without injury to blood vessels and the brain. Meningeal blood vessels may have been torn, and this will lead to extradural, subdural or subarachnoid hemorrhage. Concussion or contusion of the brain is a frequent concomitant. A compound fracture implies that there is communication with the outside because of a scalp wound, predisposing to infection of the bone and cranial contents. The scalp wound is cleansed thoroughly, débrided* and repaired as soon as the patient's condition permits to reduce the possibility of infection. A depressed fracture is one in which the fragments are driven inward, compressing or piercing the meninges and brain. As well as direct injury to the cranial contents at the site of the fracture, there is likely to be a rapid increase in the intracranial pressure affecting total brain functioning. This type of skull fracture requires early surgical treatment in which the fragments are elevated and any loose pieces or splinters are removed. In some instances, the surgeon may find it necessary to remove a portion of the skull which has been severely fragmented. Later, a cranioplasty may be done in which a "plate" of inert material, such as vitallium, may be inserted to protect the brain and improve the patient's appearance. The care of the patient following skull decompression is similar to that cited on page 637.

The bone is thinner in some areas of the base of the skull, making it less resistant to force. Basal fractures are more hazardous because they may open into paranasal sinuses or the middle ear, predisposing to infection. In some instances, the drainage of blood and cerebrospinal fluid from the nose and external ear may occur. Cranial nerves emerging through the skull may be injured, or if the fracture is adjacent to the medulla oblongata, vital centers may be seriously damaged.

---

*Débridement is the removal of foreign material and macerated, devitalized tissue.

Rarely, a skull fracture results from an indirect blow. The commonest cause is a fall from a height in which the person lands on his feet or buttocks. The impact of the spine against the head may produce a serious basal fracture.

Brain Injury. Slight or severe brain injury may result from a blow to the head and may or may not be associated with a fracture of the skull. A head injury may cause concussion, contusion, laceration, hemorrhage and compression. Injury may occur on the same side of the brain as the site of the impact and on the opposite side as well. The injury on the opposite side is due to the wave of pressure created by the blow, compressing the soft gelatinous-like brain substance against the bony ridges and opposite cranial wall. For instance, a fall on the back of the head may cause injury to the frontal and temporal cerebral lobes. Superficial and deeper cerebral vessels may be ruptured, meninges may be torn, and the brain tissue may be bruised, lacerated or compressed. The brain injury may be mild and reversible or may be severe and irreversible, leaving residual neurological deficits and disabilities if the patient survives. Cerebral edema and intracranial hemorrhage increase the intracranial pressure which, if severe, may compress the brain stem and its vital centers.

Concussion is characterized by a brief period of unconsciousness due to jarring of the brain and its sudden forceful contact with the rigid skull. Normal brain activity is temporarily interrupted, including the reticular-activating system of the brain stem which normally maintains the conscious state. The period of unconsciousness varies from a few minutes to several hours, depending on the severity of the injury. The patient presents a picture of shock; the face is pale, the pulse rate and respirations are depressed, the skin is cold and clammy and reflexes are diminished. Concussion is usually spontaneously reversible, leaving no permanent damage. When the patient regains consciousness he may be dazed, confused, restless and unable to recall what happened preceding the accident. Pulse and respirations improve and muscle tone and reflexes return. Vomiting is common in this recovery period, and the patient usually complains of headache.

Contusion (bruising) of the brain causes small, diffuse venous hemorrhages. The area in the region of the offending force becomes edematous and swollen, and intracranial pressure increases. The patient may recover from the associated concussion, but then he progressively regresses as the bleeding continues and intracranial pressure increases. Recovery from contusion may take several weeks. Permanent tissue damage and scarring may result in impaired motor, sensory and intellectual functions, or epilepsy.

Cerebral lacerations may occur when the brain is forced against rough and sharp ridges of bone. Meninges and vessels are torn, and intracranial hemorrhage follows, causing pressure.

Compression of the brain may result from a depressed fracture, edema and swelling of the brain and intracranial hemorrhage, which may be epidural, subdural, subarachnoid or intracerebral. The patient manifests progressive deepening of unconsciousness and symptoms of increasing intracranial pressure (see p. 630).

To summarize, the signs and symptoms associated with a head injury depend on the nature and severity of the tissue damage. They may appear immediately following the accident or several hours afterward as a result of cerebral edema, swelling of the brain or intracranial bleeding and the ensuing elevation in intracranial pressure. The symptoms may include: unconsciousness, which may develop at the time of injury and last for a varying length of time or may occur following a lucid interval and progressive drowsiness and stupor due to intracranial hemorrhage; headache and dizziness; disturbed vision; dilation and failure to react to light of one or both pupils; changes in vital signs, which may be characteristic of shock at first (low blood pressure, weak pulse and shallow respirations), then indicative of increasing intracranial pressure (abnormal elevation in blood pressure, slowing of the pulse); disorientation and confusion; motor and sensory deficits; convulsions; speech impairment; nuchal rigidity (stiffness of the neck) and hyperextension due to meningeal irritation; the escape of blood and cerebrospinal fluid through the nose or external ear; and hyperthermia due to interference with the heat-regulating center in the hypothalamus.

Treatment and Nursing Care

EMERGENCY CARE. As in all emergencies, the first consideration is to ensure a clear airway for respiratory exchange. The brain cells are very dependent upon a continuous oxygen supply, and if injured, adequate provision becomes even more imperative. A clear airway is also important because obstruction tends to increase cerebral venous congestion and intracranial pressure. Keeping the spine straight, the patient is carefully turned to a lateral or semiprone position to minimize the danger of aspiration. Flexion or hyperextension of the head is avoided in case there is a cervical vertebral fracture or dislocation that could seriously damage the spinal cord with movement. An open scalp wound is covered with available clean material. The victim is covered and kept quiet and undisturbed while arrangements are made to transport him to the hospital, even if he remains conscious.

On arrival at a hospital, further consideration is given to the airway; suctioning may be used to remove mucus, blood or vomitus; and an intratracheal tube may be introduced, or a tracheostomy may be done immediately. A mechanical respirator may be used if there is respiratory depression and insufficiency. The patient receives a quick, complete examination to determine the extent of the total injuries. Intravenous solutions, a blood transfusion and a vasopressor drug such as levarterenol (Levophed) may be necessary for shock. If there is an open wound, tetanus antitoxin or a reinforcing dose of tetanus toxoid may be ordered (see p. 39). X-rays of the skull are taken as soon as the initial emergency treatment is completed, and a lumbar puncture may be performed to determine if there is blood in the cerebrospinal fluid. If there is a compressed or compound fracture, or there are indications of a developing hematoma, immediate surgery may be necessary (see the care of the patient with intracranial surgery, p. 637).

The patient who has what appears to be a minor injury and who did not lose consciousness or recovered it within a few minutes of the accident may be permitted to go home after being examined by the physician. A family member or friend should remain with the patient and is advised to rouse and observe him hourly. The doctor should be notified or the patient taken to the hospital if he becomes abnormally drowsy or dizzy, vomits or experiences headache of increasing severity, visual disturbance or loss of strength in a limb.

Care of the nonsurgical patient with a head injury includes the following considerations.

OBSERVATIONS. Observation is an extremely important nursing responsibility in the care of the patient with a head injury so that significant changes and complications may be recognized in the early stage and treated promptly. On admission to the hospital, an assessment and recording are made of the patient's vital signs, level of consciousness, comprehension, orientation, responses to stimuli and commands, motor power of the limbs, and pupillary size and reaction. These initial observations serve as a guide in planning the nurse care and as a base line so that even slight changes may be readily recognized. The neurological evaluation is repeated usually at half-hour intervals for 24 hours. The physician is notified promptly of changes such as an increase in the blood pressure, decrease in pulse rate, dulling or loss of consciousness, inequality of pupils, and loss of strength in one or more limbs. The interval is gradually lengthened to 1 hour, then to 2, 3 and 4 hours as indicated by the physician on the basis of the patient's progress. The rectal temperature is usually recorded every 2 hours from the onset unless hyperthermia develops, making hourly recordings necessary. Some neurological units have a special form on which the frequent observations are recorded. In some situations, provision may be made for continuous monitoring of the heart action (electrocardiograph), cerebral activity (electroencephalogram), blood pressure and temperature.

When consciousness is regained soon after the injury, the patient is aroused gently and slowly every hour, if he goes to sleep, to determine his level of consciousness and to examine him for possible changes.

POSITIONING. If the patient is unconscious, he is kept in a lateral or semiprone position to prevent aspiration. Unless contraindicated by his particular injury, he is turned from side to side at least every 2 hours. The uppermost limbs are supported in order to prevent strain on the joints (see Positioning, p. 103). The neck is kept straight and is aligned with the spine. When the patient regains consciousness, the head of the bed is usually elevated slightly to encourage cerebral venous drainage.

PROTECTION FROM INJURY. Emergence from coma may be accompanied by restlessness and confusion, which may last for a brief period or for several days. Crib sides are used, and a nurse, nursing aide or relative remains in constant attendance to prevent self-injury. Restraints only tend to further agitate the patient and increase his thrashing about. A tranquilizer (e.g., chlorpromazine hydrochloride), barbiturate (e.g., phenobarbital) or paraldehyde may be ordered if absolutely necessary to prevent exhaustion from extreme restlessness. The use of strong sedatives and narcotics is avoided because they tend to mask neurological symptoms, and therefore their use may result in serious changes going unrecognized.

MIMIMUM OF STIMULI. The patient is kept as quiet as possible, being disturbed only for essential care. The blood pressure cuff is left on the arm between recordings. A semidarkened room and restriction of visitors help to reduce external stimuli.

FLUIDS AND NUTRITION. The patient may have to be supported by intravenous fluids or nasogastric tube feedings for a period of time. When conscious, oral fluids and a soft diet are given and increased to a light diet as soon as tolerated. The 24-hour volume of fluid may be limited if the patient manifests any signs of increased intracranial pressure. The intake and output are measured and recorded, and the balance is noted.

ELIMINATION. Occasionally, retention of urine may be present and may be responsible for the patient's restlessness. More often, incontinence of urine occurs. An indwelling catheter may be passed to protect the skin and to insure that an accurate record may be made of the urinary output. A mild laxative or a glycerin or bisacodyl (Dulcolax) rectal suppository may be ordered after 2 to 3 days if the bowels have not moved. Constipation, straining at stool and impaction must be prevented to avoid increasing the intracranial pressure. No enema is given without a physician's order.

SKIN CARE. While the patient is unconscious and during the period in which he is confined to bed on restricted activity, pressure areas require special attention to prevent decubitus ulcers. The usual measures of frequent change of position, keeping the skin clean and dry, massage and the use of soft resilient material under pressure areas or an air mattress are necessary. If the patient is restless, the elbows, knees and heels may require extra protection by the application of soft pads and bandages to prevent excoriation.

MEDICATIONS. A mild sedative or tranquilizer may be ordered to prevent exhaustion if the patient is extremely restless. Examples of drugs used are chlorpromazine hydrochloride (Thorazine), a barbiturate preparation such as phenobarbital, chloral hydrate and paraldehyde. The use of strong sedatives and narcotics is avoided, since they tend to mask neurological symptoms, and as a result, serious changes may not be recognized.

If the patient has received some brain injury, dexamethasone (Decadron) may be ordered to reduce possible cerebral edema by controlling the inflammatory process. Increased intracranial pressure may also be treated by inducing osmotic diuresis by the intravenous administration of mannitol (Osmitrol) or a hypertonic solution of urea and glucose (Urevert).

An anticonvulsant drug such as diphenylhydantoin sodium (Dilantin) or phenobarbital (Sodium Luminal) may be ordered parenterally if the patient has a seizure.

OTHER CONSIDERATIONS. If there is intracranial hemorrhage, the patient may develop a convulsion. The pillows are removed and the patient is placed in a lateral or semiprone position. He is restrained only sufficiently to prevent injury. It is important to note the parts of the body involved and which area was involved first, if the head and eyes turned to one side, the duration of the convulsion, and the condition of the patient following the seizure. (See p. 662 for care of the convulsive patient.)

The patient with a head injury commonly experiences a severe headache for several days following the accident. An ice bag may provide some relief and acetylsalicylic acid (Aspirin) may be prescribed.

If bleeding and the escape of cerebrospinal fluid from an ear or the nasal cavities occur with a fracture of the base of the skull, dry sterile absorbent cotton is placed loosely in the external orifice and is changed frequently. The amount and color of the drainage is noted and recorded. Under no circumstances should either area be packed tightly or any fluid introduced.

While the patient is unconscious, the eyes are examined closely once or twice daily for possible dryness of the cornea and failure of the eyelid to close. Brain injury may result in impaired nerve function, causing exposure of the eye and diminished secretion. Regular irrigation of each eye with sterile normal saline, the instillation of an oil and a protective eye shield may be necessary. Any sign of irritation is promptly brought to the physician's attention. Occasionally periocular edema, bleeding into the tissue and swelling are associated with a head injury. Iced compresses or a small ice bag may be applied. The fluid is usually absorbed, and the swelling is relieved in 3 or 4 days.

Hyperthermia may develop following an injury and is due to disturbance of the temperature-control center in the hypothalamus or infection. If the patient manifests an elevation of 38.6° C. (101° F.), the patient is covered only with a light cotton sheet, and fans or air-conditioning are used to keep the room temperature at 65° to 68° F. if possible. If the fever continues to rise, cold sponges are given and ice bags may be placed in the axillae and groin and along the sides of the trunk, or hypothermia may be ordered (see p. 71). Acetylsalicylic acid (Aspirin) may be ordered by mouth or may be given by rectum if the patient is unconscious. A progressive elevation of temperature is an unfavorable sign.

THE FAMILY. The family can be expected to be greatly concerned for the patient. The nurse has a responsibility to assist them and provide support by talking with them at intervals, acknowledging their anxiety, keeping them informed as to the patient's treatment and progress, and making suggestions in the interest of their own welfare as well as to how they can be most helpful to the patient. When the patient is well enough to leave the hospital, at least one member of the family is advised of the prescribed plan for continuity of care and rehabilitation. In some instances, when the accident victim has been the family provider, a referral to a social service or welfare agency may be necessary.

REHABILITATION. Following a head injury and brain damage, the patient may have some residual disability. He is evaluated, and a rehabilitation program of physical exercises and retraining is planned and started as soon as his condition permits. Progress may be slow, and the patient tends to become easily discouraged. The nurse plays an important role in providing reassuring support and encouraging him to keep trying. It requires patience and judgment to stand by and let the patient proceed, even though it may at times seem like a "cruel struggle." Activities are stopped if the patient manifests fatigue or complains of headache or dizziness. Before discharge from the hospital, the planned regimen of daily activities is outlined and reviewed with the patient and a member of his family.

Nursing Care of the Patient Treated by Intracranial Surgery

Operation. Intracranial surgery necessitates an opening in the skull. The size and location of the opening depend upon the nature and site of the lesion and the amount of exposure needed for the anticipated procedure. If the lesion is in the cerebrum, it is referred to as being supratentorial,* and the incision is usually well above the hairline. If it is in the cerebellar or brain stem regions, it is designated as infratentorial, and the incision is usually in the occipital region. The surgery may involve a craniectomy or a craniotomy. A craniectomy refers to the excision of a section of the skull and may vary from a small burr hole to a sizeable area of several centimeters. A craniotomy provides a relatively large opening and entails the freeing of a portion of the skull referred to as a bone flap. The flap is usually left attached to the muscle tissue and turned

---

*The tentorium is a fold of the dura mater between the cerebellum and the occipital lobes of the cerebrum.

back but may in some instances be freed, set aside and replaced at the completion of the operation. When the bone section is replaced, the procedure is referred to as an osteoplastic craniotomy. If it is not replaced because of needed decompression, a cranioplasty may be done later in which a plate of an especially prepared synthetic (vitallium or tantalum) or a bone graft is placed in the opening to provide protection for the brain and for cosmetic reasons.

Intracranial surgery may be done to obtain a tissue specimen for biopsy; to aspirate fluid; for exploratory purposes; to remove a neoplasm, hematoma, scar tissue which is causing seizures, or a specific area of tissue for the relief of tremors (e.g., pallidectomy or thalamotomy); to correct an aneurysm or vascular anomaly; to treat a decompressed or compound fracture; to drain an abscess; to relieve intracranial pressure; or to remove a foreign body (e.g., bullet).

Preoperative Preparation. If the patient is oriented and aware of his situation, he is likely to be quite apprehensive when advised of his need for surgery by his physician. Any impending surgery causes some anxiety, but that involving the brain is even more threatening. The alert patient is usually very fearful of permanent changes and disability, loss of competence, and death. The nurse conveys her understanding of his concern and encourages the patient to talk about his fears and ask questions. Verbal expression of his anxiety and sharing his problems help to reduce his tension. He should not be left alone for long periods. Investigative procedures and that which is likely to take place at the time of surgery and afterward are explained.

CONSENT FOR OPERATION. Surgery on the brain may carry the risk of a permanent change in appearance or function; this is explained to the competent patient and his family by the physician before the consent for operation is signed. It is the policy of most neurosurgeons and hospitals to require the signature of the patient and a close relative on the consent form. If the patient is not conscious or oriented, two relatives sign. The nurse must be familiar with the policy of the institution as to who may witness the signing of the consents.

IMPROVING THE PATIENT'S CONDITION. As with all surgery, the nutritional and hydrational status of the patient receives attention during the preoperative period, and any secondary or concomitant condition (e.g., infection, anemia) is corrected so that he goes to operation in the best possible condition. This includes the need for observing the patient's emotional reactions to the situation and making every effort to reduce his anxiety. As well as causing suffering and distress for the patient, fear may alter vital physiological activities through its effect on the autonomic nervous system and may influence his ability to cope with the stress of surgery. During this period of preparation, the patient is encouraged to remain ambulatory if his condition permits. If his lesion is such that his balance and mobility are impaired, safety precautions are taken to prevent falls.

OBSERVATIONS. The patient is observed for possible changes from day to day which may indicate a worsening of his condition. The nurse follows the vital signs closely; checks the pupils regularly for size, equality and reaction to light; and notes the patient's alertness, level of consciousness, orientation, sensory perception, motor ability and strength of the limbs. The final preoperative summary of these is essential for evaluating the patient's condition after the operation.

ELIMINATION. An enema is not usually ordered if the patient's bowels have been moving satisfactorily. If one is necessary, it is given slowly and the patient must be cautioned against straining to guard against increasing intracranial pressure. The bladder must be empty when the patient goes to the operating room. Frequently an indwelling catheter is passed the morning of operation to prevent postoperative incontinence and so that the output volume can be measured accurately.

SKIN PREPARATION. The hair is clipped and the head shampooed with an antiseptic such as hexachlorophene (pHisoHex) the afternoon or evening before operation. The cutting of the hair can be quite disturbing to the patient, since it alters his appearance. Before starting the preparation, a careful explanation is made to the patient as to why it is necessary, and suggestions are made to the female patient as to the wearing of colorful turbans or a wig later. In the case of a female, the hair is saved, being carefully placed in a bag and labeled in the event that the patient may wish to have a wig made later. Any rash, infection or abrasion of the scalp is brought to the surgeon's attention. Shaving and further cleansing of the operative site are usually done in the operating room. This more immediate preparation lessens the possibility of contamination. If the site necessitates exposure of an ear, a piece of sterile absorbent is placed in the external auditory canal following its cleansing with an antiseptic.

BLOOD TYPING. The blood loss may be considerable because of the vascularity of the scalp and brain. The patient's blood is typed and cross matched, and 1000 to 2000 ml. of blood is made available. An intravenous infusion may be started before the patient goes to the operating room so that blood, or a dehydrating preparation such as dexamethasone (Decadron) or mannitol (Osmitrol), may be readily administered during operation.

FOOD AND FLUIDS. No food is given after the evening meal the night before operation, and no fluids are taken by mouth within the 4- to 6-hour period preceding the scheduled time of surgery.

MEDICATIONS. A mild sedative may be ordered at bedtime the night before operation to ensure a good night's rest. Atropine sulphate may be prescribed to control respiratory secretions during inhalation anesthesia, but a narcotic is not usually given because of its depressing effect on respirations. Dexamethasone (Decadron) may be given to counteract subsequent brain edema and swelling.

THE FAMILY. It is natural that intracranial surgery creates a long, anxious period for the family. The doctor explains the patient's condition and what will be done at operation, and they are advised of any possibility of residual change in the patient's function, personality and appearance. The nurse acknowledges their concern, talks with them, answers their questions and keeps them informed about the patient's condition, giving them as much support and assistance as possible.

The day of operation, one or two family members are usually permitted to visit the patient briefly before he is taken to the operating room. Knowing they are near is reassuring to the patient. They are advised of the need to control their emotions when

with the patient as he is in need of their support. When he leaves the ward, they are told how long the operation might be (3 to 5 hours, depending on what is done) and are directed to a waiting room. The nurse visits them at intervals and suggests where they may go to have coffee or lunch. Appreciation of their concern increases their confidence in those caring for the patient.

Preparation to Receive the Patient. Preparation of the unit to receive the patient after operation includes the assembling of the following equipment:

The bed should have a low head piece so that the patient's head will be readily accessible.

The bed is made up with cotton sheets because of the neurosurgical patient's tendency to develop a high body temperature

Crib sides

Tongue forceps

Suction tubing and catheters

Airway (oropharyngeal and intratracheal) tubes

Tracheostomy tray

Sphygmomanometer and stethoscope

Flashlight

Rectal thermometer

Special neurological recording sheets

Intravenous pole

Urine drainage receptable

Mouth care tray

If the temperature of the room is thermostatically controlled it is usually set at 65° to 68° F. A hypothermic blanket should be available (see p. 71).

Postoperative Care. Care following the operation includes the following considerations (obviously these are modified according to the findings and what was done at operation and the surgeon's orders).

POSITIONING. The patient is placed in a lateral or semiprone position. A small pillow is placed under the head to maintain good neck alignment. The pillow is positioned so that the mouth is dependent at the edge of the pillow to allow free drainage of secretions and vomitus. The limbs are positioned and supported as for any unconscious patient (see p. 103). The surgeon's orders will indicate if the head of the bed is to be elevated or kept flat. If the surgery has been on the cerebrum, the head of the bed is usually slightly elevated unless contraindicated by shock. Following infratentorial surgery (cerebellum or brain stem), the bed is generally kept flat for 2 to 3 days.

The patient's position is changed from side to side to back (only if conscious) to side every 2 hours unless contraindicated. If a relatively large space-occupying lesion has been removed, he is usually not permitted to lie on the operative side in order to prevent a shifting of the brain into the remaining space. In the case of surgery in the occipital region, restrictions are usually placed on the dorsal recumbent position for 2 to 4 days, since the brain stem may have been affected, resulting in a dulling of the gag and swallowing reflexes, predisposing to aspiration. Keeping this patient off his back also prevents pressure on the incision as well as possible forward flexion of the head which places a strain on the incision. It is helpful in avoiding mistakes if a notice indicating the restricted position is posted in a prominent place on the head of the bed.

When the patient is repositioned, he is turned slowly and with adequate support for the head so that it and the trunk are turned as if they were one single unit. Sudden movement and jarring are avoided at all times. Particular attention is paid to bony prominences and pressure areas each time the patient is turned to prevent pressure sores. The bedding must be kept dry and free of wrinkles. An air mattress may be used, and pieces of soft, resilient material are placed under vulnerable areas.

OBSERVATIONS. The blood pressure, pulse and respirations are recorded, and the size, equality and reaction to light of the pupils and the level of consciousness are noted at regular frequent intervals. If the patient is conscious, his alertness and orientations as well as the motion and strength of his limbs are also checked. The required frequency of these observations is indicated by the physician but usually begins with 15-minute intervals which are lengthened to one-half hour and then one hour if the signs remain stable. Other significant observations include the color, condition of the skin (dry or moist and the temperature) and the fluid balance (fluid intake and output). Careful scrutiny is made of the dressing frequently for moisture and blood stains.

CLEAR AIRWAY. As well as lateral or semiprone positioning to maintain a patent airway, it may be necessary to remove secretions from the mouth and nose by means of suctioning. The catheter is moistened in normal saline or water before introducing it and is used gently to prevent injury to the mucous membrane lining. The respirations are checked frequently for any manifestations of an obstructed airway or respiratory distress. The lower jaw and tongue must be forward to prevent blocking of the pharynx.

If there are indications of accumulated secretions in the lower respiratory tract or that the patient is having respiratory difficulty, a tracheotomy may be performed to permit deep suctioning of the trachea and bronchi with a sterile endobronchial catheter. The catheter is pinched while being introduced to avoid injury of the mucous membrane which may incur bleeding and the formation of clots, which would interfere with the passage of air. A special nebulizer may be used to provide moistened air or oxygen for inhalation through the tracheotomy tube. (See p. 284 for tracheotomy care.)

If the patient is capable of responding, he is required to take 7 to 10 deep breaths every 2 to 3 hours. Coughing is used as a part of the chest routine only if approved by the doctor because of the danger of increasing intracranial pressure.

HEAD DRESSING. If the dressing becomes moist or blood stained, it is promptly reinforced with sterile pads and reported. Depending on the operative procedure, a drain may have been inserted and is usually removed in 24 to 48 hours. Following an infratentorial operation, the head may be slightly hyperextended when the dressing is applied. Long strips of adhesive may extend from the head down to the scapular region. This immobilizes the head and prevents lateral and forward flexion which would place a strain on the incision.

The initial dressing is usually changed in approximately 5 days by the surgeon. The sutures may be removed then or on the sixth or seventh postoperative day. The area may then be left exposed. The scalp may be cleansed with hydrogen peroxide to remove old blood. An application of oil or petrolatum jelly will soften any crusts that may have formed and the scalp may then be washed with an antiseptic solution. The incision is inspected once or twice daily and is cleansed with a prescribed antiseptic.

RESTLESSNESS. Restlessness is usually associated with cerebral disturbances, but it should be kept in mind that it might also be caused by head bandages being too tight, retention of urine, or feces in the rectum. To prevent the restless or disoriented patient from dislodging tubes (nasogastric, catheter, tracheotomy, intravenous) or his head dressing, restraint mitts may be applied. Dressing pads are placed between the fingers which are slightly flexed over a roll of dressing placed across the palm of the hand. A large dressing pad is then wrapped over the fingers and the hand bandaged, usually with flanelette for security. A piece of tubular stockinette is then pulled over the bandaged hand and secured with adhesive. Mitts are changed daily; the hands are washed and lightly powdered and the fingers and thumb massaged and passively moved several times through their range of motion. Ordinary restraints are not used because straining against them only tends to further agitate the patient and may also raise the intracranial pressure.

If the patient is extremely restless, the skin will require additional care. Friction areas may be lightly oiled or powdered at frequent intervals, and the elbows and heels may have to be padded and bandaged for protection. Crib sides may have to be padded to prevent injury.

Crib sides are kept in position unless someone is at the bedside with the patient. This applies for a considerable period of time even though the patient has regained consciousness and is oriented. Following intracranial surgery, patients frequently are subject to spells of dizziness and lapses of orientation or may be slow in regaining their postural reflexes.

FLUIDS AND NUTRITION. Fluids are generally given intravenously for the first 24 to 48 hours. The amount is specifically limited (usually 1000 to 2000 ml.) and is given slowly to avoid a rapid increase in the intravascular volume and an ensuing rise in blood pressure. If the patient remains unconscious or semicomatose for several days, nasogastric feedings are given every 3 to 4 hours to provide necessary fluid and nutri-

tion. When oral fluids are permitted, only a small amount is given at first through a drinking tube, and the patient is observed closely for any depression of the swallowing reflex. Following certain operations, especially those that are infratentorial, the ability to swallow may be impaired. If there is no difficulty in swallowing and no vomiting, fluids are given freely unless limited to a certain volume per 24 hours because of cerebral edema and increased intracranial pressure. The diet is gradually increased to include soft solid foods and is progressed to a full diet as tolerated. The patient is fed for the first few days to avoid fatigue and ensure an adequate intake.

ELIMINATION. Since these patients may be incontinent or may have retention of urine, an indwelling catheter may be passed previous to surgery or after the patient is returned to the neurosurgical unit. Because a retention catheter predisposes to bladder infection, a continuous drip of an antimicrobial solution may be attached to the catheter which is connected also to a closed drainage system. In the case of a male patient who is incontinent, the doctor may prefer the use of an external penile sheath (condom) to the indwelling catheter. The sheath is connected by tubing to a urine receptacle. The urinary output is measured every 8 or 12 hours and is compared with the fluid intake to determine the fluid balance.

MOUTH AND EYE CARE. Following intracranial surgery, especially during the unconscious period, one or both eyelids may remain open, exposing the conjunctiva and cornea to drying and injury. A special eye shield (not a pad) may be applied for protection. The eyes are bathed with sterile normal saline or water at regular intervals, and the instillation of an oil or ointment may be prescribed. The eyes are carefully inspected for any irritation, blood streaks and discharge which, if present, are brought to the physician's attention.

It is important, especially if the patient is on restricted fluids, that the teeth and mouth receive frequent cleansing to prevent drying and the accumulation of sordes, which predispose to infection (e.g., parotitis).

Bowel elimination is usually disregarded for 3 or 4 days postoperatively. A mild laxative such as mineral oil or milk of magnesia may be ordered on the third day. If this is ineffective, a small enema may be prescribed, depending on the patient's condition. The patient must be cautioned against straining at stool, since this raises intracranial pressure.

MEDICATIONS. Sedatives and analgesics are not usually used because they may mask important neurological symptoms and depress respirations. Discomfort and headache may be controlled by acetylsalicylic acid (Aspirin) or a small dose of codeine. If the patient is extremely restless or develops a convulsive seizure, sodium phenobarbital or diphenylhydantoin sodium (Dilantin) may be ordered parenterally. Dexamethasone (Decadron) is frequently given to counteract cerebral edema resulting from the inflammatory process incurred by the trauma of surgery.

EXERCISE AND AMBULATION. The limbs are passively moved through a full range of motion 2 or 3 times daily to preserve joint mobility. Active limb exercises are begun when indicated by the physician. The patient is assisted out of bed as soon as his condition permits. Before this takes place, the head of the bed is gradually elevated, and the patient is observed for any untoward reactions. When up in a chair, a draw sheet may be secured around the waist and the back of the chair to prevent a possible fall should the patient develop dizziness or sudden weakness. A nurse remains with the patient, closely observing his reactions. If he complains of headache or dizziness or shows signs of fatigue or a fall in blood pressure, he is returned to bed. The time he remains up is gradually increased as tolerated. When he begins to walk, someone must accompany him until he is quite safe on his feet and sure of his balance.

PERSONAL APPEARANCE. The female patient may be very self-conscious about her appearance without her hair. She is encouraged to use colorful scarves as turbans. The suggestion of a wig may also be made.

If the patient is lethargic and disinterested in appearance and dress, he is urged to improve his grooming and to dress when he is well enough to be up most of the day, rather then spend the day in a dressing gown. Gradually this tends to improve the patient's morale.

REHABILITATION. Following intracranial surgery, the patient is quite dependent upon the nurse for complete care for a few days, but as soon as he is well enough, he is encouraged to perform self-care activities. In some instances, there may be loss of movement in one or more limbs or impairment of speech and intellectual ability. A rehabilitation program is planned and instituted as soon as possible with the goal of restoring the patient to independent, useful living within his potentialities. This may involve the physiotherapist, speech therapist and social worker as well as the physician and nurse. The patient may have to relearn the performance of ordinary daily activities and progress from the simple to the more complex, much as the child learns. It is frequently a slow process, and both the patient and his family are likely to have periods of depression and discouragement. The nurse must maintain an optimistic attitude and patience, providing support and encouragement for both the patient and his family, but at the same time appreciate and acknowledge their problems. Emphasis is placed on the positive, and the patient is praised when he accomplishes certain activities. He may not be able to resume his former occupation, and eventual retraining for a different type of work may be undertaken as part of the rehabilitation. The social worker may help the family with the socioeconomic problems resulting from this illness.

Before the patient is discharged from the hospital, he and his family are informed about the exercises and activities that are to be continued. It is helpful if a day's schedule is given to them in writing. A referral is made to the visiting nurse agency so that guidance and support are continued. A referral may also be made to a rehabilitation center, or the patient may remain under the supervision of the hospital rehabilitation department.

Complications. The most common complications that may develop after intracranial surgery include hyperthermia, increased intracranial pressure, respiratory failure and convulsive seizures.

Following intracranial surgery, the patient tends to develop an elevation of temperature due to a disturbance of the temperature-regulating center and mechanisms in the hypothalamus and brain stem. To counteract this tendency, if his temperature is normal, the room temperature is kept at 65° to 68° F. and only a cotton sheet and spread are used as covers. If the patient's temperature rises above 38° C. (100° F.), it is reported to the physician. The spread is removed from the bed, and the sheet is arranged to cover only the lower half of the body. Acetylsalicylic acid (Aspirin) by rectal suppository and an increase in the fluid intake may be ordered. If the temperature continues to rise, especially if it exceeds 39° C. (102° F.), cool temperature sponge baths, the breeze of an electric fan directed on the patient, and the application of ice bags to the axillae, groins and lateral surfaces of the trunk may be employed. If the room temperature cannot be controlled satisfactorily, it may be helpful to place the patient in an oxygen tent. If these measures are not successful in controlling the hyperthermia, a hypothermia blanket with iced water circulating through the coils may be used.

Edema of the brain resulting from the trauma and inflammation incurred by surgery is generally the cause of postoperative increased intracranial pressure, but it may also develop as a result of hemorrhage. The signs and symptoms have been cited previously on page 630. Close observation of the patient and prompt reporting of any significant changes may prevent compression of brain tissue and death of the patient. The head of the bed is elevated to promote cerebral venous drainage, the fluid intake is restricted, and drugs are given to dehydrate the brain. The drugs administered are principally hypertonic solutions which are given intravenously. They cause the transfer of fluid from the brain tissue into the vascular compartment by osmosis and increase the urinary output. Those most commonly used are mannitol (Osmitrol) and urea (Urevert). Fifty per cent glucose may also be used. A saturated solution of magnesium sulfate given as a retention enema is rarely used. Dexamethasone (Decadron) which is anti-inflammatory is given postoperatively to reduce the incidence and severity of cerebral edema. A larger dose may be ordered for parenteral administration if the patient manifests increased intracranial pressure. If the prescribed dehydrating drug is not effective, a lumbar puncture may be done to remove some cerebrospinal fluid.

Respiratory failure may result from compression of the respiratory center in the brain stem (medulla). It is more likely to occur following surgery in the cerebellar and brain stem regions. The patient's respirations may be rapid and stertorous for a period; then gradually they may change and become Cheyne-Stokes or slow and shallow. Any change in the respirations is reported immediately.

The patient may develop convulsive seizures following intracranial surgery as a result of brain irritation, compression or scar tissue. It may be preceded by restlessness and twitching or may occur suddenly without warning. Pillows are removed and the patient is turned on his side as soon as possible to prevent obstruction of the airway and facilitate the drainage of accumulated oropharyngeal secretions. It may be possible to place a folded washcloth between the patient's teeth to prevent biting of the tongue, but if the teeth are clenched, no attempt should be made to pry them open, since fracture of a tooth or injury to the gums might occur. Only sufficient restraint to prevent injury is used. He must not be left alone, but someone is dispatched to notify the doctor as soon as possible. The nurse notes the nature of the onset, the initial or focal site of involvement, the direction in which the head and eyes are turned, whether the muscle responses are tonic or clonic, the duration of the seizure and the condition of the patient following the convulsion (stuporous, oriented, memory of what preceded the incident and vital signs). Sodium phenobarbital or diphenylhydantoin sodium (Dilantin) may be ordered parenterally.

If the seizure occurs when the patient is in a chair, he is gently eased to the floor. A folded towel or whatever is available is placed under his head to prevent injury.

If the family or visitors were present at the onset of the seizure, they are given an explanation and are assured that the convulsive movements have ceased. If there are other patients in the room, a screen is placed around the patient as soon as possible, since they may become quite disturbed and frightened.

Spinal Cord Injury

Accidental injury to the spinal cord is most commonly associated with a fracture of one or more vertebrae. The fracture may be the result of sudden forceful angulation of the spine (hyperflexion or hyperextension), excessive force applied along the axis of the spine (e. g., landing on the feet or buttocks from a height) or a direct blow. In some instances, rupture and posterior extrusion of the intervertebral disk may also occur. The degree of damage sustained by the cord varies, depending mainly on whether or not the fracture fragments are displaced (fracture dislocation). The cord may be contused, lacerated, or subjected to compression. Bleeding into the tissue and edema may occur, causing swelling and compression of the nerve tracts. The damage may be slight and completely reversible, or it may leave a minor degree of residual impairment. A laceration which transects the cord or causes severe compression may result in complete, irreversible interruption of ascending or descending tracts. Interruption of ascending tracts causes loss of sensation below the site of injury. Interruption of descending tracts results in paralysis of the parts deriving their innervation from the cord below the level of the lesion. Autonomic nervous function may also be disturbed.

Manifestations. The symptoms of cord injury depend on the level and degree of damage. The patient may complain of pain in the neck or back or in areas supplied by the nerves leaving the injured spinal region. Angulation of the spine may be evident. There is likely to be loss of sensation, motor ability (weakness or paralysis) and reflexes below the level of the lesion. The bladder is atonic, resulting in retention of urine, and vomiting and abdominal distention may develop as a result of paralysis of intestinal peristalsis (paralytic ileus). There may be a lack or excess of perspiration by the skin below the lesion due to disturbed autonomic innervation.

Cervical cord injury may cause paralysis from the neck down (quadriplegia). Respiratory insufficiency or complete failure occurs if there is involvement of the nerve supply to the diaphragm and intercostal muscles. Injury below the cervical region may cause paralysis of the lower limbs, bladder and rectum (paraplegia). Any recovery usually occurs within 1 to 2 weeks; if the loss of function persists beyond this period, the damage is usually irreversible. The cord

and its tracts are not capable of regeneration, but regeneration of the nerve roots (outside of the cord) can occur if the neurilemma is not severely damaged (see p. 590). Spasticity of the paralyzed muscles and exaggerated tendon reflexes usually follow the initial flaccidity of the first few days in cord injury. The bladder becomes hypertonic and frequent automatic emptying develops. When paralysis occurs as a result of injury to the cauda equina (lumbar or sacral region), flaccid paralysis and an absence of reflexes persist.

Treatment and Nursing Care. When a spinal injury is known to have occurred or is suspected, the handling and transportation is of great importance in the prevention of cord damage or additional impairment.

EMERGENCY CARE. At the scene of the accident, the victim is advised to lie still. To determine if there is cord injury and the level, he may be requested to move his toes and fingers. Loss of sensation may be assessed by gentle pinching at various levels. He is covered and kept flat while other immediate emergencies (respiratory insufficiency and bleeding) are cared for, and movement and transportation are quickly organized. A firm, flat improvised stretcher such as a door or wide plank is provided. Five or 6 persons are recruited to lift the patient and are instructed that he must be moved as a single rigid unit; even slight flexion and twisting of the spine may cause irreversible cord damage. Slight traction is applied to the head and lower extremities as he is lifted to the stretcher. Straps or strips of cloth are placed over the patient and around the stretcher to secure the patient and prevent movement. Something firm is placed at either side of the head and someone remains at the head of the stretcher providing additional support to prevent any movement of the neck in transit.

On arrival at the hospital, the patient remains on the stretcher during examination and x-rays and while the treatment bed or frame which is to be used is prepared to ensure a minimum of movement.

TREATMENT. The treatment depends on the location of the fracture and whether or not there is dislocation and indications of cord compression. Traction or hyperextension may be used to reduce the fracture. Cervical spinal injury is usually treated by skeletal traction of 10 to 30 pounds, which is applied by means of tongs (Crutchfield or Barton) that are inserted into the skull at approximately the midlateral line, a short distance above the ears. The sites of insertion of the tongs are inspected daily for signs of inflammation and infection, and following cleansing with a prescribed antiseptic, fresh sterile dressings are applied. If only slight traction is required, a halter-like arrangement may be used in place of the tongs, but prolonged continuous application usually causes considerable discomfort and skin irritation for the patient by the pressure and pull of the straps, especially under the chin. The patient may be on an ordinary bed with his head at the foot. A second mattress is added so that the traction will clear the head of the bed. The upper end of the bed may be raised on shock pins or blocks to prevent the patient from sliding down because of the traction. The Foster turning bed may be used in place of an ordinary bed; it provides a pivoting device which permits turning without interference to the appliance or traction. When reduction and sufficient healing are achieved, the patient is fitted with a neck brace or plastic collar to provide cervical immobilization and support, and he is ambulated slowly and progressively.

When there is a thoracic or lumbar spinal fracture without dislocation of the fragments, the patient may be placed flat on a firm mattress and fracture board on an ordinary bed or on a turning bed for several weeks. If the ordinary bed is used, specific directions are received as to whether the patient must remain on his back at all times. If turning is permitted, precautions are taken to ensure good alignment and avoidance of movement and displacement of the fragments. When the patient must remain on his back continuously, a sponge rubber mattress may be placed on top of the firm mattress. This facilitates the changing of the lower bed linen and the giving of frequent back care. A nurse on each side of the bed, working from the head down, uses one hand to depress the mattress while caring for the skin or changing the linen with the other one. When there is sufficient healing, the patient is gradually ambulated. A brace or firm corset may be necessary for several months to provide support and immobility of the spine.

A fracture dislocation of thoracic or lumbar vertebrae may be treated by hyperextension of the spine which may be achieved by various methods. The patient may be placed on the regular gatch bed and the gatch raised in line with the fracture. This may necessitate placing the patient's head at the foot of the bed. An alternative method is the placing of a firm roll or sandbag across the bed under the mattress to provide the required angulation. Fracture boards are placed on the springs, and a very firm mattress is used on which a sponge rubber mattress is placed, since the patient must remain in the supine position.

In some instances a plaster cast is used to immobilize the spine following a fracture in the thoracic or lumbar region. It usually extends from the shoulders to below the hips. An opening may be cut in the cast over the abdomen to prevent pressure and discomfort in that area. The cast edges are bound by the stockinette, which is under the cast, being turned back and secured with adhesive. The skin areas at the borders of the cast are examined daily for possible irritation. The cast is cut back over the buttocks sufficiently to accommodate the use of the bedpan without soiling of the cast. Extra precautions are taken to protect it by the use of pieces of waterproof material such as plastic.

Surgical treatment may be necessary in some spinal injuries to relieve compression of the cord or if the dislocation cannot be reduced by traction or hyperextension. The operation may involve a laminectomy and spinal fusion (see p. 651 for nursing care).

NURSING THE PATIENT WITHOUT CORD INVOLVEMENT. If the spinal cord is intact and undamaged in the case of a spinal fracture, nursing care is directed toward: the maintenance of alignment and stability of the spine to prevent cord and nerve damage and promote healing of the fractured vertebra; the prevention of complications such as decubitus ulcers and respiratory disease; and general supportive care (psychological and physiological).

The patient is observed closely for signs of cord compression. Any loss of motor strength or ability, loss of sensation, respiratory distress, retention of urine or incontinence, or vomiting and abdominal distention which might be indicative of paralytic ileus

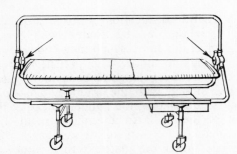

Figure 22–16 The Stryker frame, which facilitates the turning of certain patients (e.g., those who have had spinal injury or surgery or who have sustained severe burns). (From Sutton, A. L.: *Bedside Nursing Techniques,* 2nd ed. Philadelphia, W. B. Saunders Co., 1969, p. 198.)

must be reported promptly. During the period of immobilization, pressure areas require frequent attention and are inspected 2 or 3 times daily for early signs of irritation and breaks in the skin. Usually, the patient is restricted to the supine position if on an ordinary bed; frequent changing of lower sheets is achieved by 2 nurses working together as cited previously. If there is a possibility of restlessness or of the patient moving, a draw sheet placed over the patient and secured at the sides may deter moving and turning, or long sandbags placed along either side of the patient may be necessary, especially during the night. If the physician sanctions turning, sufficient persons are necessary to maintain alignment and stability of the spine while turning the patient as one immovable unit.

Having the patient on a turning bed (Stryker frame or Foster bed) has several distinct advantages. It facilitates turning the patient from the supine to prone position and vice versa with minimal risk of movement of the vertebrae and reduces the discomfort and strain for the patient in the process. It allows more frequent turning to protect the skin and the use of a bedpan without the patient having to be raised as well as eliminating the need for more than 2 nurses to turn the patient (see Fig. 22–16).

The turning bed has 2 metal frames to which sheets of canvas are firmly attached. The patient's position is changed by turning the whole frame on which he lies. This is possible by pivots at each end of the frame which are locked except during the turning. The frame that is used when he is on his

back (posterior frame) has an opening in the canvas in the buttocks and perineal area which permits the use of a bedpan that is placed on a rack beneath the opening when necessary. One end of a piece of waterproof material may be tucked under the buttocks while the other end is placed in the bedpan to direct the flow of excreta and protect the canvas. Following the use of the bedpan, the patient may be turned to thoroughly clean and dry the perineal area and buttocks. A strip of canvas attached to one side of the frame is brought across the opening in the frame and secured when the patient is not using the bedpan.

The sheets used to cover the frames must be free of wrinkles and are secured usually by large safety pins on the undersurface. In the case of the posterior frame, 2 sheets are used, 1 above and 1 below the opening. A narrow strip of sheeting is used over the canvas covering the opening.

In the supine position, a small flat pillow may be permitted under the head. A small bolster of foam rubber or toweling may be placed under the knees to provide support without flexion. A footboard attaches to the frame to support the feet in dorsiflexion. The arms are supported on arm rests to which sponge rubber pillows are secured. In the case of weakness or paralysis of the arms, additional support may be necessary. The patient's gown is usually left open at the back and tucked against his sides to avoid his lying on wrinkles. Sufficient light top covers are used to keep the patient comfortable. If the patient finds the canvas too hard, the doctor may permit the use of a thin layer of sponge rubber on each frame. This is usually enclosed in cotton to which tapes are added for securing the mattress to the frame.

To turn the patient from the supine to prone position, the arm and foot supports and top bedding are removed, and the anterior frame is placed over the patient and secured to the "bed" frame at either end by means of heavy screws. Unnecessary exposure is avoided at all times; the pubic area is covered with a towel or draw sheet that can be easily removed after turning. Two or three straps are then securely placed around the frames and the spring lock released at each end. The frames are then turned quickly and smoothly. The spring locks automatically when the frame bearing the patient is in the correct position but should be tested before the turners' holds are released. The posterior frame is then removed and the arm rests are replaced. The upper border of the canvas on the anterior frame only extends to the neck. The head is supported by a strip of canvas on which the forehead rests. This leaves the patient's face free. A rack placed below the head will hold a book, meal tray or other personal articles which should be readily accessible to the patient. A pillow is used under the ankles, and the feet are suspended over the end of the canvas.

The turning bed is not used when the spinal lesion is treated by hyperextension or in the case of a cervical injury without the use of tongs. Rarely, it is not appropriate because of the patient's excessive height or weight or persisting fear of the turning.

During the prolonged period of immobility, a high-protein, high-vitamin diet is recommended to prevent pressure sores, promote healing, maintain resistance to respiratory complications and prevent a negative nitrogen balance. Prolonged immobilization predisposes to the movement of calcium out of the bones and ensuing hypercalcemia. This favors the formation of renal and bladder calculi. The patient is encouraged to take a minimum of 3000 ml. of fluid daily to prevent concentration and stasis of the urine. His daily calcium intake, mainly in the form of milk and milk products, may have to be restricted to some degree. Swallowing is difficult for the patient who must remain flat on his back or in a position of spinal hyperextension; choking and aspiration may occur readily. Suction should be readily available in the event of aspiration, since he cannot be turned or raised. The patient is fed slowly, and only small amounts of food and fluid taken into the mouth at one time.

The patient is urged to practice brief periods of deep breathing several times a day; coughing may be contraindicated, since it raises the intraspinal pressure and is also likely to jar the fracture site. With the doctor's permission, a daily exercise regimen may be established. The limbs are gently moved through their full range of motion, and isotonic and isometric active exercises may be gradually introduced.

These activities are important in maintaining joint mobility and muscle tone and in stimulating circulation.

Constipation may be a problem because of the inactivity; dietary adjustments such as the inclusion of increased roughage and fruit juices may be necessary. A mild laxative or glycerin or bisacodyl (Dulcolax) suppositories may also be used.

Some provision is made for diversion, for the hours and days generally pass slowly for the patient. A mirror attached to the head of the bed may permit him to see what is going on about him. Special prism glasses may be provided for reading, and visitors are encouraged to spend time with him.

When the patient is allowed up after such a prolonged period of immobility, he assumes the upright position slowly and gradually, and someone should be with him in case fainting or dizziness is a problem. The patient may be required to wear a brace or corset for a considerable period of time. A good walking shoe or a firm slipper with a heel should be worn when beginning ambulation. He is instructed how to prevent strain on his spine; lifting and bending are avoided usually for several months and previous activities are resumed gradually.

NURSING THE PATIENT WITH CORD DAMAGE. The most obvious disability in cord injury is paralysis of limbs (paraplegia or quadriplegia), but it is only one of a number of dysfunctions, some of which are a direct result of the cord damage while others are secondary consequences.

Direct neurological effects include loss of voluntary movement, varying degrees of muscle spasm in the paralyzed parts, impairment of sensation which interferes with the patient's adaptation to his environment, and disturbance of some autonomic functions. Interference with autonomic nerve pathways may be manifested by an excess or absence of perspiration which may cause impairment in body temperature regulation. Lack of vascular responses may also occur which may cause postural hypotension, posing a problem later when the patient assumes a sitting or standing position.

The secondary or extraneurological effects of cord injury include bladder and bowel dysfunction, pressure sores which may develop very rapidly due to the immobility, loss of sensation and alterations in local circulation, mobilization of bone calcium, negative nitrogen balance, and emotional reactions to the disabilities and their implications.

The care of the patient with spinal cord involvement is planned according to the amount of damage and the individual patient's reactions and specific needs. He is nursed on a turning bed if possible to facilitate frequent turning. The paralyzed limbs are tested and observed for signs of any return of sensation and movement. A close check is made of the urinary output, and the amount of perspiration on parts below the level of the lesion is noted. The vulnerable pressure areas are examined frequently for discoloration, edema and broken areas, and the patient's psychological reactions are observed.

The bladder generally goes through 3 stages: it is atonic at first, causing a complete retention of urine without the patient experiencing any discomfort or sensation of needing to void; then hypotonicity develops, manifested by retention with overflow, and the patient involuntarily voids small amounts frequently. Later, the bladder becomes hypertonic; its capacity is diminished, and frequent reflex voiding develops. Bladder infection leading to pyelonephritis and eventual renal insufficiency is probably the most serious complication of paraplegia and the greatest constant threat to the patient's life. Stasis and residual urine predispose to infection and the formation of calculi. The bladder should be completely emptied at regular intervals, and the patient should have a minimal fluid intake of 3000 ml. daily. Strict aseptic precautions in catheterization and a sterile closed drainage system are extremely important in preventing infection.

An indwelling catheter is introduced soon after admission to prevent bladder damage by overdistension and involuntary voiding with ensuing skin irritation and maceration. Continuous drainage is used at first; then later, the catheter is clamped for stated intervals to counteract the hypertonicity and diminished bladder capacity. An antiseptic bladder irrigation may be ordered 3 or 4 times daily, or a continuous drip may be used as a prophylactic measure. Frequent change of position also helps to prevent residual urine and calculus formation.

Tidal (Munro) drainage may be instituted which simulates physiological functioning of the bladder. A prescribed solution enters the bladder by gravity at the rate of 40 to 60 drops per minute. The bladder fills with urine and the solution to a predetermined volume, and then drainage is initiated by siphonage. The volume allowed to collect in the bladder is indicated by the physician on the basis of the intravesical pressure and controlled by the height at which the loop of the drainage tube is fixed. The higher the loop is above the drainage, the greater will be the volume that collects in the bladder before siphonage drainage is initiated, and vice versa. (For details of the apparatus, see a nursing procedure text.) Tidal irrigation may be used to prevent the overstretching of a hypotonic bladder or the diminished capacity if it is hypertonic. As soon as possible, the catheter is removed and training to establish automatic control is begun (see p. 16).

Loss of the sensation for the need for defecation is lost, and the lower bowel functions reflexly, causing involuntary stools. Because of the immobility and loss of tone, the paralyzed patient is predisposed to constipation and impaction, especially in the early stages of his illness. An enema or suppository may be used daily or every other day to evacuate the bowel at first; then, as the patient's general condition improves and his diet becomes more normal, involuntary stools occur. The diet may be adjusted to the stool consistency and frequency to help in regulation. A regular hour for bowel elimination is established by using a glycerin or biscodyl (Dulcolax) suppository or by inserting a lubricated gloved finger to initiate defecation (see p. 15). Following a high cord injury, intestinal peristalsis may be depressed, causing severe abdominal distention and vomiting (paralytic ileus). A Miller-Abbott tube may be passed and gastrointestinal suction established (see p. 338). A peristaltic stimulant such as neostigmine (Prostigmin) and bethanecholchloride (Urecholine) may be prescribed, and a rectal tube is inserted or an enema given. During this period the patient is sustained by intravenous solutions.

A high-protein, high-vitamin diet is important to combat the tendency to a negative nitrogen balance due to immobility and to promote tissue resistance and healing power. An adequate intake may be a problem as a result of the patient's emotional reactions and inactivity. Dietary supplements between meals may be given to meet the patient's needs. Food is placed conveniently within reach, and the paraplegic is encouraged to feed himself as soon as his general condition permits. The quadriplegic needs to be fed until appropriate assistive devices are available. Food and fluids with a high calcium content (e.g., milk and milk products) may be restricted because of the tendency to renal and bladder calculi formation. If a stone develops, the patient may be placed on an acid-ash or alkaline-ash diet, depending on the composition of the calculus.

To prevent pressure sores to which paraplegic and quadriplegic patients are especially predisposed, frequent skin care must begin within a few hours of the injury. The patient is turned every 1 or 2 hours, day and night. The skin is kept clean and dry, and circulation is stimulated by gentle massage, especially the vulnerable areas such as the sacrum, buttocks, scapulae, heels and ankles (malleoli). The bedding is kept free of wrinkles, crumbs, pieces of tissues, etc. Pieces of resilient material such as sponge rubber and synthetic sheepskin may be used under pressure areas. If the patient is on an ordinary bed, an alternating pressure mattress is helpful. Alcohol is used to toughen the skin, but if it is too drying, a small amount of oil or lanolin may be applied. Talcum powder is used sparingly; an excess may form granules, especially if the patient's skin is moist, and cause irritation. If a decubitus ulcer develops, various methods of treatment are used. Whatever the physician's choice (e.g., compresses of hygeol, antimicrobial preparation, cleansing with hydrogen peroxide and the application of vaseline gauze, heat lamp therapy, gelfoam sponges), nursing aims are to keep the wound clean, as dry as possible, free of infection and to promote healing. If the area is large and resists healing, débridement and skin grafting may be necessary. With a large open area there is a marked loss of serum and protein. The patient's protein and vitamin C intake is increased to replace the loss, increase resistance to infection and promote healing.

Each time the patient is turned, the nurse checks the position of the paralyzed limbs to ensure good alignment. Trochanter rolls and supports may be necessary to prevent contractures and deformities that may develop with spasticity in the affected limbs. With the doctor's approval, limbs are moved through their full range of motion 2 or 3 times daily. Active exercises of nonparalyzed limbs are introduced when the patient's condition permits and are progressively increased in preparation for rehabilitation. The patient may require mild analgesics (e.g., acetylsalicylic acid, codeine) for pain.

Understandably, the disabilities associated with spinal cord injury and their implications are a severe shock to the patient and his family. Each patient will react in his own particular way. The nurse, by nonverbal and verbal communications, conveys understanding and appreciation of what the patient is feeling about his situation and is alert for the patient's readiness to talk about his condition and future. As soon as the patient is well enough, an active rehabilitative program is planned and instituted, beginning with simple self-care activities which can be incorporated into the regular plan of care for the patient. The reader is referred to Chapter 2 on rehabilitation. The quadriplegic patient's problems are greater than the paraplegic's; many of the activities of daily living may be impossible for him, and he remains greatly dependent on others for the remainder of his life.

Ruptured or Herniated Intervertebral Disk

The bodies of the vertebrae are separated by fibrocartilage disks that serve as cushions and shock absorbers. Each disk consists of a tough, firm outer capsule and a central core of resilient pulpy material referred to as the nucleus pulposus. The capsule is attached to the bodies of the adjoining vertebrae and the anterior and posterior longitudinal ligaments. If injury or degenerative change causes tearing or a weakened area in the capsule, the nucleus pulposus extrudes, resulting in a protrusion that may press on a spinal nerve root, giving rise to symptoms.

Heavy lifting and chronic strain on one or more disks bring about degenerative changes. Poor body mechanics, especially lifting with the trunk in acute flexion are frequent precipitating causes in herniation and rupture. Injury may be the initiating factor in degenerative changes; the immediate symptoms at the time of injury are not usually significant but signs of nerve compression appear months or years later when the disk becomes weaker and less resilient with the tissue changes.

There is a high incidence of herniated and ruptured disks. As a result, many persons suffer a good deal of pain and discomfort and become restricted in their activities. The nurse has the responsibility to practice and teach good body mechanics, which play a significant role in the prevention of disk problems. The following factors are of particular importance in avoiding undue strain on back muscles and ligaments. When picking up objects from the floor, working at a lower level or lifting heavy objects, the knees and thighs should be flexed and the back kept straight so the greater strain is placed on the muscles of the thighs and buttocks. Bending at the waist with the knees straight and twisting of the spine are avoided. Heavy objects are carried close to the body. Pulling taxes the back muscles less than pushing. Objects with which one is working should be kept at a comfortable level and close enough to avoid the strain of reaching. When sitting, the hips should be well back in the chair so that the weight is on the thighs and lower part of the buttocks, and the back is kept straight. Exercising the trunk muscles (especially the abdominal and gluteal) to promote strength and tone contributes to the patient's ability to function with a minimal risk of strain and injury to the disks.

Manifestations. The patient with a ruptured or herniated intervertebral disk experiences pain in the back and in the area of distribution of the involved nerve. The pain is usually worse on bending, lifting, straight-leg raising and with sneezing and coughing. The condition may occur at any level of the spine but the lumbar and lumbosacral disks are most frequently affected, causing pressure on the sciatic nerve. The patient complains of pain in the lower back which radiates into one buttock and down the posterolateral aspect of the thigh and leg. Continued pressure may produce degenerative changes in the involved nerve;

decreased or absence of tendon reflexes, loss of sensation, weakness of the urethral sphincter, resulting in incontinence, and muscular weakness may develop. There is restricted motion of the spine and postural deformity may be evident due to muscle spasm. Compression of a nerve by a cervical disk causes pain and disturbed sensations in the arm and hand, and limitation of neck movement. The onset of symptoms may be sudden, following severe strain or twisting, or may develop gradually. The distress may be continuous or intermittent.

Investigative procedures to confirm the diagnosis and locate the lesion may include a lumbar puncture to determine if the protrusion is blocking the flow of cerebrospinal fluid in the subarachnoid cavity, an x-ray which may reveal abnormal curvature of the spine and flattening of the intervertebral disks, and a myelogram (see p. 609).

Treatment and Nursing Care. The patient with a ruptured or herniated disk may be treated conservatively or by surgery. Surgery is usually reserved for those patients who do not respond to conservative therapy and are experiencing continuous pain and increasing signs of nerve or cord compression and disability.

Conservative treatment usually consists of rest, heat, exercises and some form of back support on ambulation. In the acute phase, the patient is placed at rest on a firm mattress and fracture board. The patient may be comfortable absolutely flat or may find that slight elevation of the legs and thighs reduces the tension of the back and thigh muscles. If the patient is flat, a small roll or pillow may be used under the knees for support, but it must be small enough to avoid flexion. Intermittent applications of heat may be prescribed, and passive and active exercises are introduced gradually as the acute phase subsides. The exercises which are done in a warm pool may help to reduce the associated muscle spasm and discomfort.

Observations are made from day to day for any motor or sensory changes. Precautions against burning are necessary when using local heat applications, since the patient may have some sensory dulling or loss. The patient is advised of the importance of maintaining good alignment of his spine and is taught to roll like a log onto his side with the uppermost leg flexed when turning. He is also warned to avoid sudden movements and twisting his trunk. A fracture bedpan is used if the patient is not allowed to go to the bathroom or use a commode at the bedside. A rolled towel placed behind the bedpan helps to reduce the strain on his back.

Constipation is a common problem and the patient is cautioned against straining at stool which increases intraspinal pressure and pain. A mild bulk-producing laxative and increased roughage and fluids in the diet are used to promote soft stools and regular elimination. A mild analgesic such as acetylsalicylic acid (Aspirin) and propoxyphene hydrochloride (Darvon) may be ordered for the relief of pain. In some instances, muscle spasm is responsible for much of the patient's discomfort and a muscle relaxant such as methocarbamol (Robaxin) or chlorzoxazone (Paraflex) may be prescribed.

When ambulated, the patient may be required to wear a brace or therapeutic corset to provide spinal support and immobilization. The principles of body mechanics to be observed in posture and activities are taught and demonstrated. He is also advised to always use a straight chair rather than a large overstuffed one and to avoid quick, jerky or twisting movements. In some instances, the physician may advise the patient against resuming his occupation. This may cause considerable concern for the patient. A social worker may be brought in to advise and assist him in obtaining suitable employment, or his previous employer may be contacted and asked to make some adjustment. The importance of the prescribed exercise regimen in the prevention of recurring attacks is emphasized when preparing the patient for discharge from the hospital.

In the case of a herniated cervical disk, intermittent or continuous traction may be applied by means of a halter. After a period of rest and traction, the patient resumes activities gradually and usually wears a plastic collar or a firm cuff for support and to limit neck movements.

If conservative treatment fails to provide the necessary relief, acute attacks are recurring more frequently, or there are signs of increasing neurological deficit due to compression, surgical therapy is undertaken.

A laminectomy is done, followed by decompression of nerve roots or the cord by excision of the herniating disk tissue. If more than one disk is involved, the spinous processes of several vertebrae in the region may be fused by bone grafts for stabilization and immobilization of the area. The grafts may be taken from an iliac crest or tibia. If a fusion is done, the patient's movement following the operation is more restricted, and he is usually required to remain in bed for a longer period. A bivalve body cast extending from the axillae to below the sacrum is sometimes applied on completion of the operation or later, before the patient is ambulated. When the cast is removed, he is fitted for a brace or therapeutic corset, which he is required to wear for at least 6 months. For nursing care following spinal surgery, see the section that follows.

Nursing Care Following Spinal Surgery

Spinal Operations. Spinal surgery is most often performed for the removal of a neoplasm, a herniated or ruptured intervertebral disk, or bony fragments following injury; the reduction of a fractured vertebra and decompression of the cord following injury; or the relief of intractable pain or spasticity and involuntary movements. In most instances these procedures involve a laminectomy (the removal of one or more laminae) to obtain access to the lesion.

A cordotomy is the neurosurgical procedure used to interrupt the spinothalamic tract in the anterolateral portion of the cord, which carries pain impulses from the trunk and lower limbs. The tract is usually severed in the high thoracic region of the cord for the relief of severe intractable pain associated with terminal disease, generally cancer. Spinothalamic cordotomy also abolishes the temperature sense and may be unilateral or bilateral, depending on the involvement of the patient's pain. More recently a simpler procedure has been developed that may be used in place of open surgery. Interruption of pain impulses is achieved by producing a lesion in the spinal cord. A spinal needle is introduced in the high cervical region and directed, under x-ray, into the appropriate region of the cord. An electrode is passed through the needle, and radiofrequent currents are discharged into the tissue to destroy the tract fibers.

A rhizotomy consists of surgical interruption of spinal nerve roots within the spinal canal. Depending on the purpose, it may involve division of the anterior or motor spinal nerve fibers to check involuntary skeletal muscle contractions or spasticity which increase the patient's handicap and pain. Interruption of posterior or sensory spinal nerve fibers may be done for the relief of intractable pain in the areas which the nerves supply.

Diskectomy implies the removal of herniated disk tissue. Spinal fusion is the immobilization of vertebrae by the overlay of pieces of bone taken from another bone.

Preoperative Preparation. The patient who is advised of the need for spinal surgery generally becomes quite apprehensive; in most cases the patient is fearful about pain and helplessness. The nurse explains in detail what he may expect following the operation, takes time to answer any questions that he and his family may have, and encourages the patient to talk about his concerns. His condition may be such that he may have a prolonged period of bed rest and convalescence before resuming former activities. This may create socioeconomic problems, especially if the patient is the wage earner and the chief support of the family. The nurse may be able to have a social service worker visit the patient and assist in arrangements for necessary help. Less apprehension and fewer worries contribute to relaxation and more favorable progress postoperatively.

If there is a risk or anticipation of any permanent changes in functional ability or appearance associated with the planned surgery, these are explained to the family and patient by the surgeon, and the signature of a close relative as well as the patient's may be necessary on the consent for operation.

The importance of maintaining spinal alignment following surgery and how it is achieved are explained. Turning as though the body were one unsegmented unit (log rolling) is discussed and practiced. The patient is advised of the deep breathing and graduated exercises (isometric and active) that he will be required to do and of how his various needs will be met (nutrition, elimination, etc.). If a turning bed is to be used, it is described or demonstrated. Other factors, such as nutritional and hydrational status, that are cited in general preoperative care (Chapter 10) are also applicable.

Spinal operations are usually lengthy procedures, producing greater predisposition to shock. The patient's blood is typed and cross matched, and blood is made available. He may be fitted preoperatively for a back brace or therapeutic corset which will be worn when he is ambulated, or a bivalve cast (anterior and posterior shells) may be made which will be used immediately after surgery to facilitate immobilization of the spine and turning. Provisions are made with padding on its inner surfaces to protect the wound and bony prominences. Straps are provided to hold the cast in position when they are applied.

Local skin preparation entails shaving and thorough cleansing of the back from the shoulders to the lower border of the buttocks and from side to side. Surgery in the cervical region necessitates higher preparation and may require clipping of the lower hair and shaving of the lower posterior scalp. If a spinal fusion is anticipated, the surgeon may also require similar preparation of the leg or iliac crest region from which the grafts are to be taken. A cleansing enema is given the afternoon or evening before operation, and an indwelling catheter may be passed the morning of operation. Retention is a common problem for a few days following operation, especially if activity is restricted.

A summary is made of the vital signs and of the patient's sensory and motor status to serve as a comparison in assessing the patient postoperatively.

PREPARATION TO RECEIVE THE PATIENT. It should be determined preoperatively from the surgeon whether the patient is to be cared for on a turning bed (Stryker frame or Foster bed) or the ordinary bed so that it will be ready to receive the patient. If the ordinary bed is used, fracture boards and a firm mattress are necessary, and a footboard, cradle, bolsters, extra pillows for placing under the full length of the lower limbs, and long sandbags or firm rolls to prevent outward rotation of the lower limbs are convenient for positioning after the patient is in bed. Suction should be available, and if the surgery is in the cervical region, a respirator, oxygen and tracheostomy tray should be at hand. A sterile tubing and closed receptacle are assembled to attach to the indwelling catheter for urinary drainage. The remainder of the equipment is the same as that cited in Chapter 10.

Postoperative Care. The care following spinal surgery varies with the particular surgery done, the patient's response to it and the individual surgeon. For example, some patients are immobilized for weeks while others are ambulated a day or two following the surgery. An understanding of what was done and specific directives are necessary in planning care, especially in relation to positioning and movement.

POSITIONING. Unless the patient is on a turning bed, he may be required to remain in the supine or prone position for 8 to 12 hours after operation without being turned. If he is restless, sandbags along either side may be indicated for immobilization. When the surgeon permits turning, it is usually done every 2 hours. The patient is reminded of the instructions received preoperatively regarding turning and is cautioned not to take an active part except to maintain a rigid straight line. The major principles to be observed are the maintenance of spinal alignment and prevention of strain on the back muscles. Twisting, jerking and angulation of the spine must be avoided. The use of a draw sheet under the full length of the spine and buttocks is helpful as a turning sheet. The patient's arms are placed at his sides or folded across his chest. The turning sheet is rolled tightly toward the patient from each side, and with the lifters keeping the sheet taut to provide the necessary support, the patient is eased to one side of the bed. The sheet on that side is then grasped by the nurses on the other side of the bed and steadily pulled to roll the patient toward them. An adequate number of personnel is necessary so that one person may turn the lower limbs and support the uppermost leg to prevent any dragging weight being placed on the back during the process. In the supine position pillows may be permitted under the full length of the lower limbs, without flexion of the knees, to reduce strain. If pillows are not used, a small bolster may be placed under the knees to prevent hyperextension, but again, it is important to guard against flexion. In the prone position, a pillow is placed under the ankles. When

lying on the side is permitted, supports are placed under the uppermost limbs. In the case of high thoracic or cervical spinal surgery, a pillow under the head is not permitted. A small sponge rubber pillow may be allowed under the neck for support, and the head and neck may be immobilized with sandbags. A footboard is used to maintain a dorsiflexion position of the feet, and the heels are protected from pressure. Sandbags or firm rolls extending laterally along the outer surface of the lower limbs from above the hip joint to below the knee may be necessary to prevent outward rotation.

If the patient is placed in the bivalve cast mentioned previously or on a turning bed, turning is facilitated and there is greater assurance of maintaining immobilization. For details of the turning bed, see page 646.

OBSERVATIONS. The patient's vital signs, color and responses are checked at frequent intervals for signs of shock or bleeding. If he is in the lateral or prone position, the dressings are examined for indications of possible bleeding or leakage of cerebrospinal fluid. Edema or bleeding at the site of the surgery may cause cord or nerve compression and interference with sensory and motor functions. Sensation and motor ability of the extremities are tested every 2 to 3 hours during the first 2 or 3 days to detect any change from the preoperative status. Any complaint of tingling or numbness is recorded and reported. The color and temperature of the extremities are also noted in case of circulatory stasis. Pressure areas are examined for irritation and edema whenever the patient is turned. The urinary output is noted; less than 15 to 20 ml. per hour is reported, since it may indicate hypotension, dehydration or renal insufficiency. If an indwelling catheter is not used, the frequency of voiding and the amount of urine are checked. The lower abdomen is examined for possible urinary retention and bladder distention if the output seems inadequate.

When the surgery is in the cervical region, the patient is watched closely for any signs of respiratory distress or failure. Trauma or edema of the cervical cord or nerves may temporarily cause paralysis of the respiratory muscles.

NUTRITION AND FLUIDS. The patient frequently receives blood during the operation and immediately following. The nurse sees that the flow is maintained and observes the patient for early signs of possible reaction (chill, urticaria, dyspnea or complaints of pain in the back). Intravenous fluids may be given for the first day or two or until the patient is taking adequate amounts orally. He should have 2500 to 3000 ml. daily unless contraindicated. Solid food is introduced as soon as it is tolerated, and the patient is encouraged to take sufficient amounts to promote normal intestinal peristalsis. The patient will probably have to be fed for the first 2 or 3 days because of his position and restricted movement. Precautions are necessary to prevent choking and aspiration if the patient is in the supine position. He is fed slowly, and only small amounts are given at a time.

SKIN CARE. Because of the immobilization, the skin requires special attention. Vulnerable areas are gently rubbed with alcohol every 2 hours or each time the patient is turned. If the skin is dry, a small amount of oil or lanolin may be used to prevent cracking. Resilient material may be placed under pressure areas for protection as long as they do not interfere with body alignment. The bottom sheets are kept clean, dry, and free of wrinkles and crumbs. If a bivalve cast is applied, sufficient padding is necessary to protect bony prominences. A vest or piece of stockinette is worn under a brace or therapeutic corset to protect the skin and also keep the appliance clean.

RELIEF OF PAIN. The patient will probably complain of considerable pain in the operative area and may also experience some pain and spasm in the muscles of the back and lower limbs due to irritation and trauma of spinal nerves at the time of surgery. An analgesic such as morphine or meperidine hydrochloride (Demerol) is given as ordered. If the surgery has been in the cervical region, morphine is not given because of its depressing effect on respirations. After 2 or 3 days, the patient should require less analgesic, and a milder form may be ordered, reducing the danger of addiction. A change of position or gentle exercise of the limbs when permitted may provide the necessary relief. The patient's position should also be rechecked for possible strain and inadequate support.

ELIMINATION. Urine retention is a common problem in patients following spinal surgery because of the possible trauma and edema of the cord or nerves in the operative site. As cited previously, in anticipation of possible retention an indwelling catheter is generally passed before or immediately after operation. Continuous drainage in a closed sterile system is usually permitted for the first 24 to 48 hours; then the surgeon may suggest clamping the catheter for intervals so that normal bladder tone and capacity may be maintained. The volume of the urinary output is measured and recorded every 8 hours. A minimal daily fluid intake of 2500 to 3000 ml. is important to prevent concentration and stasis of urine and bladder infection. If a catheter is not used, a female urinal or emesis basin may be used to collect the urine to avoid having to raise the female patient onto a bedpan.

No laxative or enema is given without the surgeon's order. Straining at defecation must be avoided. If abdominal distention occurs, it is reported. A rectal tube may be inserted and an intramuscular injection of a peristaltic stimulant such as neostigmine (Prostigmin) may be prescribed. A laxative or enema may be ordered after the third or fourth postoperative day. To place the patient on a bedpan, the patient is turned onto his side, a fracture pan is positioned, and a small pillow or padding is placed behind it to support the back. He is then rolled back onto the pan.

WOUND CARE. If the dressing remains dry, it usually remains undisturbed for several days or until the sutures are removed. The first dressing and the removal of the sutures are done by the physician. If the patient develops an elevation of temperature or there is reason to suspect possible wound infection, the dressing may be removed earlier for wound inspection. Protection of the incision by a dressing may be used for a longer period than with other wounds because of the pressure it may be exposed to when the patient is in the supine position or when wearing a cast or brace.

Following a fusion, the donor site of the grafts will also require attention. The area is checked for bleeding in the immediate postoperative period. When the tibia has been used, the leg is handled carefully, avoiding movement of the knee, and it is supported on a pillow. When the patient is allowed up, a crepe or elastic bandage may be applied for support.

EXERCISES AND AMBULATION. Beginning on the day of operation, the patient is encouraged to take 5 to 10 deep breaths every 3 or 4 hours to increase lung expansion and pulmonary exchange. The patient may find this painful because of the strain placed on the operative site. The nurse explains its importance and remains with the patient to provide necessary encouragement and support. When possible it may be timed with the administration of the prescribed analgesic to reduce the discomfort. Coughing is usually contraindicated.

Passive movements of the limbs may be restricted for the first few days. When they are begun they must be done smoothly and gently to prevent any jerking and twisting of the spine. Periodic massage of the limbs during the period of immobilization frequently proves comforting and relaxing to the patient. A specific directive is received as to active exercises; these may be started quite early with some patients; with others, especially fusion patients, active exercises may be prohibited for 2 or more weeks. After the sutures are removed and there is sufficient wound healing, the patient may be lowered into a warm pool for passive and active exercises. This type of therapy is usually quite helpful if the patient is experiencing considerable muscle spasm.

When ambulation is permitted, the patient may be raised gradually on the gatch frame to guard against hypotension. When he is ready to be assisted out of bed, a bivalve cast or brace may be applied for support. He is rolled onto his side and his legs are lowered over the side of the bed as he assumes the sitting position. He wears firm, supportive walking shoes and is slowly assisted to his feet. While up, he sits in a straight chair with his feet resting flat on the floor. Someone remains with the patient and notes his reactions the first few times he is up. The frequency and length of his time up are gradually increased. Activities and self-care are introduced and increased according to his capacity and responses.

REHABILITATION. The resumption of former activities and the required rehabilitation program must be individualized on the basis of the nature of the patient's surgery, his response and capacity and whether there are residual disabilities. Self-care and independence are encouraged as soon as his condition permits. In many instances, the patient is fearful of "undoing" the surgery by resuming activities and tends to become overdependent. The nurse must be alert for this and provide the necessary reassurance and encouragement as well as the opportunities for him to regain his confidence and independence. What he may and may not do, the therapeutic exercise regimen to be followed, and the continued wearing of a brace or corset are usually outlined by the doctor. Detailed explanations of these and assistance in planning necessary adjustments are given to the patient and his family by the nurse. The patient is usually followed closely by regular visits to the clinic or the doctor's office for a period of 6 months to a year. If necessary, when the patient is discharged from the hospital, a referral may be made to a visiting nurse agency for guidance and supervision at home. Assistance may be necessary in making arrangements to transport the patient several times weekly to a rehabilitation or physiotherapy center.

NEUROPATHIES

Disorders of the cranial nerves are frequently secondary to other diseases, but a few are primary to specific nerves. These few disorders include trigeminal neuralgia and Bell's palsy. Peripheral nerve dysfunction may be incurred by direct local trauma (pressure, severance, infection and inflammation) or may be secondary to a variety of general conditions such as malnutrition, alcoholism and chemical poisoning.

Trigeminal Neuralgia (Tic Douloureux)

The trigeminal nerve (fifth cranial) has both sensory and motor fibers. The sensory fibers transmit impulses from the corresponding side of the face and anterior half of the skull. The nerve has three main divisions: the ophthalmic, whose fibers are distributed to the anterior part of the scalp, the forehead, eye and nose; the maxillary, which supplies the skin of the cheek, upper lip, upper jaw and teeth, and palate; and the mandibular, consisting of sensory fibers which carry impulses from the lower lip, chin, lower jaw, teeth, and the tongue, and motor fibers which innervate the muscles of mastication. The sensory fibers of all three divisions pass to the gasserian ganglion which lies in a fold of the dura mater in the temporal region. From the ganglion, the sensory impulses are transmitted along fibers (axons) which terminate in a nucleus in the pons. The motor fibers originate in a small nucleus of neurons also situated in the pons and join the sensory fibers of the mandibular division just beyond the ganglion.

Trigeminal neuralgia* is characterized by brief, recurring attacks of agonizing pain along the distribution of one or more divisions of the nerve. The mandibular branch is most often affected. Abnormally hypersensitive areas occur along the pathway of the nerve (trigger zones) which, on very slight stimulation, initiate the paroxysms of pain. The patient may describe the pain as "stabbing," "knife-like," "searing" or "burning." Usually, the attack is very brief, lasting only seconds to 2 or 3 minutes. It may be followed by dull aching and frequent, recurring acute spells over a period of days or weeks after which there may be a remission of varying length (weeks or months). Generally, exacerbations become progressively more frequent in the sixth and seventh decades.

The onset of trigeminal neuralgia may occur spontaneously or may coincide with movement of the face or exposure to a draft. The patient may relate the precipitation of pain to eating, talking, cleaning the teeth, or washing or shaving of the face. As a result, he tends to avoid these activities and becomes withdrawn and occupied with preventing an attack. During the intense pain, twitching, grimacing, frequent blinking and tearing of the eye may be observed.

The cause of the neuralgia is not known; because it usually occurs in later life, it is thought it may be the result of some "aging" change in the sensory nerves but no significant organic factor has been identified. The sinuses, teeth and mouth are usually examined for possible local infection as an aggravating factor. The incidence of the disease is not great. It occurs more often in women, usually appearing between the ages of 40 and 60.

Treatment and Nursing Care. Various forms of medical treatment are used in the early stages of the condition, but eventually surgical section of the sensory nerve roots of the affected division(s) usually is necessary to provide relief. Medications which may be used in conservative treatment include analgesics, inhalations of trichlorethylene (Trilene), cyanocobalamin (vitamin B_{12}), niacin (nicotinic acid), thiamine (vitamin B_1), sodium diphenylhydantoin (Dilantin) and a tranquilizer such as chlorpromazine hydrochloride (Thorazine). There is no specific drug for the condition; what may provide relief or shorten an attack for one patient may prove of little or no value to another. Injection of absolute alcohol into the affected nerve branch may be done to interrupt the sensory impulses and usually provides relief for several months. During the period of effectiveness the patient experiences loss of sensation and feelings of numbness, stiffness and heaviness in the areas of distribution of the injected nerve branches.

Surgical therapy involves sectioning the sensory nerve roots of the affected divisions of the nerve between the gasserian ganglion and the brain. The ophthalmic division is spared whenever possible, since severance of it produces a loss of sensation in the respective cornea, abolishing the corneal reflex and predisposing the patient to drying of the cornea, keratitis (inflammation of the cornea) and ulceration of the eye. If the ophthalmic trigeminal division is also affected, necessitating its section, special protective measures will be necessary afterward.

During an exacerbation of the patient's disease, factors which are likely to precipitate an attack of the severe pain are avoided. He is protected from exposure to cold and drafts. Food and fluids are served lukewarm. Solid foods requiring chewing may be replaced by puréed foods, and concentrates may be added to liquids to increase the patient's caloric intake. He is kept undisturbed and as quiet as possible. Jarring of the bed and unnecessary activity around him are avoided. Because of the fear of aggravating his condition, the patient may evade the usual care of his face, hair and teeth. Understanding and tact are necessary on the part of the nurse; it may be helpful to provide warm water and a very soft cloth

---

*Neuralgia is defined as pain in a nerve.

or absorbent cotton and suggest to the patient that he might like to wash his face. The importance of mouth hygiene in preventing complications is explained, and a warm mouthwash is provided. The opportune time for these activities may be following the administration of an analgesic.

If a nerve section is to be done, the preparation of the patient includes an explanation of its permanent effects (loss of sensation, numbness, stiffness and heaviness) and the protective measures that he will have to observe. Some surgeons prefer the patient to have had treatment by alcohol injection previously so that he can appreciate what the permanent effects of surgery will be. Specific orders are received as to the preparation of the operative area. The approach is usually in the temporal region in front of the ear. A minimal amount of hair is removed, and the area is cleansed and shaved. In the case of a female, the remainder of the hair is brushed away from the area and secured.

The general principles of postoperative care are applicable following the surgery. As soon as the patient responds, the head of the bed is gradually elevated. He is usually ambulated in 24 to 48 hours and progressively increases his activities. Observations are made for signs of difficulty in mastication due to possible interference with the motor fibers of the mandibular nerve and for temporary facial paralysis on the operative side that may result from trauma of the facial (seventh cranial) nerve. It is not uncommon for the patient to develop herpes simplex (cold sores) around the mouth.

A full diet is introduced as soon as the patient can tolerate it. He is advised to place the food in the unaffected side of his mouth and to avoid hot foods because he would be unaware of burning in the desensitized area. Special attention to oral hygiene is necessary because of the possible accumulation of food particles on the insensitive side. The teeth should be cleansed and a mouthwash used after meals and at bedtime. Since dental problems in the desensitized area will not produce the usual warning by pain, the importance of a dental checkup every 6 months is stressed in discussions with the patient.

If surgery involves section of the ophthalmic division of the trigeminal nerve, leaving the conjunctiva and cornea insensitive to foreign particles and injury, irrigation of the eye with normal saline 2 or 3 times daily is usually ordered. The patient is taught to do this as he will be required to continue the care at home. The importance of examining his eye at least twice daily for redness and irritation and of voluntarily closing his eyelid frequently to keep the surface lubricated is explained. Glasses should be worn for protection.

Bell's Palsy

This condition is due to dysfunction of one of the facial (seventh cranial) nerves which have both motor and sensory components. The motor fibers of each nerve originate in the pons and innervate the facial muscles and submaxillary and sublingual salivary glands on the corresponding side. The sensory fibers of the facial nerve transmit impulses from taste buds of the tongue to the geniculate ganglion in the temporal bone and then into the brain stem (medulla).

Bell's palsy is manifested by a loss of the ability to move the muscles on one side of the face that occurs independently of other conditions such as stroke, intracranial tumor and injury. The cause is unknown, but it is suggested that it may be due to compression of the nerve fibers by edema associated with inflammation as a result of virus infection. The patient may complain of pain posterior to the ear for a day or two; then paralysis of one side of the face appears. The affected side of the face becomes flaccid, the mouth is drawn to the unaffected side, drooling occurs, and the patient is unable to wrinkle his brow, whistle, or retract the corner of his mouth. The eyelid on the affected side does not close, and when the patient attempts closure, the eyeball rolls up. The taste sensation is lost over the anterior two-thirds of the tongue on the respective side. Herpes lesions may appear on or in the corresponding ear.

Treatment and Care. An adrenocorticosteroid preparation such as dexamethasone (Decadron) may be administered to reduce the inflammation and edema and the resulting nerve compression. The head is protected from exposure to cold and drafts which aggravate the symptoms. Massage and electrotherapy of the face are used to stimulate circulation and muscle tone and prevent muscle atrophy. The patient is encouraged to take an adequate diet and is instructed to direct his food into the unaffected side of the mouth for mastication. Oral hygiene is emphasized to prevent the accumulation of residual food in the affected side of the mouth which predisposes to sordes and parotitis. If there is loss of the ability to close the eyelid, measures are used to prevent drying, infection and ulceration of the conjunctiva and cornea. Irrigations of normal saline and the instillation of a protective oil or ointment may be prescribed. Protective glasses or a shield may be worn.

The affected muscles usually begin to regain tone in a few weeks, and movement is generally progressively restored over a period of months. When recovery is evident, the patient is instructed to carry out a regimen of active facial exercises several times a day. Some residual deficit may occur, and rarely, permanent paralysis results from nerve degeneration.

Polyneuritis (Multiple Peripheral Neuritis)

Although neuritis implies inflammation, it is more frequently applied to dysfunction and painful conditions of peripheral nerves that are not inflammatory. Polyneuritis is a condition in which there is pain and impaired function along the distribution of many peripheral nerves. It is usually symmetrical and is manifested by both sensory and motor disturbances in the involved parts. The symptoms generally start in the parts supplied by the distal portions of the nerves and spread proximally. The patient usually experiences pain, "pins and needles," tingling and weakness first in the hands and feet. There may be a progressive loss of sensation, diminished tendon reflexes and inability to perform finer movements. The areas are tender and sore when subjected to even light pressure.

The condition is most commonly associated with vitamin B deficiency, malnutrition, alcoholism, prolonged gastrointestinal disease or chemical poisoning. It may also occur in uncontrolled diabetes or peripheral vascular disease (arteriosclerosis) or as a result of toxins produced in an infection (e.g., diphtheria).

The cause is determined and treated. Vitamin B complex is administered, and the patient's nutritional status improved. The patient tends to immobilize the affected parts because of the pain and weakness. Limbs are supported in the optimum position, and a cradle is used to protect the feet and legs from the weight of the bedding. The limbs are gently moved through their range of motion 3 or 4 times daily to prevent ankylosis of joints. Heat therapy (e.g., infrared lamp) may be prescribed but must be used cautiously because of the danger of burns due to the patient's reduced sensitivity. Gentle massage may be helpful unless the areas are excessively tender. Analgesics are generally necessary to control the pain in the acute stage.

NURSING IN CONVULSIVE DISORDERS

A convulsive seizure is a manifestation of sudden brain dysfunction in which there is an uncontrolled, rapid and excessive release of impulses by a group of neurons. The electrical discharge spreads into adjacent areas, and the propagation may be sufficient to involve the whole brain. Depending on the origin and pattern of spread of the abnormal neural activity, the effects may vary from momentary suspension of activity and awareness to complete motor, sensory, autonomic and psychic disturbances, including complete loss of consciousness.

Etiology and Incidence

Robb states that "in the normal brain, a certain stability exists between the processes of excitation and inhibition."[13] When a seizure occurs, the ability to suppress abnormal neural activity may be impaired or lost, or there may be an increased excitation within the neurons. The normal seizure level or threshold is lowered, resulting in an uncontrolled discharge of impulses in response

---

[13]Preston Robb: "Epilepsy and Its Medical Treatment." Canad. Nurse, Vol. 61, No. 3 (Mar. 1965), p. 172.

to minimal stimuli. The abnormal neural activity may occur in a small group of neurons and remain relatively localized or may spread to involve extensive areas of normal neurons. In some seizures, no focal origin of discharge is identified; large areas of the brain appear to be involved simultaneously.

Seizures may be caused by almost any intracranial, pathologic condition and by many general systemic disorders. They may be a manifestation of increased intracranial pressure or brain damage associated with a head injury, cerebral edema, or an intracranial space-occupying lesion, hemorrhage or infection. They may be a sequel to brain injury or infection that has caused tissue damage and scar tissue formation.

General systemic conditions in which seizures most commonly occur include hypoglycemia, hypocalcemia (tetany), renal insufficiency (uremia), hypoxia, high fever (especially in children), toxemia of pregnancy and chemical poisoning (e.g., alcohol, strychnine, amphetamines, lead, some insecticides). Seizures associated with conditions such as these do not recur when the causative factor is corrected and homeostasis is restored.

When seizures tend to recur independently of any concomitant craniocerebral or systemic disease, the condition is designated as epilepsy.* If the epileptic seizures are due to a residual structural or physiological defect following a previous craniocerebral injury or disease, the condition is classified as symptomatic epilepsy. In the majority of instances, however, the cause remains obscure and the epilepsy is referred to as being idiopathic, essential or primary. An inherited predisposition is thought to play a role in idiopathic epilepsy. This theory is based on clinical evidence that "a history of epilepsy in other members of the family is obtained twice as commonly in patients with idiopathic epilepsy as in those whose seizures are symptomatic."[14] Studies of epilepsy in identical and fraternal twins report a much higher incidence in both identical twins as compared with its occurrence in both fraternal twins. Identical twins have the same genetic pattern; that of fraternal twins may be quite dissimilar.[15] It has also been revealed that relatives of an epileptic frequently have an abnormal electroencephalographic tracing although they may not be subject to seizures.

Epilepsy has an incidence of approximately 1 per 200 of the population.[16, 17] The greater majority of patients develop their recurring seizures before the age of 20. If the onset takes place after the age of 20 to 30, an organic lesion or previous tissue damage is suspected.

Unless the patient's seizures are secondary to an established systemic disease, he undergoes an extensive physical and neurological examination to determine if there is organic disease. The neurological investigation may include skull x-rays, a lumbar puncture and examination of the cerebrospinal fluid, cerebral arteriogram and a ventriculogram. An accurate, detailed description of a seizure and an encephalogram are important in making the diagnosis. See page 606 for neurological diagnostic procedures.

Types of Seizures

The seizures which characterize epilepsy vary in form and length, depending on the origin of the abnormal neural activity and the extent and course of its spread within the brain. The symptoms may include loss of consciousness, changes in behavior, involuntary uncoordinated movements, abnormal sensations and alterations in visceral function. The seizures may vary in length from a brief transitory phase of a few seconds to several minutes.

Grand Mal or Major Seizure. In many patients, the grand mal seizure is preceded by a momentary warning of the attack (aura) which may take the form of a sensory hallucination, a disturbed mental state or compulsive movement. The sensory aura may

*Some authors refer to the complex of convulsive seizures as the epilepsies, probably because the word epilepsy means seizure. In clinical practice, the use of the word epilepsy is generally reserved for the condition indicated above.

[14] The Late Lord Brain, and J. N. Walton: Brain's Diseases of the Nervous System, 7th ed. London, Oxford University Press, 1969, p. 923.

[15] R. P. Schmidt, and B. J. Wilder: Epilepsy. Philadelphia, F. A. Davis Co., 1968, p. 48.

[16] Brain and Walton, *op. cit.,* p. 923.

[17] T. Rasmussen: "Epilepsy Today." Canad. Nurse, Vol. 61, No. 3 (Mar. 1965), p. 170.

be referred to one of the special senses (auditory, visual, gustatory, olfactory), or the patient may experience numbness or tingling in an area of the body or distress in the epigastric region. The aura is specific for each patient and relates to the function of the focal area of involvement. It coincides with the beginning of the abnormal neural activity.

The first objective symptom may be an involuntary cry caused by the sudden contraction of the thoracic and abdominal muscles, forcing air through the spastic glottis. The person loses consciousness and falls. The convulsive phase of the seizure commences with a strong tonic spasm of the muscles, causing rigidity and distortion of the body. The head and eyes may be turned to one side; the deviation is always to the same side with each seizure. Respirations are arrested, and the patient may become cyanosed. After a few seconds, the sustained, rigid contraction of the muscles is replaced by clonic convulsive movements which are irregular and jerky. Breathing is re-established and is stertorous. There may be foaming at the mouth and some evidence of bleeding due to the tongue being bitten in the clonic phase. The pupils are dilated and do not react to light. Incontinence of urine is common, and rarely, fecal incontinence occurs.

The convulsive movements gradually become less frequent and finally cease. Consciousness is usually regained soon after the cessation of the muscular contractions. The patient may be confused or dazed or may respond normally. He generally drops off into a deep sleep which may last several hours. On waking, he has no memory of the previous conscious interlude. Headache and physical weakness are common after a seizure.

Major seizures vary greatly in frequency from one patient to another. Some experience only a single seizure in a year or two; in others they occur with much greater frequency at irregular intervals.

Petit Mal or Minor Seizure. This type of seizure is characterized by a sudden, brief, transitory cessation of awareness and motor activity. The person stares blankly into space, the eyes usually roll upward and he stops what he is doing. Objects he was holding may be dropped. It lasts only 2 or 3 seconds and may pass unnoticed. The patient resumes his activities, often unaware that there has been an interruption. Occasionally, the attack is accompanied by a few involuntary jerky movements and falling. Petit mal seizures are sometimes referred to as absence seizures, which imply loss of awareness unaccompanied by convulsive movements. They almost always begin in early childhood or early adolesence and tend to recur with greater frequency than the major type seizures.

Psychomotor Seizures. This category of seizures is characterized by automatisms, psychosensory disturbances, and a clouding of consciousness. The person, in a trance-like state, usually carries out a stereotyped, inappropriate action which may be quite bizarre. Rarely, violent or unlawful acts may be performed. Following the attack, the victim is totally unaware of what took place. He may also experience various psychosensory symptoms. These may include hallucinations of hearing, smell, taste or vision; a disordered sense of reality and a sense of detachment from his surroundings; feelings of familiarity with strange persons, objects or situations, or a sense of strangeness with familiar persons, objects or events; or an abnormal sense of well-being or fear. The attack may last from one to several minutes. During the psychomotor disturbances, the patient is unresponsive to any effort on the part of the observer to check his actions.

Jacksonian or Focal Seizure. Seizures of this type usually have a well-defined focal origin in the cerebral cortex and are generally considered a symptom of an organic brain lesion. The manifestations are usually motor but may be only sensory or both. Clonic convulsive movements begin in one part of the body, the most common sites being the thumb and index finger, the great toe, and the angle of the mouth on the side of the body opposite to the cerebral focus of onset. It spreads to involve the entire extremity or face and other parts of the same side. In some instances it becomes bilateral, producing a major seizure with loss of consciousness.

Status Epilepticus. This is a serious condition characterized by a rapid succession of seizures without any intervening period of consciousness. Unless the seizures can be arrested, hyperpyrexia develops, coma deepens, the patient becomes exhausted and death may occur.

Excitatory Factors

Certain factors tend to precipitate seizures in some persons. These may be external stimuli such as sudden loud noises, intermittent flashing lights, some types of music or prolonged television viewing, especially if the picture is flickering or is particularly exciting. The seizure may consist of rapid, jerky muscular contractions without alteration in consciousness and ceases when the stimulus is interrupted. This type of disturbance may be referred to as reflex epilepsy.

Excitatory factors also include emotional stress, excitement, fatigue, ingestion of alcohol, fever, alkalosis and menstruation.

Precursory Symptoms of Seizures

Some epileptics manifest or experience preseizure symptoms several hours or days before an attack; many have no precursory changes. The symptoms may include irritability, depression and withdrawal, headache, light flashes, dizziness, muscular twitching or isolated jerky contractions in the limbs, or a voracious appetite.

Physical, Psychological and Social Factors

Occasionally, an epileptic receives a physical injury during a seizure. A head injury or fracture of a limb may occur with the sudden fall, or trauma or a burn may result if he falls against a machine in operation or a hot object. Fortunately, such accidents have been rare in recent years with the improved anticonvulsant therapy. A few patients may recognize the onset by the aura they experience and have time to move to a safe area and lie down. Some mental deterioration due to organic changes may develop in patients who experience frequent, severe grand mal seizures. This is generally attributed to the brain being repeatedly subjected to hypoxia incurred by the seizures.

In most instances, the most serious problems faced by the epileptic arise from the misconceptions and biases in our society in relation to his condition. Although attitudes have shown considerable improvement in the last two decades, many persons still equate epilepsy with impaired mentality and ability, and attach a stigma which has been prevalent since ancient times. The mental capacity, talents and abilities are as varied in epileptics as in the general population. Yet, all too often, the person who has epilepsy is an object of pity and rejection, mistrusted and feared, and is not given the opportunity to develop and use his potential attributes. It is frequently necessary and often helpful to remind the patient and prejudiced persons, as well as ourselves, that many famous people in history were subject to seizures. A long list of such persons includes Julius Caesar, William Pitt, Lord Byron, Charles Dickens, Martin Luther, V. Van Gogh, L. Beethoven, G. Handel, Peter Tchaikovsky and A. Nobel.

Abilities will vary in epileptics just as they do in nonepileptics; each one's capabilities and liabilities must be assessed on an individual basis. The fact that epilepsy is not synonymous with mental retardation or psychosis requires emphasis. The condition is not incompatible with normal or even superior intellect, independence and a normal satisfying life free of undue limitations. Today it can be successfully controlled in the majority of affected persons just as the diabetic's disease can be controlled. The person should receive the educational opportunities warranted by his actual intelligence and capabilities; he should be considered employable, encouraged to participate in safe recreation with others, and treated as a respected citizen.

Because of the attitudes and rejection with which so many epileptics have met, many tend to conceal their condition and do not seek assistance from available sources of help. The person lives in a constant state of anxiety, fearful of a seizure revealing his secret.

There is no characteristic personality associated with epilepsy. The same range of personality differences exists in persons with epilepsy as in nonepileptics. Personality and behavioral disturbances are more likely to be associated with seizures caused by an organic lesion (e.g., psychomotor epilepsy). However, the person with epilepsy frequently does undergo personality changes and may become resentful, moody, emotionally unstable and suspicious. These traits observed in the so-called epileptic personality are not the direct result of his disease per se, but usually develop because of the injustices, rejection and frustrations to which the person has been subjected.

One of the most difficult problems experienced by the epileptic is that of employment, even though his seizures are well controlled. Many employers associate impaired ability with epilepsy and are unwilling to accept the fact that the majority of these persons receive successful anticonvulsant therapy. They are fearful of absenteeism and of accidents to the epileptic and others. Frequently, there is concern about increased insurance rates for the workmen's compensation, yet increased absenteeism and accidents due to epilepsy are not substantiated in studies that have been done in the United States.[18] The regulations of workmen's compensation boards do not preclude the employment of epileptics in industry. As cited previously, each one must be evaluated individually. Selection of an occupation or job depends on the type of seizures and the degree of control which the person has, but a wide range of employment remains open to most epileptics without jeopardizing their safety or that of others. Granted, there is a relatively small group whose seizures cannot be sufficiently controlled to permit employment other than in sheltered workshops.

A great deal remains to be done in educating society about epilepsy. Certainly, considerable progress has been made and much credit is due the epilepsy associations[19] in this respect. As well as counseling and assisting epileptics and their families, they provide information on epilepsy in various ways for the general public, employers, teachers, police and other interested groups.

---

[18]Occupational Health Division—Information Services Division, Department of National Health and Welfare Canada: The Employable Epileptic. Occupational Health Bulletin, Vol. 22, N 11–12, 1967, p. 1 (Queen's Printer, Ottawa.).

[19]Canadian Epilepsy Association, Toronto, Canada. (There is a local organization in most of the larger cities such as the Epilepsy Information Centre for Metro Toronto, 90 Eglinton Ave. E., Toronto, Canada.)

National Association to Control Epilepsy, Inc., New York, N.Y.

National Epilepsy League, Inc., Chicago, Ill.

Treatment and Nursing Care

When the patient's seizures are a symptom of identifiable organic disease (e.g., uremia or brain tumor), treatment is directed toward eliminating the cause and may include the administration of an anticonvulsant drug. Regular administration of one or more anticonvulsant drugs remains the most effective method of treating patients with epilepsy. This does not cure their disease, but with the majority, seizures are sufficiently controlled to permit them to be self-supporting and live a relatively normal social life. The patient's acceptance of his condition and general pattern of living play an important role in successful control. Surgical treatment may be helpful to a small number of epileptics whose disease has certain characteristics.

Care During a Convulsive Seizure. When a patient has a seizure, the most important functions of the nurse are, first, to protect the patient from injury and, secondly, to make a close observation of exactly what is happening to the patient. An accurate detailed description of the seizure may be important in determining whether the patient has an organic lesion or focal or generalized epilepsy. One cannot stop a convulsion once it has begun; it is self-limited and no immediate treatment will shorten it.

If the patient is in bed, the pillow is removed and the top bedding turned back so that the convulsive movements can be observed. If the patient falls to the floor, a folded blanket or thick towel is placed under his head to prevent him banging his head during the clonic phase. If nothing is within reach, his head may be supported on the nurse's thigh. Any restrictive clothing at the neck is loosened, and the immediate area is cleared of anything that might contribute to injury (e.g., furniture, electric fan, inhalator). The patient must not be left alone. Only sufficient restraint is used to prevent the patient from injuring himself. For example, the arms may be held loosely to prevent them from striking a hard surface. Rarely, the onset may be recognized before the jaws become clenched, permitting the introduction of a folded washcloth or handkerchief or a padded tongue depressor between the teeth to prevent biting of the tongue. Once the jaws are clenched, no attempt should be made to insert a protective device between the teeth; the damage to the tongue has probably already occurred, and the effort is likely to result in injury to the gums and teeth.

A seizure can be very frightening and upsetting to those who have never seen one. If there are others in the room, the patient is screened as soon as possible, and they are reassured later that he has recovered. It is also comforting to the patient when he regains consciousness to find he has been screened from exposure to others.

The following observations are made and recorded:

The time of onset and duration of the convulsion

The mode of onset: did the patient cry out; was there deviation of the head and eyes; did the muscular contractions start in one part of the body and, if so, what course did the spread take; was there a tonic phase; did the patient become cyanosed?

Symmetrical or asymmetrical movements

Dilation and size of both pupils

Incontinence

Frothing at the mouth

The condition of the patient when the seizure terminates and he regains consciousness: was he oriented; was he able to move his extremities and, if so, was the motor power normal; was there a compulsive act (automatism); was his speech normal; did he fall asleep?

When he has recovered sufficiently, the patient may be asked what he was doing at the time of onset and to describe any warning (aura) he may have had.

After a seizure, the patient is made comfortable and allowed to rest. Fluids containing sugar are encouraged to ensure an adequate supply of glucose to the cerebral neurons.

Anticonvulsant Therapy. Seizures may be prevented or their frequency and severity significantly diminished by regular anticonvulsant drug therapy. The drugs are thought to raise the seizure threshold, thus preventing the abnormal foci from discharging in response to minimal stimuli. There are many anticonvulsant preparations; for a complete listing and details of the various preparations, the reader is referred to a pharmacological textbook. Those most commonly used include diphenylhydantoin (Dilantin), paramethadione (Paradione), trimethadione (Tridione), phensuximide (Milontin), mephenytoin (Mesantoin), primidone (Mysoline) and phenobarbital (Luminal). The patient frequently has to try several drugs before the one which provides effective control of his seizures is identified. One preparation may provide satisfactory control for one patient but may prove ineffective with others. The selection is also based on the patient's type of seizures (major, minor or psychomotor).

Treatment usually begins with minimal doses of one drug. The dosage is slowly increased within maximal limits until control is achieved or until side effects appear and preclude its use, necessitating a second choice. Occasionally a combination of two drugs is used; for example, diphenylhydantoin may be given 4 times a day and phenobarbital ordered to be taken with the bedtime dose to provide a greater depressive effect during the night. Since the epileptic will be responsible for taking his own medication after hospitalization, it is better to give it at mealtimes. He is more likely to remember it at these hours than at in-between hours, and it also reduces the possibility of gastric irritation.

Strict adherence to the drug and dosage as prescribed is emphasized to the patient and his family. The medication must not be decreased or omitted except on the doctor's directive. Irregular dosage or abrupt withdrawal may provoke recurring seizures. The effective drug or combination of drugs may be continued for 1 to 3 years. If the patient remains free of seizures during this period, the doctor may gradually decrease the dosage and eventually discontinue it.

Whenever anticonvulsant drugs are used, the nurse must be alert for early manifestations of side effects. Some are more likely to produce toxicity than others, and tolerance varies with individuals. The side effects which may develop include inflammation and hyperplasia of the gums (especially diphenylhydantoin), headache, excessive drowsiness, dizziness, photophobia, ataxia, gastric irritation, skin eruptions (particularly mephenytoin), agranulocytosis, and kidney damage (mainly with paramethadione and trimethadione). The patient and his family are warned to promptly report any unusual signs and symptoms. Routine blood examinations and urinalyses are done.

General Care. The nurse has an important role in assisting the patient and his family to accept the diagnosis of epilepsy and make the necessary adjustments. The aims of care are to prevent seizures and set realistic goals toward a self-supporting, satisfying social life. Both the patient and his family are encouraged to talk about the condition. This is likely to bring misconceptions and anxieties out into the open, giving an opportunity for clarification and suggestions for managing the patient's life. They are advised that persons with epilepsy may be found in many fields of occupation; it does not necessarily preclude education, usefulness, employment and socialization. A reasonable amount of activity is actually considered to contribute to the prevention of attacks.

Persons with epilepsy are generally advised to avoid activities and occupations which, in the event of a seizure, could be dangerous for them and others. These include climbing, swimming (unless with someone who knows about the condition and could handle the situation), working at a height or with certain machinery, riding a bicycle or a horse, and driving a car. In reference to driving, the law pertaining to a driver's license varies from one province or state to another; the majority now provide a permit for the person if he has been completely free from seizures for 2 or 3 years. The forms of occupation and recreation considered safe for the epileptic are decided by the physician on an individual basis, depending on the type, frequency and severity of the seizures. Limitations are kept to a minimum so that feelings of being "different," or resentment and undesirable outlets are less likely to develop.

The patient and his family are informed about the epilepsy association and its services and are urged to become members of a local branch. Moderation and normality in the general pattern of living for the epileptic are emphasized in discussions. Seizure-provoking factors which should be avoided are reviewed with them. The use of a firm bed pillow is suggested in case a seizure occurs at night. The family and friends are instructed on the care of the epileptic during a seizure and cautioned that

overprotection and rejection must be avoided. The nurse explains to the patient the importance of always carrying an identification card which indicates his name and address; the name, address and telephone number of his next of kin; his condition and medication; what to do if he has a seizure; and the doctor or clinic to be called for a directive.

In the case of a child, parents are urged to have him continue at school. The teacher should be advised of the possibility of seizures, what to do if one occurs and of any restrictions made by the doctor on sports or physical education. The epilepsy associations have excellent programs and several helpful brochures for teachers which provide an understanding of epilepsy and their role with epileptic children. If frequent attacks preclude the child's attendance at a public school, arrangements may be made for a visiting teacher or enrollment in a special class.

The epileptic adult may be concerned about the hereditary aspects of epilepsy. There is some evidence that a predisposition to the development of epilepsy may be attributed to genetic factors. A child of an epileptic is more likely to develop the condition.[20, 21] If questioned about the role of heredity, the nurse should suggest that the person talk with his physician or consult a genetic counseling clinic.

Status Epilepticus. A succession of recurring convulsive seizures without the patient regaining consciousness is a critical situation requiring prompt medical treatment and constant nursing observation and attention. External stimuli are reduced to a minimum. The patient is kept flat and in the prone or semiprone position if possible to prevent aspiration of the oropharyngeal secretions. Suction is used to clear the mouth and pharynx of mucus between seizures and the mouth is cleansed with swabs moistened with an antiseptic. A light application of petrolatum oil or jelly may be made to the lips. The crib sides are padded to prevent the patient from injuring himself. The vital signs are recorded frequently; fever commonly develops, and respiratory and cardiac

---

[20]Schmidt and Wilder, *op. cit.,* pp. 45–51.
[21]W. R. Gowers: Epilepsy. New York, Dover Publications, Inc., 1964, pp. 241–242.

failure may occur as a result of extreme exhaustion. Oxygen administration may be necessary. If unconsciousness is prolonged, fluids and nutrients are usually administered by a nasogastric tube. The skin requires special attention because of the friction to which it is subjected. Soft undersheets are used and may be powdered to reduce the friction.

An anticonvulsant is given intravenously; phenobarbital (Luminal), amobarbital (Amytal), diphenylhydantoin (Dilantin) or diazepam (Vallium) may be used. Paraldehyde by intramuscular injection may be prescribed. If the patient does not respond to these drugs, an anesthetic such as sodium thiopental (Pentothal sodium) by intravenous injection, or tribromoethanol (Avertin) by rectum may be administered.

Surgical Treatment. Surgery is employed in the treatment of a small number of epileptics whose disease has certain characteristics. It is reserved for patients with well-defined foci of abnormal activity in the brain whose seizures cannot be adequately controlled by anticonvulsant drug therapy and whose cerebral focal areas can be removed without resulting in a serious neurological deficit.

The operation consists of excision of the cerebral cortex, which has been identified as the focus of abnormal neural activity, and is performed under local anesthesia. The preoperative and postoperative care are similar to that of the patient having intracranial surgery (see p. 637). Very close observation for signs of increasing intracranial pressure and seizures is continued for several days. An anticonvulsant drug is prescribed and continued for at least 1 year. If the patient remains free of seizures during that period, it is gradually discontinued.

INFECTIONS OF THE NERVOUS SYSTEM

Poliomyelitis (Anterior Poliomyelitis, Infantile Paralysis)

Poliomyelitis is an acute infectious disease caused by a group of related viruses which have a predilection for the motor neurons of the spinal cord and brain stem. The causative virus is found in the nasopharyngeal secretions and feces of infected persons. The main portal of entry is considered to be the mouth, and viral growth begins in the oropharynx and gastrointestinal tract. The infection may be spread by personal contact or by contaminated food, milk or water. The incubation period is 7 to 14 days, and the most communicable period is during the latter part of this period and the first week of the acute illness. Antibody formation may confine the viruses sufficiently to prevent their invasion of the nervous system and the more serious forms of the disease.

Incidence and Prevention. The disease has a higher incidence during the summer and early autumn and among children and young adults. It may occur sporadically or in epidemics. There has been a sharp decline in the incidence of this disease since 1955 as a result of the widespread usage of poliomyelitis vaccine.

Preventive measures include isolation of infected persons during the communicable stage and immunization by means of a series of doses of a vaccine. Two types of vaccine are available: the Salk vaccine, which is a solution of killed viruses that is given intramuscularly (see immunization program, p. 45); and the Sabin vaccine, which is a preparation of attenuated living viruses that is administered orally.

Manifestations and Course. The severity and course of poliomyelitis vary markedly, depending on whether or not the nervous system is invaded and according to the level of involvement and degree of damage to motor neurons.

THE ONSET. Early symptoms are nonspecific and include headache, fever, malaise, sore throat and gastrointestinal disturbances. The infection may go unrecognized at this time or may be suspected only by reason of known contact or epidemic. The disease may not progress beyond this stage and is then classified as abortive poliomyelitis.

NONPARALYTIC PHASE. In this stage of the disease the symptoms cited above usually become more intense. Due to invasion of the nervous system by the viruses, the patient manifests restlessness, limited spinal flexion and tenderness in the muscles and usually complains of pain in the back and limbs. Positive Kernig's and Brudzinski's signs may be demonstrated and are characteristic of meningeal irritation. Kernig's sign consists of resistance to straightening of the knee when the patient's thigh is flexed on the abdomen. Brudzinski's sign is reflex flexion of a thigh when the opposite one is passively flexed and the reflex flexion of both hips and knees in response to passive flexion of the neck. Examination of the cerebrospinal fluid reveals an increase in the number of leukocytes and the protein content.

The symptoms may subside within a week or two without further development of the disease, and the patient is said to have had nonparalytic poliomyelitis.

PARALYTIC PHASE. The patients who progress to this stage develop paralysis of one or more parts of the body as a result of dysfunction or destruction of motor neurons. The parts which become paralyzed vary with the level of the lesions. If the paralysis occurs in muscles innervated by motor neurons in the cord, the condition is referred to as spinal paralytic poliomyelitis. When motor neurons in the brain stem are attacked, the disease is classified as bulbar poliomyelitis. Involvement of neurons in both the brain stem and cord is designated as bulbospinal poliomyelitis. Rarely, neurons at a higher level than the brain stem are affected, producing encephalitic poliomyelitis.

Spinal paralytic poliomyelitis is more commonly seen than the other types. The paralytic phase is characterized by pain and tenderness of varying severity, loss of reflexes and the development of weakness or flaccid paralysis in the affected muscles. The site of the paralysis varies; the disease may be patchy and asymmetrical in distribution.

Involvement of the lumbar portion of the cord may cause paralysis of one or both lower limbs and weakness of the lower abdominal and back muscles. The urinary bladder may also be affected. Disease of the thoracic level of the cord may produce weakness of the chest and upper abdominal and back muscles. The affected thoracic muscles may result in reduced respiratory sufficiency. Infection of the cervical cord is critical, since it may result in weakness or paralysis of the diaphragm as well as the muscles of the neck and one or both arms and shoulders.

Bulbar poliomyelitis may attack the neurons of various cranial nerve nuclei and regulatory centers of vital functions (respiratory, cardiac, vascular) which are situated in the brain stem. The patient may manifest dysphagia, weakness of the jaws and facial muscles, inability to cough, and respiratory and cardiac arrhythmias and insufficiency.

The paralysis may be temporary or permanent. Neurons may recover as the disease process is arrested, and hyperemia and edema disappear. The return of muscle power may slowly take place over several months. In some instances, maximal recovery requires a year or two. If the neurons are irreversibly damaged and replaced by glial scar formation, the disability is permanent. The affected muscles atrophy; in the case of a limb, its growth is stunted; it remains flail-like and vasomotor disturbances frequently persist, resulting in coldness and mottling.

Treatment and Nursing Care. There is no specific treatment for poliomyelitis. The care is principally symptomatic and is directed toward minimizing pain, paralysis and deformities and the promotion of maximum rehabilitation if there is permanent disability.

Isolation precautions are necessary for 7 to 10 days after the onset of symptoms, or longer if the temperature remains elevated. The stools are disinfected before disposal, and the bedpan is disinfected after each use. The patient's dishes and cutlery are disinfected after use, and his bed linen is also disinfected before laundering. Precautions are necessary in the handling and disposing of any articles which may be contaminated by nose and mouth secretions or excreta.

During the preparalytic stage, it is important to keep the patient at rest, since the extent and severity of paralysis are thought to be increased by muscular exercise in this period. An analgesic and sedative may be necessary to relieve the pain and reduce restlessness. The patient is observed closely for indications of muscular weakness and paralysis. He is allowed up when he is symptom-free and there is no evidence of paralysis. The physician usually recommends that the patient who has had nonparalytic poliomyelitis be followed for at least 2 or 3 months after recovery for assessment of muscular function.

The patient who progresses to paralytic poliomyelitis requires more intensive, supportive care. The mattress should be firm or a fracture board may be used, and good body alignment is maintained. When the affected limbs are moved, they must be handled very gently to prevent precipitating a spasm and pain, and the joints are supported to prevent overstretching of muscles and tendons. Appropriate supports (footboard, pillows, sandbags and bolsters) are used to maintain a neutral position and relaxation of the paralyzed muscles and to prevent foot drop, outward rotation of the lower limb, hyperextension of the knee, wrist drop and contractures of the involved parts. A cradle may be used to relieve the weight of bedding on the hypersensitive limbs.

Hot moist packs or dry heat may be used to reduce the pain due to muscle spasm. Changes of position may also contribute to relief of pain as well as to the prevention of pressure sores and respiratory and cardiac complications. Splints may be applied to assist in preventing stretching, injury and contracture of the weak or paralyzed muscles.

The patient is observed closely for signs of respiratory difficulty, especially if the arm muscles are weak or paralyzed which indicates involvement of the cervical portion of the cord. Equipment for suctioning the patient and a cabinet (iron lung) type respirator should be readily available. The nurse must also be alert to the possibility of urinary retention.

In order to keep the muscles in as good condition as possible and preserve range of motion, an exercise program is begun as soon as the acute pain and muscle tenderness subside and the temperature remains normal. Passive movements, assistive and active exercises and exercise against resistance are used in and out of water to strengthen weakened muscles and minimize muscle atrophy and shortening. Residual disabilities such as foot drop may require the use of a brace to facilitate ambulation. Surgical intervention may eventually be considered necessary to correct problems such as a contracture or a foot or wrist drop which increase the patient's handicap. For example, the foot drop associated with flaccid paralysis of a leg may be corrected by an ankle arthrodesis (surgical ankylosis or fixation of a joint). A tendon transplant may be done so that a functioning muscle may take over the work of the paralyzed muscle. Muscle re-education and rehabilitation of the patient with paralysis generally requires long-term care. He may be faced with many of the physical, psychological and socioeconomic problems cited in the discussion of rehabilitation of the handicapped in Chapter 2.

In bulbar poliomyelitis, constant nursing attention is necessary. If the patient's swallowing is impaired, secretions collect in the pharynx and may be aspirated. Frequent suctioning and positioning to promote oral drainage are necessary. The foot of the bed may be elevated, and the patient is kept in the semiprone position. A nasogastric tube is passed so that fluids and nutrition may be administered.

The vital signs are recorded frequently so that early signs of involvement of vital centers are recognized. If respiratory insufficiency develops, a mechanical respirator may be necessary (see p. 286). A tracheostomy may be done if the airway is occluded by secretions or laryngeal spasm (see p. 281).

A diagnosis of poliomyelitis creates considerable anxiety for the patient's family; they require the nurse's support and need to be kept informed about the patient's condition. They should be advised that the paralysis may not be permanent and that it may take several months for the return of function. The exercises and physiotherapy program are explained, and suggestions are made as to their role in supporting and assisting the patient. If he is the wage earner, the family may be referred to a service or social welfare organization for assistance with their social and economic problems.

Meningitis

This is an inflammatory disease of the pia and arachnoid meningeal membranes.

Etiology and Incidence. Meningitis may be caused by the invasion of any pathogenic organism that gains entrance to the intracranial or intravertebral spaces. The most common offenders are viruses, influenza bacillus, tubercle bacillus, meningococcus, staphylococcus, streptococcus and pneumococcus. When it is caused by one of the last 3 bacteria, it is usually secondary to infection elsewhere in the body but may be the result of direct invasion through a cranial or spinal wound. The meningococcal type is communicable, being spread by droplet infection. In tuberculous meningitis, the bacilli are transmitted via the blood from a lesion in another part of the body (e.g., lung, bone).

Viral meningitis is now the most common type; incidence of that caused by other organisms has been rare since antibiotics became available. The disease may occur at any age but is seen more commonly in children.

Symptoms. The onset tends to be insidious in viral and tuberculous meningitis and is more sudden and acute in the other types. The patient complains of headache of increasing severity, pain in the back and limbs, and photophobia. The temperature is elevated, and there is marked neck rigidity. Kernig's and Brudzinski's signs, characteristic of meningeal irritation, are present (see p. 665). The patient tends to remain in a lateral position with the back arched and the head retracted. He is drowsy and probably confused, and coma may develop later. Convulsions are common in children. The cerebrospinal fluid is under increased pressure, is cloudy and has a high leukocyte count, high protein content and reduced concentration of glucose. The leukocyte blood count may show an elevation, depending on the causative organism which is identified through examination of the cerebrospinal fluid.

Treatment and Nursing Care. There is no specific treatment for viral meningitis; the patient is kept at rest and is given supportive care. Tuberculous meningitis is treated with isoniazid (orally), para-amino-salicylic acid (PAS) (orally) and streptomycin (intramuscularly). These medications are continued over a prolonged period. The dosage is usually high for 2 to 4 weeks, depending on the patient's response, and then decreased and continued for as long as 1 to 3 years. In severe cases, a special preparation of isoniazid may be injected into the subarachnoid cavity (intrathecal injection). When the disease is due to other types of organisms, antibiotics may be administered intrathecally as well as parenterally.

Isolation precautions are necessary if the patient has meningococcal (epidemic) meningitis. Those caring for the patient should know that nasal and oral secretions are contaminated. Frequent mouth care is necessary because of the fever and vomiting.

The room is darkened because of the patient's photophobia. An ice bag may help to relieve the headache, and analgesics are usually necessary for the relief of pain. Temperature sponges may be used if the fever is high. The fluid intake is increased to a minimum of 3500 ml., and the fluid balance is noted. An adequate fluid and caloric intake may be a problem because of nausea and vomiting or anorexia. Intravenous fluids and nasogastric feedings may be necessary.

Side rails are used in case of disorientation. Frequent observations are made for changes in vital signs, level of consciousness and neurological deficit such as impaired hearing, vision or motor weakness.

Tetanus (Lockjaw)

This disease is caused by the effects on the nervous system of the exotoxin released by tetanus bacilli (*Clostridium tetani*). It is characterized by hypertonicity of the skeletal muscles and recurring attacks of intense tonic spasms. The organism is spore-forming and anaerobic and is found in the fecal discharge of animals and man as well as in soil. The spores or bacilli enter the body via a wound where they germinate and multiply in anaerobic conditions. Wounds contaminated with soil, deep penetrating wounds and those in which there is necrotic tissue and a reduced concentration of oxygen are more prone to develop tetanus. The bacilli remain localized but produce a toxin which is thought to be absorbed into the blood stream. The tetanus exotoxin acts on the neuromuscular junctions and the motor neurons of the spinal cord and brain stem, producing muscular spasm.

The incubation period, which may vary from 2 days to several weeks, usually falls within the range of 6 to 14 days. The disease is not communicable except by transmission of discharge from the patient's wound to an open wound of another person. It may be prevented by active or passive immunization. Active immunization is conferred by a series of doses of toxoid. It is now usually given to children in combination with other vaccines (see p. 45). If the patient has not had a booster dose of toxoid within the past 5 or 6 years and the wound is heavily contaminated with soil, the patient is given passive immunization with 250 to 500 units of human immune globulin as well as a booster dose of toxoid. The patient with an accidental wound who has not had previous active immunization is given 1500 units of tetanus antitoxin subcutaneously. If the wound is heavily soil-contaminated or the treatment has been delayed, the physician may order 3000 units. Before giving the antitoxin, a small intracutaneous dose is given to determine if the patient is hypersensitive to serum (see p. 39). He is questioned as to whether he has any allergy or has ever had asthma or eczema. Any such history is reported to the doctor before giving the prescribed antitoxin. The prevention of tetanus also includes prompt cleansing and débridement of wounds.

Manifestations. The first symptom is usually hypertonicity of the jaw muscles. The patient complains of difficulty in opening his mouth and in chewing. This progresses to painful spasms (trismus) in which the jaws are rigidly clamped. The spasticity of the facial muscles distorts his expression. The throat and tongue muscles are affected, making swallowing and speech difficult. Eventually, the tonic rigidity spreads to involve all the skeletal muscles. Periodic spasms of increased intensity occur and are extremely painful and exhausting. During these attacks, the head is sharply hyper-extended and the back may be arched off the bed (opisthotonus); respirations are arrested because of spasm of the larynx and respiratory muscles, cyanosis develops, and there is danger of asphyxiation.

The patient's temperature is elevated, and he perspires freely with the energy expenditure. The patient remains conscious and oriented unless severe exhaustion, hypoxia or complications such as pneumonia intervene. The severity of the paroxysmal muscle spasms gradually decreases in frequency and severity after a week or 10 days, but it may take several months before normal muscle tone is sustained.

Treatment and Nursing Care. If the patient does not manifest a hypersensitivity response to a small intracutaneous dose of tetanus antitoxin, he is given large doses intramuscularly and intravenously to neutralize toxin before it reaches the nervous structures. One cc. of epinephrine (Adrenalin) 1:1000 may be added to the intravenous injection to counteract possible serum

reaction. The wound is cleansed and debrided, and the surrounding area is infiltrated with tetanus antitoxin because of the high concentration of the toxin in this region. An antibiotic such as penicillin or tetracycline is given to destroy the tetanus bacilli. Sedatives, tranquilizers and muscle relaxants are prescribed; phenobarbital (Sodium Luminal), chloral hydrate, paraldehyde, chorpromazine (Thorazine), methocarbamol (Robaxin) are examples of drugs which may be ordered. A tracheostomy may be done because of laryngeal spasm and the accumulation of excessive secretions. It facilitates deep suctioning and oxygen administration (see p. 284 for care).

The patient requires constant nursing attention in a quiet, darkened room. All external stimuli are kept to a minimum. Disturbances such as a sudden noise, jarring of the bed and quick handling of the patient may precipitate a tonic spasm of the muscles. Everything must be done as gently as possible; a calm, low voice is used when speaking within the patient's hearing, and he is advised when he is going to be moved or touched.

If a tracheostomy is not done, frequent suctioning is necessary to remove oropharyngeal secretions, and the foot of the bed may be elevated to promote postural drainage. Padded side rails are used on the bed to prevent the patient from injuring himself during a spasm. Mouth and skin care are important in preventing sordes, parotitis and pressure sores. Care is given following the administration of a sedative or muscle relaxant to lessen the possibility of precipitating a spasm. A foam rubber mattress helps to protect the skin. Fluids may be given intravenously, and as soon as the convulsive spasms can be sufficiently controlled, nasogastric feedings are introduced. These are of high caloric value because much energy is expended by the muscle contractions. The patient is observed for retention of urine; catheterization may be necessary. Constipation is a common problem, and enemas may be used to prevent fecal impaction.

Herpes Zoster (Shingles)

Herpes zoster is an acute infectious disease caused by a virus similar to that which causes chickenpox (varicella). It is thought that in many instances the virus is reactivated after having remained dormant in the body for varying lengths of time. It has an affinity for the sensory neurons of the dorsal root ganglia of the spinal nerves and the ganglia associated with the sensory divisions of the cranial nerves. It rarely occurs in children and increases in incidence and severity in the older age group. Fatigue, illness and malnutrition are predisposing factors.

Manifestations. Herpes zoster is characterized by hypersensitivity, pain and a vesicular rash along the course of the sensory nerves emanating from the affected ganglia. The vesicles usually crust and dry up in a few days, but the area may remain painful for much longer. Fever and general malaise may accompany the onset. The lesions are generally unilateral. The gasserian ganglion of the trigeminal (fifth cranial) nerve is not infrequently affected. Lesions along the distribution of its ophthalmic division involve the eye; vesicles develop on the cornea which may lead to ulceration, scarring and permanent impairment of vision.

Treatment and Nursing Care. There is no specific treatment for herpes zoster; treatment and care are directed toward the relief of pain and the prevention of secondary infection of the vesicles. Acetylsalicylic acid (Aspirin), codeine and, rarely, stronger analgesics are used for the relief of pain. A calamine preparation may be applied to the local skin lesions and, if they are on the trunk, may be protected from clothing by a light, soft cloth or petrolatum gauze. If the eye is involved, an adrenocorticoid preparation may be instilled to decrease the inflammation and ensuing ulceration and scarring.

The patient is not usually confined to bed unless the fever is high or the herpes is a complication of another disease. Well-balanced meals which are high in vitamins and extra rest are encouraged.

References

BOOKS

American Rehabilitation Foundation: Rehabilitative Nursing Techniques:
    No. 1.   Bed Positioning and Transfer Procedures for the Hemiplegic.
    No. 2.   Selected Equipment Useful in the Hospital, Home or Nursing Home.
    No. 3.   A Procedure for Passive Range of Motion and Self-assistive Exercises.
    Minneapolis, American Rehabilitation Foundation.
Brain, The Late Lord, and Walton, J. N.: Brain's Diseases of the Nervous System, 7th ed. London, Oxford University Press, 1969.
Carini, E., and Owens, G.: Neurological and Neurosurgical Nursing, 5th ed. St. Louis, The C. V. Mosby Co., 1970.
Chusid, J. G., and McDonald, J. J.: Correlative Neuroanatomy and Functional Neurology, 12th ed. Los Altos, California, Lange Medical Publications, 1964.
Gardner, E.: Fundamentals of Neurology, 5th ed. Philadelphia, W. B. Saunders Co., 1968.
Gatz, A. J.: Manter's Essentials of Clinical Neuroanatomy and Neurophysiology, 3rd ed. Philadelphia, F. A. Davis Co., 1966.
Gowers, W. R.: Epilepsy and Other Chronic Convulsive Diseases. New York, Dover Publications Inc., 1964.
Hooper, R.: Neurosurgical Nursing. Springfield, Charles C Thomas, Publishers, 1964.
Krenzel, J. R., and Rohrer, L. M.: Paraplegic and Quadriplegic Individuals—Handbook of Care for Nurses. Chicago, The Paraplegic Foundation, 1966.
Luhan, J. A.: Neurology. Baltimore, the Williams and Wilkins Co., 1968.
Scott, D.: About Epilepsy. London, G. Duckworth Co., 1969.
Smith, B. H.: Principles of Clinical Neurology. New York, Year Book Medical Publishers Inc., 1965.
Sorenson, L., et al.: Ambulation—A Manual for Nurses. Minneapolis, American Rehabilitation Foundation.
Sutton, A. L.: Bedside Nursing Techniques in Medicine and Surgery, 2nd ed. Philadelphia, W. B. Saunders Co., 1969. Chapter 17.

PERIODICALS

Barager, F. D.: "Cerebrovascular Accident." Canad. Nurse, Vol. 62, No. 5 (May 1966), pp. 35–37.

Bertrand, C., and Martinez, S. N.: "Herniated Discs." Canad. Nurse, Vol. 61, No. 3 (Mar. 1965), pp. 200–203.

Bertrand, C., and Martinez, S. N.: "Parkinson's Disease." Canad. Nurse, Vol. 61, No. 3 (Mar. 1965), pp. 188–190.

Branch, C.: "Surgical Treatment of Epilepsy." Canad. Nurse, Vol. 61, No. 3 (Mar. 1965), pp. 174–177.

Buck, McK.: "Adjustments During Recovery from Stroke." Amer. J. Nurs., Vol. 64, No. 10 (Oct. 1964), pp. 92–95.

Carozza, V. J.: "Understanding the Patient with Epilepsy." Nurs. Clin. North Amer., Vol. 5, No. 1 (Mar. 1970), pp. 13–22.

Coderre, L.: "Speech Therapy." Canad. Nurse, Vol. 59, No. 3 (Mar. 1963), pp. 239–241.

Editors: "Changing the Outlook for Parkinson Patients." Med. World News, Vol. 9, No. 48 (Nov. 29, 1968), pp. 32–35.

Forster, F. M. (Ed.): "Symposium on Neurologic Disturbances." Med. Clin. North Amer., Vol. 47, No. 6 (Nov. 1963).

French, J. D.: "The Reticular Formation." Sci. Amer., Vol. 196, No. 5 (May 1957), pp. 54–60. (Available in Reprint.)

Griffin, C.: "Social Factors in Epilepsy." Canad. Nurse, Vol. 61, No. 3 (Mar. 1965), pp. 185–187.

Hilkemeyer, R., et al.: "Nursing Care of Patients with Brain Tumors." Amer. J. Nurs., Vol. 64, No. 3 (Mar. 1964), pp. 81–83.

Hudson, W. J., et al.: "Hospital Management of Hemiplegia." Canad. Nurs., Vol. 62, No. 7 (July 1966), pp. 21–23.

Hunkle, E., and Lazier, R.: "A Patient with Fractured Cervical Vertebrae." Amer. J. Nurs., Vol. 65, No. 9 (Sept. 1965), pp. 82–86.

Huxley, H. E.: "The Contraction of Muscle." Sci. Amer., Vol. 199, No. 5 (Nov. 1958), pp. 66–82. (Avail- in Reprint.)

Illerbrun, D.: "The Aphasic Patient." Canad. Nurse, Vol. 62, No. 9 (Sept. 1966), pp. 33–35.

Karnes, W. E.: "Medical Treatment for Convulsive Disorders." Med. Clin. North Amer., Vol. 52, No. 4 (July 1968), pp. 959–987.

Katz, B.: "The Nerve Impulse." Sci. Amer., Vol. 187, No. 5 (Nov. 1952), pp. 55–64. (Available in Reprint.)

King, I. M. (Ed.): "Symposium on Neurologic and Neurosurgical Nursing." Nurs. Clin. North Amer., Vol. 4, No. 2 (June 1969).

Large, H., et al.: "In the First Stroke Intensive Care Unit." Amer. J. Nurs., Vol. 69, No. 1 (Jan. 1969), pp. 76–80.

Leavens, M. E.: "Brain Tumors." Amer. J. Nurs., Vol. 64, No. 3 (Mar. 1964), pp. 78–80.

Lougheed, W. M.: "Intracranial Berry Aneurysms." Canad. Nurse, Vol. 61, No. 3 (Mar. 1965), pp. 213–214.

Moody, L.: "Care of Parkinsonian Patients." Canad. Nurse, Vol. 61, No. 3 (Mar. 1965), p. 199.

Moody, L.: "Nursing Care: Patients with Herniated Discs." Canad. Nurse, Vol. 61, No. 3 (Mar. 1965), pp. 204–206.

Robb, P.: "Epilepsy and Its Medical Treatment." Canad. Nurse, Vol. 61, No. 3 (Mar. 1965), pp. 171–173.

Robertson, M. E.: "A Patient with Back Injury." Canad. Nurse, Vol. 61, No. 8 (Aug. 1965), pp. 641–647.

Selkert, R. E. (Ed.): "Symposium on Neurologic Disorders." Med. Clin. North Amer., Vol. 52, No. 4 (July 1968).

Sidell, A. D., and Daly, D. D.: "Electroencephalography in Epilepsy." Med. Clin. North Amer., Vol. 47, No. 6 (Nov. 1963), pp. 1541–1577.

Tasker, R. R.: "Increased Intracranial Pressure." Canad. Nurse., Vol. 61, No. 3 (Mar. 1965), pp. 207–208.

Thorpe, E. L. M., and Coull, E. G.: "Nursing the Patient with Cerebrovascular Accident." Canad. Nurse, Vol. 62, No. 5 (May 1966), pp. 38–41.

Ullman, M.: "Disorders of Body Image after Stroke." Amer. J. Nurs., Vol. 64, No. 10 (Oct. 1964), pp. 89–91.

Wilcoxson, H. L.: "Cerebrovascular Accident: The Role of the Public Health Nurse." Nurs. Clin. North Amer., Vol. 1, No. 1 (Mar. 1966), pp. 63–71.

Wilson, V. J.: "Inhibition in the Central Nervous System." Sci. Amer., Vol. 214, No. 5 (May 1966), pp. 102–110.

Young, J. F.: "Nursing Care: Ruptured Cerebral Aneurysm." Canad. Nurse, Vol. 61, No. 3 (Mar. 1965), pp. 215–218.

Young, J. F.: "Recognition, Recording and Significance of the Signs of Increased Intracranial Pressure." Canad. Nurse, Vol. 61, No. 3 (Mar. 1965), pp. 209–214.

BOOKLETS AND PAMPHLETS

Cerebrovascular Accident:
   Strokes – A Guide for the Family
   Strike Back at Stroke

Up and Around
Self-help Devices for the Stroke Patient
Aphasia and the Family
Distributed by the local branches of the American Heart Association and Canadian Heart Foundation.
Epilepsy:
Facts about Epilepsy
What the Teacher Can Do for the Student with Epilepsy
The Nurse's Role in Epilepsy
Handbook for Parents
Distributed by the local epilepsy information centers and national epilepsy associations.
Multiple Sclerosis:
Multiple Sclerosis (G. A. Schumacher)
The R.N. and M.S.
M.S.—The Need—The Disease—The Organization
A Home Program for the Care of Bed Patients
A Home Program for Independently Ambulatory Patients
A Home Program for Patients Ambulatory with Aids
Distributed by the multiple sclerosis societies of Canada and United States.
Myasthenia Gravis:
20 Questions and Answers about Myasthenia Gravis
Myasthenia Gravis—The Mysterious Disease of Weakness
Distributed by The Myasthenia Gravis Foundation, Willowdale, Ontario, Canada.

23
Nursing in Bone Disorders

STRUCTURE AND FUNCTION OF BONES

BONE TISSUE

Bone is a rigid connective tissue consisting of bone cells, calcified collagenous intercellular substance and marrow. Each bone, except at joint surfaces, is covered by a tough, supportive membrane called the periosteum. It is firmly attached to the underlying bone by penetrating fibers, and its blood vessels give off many branches which enter the tissue to provide the essentials for growth, repair and maintenance. The inner layer of the periosteum gives rise to the osteoblasts, which function in the development and replacement of bone. The shaft of the long bones is hollow and is lined with a comparable membrane referred to as the endosteum. Although approximately two-thirds of bone tissue is inorganic mineral substance, which gives it the characteristic hardness and inert appearance, it is viable tissue undergoing constant metabolic processes, just as other tissues.

Bone tissue contains a network of minute anastomosing canals and spaces which contain blood vessels, lymphatics, lymph and bone cells. The rigid intercellular substance is formed in scale-like sheets or layers (lamellae) around the canals and spaces. It is composed of a tough collagenous network of fibers which becomes impregnated with mineral salts, principally tricalcium phosphate and calcium carbonate. There are 3 types of bone cells—namely, osteoblasts, osteocytes and osteoclasts. The osteoblasts are found beneath the periosteum on the surface of growing bones and in developmental or ossification areas within the bones. They are responsible for the formation of the collagenous fibers and the deposition of the mineral salts. The osteocytes are matured osteoblasts which become imprisoned in small spaces by the intercellular substance. The osteoclasts are considered responsible for the breaking down and reabsorption of bone tissue. Guyton states: "Normally, except in growing bones, the rates of bone deposition and absorption are equal to each other so that the total mass of bone remains constant."[1] This continuous breaking down, reabsorption and new bone formation are necessary, since old bone becomes weak and brittle. The bone cells respond by internal reconstruction according to the forces acting upon the tissue. The mineralization and strength of the bones are influenced by the amount of weight bearing and muscle pull to

---

[1] A. C. Guyton: Textbook of Medical Physiology, 4th ed. Philadelphia, W. B. Saunders Co., 1971, p. 934.

which they are subjected. Those of the active person and of an athlete are stronger and more resistant to stress than the bones of nonactive persons. One of the complications of prolonged bed rest is the decalcification and weakening of the bones. In older persons the bones tend to become brittle and less resistant to stress, increasing the possibility of fractures. This is due to the general decline in cell reproduction which results in a slower rate of production of the collagenous matrix and mineralization as well as of reabsorption.

Types of Bone Tissue

Each bone is composed of 2 types of tissue—compact and cancellous. Outer layers consist of dense, compact tissue, and the interior is of a spongy or porous nature (cancellous). The numerous larger spaces of cancellous tissue contain red bone marrow. The thickness of each type of tissue varies in different bones as well as in parts of the same bone.

In the long bone (e.g., humerus, tibia, femur), the extremities have a thin outer layer of compact tissue enclosing a larger mass of cancellous tissue. The shaft is formed mainly of 2 thick layers of compact bone separated by a small amount of porous tissue. The central hollow portion of the shaft forms the medullary canal, which is filled with fatty, yellow marrow. Flat bones (e.g., skull bones, scapula, ribs) have a thicker layer of cancellous tissue lying between 2 relatively thinner layers of compact tissue. Short and irregular bones such as those of the wrist and ankle have a thin shell of compact tissue enclosing a fair thickness of cancellous tissue.

Functions of Bones and Contained Marrow

The bones are bound together by ligaments and collectively form the skeleton, which provides a supporting framework for the body and protection for vital structures. They assist in body movement by providing attachment for muscles and leverage for their action. The bones also serve as the body's store of calcium. A constant level in the blood and tissue fluids is necessary for several physiological processes (e.g., blood clotting, normal muscular activity, normal heart action). If the blood calcium falls below the normal level, the deficit is met by the withdrawal of calcium from the bones. Conversely, any excess in the blood is deposited in bone tissue.

The red bone marrow is a highly vascular hematopoietic tissue contained within the spaces of cancellous tissue. It produces erythrocytes, granular leukocytes and thrombocytes (blood platelets). During childhood, all cancellous tissue contains red marrow. In the adult, much of this is replaced by yellow marrow, and the cancellous tissue of the ribs, sternum, skull bones, vertebrae, pelvic bones and the proximal ends of the long bones play the major role in hematopoiesis. Yellow bone marrow consists mainly of fat cells and blood vessels; the largest amount is found in the medullary canals of long bones.

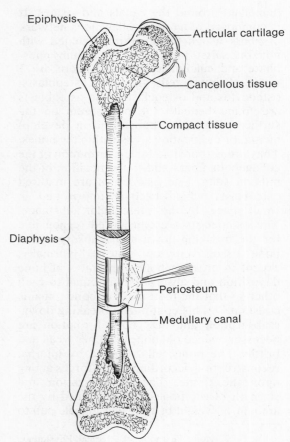

Epiphysis

Articular cartilage

Cancellous tissue

Compact tissue

Diaphysis

Periosteum

Medullary canal

Figure 23–1 Diagram of a long bone.

The Development and Growth of Bones

The development of the bones begins early in embryonic life and is not normally completed until the late teens or early twenties. They are preformed of membranous connective tissue or cartilaginous tissue, which is gradually replaced by bone in the process of ossification.

The cranial bones and the mandible (lower jaw) develop by intramembranous ossification. There is a marked increase in the vascularity of the membranous tissue. This is followed by the appearance of localized centers of ossification from which bone formation proceeds to the periphery. Radiating bundles of fibers and osteoblasts appear between the blood vessels, followed by the development of the collagenous fibrous matrix which becomes impregnated with calcium salts. The original membrane becomes the periosteum. As the conversion to bone proceeds outward, the edges of the membranous tissue continue to grow. When ossification overtakes the growth of the membranous tissue, the full size of the bone has been reached. The continued growth of the membranous tissue of the cranial bones accounts for the "soft" areas or fontanels in the skull in the infant.

The bones which are preformed of cartilage undergo intracartilaginous (endochondral) ossification, which involves destruction of the cartilage and its replacement by bone tissue. Osteoblasts develop at the surface of the cartilage and initiate the formation of surface layers of bone tissue by producing a collagenous fibrous matrix in which mineral salts are deposited. Then osteoblasts, osteoclasts and blood vessels invade internal areas of the cartilage, setting up ossification centers around which cartilage is progressively removed and replaced by bone tissue.

In long bones, an ossification center appears within the shaft (diaphysis) and later in each end (epiphysis). An ossification proceeds, growth of the cartilage continues, resulting in a persisting thin strip of cartilaginous tissue between each epiphysis and the diaphysis, which is referred to as the growth or epiphyseal plate. The bones continue to grow as long as new cartilage develops to maintain this plate. Cessation of growth occurs when it becomes ossified, and the epiphyses are fused with the diaphysis. Bones grow in circumference by the formation of layers of bone beneath the periosteum.

Factors in Bone Development, Growth and Repair

Several factors influence the development, growth and maintenance of normal bone structure. A diet which is adequate in calcium and phosphorus is essential for ossification and the constant formation of new bone to replace that which was reabsorbed. Vitamin D is necessary for the absorption and utilization of the minerals. A deficiency of any one of these substances in children may lead to rickets, which is characterized by soft deformed bones, failure of closure of the fontanels, soft and poorly developed teeth, bleeding tendency and muscle spasms. In adults, a deficiency of calcium and phosphorus or vitamin D may cause a weakening of bone structure referred to as osteomalacia. Milk and milk products provide an abundant source of the minerals. Vitamin D may be formed by exposure of the skin to sunlight, which acts on a sterol (7-dehydrocholesterol) which is a component of the skin. To ensure an adequate supply of vitamin D, a preparation of a fish liver oil (e.g., cod liver oil) or of ergosterol which has been exposed to ultraviolet rays (Calciferol) is usually administered to infants and young children. The nurse must be cognizant of the fact that excessive amounts of vitamin D can cause hypercalcemia, which may be manifested by anorexia, nausea, vomiting, drowsiness, headache, bladder irritation and renal calculi.

Adequate dietary amounts of protein and vitamin C are necessary to bones for the formation of the collagenous, fibrous, intercellular matrix in which the minerals are deposited. Vitamin A, which is essential to all tissue growth, is also necessary.

Bone growth and ossification are also influenced by certain hormones—namely, the somatotrophic or growth hormone produced by the adenohypophysis (see p. 534), thyroxine (see p. 540) and the parathyroid hormone (see p. 550).

In addition to the above factors, the demand placed on the bones by weight bearing and muscle pull plays an important role. Inactivity and less than the normal demand weakens the structure; calcium and phosphorus are lost from the bone, and the condition known as osteoporosis may develop. Osteoblastic activity is slowed, and bone deposition is depressed. Muscle pull and the degree of stress influence the shaping of the bone. For example, processes such as the greater and lesser trochanters of the femur, the tibial tuberosity of the tibia, and the deltoid tuberosity of the radius develop as the result of muscle pull when the bones are developing and growing.

NURSING IN BONE DISORDERS

FRACTURES

A fracture is a break in the continuity of a bone, separating it into 2 or more parts, which are referred to as fragments.

Causes

The majority of fractures are due to violence incurred by falls, blows or twisting. The force, in excess of the bone's resistance, may be applied directly or indirectly. In direct violence, the fracture occurs at or near the site of the applied force. When indirect violence is the cause, the force is applied at a point remote from the site of the fracture. For example, in a fall on the outstretched hand, the stress may be transmitted to the radius, ulna, humerus or clavicle. A fracture may also be due to a sudden, forceful contraction of attached muscles.

Occasionally, a fracture occurs as the result of disease of the bone which has weakened its structure to the point that it cannot withstand the normal degree of stress. Metastases, primary tumors (e.g., sarcoma, osteitis fibrosa cystica due to hyperparathyroidism), osteogenesis imperfecta (a congenital condition affecting the formation of osteoblasts) and osteoporosis are examples of diseased conditions of bone that may lead to spontaneous fracture.

Types of Fractures

Traumatic or Pathological. The fracture may be designated as traumatic when it is the result of violence or as pathological or spontaneous if it is due to disease of the bone.

Complete or Incomplete. A fracture is complete if the bone is separated into 2 distinct parts or incomplete if the break is not all the way through the bone. The greenstick fracture seen in children is an incomplete fracture in which the bone is broken on one side and bent or crumpled on the opposite side.

Simple or Comminuted. A fracture may be described as simple if it produces only 2 fragments or as comminuted if it consists of 3 or more fragments.

Open (Compound) or Closed. An open or compound fracture is associated with an open wound in the overlying skin which establishes communication between the fracture site and the outside air. This type of fracture is potentially infected. The skin wound may be produced by the force that inflicted the fracture or by a fragment of the bone. Conversely, in a closed fracture the overlying skin remains intact and there is no communication with the outside.

According to the Direction of the Fracture Line. The break may be described as transverse, longitudinal, oblique or spiral, according to the direction of the fracture line in relation to the longitidinal axis of the bone. When one fragment is driven into the other one, the fracture is referred to as impacted.

Special. A few fractures have been named for physicians associated with studies of fractures in certain areas. The commonest of these are the Colles' and Pott's fractures. In a Colles' fracture, a break occurs in the distal portion of the radius and possibly in the styloid process of the ulna. A Pott's fracture involves a break through the distal ends of the tibia and fibula. An epiphyseal separation or fracture occurs when the break is through the epiphyseal or growth plate. When a ligament or tendon under excessive stress fractures or tears away its bony attachment, the break in the bone is described as an avulsion fracture.

Effects and Manifestations

Local Effects. A fracture is always accompanied by some degree of damage to the contiguous soft tissues. Blood vessels within the bone, the periosteum and surrounding tissues are torn, resulting in hemorrhage and then the formation of a hematoma. The periosteum at the site may be stripped from the underlying bone tissue, interrupting the blood supply into the area and thus contributing to the death of bone cells. There may also be hemorrhage into adjacent muscles and joints and damage to ligaments, tendons and nerves. Soon after a fracture occurs the muscles in the area go into spasm, causing severe pain and possible displacement of a fragment due to tendon pull.

Depending on the location of the fracture, visceral injuries may occur, actually provoking a threat to the patient's life. Examples of such injuries are rupture of the bladder by a fractured pelvis and rupture of the spleen or perforation of a lung by a fractured rib.

Systemic Effects. The patient suffers varying degrees of shock, influenced by the severity of the injury, the amount of soft tissue damage, his age and his general condition at the time of injury. (see p. 239 for predisposing factors and manifestations of shock.) Usually a slight elevation of temperature and leukocytosis occur in the first 2 or 3 days.

Manifestations. The symptoms of a fracture vary with its location, type, the amount of displacement of the fragments and degree of damage to soft tissue structures.

The patient or an observer usually relates a history of a fall, blow or sudden forcible movement, and the victim may actually say that he heard the bone break. Sudden severe pain at the site is experienced which may or may not persist. Frequently, because of injury and shock, nerve function is impaired, and pain may be absent for a brief period following the injury. As function returns, muscle spasm in the area, as well as tissue damage, accounts for much of the pain, which becomes worse with any movement. Obvious deformity may be present as a result of displacement of the fragments, and there may be shortening of the affected limb due to contraction of attached muscles. Impaired mobility and loss of mechanical support occur, and in the case of long bones, there may be obvious movement in a part that is normally rigid. Complete loss of function may result from nerve compression

by displaced fragments; this is usually restored when the fracture is reduced and the fragments are placed in normal opposition. Crepitus (grating sound produced by movement of the ends of the fragments) may be noted if the patient moves the part. Under no circumstances should any attempt be made to elicit the symptom of crepitus because of the possibility of further serious damage to soft tissues (e.g., blood vessels and nerves), unnecessary displacement of fragments and the production of an open fracture. Swelling may develop rapidly over the site of the fracture because of bleeding and the escape of fluid into the tissue. After 2 or 3 days this area frequently becomes discolored (ecchymosis).

In the case of the rupture of viscera by a fragment, symptoms of impaired function of the damaged organ appear. With rupture of the bladder by a fractured pelvis, extravasation of urine gradually becomes evident, and blood appears in the urine. Rarely, perforation of the intestine is associated with pelvic fracture and causes severe shock and peritonitis. A serious complication of a rib fracture may be puncture of a lung. The patient manifests severe shock, respiratory distress, coughing and hemoptysis.

Some fractures, especially those which are incomplete or of short bones, may produce few signs and symptoms. The fracture may be suspected only on the basis of the history of violence, tenderness on pressure over the site or the patient's complaint of pain upon use of the part or weight bearing on it. Again, no attempt should be made by the first aider or a nurse to elicit symptoms by having the person move or stand. The patient is treated as having a fracture if there is any doubt.

The physician bases his diagnosis of a fracture on the history of the accident, physical examination of the patient and roentgenograms of the affected part.

Fracture Healing

Bone is different from many of the specialized tissues because of its ability to regenerate and bridge a gap to unite broken bones. Many tissues heal by laying down nonspecialized fibrous scar tissue.

Immediately following a fracture, the space between the fragments and around the fracture line is filled with blood and inflammatory exudate. The blood clots and the exudate are invaded by fibroblasts and capillaries from adjacent connective tissue and blood vessels, forming granulation tissue. The fibroblasts differentiate to form fibrous tissue and cartilage. Simultaneously, osteoblasts proliferate, mainly from the inner surface of the periosteum (and endosteum in a long bone), and invade the granulation tissue and cartilage. Calcium salts are deposited, forming a loosely woven, bone-like tissue referred to as a callus. It forms a "collar" around the bone at the fracture site, giving it greater thickness than the original bone. The callus unites and helps to stabilize the fragments but is not strong enough to bear weight or withstand stress. As the bone-forming cells increase, the callus is gradually restructured and remodeled by ossification (production of a collagenous fibrous network which becomes impregnated with mineral salts) to form true bone tissue.

In some instances, a fracture is complicated by delayed healing or nonunion. Delayed healing simply implies that the fracture is not healing as rapidly as is normally expected. In nonunion, the granulation tissue that formed between the fragments following the fracture is converted to dense fibrous tissue instead of normal callus and bone tissue. Causes of delayed union or nonunion include too wide a gap between the fragments, the interposition of soft tissues or a foreign body between the fragments, inadequate immobilization, poor blood supply to the site, loss of the hematoma by the escape of blood through an open wound or surgical intervention, infection of the bone and malnutrition.

General Principles and Methods of Treatment of Fractures

Emergency Care. The first aid treatment that the patient with a fracture receives is very important; movement on the part of the patient or improper handling may cause serious tissue damage and increased pain, hemorrhage and shock. The patient's general condition and the extent of his injuries are quickly evaluated, and priorities are set. Respiratory insufficiency, hemorrhage or shock may be evident, requiring immediate attention.

If a fracture is obvious or suspected, care at the site of the accident and during transportation to a hospital is directed toward preventing further tissue damage, visceral injury, and a closed fracture from becoming open. The patient should receive a minimum of handling; unless there is danger of further injury, he is left where he is until lifted onto a stretcher or into a vehicle for transportation to the hospital. Before moving the patient, the fracture site and the joint above and below are immobilized. A splint is made from whatever is available (e.g., a board, 2 or 3 thicknesses of cardboard, a folded quilt or blanket, pillows). In the case of a board, the surface applied to the patient must be padded (towels or clothing may be used) to prevent pressure. If the limb is in an abnormal position, it is splinted in that deformed position; no attempt is made to reduce the fracture or restore the limb to a normal position. If splint material is not available, a lower limb may be immobilized by placing a pillow or folded blanket between the legs and tying them together. The uninjured limb serves as a splint. In the case of an arm, it may be secured against the trunk by binders or bandages. If it is an open fracture, the wound is covered with the cleanest material available (e.g., a clean handkerchief). If the bone is protruding from the wound, no attempt is made to replace it or reduce the fracture. Nothing is given by mouth in case a general anesthetic will be necessary.

When the patient arrives at the hospital, a quick examination is made of his general condition, and if there is respiratory distress, bleeding or shock, appropriate treatment is instituted before the fracture receives attention. When the general condition is satisfactory, roentgenograms are made of the fracture area. Clothing is removed from the uninjured side of the body first. When it is necessary to cut the clothing on the injured side, this is done along a seam if possible so the garment may be repaired later.

Treatment. The treatment of a fracture usually involves reduction, immobilization of the part while the bone heals, and then a period of physical therapy to restore normal function.

REDUCTION. This is the procedure by which fragments are brought into their pre-injury position so that the normal shape and length of the bone are restored and union is promoted. Obviously, reduction is only necessary if there is some displacement of the fragments. It is carried out as soon as possible. A delay makes it more difficult to obtain satisfactory alignment because of the rapid organization of the blood clot and the associated muscle spasm. Also, there is likely to be less tissue trauma with early reduction.

A fracture may be reduced by closed manipulative reduction, traction applied distal to the fracture, or open (internal) reduction. In closed reduction, the physician manipulates the fragments into position by manual traction, pressure, and/or rotation. In fractures in which one fragment is overriding the other and there is considerable muscle pull, continuous traction may be applied to the distal fragment to bring it into apposition and to maintain the alignment. This method of reduction is used most often in fractures of the femur because the pull of the strong thigh muscles tends to displace the fragments and cause overriding. The traction may be applied to the skin (skin traction) or directly to bone (skeletal traction). (See the discussion of traction under Immobilization.) In some fractures, reduction can only be achieved through an open surgical incision.

Reduction may necessitate a general anesthetic. The nurse determines from the patient when he last had food and fluid and what was taken. This is reported to the physician. Reduction may have to be delayed a few hours to allow the stomach to empty and reduce the risk of vomiting and aspiration.

IMMOBILIZATION. Various methods are used to maintain reduction and immobilize the fragments. They may be categorized as external fixation, traction or internal fixation.

External fixation is most commonly achieved by enclosing the part in a plaster cast. A plaster cast is made by the application and molding of moist plaster of Paris bandages to the affected part. The bandages are strips of crinoline impregnated with gypsum (anhydrous calcium sulfate). They are immersed in warm water, 21° to 24° C. (70° to 75° F.), for a few seconds and then are lightly compressed by pushing both ends toward the middle to remove excess water before application. The addition of water to the bandage causes the gypsum to crystallize, making it possible to mold the soft moist bandage to the affected body part. As it is applied, each layer is rubbed into that below to prevent separation of the cast into layers. As the water evaporates from the bandages, the plaster hardens and the application becomes rigid.

Before the cast is applied, the skin is cleansed and examined for any contusions or abrasions. The part is then enclosed in circular stockinette for skin protection. Extra padding is used over bony prominences or to fill in spaces which might weaken the cast.

When the application of the plaster bandages is completed, the stockinette which extends beyond the cast is turned back over the cast edges and is secured by incorporation into the cast or with adhesive tape. The cast applied to a limb may be referred to as a circular cast. A walking cast may be applied with simple fractures of the tibia and fibula. A stump or walking iron is incorporated into the cast which encloses the leg and most of the foot. This device permits the patient to be up, walk and bear his weight on the limb. If a stirrup is not used, additional layers of plaster on the sole may be used. A spica cast is applied to the trunk and one or both lower or upper limbs (e.g., shoulder spica, hip spica). A cast which is applied to the trunk is called a jacket or body cast. A bivalve cast is one which has been molded to the limb or trunk, allowed to dry, and then cut down each side so it may be removed for brief periods to allow skin or wound care or other treatment. The sections are held in position by bandages or straps. See the discussion of nursing care of the patient with a cast on page 683.

A splint is occasionally used as a means of external fixation and may be of wood, metal, plastic or molded plaster of Paris. It must be long enough to immobilize the joints immediately above and below the fracture and is shaped or molded according to the part to which it is applied. Padding is placed between the skin and the splint to prevent irritation and pressure and to fill in spaces. The splint is secured by straps or firm bandages. Precautions are necessary in order to have the splint held stationary without interfering with circulation. Any swelling, discoloration, coldness or numb-

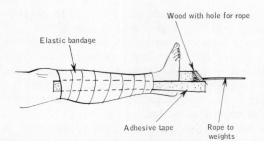

Figure 23–2 Skin traction on a lower limb. (From Sutton, A. L.: Bedside Nursing Techniques, 2nd ed. Philadelphia, W. B. Saunders Co., 1969, p. 190.)

ness of the distal parts of the limb is reported immediately so the splint may be loosened.

Traction is most commonly used to maintain reduction in fractures of the lower limbs.* It involves the application of a force along the long axis of the bone distal to the fracture. Countertraction (a force in the opposite direction) is necessary and is provided by elevating the foot of the bed in the case of a lower limb; the weight of the body on the incline supplies the required countertraction. A fracture board is placed under a firm mattress to prevent sagging which could change the direction of the force being applied and interfere with alignment of the fragments.

As cited in reduction, traction may be applied to the skin or directly to the bone. Skin traction is established by the application of moleskin or adhesive tapes to the medial and lateral surfaces of the limb. These are secured by a firm cotton or flannelette bandage. The adhesive strips extend beyond the foot and attach to a plate, bar or block (spreader) wide enough to prevent the tapes from contacting the malleoli. A rope connected to the spreader is carried over a pulley on a crossbar at the foot of the bed and suspends a prescribed weight (usually 8 to 10 pounds for an adult) to exert the traction force (see Fig. 23–2).

Skeletal traction is obtained by the insertion of a metal wire (e.g., Kirschner's wire) or pin (e.g., Steinmann's pin) through the bone distal to the fracture. A special traction stirrup or bow is fastened to the pro-

truding ends of the wire or pin and then attached to a rope leading to a pulley and weight system. When skeletal traction is used, the limb is usually suspended on a special splint (see Fig. 23–3).

Various arrangements are used in applying traction to the lower limbs. Those commonly employed are Buck's extension, Bryant's traction (gallows suspension), Russell traction and balanced or suspension traction.

Buck's extension involves simple skin traction by means of adhesive strips applied to the sides of the leg and their attachment to a spreader which in turn attaches to a rope leading to a pulley and suspended weights.

It is usually only used temporarily for reduction of a fracture. The skin should be clean and dry before the traction tapes are applied. The physician may or may not

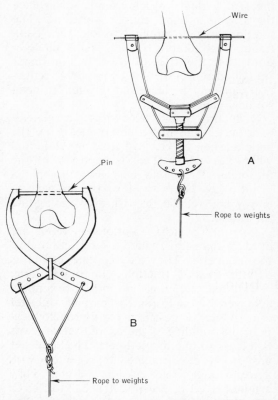

Figure 23–3 Skeletal traction may be applied by Kirschner wire and traction stirrup (*A*) or Steinmann pin and traction stirrup (*B*). (From Sutton, A. L.: Bedside Nursing Techniques, 2nd ed. Philadelphia, W. B. Saunders Co., 1969, p. 191.)

---

*Note: Traction may also be employed to correct a deformity, relieve pressure on a spinal nerve or prevent a contracture deformity in cases in which there is muscle spasm.

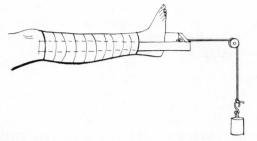

Figure 23–4 Buck's extension. (From Sutton, A. L.: Bedside Nursing Techniques, 2nd ed. Philadelphia, W. B. Saunders Co., 1969, p. 191.)

want the leg shaved. Some consider that shaving removes epithelium, leaving the skin more vulnerable to irritation by the adhesive. An application of tincture of benzoin may be ordered to protect the skin and provide better adherence of the tapes. The tapes may be nicked (approximately ¼ inch) every 1 to 1½ inch along the edges; this provides better adherence by allowing the adhesive to closely follow the contour of the leg. The knee is usually held in slight flexion during the application of the adhesive to avoid hyperextension when the weight is attached. The adhesive is not applied over the malleoli or foot but is extended unattached to the spreader beyond the sole of the foot. If the lateral tape is applied over the head of the fibula, precautions are taken to place a pad over the area under the tape to prevent compression of the peroneal nerve which lies close to the surface. Damage to the nerve could result in interference with normal ankle movement. A pillow is usually placed lengthwise under the leg and knee for support, leaving the heel suspended, free of pressure.

Bryant's traction is used in a fracture of the femoral shaft of a young child (under 6 years). Two overhead bars extend the length of the bed. Each has 2 pulleys, one in line with the child's pelvis and the other one just beyond the foot of the bed. Tapes and bandages similar to those used in Buck's extension are applied to both limbs, which are suspended at right angles to his body. Ropes from the spreaders are carried over the pulleys and suspend sufficient weight to lift the buttocks just clear of the bed. A restraining jacket is usually necessary to keep the child in position. The dorsum of the foot and the heel are examined frequently for

pressure from the bandage. Any discoloration, edema, loss of motion or sensation, or coldness indicating interference with circulation is reported promptly.

Russell traction is also used in the treatment of a fracture of the shaft of a femur. Vertical traction is applied at the knee at the same time a horizontal force is exerted on the tibia and fibula. The pull on the leg bones is exerted to counteract the contraction of the thigh muscles (quadriceps femoris and hamstring) which insert on the leg bones. Considerable spasm of these strong muscles occurs with a fracture of the femur, causing displacement and overriding of the fragments. The horizontal force is exerted on moleskin or adhesive tapes applied to the medial and lateral surfaces of the leg. The tapes are applied from just below the knee to about 1 inch above the malleoli. They are carried beyond the foot and attached to a spreader. A circular bandage is used to secure the tapes as in Buck's extension. The lateral tapes are terminated just below the head of the fibula to avoid compression of the peroneal nerve. Figure 23-5 illustrates Russell traction.

An overhead bar (Balkan frame) is attached to the bed in line with the affected limb. A cross bar is provided at the foot of the bed to hold the necessary pulleys. One pulley is attached to the overhead bar in line

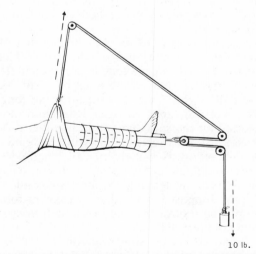

10 lb.

Figure 23–5 Russell traction, which may be used in the treatment of a fracture of the shaft of the femur. (From Sutton, A. L.: Bedside Nursing Techniques, 2nd ed. Philadelphia, W. B. Saunders Co., 1969, pp. 191 and 192.)

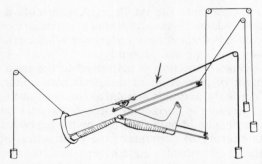

Figure 23–6 Balanced suspension traction using a Thomas splint with a Pearson attachment in the treatment of a fracture of the shaft of the femur. (From Sutton, A. L.: Bedside Nursing Techniques, 2nd ed. Philadelphia, W. B. Saunders Co., 1969, p. 192.)

with the tubercle of the tibia; two are secured to the bar at the foot of the bed, one several inches above the other; and a fourth is attached to the spreader plate to which the traction tapes on the leg are attached. A sling or hammock is placed under the knee and attached to a rope that leads vertically to the overhead pulley and then to the uppermost one on the cross bar. From there the rope passes over the pulley on the foot spreader and back to the lower pulley on the cross bar. It then attaches to weights which hang suspended well above the floor. The weight used with an adult patient is usually 8 to 10 pounds. The level of the pulleys on the bar at the foot of the bed is such that the heel is kept clear of the bed to prevent a pressure sore.

The force exerted by the sling is that of the weight at the end of the rope. The horizontal pull on the legs is approximately twice that exerted on the knee by virtue of the pull of the 2 parallel ropes at the foot. The vertical and horizontal traction are exerted on the same point and together produce a resultant force in line with the femur. A thin pillow is usually placed lengthwise under the thigh, and a second pillow is used under the leg, leaving the heel suspended. A foot support is provided to prevent foot drop. The foot of the bed is elevated to provide countertraction.

Balanced suspension traction is an arrangement in which skin or skeletal traction is applied, and the limb is supported on a splint suspended by a system of ropes, pulleys and weights. It is most commonly used in fractures of the shaft of the femur in conjunction with skeletal traction. A Thomas splint with a Pearson attachment is used (Fig. 23–6).

Firm cotton slings are secured to the upper part of the Thomas splint to support the thigh and to the Pearson attachment to support the leg. The Thomas splint extends from the groin to beyond the foot in line with the femur. The knee is in a neutral position, that is, slightly flexed to prevent stretching of the posterior knee capsule and ligaments and subsequent joint instability. The heel is suspended beyond the slings to avoid pressure, and some provision is made to support the foot to prevent foot drop. The skeletal traction is usually applied to the upper portion of the tibia. The pull is exerted in line with the femur by means of a rope attached to the bow or stirrup that is fitted to the protruding ends of the wire that passes through the bone. The rope passes over a pulley and suspends a weight. The proximal and distal ends of the splint are suspended by cords, pulleys and weights. When the patient moves up or down in bed the splint moves with him, and traction is maintained. The patient has greater freedom of movement and is usually more comfortable in this system of traction. It also has the advantage of allowing a certain amount of movement in adjacent joints.

See nursing care of the patient in traction on page 685.

Some fractures require internal surgical reduction and fixation. Various types of internal fixation devices are used. These include stainless steel or vitallium wire, screws, plates, rods and pins. They may be secured to the sides of the bone, placed through the fragments or passed through the intramedullary cavity of the bone. Internal immobilization is frequently reinforced after the wound is closed by the application of a cast or splint. If a cast is used, a "window" may be made over the wound area to avoid pressure on the incision and promote healing. See nursing care of patients who have had bone surgery on page 688.

Following any method of reduction and immobilization, roentgenograms are made periodically to determine whether reduction is satisfactory and healing is occurring. In the case of traction, some adjustment in the amount of weight being used may be necessary. For instance, the x-ray may demonstrate too wide a separation of the fragments which would prevent healing and necessitate a reduction in the weight used.

OPEN (COMPOUND) FRACTURES. The patient with an open fracture requires special treatment as soon after the accident as possible. The site is potentially infected, and there is usually a greater amount of soft tissue damage and destruction. Infection and necrosis impede union and may result in serious crippling. As soon as the patient's general condition permits, the physician examines and cleanses the open fracture wound. Gross contaminants and foreign material are removed, and the open wound is covered. The surrounding skin is then cleansed thoroughly with a solution of hexachlorophene (pHisoHex) or a surgical detergent such as benzalkonium chloride (Zephiran chloride). After this initial cleansing, the skin may require shaving, which is then followed by a second cleansing. The open wound may then be irrigated with sterile normal saline. The surgeon explores the wound and a débridement* is done if necessary. The repair of severed or torn tendons or nerves may be necessary. The fracture is reduced and then immobilized. If there has been gross contamination, the wound may be packed and left open until the danger of infection is past.

Before the administration of the anesthetic, it is determined if the patient has had previous immunization for tetanus. If he had, a booster dose of tetanus toxoid may be ordered. If he has not been immunized, an intracutaneous test dose (0.1 ml.) of tetanus antitoxin is given. If there is no reaction in 15 to 20 minutes, the usual prophylactic dose of 1500 units of tetanus antitoxin is given. Antibiotic therapy may be prescribed.

Care of the Patient in a Cast

The care of the patient following the application of a cast requires the following considerations.

Drying of the Cast. Complete drying of a cast following its application may take several hours or days, depending on its thickness, the temperature, humidity and circulation of the air, and whether slow, medium or fast-setting plaster of Paris bandages were used. During this period, support of the cast and handling are very important, since the cast is vulnerable to pressure and cracking which could alter its shape, cause indentations that result in undue pressure on an area of the body or make it ineffective. When lifting the part, it is supported on the palms of the hands to avoid making indentations by the finger tips. In the case of a body or long leg cast, a fracture board is placed under the mattress to prevent sagging. Pillows with plastic or rubber undercovers are placed under the part encased in plaster so that the cast is not subjected to pressure by the firm mattress. Since it is molded to the contours of the part to which it is applied, support by an extra pillow or folded flannelette sheet may be necessary under such regions as the lumbar or popliteal area.

Drying is promoted by exposure to dry, warm, circulating air which evaporates the moisture from the cast. The bedding is arranged so that the cast is left uncovered. A heater with a fan (similar to a hair dryer) may be placed approximately 18 inches from the cast. Unless otherwise indicated by the physician, the patient is turned every 4 to 6 hours to facilitate drying of the complete cast. He is turned toward his uninjured side by 2 or 3 persons acting in unison to avoid strain on any part of the plaster. A moist cast has a dull gray appearance and produces a dull sound on percussion. When dry, it appears white and shiny and is resonant on percussion.

Observations. Following the application of the cast, the patient's general condition is noted at frequent intervals; occasionally, a patient develops delayed shock manifested by sudden weakness, fainting, pallor and weak pulse. During the first 24 to 48 hours, swelling in the area of the fracture may occur, resulting in constriction by the cast. A frequent check is made of the parts distal to the cast (e.g., fingers, toes) for any indication of interference with circulation or pressure on a nerve. Any blanching, discoloration, coldness, swelling, edema, or loss of sensation or motion is reported immediately. Any complaint of pressure or pain must be reported and recorded.

---

*Débridement is the removal of foreign material and excision of devitalized tissue.

A daily inspection is made of the complete cast for softened areas, and the skin at the cast edges and over pressure areas is examined frequently for any signs of irritation or abrasion. After a few days, if the cast appears to have become loose and less effective, it is drawn to the doctor's attention. This may occur as a result of reduced swelling or loss of weight. The nurse is alert for any odor arising from the cast. In some instances, the only indication of a pressure sore having developed under a cast is the offensive, musty odor characteristic of tissue necrosis. If there is a known surgical or accidental wound under the cast, the area is checked frequently for signs of bleeding, infection and drainage. Infection may be detected by an odor or suspected because of an elevation of temperature.

Protection of the Cast. Care must be taken during bathing to prevent wetting of the cast. If it approximates the buttocks and perineal area, it requires protection from soiling and wetting when the patient uses the bedpan. Sheets of plastic or other waterproof material may be tucked in well under the edges of the cast, turned back over the outside and secured with adhesive tape. When the patient is placed on the bedpan, pillows are placed under the shoulders and back so that the upper part of the body is level with or slightly higher than the hips and bedpan. The nurse makes sure the patient is thoroughly cleansed and dried following voiding or defecation and that the protective plastic is changed when it becomes soiled. If the cast edges are so close to the perineum that they interfere with adequate care, the doctor may permit the cast to be cut back to provide greater exposure.

A coat of shellac or plastic spray may be applied to the total cast when it is dry to help keep it dry and clean. Superficial soil may be removed with a damp cloth and abrasive powder. If the patient is up and around, the cast may be protected by stockinette or a sock or stocking.

Skin Care. If the patient is confined to bed, frequent skin care, especially of pressure areas, is necessary. The bed is kept free of wrinkles and crumbs. The leg is supported on a pillow to prevent constant pressure on the heel. The crumbling of cast edges can be a source of much discomfort and irritation; the binding may require changing or reinforcing from time to time. The fingers or toes distal to a cast may become irritated by dry, scaly skin; they are bathed, lightly oiled and massaged at least once daily, and frequent active exercise is encouraged.

Nutrition. The patient is encouraged to take a regular, well-balanced diet to provide the essentials for tissue healing as well as to maintain normal physiological processes. If his activity is restricted, the roughage content may have to be increased to control bowel elimination. If, in the case of a hip spica or jacket cast, intestinal distention becomes troublesome, gas-forming foods may have to be avoided. If the discomfort keeps recurring, the physician may cut a "window" in the cast over the abdominal region.

Exercise. Exercise is important in the care of the fracture patient to stimulate circulation and to prevent muscle atrophy, loss of strength and stiffness of uninvolved joints. The purpose and details of the exercises are explained to the patient. Uninvolved joints are put through their full range of motion several times daily, and he is encouraged to exercise the unaffected limbs and use them in self-care, turning and raising as much as possible. An overhead trapeze is provided so he can move and lift himself. A schedule of deep breathing and coughing is established for inactive and older persons who are predisposed to pulmonary complications.

The muscles of the immobilized limb are exercised as soon as the doctor permits by having the patient contract those muscles immediately above and below the fracture (isometric exercise) frequently without moving the joint. These exercises may be demonstrated on the unaffected limb so that the patient sees that the muscles can be contracted without moving the limb. For quadriceps setting, the nurse places her hand under the knee and instructs the patient to push down. If it is an arm that is encased in plaster, isometric exercise of the arm muscles is done by having the patient make a fist. The fingers or toes distal to the cast should be exercised several times daily.

Discharged Home with Cast. Frequently the patient is allowed to go home as soon as the cast is dry. The patient and his family are advised that the limb should be elevated for the first 24 to 48 hours. Instructions are given to examine the toes and fingers frequently and to immediately report to the physician or the clinic any swelling, blueness, coldness, numbness or inability to move the digits. Persisting pain of the limb or any crack or softening of an area in the cast should also be reported.

The arm with the cast may be supported in a sling when the patient is up. It is important that the sling support the hand to prevent strain and pressure on the wrist. The knot of the sling at the back of the neck is placed lateral to the cervical vertebrae, and a pad may be placed between the sling and the neck to prevent pressure and irritation.

The patient who is discharged with a cast on his leg must know whether or not he may bear any weight on the limb. If he has a walking cast, he is advised as to when he may start to bear weight on it, how to protect the cast, and the necessary precautions to avoid falls. If the patient is to use crutches, they are selected according to the patient's height, and instructions are given in their use (see p. 694).

An appointment is usually made for the patient to have the limb and cast checked in 2 or 3 days and then to return in approximately 10 to 12 days for an x-ray to determine if the callus formation and healing are satisfactory.

Removal of the Cast. When the cast is taken off, the rigid support to joints which have been immobilized for a considerable period of time is removed. The patient is likely to be discouraged by the stiffness, instability and weakness which he encounters and requires reassurance that with exercise and progressive use function will be restored.

The cast is removed by special cast cutters. Soaking the cutting line with acetic acid (vinegar) softens the plaster, making the cutting less difficult. The limb must be handled gently and with support under the joints. The skin is bathed gently, and an application of oil or lanolin is made to soften the accumulation of dry, scaly skin. Vigorous rubbing is discouraged to avoid skin irritation and abrasions.

A regimen of passive and active exercises and massage is established to restore joint and muscle function. Weight bearing and activities are gradually resumed. When the cast is removed and the limb becomes dependent, edema and swelling are likely to occur. The patient is advised to elevate the limb when sitting and lying, and an elastic or crepe bandage may be applied when he is ambulatory to control the edema which gradually becomes less troublesome as muscle tone improves and there is increasing activity.

Care of the Patient in Traction

It is important that the nurse be familiar with the purpose of the traction and that she understand how the appliances being used are designed and applied to achieve this purpose.

Responsibilities in Relation to the Applied Traction. Traction must be constant to be effective in the treatment of fractures. The complete traction system is inspected frequently as well as after any movement or treatment of the patient to detect possible interference with the traction or the direction of its pull. Ropes must be taut, ride freely over pulleys and be kept free of bedding. Knots are examined frequently for security, and the weights, which must never be lifted or changed, are checked for free suspension. Areas that may be subjected to irritation by adhesive tapes, constriction by circular bandages, or pressure or friction by contact with a part of the appliance are examined several times daily, and any interference with circulation or skin irritation is reported and recorded promptly. Distal portions of the extremity are checked for discoloration, coldness, swelling, edema, and loss of sensation or movement. The nurse is alert for any sign of discharge or a musty odor that might indicate skin necrosis in an area covered by adhesive tapes or bandages. Any change in the alignment of the limb, such as outward rotation, hyperextension or foot drop, is brought to the physician's attention. Every complaint of pain or discomfort deserves investigation and reporting.

Countertraction is maintained by elevation of the bed under the part to which the traction is applied and by preventing a change of position that allows the foot plate or bar to rest against the foot of the bed or a cross bar. The heel, which is so vulnerable to pressure, must remain suspended, and the foot is supported to prevent plantar flexion (foot drop). If the limb is supported in a ring splint (e.g., Thomas' or Thomas-Pearson splint), the ring should not cause undue pressure in the groin. The skin under the ring is bathed frequently, thoroughly dried and lightly powdered. If the patient keeps "sliding into the ring" or if skin irritation occurs, the weights may require adjustment by the physician. When the Pearson attachment is used with a Thomas' splint in suspension traction to support the leg from the knee down, the patient's knee should rest over the point of attachment of the Pearson extension.

When skeletal traction is used, the wounds are covered with small sterile dressings. The surrounding skin is inspected daily for any redness or discharge that may indicate infection. The protruding ends of the wire or pin are covered with cork or adhesive tape.

Positioning, Skin Care and Exercises. The patient in traction is required to remain on his back; this becomes tiresome and is a source of discomfort for the patient. An explanation is made to the patient of the reason the dorsal position is necessary, and he is told that turning would prevent immobilization of the fracture which is essential to healing. A directive is obtained from the physician as to how much movement is permitted. Good body alignment is important; a firm mattress on a fracture board is used. The upper part of the body is kept straight; if the patient lies diagonally, it may alter the desired position of the affected limb and the direction of the pull on it. The patient in traction frequently has a tendency to keep his unaffected leg in flexion. He may need to be reminded to extend it for intervals to prevent shortening of the flexors.

Frequent skin care (at least every 2 to 3 hours) of the back, buttocks and the heel of the unaffected leg is very important to prevent pressure sores, especially in elderly persons. Brisk massage with the application of alcohol helps to stimulate circulation in the areas and increase the resistance of the skin. An occasional application of lanolin or oil is usually necessary to prevent excessive drying and possible cracking of the skin. Squares of synthetic sheepskin or sponge rubber are placed under the vulnerable areas. Thorough cleansing and drying

following the use of the bedpan and keeping the bedding clean, dry and free of wrinkles and crumbs are important nursing measures. Vulnerable areas are carefully inspected frequently for any discoloration, mottling, edema or break in the skin. A second person is necessary to assist with the raising of the patient while back care is given and the lower bed linen is changed. If the patient cannot be raised, the person assisting pushes down on the mattress, permitting the nurse to slide her hand in to give the necessary care. The patient may be permitted to raise himself slightly by pulling on a trapeze suspended from the overhead frame. Linen changes are made by working from the unaffected side toward the affected side or from the top of the bed toward the foot. The method which proves easier and least disturbing for the patient is used. The top bedding is arranged to avoid interference with the traction. Small lightweight blankets may be used over the limb in traction for warmth. If suspension traction is used, the patient usually has greater freedom of movement and can be raised with less danger of disturbing the fracture site. When slight turning of the trunk is permitted for care, the turning is toward the leg in traction.

The patient is required to practice deep breathing and coughing every 1 to 2 hours to prevent pulmonary complications. To stimulate his circulation and prevent muscle atrophy and joint stiffness, active exercises of uninvolved limbs are carried out several times daily. Self-care activities are encouraged and an explanation of their role in his progress is made to the patient. He is also taught to practice static exercises (isometric contractions or muscle setting) of the abdominal and gluteal muscles.

Nutrition. A well-balanced diet is provided, and the patient is advised of his need for adequate nutrition to provide the essential materials for healing of the fracture and to maintain his resistance. His protein and vitamin C (ascorbic acid) intake receive special attention; a deficiency of these elements predisposes the skin to pressure sores. The reduced activity and subsequent constipation may necessitate increased dietary roughage. Immobilization causes some decalcification of the bones and resultant hypercalcemia, predisposing to the formation of renal and bladder calculi. The patient is encouraged to take 2500 to 3000 ml. of fluid daily (unless contraindicated) to promote elimination of the excessive blood calcium. He may have to be fed at first but should gradually be encouraged to do this for himself. The nurse makes sure that the food is within easy reach of the patient and that he receives the necessary assistance in cutting his meat, buttering bread, pouring coffee, etc.

Elimination. The use of the bedpan by the patient in traction frequently presents some difficulty, mainly because of the elevation of the foot of the bed for countertraction. Unless contraindicated, the patient assists in raising himself on to the fracture pan by using the trapeze and unaffected leg. A pillow may be placed under the back and shoulders so that the patient is more level with the bedpan. For voiding, a female urinal or an emesis basin may be used for female patients. The nurse must see that the patient and bed are left clean and dry.

As cited previously, the enforced inactivity may give rise to constipation and flatulence. If the problem is not corrected, fecal impaction may develop, necessitating digital disimpaction and cleansing enemas, which are distressing and exhausting for the patient. Dietary adjustments and a mild laxative may prevent this problem.

Diversion. The fracture patient is usually in traction for several weeks; time passes slowly, and he is likely to be discontented, depressed and unable to sleep. The provision of diversion and some form of occupation is an essential part of the nursing care plan. The patient's need for socialization, interest and occupation may be discussed with his family and friends. It may be suggested that they plan their visits so that he is not alone for several days and then visited by everyone at the same time. The patient's interests should be determined; reading material, a radio or television (if permitted by the hospital) and small handicrafts frequently prove helpful. In the case of a housewife and mother, her family might be encouraged to have her participate in planning and decision-making regarding home matters so that she feels that she is still maintaining her role. Similarly, it is psychologically beneficial to the father or businessman to be consulted. Mental and purposeful physical activity help to produce normal fatigue; the

patient is likely to sleep and rest better at night and will require less sedation.

Convalescence and Rehabilitation. When the traction is removed, the patient will probably be surprised and depressed by the weakness and joint instability in the limb. Before he is allowed up, the head of the bed is elevated so he may adjust to having his head and trunk in an upright position after being flat and in the countertraction position for so long. The elevation is gradual; otherwise he may experience faintness.

Passive, active and resistive exercises of the affected limb are introduced. These may be planned and supervised by a physiotherapist, but the nurse must be familiar with the plan so that the necessary assistance is provided when the therapist is not at the bedside. In some situations the nurse may have to assume responsibility for teaching the exercises and for helping the patient to resume walking. Arm and shoulder exercises are continued to strengthen the upper limbs in preparation for the use of a walker or crutches. When the patient is allowed up the casters are removed from the bed; having it lower makes it easier and safer for him to get in and out. Specific orders are received from the physician as to when weight bearing and ambulation may begin. Depending on the strength and age of the patient, a walker may be used before crutches or canes are introduced. It is usually used with elderly and debilitated patients because there is less danger of falls and they feel more secure. Firm, low-heeled walking shoes should be worn, preferably an oxford with a rubber heel. When the patient's ability and confidence increase, he may then progress through crutch walking to a cane. When relearning to walk, he may need prompting to maintain an erect posture (avoid bending forward) and to increase the degree of flexion of his thigh and leg when raising a foot off the floor to take a step in order to overcome the tendency to shuffle. Most patients requre a good deal of encouragement and reassurance from the nurse. Physical assistance and support are gradually withdrawn, but the nurse remains with the patient when he is getting in and out of the bed or a chair until it is evident that he can safely manage on his own. Before he is discharged, it is important to know the home situation in order to suggest necessary adjustments. Will he have to use stairs to get to the apartment or to the bathroom? Will there be someone there with him all the time? The necessary information may be obtained from the patient or his family, or a visit may be made by a visiting nurse to assess the situation and suggest adjustments in the environment and arrangements for care. It may be necessary for him to spend an interim period in a convalescent home. When he goes home, a referral may be made to the visiting nurse agency so that he receives regular assistance and supervision. Resumption of his former occupation and activities will depend on his progress in relation to mobility and independence. He is seen at frequent intervals in the clinic or by his physician until fully rehabilitated.

Nursing the Patient with Internal (Surgical) Fixation

Preoperative Preparation. How soon the operation for internal fixation is performed after a fracture has occurred depends on the patient's condition and whether there are associated injuries or health problems. It is usually done as soon as possible but may have to be delayed because of shock or because the patient had eaten recently and as a result should not have a general anesthetic until the stomach empties. During the preoperative period, some temporary form of immobilization may be applied to the injured part (e.g., sandbags, splint or Buck's extension). It must be handled as little as possible to prevent movement of the fragments and further tissue damage. An analgesic such as morphine, meperidine hydrochloride (Demerol) or codeine may be ordered for relief of pain. Older patients may not tolerate these drugs and following each administration must be observed closely, especially for respiratory depression, shock and disorientation. Crib sides are placed on their beds as a precautionary measure, and their condition may necessitate constant attendance at the bedside. The patient's blood is typed and cross matched, and blood is given to counteract shock or hemorrhage. If the patient manifests dehydration, intravenous infusions of electrolyte and glucose solutions are administered. If the patient is elderly, as so many are who have internal fixation, intra-

venous solutions (including blood) are given slowly to avoid an excessive demand on the heart caused by a rapid increase in the circulating intravascular volume. The urinary output and fluid intake are measured, and the balance is determined so that any renal insufficiency may be detected and reported. The preoperative assessment may include blood tests and an electrocardiogram. If the period between the accident and the operation is more than a few hours, the patient is required to cough and breathe deeply every 1 to 2 hours. Frequent special skin care may also be necessary because of the immobility and constant dorsal position.

Because of bone tissue's susceptibility to infection and the difficulty in bringing it under control if it occurs, meticulous preoperative cleansing of the skin is very important. Specific directions are usually received from the surgeon. A large area is carefully shaved and cleansed with a solution of hexachlorophene (pHisoHex) or benzelkonium chloride (Zephiran chloride). The cleansing may be repeated, depending on the amount of time available. If the surgery is to be performed on a limb, special attention is paid to the skin between digits and to the nails.

Postoperative Care. Following internal reduction and fixation, the general principles of postoperative care are applicable (see p. 115). The patient is observed closely for any changes in color, blood pressure, pulse and respirations that may reflect shock, hemorrhage or cardiac failure. If the surgery was performed on a limb, the extremity is elevated on pillows to prevent edema. The operative site may be enclosed in a cast, making it difficult to detect early signs of external bleeding. The area is checked for any staining of the cast or oozing from its edges. The initial area of staining may be encircled with a pencil mark so that continued bleeding may be recognized and assessed. As with any plaster application, the part of the limb distal to the cast is examined frequently for any nerve compression or interference with circulation. After the cast is dry, the surgeon may order a "window" to be cut out over the incision. This allows for a change of dressing, if necessary, and permits exposure to air, which helps to keep the wound dry.

The limitations of positioning and activity

are determined by the surgeon. During the period of confinement to bed, exercises of uninvolved parts of the body and self-care activities are usually encouraged to maintain the normal range of joint movement and muscle tone. A trapeze attached to an over-the-bed bar (Balkan frame) allows the patient to move and shift his weight. He is instructed to cough and take 8 to 10 deep breaths every 2 to 3 hours if activity is restricted. When crutch walking is anticipated, exercises to strengthen the arms and shoulders are introduced (see p. 693). Frequent skin care, especially to susceptible pressure areas (scapular areas, sacrum, heels), is necessary. If turning is permitted, the patient is turned onto the unaffected side; the affected limb is supported during the process and is positioned on pillows to maintain good alignment and prevent strain. A crib side on the side of the bed toward which he turns provides something for him to grasp when turning.

The patient may be allowed out of bed, but in the case of surgery on a lower extremity, he is not usually permitted to bear any weight on it for several weeks. He may be allowed the use of a wheelchair and is gradually introduced to the use of crutches (see p. 694). When sitting in either a stationary chair or a wheelchair, provision is made for elevation and support of the affected limb. Precautions against pressure sores and slumping posture are necessary when the patient is allowed up in a chair for long periods. He is returned to bed for skin care at regular intervals or may be taught to shift his weight frequently so that no one area is subjected to continuous pressure. Adjustments may also be necessary to avoid prolonged pressure on the popliteal area of the unaffected, dependent leg and to prevent forward sagging of the shoulders.

Exercises of the affected part are started as soon as the doctor permits. They may be limited to isometric contractions for a period, followed by the gradual introduction of passive and active movements and resistive exercises. In the case of a lower extremity, weight bearing is not introduced until roentgenograms indicate satisfactory healing. The overambitious patient is cautioned not to attempt standing or walking without the assistance of a physiotherapist or nurse. He should have a firm, rubber-heeled pair of walking shoes and be assisted first to stand. The nurse stands facing the patient and places her hands to the sides of his lower chest. She encourages him to stand erect, knees extended and head up. When he is sure of his balance in the upright position, he is then assisted with the next step, which may be the use of crutches, a walker or simply walking with only the assistance of the nurse. If the nurse provides the only assistance, support is given to the affected side.

Fracture of the Hip. This refers to a fracture of the proximal extremity of the femur and may be classified as intracapsular or extracapsular. The intracapsular fracture occurs through the neck of the femur and is slower in healing because frequently there is an associated interruption of the blood vessels in the medullary canal which are the main blood supply to the head of the bone. The extracapsular hip fracture may pass through either the greater or lesser trochanter or the intertrochanteric area. A fracture of the hip is usually treated by internal (surgical) reduction and fixation. A variety of metallic nails, plates and screws are available as fixation devices (e.g., tri-flanged Smith-Peterson nail, Neufeld nail and plate with screws). The selection depends on the location and angle of the fracture. If the intracapsular fracture is comminuted, if satisfactory reduction cannot be obtained, or if the surgeon suspects that avascular necrosis and nonunion are likely to develop because of injury to blood vessels, the femoral head may be removed and replaced by a metal (vitallium) prosthesis. It has a ball-shaped head which fits into the hip socket (acetabulum) and a lower intramedullary rod which is fitted into the lower neck and upper part of the shaft of the femur.

The majority of patients who suffer a fracture of the hip are elderly persons. They do not tolerate the prolonged immobilization and bed rest imposed by traction and spica casts; under such treatment they are prone to develop pulmonary and circulatory complications, pressure sores and rapid debilitation. Internal fixation makes it possible to have the patient exercise and be out of bed much earlier than with traction, thus reducing the risk of serious complications.

Following the surgical reduction and fixation, constant nursing attention and close observation of the vital signs are necessary; the older person is more likely to develop shock, respiratory depression and cardiac failure. The patient is placed on a firm mattress on a fracture board to prevent sagging and flexion of the hips. The surgeon may order the affected limb supported on pillows the full length of the extremity. When the patient is in the dorsal position, alignment is maintained by sandbags placed along the lateral aspect. Occasionally, traction is applied for 2 or 3 days to overcome muscle spasm.

Postoperative disorientation and restlessness are common with elderly persons. Crib sides are placed on the bed for protection. Analgesic drugs and sedatives are used judiciously; the patient must not be allowed to suffer unnecessarily, but the reduced tolerance of older persons for these drugs, especially opiates and barbiturates, may depress respirations and cause disorientation.

As soon as the patient regains consciousness, a schedule for frequent coughing and deep breathing is established. He is turned frequently as soon as possible to help prevent pulmonary congestion. Change of position may be restricted to turning on the unaffected side for a few days. The affected limb is supported during the process and is positioned on pillows, keeping the hip and knee in the same plane to prevent strain on the operative site.

Retention of urine or incontinence may be experienced in the early postoperative period. An indwelling catheter may be passed as part of the preoperative preparation, or it may be introduced following the operation. Its use should be limited to as brief a period as possible because of the danger of bladder infection. The catheter is usually clamped for stated periods, allowing a normal volume of urine to collect in the bladder to promote tone and normal capacity. A fluid intake of approximately 2500 ml. is encouraged unless contraindicated by circulatory or renal insufficiency. When the catheter is removed, the bedpan is given every 2 hours until normal bladder function and control are established. Constipation is a common problem, and fecal impaction is prone to develop. A mild laxative such as milk of magnesia or psyllium hydrophilic mucilloid (Metamucil) may be ordered, and

the diet is adjusted to include increased roughage.

Exercises of the unaffected extremities are started as soon as possible, and the patient is encouraged to alternately flex and extend the toes and ankle of the affected extremity to stimulate circulation. The surgeon may order the application of elastic or crepe compression bandages to the lower extremities to prevent venous stasis, which predisposes the patient to thrombophlebitis. Specific exercises are prescribed for the affected limb; passive movements may be introduced first, followed by active exercises. The patient is assisted or lifted out of bed into a chair on the second or third day. The affected leg is usually extended and supported the first few days unless otherwise indicated by the surgeon, then lowered and observed for swelling and discoloration. The patient is taught to stand on the unaffected extremity and to transfer to a chair without bearing any weight on the affected limb. He may then be permitted early ambulation with crutches. In most instances, the elderly patient is not taught crutch walking because of the danger of his falling. Weight bearing on the affected leg is not allowed until there is x-ray evidence of satisfactory healing. When permitted, the older patient is taught to use a walker.

Continued pain or muscle spasm is reported and recorded; it may be due to unsatisfactory reduction or avascular necrosis of the head of the femur. When a prosthesis has been implanted, unless the limb is in traction, a specific directive is received as to the positioning of the patient and the affected extremity. It varies with the location of the operative approach through the joint capsule. If it has been posterior, the patient lies flat, and the leg is abducted and positioned in external rotation; if the approach through the capsule was anterior, the limb is internally rotated, and the patient is permitted to sit up.

Firm healing of the bone following a hip fracture and the resumption of walking is a long slow process. Periods of discouragement and depression are common. The patient requires a good deal of support. Self-care activities are promoted to reduce his feelings of dependence as well as to maintain muscle tone. Various forms of diversion in which he is interested are provided. The patient may be permitted to go home before weight bearing is allowed. Adjustments in the home environment and care of the patient are discussed in detail with members of the family. A referral may be made to a visiting nurse agency.

AMPUTATION OF A LIMB

The incidence of amputation of a part of a limb has been reduced in the last 2 to 3 decades. This is attributed to the medical progress made in vascular surgery, the treatment of infection and the control of diabetes mellitus. For those for whom an amputation is a necessity, the loss of the limb has become less obvious and less disabling as a result of improved prostheses and rehabilitation programs.

An amputation is done to preserve the patient's life or may be undertaken to improve function and usefulness. A lower extremity is more frequently involved, and amputation occurs more often in males. The conditions which necessitate amputation include: insufficient blood supply to the part and resulting gangrene; severe, uncontrollable infection such as gas gangrene (*Clostridium perfringens* infection) or chronic osteomyelitis in which there is marked bone destruction; malignant neoplasm (e.g., osteosarcoma); an injury that has resulted in irreparable crushing of the limb or laceration of arteries and nerves; and a handicapping deformity.

Level and Types of Amputation

When possible, the level of the amputation is decided before operation so that the patient may be informed of the anticipated extent of the loss. The decision as to the level is based on achieving complete removal of the diseased tissue, an adequate blood supply to the remaining part of the limb, and a stump that will allow for a satisfactory fitting and functional movement of a prosthesis.

Two types of operative procedures are used: the closed or flap type of amputation and the guillotine amputation.

In the flap type of procedure, fascia, probably muscle, and full-thickness skin flaps are brought over the end of the bone. In a lower limb amputation, the anterior flap is usually longer in order to bring the suture line to the posterior aspect. This arrangement prevents direct pressure on the scar by the prosthesis in weight bearing. When it is an upper limb that is involved, the anterior and posterior flaps are generally equal in length, producing a terminal scar. The skin flaps are dissected to provide a smooth surface over the end of the stump, free of wrinkles and folds, and the skin edges are sutured in apposition with a minimum of tension.

A guillotine or open amputation is reserved for emergency cases in which the limb has been severely traumatized and contaminated or in which gas gangrene has already developed. The skin and other soft tissues are severed at the same level as the bone. The wound is left open and closed later when infection is brought under control. Traction may be applied to the skin while it remains open to prevent retraction of the soft tissues.

Preoperative Nursing Care

Psychological Preparation. When the amputation is an elective procedure, the surgeon advises the patient and his family of the need for the operation and the level at which the limb will be removed. The information is likely to be a shock, causing considerable emotional disturbance. The patient's body image and independence are seriously threatened, and he needs the support of an understanding nurse. He is encouraged to verbalize his feelings, and through listening, the nurse identifies his particular fears and concerns. These and the reactions vary among patients, depending on their personality, life situation and ability to handle crises. For example, the wage earner is likely to be greatly distressed about a loss of earning power to support his family. For another, an amputation may mean a complete change in his accustomed activities and occupation. The patient and his family receive explanations of how the problems associated with the loss of a limb may be handled through a planned rehabilitation program. The knowledge that the interest and assistance of specialists in this area are available helps the patient to develop a hopeful and positive attitude toward overcoming the handicap. Opportunities are provided for questions and discussions about what is likely to take place before and after the operation. The patient may derive support from a visit by someone who has had a similar amputation and has been successfully rehabilitated.

The policy relating to the operative consent for an amputation may vary from that used generally. Some institutions and surgeons require the signature of the patient and the closest relative. If the patient is confused and his responsibility questionable, two of his next of kin may be required to sign the consent.

Physical Preparation. During the preoperative period the patient is taught deep breathing and coughing. If his condition permits, exercises are introduced which will facilitate his postoperative mobilization and rehabilitation. These include active exercises of the unaffected limbs to prevent loss of muscular strength. If crutch walking is anticipated, push-ups may be introduced to strengthen the shoulder and arm muscles. Frequent skin care and change of position are necessary to prevent pressure sores, since the patient often tends to remain immobile to reduce pain. Overprotection of an affected lower limb usually results in continuous flexion of the hip and knee joints, leading to contractures. This is discouraged by having the patient assume the prone position several times a day.

Attention is directed toward promoting optimum nutritional and hydrational status. The importance of adequate protein, vitamins and fluids in postoperative progress is explained to the patient. If the patient is overweight, his caloric intake may be moderately reduced, since excess weight may retard his postoperative ambulation and rehabilitation. Too restricted a caloric intake (below 1000 to 1200 calories) and a rapid weight loss are avoided because of the danger of causing acidosis, especially postoperatively. Blood typing and cross matching are done, and blood is made available. A transfusion may be given during the preoperative period to improve the patient's general condition as well as during and following the operation. The blood pressure and the pulse rate and volume are noted to serve as a base line in postoperative care.

Preoperative preparation of the skin involves the usual shaving and thorough cleansing well above and below the anticipated level of amputation.

Preparation to Receive the Patient After Amputation

In preparing the postoperative bed, a fracture board is placed beneath a firm mattress to assist in maintaining good body alignment, facilitate postoperative exercises and prevent sagging of the bed at hip level which predisposes to flexion contracture. Obviously, amputation necessitates the severing and ligation of large blood vessels. A heavy tourniquet is placed at the bedside and is ready for immediate use in the event of hemorrhage. Provision is also made for elevation of the foot of the bed in case of hemorrhage or shock. Blood, fluids and equipment are made available for prompt intravenous infusion.

Postoperative Nursing Care

Observations. The blood pressure, pulse and respirations are recorded, color noted and the stump examined at frequent, regular intervals for the first 48 hours for early signs of shock and hemorrhage. The patient is observed for general apathy and psychic trauma following the amputation. Even though he was prepared for and consented to the operation, the actual loss of the limb may cause severe depression. The nurse is also alert for any indications of infection such as fever, increased pain, reddened streaks or areas and wound discharge.

Care of the Stump. Any blood staining of the dressing is reported immediately, and the tourniquet is applied if necessary until the bleeding is brought under control by the surgeon. A tissue drain is usually placed in the wound at the time of operation; if serous drainage soaks through, the dressing is promptly reinforced. The drain is removed in 2 to 3 days and the sutures in 10 to 12 days.

The surgeon may order the stump elevated on a pillow for the first 24 to 48 hours, or in the case of a lower limb, the foot of the bed may be elevated for approximately 24 hours. Prolonged use of the pillow under the stump with the patient in the supine position leads to flexion contracture and later difficulty in mobility and the fitting of a prosthesis. With an arm amputation, precautionary measures are used to prevent contracture of the shoulder adductor and inward rotator muscles. Following an amputation above the knee, the nurse must guard against shortening of the hip flexors and abductors. In an amputation below the knee, the patient is encouraged to maintain extension of the knee to avoid contracture of the hamstring muscles.

When the wound has healed, a compression bandage (elastic or crepe) is applied to the stump to reduce edema and promote firming and molding of the tissue in preparation for a prosthesis. A generous number of long, recurrent, vertical folds are made over the end of the stump and are secured by circular turns. The bandage must be sufficiently firm to compress and shape the soft, flabby tissue, but one must guard against any interference with the blood supply by excessive tightness. The bandage is removed and reapplied 3 or 4 times daily. While it is off, gentle massage of the tissue may be prescribed to stimulate circulation and prevent adherence of the scar tissue to the bone. The patient or a member of the family is taught the care of the stump and the correct application of the bandage. The stump is bathed daily with a mild soap and rinsed and dried thoroughly. Nothing is applied to the skin unless it is prescribed by the physician. Certain activities may be ordered which apply pressure to the stump in preparation for the use of a prosthesis and weight bearing. Contact is first made with something quite soft, and as tolerance is developed, the firmness and resistance of the contact surface and pressure are progressively increased. If the patient complains of muscular spasms and discomfort, heat and massage to the stump may provide relief.

Safety Precautions. Crib sides on the bed are a necessary precaution, especially with older patients. They may become disoriented or, in turning, may readily lose their balance and fall out of bed.

Pain and Depression. An analgesic is necessary the first 2 or 3 days to control the pain and is then usually tapered off gradually to discourage drug dependency. Some patients experience pain or other sensations which are interpreted as originating in the portion of the limb which has been removed. This is referred to as phantom pain (see p. 77). It may be temporary, but if it persists, the nerve endings in the stump may be injected with alcohol or resected.

The nurse may assist the patient in overcoming his despair by conveying an understanding of his feelings and by making positive references to his future activity, mobility and rehabilitation.

Fluids and Nutrition. Intravenous fluids may be necessary during the first 24 to 48 hours to maintain an adequate intake. Oral fluids are given freely, and the patient progresses to a regular diet as soon as it is tolerated. An explanation is made, if necessary, of the importance of adequate nutrition in maintaining and promoting his muscular strength for the exercises that will assist in rehabilitation.

Exercises. An hourly routine of coughing and deep breathing and frequent change of position are necessary until the patient is allowed up and becomes sufficiently active to prevent limited ventilation and circulatory stasis.

As soon as he is well enough, a daily regimen of exercises is introduced to maintain and promote the muscular strength and joint mobility that are needed for rehabilitation. The tone of the trunk muscles receives attention as well as that of the limb muscles, since adjustments and compensation are necessary for the amputee to maintain his balance. If the lower limb has been amputated above the knee, the hip extensors and adductors play an important role in remobilization. To prevent flexion contracture of a thigh stump, the patient lies in the prone position for one-half hour every 3 or 4 hours. A pillow may be placed under the abdomen, under the stump and under the ankle if the foot is not suspended over the edge of the mattress. While in the prone position, he is encouraged to do push-up exercises to strengthen the shoulder and arm muscles. If the leg is removed below the knee, the quadriceps of that limb is exercised. Following the amputation of an arm, the shoulder muscles of that limb are exercised.

Rehabilitation. The patient is allowed out of bed as soon as possible. Assistance must be available until he can maintain his balance and is able to maneuver safely. In the case of a lower limb, the patient first learns to stand, get up from a chair, to get in and out of bed and to walk with crutches (see below). Attention is paid to his posture; any tendency to lean forward or to one side should be corrected.

When an upper limb has been amputated, the patient is assisted and encouraged to begin self-care activities with his one arm as soon as possible. Certain simple adjustments in the serving of his food, clothing fasteners, etc. are made to facilitate his independence.

When the stump has sufficiently shrunk and is conditioned, measurements are taken, and a prosthesis is made. A special wool stump sock is worn with the prosthesis, and the patient is instructed on the importance of it being well-fitting, free of wrinkles and changed daily. He is also advised to inspect the stump daily for redness, swelling, irritation and calluses. If any symptoms develop, he should avoid weight bearing on the area and consult his physician.

When learning to use a lower limb prosthesis, the patient first uses crutches for support, then progresses to canes, and finally when he achieves a satisfactory stable gait, he is encouraged to discontinue the use of a cane. All of this takes considerable time and perseverance; the amputee will require encouragement and support from his family and those working with him in rehabilitation. If the patient is elderly and adjustment to a prosthesis is too difficult, he is instructed in wheelchair activities.

Immediate Postsurgical Prosthetic Fitting. In recent years, early crutch walking with partial weight bearing on a prosthesis has been introduced. On completion of the amputation, a plaster of Paris cast is applied over the well-padded stump, and a fitting for a prosthesis is made. If the patient's general condition is satisfactory, the prosthesis is attached after 24 hours, and he is assisted to stand putting some weight on the artificial limb and using crutches, a walker, or canes for support. He is then encouraged to walk, progressively increasing his activity. The cast is usually changed in 10 to 14 days, and then removed in 3 to 4 weeks. A more permanent prosthesis is then provided, and gait training continues. This procedure is used most often with a below-the-knee amputation.

Crutch Walking

Crutch walking may be a permanent or temporary means of ambulation when one or both lower limbs are disabled. The initial instruction in the use of crutches is usually done by a physiotherapist with support, assistance and reinforcement of instructions provided by the nurse. In some instances, the nurse may have to assume full responsibility. In either situation, she must understand the principles involved and have a knowledge of the various gaits which may be used.

Ambulation through the use of crutches may mean that the patient becomes mobile much faster than would otherwise be possible. Preparation, physical and emotional, begins long before the actual event. Maintenance of good body alignment during the period of bed rest helps to ensure good posture and balance when the upright position is resumed. Joints are put through their full range of motion daily, and active exercises are encouraged in order to maintain joint mobility and muscle strength. These activities prevent restricted movement, weakness and deformities, such as foot drop, which could interfere with walking.

It is necessary to strengthen the extensor muscles of the upper arm, namely the triceps, in readiness for crutch walking. Several exercises can be done by the bed patient to achieve this. The patient lies on his abdomen and lifts his chest off the bed using both arms; he lies flat on his back and straightens his elbows several times while holding a weight in each hand; or, while sitting on the side of the bed with his feet dangling over the edge, he presses down on the mattress with both hands and lifts his hips off the bed. This last exercise also gets the patient used to bearing his weight on the palms of his hands. Quadriceps muscles may be strengthened while the patient is sitting by having him straighten his knee or lift his stump off the mattress. These exercises may be done 2 or 3 times daily but always with sufficient support and not to the point of undue fatigue.

The patient's prognosis, physical condition and emotional make-up will greatly influence his progress in the use of crutches. It is a slow process which requires considerable physical effort and can quickly lead to feelings of discouragement and hopelessness. A nurse who is sincere in her interest, patient in giving instruction, who encourages the patient to express his feelings and willingly provides reassurance to him and his family is of great value. Care is taken that both patient and nurse understand the doctor's direction. The plans for teaching the skill are adapted to the patient according to his future activities, attitude, age, weight and strength. Setting attainable goals, such as walking to the window, for each session will help to combat frustration and perhaps stimulate some interest in what goes on beyond his bed. Enlisting the patient's help in planning his daily progress helps to maintain his enthusiasm.

Selection of proper crutches is of the utmost importance. There are several ways in which the length is determined. One method is to measure the patient while he is lying flat with his arms at his sides from the axilla to a point 6 inches out from the side of his foot, allowing three-quarters of an inch that will be added by the crutch tip. Another is to subtract 16 inches from the patient's height. With children, crutches must be changed periodically to allow for normal growth. The hand bars on which the palms of the hands bear the weight must allow for flexion of the elbow at a 30° angle, or almost complete extension of the arm. A third factor in the selection of crutches is to allow space between the crutch top and the axilla. Undue or prolonged pressure here can cause severe, and occasionally permanent, paralysis of the radial nerve. The axillary bar may be padded with material such as sponge rubber wrapped in soft cloth.

Some minor adjustments may be necessary after the patient becomes more skilled in crutch walking. Good quality rubber tips on the ends of the crutches are imperative for safety. These must be checked frequently. A suction cup tip is available which is particularly helpful for those who are severely disabled and must place their crutches at a wide angle for good balance.

The efforts of all concerned are directed toward assisting the patient to use crutches to walk smoothly and evenly while maintaining good posture. The patient's disability and strength will determine which gait he is to use—the swinging, the 4-point, 3-point or 2-point. Lessons should be in an environment that avoids crowding, has a smooth floor surface, is free of hazards such as electric cords or rugs, and which is equipped with a full-length mirror if possible.

When only one leg can bear weight, the patient may use the swinging gait. Both crutches are placed at an equal distance in front of the patient's good leg. He then swings his good leg slightly ahead of the crutches and repeats the sequence. Smoothness and speed will increase with practice, and emphasis is placed on the maintenance of good balance and a short stride. The 4-point gait is used when both lower limbs are affected but can bear at least part of the patient's weight. One crutch is brought forward, then the opposite leg, then the second crutch and the other leg. Having the patient count to 4 may aid in achieving smoothness. This method provides stability since there are always 3 points of contact with the floor.

If one leg is affected but partial weight bearing is allowed, the 3-point gait may be taught. Both crutches and the weak leg are brought forward, and then the good leg is advanced. Emphasis is placed on taking steps of equal length to avoid a limp that may persist even after crutches are discarded. As his strength increases, the patient may progress to the 2-point gait, which is more rapid and appears closer to the normal. Weight is borne on one crutch and the opposite leg while the other crutch and leg advance; then the weight is shifted to the latter pair, and the process is repeated.

OSTEOMYELITIS

When bone tissue becomes infected the condition is known as osteomyelitis. The pathogenic organisms may be introduced directly through an open fracture or from infected contiguous tissue but are more commonly carried by the blood to the bone from a distant primary focus such as boils (furuncles), an abscessed tooth or infected tonsils. When the infection is blood-borne, the condition is referred to as hematogenous osteomyelitis. The most common bacterial offender is the *Staphylococcus aureus,* but the disease may also result from the invasion of streptococci, pneumococci or other strains of staphylococci.

Growing bone is more susceptible to hematogenous osteomyelitis, and as a result, the incidence is highest in children and adolescents. The infection usually develops in long bones at the diaphyseal side of the growth plate. Unless it is checked at the onset, the inflammatory process forms a purulent exudate that collects in the minute canals and spaces of the bone tissue. The pressure of the exudate builds up because of the resistant, rigid bone and presses upon the blood vessels, causing thrombosis and occlusion. The accumulation under pressure eventually breaks through the cortex of the bone into the subperiosteal space. The periosteum at that site becomes elevated and stripped from the bone, interrupting the blood vessels that lead into the bone. Interference with the blood supply results in an area of dead bone tissue, which is called a sequestrum. The periosteum may rupture, and the infection may then extend into the adjacent soft tissues, forming a sinus tract that discharges onto the skin surface. Small sequestra, separated from the living bone tissue, may escape with the exudate through the sinus. The infection may destroy the growth plate (epiphyseal line), leading to reduced growth of the limb, or it may extend into the adjacent joint with ensuing permanent loss of joint function. The periosteum initiates the formation of new bone tissue around the affected area. The new tissue is called the involucrum* and may enclose and trap sequestra and infecting organisms. These organisms continue to grow in the confined area and the osteomyelitis becomes chronic, characterized by recurring abscess formation and sequestration.

Signs and Symptoms

The onset of acute osteomyelitis may be manifested by a chill, high fever and rapid pulse. The patient has the appearance of being acutely ill; he perspires freely, is restless and irritable and may be nauseated and vomit. Severe pain develops as a result of the pressure by the accumulating exudate and the destruction of bone. The pain is aggravated by slight movement or jarring of the bed. The patient protects the limb by avoiding weight bearing and movement and usually holds the adjacent joint in flexion. The local area is very tender on slight pressure and becomes red and swollen when the infective process reaches the subperiosteal area and surrounding soft tissues.

There is a marked increase in the leukocyte count, and the erythrocyte sedimentation rate is elevated. After 1 to 2 weeks, roentgenograms reveal destructive bone changes and periosteal elevation and reaction.

---

*Involucrum—a membranous covering or envelope.

Treatment and Nursing Care

Antimicrobial drug therapy and rest in the early stage of osteomyelitis may bring the infection under control with minimal bone damage. In more advanced cases, surgery may be necessary to provide drainage to relieve the pressure within the bone and periosteum and to remove dead bone tissue.

Efforts are made to identify the infecting organism by making cultures of the blood, nose and throat secretions and discharge from any skin lesions (e.g., boils). If a positive culture is obtained, sensitivity tests may then be made to determine the most effective antibiotic therapy.

Large doses of antibiotic are given usually by parenteral channels. If the response is favorable and the infective process controlled, antimicrobial therapy is generally continued for several weeks to ensure destruction of the organisms.

The patient is placed at rest, and the affected limb is handled very gently. It is positioned and supported to prevent contractures and deformities. A splint may be used to immobilize the adjacent joint. The patient tends to remain in one position because of fear of pain. He must be assisted to turn at frequent intervals to guard against pressure sores and respiratory complications. Fluids are given liberally because of the fever and blood infection. A high-calorie, well-balanced diet is encouraged to increase the patient's resistance. If nausea and vomiting are a problem, intravenous infusions of parenteral fluids and a blood transfusion may be necessary.

If surgical drainage or a sequestrectomy is performed, the wound is packed and allowed to heal by granulation from within toward the surface. Antibiotic or sulfonamide preparations may be introduced locally into the wound. The dressing is changed often enough to keep the wound clean and to prevent the development of an offensive odor that may become very distressing to the patient and those in his environment. Precautions must be taken to observe aseptic technique when dressing or treating the wound to prevent the introduction of secondary infection and to prevent the transmission of the patient's infection to others.

When the patient is allowed up, he must be cautioned against falls and injury to the limb. The loss of bone substance may weaken the bone structure, predisposing it to fracture when subjected to even slight injury or pressure. In the case of a lower extremity, weight bearing may be contra-indicated for many weeks while new bone tissue is being formed. The patient may then have to be taught to use crutches. He may be discharged from the hospital but is likely to require guidance and supervision for a considerable period of time.

As cited earlier, hematogenous osteo-myelitis is seen most often in children as a result of infection in some area of the body, and unless treated early, it may lead to a long illness and serious crippling. Nurses (especially those visiting in homes and schools) and parents must be constantly alert to the possible significance of focal and recurring infections, such as boils. Medical treatment should be sought for the child. Any complaint of tenderness or pain in a limb, especially if it is associated with fever or general malaise, requires prompt attention.

OSTEOPOROSIS

This condition is characterized by de-creased density and strength of bone tissue due to decreased bone formation by the osteoblasts. There is a diminished produc-tion of the collagenous matrix in which calcium and phosphorus are deposited; as a result, bone tissue is worn down more rapidly than it is replaced. The trabeculae are fewer, and the tissue is rarefied as com-pared to normal bone. The calcium and phos-phorus levels of the blood are normal or may be elevated if the intake is normal.

The weight-bearing vertebrae (lower tho-racic and lumbar) and pelvis are usually the first bones to be involved. As the disease becomes more advanced, the long bones, ribs and skull are affected. Osteoporosis has a higher incidence in females, especially after menopause, and is commonly seen in elderly persons.

The cause of osteoporosis may be the decreased demand and strain associated with immobilization or sedentary life that reduces the stimulation of osteoblastic activity, a diminished secretion of anabolic sex hor-mones (e.g., estrogen) as occurs after the climacteric and in senility, or a deficient protein intake. The disease may be second-ary to some endocrine disturbances such as hyperthyroidism and Cushing's syndrome (adrenocortical hyperfunction) or may be the result of therapeutic doses of corticoids.

Signs and Symptoms

The initial symptom in most patients is usually pain in the back due to a flattening or collapse of vertebrae and resulting pres-sure on spinal nerves. Muscle spasm and limited movement may also develop. Remis-sions occur, and frequently, exacerbations are precipitated by lifting or stooping. Kyphosis (forward curvature of spine), loss of the normal lumbar curve and loss of stature may become apparent. The bones fracture more readily and osteoporosis con-tributes to the high incidence of fracture of the hip in older persons. In many instances, the condition goes unrecognized until the person receives a fracture in a simple fall and the x-rays reveal a loss of density in bone tissue.

Treatment and Nursing Care

During an acute episode, the patient is placed on bed rest and given analgesics such as acetylsalicylic acid (Aspirin) or dextro-propoxyphene (Darvon) to relieve the pain. A firm mattress on a fracture board is im-portant. As soon as the pain and muscle spasm are reduced, the patient is mobilized, for prolonged bed rest only contributes to further weakening of the bone structure and muscles. A liberal fluid intake is recom-mended, especially if the serum calcium level is elevated, to reduce the possibility of hypercalciuria and ensuing renal or bladder calculus formation. The patient is encour-aged to take additional amounts of protein, and in some instances, because of a negative calcium balance, an increased intake of cal-cium-containing foods is prescribed. A me-dicinal preparation of calcium may also be ordered (e.g., calcium gluconate). The ca-loric intake is controlled to avoid overweight, which places added strain on the weakened bone structure.

Activity is encouraged to stimulate osteo-blastic activity, and a daily exercise regimen is frequently prescribed. Some patients may receive estrogen (e.g., diethylstilbestrol) or androgen (e.g., testosterone propianate) orally. In the case of a female receiving estrogen therapy, close observations are made for any sign of vaginal bleeding, which is reported promptly.

The patient is instructed to avoid lifting heavy objects and to keep his spine straight and flex his thighs and knees when he wants to reach something at floor level. Older patients who are predisposed to osteoporosis are cautioned against falls. Scatter rugs, footstools or other objects in their environment that might lead to a fall are removed. For comfort and mobility, a few patients may require a spinal support or brace.

Osteomalacia

Osteomalacia is an adult disorder comparable to rickets in children, and for this reason it is occasionally referred to as adult rickets. It is characterized by an insufficient plasma concentration of calcium and inorganic phosphate for normal calcification of bone tissue. The bones become soft and weak. The person complains of tenderness and an aching pain in the bones. Some bowing of long bones and deformities may develop. A loss of weight and muscular strength may be manifested, and if the calcium deficiency is marked, tetany may be exhibited (see p. 59).

Osteomalacia may be the result of an insufficient amount of calcium reaching the plasma or an excessive urinary excretion of the mineral. In the first instance, the deficiency of calcium may be due to a lack of calcium-containing foods in the diet, insufficient absorption of the mineral from the intestine (caused by steatorrhea or prolonged diarrhea), or a deficiency of vitamin D, which is necessary for normal absorption of calcium and its deposition in bone tissue. Osteomalacia may also occur during pregnancy if the woman does not receive additional calcium to meet the increased demand incurred by the developing fetus.

The second major cause of the disease — that is, of an excessive urinary excretion of calcium — is usually the result of acidosis associated with renal failure or of renal tubular damage and malfunction.

The treatment consists mainly of the administration of calcium and vitamin D. If the serum calcium concentration is markedly low, calcium (e.g., calcium gluconate 10 per cent) may be given intravenously.

References

BOOKS

Burgess, E. M., Romano, R. L., and Zettl, J. H.: The Management of Lower Extremity Amputations (Prepared for the Prosthetic and Sensory Aids Service, Veterans' Administration). Washington, D.C., United States Government Printing Office, 1969.

Cole, W. H., and Zollinger, R. M.: Textbook of Surgery, 8th ed. New York, Appleton Century-Crofts, 1963. Chapter 22.

Davis, L. (Ed.): Christopher's Textbook of Surgery, 9th ed. Philadelphia, W. B. Saunders Co., 1968. Chapter 31.

Gius, J. A.: Fundamentals of General Surgery, 3rd ed. Chicago, Year Book Medical Publishers, Inc., 1966. Chapter 29.

Kerr, A.: Orthopedic Nursing Procedures, 2nd ed. New York, C. P. Springer Publishing Co., Inc., 1969.

Larson, C. B., and Gould, M.: Orthopedic Nursing, 7th ed. St. Louis, The C. V. Mosby Co., 1970.

Ralston, E. L.: Handbook of Fractures. St. Louis, The C. V. Mosby Co., 1967.

Salter, R. B.: Textbook of Disorders and Injuries of the Musculoskeletal System. Baltimore, The Williams and Wilkins Co., 1970.

Sweetman, R. (Ed.): Will's Fractures, Dislocations, Sprains, 2nd ed. London, J. and A. Churchill Ltd., 1969.

PERIODICALS

Bitenc, I.: "Hip Arthroplasty." Canad. Nurse, Vol. 60, No. 5 (May 1964), pp. 463–466.

Burnham, P. J.: "Amputation of the Lower Extremity." Clin. Symp., XVI, No. 1 (Jan.–Mar. 1964), pp. 3–18.

_____ "Amputation of the Upper Extremity." Clin. Symp., XIII, No. 1 (Jan.–Mar. 1961), pp. 3–33.

Calderwood, C.: "Russell Traction." Amer. J. Nurs., Vol. 43, No. 5 (May 1943), pp. 464–469.

Jones, G. P. (Ed.): "Symposium on Orthopedic and Surgical Nursing." Nurs. Clin. North Amer., Vol. 2, No. 3 (Sept. 1967), pp. 383–435.

McKay, J.: "The Long Road Home." Canad. Nurse, Vol. 60, No. 5 (May 1964), pp. 466–470.

Moncrieff, M. J.: "Problems, Principles and Practices in the Care of Patients in Plasters." Canad. Nurse, Vol. 59, No. 11 (Nov. 1963), pp. 1040–1052.

Monteiro, L. A.: "Hip Fracture: A Sociologist's Viewpoint." Amer. J. Nurs., Vol. 67, No. 6 (June 1967), pp. 1207–1210.

Newton, K.: "Orthopedic Problems of Older People." Amer. J. Nurs., Vol. 48, No. 8 (Aug. 1948), pp. 508–511.

Schewchuk, M., and Young, Z.: "The Amputee and Immediate Prosthesis." Canad. Nurse, Vol. 65, No. 5 (May 1969), pp. 47–49.

24
Nursing in Joint and Collagen Disease

JOINT STRUCTURE AND FUNCTION

A joint, or articulation, is formed at the junction of 2 bones. Joints may be classified according to their structures or the degree of movement they permit. Synarthroses or fibrous joints are immovable and have a layer of connective tissue which unites the bones. The cranial bones form synarthroses. Amphiarthroses or cartilaginous joints are slightly movable; the bones are separated by a layer of fibrocartilaginous tissue which allows a limited amount of bending or twisting. The symphysis pubis of the pelvis and the joints between the vertebral bodies form amphiarthroses.

Most of the articulations of the skeleton are diarthroses or synovial joints, which are freely movable. The bones are separated by a small cavity enclosed in a tough fibrous capsule which is continuous with the periosteum of the bones. This arrangement serves to stabilize the joint and keep the bones in normal apposition. The joint may be further reinforced by ligaments extending from one bone to the other. The capsule is lined with a synovial membrane that se-

cretes a lubricating fluid called synovia. The joint surfaces of the bones in diarthroses are covered by a layer of cartilage. In addition, some diarthrotic joints have flat, crescent-shaped pieces of cartilage lying in the cavity between the ends of the bones (e.g., knee). These and the layer of cartilage on the joint surfaces buffer the impact of the rigid bone as well as cushion and protect the bone tissue.

Shapes of the articulating surfaces vary with the particular type or types of movement required of that area of the skeleton. For instance, the shoulder and hip joints are ball-and-socket in structure to allow all types of movement. The elbow and knee are hinge-like, allowing only flexion and extension.

Bursae

A bursa is a protective structure consisting of a small, flat, fibrous sac lined with synovial membrane. Bursae are located in areas subject to friction or pressure, such as between a bone and overlying tendon or portion of skin. Bursitis may develop in response to injury or infection. The bursae most commonly encountered clinically in

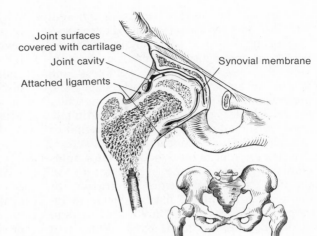

Figure 24–1 Diagram of a freely movable joint (diarthrosis).

bursitis are those situated between the olecranon process of the ulna and the skin, the patella and the skin, the shoulder muscles or their tendons and the head of the humerus or scapula, and the tendon of Achilles and the calcaneus (heel bone).

RHEUMATIC DISEASES

Rheumatism and rheumatic disease are general terms which are commonly applied to joint disturbances but which currently include a wide variety of disorders that have more diffuse involvement of the collagenous component of connective tissue.[1] In some rheumatic diseases the dominant clinical manifestations are localized joint disturbances; the condition is then referred to as arthritis. In others, the symptoms are systemic and are manifested more generally throughout the body. Those diseases most commonly seen and selected for discussion here include rheumatoid arthritis, ankylosing spondylitis, osteoarthritis and systemic lupus erythematosus.

RHEUMATOID ARTHRITIS

Rheumatoid or atrophic arthritis is a chronic inflammatory disease of connective tissues; the dominant site is the joints.

The disease is a major health problem,

---

[1]The Committee of the American Rheumatism Association: Primer on the Rheumatic Diseases. New York, The Arthritis Foundation, 1964.

being responsible for much of the existing chronic illness and crippling incapacity of adults. The incidence is 3 times higher in women than in men. It may have its onset at any age but most commonly begins in the fourth or fifth decade.

The cause of rheumatoid arthritis remains obscure. Several etiological factors such as heredity, infection and nutritional deficiencies have been suspected from time to time, but none have been substantiated. In recent years, attention has been focused on the possibility of an autoimmune or hypersensitivity reaction being the causative factor. Currently, this theory receives considerable support because of the presence of the rheumatoid factor in the blood of 70 to 80 per cent of persons with rheumatoid arthritis. This is a large antibody-like protein molecule which is thought to be produced in response to an altered gamma globulin in the connective tissues.

Clinical Course and Features

The onset is usually insidious; the person experiences a period of general fatigue, nonspecific illness, and morning stiffness and tenderness in some joints. The small joints of the hands or feet or of the wrists, elbows or knees are generally the first to be involved. The disease develops symmetrically, and as it progresses, the affected joints become swollen, painful, red and increasingly difficult to move. Their range of motion is reduced. The overlying skin may take on a stretched, smooth glossy appearance. The severity of the disease varies in different persons, and remissions and exacerbations may occur. Physical or psychological stress may be a precipitating factor or may aggravate the disease. Muscle weakness and spasm are common in the early stages and are frequently followed by marked muscular atrophy. Unless early treatment is instituted, joint tissue destruction and deformities develop. Partial dislocation (subluxation) and flexion contractures occur. Deformities commonly seen include hyperextension of the distal phalanges, flexion contracture or ulnar deviation of the fingers due to metacarpal-phalangeal joint involvement, and flexion contraction of the wrists, knees and hips. Subcutaneous nodules (rheumatoid nodules) appear principally on extensor surfaces or areas subjected to pressure. These are composed mainly of fibrinoid material (degenerative tissue cells) and granulation tissue.

The initial pathological changes within the joints are inflammation and swelling of the synovial membrane and joint capsule. The process is reversible in the early stage, and the joint may be left undamaged and functional. If the inflammation continues, granulation tissue forms and spreads as a pannus over the cartilaginous surfaces of the articular ends of the bones. The pannus cuts off the nutrients normally available to the cartilage from the synovial fluid. The cartilage is gradually eroded. Fibrous scar tissue and adhesions develop between the opposing joint surfaces, leading to fibrous ankylosis of the joint. The exposed, roughened ends of bone tissue may eventually proliferate bone cells into the joint cavity, resulting in calcification and bony ankylosis.

The patient with rheumatoid arthritis may also have diffuse involvement of nonarticular connective tissue. Degenerative lesions of the collagen component of the connective tissue may develp in muscles, tendons, blood vessels, pleura, heart or lungs.

General constitutional disturbances are manifested; the patient is pale and looks ill. He experiences anorexia, loss of weight and energy, and mental depression. Low-grade fever, tachycardia, anemia and a mild leukocytosis may be present. The erythrocyte sedimentation rate is usually elevated (normal: Westergren, 15 mm. per hour; Wintrobe, 0 to 9 mm. per hour for males and 0 to 20 mm. per hour for females), and later in the disease, a blood examination may reveal the presence of the rheumatoid factor. When rheumatoid arthritis develops in children, it may be referred to as Still's disease. In addition to the symptoms mentioned for adults, they usually have some enlargement of the lymph nodes.

Treatment and Nursing Care

The care of the patient with rheumatoid arthritis is directed toward the suppression of the inflammatory process, the prevention of deformities, and the maintenance and promotion of joint function. The earlier treatment is instituted, the less advanced and less crippling the disease is likely to be. The patient may be hospitalized during the initial investigative and therapeutic period and is then followed at home by a visiting nurse or at the clinic. Bed rest may be prescribed when many joints are acutely inflamed and when systemic disturbances such as fever, anemia and severe fatigue are manifested.

Drug Therapy. Various drugs are used in the treatment of rheumatoid arthritis and include salicylates, gold salts, antimalarial preparations, corticosteroids and phenylbutazone.

The salicylate preparation most commonly used is acetylsalicylic acid (Aspirin). It is prescribed in relatively large doses and must be taken regularly at the stated intervals in order to maintain effective antirheumatic levels in the plasma. Salicylates may produce some adverse effects for which the nurse must be alert. The patient may complain of gastrointestinal disturbances, tinnitus (a ringing or roaring in the ears) and loss of auditory acuity. Since they frequently cause gastrointestinal irritation, the prescribed salicylate is more likely to be tolerated if taken with or soon after meals or with milk or some bland food between meal hours. Gastric or intestinal bleeding is not an uncommon side effect, and patients with any history of peptic ulcer do not usually receive salicylate therapy.

When a preparation of gold salts such as gold and sodium thiomalate (Myochrysine) is given, the patient is observed closely for signs of toxic reactions. Such signs may be reflected as stomatitis (inflammation of the oral mucous membrane), dermatitis, renal damage and bone marrow depression leading to severe anemia, leukopenia (agranulocytosis) and thrombocytopenia. Gold therapy usually involves a weekly intramuscular injection over 4 to 6 months. Urine analysis and blood cell counts are usually done weekly, and the patient is checked for possible signs or symptoms of adverse side effects.

The antimalarial drugs such as amodiaquine hydrochloride (Camoquin), chloroquine phosphate (Novaquine or Aralen) and hydroxychloroquine sulfate (Plaquenil) may be prescribed over a period of several months for some patients. Toxic effects that may develop include skin eruptions, headache, anorexia, nausea, vomiting and auditory or visual disturbances. Frequent blood cell counts are done because occasionally bone marrow depression occurs.

Adrenal corticosteroids are now usually reserved for patients whose rheumatoid arthritis is rapidly progressing, is very painful and has not responded to therapeutic courses of other antirheumatic drugs. The preparations frequently used are prednisone (Meticorten) and prednisolone (Delta-Cortef). The dosage is individualized and kept to a minimum because of the unfavorable side effects which may develop. It is important that the patient understand that the drug will be given only for a limited period. The dosage is gradually reduced and then completely withdrawn. Adverse side effects which are likely to develop with overdosage or prolonged therapy include reduced lymphocyte and antibody production leading to increased susceptibility to infection, sodium and water retention, excessive potassium excretion, mood swings or euphoria, restlessness or overactivity, hyperglycemia and glucosuria, fullness or rounding of the face (moon face), and growth of hair on the face in the case of a female. The patient who has experienced increased appetite, a marked sense of well-being and some remission of his disease while receiving a corticosteroid may feel quite depressed and letdown when the drug is withdrawn; he will require considerable emotional support from the nurse.

When only one or two joints are affected, intra-articular injections of a corticosteroid may be made to arrest the inflammatory process.

Phenylbutazone (Butazolidin) is occasionally prescribed, and unfavorable effects may be reflected in skin eruptions, bone marrow depression or gastrointestinal irritation.

Positioning and the Application of Splints. During the acute inflammatory stage, the affected joints are especially painful on movement. The involved part usually assumes the flexed position because of spasm of the dominant flexor muscles, and contracture deformity is likely to develop. Limb joints may be placed at rest and immobilized in a neutral position by the application of padded splints to reduce the severity of pain and prevent contractures and deformities. At first, these may only be removed during the daily exercise or heat therapy periods. Later, as the muscle spasm lessens, the splints are left off for most of the day and may only be necessary during the night.

To prevent hip and spinal flexion a fracture board is placed under the mattress and the patient is encouraged to use only a small pillow to maintain good cervical alignment. If the patient is confined to bed for a period longer than 24 hours, he is advised to change his position frequently. Two or three periods of one-half hour or more should be spent in the prone position to prevent flexure contraction at the hips. A footboard is provided to keep the feet at right angles while in the dorsal position. When positioning or assisting the patient, the affected parts must be handled very gently, and support is given to the joints. Jarring and quick, jerky movements are avoided. Independence and active movements are encouraged; the patient moves slowly and the nurse and his family must learn to be patient and allow him the necessary time.

When up, attention is paid to the arthritic's posture. He is encouraged to stand erect and "sit straight" to avoid forward flexion of the trunk and drooping of the shoulders.

Heat Applications. Various forms of heat applications are used to help to reduce muscle spasm, pain, joint stiffness and swelling. Soaks in water at 38° to 39° C. (100° to 102° F.) or the application of dry heat (hot water bottle, electric heating pad or infra red heat lamp) may be prescribed. Hot paraffin immersion is also used. Paraffin mixed with mineral oil (3½ pounds of paraffin to 1 cup of mineral oil) is heated to 51.4° to 54° C. (125° to 130° F.). The affected limb is repeatedly dipped in the solution until 6 to 8 coats are applied and then wrapped in paper and a thick bath towel. If the affected joint cannot be immersed in the paraffin, several layers may be quickly applied to it with a paint brush. The wax coating is left for approximately 1 hour and then is peeled off and reused.

Whatever form of heat is used, precautions must be used against burning; the skin over acutely inflamed joints is more sensitive and is readily burned. Heat is not used if there is any break in the skin.

Exercises and Activity. As soon as possible, a daily exercise schedule is introduced to achieve and preserve the most complete range of motion possible as well as to maintain muscle strength. Exercises are planned and prescribed on an individual basis and are carefully supervised by a physical therapist or nurse until they are understood and are familiar to the patient. Indiscriminate movements or overstretching may cause a dislocation or torn tendons.

When acute inflammation, swelling and severe pain preclude joint movements, isometric exercises are recommended. Joint exercises may be passive or active-assisted to start with and are gradually progressed to active and resistive exercises within the limits set by the physician. The exercises are only of value if carried out at regular intervals. The patient's reaction to the exercises is noted; excessive fatigue or increased pain necessitate some modification in the exercise program. An explanation is made to the patient and his family of the purpose and importance of the exercise regimen. The exercises may be performed with less difficulty if preceded by some form of heat application which promotes muscle relaxation. Special shoes, canes, a walker or braces may be recommended to assist with weight bearing and mobility.

Self-care and the activities of daily living are encouraged. If the range of motion is limited because of joint destruction or ankylosis, self-help devices may be provided to promote maximum independence in such activities as dressing, grooming and feeding. Good grooming and taking pride in appearance are encouraged by providing the essentials and commending the patient.

Surgical Treatment. Surgery is playing an increasing role in the treatment of rheumatoid arthritis. The thickened inflamed synovium is removed (synovectomy) from the affected joint(s) early in the disease, prior to cartilage and bone destruction or the formation of fibrous adhesions and ankylosis.

In more advanced disease in which there has been irreversible joint damage that has led to deformity and loss of function, various surgical procedures may be undertaken to reduce the handicap. Arthrodesis (fixation of the joint) to provide joint stability or arthroplasty (reconstructive procedure) with the use of prosthetic devices may be done. A rigid exercise program following surgery is usually very necessary to ensure functional improvement for the patient.

General Supportive Measures. In planning care for the arthritic, the nurse also gives consideration to the psychological support, rest and nutrition needed by the patient.

The diagnosis of rheumatoid arthritis is likely to produce considerable emotional response in the patient because of the chronic nature of the disease and because the possible crippling effects are common knowledge to most persons. The patient may become resentful or depressed and uncooperative. The nurse, recognizing the patient's reactions as normal responses to threatening situations, accepts them and watches for opportune situations to convey her understanding of his feelings and to encourage him to talk about his problems, at which time she may offer explanations as to the available assistance and suggestions as to how he may adjust. He is advised of the variability in the severity and rate of progress and should be reminded that many patients lead a normal, useful life with only slight modifications in their pattern of living. Some activities which previously seemed very simple and were taken for granted may become quite a chore and time-consuming. Adjustments in his daily routine may be made to allow more time for such tasks. Many of the patients afflicted with rheumatoid arthritis are in what are referred to as the most productive years. Restricted employment, reduced earning capacity and limited social and recreational activities add considerable stress to the situation and are frequently a source of great concern for the patient and his family. A social worker's assistance, a chaplin's counsel and the assurance that there is a planned therapeutic and rehabilitation program will help with emotionally disturbing factors. Successful adjustment in the initial stage of the disease is important. If the patient accepts and follows the prescribed modifications and treatment regimen at the onset, he is usually less distressed and more likely to respect the necessary adjustments during an acute recurrence.

The person with rheumatoid arthritis generally requires extra rest. The amount depends on the severity of his disease. His daily schedule may require modification to allow a rest period in the middle of the day and more hours in bed at night. The arthritic must appreciate that rest alone or exercise alone is not good, but rather that both are essential. Controlled activity and exercise must be balanced with an appropriate amount of rest. The amount of each is recommended by the physician but is an individual factor, frequently requiring modification from time to time.

A well-balanced diet, similar to that essential to the health of all persons, is recommended for the arthritic. The total caloric intake may require some adjustment with a view to achieving or maintaining the person's normal weight. Overweight is avoided, for it increases the strain on joints and may also reduce motivation in exercise.

Instruction and Rehabilitation. The long-term goal in planning and implementing care for the person with rheumatoid arthritis is to have him be as independent and as useful as possible, gainfully employed and living as normal a social and family life as possible.

It is important for the patient and his family to understand the nature of rheumatoid arthritis and that much of the disability and deformity commonly associated with the disease can be prevented if early treatment is instituted and the prescribed regimen followed. The nurse's explanation can be reinforced by providing them with booklets especially prepared for patients and the public by the national arthritis and rheumatism societies.[2]

---

[2]The Canadian Arthritis and Rheumatism Society, Toronto, Canada.

The Arthritis and Rheumatism Foundation, New York, N.Y.

The Diabetes and Arthritis Program of the Division of Chronic Diseases, Public Health Service, United States Department of Health, Education and Welfare, Washington, D.C.

Rehabilitation depends largely on the severity of the patient's disease and whether or not the pathological process in the joints is arrested. Obviously if the disease is severe and more and more joints are progressively involved, the patient is less likely to be well enough to return to his former occupation and will require a more active and closely supervised care program. Many patients are well enough to go to work and adjust their daily life to provide for extra rest as well as continuance of a daily physical exercise regimen. Some find it necessary after the onset of arthritis to change their former type of work. This may necessitate assistance in finding suitable employment or in interpreting the patient's condition to his employer, who may be persuaded to employ him in another type of job. A period of vocational training may be necessary before the arthritic can be re-employed.

Before leaving the hospital, the patient is given a written outline of his exercises. These are reviewed and discussed with him and a family member. If there is some restriction in the range of motion of some joints, interfering with self-care activities, arrangements are made for the provision of self-help devices. The family members are made aware of the importance of encouraging the patient to do things for himself. They are advised that he may be very slow in achieving various activities which seem very simple to them. They should appreciate the need for additional patience and for planning that will provide the required extra time.

If drug or heat therapy is to be continued as well as the exercises, or if the patient is sufficiently handicapped to require physical care, a referral may be made to the visiting nurse agency. The visiting nurse frequently is of assistance in assessing the home situation and making recommendations for adjustments that will simplify the care of the patient and will increase his mobility and independence. For example, suggestions may be made for reorganizing the kitchen in order to make equipment more readily available and lessen the demands on the worker. Such recommendations for simplification of household chores may enable a woman with arthritis to carry on the care of her home.

The importance of maintaining good body alignment is stressed; as well as fracture boards and footboards for the bed, a comfortable straight chair of appropriate height and good walking shoes are needed.

The patient and his family are acquainted with the services of the Arthritis and Rheumatism Foundation and its publications, which may be helpful, are provided. Transportation is frequently a problem for the arthritic. If he is required to go regularly to a physical therapy clinic or rehabilitation unit, the society will usually provide transportation if requested.

In discussing the necessary care, emphasis is placed on the avoidance of becoming overtired, emotionally upset about things that cannot be corrected and exposed to cold. The patient is also reminded to minimize as much as possible the strain and pressure normally placed on the affected joints. He and his family are cautioned against quack or folk remedies and the taking of unprescribed drugs. Regular attendance at a clinic or the physician's office is essential for repeated ongoing evaluation and appropriate adjustments in treatment.

The nurse is alert for economic problems that may be imposed by the illness, and a referral is made, when necessary, to a welfare or service agency for assistance.

ANKYLOSING SPONDYLITIS

This is a chronic disorder characterized by inflammation and ensuing ankylosis of the sacroiliac joints and spinal articulations. It may also be designated as Marie-Strumpell arthritis or rheumatoid spondylitis. The pathological process is similar to that seen in rheumatoid arthritis, but there is a greater tendency toward calcification. In most instances the disease remains confined to the joints cited above but occasionally does spread to peripheral joints.

The highest incidence is in young men, the onset occurring most often in the late teens or twenties. The cause is unknown, but heredity is suspected of having a role, since a large majority of those afflicted have a family history of some form of inflammatory arthritis.

Clinical Features

The onset of this disease is usually insidious; the patient first complains of stiff-ness of the back in the morning or following a period of inactivity. Progressively, this becomes more noticeable; limitation in the range of spinal flexion develops, and there is low back pain radiating to the buttocks and thighs along the sciatic nerve pathways. General systemic symptoms are usually absent or are limited to unusual fatigue and probably some weight loss. Remissions and exacerbations of acute disease are common. In more advanced stages, some patients develop some peripheral rheumatoid arthritis. A few develop circulatory complications due to aortitis and aortic valvular insufficiency.

Progressive involvement of spinal segments may continue over a period of years and eventually leave the patient with practically his whole spine firmly ankylosed, producing what may be referred to as a poker back or poker spine. Rarely, rheumatoid spondylitis has an abrupt, acute onset and spreads rapidly through the lumbar, thoracic and cervical segments, leaving the patient with a poker spine in a relatively short period.

Treatment and Nursing Care

Care of the patient with ankylosing spondylitis is directed toward the relief of pain, the maintenance of good spinal alignment and the preservation of maximum spinal function.

During acute phases, the patient usually receives acetylsalicylic acid (Aspirin), phenylbutazone (Butazolidin) or indomethacin. Radiation therapy over affected spinal areas may occasionally be used.

Proper positioning at rest and good posture at all times are extremely important so that ankylosis of the affected joints occurs while they are in the normal neutral position, thus preventing deformity and handicap. The patient is advised of the need for constant attention to proper posture when he is up, emphasizing contraction of the buttock and lower abdominal muscles and keeping his chest up, shoulders back and head erect. In some instances, he is fitted with a back brace to maintain optimum alignment of the affected joints. A fracture board and a firm mattress are placed on his bed, and it is suggested that he use no pillow or only a very small one. The small of the back may be supported by a small pillow, but hyperextension is avoided. The patient is advised to sleep on his back as much as possible to discourage possible flexion of the spine.

A daily physical exercise program is usually prescribed with the objective of strengthening the muscles which help to support the spine and maintain good alignment. Since ankylosis of the costovertebral joints may occur and reduce the ventilatory capacity, breathing exercises may also be included in the suggested exercise regimen.

Heavy lifting and activities which place strain upon the back are restricted. The patient assists in determining his level of tolerance of physical activity; that which produces pain should be avoided. His disease may necessitate a change of occupation and vocational retraining before suitable employment can be found.

OSTEOARTHRITIS

Osteoarthritis is a common degenerative joint disorder that may also be called hypertrophic arthritis, senescent arthritis or degenerative arthritis. The cartilage on the articular ends of the bones becomes thin and worn and gradually breaks down, leaving the underlying bone exposed. Outgrowths of bone develop from the joint margins, resulting in thickening of the ends of the bones and protruding ridges and spurs (osteophytes) which impair joint movement.

The weight-bearing joints, such as the spinal, hip, knee and the interphalangeal joints, are most frequently the site of degenerative joint disease. It may develop in both males and females; the early symptoms appear in the middle or later years of life. The principal cause is thought to be the cumulative strain and wear on the joints through the preceding years. Trauma of the joint, overweight, and malalignment, probably due to poor posture, may be causative factors.

Signs and Symptoms

The patient complains of stiffness, soreness and pain in the affected joints, and crepitus may be felt or heard on movement. The range of motion becomes increasingly limited because of pain, muscle spasm and

the bony outgrowths. Joint enlargement and instability develop. The joints feel hard and irregular. Bony outgrowths on the dorsal surface of affected interphalangeal joints give the knuckles a knobby or gnarled appearance. These knobby protrusions are referred to as Heberden's nodes.

Care of the Patient

The strain on the affected joints is kept to a minimum. The patient may have to change his occupation and give up any strenuous sport or other form of recreation. If overweight, the patient is urged to lose weight. During periods of acute pain, a brief period of bed rest, heat applications and a course of acetylsalicylic acid (Aspirin) or aspirin and codeine compounds may be necessary. Appropriate corrective exercises may be prescribed to maintain muscle tone and movement and promote good alignment and joint stability. The patient is encouraged to be posture conscious. A fitted brace may be of value to immobilize and provide support in the case of degenerative changes in the spine. Surgery may be used to relieve pain and improve function in degenerative disease of a hip or knee (e.g., arthroplasty).

GOUT

Gout is a disorder of uric acid metabolism, characterized by recurring episodes of acute inflammation, pain and swelling in a joint. Any joint may be affected, but those of the foot are more susceptible; the condition usually develops first in the great toe. Gout occurs more commonly in men over 40 years of age and is rarely seen in females.

The disorder is thought to occur as the result of a genetic defect in the metabolism of purine. It causes an excessive concentration of uric acid in the plasma (hyperuricemia) which may be brought about by an overproduction or faulty disposal. Urate crystals may be precipitated and deposited within joint tissues, setting up irritation and a local inflammatory response. The small masses of crystals, which are called tophi, may also form in cartilage or soft tissues in other areas of the body.

Secondary gout may develop in disorders such as blood dyscrasias in which there is a marked breakdown of cellular nucleic acid.

Signs and Symptoms

Acute episodes are characterized by the sudden onset of excruciating pain in the affected joint. It becomes very tender, red, hot and swollen. Veins in the area stand out because of distention. The patient may also experience anorexia, headache, fever and constipation. The blood uric acid concentration is elevated (normal: 2.5 to 5 mg. per cent). Subcutaneous tophi are frequently apparent in the ears or over joints or knuckles. Precipitations of urates may occur in kidney tissue, leading to impaired renal function. In some patients, the excessive concentration of uric acid results in the formation of kidney stones.

The acute attack usually subsides in a few days, and in the early stages of the disease the joint returns to normal. Remissions may gradually become shorter, and the disease becomes chronic. More joints become involved, and there are irreversible changes, leading to deformity and loss of function.

Treatment and Nursing Care

During an acute attack of gout, the patient is placed on bed rest, and drug therapy is promptly instituted. The preparation that has proved most effective to date and is most commonly used is colchicine. It may be administered orally or intravenously. If it is given intravenously, precautions are taken to avoid any of the drug being deposited in the subcutaneous or extravascular tissues because of its local irritating effect. Side effects include nausea, vomiting, abdominal discomfort and diarrhea. The drug generally relieves the pain fairly quickly but does not lower the hyperuricemia. If the patient cannot tolerate or does not respond to colchicine, phenylbutazone (Butazolidin) or an adrenal corticosteroid preparation such as prednisone may be prescribed. For possible side effects of these, see page 703.

Hot or cold applications to the affected joint(s) may provide some relief, but frequently the patient cannot tolerate either. His discomfort is usually less when the part is protected as much as possible from any direct contact with applications and bedding.

A fluid intake of 2500 to 3000 ml. is encouraged to promote dilution and renal elimination of the uric acid. The urinary output is recorded, and the fluid balance is determined.

The diet is generally restricted to fluids for the first day or two; then it is gradually increased as tolerated to include mainly soft carbohydrate foods. The protein and fat contents are kept low and then are added in specified, limited amounts. He is then progressed to a well-balanced diet that is low in fat and has a controlled protein content, which he is advised to follow during remissions. The prescribed diet prohibits foods high in purines such as organ meats (liver, kidneys, heart, sweetbreads), shellfish, sardines and meat extracts. If the patient is overweight, the caloric intake is adjusted to promote a gradual reduction to his optimum weight. Some physicians recommend that the patient subject to acute attacks of gout should abstain from drinking alcohol. Others permit their patients to have a limited amount. The importance of a high fluid intake is explained to the patient, and a minimal daily intake of 2000 to 2500 ml. is continued during remissions.

Patients who are having frequent and severe attacks may receive a uricosuric drug routinely. This type of preparation promotes the urinary excretion of uric acid by inhibiting renal tubular reabsorption. The patient must have a high fluid intake, and an effort is made to keep his urine alkaline. These measures are used to prevent the formation of urinary calculi. The patient is taught to take alkaline-producing foods and fluids or sodium bicarbonate tablets and to test his urine. If the urine reaction is acid while he is receiving the drug, it is reported to his physician. The uricosuric drugs include probenecid (Benemid) and sulfinpyrazone (Anturane). Salicylate preparations are not administered when the patient is receiving a uricosuric agent, since they counteract the desired effect.

SYSTEMIC LUPUS ERYTHEMATOSUS

This disorder is classified as a collagen disease because it is characterized by diffuse inflammation and biochemical and structural changes in the collagen fibers of the connective tissue in organs and tissues throughout the body. Originally, lupus erythematosus, dermatomyositis and scleroderma comprised the collagen diseases. In recent years, some references include rheumatoid arthritis, rheumatic fever and polyarteritis nodosa in the classification of collagen disease.

Systemic lupus erythematosus (SLE) is poorly understood. It usually runs a chronic, irregular course and may prove fatal. The cause is not known, but an autoimmune mechanism is suspected of playing a role.

The disease may begin at any age in either sex but is seen most often in young women. The signs and symptoms, especially at the onset, vary greatly from one person to another. Those most commonly seen include fever, general malaise, excessive fatigue, weakness, anorexia, weight loss and joint pain. A skin rash may be evident on the face, neck or the extremities. The erythrocyte sedimentation rate is elevated (normal: Westergren, < 15 mm. per hour; Wintrobe, 0 to 9 mm. per hour for males and 0 to 20 mm. per hour for females), and anemia is a frequent development. The presence of the LE cell or factor in the serum facilitates diagnosis. The LE cells are polymorphonuclear leukocytes which are enlarged as the result of "ingested" nucleoprotein that has been released by damaged leukocytes in an antigen-antibody reaction. As the disease progresses, serious visceral involvement and ensuing dysfunction are likely to develop. Impaired pulmonary, cardiovascular and kidney function are common. Renal failure is the most frequent cause of death of the patient with SLE.

During an acute exacerbation, adrenal corticosteroids may be prescribed for a brief period, then gradually they are reduced and withdrawn. The care of the patient is mainly supportive and symptomatic. In remissions the patient is advised against exposure to sunlight, infection and excessive fatigue which are thought to predispose or precipitate an exacerbation of the disease process.

DERMATOMYOSITIS

In this form of collagen disease, the skin and voluntary muscles are the principal focal sites of the pathological process. The onset is insidious and may be manifested by an erythematous skin rash, subacute fever, and tenderness and weakness of the muscles. Contracture of the skin and muscles, due to scar tissue, may lead to tightly drawn skin in the affected areas, muscle contracture and loss of function. Involvement of the respiratory muscles may cause respiratory insufficiency. In some instances, the condition is confined to muscle tissue and is referred to as chronic polymyositis. Either form of this collagen disease may be treated with an adrenal corticosteroid preparation, but the outlook may be unfavorable.

SCLERODERMA

This is a chronic collagen disorder in which the collagen component of the skin undergoes degenerative changes and becomes sclerotic. The dermal changes and contraction give rise to deformities and restricted movement. The condition may spread to viscera, causing systemic disturbances and organ dysfunction similar to those that may occur in systemic lupus erythematosus.

POLYARTERITIS NODOSA

This disorder is characterized by diffuse inflammatory and necrotizing lesions in the walls of smaller arteries. The vessel wall is weakened at the site of the lesion, and an aneurysm may develop. In other instances, thrombosis within the lumen of the vessel may lead to occlusion. Vague and varying signs and symptoms occur as with other collagen diseases. If the arteries in vital organs, such as the kidneys and heart, are attacked, essential life-supporting functions may be threatened. Similar to other collagen diseases, there is no specific treatment; adrenal corticosteroids may be administered and may provide a temporary remission.

References

BOOKS

Bland, J. H.: Arthritis, Medical Treatment and Home Care. New York, Collier Books, 1963.
Committee of the American Rheumatism Association: Primer on the Rheumatic Diseases. New York, The Arthritis Foundation, 1964.
Davidson, Sir Stanley: The Principles and Practice of Medicine, 9th ed. Edinburgh, G. & S. Livingstone Ltd., 1970, pp. 538–572.
Falconer, M. W., et al.: The Drug, The Nurse, The Patient, 4th ed. Philadelphia, W. B. Saunders Co., 1970. Chapter 21.
Harrison, T. R., et al. (Eds.): Principles of Internal Medicine, 4th ed. New York, The Blakiston Division, McGraw-Hill Book Co., Inc., 1962, pp. 1902–1923.
Sodeman, W. A., and Sodeman, W. A., Jr.: Pathologic Physiology, Mechanisms of Disease, 4th ed. Philadelphia, W. B. Saunders Co., 1967. Chapter 32.

PERIODICALS

Bland, J. H. (Ed.): "Symposium on Rheumatoid Arthritis." Med. Clin. North Amer., Vol. 52, No. 3 (May 1968).
Calabro, J. J., and Maltz, B. A.: "Current Concepts on Ankylosing Spondylitis." New England J. Med., Vol. 282, No. 11 (Mar. 12, 1970), pp. 606–610.
Clark, W. S.: "Arthritis and Rehabilitation." J. Rehab., Sept.-Oct. 1965, pp. 10-12.
MacGinnis, O.: "Rheumatoid Arthritis—My Tutor." Amer. J. Nurs., Vol. 58, No. 8 (Aug. 1968), pp. 1699–1701.
Margolis, H. M.: "Rheumatoid Arthritis." Amer. J. Nurs., Vol. 47, No. 12 (Dec. 1947), pp. 787–793.
Marmor, L., et al.: "Rheumatoid Arthritis—Surgical Intervention." Amer. J. Nurs., Vol. 67, No. 7 (July 1967), pp. 1430–1433.
Potter, T. A., and Nalebuff, E. A. (Eds.): "Symposium on the Surgical Management of Rheumatoid Arthritis." Surg. Clin. North Amer., Vol. 49, No. 4 (Aug. 1969).
Walike, B. C., et al.: "Rheumatoid Arthritis." Amer. J. Nurs., Vol. 67, No. 7 (July 1967), pp. 1420–1426.
Walike, B. C.: "Rheumatoid Arthritis—Personality Factors." Amer. J. Nurs., Vol. 67, No. 7 (July 1967), pp. 1427–1430.
The Canadian Arthritis and Rheumatism Society, Toronto.
  Booklets: Arthritis and Rheumatism
  Nursing Care of the Arthritic Patient
  Osteoarthritis, A Handbook for Patients
  Rheumatoid Arthritis, A Handbook for Patients

25
Nursing in Skin Disorders and Burns

STRUCTURE AND FUNCTIONS OF THE SKIN

The skin (integument) is composed of 2 layers: a thin, avascular, epithelial layer called the epidermis and a supporting layer of connective tissue on which the epidermis rests, called the dermis, or corium. The epidermis has several layers of cells which differ in shape and composition from layer to layer. The cells are produced in the basal (germinating) layer and then gradually move through the other layers to the surface. As they ascend, they progressively undergo degenerative changes. The nuclei disintegrate, the cell substance changes to a water-repellent, waxy, protein-like substance called keratin, and the cells become flat. They are continuously reproduced in the basal layer and cast off from the surface. It is thought that normally they reach the surface in approximately 27 to 30 days. The cells that are shed disintegrate, leaving their keratin on the surface; this keratin helps to protect the skin. The germinating layer is supported by the diffusion of nutrients from capillaries in the dermis.

The thickness of the epidermis varies in different areas of the body, being thickest on the soles of the feet and palms of the hands and thinnest on the lips and eyelids.

The dermis, consisting of fibrous and elastic connective tissue, contains many blood vessels, lymphatics, nerves and their end-organs, sebaceous and sweat glands, ducts and hair follicles. The under-surface merges with the loose, fatty subcutaneous tissue.

Lying between the epidermal, germinating layer and the dermis are the melanocytes, which produce the pigment melanin and deliver it to the epidermal cells. The amount of pigment is mainly determined by the person's genetic inheritance. The activity of the pigment-producing cells may also be influenced by the melanin-stimulating hormone (MSH), which is released by the pituitary gland, and by exposure to sunlight and friction.

The sebaceous glands secrete an oily substance (sebum) which reaches the skin surface via the hair follicles. The secretion prevents drying of the hair and skin and helps to keep the skin soft and pliable. Blackheads are discolored accumulations of sebum in hair follicles and frequently provide a medium for organisms, causing pimples or the condition acne. Sebaceous gland activity increases at puberty and decreases in later life due to the influence of gonadal hormones on the output of sebum. The growth of hair on certain areas of skin

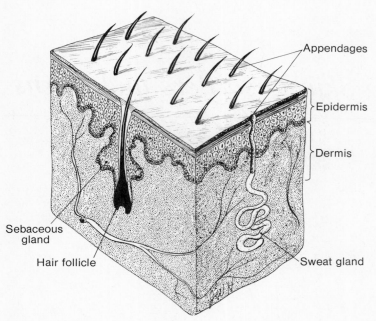

Appendages

Epidermis

Dermis

Sebaceous gland

Hair follicle

Sweat gland

Figure 25–1 Section showing layers of skin.

is also stimulated by gonadal hormones, principally the androgens.

The skin has five important functions — protection, sensation, heat regulation, absorption and storage.

The skin protects the internal structures from injury, drying and the invasion of organisms by the water-repellent, waxy nature of the surface cells, desquamation (separation of the superficial cells), and the acid pH (4.5 to 6.5) of the secretion on the surface; this secretion has a bactericidal effect on many organisms.

The abundance of sensory receptors and nerves in the skin function in the sensation of touch, pressure, pain and temperature. These sensations serve as an important protective mechanism for the body and also convey impulses that contribute information about the external environment. For example, through touch we can appreciate shape, composition and texture.

The skin plays an important role in regulating body temperature by varying the caliber of its blood vessels and the activity of the sweat glands. These controlled mechanisms may promote the dissipation of the body heat or conserve it according to the need indicated by the heat-regulating center in the hypothalamus. For further details of temperature regulation, see Chapter 6.

The absorptive function of the skin is mainly limited to the absorption of ultraviolet rays from the sun or special lamps; it then converts sterol substances in the skin to vitamin D. A few drugs which may be included in ointments or lotions may be absorbed in small amounts.

The dermis and subcutaneous tissue may act as a storage place for water and fat. For instance, when an excess of water is retained in the body, the accumulation in these tissues becomes evident as edema. The subcutaneous tissue serves as one of the main fat depots.

With advancing years, the sebaceous and sweat glands become less active as a result of the decreased production of hormones, and the skin becomes dry. Degenerative changes occur in the elastic tissue and collagenous component of fibrous tissue, and the skin becomes wrinkled. Frequently, areas of melanocytes produce more pigment, and "brown spots" characteristic of aging skin appear.

DISORDERS OF THE SKIN

Skin disorders may be primary or may be secondary to a systemic disease or reaction. It is not the author's intention to present a discussion of many specific skin disorders but, rather, to offer a brief description of common manifestations, general principles of nursing care of patients with skin disorders, and a discussion of a few conditions that are more frequently encountered.

Manifestations

Lesions. Various changes in areas of the skin may occur, and the exact nature of these is important in diagnosis and treatment. Characteristic primary lesions in which the skin is usually intact include the following:

Erythema—an area in which the blood vessels become dilated, causing redness, warmth and increased firmness of the skin.

Macule—a circumscribed, smooth, flat, discolored area.

Papule—a small circumscribed elevated area that may or may not be discolored and is not more than 0.5 cm. in diameter.

Vesicle—an elevated area that contains clear fluid.

Pustule—a small elevation of the skin that contains pus.

Nodule—an elevation larger than a papule, usually involving both the skin and subcutaneous layers.

Wheal—a localized, elevated, edematous area which is red at the margins with a blanched center.

Bulla—a large elevation of superficial skin layers containing serous or purulent fluid.

Secondary lesions are those that develop as a result of a break in the skin and destruction of cells. These include:

Crust—a rough, dry area formed by the coagulation and drying of plasma and exudate over a primary lesion.

Scales—thin, flat, minute plates of dried epidermal cells which have not completely undergone the normal keratinization process before being separated. Desquamation is the term which refers to the separation of scales or patches of cells.

Fissure—a split or crack in the surface, extending through the epidermal layers and possibly into the dermis. If it extends into the dermis, bleeding occurs. This type of lesion is most likely to occur in a natural skin or surface crease such as those located over knuckles, at the angles of the mouth, in the groins, between the buttocks and behind the ears.

Excoriation—an abrasion in which the epidermis is removed.

Ulcer—a denuded area due to necrosis of superficial tissue extending into the dermis.

Lichenification—the thickening and hardening of skin as a result of continued irritation.

Leukoplakia—a white plaque which is seen most commonly in the mucous membrane of the oral cavity or tongue but may occur on the lips and, rarely, on other atrophied skin areas.

Pruritus. Generalized or localized itching is a common complaint in skin disorders. The sensory nerve endings or end-organs are irritated, giving rise to the desire to scratch. The patient is hard-pressed to refrain from scratching, which further irritates the area and is frequently responsible for fissures and abrasions and subsequent secondary infection.

Pain. The pain associated with skin lesions may be described as prickly or burning. It may be caused by chemical or pressure irritation of the cutaneous sensory nerves, actual cellular damage or exposure of the nerve endings due to tissue destruction and erosion.

Redness. Erythema or redness of the skin indicates vasodilation and hyperemia in the area. Erythematous lesions are initially macular but frequently become papular because of the edema or developing exudate in the affected tissues.

Swelling. A puffy swollen area of the skin is usually due to localized edema, resulting from increased permeability of the capillaries, or to localized inflammatory reaction.

Fever. An elevated temperature is likely to be present if the skin disorder is associated with either a localized or systemic infection.

General Principles in Nursing Patients with Skin Disorders

The nursing care varies greatly with these patients. The extent of the skin involvement as well as the nature of the condition determines whether or not the patient continues activities, is ambulatory and is treated at home. The following are general considerations which will require adaptation and modification according to the individual;

this, of course, is true of all nursing.

Psychological Support. The patient with skin lesions is likely to be quite sensitive and become emotionally disturbed over his condition. Many are self-conscious about their appearance, worry constantly and tend to withdraw. The disease may be such that it persists over a long period, interfering with the patient's ability to work or go out socially. The understanding nurse guards against any reluctance on her part to care for the patient and any expression of displeasure or revulsion because of his appearance. An effort is made to convey to the patient an appreciation of his feelings, to have him aware that he is accepted and to provide the necessary support and care which will help to reduce the patient's anxiety.

Cleansing. A specific directive is received from the physician regarding the cleansing of the skin or affected area(s). In some instances the application of soap and water may be contraindicated, and an alternative method of cleansing is necessary. For example, it may be necessary to cleanse the skin with a vegetable oil. If soap is permitted, it should be mildly alkaline and used very sparingly. A soft washcloth is preferable, and the surface is washed lightly and gently to discourage an increased blood supply. If there are open, discharging lesions, sterile absorbent may be used in place of a washcloth, and the nurse may be instructed to wear rubber or polyethylene gloves. Special local or general therapeutic baths may be prescribed. These may be used to relieve itching, remove scales or crusts, or apply medications as well as for cleansing purposes. Caution is used against having the water or solution hot; a temperature higher than 35° to 38° C. (95° to 100° F.) is likely to be too hot for the sensitive areas. Also, the heat is likely to promote hyperemia and itching. Various preparations may be added to the bath according to its purpose. The patient is usually encouraged to remain in the prescribed bath for 10 to 20 minutes, and an attendant remains with the patient or close by, depending on his condition and age. Assistance is provided while he gets into and out of the tub. Measures are taken to prevent the patient from slipping, since many of the preparations used (e.g., oatmeal, bran, emollients) make the surface of the tub especially slippery.

Moist Compresses. Wet dressings may be applied over lesions, especially if they are open and discharging. The compresses are generally left uncovered and dry out very quickly, necessitating frequent changing. The prescribed solution is usually used at room temperature.

Drug Therapy. Many different drug preparations are used in the treatment of skin disease. Topical applications may be in powder, paste, lotion or ointment form. They may be applied to relieve itching or pain (antipruritic or anesthetic), to produce an antimicrobial effect (antiseptic), to soften crusts or thick scaly skin (emollient or keratolytic), or to protect the areas (protective).

Systemic drugs which may be ordered for certain skin conditions include: antihistamine preparations, such as chlorpheniramine (Chlor-Tripolon) and diphenhydramine (Benadryl), for the relief of pruritus; antimicrobial drugs, such as the antibiotic penicillin, if infection is involved; and adrenal corticosteroid preparations, such as prednisone. Prednisone is used for only a brief period, but the anti-inflammatory effect and the reduction of tissue sensitivity produce a rapid, favorable response in the patient. Rarely, a sedative or tranquilizer is ordered to reduce the patient's emotional responses and provide much-needed sleep and rest. Examples of drugs used for this purpose are chlordiazepoxide hydrochloride (Librium), meprobamate (Equanil), amobarbital (Amytal) and phenobarbital.

Observation. Following each cleansing and before each local therapeutic application, the lesions are examined carefully. Any change in size, color or appearance is noted and reported. The nurse is constantly alert for factors in the patient's environment (e.g., contacts, diet, drugs) with which exacerbations of his condition may be associated.

Nutrition. Attention is paid to the patient's nutritional status and to whether he is taking sufficient food. Frequently severe anorexia is a problem with the dermatological patient because of the skin irritation he experiences as well as the emotional disturbance. Dressings, ointments, lotions or similar applications on their hands may preclude his feeding himself.

Instruction. In the clinic or during preparation for discharge from the hospital, the patient and a family member are advised of the day-to-day care required and precautionary measures applicable to the prevention of an exacerbation. Verbal and written directions are given about the application or taking of medicinal preparations. For example, adrenal corticosteroid preparations in the form of an ointment or cream are used topically to suppress inflammation and reduce sensitivity of the tissues. The patient must be cautioned to apply the corticoid preparation sparingly. If compresses or therapeutic baths are to be continued, specific details of the preparation, temperature and application are outlined and demonstrated if necessary. In the case of contact dermatitis, the patient may not be able to return to his former occupation. A referral to the social service may be helpful in finding a suitable job.

URTICARIA

Urticaria is a skin disorder which is characterized by itching wheals of varying size which may develop very rapidly and become widespread. The lesions are a reaction to an external agent or to an irritating substance reaching the skin via the blood stream. The reaction consists of dilatation and increased permeability of the capillaries and arteriolar dilatation. The combination of these is referred to as the triple response. The lesions usually disappear in a few hours when the blood vessels return to normal. The condition is commonly referred to as hives. Urticaria may be a manifestation of an allergic reaction to a food, drug, vaccine or serum, or it may be caused by insect bites, contact with certain plants or chemicals or prolonged exposure to heat, cold, pressure or sunlight.

Urticaria is treated by the administration of an antihistamine preparation, or if it is widespread and is causing considerable irritation, epinephrine (Adrenalin) 1:1000 may be ordered subcutaneously and usually provides immediate relief. The application of calamine lotion or a cream of calamine, diphenhydramine and camphor (Caladryl) may be useful in reducing the itching and local response. Unless the cause is definitely known, an investigation is made to identify the offending substance. Intracutaneous or scratch sensitivity tests may be done (see p. 37).

DERMATITIS

The term dermatitis obviously implies some type of inflammation of the skin, but its use is generally reserved for the inflammatory reaction of hypersensitive skin to an internal or external substance. The causative agent would not excite the skin of a "normal" person. The lesions usually progress through various forms, beginning with an erythematous area on which small papules develop and rapidly progress to vesicles. The vesicles may rupture and discharge their contents. Those vesicles which do not rupture dry and form crusts or scales. The affected areas may become denuded, leaving a red glazed surface which probably oozes a serous discharge, giving rise to what is referred to as "weeping eczema." As the denuded areas are recovered by regenerated epidermis, more lesions may develop so that various stages (papular, vesicular, scaly, weeping, healing) exist at one time unless the reaction is corrected in the early stages. The patient experiences itching and burning, and scratching may result in infected lesions. The affected areas may remain localized to certain parts of the body or become disseminated.

Local applications such as wet compresses, creams and ointments are used to reduce the itching and tissue response and provide protection. If lesions are extensive, involving large areas of the body, therapeutic baths are used. An antibiotic ointment may be prescribed if there is infection.

A systemic drug may also be ordered for the relief of itching (e.g., diphenhydramine), and adrenal corticosteroid (e.g., prednisone) may be administered to reduce the tissue response and inflammation. The patient is advised of the importance of avoiding scratching. The application of arm splints or mittens may be necessary to control scratching in children.

The patient undergoes an investigation to determine the precipitating factor or allergen (see p. 37). It should be remembered that dermatitis may be aggravated by emotional disturbances. Kind, sincere attention by the nurse may reduce the patient's tension or lead to discussions that reveal his concerns and disturbances.

Dermatitis is sometimes classified as: contact dermatitis, which implies the cause is external contact with a substance to which the patient is sensitive; drug dermatitis, because of the obvious cause; exfoliative dermatitis, which is characterized by extensive scaling and thickening of the skin; infantile dermatitis, or eczema; or infective dermatitis, because infection has been superimposed.

PSORIASIS

Psoriasis is a relatively common, chronic skin disorder characterized by remissions and exacerbations and dry, scaly lesions. These lesions develop initially as dull, red papules on which silvery white, waxy scales accumulate in layers. The lesion gradually increases in size, and several may coalesce, forming large, prominent, scaly plaques. Removal of the scale produces small, pinpoint bleeding areas. The patient may or may not experience itching. Any skin area, including the nails, may be involved, but common sites are the extensor surfaces of the arms and legs (especially pressure areas such as the knees and elbows), the scalp, and the lumbar and sacral regions. The amount of involvement varies from one attack to another, and chronic patch areas vary in individuals; that is, it may always appear first on the fronts of the knees, the backs of the elbows or the back. If the nails become affected, they usually manifest pitting, discoloration and separation from the underlying tissue, which tends to become thick, dry and hard (keratosis).

The onset may be gradual or sudden. The lesions may persist for weeks or months and then may disappear spontaneously.

The cause of psoriasis is not known, but "there is general agreement, however, that it is an autosomal, inheritable disorder which frequently flares or appears following pathophysiological, mechanical, or psychic stress."[1] Males and females are equally affected, and the incidence is much higher in temperate climates. The onset of the disease may be at any age but most commonly occurs in adolescence. Psoriasis is occasionally seen in persons with rheumatoid arthritis. Exacerbations are more prevalent in winter months. Patients who move from a cold, wintery

climate to a warm, sunny climate have found that their psoriasis usually clears spontaneously and quickly.

The treatment consists principally of local applications. One preparation may prove effective for one patient and not for another. The treatment is individualized—this must be impressed on the patient. Various preparations in the form of ointments or creams are used and include derivatives of coal tar and adrenal corticosteroid. The patient has a daily therapeutic bath, remaining in it 20 to 30 minutes to soften and promote separation of the scales. The lesions may be gently scrubbed, using a soft brush or rough terry cloth. When there are only one or two lesions, an intralesional injection of triamcinolone may be made by the physician.

Vitamin A to be taken orally may be prescribed and may help some persons. Methotrexate (Aminopterin) given orally may be used rarely. It is an antimetabolite (a folic acid antagonist) and has proved effective with some patients. Exposure to sunlight or ultraviolet light rays may prove beneficial, but the daily exposure time must be gradually increased to avoid burning.

CANCER OF THE SKIN

Carcinoma of the skin has a high incidence and occurs more often in males. The prognosis in skin cancer is usually more favorable than when the disease is located in other tissues and organs. Malignant skin lesions are readily discovered, resulting in early treatment, and generally progress quite slowly.

The symptom that most frequently prompts the patient to seek medical advice is a discolored lesion which persists and progressively increases in size or an open sore (ulcer) which does not heal and progressively becomes deeper. The nurse should be alert for lesions that frequently precede malignant changes. Most significant are soft black moles that tend to increase in size, leukoplakia (white patches) and a sore which does not heal.

Epithelioma is the type of skin cancer most commonly seen. The primary nodular lesion most often develops on the face, slowly enlarges and ulcerates, and is referred to as a rodent ulcer. The lesion may be treated by excision or radiation. The

---

[1] H. L. Wechsler: "Psoriasis." Amer. J. Nurs., Vol. 65, No. 4 (Apr. 1965), p. 85.

neoplastic cells rarely metastasize, and the disease remains controlled.

Squamous cell carcinoma develops in the skin occasionally and is more serious than the epithelioma type because it tends to invade surrounding tissues and metastasize more readily. The primary lesion ulcerates and enlarges. The common sites are similar to those of epitheliomas—namely, the face, lips, nose, forehead and arms. The treatment is also similar, and the patient is followed closely for possible metastases.

Malignant melanoma usually arises from a pre-existing mole and is a rapidly spreading cancer that readily metastasizes and presents a grave prognosis. Wide excision of the primary lesion is done, and the regional lymph nodes may also be removed. The surgery is followed by radiation therapy.

NURSING THE BURNED PATIENT

Burns continue to be a major cause of suffering, disfigurement, disability and death, and a large proportion of those that occur are due to carelessness and could be prevented. More emphasis on safety measures, especially in the home, seems necessary. Through increased public education by the use of such aids as mass media and printed pamphlets, we have been able to alert the public to the danger signals of cancer and the importance of early treatment. A comparable program relating to burn statistics, causes of fires and safety measures might produce greater caution in homes and elsewhere.

Causes of Burns

A burn may be inflicted by dry or moist heat, irradiation, electrical current or chemicals. The burn that is caused by dry or moist heat may be referred to as a thermal burn and is the type of greatest incidence. The discussion that follows pertains to the burn incurred by heat.

Classification and Assessment of Burns

Burns may be classified according to cause (thermal, electrical, chemical or irradiation), the extent of the body surface burned, and the depth of tissue damaged or destroyed. The assessment of the severity of a burn is made principally on the last two factors. The seriousness is also influenced by the patient's age, health at the time of the accident and whether or not any other injury was incurred at the same time.

The most accurate estimation of the percentage of body surface burned may be based on the Lund and Browder chart (see Fig. 25–2). The chart assigns a certain percentage to various parts of the body and includes a table indicating the adjustments necessary for different ages, since the head and trunk represent relatively larger proportions of body surface at different stages of development. Copies of these charts may be kept available in the emergency department or intensive care unit so that the burned areas can be mapped out when the patient is examined and the percentage is estimated.

If the Lund and Browder chart is not available, a quick approximate estimate of the percentage of body surface burned may be made on the Rule of Nines (see Fig. 25–3). The body is divided into areas, each of which represents 9 per cent. The apportionment is as follows: an arm is 9 per cent, a thigh 9 per cent, a leg (below the knee) 9 per cent, the anterior chest 9 per cent, the posterior chest 9 per cent, the abdomen 9 per cent, the lower half of the back (lumbar and sacral regions) 9 per cent, the head and neck 9 per cent, and the perineum 1 per cent. It should be remembered that in infants and children the head represents a relatively large percentage, but the extremities comprise a smaller portion of the body surface.

If approximately 10 per cent or more of the body surface of a child or 15 per cent or more of that of an adult is burned, the injury is considered to be a major burn. The patient requires hospitalization and fluid replacement.

The depth of tissue damage and destruction in a burn is indicated by the classification as first, second, or third degree. A first-degree burn is characterized by erythema with destruction of only superficial layers of the epidermis. It may be quite painful for a short time but heals quickly without residual evidence of tissue injury. Systemic effects may accompany a first-degree burn if a large percentage of the body surface is involved.

Second-degree burns involve the destruction of several layers of the skin, but suffi-

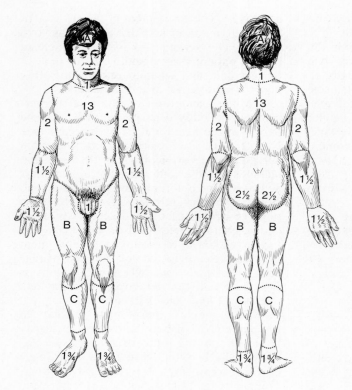

For body areas marked A, B and C in the figure, use the table of percentages below. The percentages reflect different rates of growth of different body parts.

AGE IN YEARS

	0	1	5	10	15	*Adult*
A — ½ of head	9½	8½	6½	5½	4½	3½
B — ½ of one thigh	2¾	3¼	4	4¼	4½	4¾
C — ½ of one leg	2½	2½	2¾	3	3¼	3½

Figure 25–2 The Lund and Browder burn chart.

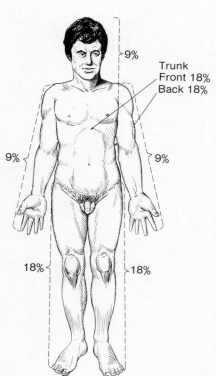

Figure 25–3 Rule of Nines; used for estimating the percentage of body surface burned.

cient viable dermal tissue remains to promote regeneration of the cells to replace those burned. Separation of epidermal layers occurs by the collection of fluid in the tissues, forming blisters which are characteristic of second-degree burns. This type of burn may also be described as being one of partial thickness.

A third-degree burn is characterized by the destruction of the full-thickness of the skin and its appendages. Underlying tissues such as the subcutaneous fat, muscles, tendons and bone may also be burned. The sensitivity of the area is reduced because of the destruction of sensory nerve endings. The injured area may be charred or have an opaque white appearance. Because the burn is of full-thickness depth, spontaneous regeneration and replacement of the skin is not possible. The area may be slowly filled in with granulation tissue, then fibrous scar tissue, proliferated from marginal or underlying connective tissue, or it is recovered by skin grafting.

The age of the patient is an important factor in the seriousness of a burn. The

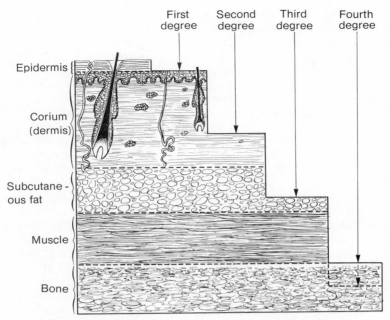

Figure 25—4 Classification of burns according to depth.

severity of the burn increases with age when the patient is over 55 to 60 years old. The person of 40 withstands a burn much better than the patient of 60, even though the percentage of body surface burned and the degree are the same in both. Infants and young children also tolerate burns less well than those who are more mature.

Effects of Burns

The patient who suffers a major burn manifests shock which, in some cases, may be irreversible. Immediately following the injury, the intense pain and fear which may be experienced by the injured person are considered to be responsible for widespread vasodilation and subsequent hypotension and impaired circulation. This phase may be referred to as primary or neurogenic shock. The duration varies; it may be brief or may persist to become a part of the hypovolemic (oligemic) shock that develops rapidly as a result of the loss of fluid from the circulating blood volume. Increased permeability and dilation of the capillaries in the burn area result in a shift of protein-rich fluid out of the vascular compartment into the interstitial spaces, causing the formation of blisters and edema. Large volumes of fluid

which is similar in composition to plasma may seep into the tissues. Some is carried away via the lymphatics, but an amount in excess of what can be drained into the lymphatic system accumulates. The edema is also promoted by the loss of blood proteins with the fluid and the ensuing reduction of the intravascular colloidal osmotic pressure. In a third-degree burn, the fluid loss is extensive, and in areas of greater vascularization, such as the face, the edema and swelling may be very severe.

The blood volume diminishes, the blood pressure eventually falls, the cardiac output is reduced, and the blood flow through the tissues is reduced. Hypovolemic shock develops unless there is adequate fluid replacement. The reduction in the intravascular volume produces a corresponding hemoconcentration, evidenced by an increase in the hematocrit and hemoglobin levels (Normal hematocrit: 40 to 50 per cent; normal hemoglobin: 12 to 16 Gm. per cent). The greater concentration of cellular elements in the blood increases the demand on the heart and predisposes to thrombosis and circulatory insufficiency.

A decrease in the number of red blood cells occurs especially in deep burns, due to trapping and heat injury of those in the skin capillaries at the time of the injury. If a large erythrocyte mass is destroyed, hemoglobinuria may be manifested as the cells hemolyze. Normal production may also be reduced because of toxic depression of the bone marrow.

The urinary output is decreased as a result of the decreased intravascular volume and subsequent hypotension. Diuresis and increased sodium excretion occur in 3 to 5 days and are favorable signs. If the blood supply is markedly reduced in the shock phase, renal tubular damage may result. In severe burns gastrointestinal peristalsis is depressed; nausea, vomiting and abdominal distention may occur.

Toxemia may develop in 3 to 5 days, especially with a large surface area burn. This is attributed to absorption of decomposition products of dead tissue.

Electrolyte imbalances develop because of the burn edema, loss of fluid through the open wound, impaired renal function in the associated shock, and excessive release of potassium by the damaged tissue cells and erythrocytes. The disturbances are also influenced by the adrenocortical response (increased secretions) to the stress which produces sodium retention and increased potassium excretion by the kidneys if they are functioning satisfactorily. The adrenocortical hyperactivity also accelerates protein catabolism, resulting in a negative nitrogen balance.

The effects of the heat at the site of the burn depend on the intensity of the heat. The layer of burned tissues may present a dry, charred, coagulated surface, called an eschar, or a soft, moist noncoagulated area. Inflammation and edema develop at the wound margins and below the layers of dead tissue. Many small blood vessels below the devitalized tissue may be thrombosed, promoting further cellular destruction. The decomposition of dead tissue and sloughing produce a favorable culture medium for organisms. Most major burns are mixed in depth; some areas will have partial-thickness skin loss while other areas suffer full-thickness destruction.

Treatment and Nursing Care

Treatment and care are directed toward the following: the prevention of shock, or its reversal should it occur; the prevention of wound contamination and the treatment of infection; the prevention of contractures and deformities; and maximum rehabilitation of the patient.

First Aid. The initial move in the case of burning due to flames is to smother the fire if possible or remove the victim from exposure to it. If his clothes are on fire, he should remain stationary, for movement fans the flames, and lie down on the floor or ground. This position may prevent the igniting of his hair and the inhalation of flames with subsequent respiratory damage. He is quickly rolled in a rug, blanket or something comparable to smother the flames or is doused freely with water. If nothing is quickly available, the flames may be extinguished if he rolls on the ground.

The immediate application of cold either by holding the part under cold running water, immersion, or the application of cold, moist towels or compresses is recommended as a valuable first-aid measure by Artz and Moncrief. The cold reduces pain and "may have some value in arresting the effect of heat on the tissues."[2]

Oils, ointments, lotions and other preparations should not be applied, and no attempt is made to remove clothing that is adherent. The burn area is covered with the cleanest material available to exclude air, which stimulates pain, and to reduce contamination. While awaiting transportation, the patient is kept at rest. A minimal amount of movement and handling is important, but any constricting shoes, clothing and jewelry are loosened or removed.

In the case of chemical burns, the area is washed with generous amounts of water. The patient's clothing is removed, since it is most likely holding some of the offending substances.

Most first- and second-degree burns involving approximately less than 10 per cent of body surface are treated at home or in the clinic. Systemic effects in such cases are minimal and are not considered sufficiently significant to require hospitalization. However, it should be remembered there are variables; concomitant disease or injuries,

---

[2]C. P. Artz, and J. A. Moncrief: The Treatment of Burns, 2nd ed. Philadelphia, W. B. Saunders Co., 1969, p. 89.

the patient's reactions and availability of home care are a few examples of factors which may influence the decision as to whether he requires hospitalization.

Preparation to Receive the Burned Patient. If notified of the imminent admission of a burned patient, preparations include the assembling of the following equipment for prompt use:

Tray and tubes for a tracheostomy

Oxygen and mechanical respirator

Intravenous infusion and blood transfusion sets, including equipment for venous cutdown

Colloidal and electrolyte intravenous solutions

Equipment for taking blood specimens for typing and cross matching, hematocrit, hemoglobin and electrolyte determinations

Sphygmomanometer, stethoscope and a central venous pressure set

Catheterization tray with indwelling catheter (Foley catheter), tubing and drainage bag

Sterile gowns, masks and gloves for physicians and nurses

Appropriate instruments, sterile towels, dressings and bandages

Solutions for cleansing the area (e.g., sterile water, normal saline, hexachlorophene [pHisoHex], mild liquid soap)

Burn applications (antimicrobial topical preparations such as Sulfamylon and silver nitrate 0.5 per cent)

Tetanus toxoid, tetanus antitoxin and analgesics such as morphine and meperidine hydrochloride (Demerol) and injection equipment

Bed made with sterile sheets and cradle. If the victim is known to have received major trunk or circumferential burns, a Stryker frame or CircOlectric bed is prepared to receive the patient following the initial assessment and treatments.

On Admission. An immediate assessment of the patient's general condition is made by the physician before attention is directed to the burn wound. Damage to the respiratory tract and respiratory insufficiency demand prompt attention. Respiratory impairment is frequently associated with burns of the face or neck and may be the result of the inhalation of smoke, a gaseous chemical or flames. A tracheostomy may be considered necessary if edema of the respiratory mucosa is likely to develop. If there is marked insufficiency, a mechanical ventilator may be used in conjunction with the tracheostomy tube. Frequent estimations of the blood gases and expiratory or tidal volume may be done. See Chapter 14 for the care required in respiratory insufficiency and tracheostomy.

Respiratory insufficiency may develop later in circumferential or severe chest burns due to restricted respiratory excursion as a result of the firm unyielding coagulum or eschar. The physician may make several incisions in the eschar to relieve the thoracic restriction.

Relief of Pain and Anxiety. Unless contraindicated by respiratory impairment or depression, the patient is usually given an analgesic on admission to relieve pain and reduce his anxiety, since both contribute to shock. A small dose of morphine, codeine or meperidine hydrochloride (Demerol) is generally given intravenously by the physician. This route is used because the circulatory disturbance, shock and edema reduce absorption of subcutaneous injections.

An analgesic may be necessary 3 or 4 times in 24 hours for 2 or 3 days to keep the patient reasonably comfortable. Some patients require the administration of the prescribed narcotic only before the daily dressing of the burn areas. The nurse must be alert for signs of addiction; generally, the drug order is changed to a tranquilizer or milder sedative after 3 or 4 days.

Fluid Therapy. The control of shock resulting from the loss of intravascular volume in a severe burn is dependent upon prompt, adequate fluid replacement. A venous cutdown and the insertion of a polyethylene cannula or catheter is usually done immediately on admission to establish a reliable intravenous route. The solutions administered may include colloidal solutions,* such as plasma, whole blood and plasma expander (e.g., dextran), or a solution of electrolytes (e.g., lactated Ringer's solution) and glucose 5 per cent in distilled water. The volume, composition and rate of flow of the intravenous fluids are based principally on the hourly urinary output, arterial blood pressure, central venous

---

*A colloidal solution contains large nondiffusible particles of solutes which will not leak out of the capillaries.

pressure, hematocrit, hemoglobin and serum electrolyte concentrations, especially potassium and sodium.

Fluid is given orally when tolerated and may be restricted to the following formula: sodium chloride 4 Gm. (level tablespoonful) and sodium bicarbonate 1.5 Gm. (level teaspoonful) dissolved in a liter of water. The solution is chilled and may be flavored with fruit juice. Generally, after the first 24 to 36 hours, fluid extravasation into the tissues ceases and the intravascular volume tends to be stabilized. The intravenous fluid therapy is gradually reduced and may be discontinued when laboratory studies indicate satisfactory concentrations and the patient is able to take adequate amounts orally. He is observed closely for signs of circulatory overload, since much of the fluid in the interstitial spaces is reabsorbed into the intravascular compartment. Overloading of the circulatory system may be manifested by pulmonary edema, a central venous pressure in excess of 13 cm. of water and a weak pulse. If renal function is normal, the excessive amount is taken care of by diuresis. A blood transfusion may be necessary later if the hematocrit or red blood cell count point to anemia.

Indwelling Urinary Catheter. An indwelling (Foley) catheter is passed as soon as the patient is admitted so that the hourly urinary output may be noted. This serves as a guide in determining intravenous fluid requirement. It also provides information about the patient's general circulatory status and renal function. The urinary output should be at least 25 to 30 ml. per hour for an adult, 20 to 25 ml. per hour for a child and 10 to 20 ml. per hour for an infant. A volume below the minimal normal is reported promptly.

Observations. The patient is observed closely during the early postburn period for shock. His blood pressure, pulse and level of consciousness are noted every 15 to 30 minutes, and the urinary output per hour is recorded. A diminishing intravascular volume and subsequent circulatory failure may be reflected by a fall in blood pressure, weak pulse, abnormal drowsiness, disorientation and a urinary output of less than 30 ml. per hour. A long venous catheter may be passed via the cephalic vein into the vena cava so that the central venous pressure may be monitored hourly. It is a guide to the volume and rate of intravenous fluid administered. If it is significantly elevated, intravenous infusion is reduced (normal central venous pressure: 10 to 15 cm. of water).

Frequent hemoglobin and hematocrit determinations are made; abnormal elevations point to hemoconcentration due to loss of intravascular fluid into the tissues. Serum protein and electrolyte concentrations are also obtained frequently and serve as a guide for the type of intravenous solutions required. An accurate record of the fluid intake (oral and intravenous) and the output is necessary. The patient is weighed daily as soon as his condition permits. At first, a gain is manifested because of the increased extracellular fluid and the intravascular infusion. Then a marked weight loss accompanies the diuresis that corresponds with his recovery from shock. During this period he is observed closely for any sign of overhydration. Much of the fluid which escaped into the interstitial spaces is reabsorbed into the vascular compartment. If the intravenous infusion is continued at the previous rate of administration at this time, the vascular system may become overloaded, placing an excessive demand on the heart and causing pulmonary edema. The reabsorption of the tissue fluid can usually be recognized by a marked increase in the urinary output. Pulmonary edema is manifested by dyspnea, râles, cough and the expectoration of frothy mucus.

After the initial period, the nurse is alert for an elevation of temperature, rapid pulse, leukocytosis, odor and discharge from the burned area which may indicate infection.

The patient's position, especially that of the burned parts of the body, is checked frequently during the day and night for optimum alignment. Flexion contracture may develop very quickly and preclude restoration of function.

Psychological Support. Following a severe burn, the patient and his family experience considerable emotional disturbance. As with any psychological concern, the reactions and adaptive mechanisms may vary markedly from one person to another, depending mainly on the particular situation and past experiences of each person. Factors which generate fear and anxiety in both the patient and his family include the actual threat to life, permanent incapacity and disfigurement, the prolonged period of treatment necessitating dependence as well as separation, and the uncertain future. An understanding of the problems of the patient and his family should be appreciated by the nurse in order to convey understanding support and to help the patient to work through to acceptance and a more positive outlook. He may have guilt feelings about the accident, especially at first. Withdrawal, depression and resentment are commonly manifested. Long periods of the patient being alone are avoided; the visitors he is permitted to have are encouraged to visit regularly. Reading material and a radio or television usually help, and as he improves, constructive activities in which he may be interested are gradually introduced by the occupational therapist.

It is important that the patient be given honest, realistic explanations of his progress and of the plans for treatment (e.g., skin grafting) and his rehabilitation. It is more supportive when the patient and his family can relate to one or two key persons in his therapeutic team throughout the entire course of his illness. Constant change of personnel can be very disconcerting and may undermine the patient's confidence.

Wound Care. Infection is a serious hazard in severe burns and is a major cause of death of burned patients. The skin, which is damaged or destroyed, is the normal protective barrier against environmental organisms as well as those commonly found on the skin, in hair follicles and in sweat and sebaceous ducts. Thrombosis and damage of local vessels and stasis of circulation in the burn area frequently prevent antibodies and systemic antimicrobial medications from reaching the wound to destroy organisms. At the same time the patient's ability to produce antibodies may be reduced.

Various forms of local treatment are used to prevent further wound contamination and tissue destruction, suppress the growth of bacteria in the area, and promote separation of the devitalized tissue and its replacement with skin.

Initially, the burn is cleansed of dirt, foreign substance and detached epithelium, using a mild soapy solution, water or normal saline. The cleansing must be very gentle to avoid damage of exposed viable tissue, and the area is rinsed with generous amounts of water or saline.

First-degree burns may be left exposed or may receive an application of an ointment. The ointment frequently contains a local anesthetic for the relief of pain; an example is dibucaine hydrochloride ointment (Nupercaine). Cold, moist applications for the first few hours will also provide relief of pain.

In second-degree burns, opinion differs as to whether blisters are better left intact or should be opened and the overlying devitalized tissue removed.[3, 4, 5] Furnas states that healing occurs more quickly under intact blisters. However, Artz and Moncrief suggest that the dead tissue and the fluid encourage infection. There is a consensus, however, that blisters on the palms of the hands, where the skin is thick and not easily ruptured, should be left intact.

The more common, current methods of local treatment of major burns include silver nitrate dressings, mafenide (Sulfamylon) applications, exposure and occlusive dressings. In third-degree burns, treatment following the separation of the dead tissue (eschar) usually involves skin grafting.

SILVER NITRATE DRESSINGS. After the wound has been cleansed and a débridement done, thick gauze dressings (free of absorbent) saturated with silver nitrate 0.5 per cent are applied. The patient is covered with a cotton sheet and light blanket to reduce evaporation and loss of body heat. The dressings are kept wet by the frequent addition of solution with a bulb syringe. The dressings are changed daily, and the patient is usually placed in a sterile bath, 35.5° to 37.5° C. (96° to 99.5° F.) for 1 to 3 hours to facilitate the separation of inner dressings and slough and to cleanse the area. While in the bath, the patient is encouraged to exercise his limbs to maintain joint mobility and prevent contractures. The use of silver nitrate dressings is considered one of the most effective methods in control of infection. It has, however, some disadvantages,

---

[3]Artz and Moncrief, op. cit., p. 112.

[4]D. W. Furnas: A Bedside Outline for the Treatment of Burns. Springfield, Charles C Thomas, Publishers, p. 27.

[5]L. Davis (Ed.): Christopher's Textbook of Surgery, 9th ed. Philadelphia, W. B. Saunders Co., 1968, p. 148.

the most significant one being the body losses of electrolytes into the silver nitrate dressings. Frequent checks (every 4 to 8 hours, depending on the size of the burn area) are made of the blood for sodium, potassium, calcium, bicarbonate and chloride concentrations. Deficits are made up by parenteral solutions or dietary supplements. A second problem with the use of silver nitrate is its dark staining of the skin (argyria) and of linen. Adequate protection of the bed must be ensured, and old linen should be used. The nurses and physicians giving wound care wear masks and sterile gloves and gown to protect the patient. The gowns also protect them from the staining. When the wound appears clean and free of dead tissue and shows the development of granulation tissue, skin grafting is generally undertaken.

MAFENIDE (SULFAMYLON) APPLICATIONS. Following the initial cleansing, mafenide hydrochloride (Sulfamylon Hydrochloride) or mafenide acetate (Sulfamylon Acetate) may be applied freely to the burn, which is then left exposed. The creamy preparation of sulfonamide is in a water-soluble base and diffuses readily through the sloughing tissue. It is considered quite effective in controlling the major skin pathogens. Since a large proportion of it is water, the amount of body fluid lost by evaporation is reduced.

A thick layer is usually applied twice daily; occasionally, more frequent application is necessary if some has been rubbed off on the bedding. It is applied with a sterile gloved hand. The wound is cleansed daily, generally by the patient being placed in a bath or whirlpool bath. The agitation of the water in the whirlpool bath provides more efficient cleansing and promotes the separation of devitalized tissue. The area is examined by the surgeon after the bath, and further débridement done before re-application of the Sulfamylon. Following the first few applications of the mafenide cream, the patient may complain of a burning sensation for 15 to 30 minutes which may necessitate the administration of an analgesic.

Absorption of Sulfamylon Hydrochloride may cause a reduction in blood pH (acidosis) through interference with the normal renal tubular buffering mechanism. As a result, Sulfamylon Acetate is more commonly used for prolonged treatment.

EXPOSURE. Following cleansing and gentle drying, the burn area is left exposed. In a second-degree burn, a coagulum of serum forms, providing a dry protective crust which serves as a protective covering. Healing (i.e., re-epithelialization) takes place under the crust, which gradually separates. When a third-degree (full-thickness) burn is sustained, the nonviable tissue changes in 3 to 5 days to a hard, tough black layer called the eschar, providing a protective surface which organisms cannot penetrate as long as it remains dry and intact. The underlying dead tissue eventually sloughs, liquefies and detaches the eschar from the viable tissue. There may be considerable drainage before there is complete separation, and dressings may then be ordered. Infection frequently develops under the eschar as a result of organisms that were deep in ducts or on adjacent areas and were not destroyed at the time of the burn.

As the eschar is removed by slough or débridement, granulation tissue which consists of fibroblasts and capillaries is gradually formed. If the granulation tissue is allowed to mature to fibrous scar tissue, the natural shortening of the collagenous fibers results in contracture of the area and possible deformity or loss of function, depending on the location. Some marginal growth of epithelium may take place, but unless the burn is very small, this is usually insignificant.

The usual procedure is to apply split-thickness skin grafts to the area as soon as it is reasonably clean and there is some granulation tissue. Frequent dressings may be ordered for a period following the removal of the eschar to promote drainage and bring the infection under control in preparation for grafting.

The patient's general condition and the size of the burn area determine whether the grafting will require several stages. Priority is given to areas where scarring and contraction produce loss of movement and marked deformity. The grafts are usually laid on (not sutured) and are covered with petrolatum-impregnated gauze, pads and an elastic or crepe bandage. If the grafts are around or over a joint surface, a splint or plaster cast may be applied to immobilize the part. Unless necrosis and infection are suspected from the patient's symptoms, the dressing usually is not changed for 5 to 6 days. Further information is offered about skin grafts at the end of this discussion on the care of the burned patient.

OCCLUSIVE DRESSINGS. A bulky, resilient dressing which applies slight pressure is used principally with burns of the distal portions of the extremities, especially with nonhospitalized patients. Its purposes are to protect the area from contamination, immobilize the area and provide slight compression to reduce vascular and lymphatic stasis. The dressing is applied firmly enough to eliminate dead space and prevent irritation of viable tissue by its movement, and yet it must "give" sufficiently to avoid any possible interference with the blood supply to the part.

Gauze which has been impregnated with petrolatum or water-soluble ointment is applied directly to the skin. Digits are separated and each is completely covered with gauze to prevent any direct surface contact between them. A thick layer of fluffed absorbent gauze and then dressing pads are placed over the gauze. The dressing is held in place by stockinette or an elastic or crepe bandage. Particular attention is paid to placing the hand or foot and the digits in optimum position so contractures and deformities are prevented, and normal function of the part may be readily resumed. Prolonged periods of the limb in the dependent position are avoided, since the formation of edema would be increased. In some instances the physician may order the limb to be elevated on pillows or suspended by slings or ties.

The dressings are changed every 2 to 5 days. They are examined frequently, and if moisture soaks through to the outer surface, or there is any odor or other sign of infection, the doctor is notified.

Precautions Against Infection. If the patient with a deep burn has been immunized within the preceding 5 years for tetanus, he receives a booster dose of toxoid. The patient with no tetanus immunization is given a prophylactic dose of tetanus antitoxin. This necessitates questioning the patient or the family as to whether he has ever had asthma, eczema or any known allergy. A small intracutaneous test dose of antitoxin is given to determine possible sensitivity.

Infection of the burn area may originate with bacteria that were present in the area before the burn and survived the heat. Special protective measures are used to minimize the possibility of contamination from outside sources. Reverse-isolation technique and sterile bed linen may be used when exposure methods of local treatment are employed. Strict aseptic technique is observed in providing wound care and changing dressings. Masks and sterile gowns and gloves are worn by those participating. The patient may be moved to a special burn-dressing room or to a small operating room. Obviously, personnel with infection (e.g., cold, sore throat, skin infection) are not allowed to care for the patient. Visitors are restricted in number and are given an explanation of their role in protecting the patient. They are required to wear gowns and masks while with him.

When changing the dressing, the inner layers of gauze are removed very gently to minimize tissue bleeding and damage. Moistening of the gauze with a sterile solution or in a bath may be necessary to prevent trauma. The dressing procedure is likely to be painful and anxiety-producing for the patient, especially in the early stages; an analgesic such as merperidine hydrochloride or codeine may be ordered to be administered 15 to 30 minutes before the dressing time.

One of the most serious complications in third-degree burns is septicemia, and it generally develops during the second or third week. It may have a sudden onset, ushered in by chills and a rapid elevation of temperature, or it may gradually develop over 2 to 3 days. It is characterized by high fever which may fluctuate, rapid pulse, drowsiness and disorientation. Paralytic ileus is a common concomitant, and petechiae ecchymoses and oozing from the burn areas frequently appear, since a bleeding tendency develops. Blood cultures are done to identify the organism(s) which have invaded the blood stream. Common offenders are *Staphylococcus aureus,* hemolytic streptococcus, and *Pseudomonas aeruginosa.*

Treatment includes massive doses of antibiotics intravenously, promotion of the separation of the eschar to permit drainage and the application of a topical antimicrobial preparation, and supportive therapy. Intravenous fluids are given to sustain the patient. Gastrointestinal decompression suction is established if there is vomiting and abdominal distention. Blood transfusions may be given; and if the patient's condition deteriorates, which may be manifested by a subnormal temperature and shock, a corticosteroid preparation such as Solu-Cortef may be given parenterally or intravenously.

Positioning and Exercises. The patient is turned every 2 to 3 hours to prevent respiratory congestion and circulatory stasis. If his back is burned or the involvement is circumferential, care is facilitated if the patient is nursed on a Stryker frame or CircOlectric bed. Because of the edema, burned extremities are elevated on pillows or another form of support during the initial phase. Frequent attention is paid to body alignment; as previously cited, flexion contractures, outward rotation of thighs and foot drop must be prevented. Burned parts which involve joints are moved through their range of motion as soon as possible and as indicated by the physician. If the patient is placed in a bath, he is encouraged to exercise while soaking. As healing occurs, the activity program is progressively increased to preserve normal range of motion and function.

Nutrition. Nutrition plays an important role in the recovery of the burned patient. In the initial shock period in severe burns the patient is sustained mainly by intravenous fluids. If oral fluids are tolerated, the solution of sodium chloride and bicarbonate previously cited may be given. Following recovery from shock, if there is no vomiting or abdominal distention, the intake is progressively increased from fluids, through soft foods, to a full normal diet.

The patient develops a negative nitrogen balance as a result of tissue catabolism and the reduced intake, which increases his susceptibility to infection and debilitation and delays healing. A high-calorie, high-protein (150 to 200 Gm. per day for an adult) and high-vitamin diet is recommended to provide the essentials for tissue repair and the production of antibodies and blood cells.

Of the vitamins, C is essential in the synthesis of corticosteroids and in tissue repair, and the B complex is needed in the many cellular enzyme systems essential to normal cellular responses.

Ingenuity and resourcefulness are necessary on the part of the nurse to have the patient take the essential food. He should be advised of the important role of nutrients in his diet, and small frequent feedings of high-calorie foods are offered. Supplements of protein concentrates (e.g., Sustagen) may be added to fluids. His likes and dislikes are determined and respected, and his family is encouraged to bring in occasional "treats" in the form of his favorite foods. Adequate assistance is provided so that taking his meals does not require too great an effort. A close check is made of the patient's daily intake, and his weight is also recorded daily.

Rehabilitation. Rehabilitation of the burned patient is fostered throughout the acute stages by conscientious attention to good body alignment, the prevention of infection, and the maintenance of joint and limb mobility. Following recovery from the burn, the patient may require considerable reconstructive surgery and retraining before he can resume independent and self-supportive functioning. Rehabilitation is a lengthy process for many, and they and their families may require social guidance and financial assistance as well as psychological support throughout. Retraining for a different occupation may be necessary. In some instances the patient finds it very difficult to resume social contacts and to take his place in society because of scarring and gross disfigurement.

GRAFTS

A graft implies the placement of body tissue or other material in an area of the body where it becomes a part of the local structure, substituting for absent or damaged tissue.

Types of Grafts

Various terms are used to describe grafts and are defined as follows:

Autograft of Autogenous Graft. The autograft is obtained from the recipient's own body and may be skin, vein, artery, fascia, tendon or bone, depending on the particular recipient site and correction to be made. No tissue rejection is involved.

Isograft or Isologous Graft. This is a graft between identical twins. Because of the same germ cell origin, the graft is biologically compatible with the recipient's tissue, and there is no tissue rejection.

Homograft (Homologous Graft or Allograft). The donor and the recipient of the graft are of the same species. It may be obtained from a living person or taken from a body shortly after death. Homografts consist mainly of skin, cornea, bone or blood vessel. Homografts do not survive indefinitely because the tissue is recognized as "unlike self" and rejected. The rejection phenomenon is an immunological reaction in which the graft is an antigen and antibodies are formed by the host in response to it. The tissue is attacked, and an inflammatory process ensues, ending in a breakdown of the graft. The graft must receive nutrients and oxygen from a blood supply; therefore, donor tissue which normally requires a lesser blood supply, such as the cornea, withstands rejection for a longer period. The transplanted cornea functions for a period during which it is rejected very slowly while at the same time repair slowly replaces it. Homografting of skin may be used in extensive third-degree burns as a temporary means of providing a covering to protect the patient against massive infection and excessive loss of fluid. In donor selection, the person of closest relationship to the patient is selected if possible. The survival period for the graft varies, but it is usually 1 to 3 weeks. By this time, the patient's condition may have improved sufficiently that a series of autogenous grafting may be done.

Arterial and venous homografts are rejected slowly, and during the process, new host tissue replaces the graft wall. These grafts are frequently complicated by thromboses and closure of the vessels.

Bone homografts seem to be one of the more successful of homologous tissue transplants.

Organ transplant from one person to another is currently receiving a great deal of attention. Renal homotransplants appear to have been the most gratifying; many persons with renal insufficiency that was incompatible with life have received a kidney transplant and, with the aid of immunosuppressive drugs, are living extended, useful lives.

Homostatic Graft. The tissue in the homograft may or may not be viable when placed in the recipient. It serves temporarily as a framework for new host tissue that forms or provides materials for new host tissue when it disintegrates. Bone tissue grafts are an example.

Substitute Graft. This graft is made of inert material to which there is a minimum of tissue reaction. It may serve as a replacement for weak or destroyed tissues or as a framework for the formation of host tissue. An example of the latter is a porous teflon tube which is placed in the aorta during the correction of a coarctation. The teflon is eventually incorporated into the host tissue as the tissue grows through the pores. Other examples of substitute grafts are patches of inert material used to strengthen or correct an area (e.g., defect in the cardiac wall).

Heterograft. This implies the transfer of tissue between species and results in rapid rejection.

Skin Grafting. A large proportion of reconstructive surgery and the correction of cutaneous defects involves skin autografts. As indicated in the preceding discussion on the care of the burned patient, skin grafting is necessary in many third-degree burns to prevent handicapping and disfiguring contractures.

A skin graft may be classified as a free graft when it is completely separated from the donor site and is transferred to another area of the body. If the graft remains attached at one end to the donor site in order to maintain a blood supply, it may be referred to as a pedicle graft or a flap. The detached end is moved to the recipient area, and when sufficient blood vessels form to establish an adequate circulation between the graft and the surrounding tissue, the pedicle or flap is then separated from the donor area. The thickness of skin grafts varies. The graft may be of split-thickness, which consists of the epidermis and a portion of the dermis. A full-thickness graft includes the epidermis and complete dermis.

Types of free grafts include: the Ollier-Thiersch grafts, which are thin strips or sheets of partial-thickness; pinch or Reverdin grafts, which are very small pieces (approximately 0.5 cm. in diameter) of full-thickness; and Wolf's grafts, which are full-thickness pieces of skin that are larger than pinch grafts. The donor sites most commonly used for free grafts are the thighs and trunk. The donor site for a flap or pedicle graft must be within reach of the recipient site, since one end is attached to each site. When grafts are placed in position, they may be held in position by dressings or may be sutured and left exposed.

Nursing Care

The donor area is shaved and cleansed as for any other surgery. The recipient site may receive frequent moist antiseptic dressings or the application of a topical antimicrobial preparation to render it as free of organisms as possible. If a thick layer of granulation tissue has developed, it may be pared down by the surgeon before the application of a graft.

The patient's blood is typed and cross matched, and blood is made available for transfusion. Débridement (the removal of granulation tissue and oozing from the donor area) may result in a considerable loss of blood, which could interfere with the growth of the graft.

Unless the graft is sutured, the area is covered with fine mesh, petrolatum gauze, dressing pads and elastic or crepe bandages. If the recipient site involves or is adjacent to a joint, a splint or plaster cast is applied to immobilize the part. The dressing remains undisturbed for 4 to 6 days unless infection is suspected because of fever, leukocytosis, or an offensive odor and discharge from the area.

The donor site may be covered with petrolatum gauze for 24 to 48 hours and then exposed. This area may be painful and a greater source of discomfort than the recipient area.

References

BOOKS

Artz, C. P., and Moncrief, J. A.: The Treatment of Burns, 2nd ed. Philadelphia, W. B. Saunders Co., 1969.
Furnas, D. W.: A Bedside Outline for the Treatment of Burns. Springfield, Charles C Thomas, Publishers, 1969.
Gius, J. A.: Fundamentals of General Surgery, 3rd ed. Chicago, Year Book Medical Publishers, Inc., Chapter 8.
Harrison, T. R., et al. (Eds.): Principles of Internal Medicine, 4th ed. New York, The Blakiston Division, McGraw-Hill Book Co. Inc., 1962, pp. 1925–1939.
Ingram, J. T.: Clinical Dermatology. London, J. & A. Churchill Ltd., 1969.
Percival, G. H.: An Introduction to Dermatology. 13th ed. Edinburgh, E. & S. Livingstone Ltd., 1967.

PERIODICALS

Brown, W. A.: "Thermal Burns." Canad. Nurs, Vol. 61, No. 5 (May 1965), pp. 365–367.
Domonkos, A. N. (Ed.): "Symposium on Recent Advances in Dermatology." Med. Clin. North Amer., Vol. 49, No. 3 (May 1965).
Fitzpatrick, P. J.: "Tumors of the Skin." Canad. Nurse, Vol. 63, No. 2 (Feb. 1967), pp. 45–47.
Jacoby, F.: "Current Nursing Care of the Burned Patient." Nurs. Clin. North Amer., Vol. 5, No. 4 (Dec. 1970), pp. 563–575.
Larson, D., and Gaston, R.: "Current Trends in the Care of Burned Patients." Amer. J. Nurs., Vol. 67, No. 2 (Feb. 1967), pp. 319–327.
Margolius, F.: "Burned Children, Infection and Nursing Care." Nurs. Clin. North Amer., Vol. 5, No. 1 (Mar. 1970), pp. 131–142.
Martyn, D.: "Radiation Therapy for Skin Cancer." Canad. Nurse, Vol. 63, No. 2 (Feb. 1967), pp. 48–50.
McCrady, M., and Mitchell, C.: "Nursing Care: A Patient with Burns." Canad. Nurse, Vol. 61, No. 5 (May 1965), pp. 371–374.
Minckley, B. B.: "Expert Nursing Care for Burned Patients." Amer. J. Nurs., Vol. 70, No. 9 (Sept. 1970), pp. 1888–1893.
Waters, W. R.: "The Patient with Severe Burns." Canad. Nurse, Vol. 61, No. 5 (May 1965), pp. 367–371.
Wechsler, H. L.: "Psoriasis." Amer. J. Nurs., Vol. 65, No. 4 (Apr. 1965), pp. 85–87.

26
Nursing in Disorders of the Eye

STRUCTURE AND FUNCTION OF THE EYES

Vision, like all sensory mechanisms, requires receptors, an afferent pathway to carry the impulses into the central nervous system and an interpretive center. The eyes serve as receptors which are sensitive to light rays; the pathway is formed by the optic nerves and tracts within the brain; and the interpretive centers are composed of groups of neurons localized in the cortex of the cerebral occipital lobes (visual centers). In addition, the visual apparatus includes intrinsic and extrinsic muscles which play an important role in vision. There are also several accessory structures which function to protect the eyes.

Location of the Eye

Each eyeball rests in a cone-shaped cavity (the orbit) in the skull. The orbit is covered posteriorly by a fibrous sac lined with a smooth moist membrane which promotes smooth movement of the eye in its socket.

Accessory External Structures

The accessory structures include the eyelids, lacrimal system and the extrinsic ocular muscles.

Eyelids (Palpebrae). The upper and lower eyelids are curtain-like structures lying in front of the eyeball. They serve as protective coverings by shutting out intense light, dust and foreign bodies. The space between them is referred to as the palpebral fissure; the angles or corners where the lids meet are known as the inner (medial) and outer (lateral) canthi. Each eyelid has an outer layer of skin, a layer of firm fibrous tissue (tarsal plate), sebaceous-like glands (meibomian glands) which secrete an oily substance onto the free margins of the lids, and a mucous membrane lining called the conjunctiva. The conjunctiva is reflected over the anterior of the eyeball. The secretion of the meibomian glands prevents adherence of the lids when the eyes are closed and also prevents the overflow of normal amounts of lacrimal secretion. The eyelashes emerge from the free borders of the eyelids to protect the eye from dust and perspiration.

Lacrimal System. The lacrimal apparatus protects the eye by continuously secreting a fluid that "washes" over the anterior surface of the eyeball, keeping it moistened and cleansed. The system of each eye consists of a gland, ducts and a drainage system.

The lacrimal gland lies in a slight depression in the outer superior portion of the orbit. Several ducts carry the secretion of the gland

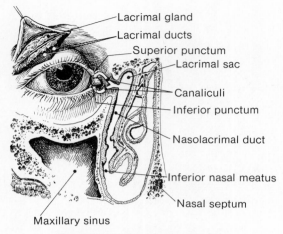

Figure 26–1   The lacrimal system.

on to the inner surface of the upper eyelid. The secreted fluid is distributed over the anterior surface of the eye and then drains through 2 small openings (puncta) in the medial canthus into 2 short canals (lacrimal canaliculi). The canals drain into a small sacular structure, the lacrimal sac, which narrows to form the nasolacrimal duct, which carries the secretion into the nasal cavity.

A volume of lacrimal secretion in excess of what the drainage system can handle results in fluid overflowing the eyelids and forming tears. Increased lacrimal secretion occurs in response to irritation of the conjunctiva or to certain emotions.

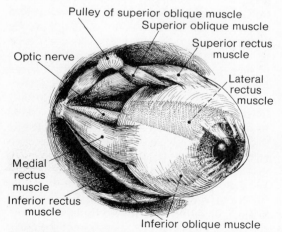

Figure 26–2   Extraocular muscles of the left eye.

Extrinsic Ocular Muscles.   Several external muscles have their origin in orbital structures and insert on the eyeball to provide movement of the eye within its socket. There are four straight muscles (recti muscles) and each is named for the direction in which it moves the eye. The superior rectus turns the eye up; the inferior rectus turns it downward; the medial rectus turns it in; and the lateral moves it in the reverse direction. In addition to the recti muscles, 2 oblique muscles (a superior and an inferior) provide rotation and modification of straight movements. For most movements, more than one external ocular muscle generally operate; various combinations of recti and oblique muscle action are necessary.

The external ocular muscles include the levator palpebrae superioris muscle which inserts in the upper eyelid. It is responsible for raising the upper eyelid (opening the eye).

Eyeball

The eyeball is spherical with a slight anterior bulge. It is composed of 3 layers of tissue which enclose the iris and special transparent, refracting structures. The tough, outer coat forms the sclera and cornea. The sclera, which covers the posterior five-sixths of the eyeball, is white, opaque fibrous tissue. The cornea is a continuation of the sclera, the anterior portion of the eye. It consists of transparent, special connective tissue and is devoid of blood vessels. The corneoscleral junction is referred to as the limbus.

Underlying and attached to the sclera is a thin, heavily pigmented, vascular coat, the choroid, which extends forward to what is referred to as the ciliary body. The pigmentation prevents the reflection of the light rays.

The ciliary body consists mainly of muscle tissue which takes its origin at the corneoscleral junction and inserts in the suspensory ligaments that are attached to the lens, holding it suspended in position. The action of the ciliary muscle influences the curvature, and thus the refractive power, of the lens. The second layer of the eyeball continues inward beyond the ciliary muscle to form the iris. The iris is composed of circular and radial muscles and pigmented

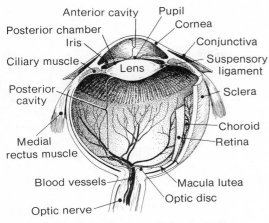

Figure 26–3 Parts of the eyeball.

cells and is perforated centrally, creating the opening referred to as the pupil. Contraction of the circular muscle fibers (sphincter pupillae) constricts the pupil; dilation is controlled by the radial fibers.

The retina is the innermost and nervous coat of the posterior two-thirds of the eyeball. It consists of several strata of cells through which light rays pass before reaching the outer layer of cells, which are light-sensitive receptors that convert luminous energy into nerve impulses. There are two types of receptor cells—namely, the rods and cones. The rods have a lower response threshold, making them more sensitive to lower levels of illumination. The cones have a higher response threshold and, as a result, function in bright light and provide color and detail vision.

In the center of the retina, a small area occurs in which the inner layers of cells are absent and only cones are concentrated. Light rays falling on this site strike the cones directly and produce the greatest visual acuity. This area is referred to as the fovea centralis and occurs as a slight depression in a small, elevated, yellowish area called the macula lutea, or yellow spot. Slightly medial to the macula, there is a pale papillary area called the optic disk, or fundus oculi. It is at this point the optic nerve and ophthalmic blood vessels leave and enter the eyeball. The disk is a blind spot, since the area is devoid of rods and cones.

The eyeball is "filled out" by contents composed of fluids (aqueous humor), a biconvex disk (lens) and a jelly-like mass (vitreous humor).

The lens is elastic and crystal clear and is suspended just behind the iris by ligaments which attach to the ciliary body. Its shape varies with age; it is spherical in infancy, gradually flattening to a disk shape. In the elderly, the lens tends to flatten and become less elastic.

Divisions of the Interior of the Eyeball. The interior of the eyeball is divided into the anterior and posterior cavities. The anterior cavity is the space between the cornea and lens and is subdivided into the anterior and posterior chambers, which are areas frequently referred to in clinical work. The anterior chamber lies posterior to the cornea and in front of the iris. The posterior chamber is situated posterior to the iris and anterior to the lens. The content of the two chambers is aqueous humor.

The posterior cavity lies posterior to the lens and is the remainder of the interior of the eyeball. It is filled with the vitreous humor, or vitreous body.

Fluid System of the Eye and Intraocular Pressure. The interior of the eyeball is filled by the aqueous and vitreous humors and the crystalline lens. The vitreous humor is a clear, jelly-like mass enclosed in a hyaloid membrane which anteriorly is continuous with the capsule of the lens. The vitreous humor fills out the larger and posterior portion of the eyeball that lies behind the lens.

The anterior and posterior chambers are filled with a clear fluid, the aqueous humor. There is a continuous flow into and out of the eye. The fluid originates from capillaries contained in processes of the ciliary body. Some fluid diffuses into the vitreous body from the posterior chamber; the greater proportion flows through the pupil into the anterior chamber. From here, a small amount of the aqueous humor continuously drains into the canal of Schlemm, from which it is carried into the venous circulation. The canal of Schlemm is a channel that circles the eye in the region of the corneoscleral junction. Small spaces (spaces of Fontana) leading to the canal occur in the tissues at the angle formed by the junction of the cornea with the anterior surface of the iris. This may be referred to as the filtration angle. The production of aqueous humor and its drainage are constant in order to maintain a normal intraocular pressure, which is 15 to 25 mm. Hg. Any interference with normal drainage of the fluid from the anterior chamber raises the pressure, leading to decreased blood supply, pain and impaired vision.

Visual Impulse Pathway

Impulses generated by the rods and cones synapse through several neurons to ganglionic cells whose axons course toward the site of the optic disk where they unite to form the optic nerve. This nerve differs from most nerves in that it has no neurilemma; thus, it is incapable of regeneration if damaged or destroyed. At the base of the brain, the nerve fibers from the medial half of the retina of each eye cross, going to the opposite side of the brain. The fibers from the lateral halves of the retinae do not cross but continue on to the corresponding side of the brain. This arrangement forms the optic chiasma (see Fig. 26-4). Within the brain, the fibers from the lateral half of the right eye and those from the medial half of the left eye continue on as the right optic tract. The fibers of each tract synapse with the lateral geniculate in the thalamus on the corresponding side. From there, the impulses are transmitted along the postsynaptic fibers (optic radiations) to the visual center in the occipital cerebral cortex of the same side where they are interpreted as sensations of light, color and form. Other cerebral areas are necessary for normal vision; correlation with information stored as memory in association areas has to occur in order to give meaning to what is seen. For example, a written word or an object may be seen, but unless the person has heard or experienced its meaning, he is unable to interpret it.

Visual Fields

The retinae of both eyes receive light rays at the same time from an object within the field of vision (binocular vision). Light rays from an object in the left outer visual field are received on the medial, or nasal, side of the left retina and on the lateral, or temporal, side of the right retina. The ensuing impulses are carried over fibers of the left and right optic nerves, but with the crossing of fibers in the chiasma, the impulses will travel along the right optic tract to the visual center in the right occipital lobe for interpretation. Conversely, rays from objects in the right visual field will fall on the lateral area of the left retina and nasal area of the right retina with the resulting impulses ending up in the visual center of the left occipital lobe. There is some overlapping between the two halves of each retina, and as a result, the central half of each is represented in each hemisphere.

If the optic nerve of one eye is destroyed, blindness occurs in that eye; but destruction of fibers of the optic tract (i.e., beyond the optic chiasma) causes blindness to occur in half of each retina, limiting the field of vision. The term for this blindness is hemianopia.

Eye Reflexes

The eye reflexes are used frequently in assessing the patient's condition. Some fibers of each optic tract terminate in a group of neurons referred to as the superior colliculus.

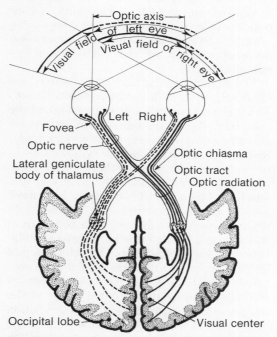

Figure 26—4 Left and right visual fields and the impulse pathway in the eye.

From here, efferent impulses originate, resulting in blinking of the eyelids, movement of the head, or dilation or constriction of the pupil.

The conjunctival and corneal reflexes are protective responses of blinking, elicited by touching these surfaces.

Pupillary reaction is observed by flashing a light into the eye; this normally results in constriction of the pupil. A second reflex that may be noted is the accommodation reflex. The pupils are observed while the person shifts his gaze from a distant to a near object. The normal response is constriction of the pupils. In some pathological conditions (e.g., syphilis), the response of the pupil to light may be absent while the accommodation reflex is present. This type of response is referred to as an Argyll-Robertson pupil.

Refraction, Accommodation, Pupillary Modification and Convergence

Several processes may be necessary to focus the light rays on the retina in order to form a clear image.

Refraction. When light rays pass obliquely from one medium to another of a different density, their velocity is altered, and they are bent or deflected. The process is referred to as refraction. If the rays pass into a medium of greater density, they are deflected toward the perpendicular; conversely, in a medium of lesser density, the rays are bent away from the perpendicular. Parallel rays striking a surface at right angles are not refracted. Parallel light rays striking the center of the cornea and lens pass through unrefracted. At either side of the center of the convex surfaces of the cornea and lens, light rays enter at an angle to the surface and are refracted toward the perpendicular. The greater the curvature or convexity of the surface, the greater is the degree of refraction.

The cornea and lens are the principal refractive media in the eye; the lens is particularly significant in that its curvature and degree of refraction can be varied according to the amount required to focus the light rays on the retina. The aqueous and vitreous humors also contribute to refraction, but they, with the cornea, remain the same. Without strain or modification, the normal eye will refract light rays from an object 20 or more feet away sufficiently to focus them on the retina. For objects that are near, refraction must be increased; and for distant objects, the eye must decrease its refraction. When greater refraction is necessary, the ciliary muscles contract and the suspensory ligaments, which are attached to the lens and the ciliary body, move forward, reducing their pull on lens. As a result, the lens increases its convexity and thickness and, thus, its refractive power. When light rays reflected by distant objects enter the eye, the ciliary muscles relax, and the suspensory ligaments exert greater tension on the lens. This reduces convexity, thickness and refractive power of the lens, and focus of the light rays on the retina is achieved.

Various errors of refraction occur which interfere with the ability of the eye to focus light rays on the retina, resulting in impaired vision.

Nearsightedness, called myopia, is the result of light rays from an object at 20 feet or more being focused at a point in front of the retina. The close objects can be seen, but distant objects are blurred.

Farsightedness (hypermetropia) is due to insufficient refraction, and as a result, light rays from an object at 20 feet or less are focused at a point behind the retina. The person sees distant objects more clearly than close ones. In the later years of life, as part of the aging process, the lens loses its elasticity and becomes thinner and flatter. This lessens the normal degree of refraction, and the person becomes farsighted. This refractive error is referred to as presbyopia.

In some persons, the horizontal and vertical curvatures of the cornea are uneven, producing differences in the degree of refraction. This results in different focal points; some light rays may be focused on the retina, but others may fall short or be carried to a point beyond the retina. This type of refractive error is known as astigmatism.

Accommodation. This is the process by which the degree of refraction by the lens is changed in order to focus rays from objects at various distances. This is made possible by the elastic nature of the lens and the action of the ciliary muscles on the suspensory ligaments as explained under refraction.

Pupillary Modification. The pupillary aperture is varied to control the amount of light entering the eye. For clear vision of near objects, the iris constricts the pupil of each eye to prevent divergent rays from entering. The opening is also reduced to restrict the entrance of excessively bright light, which may harm the retina. The iris constricts the pupil through parasympathetic innervation; sympathetic nervous stimulation produces dilation of the pupil. In dim light and when focusing on a distant, wider visual field, the iris dilates the pupil to admit more light rays.

Convergence. Although light rays from the same object(s) fall on both retinae, only single vision is experienced. This is due to light rays from the object falling on corresponding points of the 2 retinae. This is brought about by convergence, which involves the extrinsic muscles (recti and oblique). The movements of the 2 eyes must be coordinated accurately. As an object is brought closer to the eyes, convergence of their axes occurs as they turn inward. For distant objects convergence is not necessary; the eyes remain parallel. Strabismus is a defect which interferes with coordination of the eye movements, and the light rays do not fall on corresponding points of the 2 retinae. It is usually due to an abnormal extrinsic muscle. Two images result and the person "sees double"; this is termed diplopia.

Light and Dark Adaptation

Light Adaptation. When exposed to intense light, adaptation takes place by constriction of the pupils and lowering of the eyebrows, eyelids and head; the visual purple (rhodopsin) within the rods is bleached, thus reducing their sensitivity and responses.

Dark Adaptation. When a person goes from a light to a dark area, he cannot see immediately; then gradually he sees outlines of objects. This vision in dim light is due to an increased sensitivity of the rods as they produce a chemical pigment, visual purple or rhodopsin. Vitamin A is essential for the formation of the chemical; if it is deficient, the person experiences night blindness. At the same time that the rods increase their sensitivity, the pupils dilate to admit more light.

IMPAIRED VISION

Man is very dependent upon his sense of vision, since most of his knowledge of his environment is obtained through his eyes. The eyes are also used in expressing emotions. Any impairment or loss of vision is a serious threat. In many instances the ability to freely move about safely and the privilege of enjoying color, form, depth, beauty and distance are lost. Loss of vision results in reduced sensory input and stimulation; this may lead to boredom and reduced responsiveness on the part of the person unless stimuli by other channels (e.g., hearing) are increased and the person's interest maintained.

Nursing is concerned with the prevention of visual impairment, curative aspects when a disorder exists, and the rehabilitation of the patient with a loss of vision. The nurse should appreciate the incalculable value of sight and the natural anxiety and concern of the patient when it is threatened. Reduced vision affects his whole way of life socially, physically, economically and emotionally.

Factors in the Preservation of Sight

Good General Health. There is a tendency to consider the eyes as being independent of general health. The vision remains good in some serious bodily disorders, while others may have a serious effect on visual acuity. Occasionally, general body disease is discovered because of changes in the eyes and vision.

Optimum Diet. A well-balanced diet contributes to good eye health as well as to good general health. Vitamins A and B complex are considered important; a deficiency of vitamin A may cause drying and changes of the cornea and conjunctiva and a decreased production of the retinal pigment, rhodopsin, leading to night blindness. A deficiency in the vitamin B complex may predispose to retinal changes.

Protection of Children's Eyes. There is a legal requirement that a silver nitrate preparation be instilled in the eyes of every newborn infant in order to prevent possible infection, especially gonorrhea, which leads to corneal scarring and blindness. A child's eyes are not fully grown until he is at least 7 years of age. The infant's eyes require protection from prolonged exposure to direct sun and artificial light. Toys and playthings should be selected to avoid broken, sharp and pointed parts that predispose to injury. Children are taught to keep dirty fingers and other objects away from their eyes and are also instructed in the necessary precautions when old enough to play with such things as arrows, catapults and peashooters.

Avoidance of Eyestrain. Good lighting for reading and on close work is important to prevent eyestrain. Unshaded lights, glare and working with a light directly in front of the eyes are to be avoided. The rays should come from the back and one side onto the work area, which is kept free of shadows. Reading material or close work is held 14 to 16 inches from the eyes. Immobility is maintained when reading or doing close work; this precludes reading in moving vehicles.

When doing detailed and exacting work, the person should take frequent rests and look off into the distance. Close work is best avoided when fatigued.

Regular Periodic Eye Examination. Some eye diseases and changes develop insidiously without markedly reducing vision or causing pain until they are well advanced. Regular eye examination may reveal early signs, and a serious disease may be checked before it progresses to loss of vision and blindness. If glasses are necessary, only those which have been properly prescribed should be used. Lenses are individually ground for each eye according to the testing and examination findings.

Prompt Treatment. No "eyedrops" or solutions should be instilled in the eyes unless prescribed by a physician. In the event of a persisting foreign body which cannot be gently washed or wiped away, inflammation or any other disturbance in an eye, early treatment by a physician or oculist (ophthalmologist) should be secured.

Use of Protective Devices. To avoid injury by chemicals, dust, mechanical objects, wind, sun rays, and the like, appropriate safety goggles, shields or glasses should be worn.

Manifestations of Visual Disorders

The development of signs and symptoms of impaired vision varies greatly; as cited previously, the onset of changes may be very insidious; the person may continue to see well, but actually he is experiencing acute eyestrain. In others, the onset of a disorder and its manifestations may occur suddenly. One or both eyes may be involved. The symptoms may be principally objective with changes being noted by an observer.

The person may be seen holding reading material or an object nearer than 12 inches to the face or beyond the distance of 16 to 18 inches. He may scowl or have a strained expression when making an effort to see. In the case of a child, he may fail to develop at a normal rate or make normal progress at school.

Errors may be observed because of misread information or directive. The person may complain of difficulty in seeing—that persons and objects are blurred or foggy. His field of vision may be limited, the outline and size of objects may be distorted, or diplopia may be experienced. Colored halos around lights may be seen if the intraocular pressure is increased.

With some conditions, the patient may complain of flashes of light or stars, increased sensitivity to ordinary light (photophobia), spots before his eyes, itching, burning, or pain and irritation. There may be redness of the eye or lids, excessive lacrimal secretion and tearing, or serous or purulent discharge.

Eye Examinations

Tests for evaluation of eye function include the following:

Measurement of Visual Acuity. Visual acuity implies the ability to distinguish details of objects and is measured as a means of evaluating ocular function. Each eye is tested separately; the other eye is completely covered. A wall chart (Snellen chart) with rows of letters of decreasing size is used and placed 20 feet from the patient. The person is required to read the chart through to the line of smallest letters he can see. The distance from which the normal eye can read each line is known. For instance, on the Snellen chart the normal eye can read the seventh line from 20 feet away. Visual acuity is expressed as a fraction; the numerator represents the distance between the chart and the patient, and the denominator is the distance from which a person with normal vision could read the same line. Visual acuity recorded as 20/20 means normal vision. If the patient 20 feet from the chart can only read the line that the normal eye could read at 60 feet, the visual acuity is expressed as 20/60 and his vision is one-third of normal. The larger the denominator recorded, the poorer is the vision. In a person with severe impairment who can only see a hand moving in front of his face, the visual acuity may be recorded as H.M. (hand movements). If the person can only distinguish between light and dark, the recording is L.P. (light perception).

Refraction. The testing of the eyes' ability to focus the light rays on the retina is done by using a series of trial lenses as well as by assessing the person's visual acuity. In doing a refraction test, the physician may require the instillation of a cycloplegic drug such as atropine 0.5 to 2 per cent or hyoscine 0.2 to 0.5 per cent which temporarily inhibits ciliary muscle action and dilates the pupil.

Visual Field Measurement (Perimetry). A special semicircular instrument, called a perimeter, which is marked in degrees, is used to determine if the patient's visual fields are normal or restricted. Defects in the visual fields are frequently associated with intracranial lesions or damage to an optic nerve.

Ophthalmoscopic Examination. With an ophthalmoscope, the posterior, internal surface of each eye is magnified and observed. The blood vessels, retina, optic nerve and disk are examined. In order to get a wider view, the pupil is frequently dilated by the instillation of a mydriatic such as atropine 0.5 to 2 per cent.

Measurement of Intraocular Pressure. The detection of increased intraocular pressure is important; an excessive pressure is very painful and progressively causes permanent damage within the eye, leading to loss of vision. The pressure is measured by an instrument called the tonometer. A few drops of a local anesthetic (e.g., cocaine 0.5 to 5 per cent) are instilled in each eye. The tonometer is then placed on the corneal surface, causing indentation; the extent of the indentation reflects the intraocular pressure. If the pressure is high, the cornea resists indentation. The calibrated scale of the tonometer records the pressure in mm. of Hg. The normal intraocular pressure is approximately 15 to 25 mm. Hg.

Common Eye Disorders

Glaucoma. This disorder is characterized by an increase above the normal in the intraocular pressure. Normal pressure is generally maintained by a balance between the production of aqueous humor by the ciliary body and its reabsorption from the anterior chamber. If an imbalance occurs between production and drainage, the pressure increases, compressing the retina and the blood vessels within the eye. Permanent retinal damage leading to blindness results unless there is early recognition and treatment of the disease.

Glaucoma usually develops gradually and has a high incidence in persons over 40 years of age. The disease may be primary or secondary and is usually caused by some interference with the outflow of aqueous humor from the anterior chamber into the canal of Schlemm. Secondary glaucoma may be associated with inflammation, trauma, infection or a tumor within the eye. The cause of primary glaucoma is not understood, but the tendency to familial incidence points to an inherited predisposition. It may be acute or chronic.

In acute glaucoma, the intraocular pressure increases rapidly as a result of a com-

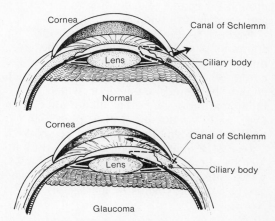

Figure 26–5 This diagram shows how a disturbance in the balance of fluid within the eyeball increases pressure in the eye and can result in glaucoma.

plete block in the outflow of the aqueous humor. The iris appears to have gradually pushed forward, narrowing the peripheral angle between it and the cornea (see Fig. 26–5), and with dilation of the pupil and the ensuing thickening of the iris, the openings in the angle which lead into the canal of Schlemm become occluded. Rapid compression of the retinal blood vessels develops, and destruction of the optic nerve cells and fibers occurs.

The patient with acute glaucoma experiences severe pain, nausea and vomiting, halos or rainbows around artificial lights and blurring of vision. On examination, the pupil is seen to be dilated, and there is evidence of congestion and a marked increase in intraocular pressure. The cornea becomes edematous and eventually loses its luster and transparency.

Prompt treatment is necessary to prevent blindness. A miotic preparation such as pilocarpine hydrochloride is instilled to constrict the pupil; this effects an increase in the peripheral angle by moving the iris away from the cornea. A drug such as acetazolamide (Diamox) or methazolamide (Neptazane) may be administered orally to reduce the formation of aqueous humor. The patient is kept on complete bed rest with his head and shoulders elevated. An analgesic is usually prescribed to relieve the pain. If an immediate, satisfactory response to drug therapy does not occur, surgical intervention is undertaken. A small section of the iris is removed (iridectomy) to prevent it from being imposed on the drainage system. Alternative surgical procedures which may be used are iridencleisis and corneoscleral trephine in which an opening is made between the subconjunctival space and the anterior chamber.

Chronic glaucoma, which is the more common form, has an insidious onset and is frequently well advanced before the person seeks assistance. His visual field progressively diminishes, and he may become aware that something is wrong when he learns of objects on either side of him that he "missed" or if he persistently sees halos around artificial lights. His condition may be discovered during a routine examination. As the condition progresses, the person may complain of some pain in the eye(s), especially in the morning on awaken-ing. If chronic glaucoma is not recognized and treated in the earlier stages, the person eventually experiences symptoms similar to those cited for acute glaucoma.

Treatment of chronic glaucoma in the early stages usually consists of a daily instillation of a miotic. Preparations are available now which have a more prolonged effect, requiring instillation only once in 24 hours. An example of such a preparation is echothiophate iodide (Phospholine Iodide). Surgical treatment may become necessary. As in acute glaucoma, an iridectomy, iridencleisis or corneoscleral trephining may be done.

Following surgery for glaucoma, the patient is usually kept flat for 12 to 24 hours and then is gradually elevated and allowed to move.

Because glaucoma accounts for such a large proportion of blindness, more effort has been directed toward informing the general public about the disease and the significance of early recognition. Clinics have been organized so that mass surveys may be made in order to identify persons in the early stages.

Glaucoma cannot be cured, but blindness can be prevented by continuous use of a miotic as prescribed and by medical supervision, if it is begun early in the disease.

An important nursing responsibility is to alert the patient to activities and situations that predispose to a rise in intraocular pressure. The condition is explained to the patient and his family, and emphasis is placed upon the need for some precautions to prevent visual damage. Emotional and stress situations are avoided as much as possible; the patient must learn to accept calmly what he cannot change. Limitations are placed on the length of periods for reading, watching television and close work. Tight clothing around the neck is avoided. Constipation is dangerous, since it leads to straining at stool which causes an elevation of intraocular pressure.

The patient and his family must appreciate the importance of regularly scheduled visits to the physician for measurement of the intraocular pressure and visual field and acuity testing. They are taught the correct method of instilling the prescribed miotic and cautioned against the use of any solution or medication that is not prescribed by the doctor. An identification card or Medic Alert pendant indicating that the person suffers from glaucoma is recommended. He is encouraged to continue his former occupation unless it requires prolonged periods of close visual concentration. If it does require such concentration, some job modification or change may be made if the employer is approached and is given an explanation of the employee's condition. Patients with advanced glaucoma and loss of vision are referred to the National Association for the Blind.

Cataract. A cataract is a cloudiness of the crystalline lens, resulting in opacity. It develops most commonly in persons over 50 years of age and is then classified as senile cataract. In a few instances it is present at birth and termed congenital cataract. It may develop secondary to trauma or disease at any age. The cause of senile cataract is not known; it is suggested that an inherited predisposition to develop the characteristic lens changes plays a role. Some deficiencies in nutrients, such as vitamins C and B, or a metabolic change have also been suggested as possible etiological factors. Cataract is frequently associated with diabetes mellitus. Congenital cataract occurs most often in infants whose mothers have a history of a viral infection (e.g., German measles) during the first trimester of pregnancy.

The opacity develops very gradually and may be localized to the center of the lens, incurring early impairment of vision, or it may start in the periphery.

The loss of the normal refractive ability of the lens prevents light rays from being focused on the retina. Vision becomes blurred and objects may appear distorted. Visual loss is very gradual and is directly proportional to the degree of opacity of the lens.

The patient with a cataract is treated by surgical removal of the lens. The procedure of choice is the intracapsular extraction in which the lens is removed, complete with its capsule. An extracapsular extraction is used principally with traumatic cataracts and those in younger persons. The anterior portion of the capsule and the lens content are removed, leaving the posterior part of the capsule because of its adherence to the vitreous body. A third procedure that may be used is discission or "needling," in which a small opening is made in the anterior surface of the lens capsule to permit the flow of aqueous humor in and out of the lens, washing away the opaque content. A newer method of extraction which has been used more recently is cryoextraction. A probe-like instrument is introduced so that it lies against the lens and is cooled to $-30°$ C. to $-35°$ C. The lens and its capsule freeze to the probe and are removed when the probe is withdrawn.

Following the operation the patient is kept at complete rest for at least 24 hours. Bed activity and elevation are gradually resumed and if the progress is satisfactory the patient is allowed up in 2 to 3 days. A dressing and shield are applied to the affected eye and in some instances the unoperated eye may also be covered for a day or two. A dressing is usually kept on the eye for 7 to 10 days. When the dressing has been taken off, the patient may experience discomfort with full exposure to the light, and some adaptation is necessary. Temporary glasses with thick convex lenses are used for approximately two months; the patient is then provided with permanent glasses.

Detachment of the Retina. Retinal detachment is separation of the retina from the choroid as a result of tears or holes in the retina. These openings permit fluid from within the eye to leak through and accumulate behind the retina, separating it from the choroid.

The cause may be degenerative retinal changes associated with the aging process, trauma or tumor. The damaged areas are usually toward the periphery of the retina. The manifestations appear suddenly and include flashes of light, blurred vision, floating particles in the line of vision, the sensation of a curtain coming in front of a part of the eye, restricted visual field and eventual loss of vision.

The patient is placed on complete bed rest, and both eyes are covered. He is positioned so that the detached area of the retina will approximate the underlying choroid. A sedative or tranquilizer is usually prescribed to reduce the patient's fear and apprehension and promote immobility. Surgical intervention is usually undertaken fairly early. Various procedures are used, but the underlying principle is scarring of the area. As the scar tissue forms, it fills in the retinal hole and provides attachment to the underlying sclera. The surgical procedures include electrodiathermy, cryosurgery, photocoagulation which involves the application of heat by means of directing a very intense light into the eye (laser beam), and scleral buckling. In scleral buckling, the accumulated fluid is removed, the area is treated to produce scar tissue, and a fold is then made in the overlying sclera, which buckles the underlying choroid and retina, bringing them in contact.

After the operation, the patient is kept in bed at complete rest with both eyes bandaged for several days. Elevation, self-care and movement are resumed very gradually. The patient must be cautioned against bumping his head, rapid eye movements, reading and close work.

Inflammation. Inflammation of the eye is usually due to infection which occurs most often in the eyelids and conjunctiva. If the infection persists, it may of course eventually extend to other structures. The source of eye infection may be foreign bodies, dust, hands, extension from neighboring infected tissues (nose, sinus, face) and contaminated equipment or solutions used in treatment.

Blepharitis is infection and inflammation of the eyelids. A purulent discharge, crusting and irritation are present.

A hordeolum, or sty, is a small abscess that develops within a marginal gland or hair follicle of an eyelash. A small, red, swollen tender area appears. Spontaneous drainage of pus may be hastened by the application of hot, moist compresses. Rarely, a small incision is necessary to drain the abscess. The patient with a sty is cautioned not to squeeze the area as this may "break down" the localization and lead to cellulitis.

A chalazion is a cyst that forms in a meibomian gland. It may remain as a small, firm, painless swelling in the lid for a long period. It may eventually become infected, frequently necessitating a small incision in the eyelid for drainage and curettage.

Treatment of these infections in the eyelids usually comprises the application of hot, moist compresses, frequent gentle cleansing of the lid margins to prevent encrustations and the application of an antimicrobial ointment.

CONJUNCTIVITIS. The symptoms of conjunctivitis may include redness, congestion, irritation, light sensitivity (photophobia), purulent discharge and increased lacrimal secretion, which may cause watering or tearing. It may be due to infection, a foreign body, trauma or allergy.

Treatment depends on the cause; if there is infection, antimicrobial drugs are used topically and generally. Warm, moist compresses or irrigations may be used. Precautions must be observed to prevent possible transmission of infection from one eye to another. The eye is left uncovered. In allergic irritation, the administration of an antihistamine preparation may be prescribed to relieve the irritation. For the care following an injury, see page 740.

UVEITIS. Inflammation due to injury or infection may develop in the uveal tract, which includes the choroid, iris and ciliary body. It may also be associated with collagen disease (e.g., rheumatoid arthritis, sarcoidosis). The patient complains of pain, photophobia, and impaired vision in the affected eye. The pupil usually remains constricted.

Treatment may include rest of the eyes and the administration of an antimicrobial drug if infection is suspected as being the cause. A mydriatic (e.g., atropine) is instilled to dilate the pupil and prevent adhesions from developing between the iris and the lens. A corticoid preparation may be given systemically to arrest the inflammatory process and scar formation, since scar formation is likely to cause loss of vision.

Keratitis. This is the term used for inflammation of the cornea and is a serious condition. It may be due to infection or trauma and is likely to lead to ulceration and scarring. These areas lose their transparency, diminishing the light rays entering the eye. Keratitis is manifested by irritation, discharge if the cause is infection, redness of the eye due to injection of the peripheral areas of the cornea by blood vessels, photophobia and tearing.

Prompt medical treatment is necessary to prevent visual damage. Keratitis frequently could be prevented by early removal of foreign bodies as well as early treatment of injuries and infection.

Treatment includes rest, the use of antimicrobial drugs, warm moist compresses, the instillation of a mydriatic and a local anesthetic solution to relieve pain. The eyes are covered to protect them from light and to keep them at rest.

Keratoplasty (Corneal Transplantation). Destruction of the cornea or loss of transparency resulting in loss of vision may be corrected by a corneal transplantation. The central portion of the cornea is removed and replaced with a cornea obtained from a cadaver. The graft may have been removed within a few hours of death or may have been preserved by freezing. The patient receives a general anesthetic for the transplant. Postoperative nursing measures are directed toward healing the graft by keeping the patient and both eyes at rest, preventing or detecting early signs of increasing intraocular pressure, and preventing infection. Bed activity is usually very much restricted for at least a week. Personal care must be provided by the nurse. Elevation and activities that are likely to cause straining are very gradually resumed.

Injury to the Eye. An eye may be traumatized by a foreign body, laceration or a chemical. Persisting pain, loss of vision and bleeding usually manifest a serious injury.

A foreign body may lodge on the conjunctiva or may be embedded in the conjunctival or corneal tissue, causing inflammation and possible ulceration. In some accidents, the injury may penetrate the lens or even the retina. If a foreign body is not easily and lightly wiped off or washed out, the patient is promptly referred to a clinic or oculist. Deep metal foreign bodies may be removed by the use of a strong electric magnet.

Lacerations of the eyeball seriously threaten vision because of the formation of scar tissue in healing and by predisposing the eye to infection. Prompt treatment and strict asepsis are very important.

Various chemicals, acids and alkalies may cause serious irritation or burns of the conjunctiva and cornea. Emergency treatment consists of washing the eye with copious amounts of water. The lids must be widely open and assistance may have to be provided in order to keep the eye open during the flushing. The person is referred to a doctor as quickly as possible.

Strabismus (Squint). Normally, both eyes perform an equal range of movement and assume corresponding lines of position when focusing on an object. Strabismus ("cross eyes") is characterized by the deviation of one eye from the position of the other; one eye (the normal or fixing eye) focuses directly on the object, but the other one (the deviating eye) appears to be focused on a different object or area. The inequality in the movement of the eyes is due to an imbalance in the function of one or more extrinsic ocular muscles. The defect may result in the eye being turned medially, producing a convergent strabismus (esotropia). If the eye is turned laterally, the condition is referred to as divergent strabismus (exotropia). The result of the unequal movement and two points of focus is double vision (diplopia). Two images are formed on the retinae and the visual centers in the brain receive two sets of impulses, each producing a separate picture.

Strabismus may also be classified as being nonparalytic or paralytic and monocular or alternating. Nonparalytic strabismus (the more common) is the result of an inherited abnormality. The defect is in the central nervous system mechanism which coordinates the movements of the eyes in order to bring them into the positions that will focus the light rays from an object on corresponding areas of the 2 retinae. The person may be able to focus the right eye on an object of attention, but the left deviates, presenting a different image. If the person has alternating strabismus, he may be able to focus first with one eye on the object, then with the other. The eye that is in the correct position is referred to as the fixing eye; the other is called the deviating eye. If it is always the same eye, the strabismus is said to be monocular.

The person with strabismus develops single vision, seeing only what the fixing or nondeviating eye perceives by involuntarily suppressing the confusing image presented by the deviating eye. Nonparalytic strabismus is generally recognized in early childhood.

Paralytic strabismus is due to the inability of the extraocular muscles to move the eye into the position corresponding to that of the other eye. As a result the person experiences diplopia. The cause of paralytic strabismus may be a defect in the muscle itself or a disturbance in the muscle innervation. The condition may be a manifestation of a disorder within the brain or orbit that interferes with the transmission of impulses by the third (oculomotor), fourth (trochlear) or sixth (abducens) cranial nerve.

Strabismus requires medical treatment; unfortunately, in some instances parents think it will correct itself as the child becomes older. A delay may result in permanent damage; constant suppression of the vision presented by the deviating eye may lead to loss of vision in that eye. The form of treatment will depend on the cause and severity of the strabismus. Obviously, if it is secondary to a lesion that is interrupting nerve impulses, the primary condition is surgically treated, if possible. Strabismus in the child may be corrected by the wearing of prescribed glasses. The good eye may be covered for periods to enforce the use of the deviating eye. Special eye exercises may be ordered (orthoptics). If the condition does not respond to these conservative forms of treatment, surgical correction may then be undertaken. The procedure may involve shortening or lengthening of one or more extrinsic eye muscles. Following the surgery, exercise and the wearing of glasses may still be necessary for a period of time. The patient requires continued medical supervision.

Enucleation. Enucleation is the removal of an eyeball and may be necessary because of a malignant newgrowth, deep infection, severe trauma or persisting pain in a blind eye. Rarely, an enucleation is done to remove a disfiguring blind eye. When an eyeball is removed, the extrinsic muscles are severed close to their insertion, and the Tenon's capsule is retained. These may be arranged around a plastic ball to provide support and movement for an artificial eye.

Occasionally, the operation performed is an evisceration in which the contents of the eyeball are removed, leaving the sclera.

A more radical procedure may be necessary in malignancy or severe trauma. The operation performed is called exenteration and involves the removal of the eyeball and the surrounding structures.

Sympathetic Ophthalmia. Following an eye injury, especially a deep penetrating one, the patient may develop uveitis (inflammation of the ciliary body, choroid and iris) in the uninjured eye. This response is not understood; it has been suggested that it may be an allergic reaction to the pigment released by the damaged eye. Any redness or tearing of the uninjured eye and any complaint of photophobia, pain or loss of vision must be reported promptly. The condition may develop soon after the injury or several months or years later. Unless the inflammatory reaction is checked promptly, loss of vision results. Corticoid preparations are used locally and generally. Rarely, the injured eye is removed to prevent the sympathetic ophthalmitis from developing.

General Considerations in Nursing the Patient with an Eye Disorder

Fear and Insecurity. Impairment and threatened loss of vision arouse considerable fear, insecurity and emotional reactions. All the implications which impaired vision may have in the present and future crowd in on the patient. Fears and worry may be greatly exaggerated, and the patient becomes panicky, which he cannot control without help. The understanding of the nurse as to what the patient may be experiencing and the provision of emotional support contribute greatly to the care of this patient.

Factors which help to reduce the patient's anxiety include the following suggestions. The patient is carefully oriented to any new environment; if he is confined to bed, the orientation is by a verbal description. If he is allowed up, the verbal description is combined with helping him to explore it. An explanation is made of how his usual daily needs will be met.

The patient is given the opportunity and is encouraged to express his concerns and to ask questions. The person who cannot see is spoken to as he is approached and is advised who it is. If the nurse is working in the room but not with the patient, he is told. Anything that is going to be done for him is outlined (e.g., treatment, investigative procedure). It means a great deal to the patient to always have his signal within reach; it reassures him that help is always at hand. He should not be left alone for long periods; he may not require a lot of physical care but still requires support and contacts. The nurse takes time to converse with the patient; the flowers, cards, and other details of the environment are described vividly. He has visual memory from which he can recall sufficiently to form a mental picture of that being described. Some appropriate form of diversion, such as a radio, visitors to chat with the patient or read to him, and records, is provided. Noisy, confusing situations are avoided; if in darkness, the patient becomes more alert and is more sensitive to sounds and voice inflections. An effort is made to anticipate the patient's needs.

Prevention of Injury. Adequate orientation and frequent observations are important to prevent accidents when the patient's vision is seriously impaired. Crib sides are placed on the bed until he is accustomed to the situation. If the patient is disoriented, it may be necessary to have someone remain with him to ensure his safety. The environment must be checked carefully for any hazards for the unseeing, ambulatory person. He should be escorted around the area until he becomes familiar with it. Stools, rugs or other such articles over which he might trip are removed. Furniture is not moved from its original position, and doors are kept closed or wide open. The person is cautioned about nearby stairs and radiators.

Observations. The nurse is required to be familiar with any specific observations that are important in certain eye disorders. Generally, significant factors that should be brought promptly to the doctor's attention include elevation of the temperature, discharge, pain, headache, retraction of the eyelid, any evidence of disturbance in the unaffected eye, drying of the cornea, and signs of bleeding in the anterior chamber.

Positioning and Activity. The position which the patient with an acute eye disorder is to assume varies with different conditions and is usually indicated by the physician. For instance, if increased intraocular pressure is a concern, as in glaucoma, the head of the bed is elevated; if detachment of the retina occurs, the patient is kept flat; following a cataract extraction, some surgeons require the patient to lie flat, and others permit the head of the bed to be elevated 30 to 45 degrees. Usually, if the patient with an eye disorder is permitted to turn, he lies on the side of the unaffected eye only. Prolonged restriction of activity is rare; patients worry less and have fewer complications when allowed up as soon as possible. If the patient is required to remain in bed, lying flat with his head immobilized, his arms and lower limbs are moved through a range of motion, and active exercises of the legs are begun as soon as the doctor permits.

Infection. Infection within the eye can be very serious and may lead to loss of vision. Strict asepsis is observed in all eye treatments. Clean dressings are done before infected ones. If both eyes are infected, separate equipment is used for each one. If only one eye is infected, precautions are taken to protect the unaffected eye. For instance, when irrigating or cleaning the affected eye, the nurse works from the inner canthus toward the outer corner, making sure no fluid escapes over the bridge of the nose into the other eye. In conjunctivitis, the eyes are left exposed; frequent cleansing may be necessary to remove the discharge and crustations.

Dressings and Instillations. In order to keep the affected eye at rest, the unaffected eye may be covered. Adaptation to light is resumed gradually; the unaffected eye may first be exposed by wearing a shield with a small central opening. This minimizes eye movement. A similar shield may also be used later on the affected eye. Extreme gentleness is used when changing dressing or doing any treatment; caution is used to avoid pressure on the eyeball.

Preparations of drugs used for instillations should be fresh; the labels carry the date of expiry. A fresh, sterile dropper is used for each solution. Drops are placed on the inside of the lower lid and not directly on the eyeball to avoid reflex squeezing of the eye.

Nutrition. The patient frequently experiences anorexia due to anxiety and because of the difficulty with taking food when he cannot see. The necessary assistance is provided, and when feeding him, the food is described; only small amounts are offered to avoid choking and coughing, since coughing raises the intraocular pressure. As soon as the patient is well enough, he is encouraged to start feeding himself and to become independent. Assistance is withdrawn gradually, not all at once.

Elimination. Constipation and straining at stool are avoided, since they tend to cause an elevation in the intraocular pressure. A mild laxative may be administered and the diet modified to encourage normal bowel evacuation.

Preoperative Preparation. The surgeon advises the patient and his family of the anticipated surgery, but the nurse is prepared to clarify the explanation and answer their questions. Many eye operations are performed under local anesthesia; the patient is told what to expect and is cautioned against squeezing the eye during operation. A cleansing enema is usually given the night before operation unless the intraocular pressure is elevated above normal. Food and fluid are withheld the morning of operation if a general anesthetic is to be used. If the patient is to have local anesthesia, a fluid or soft diet may be given at breakfast.

A specific directive is received as to the local preparation required. The area around the eye is thoroughly cleansed but not shaved, and drops (e.g., mydriatic and local anesthetic) are generally instilled 1 or 2 hours before the scheduled time.

Rehabilitation of the Blind. The patient with marked visual impairment or with total loss of vision needs a great deal of assistance in adjusting to the situation. He must be persuaded that life still holds something for him. Emphasis is placed on what he can do. He still has visual memory of form, color, and space and can learn that other senses can be put to greater use.

The development of independence is started as soon as possible, beginning with self-care (feeding, bathing, dressing and hair). He is assisted with moving about the room, then from room to room, locating furniture and necessary articles by touch.

His environment is organized to provide safety. Furniture is left in the same place unless he is advised and orientated to its new position; rugs, footstools and other such hazardous objects are removed. Doors are kept wide open or closed.

Anyone walking with a blind person allows him to take an arm rather than grasping his and pushing. Writing is practiced, beginning with the signing of his name. Differentiation by touch is also tested and practiced. The person learns to tell the time by opening the crystal of a watch.

Various forms of diversion and recreation are introduced (records of books and music, radio, games). The patient is referred to the national associations for the blind,[1] which provide vocational training, assistance in learning Braille and in finding a job, recreation, transportation, and financial assistance when necessary. The use of the white cane is introduced and the necessary guidance given on excursions beyond the house until the person is capable of safely getting around alone.

The patient and his family are advised of the financial assistance available for the blind and are assisted in making application for it. The family may require help in accepting the blind patient and in organizing the home environment in the interest of his safety and independence.

[1]The Canadian National Institute for the Blind, Toronto, Ontario, Canada.
The American Foundation for the Blind, New York, New York, U.S.A.

References

BOOKS

Flitter, H. H.: Physics in Nursing, 5th ed. St. Louis, C. V. Mosby Co., 1967, pp. 156–166.

Greau, J. H.: An Introduction to Human Physiology, 2nd ed. London, Oxford University Press, 1968, pp. 164–167.

Jacob, S. W., and Francone, C. A.: Structure and Function in Man, 2nd ed. Philadelphia, W. B. Saunders Co., 1970, pp. 274–282.

Langley, L. L.: Outline of Physiology, 2nd ed. New York, The Blakiston Division, McGraw-Hill Book Co., 1965, pp. 84–99.

Saunders, W. H., Havener, W. H., Fair, C. J., and Hickey, J. T.: Nursing Care in Eye, Ear, Nose, and Throat Disorders, 2nd ed. St. Louis, The C. V. Mosby Co., 1968, pp. 3–138.

PERIODICALS

Chodil, J., and Williams, B.: "The Concept of Sensory Deprivation." Nurs. Clin. North Amer., Vol. 5, No. 3 (Sept. 1970), pp. 453–465.

Condl, E. D.: "Ophthalmic Nursing: The Gentle Touch." Nurs. Clin. North Amer., Vol. 5, No. 3 (Sept. 1970), pp. 467–476.

Dowling, J. E.: "Night Blindness." Sci. Amer., Vol. 215, No. 4 (Oct. 1966), pp. 78–84.

Hubel, D. H.: "The Visual Cortex of the Brain." Sci. Amer., Vol. 209, No. 5 (Nov. 1963), pp. 54–62.

O'Neill, P. C.: "Understanding Your Blind Patient." Canad. Nurse, Vol. 61, No. 9 (Sept. 1965), pp. 728–730.

Rabb, M. F.: "The Present Status of Corneal Transplantation." Nurs. Clin. North Amer., Vol. 5, No. 3 (Sept. 1970), pp. 477–482.

Seaman, F. W.: "Nursing Care of Glaucoma Patients." Nurs. Clin. North Amer., Vol. 5, No. 3 (Sept. 1970), pp. 489–496.

Snyder, J.: "Newer Concepts in Ophthalmic Surgery." Nurs. Clin. North Amer., Vol. 3, No. 3 (Sept. 1968), pp. 539–541.

Warner, D. M., and Pratt-Johnson, J. A.: "The Use and Abuse of Contact Lenses." Canad. Nurse, Vol. 61, No. 9 (Sept. 1965), pp. 724–727.

PAMPHLETS

Available from:

The American Foundation for the Blind, 15 W. 16th St., New York, New York, USA.

The Canadian National Institute for the Blind, 1929 Bayview Ave., Toronto, Ontario, Canada.

27
Nursing in Disorders of the Ear

STRUCTURE AND FUNCTIONS OF THE EAR

The ear is concerned with the special sense of hearing as well as with the maintenance of equilibrium. It has three divisions: the external and middle ears for the collection and conduction of sound waves and the internal ear, which actually serves as the receptor. The eighth cranial (auditory or acoustic) nerve provides the afferent impulse pathway of the sensory unit. Part of

its fibers carry impulses to the interpretive centers for sound in the temporal lobes, and the others transmit impulses to areas of the brain stem and cerebellum associated with control of body posture.

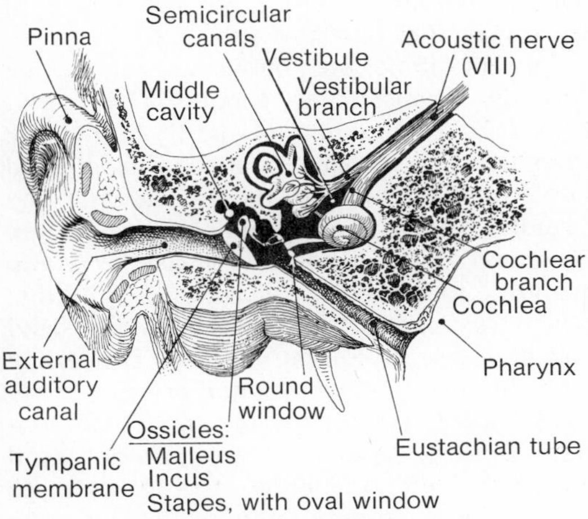

Ear Structure

External Ear. The outer ear consists of the auricle (pinna) and the external auditory meatus. The auricle is an immobile cartilaginous framework covered with skin and may contribute slightly to the collection of sound waves. The external auditory meatus is an S-shaped tube of approximately 1 inch. The tube ends at the tympanic membrane (eardrum), which separates the external and middle ears. The skin lining the canal is covered with fine hairs near the opening and has special glands which produce a yellow waxy secretion called cerumen for protection against insects and dust particles. The tympanic membrane is a thin, semitransparent membrane covered externally with skin and internally with mucous membrane which is continuous with that which lines the middle ear cavity.

Middle Ear. This portion of the ear is contained within a small cavity in the temporal bone. The cavity communicates with the nasopharynx by means of the

Figure 27–1   The parts of the ear.

eustachian or auditory tube and the mastoid cells. The eustachian tube permits the entrance of air into the middle ear; this equalizes the pressure on the internal surface of the eardrum with atmospheric pressure (that which is exerted on the external surface of the drum). The cavity is lined with mucous membrane which is continuous with that of the eustachian tube and mastoid cells. The mastoid cells are small air spaces within the posterior portion of the temporal bone. Obviously, the continuity of the lining membrane provides a ready means for the spread of infection from the throat to the middle ear and from the middle ear to the mastoid.

The middle ear cavity contains three small bones called the auditory ossicles, which are movable for the purpose of transmitting sound vibrations. The first ossicle, the malleus, is attached to the eardrum and articulates with the second ossicle, the incus. The incus articulates with the third ossicle, the stapes, which is attached to the membranous oval window (fenestra ovalis) that leads into the internal ear.

Internal Ear (Labyrinth). The inner ear consists of a system of irregularly shaped cavities which contain fluid and complex membranous structures which initiate nerve impulses as a result of sound waves or change of position. The bony (osseous) labyrinth is divided into three parts—the cochlea, vestibule and semicircular canals. Within the bony labyrinth is a membranous labyrinth which conforms fairly closely to the shape of the bony-walled cavities. The fluid contained within the osseous cavities is called perilymph, and that within the membranous cavities is known as endolymph.

The complex snail-shaped structure, the cochlea, consists of three tubes wound two to three times around a central column called the modiolus. The channels formed by the tubes are called the scala vestibuli, scala media (cochlear duct) and scala tympani. The scala vestibuli is closed at one end by the membrane of the oval window. As a result, vibrations transmitted to the membrane by the stapes set up waves in the fluid within the scala vestibuli. The scala vestibuli communicates with the scala tympani at the apex of the cochlea so that

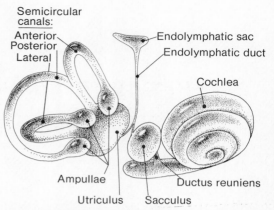

Figure 27–2 The membranous labyrinth in the ear.

when the fluid within the scala vestibuli is set in motion, the fluid in the scala tympani is similarly affected. The base of the scala tympani is closed off by the membrane covering an opening into the middle ear which is known as the round window (fenestra rotunda).

The scala media is walled off from the scala vestibuli by Reissner's membrane and from the scala tympani by the basilar membrane. The basilar membrane is composed of many fibers of varying length; it is shorter at the end nearer to the round window and becomes progressively longer toward the apex of the cochlea. On the surface of the basilar membrane are special cells with hair-like projections. Sound vibrations of the basilar membrane give rise to nerve impulses that are picked up by fibers of the acoustic nerve. These special cells of the basilar membrane comprise the organ of Corti (see Fig. 27–3).

The vestibule lies between the cochlea and the semicircular canals. The bony-walled cavity contains perilymph. The suspended membranous portion is divided into two sacs, called the utricle and the saccule, which contain endolymph. Within these cavities are hair-like projections and calcium carbonate concretions (otoliths) which respond to movements of the head and give rise to neural impulses concerned with the maintenance of equilibrium.

The third division of the inner ear consists of three semicircular canals hollowed out of the temporal bone at right angles to each other. They communicate with the

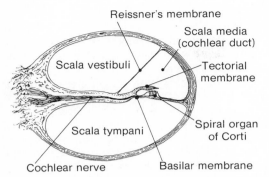

Figure 27–3 Cross section of the cochlea.

osseous vestibule and contain perilymph. Three semicircular membranous ducts suspended within the osseous canals contain endolymph and communicate with the utricle. Each membranous semicircular canal has a dilated portion at one end, called the ampulla, which contains special sensory hair cells, forming the crista acustica, or crista ampullaris. The crista is sensitive to movement of the endolymph within the ampulla, initiating neural impulses that are transmitted by the vestibular portion of the acoustic (eighth cranial) nerve to the central nervous sytem.

Auditory Pathway

Sound waves passing into the external ear strike the tympanic membrane, causing it to vibrate with the same frequency as the sound waves. This in turn results in vibrations of the ossicles in the middle ear. The stapes, being attached to the oval window, causes its membrane to move in and out. These vibrations are transferred into the perilymph of the scala vestibuli of the inner ear and in turn through the Reissner's membrane and through the endolymph in the scala media to the basilar membrane. Movements of the endolymph and basilar membrane stimulate the cells of the organ of Corti, initiating neural impulses which are transmitted via nerve fibers to a ganglion in the central core (the modiolus) of the cochlea. The axons of the ganglionic neurons form the cochlear branch of the acoustic (eighth cranial) nerve. The cochlear branch synapses with a group of neurons in the medulla (cochlear nucleus), and eventually, the impulses reach a cortical area of the temporal lobe (auditory center) where they are interpreted as sound. Each ear delivers impulses to both auditory centers.

The movements of the perilymph, initiated by the vibrations of the oval window, are transmitted through the helicotrema (communicating channel between the scalae at the apex of the cochlea) to the scala tympani and subsequently to the membrane of the fenestra rotunda (round window).

Pitch and Intensity of Sound

The pitch of a sound depends upon the frequency of the vibrations (number per second). The fibers of the basilar membrane vary in length. It is thought that different frequencies stimulate selective areas of fibers and cells of the membrane; i.e., each place on the basilar membrane is sensitive to sound waves of a certain frequency.

Figure 27–4 Schematic drawing of the cochlea.

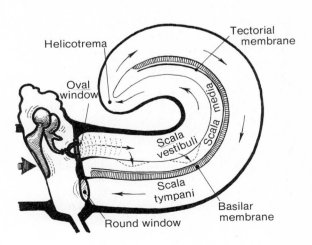

The intensity, or loudness, of a sound depends upon the amplitude or force of movement of the vibrations. The louder the sound, the greater is the displacement back and forth.

Equilibrium

When the head moves, neural impulses originate in the crista acustica of the semicircular canals and the maculae acusticae of the utricle and saccula and are transmitted by nerve fibers which form the vestibular branch of the acoustic nerve. The vestibular nerve fibers run to groups of neurons (vestibular nuclei) in the brain stem from which impulses may be delivered to the cerebellum, reticular formation, down the vestibulospinal tracts to motor neurons which innervate skeletal muscle, the oculomotor center and the thalami. The principal purpose of these impulses is to orient the person in space, and reflexly stimulate muscles so that he may assume an upright position or maintain the position he has assumed against gravity.

AUDITORY DISORDERS

Loss of Hearing

The incidence of loss of hearing in varying degrees is very high, and in many instances, the person is unaware of it until it is well advanced. Hearing limitations interfere with the ability to communicate with others which is extremely important. Obviously, the effects and problems vary with the degree of loss and the age at which it developed. In the child, it retards development, affecting the learning of speech and normal adjustment within society. It creates physical, emotional and socioeconomic problems for both the person and his family.

The degree of loss of hearing may be indicated by classifying those affected as "hard of hearing" or "deaf." The hearing is defective in those who are hard of hearing but is not totally absent. They have sufficient hearing, either with or without the use of a hearing aid, to cope with ordinary activities. Persons who are described as deaf have a marked or total loss of hearing that makes it very difficult, if not impossible, to function normally.[1]

Manifestations of Impaired Hearing. Indications of a hearing deficit may include failure to respond when addressed, frequent requests for repetition, misinterpretation of what was said, a short attention span or lack of attention, lack of interest, a strained confused expression, turning of the head to direct the "good" ear to the source of sound, irritability because of the strain and withdrawal from the group. Changes in speech, such as a lack of inflections and a low or excessive volume, may develop. A person with conductive deafness tends to speak softly; the person with nerve deafness usually speaks loudly. In the case of a child, impaired hearing may be suspected if there is a failure in the development of speech, a lack of normal progress in school, no response to voice or sound, or no interest in noise-making toys. The severity of the speech defect depends on when the hearing deficit developed and the degree of loss. If the person is partially deaf with loss for high frequency (high pitched) sounds, he may hear vowels but not consonants. The deaf child, when in need of comfort and reassurance, responds to cuddling or touch rather than to verbal expressions. He may develop and persistently use gestures to indicate his needs or wishes rather than producing vocal expressions.

Classification and Causes of Loss of Hearing. A hearing deficit may be congenital or acquired and may be classified as conductive, sensorineural, central or combined.

In a conductive hearing loss, sound waves fail to reach the internal ear as a result of some disturbance in the external ear, middle ear or the oval window (fenestra ovalis).

In sensorineural deafness, which may also be called nerve or perceptive deafness, the disorder is located in the organ of Corti, cochlear division of the acoustic nerve, or the auditory impulse pathway or center within the brain.

Central hearing loss denotes a hearing deficit resulting from disturbances within the brain, principally the auditory center in the temporal lobe.

Combined hearing loss occurs because of

---

[1] E. R. Nilo: "Needs of the Hearing Impaired." Amer. J. Nurs., Vol. 69, No. 1 (Jan. 1969), p. 115.

impairment within both the conductive and neural auditory mechanisms.

Congenital loss of hearing may be due to a prenatal malformation or lack of development of a part of the auditory apparatus. Heredity may play a role, or it may be the result of a viral infection in the mother during the first trimester of the pregnancy, the effect of a toxic drug taken by the mother during pregnancy, hypoxia or a birth injury.

Acquired impairment of hearing may be caused by obstruction of the external auditory canal by a foreign body or impacted cerumen, infection (e.g., otitis media, labyrinthitis, meningitis), a newgrowth (e.g., acoustic neuroma), an ototoxic drug (e.g., streptomycin, quinine), trauma associated with a skull fracture or excessively loud noise, obstruction of the eustachian tube, or degenerative changes in the auditory pathway frequently associated with the aging process (presbycusis).

Preservation of Hearing

Nurses, especially those working with industrial workers and school children, have an important role in the prevention of hearing loss. The public requires education about the causes and early signs of impaired hearing and significant preventive measures.

Good prenatal care and the avoidance of contact with persons with measles or other viral infections are important in preventing congenital deafness. Prompt treatment of respiratory infection and infectious diseases may allay the complication of otitis media. Prompt medical treatment and follow-up are urged for persons with an ear disorder.

The danger of introducing foreign objects into the external ear canal should be emphasized; for example, cleansing the ear with applicators, matches and hairpins is dangerous. If the wax (cerumen) becomes dry and impacted or an insect or foreign body becomes lodged in the canal, a few drops of warm oil or glycerine may be instilled and followed by a warm water or normal saline irrigation in a few minutes. If this does not remove the foreign object or impacted wax, the person is advised to promptly seek medical attention.

Routine tests of school children's hearing are important so that early recognition may be made of any impairment. Teachers and school nurses must be familiar with manifestations of a hearing deficit.

The nurse caring for a patient receiving a preparation of streptomycin or quinine must be alert for early signs of damage to his hearing.

The occupational health nurse, especially in an industry in which there is prolonged, intense noise in the work environment, must be cognizant of the possibility of noise-induced hearing loss. Frequently the employees tend to accept noise simply as a necessary part of the occupation and do not realize that hearing damage may be insidiously developing. Gradual loss of hearing usually involves, first, failure of response to high frequency sounds. Later, areas of the cochlea which respond to lower frequencies become damaged. In order to protect persons exposed to noise that endangers hearing, protective devices in the form of earmuffs, ear plugs or a special helmet are provided. Employees should receive regular hearing tests and be exposed to an active educational program.

Suggestions to Those Speaking to a Person Who Is Hard of Hearing

Do not speak until you have the person's attention. The speaker's face should be in full view of the listener so that he has the opportunity to observe lip movement.

Determine which is his better ear and go to that side of him if possible. Look directly at the listener.

Speak slowly, enunciate clearly and avoid raising the pitch of voice. The volume is increased, but actual shouting is avoided. Guard against running words together. The natural form of conversation is used rather than broken statements and incomplete sentences.

Exaggerated lip movement only confuses the listener.

If repetition is necessary, rephrasing the communication may be helpful; remember that vowels are heard more readily than consonants.

Patience, tact and understanding are needed. Avoid any irritation or annoyance; such reactions on the part of the speaker only discourage the listener.

Do not prolong a conversation unnecessarily, since the listener tires under the strain.

If a hearing aid is used, give the person time to adjust it. Do not get within 4 to 5 feet of the aid and use natural volume and tone.

A misinterpretation must not be ridiculed or treated as a joke.

When a deaf person enters a room, an effort is made to draw him into the group. He is advised of the topic of conversation and is encouraged and given the opportunity to participate. Otherwise, he tends to withdraw and become isolated.

If it is not possible to communicate verbally, write the message.

Suggestions to Those Who are Hard of Hearing

Look directly at the speaker, since observation of lip movements proves helpful.

Concentrate on the speaker; look directly at his face.

Observe the total situation, since this may give a lead to the topic of conversation.

Acknowledge your hearing deficit; do not guess at things rather than ask for repetition.

Investigative Procedures

Hearing Evaluation. In testing hearing, the examiner considers, first, the degree of hearing loss and, second, whether the impairment is conductive or neural. A variety of tests may be used.

TUNING FORK TESTS. These tests provide information about the type of hearing loss experienced by the patient. The Rinne tuning fork test involves setting the fork in vibration and holding it in turn near each ear. The patient is asked to indicate when the sound becomes inaudible. At this point, the stem of the fork is placed against the mastoid process. If the sound is again heard, a conductive hearing loss is indicated; sound waves are being conducted to the cochlea by bone vibrations.

The Weber test also distinguishes conductive and neural hearing loss. The fork is set in vibration, the stem is held against the middle of the forehead and the patient is asked if he hears the sound better in one ear than the other. If the sound is heard

better in the ear with which he normally hears less well, his hearing loss is conductive. If the reverse is true, a neural loss is implied. If the sound is equal in both ears, the hearing loss is the same in both ears.

AUDIOMETER TESTS. The audiometer is an instrument which provides an accurate measurement of hearing. The minimum intensity of sounds of varying frequencies heard may be determined. The intensity of sound (i.e., the pressure exerted by the sound waves) is expressed as decibels. The audiometer is operated to produce sounds of known intensity and frequency. Frequency implies the number of sound waves (cycles) produced per second (cps). In testing, the intensity of the sound is gradually increased from the zero level on the scale for the particular frequency being used, and the level at which the sound is just heard is noted. Zero on the scale represents the level at which the normal ear usually hears the sound. The number of decibels above the zero level at which the sound is heard indicates the degree of hearing loss. The hearing in each ear is measured separately through a range of different frequencies.

SPEECH AUDIOMETRY. Hearing loss for speech may be determined by a speech audiometer. The instrument permits the delivery of actual words by earphone and record player to the person being tested. Various intensities may be used. The zero level is taken as normal. Hearing loss for speech is recorded as the number of decibels in excess of the zero level.

DISCRIMINATION TEST. This tests the ability to distinguish between words and to understand what is heard. The persons tested for discrimination frequently are those who have said "words run together and are not clear" or "I can't grasp the separate words." Using the speech audiometer, the person listens to a list of phonetically balanced, single syllable words that are frequently used in conversation. The words are presented at an intensity that ensures hearing. A score of less than 90 per cent generally indicates some sensorineural loss of hearing.

Roentgenogram. An x-ray examination of the temporal bone may be done to determine if mastoiditis has developed.

Blood Examinations. Leukocyte and differential cell counts may be ordered if acute infection of the middle ear or labyrinthitis is suspected. In the case of acute infection and inflammation, the leukocyte count is usually above normal, the increase being principally neutrophils.

Culture. Any discharge from the ear is usually cultured as soon as observed in order to identify the causative organism. Sensitivity tests to antibiotics may also be done.

Assistance and Hearing Aids

Some persons with a hearing deficit may be helped by using a hearing aid, which is a small, battery-operated instrument which amplifies sounds. Aids are helpful to persons who have a reduced conduction of sound waves into the inner ear. Few of those with sensorineural loss of hearing receive help from hearing aids; amplification of sound does not assist with the distortion and impaired discrimination resulting from impairment of the neural elements of the auditory apparatus. Before purchasing a hearing aid, the person with a hearing deficit should be examined by a physician for evaluation of his residual hearing and identification of the type of his hearing loss. The selection of the aid is based on the patient's particular type of hearing loss. If an aid is recommended, it should be worn for a trial period to determine if it does help.

Those who are deaf or hard of hearing and their families should be familiar with the American or Canadian Hearing Association and its local branches.[2] Assistance may be provided in the form of procuring medical examination and treatment, counseling as to types of hearing aids, obtaining vocational training and employment, arranging for special classes (e.g., speech) and obtaining printed advice in pamphlets.

Common Disorders of the Ear

Otitis Media. This is an inflammation of the middle ear and is most often due to infection that has gained access through the eustachian tube. It is frequently a complication of a respiratory infection or an infectious

---

[2]The Canadian Hearing Society, 60 Bedford Road, Toronto, Ontario, Canada.
The American Hearing Society, 18th St. N.W., Washington, D.C., USA.

disease such as measles. The disorder is usually acute but may become chronic. The initial inflammatory response causes congestion and swelling of the mucous membrane lining of the middle ear, and the cavity fills with exudate. The tympanic membrane may bulge externally, and unless the infection is checked, the exudate generally becomes purulent. If the cavity is not surgically drained, the tympanic membrane may rupture spontaneously.

The patient with otitis media experiences a sensation of fullness in the ear and dullness of hearing at first, then severe pain, and increasing loss of hearing because of failure of the conduction of sound waves through the middle ear. The temperature and leukocyte count are elevated, and the patient feels generally ill. Examination of the eardrum by means of an otoscope reveals redness and external bulging or rupture and drainage in the advanced stage.

The patient is given an antibiotic, and if the infection has progressed to the suppurative stage, the eardrum is surgically opened to permit drainage. The operative procedure is referred to as a myringotomy. Incision and drainage is preferable to leaving the condition until there is spontaneous rupture of the tympanic membrane. Such delay predisposes to mastoiditis, chronic otitis media and permanent hearing loss.

The patient having a myringotomy receives a local anesthetic or a brief-acting general anesthetic. Fluid is aspirated from the middle ear cavity through the incision, and a culture is taken. Absorbent cotton is placed loosely in the outer ear to absorb the drainage. The patient is encouraged to lie on the affected side to promote drainage. A persistent elevation of temperature, pain and deep tenderness in the region of the mastoid, headache, drowsiness or disorientation is reported to the physician. These may indicate the onset of a serious complication such as mastoiditis, meningitis or brain abscess.

Mastoiditis. The small spaces (air cells) in the mastoid communicate with the middle ear cavity and are lined with mucous membrane which is continuous with that of the middle ear. As a result, infection may spread readily to the mastoid in acute or chronic otitis media. The patient experiences tenderness over the mastoid process, headache and fever. A roentgenogram of the temporal bone shows a cloudiness in the mastoid cells.

Generally, early treatment with antibiotics checks the infection and no residual damage to hearing occurs. Rarely, if the infection is neglected or is virulent and unresponsive to the antibiotic given, bone tissue of the mastoid becomes infected, necessitating surgery. A myringotomy and a simple mastoidectomy are done. A simple mastoidectomy involves an incision behind the auricle and the removal of the diseased bone by curettement.

If the patient develops chronic otitis media and chronic mastoiditis, more extensive surgery may be undertaken. A radical mastoidectomy involves the removal of the diseased mastoid tissue and the incus, malleus and remainder of the tympanic membrane, leaving the mastoid and middle ear as one large cavity. This surgery on the middle ear results in loss of hearing.

Preoperative preparation for a mastoidectomy is the same as that for any patient who is to have a general anesthetic (see Chapter 10). The scalp is shaved 1 to 2 inches around the affected ear, and the long hair is combed toward the opposite side and secured.

Postoperatively, the dressing remains undisturbed for 3 to 4 days. Packing is placed in the wound to promote drainage and remains in place until the first dressing change. The bulky dressing and trauma make it difficult for the patient to move or raise his head. The nurse provides assistance at first, but gradually the patient learns to support his head with his hands when moving. He is observed closely for nystagmus or any sign of facial paralysis. Facial paralysis is a threat in mastoidectomy because of the facial (seventh cranial) nerve's proximity to the operative site. Persisting headache, stiffness of the neck, elevation of the temperature or disorientation is brought to the physician's attention, since it may indicate a complicating brain abscess or meningitis. Fluids are given freely and a regular diet is served as soon as it is tolerated.

The patient is generally allowed up on the second day; someone remains with him at first in case of dizziness and nausea that may develop as a result of labyrinth disturbance following a radical mastoidectomy.

If the patient suffers some hearing loss, he is reassured that assistance is available.

The nurse advises him as to how he may help himself in trying to communicate with others and may also refer him to the National Association for the Deaf and Hard of Hearing.

A radical mastoidectomy may be followed by a tympanoplasty. This is a surgical procedure done to improve conduction through the middle ear. A perforated eardrum may be repaired by the application of a graft (myringoplasty). Epithelium from the ear canal, skin from the postauricular area, fascia stripped from the temporal muscle or a section of a vein may be used as a graft. More extensive plastic surgery may be done that includes a graft that extends across the middle ear cavity to contact the stapes. This provides transmission of sound waves from the tympanic membrane to the stapes and thus to the inner ear.

Tympanoplastic surgery is only undertaken if infection is controlled. After operation, the dressing is usually left undisturbed for 3 to 4 days; if necessary, the outer part may be reinforced. The patient is asked not to blow his nose to avoid forcing air through the eustachian tube into the middle ear. He is gradually elevated in bed and observed closely when assisted out of bed for dizziness, nystagmus and nausea. Some patients require an antiemetic drug such as dimenhydrinate (Dramamine) or meclizine hydrochloride (Gravol).

Otosclerosis. This is a chronic ear disease in which the stapes becomes immobilized because of progressive growth of bone tissue over the oval window, interfering with the transmission of vibrations into the inner ear. Both ears are affected. The disease appears to be hereditary and has a higher incidence in females. The ability of the stapes to vibrate progressively decreases, and the loss of hearing usually becomes apparent in the teens or twenties. The person may complain of tinnitus as the deafness becomes more marked. The testing of hearing with a tuning fork reveals that the person has good bone conduction of sound but none by air. A hearing aid may be of some help for a period of time, but a stapedectomy has proved to be the treatment of choice at present. By means of a surgical microscope, the surgeon works through the external auditory canal and the middle ear. The stapes is removed, and a prosthesis introduced to transfer the vibrations of the incus through the oval window into the inner ear. Various forms of prostheses have been used and include a wire or polyethylene tube with a section of vein, a "pad" of fat, or Gelfoam. The wire or polyethylene tube is attached to the incus while the vein, fat or Gelfoam is fitted into the oval window. Only one ear is done at a time.

Following the operation, dizziness and nausea may be troublesome because of the disturbance of the labyrinth. A specific directive is received from the surgeon about the position in which the head is to be maintained. A close check is made for any sign of infection (elevation of temperature and leukocyte count, discharge and pain); if it is suspected, an antimicrobial drug is prescribed. The patient is allowed out of bed in 2 or 3 days and is cautioned to move slowly. If vertigo is experienced, ambulation may have to be delayed. The patient requires assurance that the dizziness is temporary.

Meniere's Disease or Syndrome. This is a disorder of the internal ear characterized by recurrent attacks of severe vertigo, nausea, vomiting, tinnitus and a progressive loss of hearing. The cause is not known but an excess of endolymph resulting in increased pressure and dilation of the canals has been suspected. Vascular spasm and allergic re- action have also been suggested as possible etiological factors. The disorder usually makes its appearance between the ages of 40 and 60 and occurs more often in males.

The episodes have a sudden onset, and the patient is generally prostrated by the dizziness and nausea. The duration of an attack varies from hours to days.

During an attack, the patient remains in bed in a quiet environment. Crib sides may be necessary for safety because of the vertigo. An antiemetic such as dimenhy- drinate (Dramamine) and a sedative (e.g., phenobarbital or amobarbital) may provide some relief. In an effort to offset episodes, the patient is placed on a low sodium diet; a diuretic such as chlorothiazide (Diuril) to reduce the formation of endolymph and a vasodilator (e.g., nicotinic acid) to dis- courage vasospasm may be prescribed. Al- though the acute attacks are episodic, the hearing loss tends to be permanent.

The condition can be very incapacitating and may necessitate surgery. The procedure entails the destruction of the membranous labyrinth. More recently, ultrasonic waves have been used. This form of treatment requires a mastoidectomy to permit the application of the probe. If the patient still has considerable hearing in the affected ear, ultrasonic treatment is used because it is thought to be less hazardous for the hearing.

References

BOOKS

Flitter, H. H.: Physics in Nursing, 5th ed. St. Louis, The C. V. Mosby Co., 1967, pp. 135–142.

Green, J. H.: An Introduction to Human Physiology, 2nd ed. New York, Oxford University Press, 1968, pp. 167–169.

Guyton, A. C.: Textbook of Basic Human Physiology, 4th ed. Philadelphia, W. B. Saunders Co., 1971, pp. 441–449 and 466–469.

Jacob, S. W., and Francone, C. A.: Structure and Function in Man, 2nd ed. Philadelphia, W. B. Saunders Co., 1970, pp. 282–287.

Saunders, W. H., Havener, W. H., Fair, C. J., and Hickey, J. T.: Nursing Care in Eye, Ear, Nose and Throat Disorders, 2nd ed. St. Louis, The C. V. Mosby Co., 1968. Chapter 28.

Warren, R.: Surgery. Philadelphia, W. B. Saunders Co., 1963. Chapter 16.

PERIODICALS

Aldred, Sister B.: "Recognition, Referral, Reassurance of the Deaf Child." Canad. Nurse, Vol. 62, No. 8 (Aug. 1966), pp. 35–36.

Conover, M., and Cober, J.: "Understanding and Caring for the Hearing-Impaired." Nurs. Clin. North Amer., Vol. 5, No. 3 (Sept. 1970), pp. 497–506.

Humenik, P., Damen, M., and Vines, T.: "Rehabilitation of Children and Adults with Hearing Impair- ment." Canad. Nurse, Vol. 62, No. 8 (Aug. 1966), pp. 37–44.

Moore, M. V.: "Diagnosis: Deafness." Amer. J. Nurs., Vol. 69, No. 2 (Feb. 1969), pp. 297–300.
Nilo, E. R.: "Needs of the Hearing-Impaired." Amer. J. Nurs., Vol. 69, No. 1 (Jan. 1969), pp. 114–116.
Rubin, J. A.: "Deafness and Its Management." Canad. Nurse, Vol. 62, No. 8 (Aug. 1966), pp. 32–34.
von Békésy, G.: "The Ear." Sci. Amer., Aug. 1957.

PAMPHLETS

Available from:
The Canadian Hearing Society, Bedford Rd., Toronto, Ontario, Canada.
American Hearing Society, 18th St. N.W., Washington, D.C., U.S.A., 20006.

Index

Page numbers in *italics* indicate illustrations.